Y0-ABH-980

THE

ENCYCLOPEDIA

OF

PURE MATERIA MEDICA.

A RECORD OF THE

POSITIVE EFFECTS OF DRUGS UPON THE HEALTHY HUMAN ORGANISM.

EDITED BY

TIMOTHY F. ALLEN, A.M., M.D.,

PROFESSOR OF MATERIA MEDICA AND THERAPEUTICS IN THE NEW YORK HOMŒOPATHIC
MEDICAL COLLEGE; CORRESPONDING MEMBER OF THE BRITISH
HOMŒOPATHIC MEDICAL SOCIETY.

WITH CONTRIBUTIONS FROM

DR. RICHARD HUGHES, OF ENGLAND.
DR. C. HERING, OF PHILADELPHIA.   DR. CARROLL DUNHAM, OF NEW YORK.
DR. AD. LIPPE, OF PHILADELPHIA, AND OTHERS.

VOL. 11

B. Jain Publishers Pvt. Ltd.
NEW DELHI-110055

Reprint Edition 1995

© Copyright with Publishers

Price : **Rs. 1200.00**   12 Vols. set

Published by :
B. Jain Publishers Pvt. Ltd.
1921, St. No. 10th Chuna Mandi, Paharganj,
Post Box: 5775 new Delhi - 110 055 (INDIA)

Printed in India by:
J.J. Offset Printers
23, Kishan Kunj, Delhi - 110 092

ISBN 81-7021-501-3
ISBN 81-7021-503-X

BOOK CODE: BA-2008

LIST OF REMEDIES IN VOLUME II.

ENCYCLOPEDIA

OF

PURE MATERIA MEDICA.

AURUM.

Aurum foliatum, metallic gold. *Preparation*, Triturate pure gold with sugar of milk.

Authorities. 1, Hahnemann (Chr. Kr., 1, 214); 2, Franz, ibid.; 3, Gross, ibid.; 4, Fr. Hahnemann, ibid.; 5, Hempel, ibid.; 6, Hermann, ibid.; 7, Langhammer, ibid.; 8, Lehmann, ibid.; 9, Michler, ibid.; 10, Rummel, ibid.; 11, Wislicenus, ibid.; 12, Schulze, ibid. (reference not obtainable); 13, Eph. Nat. Cur. Cent. X, ibid. (no observation about Aur. found here); 14, Eph. N. C., Dec. II, ibid. (a casual mention); 15, Molin, proving, Bull. d. l. Soc. Med. Hom. de Paris, 1, 19; 16, Lembke, N. Z. f. H. K., 11, 17 (took the 100th); 17, Robinson, B. J., 25, 32 (took the 12th and 200th).

Mind.—Religious excitement,[15].—In a reverie he says something absurd,[1].—The child woke after three o'clock, *early* in the morning, and spoke rapidly in a strong voice, and with red face, thus: "Mother, thou art my jewel of a daughter! What sort of a dog is that? What sort of a head is that at the wall? What is running about there in the room?" and many other such foolish questions,[1].—Desire for solitude,[15].—(*Loathing of life*),[1].— *Disgust for life, suicidal tendency*,[15].—Good humor the whole day, with talkativeness and self-satisfaction (reaction),[1].—Tolerable degree of cheerfulness, agreeable ease (after two hours),[2].—Frequent weeping,[15].—[10.] *She howls and screams, and imagines herself irretrievably lost*,[1].—*Despondent*,[1].—*Melancholy; he imagines he is unfit for this world, and longs for death, which he contemplates with internal delight*,[2].—*Despondent melancholy, he imagines he cannot succeed in anything*,[11].—*Dejected, and full of melancholy*,[1].—*He is dejected, and seeks solitude*,[1].—*He imagines he has lost the affections of his friends; this makes him sad, even unto tears*,[2].—Discouraged, and out of humor with himself,[1].—The least trifle makes him discouraged,[1].—He feels discouraged and despondent; he imagines he does everything wrong, and cannot succeed in anything,[5].—[20.] He is dissatisfied with everything; he imagines obstacles everywhere in his way, partly occasioned by adverse fate, partly by himself; this latter makes him morbidly depressed,[1].—*Great anguish coming from the præcordial region, and driving him from place to place, so that he can remain nowhere*,[1].—*Excessive anguish, with palpitation of the heart*, weariness in all the limbs, and sleepiness,[1].—Great anguish, increasing unto self-destruction, with spasmodic contraction of the abdomen,[1].—Uneasiness, and hurried desire for bodily and mental activity; he cannot do anything fast enough, and cannot live so as to be satisfied with himself,[5].—He feels uneasy and uncertain, without orgasm; he constantly imagines he neglects something, and deserves reproaches in consequence; he appears to carry this uneasiness about him in his mind, and it deprives him of all energy and perseverance,[5].—While eating, the anxiety of mind leaves him,[2].—Timidity,[1].—*Apprehensiveness; a mere noise at the door made him anxious; he feared lest some one would come in; anthropophobia,[1].—Constant sullen mood and taciturnity,[7].—[30.] Unsociable mood,[1].—Weariness; causeless vexation,[15].—Some persons are offensive to him,[1].—Peevishness, and want of disposition to speak,[6].—*Peevish and vehement; the least contradiction excites his wrath,[3].—Impatience; anger,[15].—Choleric and quarrelsome,[1].—Violent anger and vehemence,[1].—Extreme disposition to feel offended; he was deeply affected and provoked by the least thing that seemed to grieve him,[5].—He becomes angry while thinking of some absent persons,[1].—[40.] He quarrels with every one, and says coarse things,[1].—She alternately weeps and laughs, as if not conscious of herself,[1].—Silent peevishness and cheerfulness, often alternate (after one and three hours),[6].—If left alone, he sits still, taciturn, apparently melancholy, in a corner by himself; but the slightest contradiction excites his wrath, which he first manifests by disputing and talking a good deal, afterwards by uttering a few detached words (after three days),[6].—The intellectual faculties are more acute, and the memory more faithful (reaction),[1].—She is anxious to reflect deeply about this or that subject; this, however, makes her quite weak, tremulous, cold, and damp over the body,[1].—Memory impaired,[15].

Head.—Confusion of the head,[6].—Confusion of the head, early on rising, with heaviness in the occiput,[11].—When standing, vertigo, forcing him to sit down,[6].—[50.] Great vertigo, when stooping,[15].—*Vertigo, when stooping, as if turning in a circle; it goes off on raising the head,[7].—*When walking in the open air, vertigo, as if he were drunk, and would fall to the left side he was forced to lie down, but even then for some time the vertigo returned on the slightest motion (after forty-three hours),[7].—His head shakes sideways and up and down,[1].—Headache as from an incipient cold,[1].—Pains in the head, caused by intellectual exertions,[15].—Headache, sometimes as from a contusion, sometimes like a painful pressure in one part of the brain, sometimes like a tearing; it has increased ever since morning, and disappears at 3 P.M. (after twenty-four hours),[1].—Burning heat of the whole head, worse at the occiput,[15].—*Rush of blood to the head,[1].—Great determination of blood to the brain (after three-quarters of an hour),[1].—[60.] Violent rush of blood to the head when stooping; it passes off after raising the head again (after eight days),[6].—A kind of hypochondriacal intoxication; the head feels full of compressed air, especially towards the nape of the neck,[1].—Boring in different parts of cranial bones,[16].—*The bones of the head pained him on lying down, as if broken, so that all his vital energy seemed affected,[1].—Stunning, pressive headache, as from violent wind,[7].—Pressive tearing in the head here and there, especially in the forehead, with feeling of vertigo,[6].—Headache, ever since morning, as from a bruised brain; when reflecting or reading, especially when talking or writing, the headache increases to the utmost violence, and a perfect confusion of ideas; when ceasing to reflect, speak, or write the headache ceases, until it disappears entirely at 7 in the evening (after six hours),[1].—Small, bony tumor on the upper part of the left side of the forehead,[1].—Burning in skin of forehead,[16].—Pressive pain on the forehead externally (after ten hours),[6].—[70.] Boring in left side of frontal bone.[16].—Boring in left side of forehead.[16].—Pressure in left side of forehead (after an hour and a half),[6].—Fine tearing in the forehead,[6].—Very frequent tearing in forehead,[16].—*Tearing headache* in front, in the forehead and temples, deep in the brain, abating in the open air,[3].—Tearing in the left side of the forehead, more violent during motion,[6].—A stitch on the frontal bone like a slow drawing (after six hours),[2].—Stitch in the centre of the forehead, where the hair begins,[1].—Prickings, as from pins, in the forehead externally (after twenty-four hours),[6].—[80.] Tingling sensation in the forepart of the head,[1].—*Small, bony tumor on the right side of the vertex, with boring pain that grows worse when the tumor is touched*,[1].—Burning in skin of right temple,[16].—Pressive pain in the temples,[1].—Pressive pain on the left temple externally (after thirty-two hours),[6].—Pressure on the left temple, worse by touch (after a quarter of an hour),[6].—Tearings in the left temple,[2].—*Severe* and constant *burning heat* on the top of the head,[15].—Tearing pressure in the left side of the vertex, more violent during motion,[6].—Tearing in the right side of the vertex (after three hours),[6].—[90.] Tearing in the left side of the vertex (after one and a half hours),[6].—Cutting tearing pain in the right side of the vertex (after seventeen days),[6].—Drawing in right side of head,[16].—Pressive tearing in the right side of the head, from the occiput to the forehead (after three hours),[6].—One-sided, sharply throbbing, hacking headache,[1].—Grinding, boring, and slight throbbing in one side of the head, early in the morning shortly after waking, increased by coughing, and bending the head backwards,[1].—Megrim returning every three or four days, with stitching, *burning*, and beating in one side of the forehead, qualmishness, nausea, and even bilious vomiting,[15].—Tearing pressure in the right occiput,[6].—*Fine tearing from the right side of the occiput through the brain as far as the forehead; more violent during motion* (after one hour),[6].

Eyes.—Prominent, protruding eyes,[1].—[100.] Sensation of weakness and pressure in the eyes,[1].—A kind of burning in the eyes,[1].—*Tension in the eyes, which makes seeing difficult* (after one hour),[6].—Excessive tension in the eyes, with diminution of sight; more violent when fixing the eyes upon something; less when closing them (after nine days),[6].—*Pressure in the eyes,* as from a foreign body,[1].—Pressure upon the left eye from without inwards (after eight days),[6].—*Sensation in his eyes when looking, as of violent heat,* as if the blood pressed upon the optic nerve,[1].—*Constant feeling of sand in the eyes,*[15].—Burning, stitching, drawing, and itching in the inner canthus of the eyes,[15].—Drawing above the right eye,[16].—[110.] Excessive spasmodic pressure in the posterior segment of the left orbit,[3].—Fine tearing in the right orbit, close to the external canthus (after five hours),[6].—Dull stitch in the lower part of the left orbit, from within outwards,[1].—Redness of the lids at the approach of the menses,[15].—Bluish appearance of the inner canthi,[1].—Swelling of the lower lids,[4].—*Morning agglutination,*[15].—Burning, stitching, and itching of the eyelids,[15].—Biting pain in the left upper eyelid,[1].—Several single stitches in the internal canthus and lid of the left eye (after thirty-six hours),[6].—[120.] Itching and burning in the right canthus,[1].—*Constant lachrymation,*[15].—*Redness of the sclerotica,*[15].—Sensation of pressing out in the internal and superior angle of the left eyeball,[2].—Pressive pain in the right eyeball, from without inwards; more violent during motion (after six hours),[6].—Dilatation of the pupils (after three hours and a half),[7].—Contraction of the pupils (after two and four hours),[7].—Indistinct sight, as if a black veil were drawn before the eyes (after six days),[6].—*Half-sightedness*, as if the upper half of the vision were covered with a dark body, *so that he can only see lower objects with the inferior half;* upper objects remain invisible,[6].—His sight is lost for a moment,[1].—[130.] Fiery sparks before the eyes,[1].—*He cannot distinguish anything clearly,* because he sees everything double, *and one object is seen mixed with the other, with violent tension in the eyes,*[6].

Ears.—Moisture behind the ears,[15].—Burning, pricking, and itching behind the ears,[15].—Boring behind the left ear,[16].—Burning and stitching in the ears,[15].—Tension in the ears,[1].—Pressive tearing in the left meatus auditorius externus,[6].—Hardness of hearing,[15].—Sense of deafness (12th),[17].—[140.] Crackling in the left ear,[1].—Humming before the left ear,[1].—Humming, whistling, and ringing in the ears,[15].—Raging and roaring in the head, as if sitting close to roaring water (after fourteen days),[1].—Roaring in the ears, early in the morning, in bed,[1].

Nose.—*Redness and swelling of the nose,*[15].—*Ulcerated, agglutinated, painful nostrils, so that he cannot breathe through the nose,*[1].—*Swelling and redness of the right nostril, and underneath,*[6].—*Swelling of the nose,* in the room, after walking in the open air,[1].—Dark, brownish-red, slightly elevated spots upon the nose, which ache only when touched (after twenty-four hours),[6].—[150.] *Crusts in the nose,*[15].—*Crusts, as from ulcers, in the right nostril,* yellowish, almost painless, and dry,[6].—Frequent sneezing,[15].—Coryza,[6].—Violent fluent coryza,[1].—Coryza, with thick discharge like white of egg,[15].—*The nostril appears obstructed, although air passes through it,*[6].—*Sense of obstruction of the nose, as in dry coryza; nevertheless, the air passes freely through the nose* (after two and a half hours),[7].—Burning and itching on the exterior of the nose,[15].—Violent burning in right wing of nose,[16].—[160.] *Burning, itching, stitching, and smarting in the nose,*[15].—Boring in cartilage of nose,[16].—*Boring in left side of nasal bone, toward upper maxilla,*[16].—*Feeling of soreness in the nose,*[6].—*Soreness in both nostrils, especially when touching them,*[1].—*The right nasal bone and the adjoining part of the upper jaw are painful to the touch, especially at the place where the infraorbital nerve comes out,*[1].—Shootings in the septum of the nose, from above downwards,[11].—Biting pain in the lower part of the nose,[6].—Biting pain in the lower part of the nose, so that the tears came into his eyes, as when desiring to sneeze, excited by strong sunlight, or exalted, pious grief, or the highest degree of pity,[2].—Itching of the nostrils,[1].—[170.] Itching titillation in the wings of the nose, as in a cold, sometimes with desire to scratch,[7].—*Sensitive smell; everything smells too strong for him,*[1].—The smoke of the lamp is offensive,[1].—Frequently, a sweetish smell in his nose,[1].—Momentary smell of brandy in the nose, with dyspnœa,[1].—*Putrid smell in the nose when blowing it,*[1].

Face.—(When speaking, he smiles involuntarily),[1].—Redness of the face,[15].—Flushed face,[15].—Red and blue spots on the face,[15].—[180.] Bloated face, shining as from sweat, with prominent protruding eyes,[1].—*Drawing tearing on the left side of the face,*[11].—Itching pricking, as from pins, on the right side of the face,[1].—Swelling of both cheeks, with swelling of the lips and nose, early in the morning,[1].—*Swelling of one cheek, with drawing and tearing in the upper and lower jaws,* and sensation of hacking, and grumbling pain in the teeth, which appear too long,[1].—Tension in the malar bone and ears,[1].—*Violent tearing in the zygoma,*[5].—Painful stitches in one cheek (after first day),[1].—*Burning stitches in the zygoma,*[1].—*Violent boring in right zygomatic process, when walking,*[16].—[190.] Burning vesicle upon the vermilion border of the lower lip,[1].—Burning in lips.[16].—Pain in a gland of the lower jaw, as if swollen,[1].—Boring in left side of upper jaw,[20].—Boring in right side of lower jaw,[10].—Tearing pressure at the right lower jaw, going off by pressing upon it,[6].—Tearing in the right half of the chin,[2].—Intermittent, dull stitches in the external border of the lower jaw,[3].

Mouth.—Looseness of the teeth, even the anterior, in sudden paroxysms,[1].—Sensation of dulness of the molar teeth (after half an hour),[1].—[200.] The upper front teeth are very painful when chewing,[1].—*Toothache caused by drawing air into the mouth,*[1].—Hacking and grumbling pain in the teeth, with swelling of the cheeks,[1].—Dull tearing in the two posterior molar teeth of the right upper jaw, excited by touch and eating, with painful swelling of the gums,[6].—*When chewing, suddenly a painful dulness in one of the upper molar teeth,*[1].—Single stitches in the teeth,[1].—Shooting pain in the upper row,[4].—Redness and swelling of the gums,[15].—Swelling of the gums of the molar teeth of the right upper jaw, with pressive soreness when touched, or when eating,[6].—Painful pustules on the gums, as if a fistula dentalis would form,[1].—[210.] Ulcer on the gums, with swelling of the cheeks (after ten days),[1].—The gums bleed easily,[15].—Violent burning in tip of tongue,[16].—Stitching and burning in the tip and on the edge of tongue, and on its under surface,[16].—Aphthæ in the mouth,[15].—Mouth blistered inside (200th),[17].—Smell from the mouth as of old cheese,[1].—*Putrid smell from the mouth,*[1].—*Fetid odor from the mouth,* in the evening and at night, unperceived by himself,[1].—Difficulty in eating,[15].—[220.] Heat and smarting in the mouth,[15].—A kind of pressure in the region of the palate, for several hours,[1].—Agreeably sweetish saliva accumulates in the mouth,[2].—The taste is insipid,[1].—Agreeable, milky taste in the mouth,[1].—Sweet taste on the anterior part of the tongue,[1].—Sometimes, sourish taste in the mouth (after two and a half hours),[1].—*Bitter taste in the mouth,* with sensation of dryness (after eight hours),[7].—*Putrid taste in the mouth, as of spoiled game, between meals,*[1].

Throat.—Frequently, phlegm in the throat, which can be hawked up, but prevents a full inspiration (after two hours),[2].—[230.] Much phlegm in the throat, for several days,[1].—Pain in the parotid glands,[15].—*The parotid gland is painful to the touch, as if pressed or contused,*[1].—Lumpy state of the throat; she wakes at night and desires to moisten it (200th),[17].—Burning, stitching, and itching in the throat, worse on swallowing,[15].—Drawing and scraping in the throat,[15].—*Dull, pressive pain, either with or without swallowing, in a gland below the angle of the lower jaw,*[1].—Throat feels pricked with needles (200th),[17].—Swallowing food causes a stinging sensation in the throat (200th),[17].—*Stinging soreness in the throat, only during deglutition,*[1].—[240.] Painful obstacle to deglutition in the left side of the pharynx,[1].—Attacks of distension of the pharynx, as in vomiting, but without nausea,[1].

Stomach.—He relishes his meal, but his appetite is not appeased; he could have eaten again, shortly after,[1].—He is forced to eat hastily, especially at the beginning of the meal,[1].—Has no appetite for anything; can only eat bread and milk,[1].—Repugnance to meat,[1].—Much thirst for six days,[4].—Burning thirst; desire for cold drinks,[15].—Desire for spirituous liquors,[15].—Great longing for coffee,[1].—[250.] Watery eructations,[15].—Eructations tasting of the drink (beer),[1].—Hiccough,[15].—Nausea,[15].—Nausea in the stomach and throat,[6].—Mental labor causes nausea, which affects his whole being,[1].—Sensation of nausea; discomfort from the stomach and in the abdomen,[1].—Inclination to vomit after eating, sometimes even while eating,[15].—Regurgitations as if the person would vomit; with pressure in the abdomen,[4].—Pain at the stomach, as of hunger,[1].—[260.] Burning at the stomach, and hot eructations (12th),[7].—Burning, drawing, and cutting pain in the stomach,[15].—*Pressure in the region of the stomach, at noon,[1].— *Pressure on the left side, near the pit of the stomach, below the cartilages of the upper false ribs; more violent during an expiration (after seven days),[6].

Abdomen.—*Burning heat and cutting pain in the right hypochondrium,[15].—Continual pressure in the hypochondria, as from flatulence, especially after food or drink, often increased by motion and walking; goes off without flatus,[1].—Stitches in the left hypochondrium, like stitches in the spleen,[1].—Painful stitch in the left hypochondrium,[15].—Rumbling in the abdomen,[1].—Rumbling in the bowels (after one hour),[6].—[270.] At night, painful accumulation of flatulence, especially in the left hypochondrium,[1]. —Emission of much flatulence (first day),[1].—Emission of much fetid flatulence (after eight hours),[6].—He is much troubled with flatulency; it becomes incarcerated under the left ribs, with lancinating pain,[1].—Discomfort in the abdomen, with sensation as if he should go to stool, especially after dinner (after thirty-six hours),[6].—Pains in the abdomen, as from labor, as if the menses would make their appearance,[1].—Heat and drawing in the abdomen,[15].—Pinching pain, here and there, in the abdomen (after twelve hours),[6].—Dull pinching and cutting in the abdomen, then diarrhœa, and after the diarrhœa, distended abdomen,[1].—Painful feeling of contraction in the abdomen,[1].—[280.] Heaviness in the abdomen, with icy-cold hands and feet,[1].—Pressure in the abdomen,[1].—Tensive pressure in the abdomen and the lumbar regions, with desire for stool (after six days),[6].—Tensive pressure in the abdomen, just below the navel, and on both sides in the lumbar regions, with feeling of fulness (after fifty-three hours),[6].—Single tearings in the right side of the abdomen, extending as high up as below the ribs, as if everything there was shattered; forces him to bend crooked, when sitting (after thirty-six hours),[2].—Cutting pain, heat, and scraping sensation in the groins,[15].—Twisting pain in the abdomen, before and during stool,[15].—Colic,[15].—Colic in the abdomen,[14].—Flatulent colic, shortly after the lightest and most moderate meals,[1].—[290.] Flatulent colic, after midnight; much flatus rapidly accumulates which does not pass, and therefore causes painful pressure, squeezing and anxiety; both when at rest and in motion,[1].—The abdomen is tender to the touch,[15].—Protrusion of an inguinal hernia, with great cramplike pain; flatus seems to get into the hernia,[1].— Rumbling in the lower abdomen,[1].—Heat and sensitiveness of the hypogastrium,[15].—Pinching pain on the inner side of the ischiatic bones,[11].—Weight on the pubis,[15].—Jerking twinges in the left side of the pelvis, causing him to jump or start,[11].—Weakness in the groin,[1].—Want of flexibility and painful stiffness in the bends of the groin and the tendons of the lumbar muscles, when walking or spreading the legs, as after a long journey on foot (after three and a half hours),[1].—Pain in the groin, as from a swollen gland,[1].—[300.] Burning pain in the abdominal ring, which is otherwise healthy,[1].—Drawing from the groin into the thighs,[1].—Pressing in the right abdominal ring, as if a hernia would protrude, when sitting and stretching the body; goes off when rising,[2].—Cutting thrusts in both groins, forcing him to draw the abdomen in and the feet up,[11].—Bruised pain in the right iliac region, when sitting; goes off when rising and drawing up the thigh (after twenty-four hours),[2].

Stool and Anus.—Sharp stitches in the rectum and anus,[6].—External hæmorrhoids, bleeding during stool,[15].—The border of the anus is painfully swollen,[1].—Burning heat and tearing pains at the anus,[15].—Heat and dull pain at the perineum,[15].—[310.] Diarrhœa,[2].—Diarrhœa day and night; green stools,[15].—Frequent diarrhœa, especially at night, with grayish-yellow stools,[15].—Nightly diarrhœa, with much burning in the rectum,[1].—(White-yellowish stool),[1].—Copious, but normal stool (after sixteen hours),[6].—Unusually copious stool, in the evening (after ten hours),[1].—Soft stool every morning, with a little pinching,[1].—Stool very large; passed with difficulty,[1].—*Very hard, knotty stool every day,[1].—[320.] Constipation for three days,[2].

Urinary Organs.—Sharp stitches, when breathing, apparently in the side of the bladder,[1].—Burning, stitching, and smarting in the urethra,[15].—Dull tearing in the urethra,[6].—Tearing stitches at the glans, when obliged to urinate (after three hours),[11].—Dysuria,[15].—Constant desire for micturition, with scanty but natural urine,[3].—He passes more urine than corresponds to the quantity he drinks,[1].—Urine greatly diminished,[15].—Infrequent discharge of scanty, yellowish urine,[15].—[330.] *Turbid urine, like buttermilk,* with much sediment of mucus,[1].—Thick urine, having a strong ammoniacal odor, and decomposing rapidly,[15].—Hot, red urine, containing sand,[15].

Sexual Organs.—(*Male.*)—Moisture around the glans,[15].—Painful twitches in the penis, from before backwards,[1].—Painful erections,[15].—Nightly erections, without emissions (first night),[11].—Erections many nights in succession,[1].—Prickings, as from pins, at the extremity of the glans; every single pricking is followed by a similar one above the navel, towards the pit of the stomach (after three hours),[11].—*Itching of the scrotum,*[1].—[340.] *Swelling of the right testicle, with pressive pain when touching or rubbing it; this symptom came on for several evenings at 6 o'clock, and ceased towards 11 o'clock (after five days),*[6].—*Pressive and tensive pain in the right testicle, as from contusion* (after three and a half hours),[7].—The sexual desire, which had been dormant in him for a long time, is roused,[1].—Much desire for coition, early, after rising, with violent erections,[1].—He was unable to sleep the whole night, on account of his sexual desire being roused; he finally had to satisfy it by coition (first night),[1].—For two nights he is full of lewd fancies, the penis being small and relaxed (second and third night),[1].—Pollutions at night (the first nights),[11].—Nightly pollutions, with voluptuous dreams (after seven days),[6].—*Nightly erections and pollutions,*[3].—Prostatic juice comes out of the penis, which is relaxed,[1].—[350.] Pollutions three nights in succession, without subsequent weakness,[1].—(*Female.*)—Drawing pain in the mons veneris,[1].—Heat, pricking, and smarting of the vulva,[15].—Redness and swelling of the labia majora,[15].—Burning and pricking in the vagina,[15].—Thick white leucorrhœa,[15].—Retarded menstruation,[15].

Respiratory Apparatus.—Husky voice (12th),[17].—Cough,[4].—Infrequent short dry cough,[15].—[360.] Frequent severe and racking cough,[15].—Cough at night, on account of want of breath,[6].—Splitting cough at night,[15].—Phlegm deep in the lungs, which is easily thrown up in large quantity; this is succeeded by free and expansive breathing, whereas generally he was asthmatic,[1].—Difficulty of raising phlegm (12th),[17].—Adhesive phlegm in the larynx, difficult to hawk up,[1].—Frequently, phlegm deep in the larynx, which he does not succeed in coughing up, even with the greatest effort,[3].—*Frequent deep breathing,*[1].—Difficult breathing,[15].—Difficulty of breathing,[1].—[370.] *Severe dyspnœa,*[1].—*Dyspnœa, also when at rest, which cannot be relieved by any position; he constantly takes deep breath, and cannot inspire air enough,*[2].—Severe dyspnœa when walking in the open air,[1].—Dyspnœa when laughing or walking fast, as if the chest were too tight for breathing and too flat in front (after forty-four hours),[3].—Dyspnœa, with dull stitches in the chest, when inspiring,[6].—Excessive dyspnœa, with difficulty of breathing at night,[.].—Sense of suffocation soon after eating,[15].

Chest.—During an expiration, râles in the upper part of the chest, descending into the abdomen and groin, succeeded by quick beatings of the heart, with weakness and apprehension; then slumber,[1].—Persistent dry catarrh on the chest, early in the morning, on waking; it is with great trouble he succeeds in hawking up a little phlegm, and even this only after rising from bed (after sixteen hours),[1].—Burning, stitching, and pricking in the chest,[15].—[380.] Tightness of the thorax, with anxiety (after three days),[6].—Drawing in left side of chest, below nipple,[16].—Oppression of chest and abdomen when coughing,[1].—A few very violent stitches in the chest, over the heart (after seventy-two hours),[1].—Intensely painful stitches under the ribs when breathing deeply (and yawning); they prevent breathing and yawning; cease on going to bed,[1].—Shuddering in the right chest, when yawning,[1].—Pressure in left wall of thorax,[16].—Pressure on the right side of the chest, with extreme anguish,[2].—Dull cutting pain on the left side, near the sternum; more violent during an inspiration (after nine days),[6].—Stitches in the left chest when breathing,[1].—[390.] Stitches under the left ribs when coughing,[1].—Fine tearing stitches on the right side, near the lumbar vertebræ, going off by pressure,[6].—Dull painful stitches and lancinations on the right side, near the sternum, under the last true ribs,[6].—Dull oppressive stitches under the cartilages of the first three ribs on the right side; they sometimes continue as a sensation of a plug inserted there; sometimes they are slowly intermittent and little felt in walking; externally, the place is red (after sixteen hours),[3].—Dull stitches on both sides of the chest, with heat in the chest and dyspnœa; increased by inspiration,[11].—Pressure on the sternum, with busy demeanor, as if something very agreeable were about to happen,[2].—Pressure on the sternum, as of something hard, with drawing tearings towards the shoulders,[2].—Sharp stitches in the sternum (after two hours),[11].—Swelling of the præcordial region and the whole upper part of the abdomen, with a painful stitch when pressing upon it or lacing it tightly,[1].

Heart and Pulse.—When walking, the heart seems to shake as if it were loose,[2].—[400.] Sometimes, one single very violent beat of the heart,[1].—Strong irregular beating of the heart,[15].—*Palpitation of the heart (after half an hour),[.].—* Violent palpitation of the heart (after four days),[6].—Palpitation when lying on the back,[15].—*Frequent attacks of anguish about the heart, and tremulous fearfulness,[13].—Heat and itching at the heart,[15].—Drawings and cutting pains at the heart,[15].

Neck and Back.—Difficulty in turning the head, as in torticollis,[15].—Tension in the neck, as if a muscle were too short, even when at rest, but more violent when stooping (after ten hours),[11].—[410.] Drawing in nape of neck towards left clavicle,[16].—Drawing in left side of nape of neck,[16].—Tearing pressure in the lower part of the right side of the neck (after fourteen days),[6].—Jerking, tearing stitches in the left external muscles of the neck (after seven days),[1].—Tearing pain on the inner side of the scapula and below it, when bending the body backwards and to the left (after eleven hours),[6].—Early in the morning, such a severe pain in the spine that he was unable to move a limb,[1].—Heat, pricking, and itching in the back,[15].—Pain in the small of the back, as from fatigue (after three hours),[.].—Drawing in the muscles of the back,[16].—Burning heat, which seems to start from the kidneys and extend to the bladder,[15].—[420.] Cutting over the small of the back when sitting, as if from pressure with a sharp instrument,[2].—Heat in the loins,[15].—Sharp piercing pain in the right loin, only during inspiration,[1].—Bruised pain in the loins,[15].

Extremities in General.—Going to sleep, numbness and insensibility of the arms and legs, early on waking, more when lying still than in motion,[1].—Shooting and drawing pains in arms and legs occasionally,[10].

Upper Extremities.—Fatigue in the arms,[15].—Difficult movement of the arms,[15].—Burning, stitching, and pricking in the arms,[15].—Heat in the axillæ,[15].—[430.] Tearing tension under the axilla,[11].—Boring in left shoulder,[16].—Boring in left shoulder, when sitting,[16].—Stitching in left axilla,[16].—Fine stitches upon the shoulder,[11].—Soreness of the shoulders, even when not touched or moved,[2].—Burning in skin of right upper arm,[16].—Drawing in skin of left upper arm,[16].—Drawing pain down the left arm, on the bone, going off by motion,[2].—Pressure on the under surface and in the middle of the right upper arm,[6].—[440.] Pressure in the left upper arm, near the periostoum (after forty-eight hours),[6].—Tearing pressure in the anterior surface of both upper arms (after fifteen days).[6].—Fine tearings in the left upper arm, most severe on uncovering it (after three hours),[11].—Severe bone-pains in the right elbow (200th),[17].—Boring in right elbow-joints,[16].—Cramplike tearing in the right elbow-joint,[3].—The forearms feel heavy when at rest, but not in motion (after twelve hours),[11].—Boring in right forearm,[16].—Pressure on the external side of the right forearm (after twelve days),[6].—Pressure on the anterior surface of the forearm,[6].—[450.] Intermittent tearing pressure on the inner side of the left forearm,[6].—Tearing in the bones of the wrist-joint (after eight hours),[6].—*Cramplike tearing in the bones of both wrists,* deep in the interior, from the upper to the lower row of the carpus, especially at night, but also by day,[3].—Stitching and pressure in wrists,[16].—Cramplike pain in the metacarpal bones of the left hand, especially the thumb, without interfering with motion,[3].—Tearing in the metacarpal bones,[6].—Tension in roots of right fingers,[16].—Boring in finger-joints,[16].—Drawing in the finger-joints,[5].—Pressure in the last joint of the left little finger, and in the right thumb-joint, during rest,[16].—[460.] Dull tearing in the joints of all the fingers, often spreading into the phalanges (after five days),[6].—Fine tearing in the right fingers,[6].—Fine tearing in the anterior joint of the right thumb,[6].—Tearing in the last joint of the left little finger,[6].—Tearing in the lowest joints of the right fingers (after four days),[6].—Acute pain in the finger-joints,[15].

Lower Extremities.—*All the blood appeared to rush from her head into the lower extremities;* they feel paralyzed and she has to sit down immediately,[1].—Uncommon paralytic pain in the hip-joint, only when rising from a seat and walking, not when sitting,[1].—Cramplike pain in the region of the hip, on the inner brim of the pelvis, increased by rubbing (after thirty-six hours),[11].—In the glutei muscles, a fine stitch, several times repeated; winds downwards (after sixteen hours),[11].—[470.] Weakness of the thigh when walking,[1].—The thigh feels paralyzed, and the tendon of the lumbar muscles is so painfully stiff, that the thigh cannot be raised,[1].—Pain in the right femur, as if broken, on laying the right thigh across the left,[2].—Cramplike drawing in the tendon of the psoas muscle, down into the thigh when sitting, going off when rising,[2].—Pressive and tensive pain in the muscles of the left thigh when walking in the open air, relieved when sitting, but not when standing or walking, or by touching the parts,[7].—Tearing in the thigh as from growing, only during motion, not when sitting (after twenty-four hours),[1].—At night, when lying down, a sore place forms on the external surface of the left thigh,[3].—When sitting, or laying the left limb across the right, the posterior muscles of the right thigh appear to be twitching,[3].—Tottering of the knees,[1].—Painful stiffness and sense of paralysis of the knees, both when at rest and in motion,[1].—[480.] Simple pain, when walking, in the right knee,[1].—Boring in left knee,[16].—*Pain in the knees as if firmly bandaged*, when sitting and walking,[1].—The right knee becomes weak from walking, so that a drawing pain is felt in it when walking, and setting the foot upon the floor (after twenty-four hours),[3].—Pressure in left knee,[16].—Stitching and pressure in knees,[16].—Hard, red swelling of the leg, from the malleolus to the calf, occasioned by the rubbing of the boots; going off again after a short rest,[10].—Boring in right tibia,[16].—Violent boring in centre of left tibia,[16].—Dull, gnawing pain in both sides of the legs, over the malleoli, together with a few sharp stitches in the tendo Achillis when at rest; they pass off during motion (after fourteen hours),[11].—[490.] Pressure on the left tibia, when stretching the leg,[2].—Burning in calves,[16].—Pressure in right ankle,[16].—Boring in left ankle,[16].—Tensive pressure near the right internal malleolus (after five days),[6].—Swelling of the feet; walking is difficult,[15].—Boring in back of right foot, toward the ankle,[16].—Boring in back of left foot,[16].—Drawing pain in the feet,[10].—The heels are painful, as from ulceration or extravasation of blood,[1].—[500.] Severe drawing in both heels, in the evening when going to sleep,[10].—Violent stitches on the dorsum of the foot, behind the toes,[1].—Pressure in the hollow of the sole of the foot, as from something hard,[1].—Tearing pain in the posterior part of the right sole (after thirty hours),[6].—Redness and burning of the toes,[15].—Drawing in the toe-joints,[10].—Paralytic drawing in the right toes,[6].—Paralytic drawing in the metatarsal bones of the big toe, as far as the tip,[6].—Fine tearing in the right toes,[6].—Violent stitching in right toes,[16].—[510.] Pain as from a bruise or sprain in the last joint of the big toe when walking,[1].—Grinding pain in old chilblains (after one hour),[1].

Generalities.—Tremulous agitation of the nerves, as in joyous hope,[2].—He trembles when he cannot express his anger,[1].—(When thinking of a motion, he makes small motions without knowing it),[1].—Inclination to move from place to place,[15].—He is constantly impelled to be in motion, and regrets his inactivity, although he cannot do any work,[2].—At night he could lie neither on the left nor on the right side,[1].—Suddenly, great lassitude, in the afternoon when sitting or lying down; he fell asleep on account of it; on waking, the lassitude had disappeared (after nine hours),[7].—Internal emptiness and weakness of the whole body,[1].—[520.] Early on waking, very feeble,[1].—Early in the morning, very tired; her legs ached so that she would have liked to lie down immediately,[1].—Mental labor wears him out; he feels exhausted,[1].—All his sensations are fine and acute,[5].—Excessive sensitiveness in the whole body; susceptibility to every sort of pain; on thinking of it, he imagines he already feels it; everything is disagreeable to him,[5].—Comfortable feeling in the whole body (reaction),[1].—Simple pain, or pain as from a bruise, early in the morning, in bed, in all the joints, especially the small of the back and knees; the pain increases by lying still; and passes off after rising,[1].—Great anguish and weakness; they think him near dying,[12].—In the afternoon, painful drawing in the veins with exhaustion,[1].—Pressure on the left side, near the lumbar vertebræ, and on the upper border of the os innominatum,[6].—[530.] Pecking, very rapid, almost stitching, between the thumb and the index,[1].—Itching and burning shootings, here and there, almost like stitches,[1].—All the joints feel bruised, early in the morning and the whole forenoon,[1].—*Pain as from bruises* in the head *and all the limbs*, early in bed, most violent when at rest; passes off immediately after rising,[1].

Skin.—Large red pimples on the face,[15].—Painless smooth pimples on the border of the right lower lid,[1].—Red pimples on the nose,[16].—Pimples on the lips, with burning, stitching, pricking, and much itching,[15].—Eruption of small white pimples all over the hairy scalp, with **heat** and itching,[15].—Indurations under the skin, like wheals, on the leg, over the heel and behind the knees, with violent itching, which can hardly be borne when walking (eleventh day),[10].—[540.] Small elevations on the leg and below the knee; when slightly rubbed, they change to thick, hard nodosities under the skin (fifth and eighth day),[10].—Small and larger elevations on the legs and calves, looking like blotches from the stinging of nettles, burning and feeling like hard knots, of a dirty yellow color, disappearing again after a few hours, and forming less in the room than in the open air,[16].—*Eruption on the face; fine pimples,* with tips filled with pus, for some hours,[1].—Eruption of fine pimples, with tips full of pus, on the neck and chest, for some hours,[1].—Pustules in the face and on the neck and chest,[1].—Sensitive pricking, as with pins, just below the right scapula, near the spine (after half an hour),[3].—Formication, here and there, over the body,[5].—Itching of the hand between the thumb and the index finger,[1].—Itching of the joints of the feet, especially when walking (seventh day),[10].—Itching of the joints and soles of the feet,[10].—[550.] Transient but intense itching of the abdomen, of the hips, knees, arms and wrists,[10].

Sleep and Dreams.—Continual sleepiness,[15].—Drowsiness by day,[1].—Slumber, with weakness of head, when sitting, by day,[1].—Invincible sleep after dinner; during this sleep his mind was thronged with ideas (after four hours),[2].—*He sobs aloud in sleep,*[3].—Uneasy sleep, during which he feels the pains,[1].—Frequent waking, at night, as by fright,[7].—After 4 o'clock in the morning, he cannot sleep well, turns from side to side, because he cannot remain long in one position, and the hand on which he lies soon gets tired,[3].—*Awake the whole night, but without pain; nevertheless, no sleepiness or lassitude in the morning,*[1].—[560.] Sleeplessness; nightly restlessness,[15].—Agreeable and sensible dreams, but which cannot be remembered,[1].—*Vivid dreams at night, which cannot be remembered,*[7].—Dreams with constant erection, every night,[1].—She dreamed the whole night that she was in darkness,[1].—She dreamed much in the evening, immediately after falling asleep, as if some one were talking to her; she was yet half awake,[1].—Dreams full of disputes,[1].—He wakes in violent dreams,[1].—Troublesome, fatiguing dreams,[15].—He dreams that he would fall from a great height,[1].—[570.] *Frightful dreams,*[1].—Frightful dreams at night,[3].—*Frightful dreams about thieves, with loud screams while asleep,*[1].—Horrid dream, at night,[1].—Dreams about dead men,[1].

Fever.—*Very sensitive to cold, over the whole body,*[1].—Horripilation over the whole body in the evening, with dry coryza, without heat or subsequent thirst,[7].—Coldness of the body, especially of the hands and feet,[1].—Coldness in the body, almost the whole day, with blue nails, insipid taste, and inclination to vomit; followed by increased warmth, but without fever,[1].—Coldness over the whole body, early in the morning, especially of the arms and hands, beginning at the shoulders; with blue nails, but without fever,[1].—[580.] Chilliness in the evening, in bed, with coldness of the legs as far as the knees; he cannot get warm the whole night; sleeps little, only half an hour at a time, with anxious dreams, which he does not recollect (after sixteen days),[1].—Chills through the whole body, as if he had caught cold in a draught; could scarcely get warm; evening, in bed (after sixteen and nineteen hours),[7].—In the evening, chills over the whole body, with coldness of the hands and warmth of face and forehead, without thirst,[7].— Shivering through the whole body, with gooseskin upon the thighs, and shaking of the brain against the frontal bone,[2].—In the evening, shiverings and chills after lying down; headache before lying down,[1].—Chilliness between the scapulæ,[1].—Chills in the back,[1].—Coldness of the hands and feet, in the evening, in bed,[1].—Coldness of the soles of the feet and patellæ, as soon as he gets into bed in the evening,[5].—*Violent orgasm, as if the blood were boiling in all the veins* (after twenty-four hours),[1].—[**590.**] Alternate chilliness and heat,[4].—Coldness of the whole body, and subsequent increased warmth, without fever,[1].—Heat in face, with cold hands and feet,[1].—Sweat early in the morning all over the body,[1].—Slight perspiration at night; only between the thighs was there real sweat (after ten hours),[1].

Conditions.—**Aggravation.**—(*Morning*), Early, after 3 o'clock, delirious talk; early, on rising, confusion of head, etc.; early, shortly after waking, grinding, etc., in side of head; early, swelling of cheeks; soft stool; early, after rising, desire for coition; early, on waking, catarrh on chest; early, pain in spine; early, on waking, going to sleep, etc., of limbs; early, on waking, very feeble; early, very tired; early, in bed, pain in joints; early, joints feel bruised; early, in bed, *pain in head, etc.;* after 4 o'clock, cannot sleep, etc.; early, coldness over whole body, etc.; sweat all over.—(*Noon*), Pressure in region of stomach.—(*Afternoon*), When sitting or lying down, great lassitude; drawing in the veins, etc.—(*Evening*), The symptoms; fetid odor from mouth; copious stool; when going to sleep, drawing in heels; horripilations over whole body, etc.; in bed, chilliness, etc.; in bed, chilliness; chills over whole body, etc.; after lying down, shivering, etc.; in bed, coldness of hands and feet; on getting into bed, coldness of soles, etc.—(*Every evening*), At 6 o'clock, swelling of testicle, etc.—(*Night*), Fetid odor from mouth; diarrhœa; diarrhœa, etc.; cough; splitting cough; difficulty of breathing; **tearing in wrist-bones;* when lying down, sore place forms on external surface of thigh; slight perspiration.—(*After midnight*), Flatulent colic.—(*Every three or four days*), Megrim, etc.—(*Walking in open air*), Vertigo; dyspnœa; pain in muscles of thigh.—(*Bending head backwards*), Grinding, etc., in side of head.—(*Bending body backwards and to left side*), Pain in one side of the scapula.—(*When blowing nose*), Putrid smell in nose.—(*Breathing*), Stitches in left chest; stitches apparently in bladder.—(*Deep breathing*), Stitches under the ribs.—(*When chewing*), Upper front teeth painful; painful dulness of a tooth.—(*Coughing*), Grinding, etc., in side of head; oppression of chest, etc.; stitches under left ribs. —(*After dinner*), Discomfort in abdomen, etc.; sleep.—(*Drawing air into mouth*), Causes toothache.—(*After drinking*), Pressure in hypochondria.— (*While eating*), Tearing in molar teeth; soreness in gums; inclination to vomit.—(*After eating*), Inclination to vomit; pressure in hypochondria; sense of suffocation.—(*When fixing eyes upon something*), Tension in eyes, etc.—(*When inspiring*), *Stitches in chest;* pain in left side; stitches in sides of chest, etc.; pain in right loin.—(*Intellectual exertion*), Causes pain in head; causes nausea.—(*When laughing*), Dyspnœa.—(*On laying right thigh across left*), Pain in right femur.—(*When laying left limb across right*), Muscles of thigh appear to be twitching.—(*When looking*), Sensation as if the blood pressed upon the optic nerve.—(*On lying down*), Bones of head painful.—(*When lying still*), Going to sleep, etc., in limbs; pain in all the

joints.—(*When lying on back*), Palpitation.—(*Between meals*), Putrid taste
in mouth.—(*Motion*), Tearing in side of forehead; *heat on top of head*; pressure on side of vertex; tearing from occiput through brain; pain in eyeball; pressure in hypochondria; tearing in thigh.—(*Pressure*), Pressure at
right lower jaw; painful stitch in præcordial region, etc.—(*When reading*),
Headache.—(*Reflecting*), Makes her weak, etc.—(*Rest*), The symptoms;
forearms feel heavy; pressure in little finger-joint, etc.; pain in sides of
legs, over malleoli, etc.—(*When rising from seat and walking*), Paralytic
pain in hip-joint.—(*In room*), After walking in open air, swelling of nose.
—(*Rubbing*), Pain in testicle; pain in region of hip.—(*When sitting*), Pain
in iliac region; cutting over small of back; boring in left shoulder; drawing in tendon of psoas muscle; muscles of thigh appear to be twitching;
pain in knees, as if bandaged.—(*When sitting and stretching body*), Pressing
in right abdominal ring.—(*When spreading legs*), Want of flexibility, etc.,
in bends of groin.—(*When standing*), Vertigo.—(*Before stool*), Pain in abdomen.—(*During stool*), Pain in abdomen.—(*When stooping*), Vertigo; rush
of blood to head; tension in the neck.—(*When stretching leg*), Pressure on
left tibia.—(*Swallowing*), Burning, etc., in throat; stinging in throat; stinging soreness in throat.—(*Talking*), Headache.—(*Touch*), *Pain in tumor on
vertex*; pressure on temple; aching in spots upon nose; soreness in nostrils;
tearing in teeth, etc.; soreness in gums; pain in testicle.—(*Uncovering the
part*), Tearings in left upper arm.—(*When walking*), Boring in zygomatic
process; pressure in hypochondria; want of flexibility, etc., in bends of
groin; heart seems to shake as if loose; weakness of the thigh; pain in
right knee; pain in knees, as if bandaged; right knee becomes weak; pain
in joint of big toe; itching on the leg; itching of joints of feet.—(*When
walking fast*), Dyspnœa.—(*When walking and setting foot on floor*), Pain in
knee.—(*When writing*), Headache.—(*When yawning*), Shuddering in chest;
stitches under ribs.

Amelioration.—(*Towards* 11 P.M.), Pain in testicle ceased.—(*In
open air*), Feels well; *tearing headache.*—(*On going to bed*), Stitches under
ribs cease.—(*When closing eyes*), Tension in the eyes.—(*Motion*), *Pain down
arm goes off; *pain in sides of legs.—(*Pressure*), Stitches on right side go
off.—(*Raising head after stooping*), Rush of blood to head.—(*On rising*),
Pressing in right abdominal ring goes off; drawing in tendon of psoas
muscle; pain in joints passes off; pain in head, etc., passes off.—(*Rising
and drawing up thigh*), Pain in iliac region.—(*In room*), Elevations on legs
form less.—(*Sitting*), Pain in muscles of thigh.

AURUM FULMINANS.

Formula, Au$_2$O$_3$4NH$_3$OH$_2$. The substance referred to by Hahnemann is
doubtful. (See Chr. Kr., 1, 242.)

Pains in the bowels (Pharmac. Wurt., II), (not obtainable).—Sinking of
strength, faintness, cold sweat on the limbs, violent vomiting, convulsions
(Hoffmann, Med. Rat. Syst., etc.), (statement of pernicious effects of A.,
leading on to death).—Forcible evacuations from the bowels (Ludovici
Pharm., etc.), (not obtainable).

AURUM MURIATICUM.

Auric chloride, AuCl₃. *Preparation*, Solution in distilled water for the lower potencies.

Authorities.   1, Hahnemann, Ch. Kr., 1, 241; 2, Mch., ibid.; 3, Molin, d. l. Soc. Med. Hom. de Paris, 1, 24; 4, Buchner, N. Z. f. H. K., 4, 208 (proving with 2d cent. dil.); 5, Eberle, ibid. (proving with the 1st, 3d, and 6th dec. dil., and solution of the crude 1 to 16); 6, "A girl," ibid. (proving with 1st, 3d, and 6th dec. dil., and the crude solution and trituration); 7, "An officer," ibid. (proving with the 6th dec. dil.); 8, Chrestien from Wibmer (effects of $\frac{1}{10}$th gr.); 9, Magendie, from Wibmer (effects of $\frac{1}{10}$th gr.).

Mind.—Excessive cheerfulness, carelessness,³.—Great sadness,⁶.—Sadness, frequent weeping,³.—Sad mood, as though a great misfortune impended (several days),⁵.—Disgust for life; inclination to suicide,³.—Unreasonable contrariety,³.—Indisposition for mental work,⁴.—Weakness of memory,⁴.

Head.—Confusion of the head,⁴.—[10.] Frequent dizziness,³.—Vertigo, and whirling before the eyes on every motion, with tearing pain over the eyes, aggravated by stooping, relieved in the open air; lasts all day, and only goes off on going to bed at night,⁶.—Frequent nodding of the head,³.— Heaviness of the head,³.—Headache, on rising, after a restless night,⁶.— Pressure on the brain, along the sagittal suture,⁴.—Throbbing headache, with heavy dreams,⁶.—Burning in the forehead,³.—Drawing headache in the forehead (after two hours),¹.—Violent pain, like a toothache, in the left frontal eminence, extending towards the supraorbital foramen (the following day in the right side),⁵.—[20.] Beatings in the left side of the forehead,³. —Tickling itching of the forehead (after one hour),¹.—Drawing pain in the left temple, extending to the vertex,⁵.—Tearing in the left temple, lasting several hours, and returning in bed,⁶.—Violent tearing from the left temple towards the ear, with vertigo and tearing over the eye,⁶.—Tearing pain in the left temporal region, extending to the right; lasts all day, and only disappears in bed,⁶.—Throbbing pain in the left temple after rising; relieved by applying cold water; returning after midnight, and lasting four hours,⁶.—Violent tearing in the right temple,⁵.—Sensation of coolness on the top of the head,³.—Burning and stitching in the back of the head,³.

Eyes.—[30.] Dryness of the eyes,⁴.—Burning, pricking, and itching of the eyes,³.—Severe pressure in the eyes in open air, and tearing in them, with complete blindness,⁶.—Tearing pain in the left eye,¹.—Tearing pain, beginning above the left eye and extending toward the right ear, where it at last comes out; the pain was so severe that she had to lie down in bed, when the pain immediately ceased,⁶.—The eye symptoms appeared periodically for some time,⁶.—If the eyes are covered with the hand the symptoms disappear,⁶.—Redness and swelling of the eyelids,³.—Morning-agglutination,³.—Difficulty in keeping the eyes shut,³.—[40.] Biting and itching in the right external canthus, obliges him to scratch,³.—Burning, stitching, pricking, and smarting of the lids,³.—Burning in the conjunctiva,⁴.—Weakness of visual power,⁴.—The letters disappear, at evening by candlelight, for some minutes; instead of the letters, the paper was white as if not printed,⁴.

Ears.—Crusts behind the ears,³.—Burning and itching behind the ears, especially at night,³.—Sensation in the left ear, as if a plug were in it (lasted for several days during the proving),⁵.—Drawing pain in the right ear,⁵.—Sticking pain in the left ear,⁵.—[50.] Deafness in the ears (after six hours).[1].—Deafness follows the ringing in the ears, as if the ears were wide internally and hollow, and so nothing could be heard distinctly,[1].

Nose.—Redness and swelling of the nose,[3].—Red swelling in the right nostril and underneath, with a painless crust of ulcers internally, and a sense of obstruction, although air passes through,[2].—*Red swelling of the left side of the nose; the nasal cavity is ulcerated deep in, with dry, yellowish scurf, and sense of obstruction,* although enough air passes through it,[1].—Redness and itching inflammation of the nose, with subsequent desquamation,[1]. —Crusts in the nose, with constant inclination to pick at them with the fingers,[3].—*A bad-smelling, watery discharge from the nose,* very irritating to the lip,[3].—Discharge of a yellow-greenish matter from the nose, without bad smell, for seven days (after ten days),[1].—Much sneezing in succession, then tearing in the left nasal bone towards the eye, with much injection of the conjunctiva and profuse lachrymation, which suddenly appears, and is so violent that the tears spirt out,[6].—[60.] Thick, yellow coryza,[3].—Fluent coryza nights,[6].—Coryza, with much tickling in the throat,[5].—Fluent coryza, with rough throat and irritation to cough,[5].—Burning and itching of the nose,[3].—Burning and itching pain on the upper part of the nose externally,[1]. —Crawling in the nose, as if something were running about in it,[1].

Face.—Red face,[3].—Lightning-like twitches in the right upper jaw,[5].

Mouth.—Jerking toothache in the anterior and upper row of teeth,[2].— [70.] Jerking pain in the teeth, partly on one side, partly in the upper incisors,[1].—Redness and swelling of the gums, especially at night,[3].—Aphthæ all over the mouth,[3].—Burning, itching, and smarting in the mouth,[3].—Flat taste, lasts all day, with great nausea, passing off at night in bed,[6].—Strong, metallic taste, with increased saliva, with frequent desire to swallow, and a feeling as if a plug were in the throat (after the undiluted solution),[5].

Throat.—Painful swelling of the submaxillary glands,[3].—Pain in the throat, and redness of the mucous membrane of the fauces,[6].—Scratching and pricking in the throat,[3].—Difficult deglutition,[3].

Stomach.—[80.] Want of appetite,[3].—Loss of appetite,[6].—Thirst,[3].— Risings having a putrid taste,[3].—Inclination to vomit after eating,[3].—Nausea and inclination to vomit, mornings fasting, disappears after breakfast,[6].— Great nausea and vomiting of the water taken after the gold, with a trace of clear blood (from a grain of *Aur. mur.* in substance),[6].—Vomiting (for a quarter of an hour), with violent retching and foul eructations, soon afterward cutting colic, and four watery stools,[6].—Violent gastritis,[9].—Slow digestion,[3].—Emptiness in the stomach,[5].—[90.] Distress at the stomach after eating,[3].—Burning, stitching, and gnawing and cutting pains in the stomach,[3]. —Painful drawing in the pit of the stomach extends to the middle of the sternum; as if a hard body were pressed into the cavity;. aggravated by stooping, eating, drinking; it appears only in paroxysms,[5].

Abdomen.—Burning in the right hypochondrium,[3].—Constant disagreeable feeling in the right hypochondrium,[3].—Stitch in the left hypochondrium, as from running too fast,[3].—Redness, heat, itching, and smarting at the umbilicus,[3].—Distension of the abdomen,[1].—Swelling and inflation of the abdomen,[3].—Much flatus passes in the afternoon,[6].—[100.] Much flatulence, with colic and a fluid stool,[6].—Drawings in the entire abdomen,[3]. —Drawing pain in the small intestines, returning the next day, relieved by fluid evacuations, eating, drinking, motion, but not by pressure with both hands on the abdomen,[5].—Dull colic,[3].—Violent constrictive colic obliges her to double up; lasts three and a half hours, and only goes off in bed,⁶.—The abdomen is tender to touch,³.—Heat and pricking in the hypogastrium,³.

Stool and Anus.—*Hæmorrhoids, with discharge of blood during stool,³.—Diarrhœa very violent for several days,⁷.—Diarrhœa, especially at night; gray-whitish stools,³.—[110.] Continued call to stool, with much rumbling in the bowels; in spite of the desire, no satisfactory stool,⁶.—Thin watery stools (immediately after taking it),⁶.—Thin frequent stools, with burning at the anus,⁵.—Frequent thin stools, with tenesmus,⁵.

Urinary Organs.—Heat and itching in the urethra,³.—Burning on urinating; feeling as if the urine was too hot and acrid,⁵.—Burning and smarting in the urethra while urinating,³.—Feeling of heat in the urethra, with tenesmus vesicæ; the urine felt too hot,⁵.—Sticking pain through the whole length of the urethra on standing,⁵.—Constant desire to urinate,⁴.—[120.] Urine increased,⁶.—Profuse urine for two and a half days,⁴.—Scanty urine; red thick urine, containing sand,³.—The urine rapidly decomposes,⁴. —Increase of urea and urates,⁴.

Sexual Organs.—(*Male.*)—Exhausting erections,⁹.—Violent itching of the glans penis wakes at night,⁵.—Drawing along the spermatic cords,³.—Swelling and tension in the testicles,³.—Painful drawing in the left testicle extends toward the inguinal ring, recurring by paroxysms,⁵.— (*Female.*)—Redness and swelling of the labia,³.—A few days before the menses, eruption of large red pimples on the labia majora,³.—**Constant running from the vulva*,³.—**Burning and itching of the vulva*,³.—**Heat and itching in the vagina*,³.—Severe itching of the pudenda, transient,⁶.—Menstruation too early, more profuse; the blood was acrid, and made her sore; before the menses she had leucorrhœa (formerly she had had it a short time only after menses),⁶.—Menses, seven days too early, lasted only two days (usually four days); blood bright (not so acrid as the last time),⁶.— **Leucorrhœa returned* (it had ceased for some time) very profusely, and lasted four days; very acrid, making the thighs sore, with itching of the genitals,⁶.—**Light-yellow leucorrhœa, especially in the morning*,³.

Respiratory Apparatus.—Tickling in the air-passages, with dry cough, as from inspired dust,⁵.—Difficult speech; deep, hoarse voice,³.— Frequent loud cough,³.—[130.] Frequent cough, especially at night,³.— Short dry cough in paroxysms, especially at night, followed by heat in the throat,³.—Frequent hard cough, with white expectoration, mingled with threads of blood,³.—Constant thick cough, with thick yellow expectoration,³. —Difficult respiration,³.—Short breathing and apparent obstruction of the larynx for a few days,¹.—On standing, heavy deep respiration, as if a stone lay on the chest,⁶.—Sense of suffocation,³.—Suffocative attacks at night,³.

Chest.—Great oppression of the chest, scarcely permitting breathing,⁵. —[140.] Spasmodic drawing between the sixth and seventh ribs, with a sensation as though some one attempted to stretch out the heart,⁵.—Burning pains in the left clavicle, transient,⁵.—Drawing pains in both sides of the chest,⁵.—The right side of the chest felt sprained on standing up; touching the pectoral muscles was painful,⁵.—Tearing in the right chest from the middle of the sternum towards the right shoulder-joint; increased by every inspiration (lasts a quarter of an hour),⁶.—Sticking tearing in the intercostal muscles of the right side, then of the left,⁵.—Sticking in the right pectoral muscles; not increased by pressure, somewhat so by deep inspiration; very much increased by motion of the upper part of the body,⁵. —Sticking in the præcordial region, extending toward the middle of the sternum, aggravated by every motion and deep inspiration (lasts four hours),[6].

Heart and Pulse.—Palpitation of the heart,[3].—Burning and pricking at the heart,[3].—[150.] Drawing and cutting pains at the heart,[3].—Wakened in the night by a sticking boring pain at the point of impulse of the apex of the heart, deep in, as if in the heart itself; it lasted some minutes; the prover felt that he could not have longer endured it; not changed by deep inspiration, but as soon as he pressed the hand tightly against the præcordial region the pain disappeared; immediately afterward a lancinating streaming pain extends from this place, and ends in the left hypochondrium; only momentarily so severe that it interrupts respiration; when he inspired more deeply, the pain disappeared,[5].—Oppression about the heart, compelling a deep breath, which relieves,[4].—A few stitches immediately over the heart,[1].

Neck and Back.—Stiffness in the neck,[5].—Burning, pricking, cutting pains and stiffness in the back,[3].—Bruised feeling in the small of the back, which makes stooping almost impossible,[5].—Painful fatigue in the loins,[3].—Pricking in the loins,[3].

Extremities in General.—Unusual prostration of the limbs,[6].—[160.] Bruised feeling of the limbs,[4].

Upper Extremities.—Stiffness in the arms,[3].—Burning and lancinations in the arms and forearms,[3].—Sensation as if the left arm were sprained,[6].—Involuntary shocks in the arms,[3].—Painful feeling in the shoulders and arms,[3].—Paralytic feeling in the left shoulder, after rising (lasts half an hour),[6].—Drawing pain in the right shoulder-joint,[5].—Drawing and boring in the middle of the right upper arm, recurring three days in succession,[5].—Tearing in the left shoulder, lasts two hours; the shoulder still, after two days, sensitive to touch,[6].—[170.] Drawing in the elbows, as if a tendon were violently drawn; frequently returning for a moment, day and night,[5].—Tearing in the right arm from the elbow-joint to the tip of the little finger, so violent that it hinders work,[6].—Difficulty in clenching the hands,[3].—Burning and itching in the hands,[3].—Violent drawing in the balls of the right hand,[5].—Stiffness of the finger-joints,[3].—Tearing pain in the middle finger, after dinner,[1].—Swelling in the wrist, without pain, if left alone; tensive only on bending the hand backwards; stitches in the wrist upon seizing anything,[1].

Lower Extremities.—Drawing tearing pain in the muscles of both hips, lasts some time,[3].—Lancinating paroxysmal pain beginning in the front and middle of both thighs, and extending toward the patellæ, so severe that he must start up,[5].—[180.] Stiffness of the thighs and legs,[3].—Swelling of the knees,[3].—Heat, pricking, and lancinations in the knees,[3].—Spasmodic tearing in the leg, beginning below the popliteal space, and extending to the middle of the calf; lasts four hours severely, and then gradually disappears,[6].—Bruised sensation in the lower third of the right leg; it becomes so painful on continuing to walk that he has to limp home; with the feeling as if it always more and more tended to the great toe, and would go off the end of it,[5].—Swelling of the feet,[3].—Burning in the feet,[3].—Redness of the toes,[3].—Tearing on the inside of the right great toe and right knee,[6].—Cutting pain in the toes when walking,[3].

Generalities.—[190.] Laziness; aversion to all work,[3].—Weariness,[3].—Weariness during the whole proving, so great that often she could hardly go about, and had to rest frequently through the day,[6].—Great fatigue,[5].—Unending feeling of prostration in the limbs, indescribable weari-

ness in the whole body; can scarcely rise from his seat,[5].—General erethism,[8].—The excited condition lasted several years,[9].—Drawing tearing
pains in various parts of the body, especially in the extremities,[5].

Skin.—Pimples on the lips, with smarting and itching,[3].—Eruption
of small red pimples above the pubis,[3].—[200.] Petechiæ-like exanthema
on both legs, with a small pimple in the centre (disappears in five days),[5].—
Boils on the buttocks and thighs,[3].

Sleep and Dreams.—Frequent yawning soon after taking a dose;
it disappears after eating, but returns and lasts two hours,[6].—Much yawning after eating,[3].—Sleepiness in daytime, even while at work,[3].—Sleepiness; deep sleep,[4].—Sleep very restless, with frightful dreams the whole
night,[5].—Waking with a start,[3].—Sleeplessness obstinate,[9].—Nocturnal
sleeplessness,[3].—[210.] Troublesome dreams,[3].—Heavy dreams of impending unhappiness,[6].

Fever.— Chilliness, with gooseflesh,[6]. — *Violent fever,*[8][9]. — Sweat increased,[8].

Conditions.—Aggravation.—(*Morning*), On rising, after a restless
night, headache; fasting, nausea, etc.; leucorrhœa.—(*Night*), Burning, etc.,
behind ears; redness, etc., of gums; diarrhœa; itching of glans penis; frequent cough; short dry cough; suffocative attacks; pain at apex of heart.—
(*In open air*), Pressure in eyes, etc.—(*In bed*), Tearing in left temple returns.—(*After dinner*), Pain in middle finger.—(*Drinking*), Drawing in
pit of stomach.—(*After eating*), Inclination to vomit; distress at stomach;
drawing in pit of stomach; much yawning.—(*Every inspiration*), Tearing
in right chest.—(*Deep inspiration*), Sticking in right pectoral muscles;
sticking in præcordial region.—(*Motion*), Vertigo, etc.; sticking in præcordial region.—(*Motion of upper part of body*), Sticking in right pectoral
muscles.—(*Periodic*), The eye-symptoms.—(*After rising*), Paralytic feeling
in left shoulder.—(*Upon seizing anything*), Stitches in wrist.—(*On standing*), Pain through the urethra; heavy, deep respiration; right side of chest
felt sprained.—(*Stooping*), Drawing in pit of stomach.—(*Walking*), Bruised
sensation in right leg; cutting pain in toes.

Amelioration.—(*Night*), In bed, flat taste, etc., passes off.—(*In
bed*), Pain in temporal region disappears; colic goes off.—(*After breakfast*),
Nausea, etc., disappears.—(*When covering eyes with hand*), Eye-symptoms
disappear.—(*After eating*), Yawning ceases.—(*Deep inspiration*), Pain at
apex of heart disappears; oppression at heart.—(*On lying down in bed*),
Pain from above eye towards ear ceases.—(*Pressing hand tightly against
præcordial region*), Pain at apex of heart disappears.

AURUM MURIATICUM NATRONATUM.

Chloro-aurate of soda. *Formula*, $NaCl,AuCl_3,2H_2O$. *Preparation*, Triturations.

Authority. 1, Lembke, N. Z. f. H. K., 11, 17, et seq., took the 3d, 2d
and a solution of the salt in water; 2, Chatterly, Dublin Press, 1852 (effect
of $\frac{1}{30}$ grain injected under the skin); 3, Cullerier, from Wibmer, general
statement of effects.

Head.—Headache,[3].—Heaviness in forehead, all day,[1].—Heaviness
and pressure in forehead,[1].—Heaviness in forehead when sitting,[1].—Wandering pains in forehead,[1].—Heat and heaviness in forehead,[1].—Violent
boring in frontal bone, especially on right side,[1].—Boring in left side of

frontal bone,[1].—Violent boring in left frontal bone, deep into left eye,[1].—
[10.] Drawing in left side of forehead,[1].—Frequent drawing in forehead,
above the eyes, with pressure and heaviness, lasting several hours,[1].—
Drawing and boring in the frontal bone,[1].—Drawing in frontal bone, when
sitting,[1].—Pressure in forehead,[1].—Violent tearing in right side of frontal
bone,[1].—Boring in left temple,[1].—Boring as with a wedge in left temple,[1].—
Violent boring in right temple,[1].—Violent boring in left temple,[1].—[20.]
Distensive pressure in temples,[1].—Throbbing in temples,[1].—Boring in right
side of vertex,[1].—Drawing diagonally across vertex,[1].—Tearing diagonally
over vertex,[1].—Violent stitching in left side of vertex,[1].—Boring in right
side of head,[1].—Tearing in the left side of the skull bone,[1].—Tearing in
left side of head,[1].—Cutting pain in a small spot of right parietal bone,[1].—
[30.] Sharp, cutting pain, while sitting, above forehead, on left side of
head,[1].—Heaviness and heat in occiput,[1].—Boring in left side of occiput,[1].—
Drawing in bones of occiput,[1].—Drawing in occiput,[1].—Drawing in left
occiput,[1].—Lateral drawing sensation in occiput,[1].

Eyes.—Forcible and involuntary closing of left eye, by a violent boring
in left side of frontal bone,[1].—Boring in right eye,[1].—Stitches in left eye,[1].—
[40.] Boring above both eyes,[1].—Violent boring in the orbital bone, above
the right eye, when walking,[1].—Violent boring in bone over left eye,[1].—
Boring above right eye,[1].—Constant boring in the bones below the eyes,[1].—
Burning in edges of eyelids,[1].—Stitching in right inner canthus,[1].—Stitches
in left outer canthus,[1].—Stitches and burning in margins of eyelids,[1].—
Stitching in right eyeball,[1].—[50.] Violent stitches in left eyeball,[1].

Ears.—Deepseated boring in neighborhood of right ear,[1].—Violent
boring in bone before left ear,[1].—Boring behind left ear,[1].—Pressure in
bone before right ear,[1].—Burning heat in the ears,[1].—Boring in depth of
right ear,[1].—Stitches in right ear,[1].—Stitches deep in left ear,[1].

Nose.—Air passes with unusual freedom through nasal passages,[1].—
[60.] Frequent sneezing,[1].—Boring in the nasal bones,[1].—Boring close to
right of nasal bone,[1].—Violent boring along left side of nose,[1].—Drawing
in nose, from tip upwards; also, on both sides of nose, with sensation as if
the organ and adjacent parts were thickened,[1].—Pressure in left side of
nasal bone,[1].—Biting pain in right wing of nose,[1].

Face.—Deepseated drawing in face and head,[1].—Heat in cheeks and
ears, perceptible externally,[1].—Heat in cheeks, and sensible burning,[1].—
[70.] Burning heat in cheeks,[1].—Burning in the cheeks, increased by
stooping,[1].—Boring deep in left cheek,[1].—Drawing in left cheek,[1].—Drawing pain from above downward, in left cheek,[1].—Drawing in right cheek
when sitting,[1].—Tearing in left cheek,[1].—Stitching in skin of left cheek,[1].—
Fine stitching in the skin of the cheeks, followed by heat,[1].—Cutting pain
on a small spot of the skin of the right cheek,[1].—[80.] Lower lip cracked
in centre, with biting, burning, and pain when touched,[1].—Burning in
under lip,[1].—Burning on the edge of the upper lip,[1].—Violent stitching in
left side of under lip,[1].—Violent stitching in the vermilion border of the
lower lip,[1].—Biting in the under lip,[1].—Pulsation in under lip, with feeling
as if its centre was thickened,[1].—Twitching about the chin, toward the lower
lip,[1].—Drawing in chin,[1].—Boring in left upper jaw,[1].—[90.] Boring in left
side of lower jaw,[1].

Mouth.—Tension in the roots of the teeth on the left side,[1].—Boring
in the roots of the teeth of the right side; also, alternating with stitches
when sitting,[1].—Drawing in the lower incisors,[1].—Cutting and boring in
lower incisors,[1].—Burning on the under surface of tongue, and below

tongue,[1].—Deepseated burning below tongue,[1].—Burning in the tip of the tongue,[1].—Persistent burning in tip of tongue, with stitching,[1].—Stitching in tip of tongue,[1].—[100.] Stitching below the tongue, with some scraping,[1]. —Biting sensation on tip of tongue, immediately after taking the medicine,[1].—Redness and painful swelling of the mucous membrane behind the upper incisors, especially when touched, and by contact with warm or salted food,[1].—The inflamed spot is like a yellow blister with a red edge, the redness extending toward the left palate; it afterwards looks rose-red, is somewhat painful to touch, and feels rough and swollen,[1].—Dryness of mouth and throat,[3].—Saliva increased,[2].—Taste partly sweetish, partly metallic, with copious flow of saliva,[1].—Long-lasting metallic taste, after each dose,[1]. —Coppery taste in mouth, with constriction of the salivary glands, clear saliva and dulness of the teeth, ceasing while eating, but afterwards commencing again,[1].

Throat.—Stitching deep in the throat,[1].—[110.] Scraping in fauces, with pretty copious flow of saliva,[1].

Stomach.—Short-lasting nausea, immediately after taking the medicine,[1].—Gastric irritation,[3].—Pressure in epigastric region,[3].

Stool and Anus.—Appearance of a hæmorrhoidal tumor, which protrudes and is painful,[1].—Stitches in the anus,[1].—Constipation or diarrhœa,[3].

Urinary Organs.—Stitching in the end of the urethra,[1].—Cutting in the end of the urethra, also on urinating,[1].—Very frequent urination,[1].— [120.] Excessive diuresis,[2].

Respiratory Apparatus.—Sudden and very violent scraping in the larynx, with violent dry cough, causing gagging,[1].—Tickling in the larynx, with dry cough,[1].—Tickling in the larynx, and as if somewhat deeper,[1].—Very violent tickling in larynx, followed by dry cough, causing gagging, when sitting and writing,[1].—Much short dry cough,[1].—Frequent short, dry cough, with scraping in the larynx,[1].—Difficult respiration, with anxiety,[1].

Chest.—Wandering pain in left wall of thorax, during rest,[1].—Boring in the left wall of the thorax, above the nipple,[1].—[130.] Drawing pain above left clavicle, towards the shoulder and nape of neck, when sitting,[1].— Pressure, outwards, from the right nipple, on the wall of the thorax, unaffected by respiration,[1].—Dull pressure between sternum and right nipple,[1]. —Tearing between the ribs, below the left nipple, when walking,[1].—Much stitching in right thoracic wall,[1].—Stitches in the wall of the thorax, below the left axilla,[1].—Stitches in the left thoracic wall, two inches below the nipple, unaffected by respiration,[1].—Transient stitches in the wall of the thorax, now on the right, now on the left, when walking,[1].—Seated pressure deep in chest, behind the sternum, and extending into the back, when walking,[1].

Heart and Pulse.—Irregular beating of the heart, with anxiety and shortness of breath,[1].—[140.] Rapid, small, irregular beats of the heart, on slight motion, with oppression,[1].—Rapid, irregular beats of the heart, when stooping,[1].—Several violent beats of the heart, with sensation of pressure while standing,[1].

Neck and Back.—Cracking in the cervical vertebræ on bending the head,[1].—Burning pain in the skin of the nape of neck,[1].—Heat in nape of neck, rising into the head and cheeks,[1].—Burning and drawing to the left of nape of neck,[1].—Tension and pressure in the muscles to the left of the nape of the neck, as far as the left clavicle, increased by bending the head to the right, at times also unbearable during rest,[1].—Boring in left scapula,[1].—Pressure in the muscles on the side of the left shoulder-blade,[1].— [150.] Drawing in the dorsal vertebræ,[1].—Pressure and drawing in the muscles on the left side of the back,[1].

Upper Extremities.—Bruised pain during rest, in the joints of the arms and in the wrists,[1].—Deepseated burning in left shoulder,[1].—Burning in skin of right axilla,[1].—Drawing in left shoulder,[1].—Drawing in the shoulders and upper arms.[1].—Drawing and boring in left shoulder,[1].— Severe and frequent pressure in shoulder-joints,[1].—Pressure and drawing in right shoulder,[1].—[160.] Violent pressure on the right shoulder-blade,[1].— Violent pressure in the left shoulder, when walking,[1].—Pressure in the right deltoid muscle, with feeling of warmth which extends into the fingers,[1].—Stitching in right axilla, during rest,[1].—Burning in the inner side of right arm,[1].—Drawing in the skin of right upper arm,[1].—Stitching in the upper portion of the left arm,[1].—Violent boring above the right elbow,[1].—Drawing in left elbow-joint,[1].—Pressure above the right elbow,[1].— [170.] Pressure in right elbow-joint,[1].—Pressure in left elbow-joint,[1].— Pressure in both elbow-joints, during rest,[1].—Violent pressure in bend of left elbow, when walking,[1].—Pressure in left elbow-joint, and into the forearm, during rest,[1].—Continual pressure in the right elbow-joint, during rest, decreasing on motion of the arm,[1].—Violent tearing in left elbow-joint, relieved by motion,[1].—Bruised pain in right elbow-joint,[1].—Pain, as from weariness, in lower part of left forearm,[1].—Constant pain as from weariness in right forearm, with increased sensation of warmth,[1].—[180.] Burning pain in skin of dorsal side of left forearm,[1].—Boring in lower part of left forearm,[1].—Violent pressure in the right forearm,[1].—Very painful pressure in both forearms, when lying quiet,[1].—Violent pressure in the forearm and elbow-joint, when sitting,[1].—Pressure in left forearm, during rest of the part,[1].—Bruised pain in right forearm, during rest,[1].—Pressure in the left wrist, then in the right,[1].—Pressure in right wrist, then in left, when sitting,[1].—Pressure in both wrists, during rest,[1].—Pressure in the right wrist, during rest of the part,[1].—[190.] Pressure in wrist and elbow-joints,[1].— Cold hands, blue nails, with heat in the face and ears,[1].—Constant sharp burning in the skin of the back of the right hand,[1].—Drawing in bones of right hand, with sensation as if they were broken,[1].—Burning in tip of left little finger,[1].—Boring in the bones of the right fingers,[1].—Boring in the roots of the left fingers,[1].—Boring in the right finger-joints,[1].—Violent boring in the first joint of the left index finger, during rest of the part,[1].— Tension in the roots of the fingers,[1].—[200.] Tension in the roots of the right fingers,[1].—Violent stretching sensation in the right fingers, when walking,[1].—Sensation of stretching apart in the roots of the left fingers, afterwards in the left wrist, when sitting,[1].—Drawing in the roots of the fingers,[1].—Drawing in the roots of the left fingers,[1].—Very painful drawing in the right fingers, when sitting,[1].—Drawing in the roots of the left fingers, when walking and sitting,[1].—Pressure in the second joint of right thumb,[1].—Pressure in the joints of the right little finger,[1].—Violent tearing in the second joint of the right thumb,[1].—Violent stitching in left finger-tips,[1].—[210.] Violent stitching, as with needles, in the tip of the right little finger,[1].—Very painful stitching in several finger-joints,[1].

Lower Extremities.—Pain as from weariness in legs when sitting, ceasing while moving them,[1].—Burning in the skin of right hip,[1].—Pressing in the hip-joint, when sitting,[1].—Stitching in the flesh on the inner side of the left thigh,[1].—Pain in right knee, when walking,[1].—Burning in the skin, above left knee, afterward above right knee,[1].—Boring in the knees,[1].—Boring in right knee,[1].—[**220.**] Violent boring in the right knee,[1].—Violent boring in right knee, when sitting,[1].—Drawing in left knee,[1].—Pressure in right knee,[1].—Pressure in left knee,[1].—Pressure in right knee, as if broken,[1].—Boring pressure in the knees,[1].—Pressing, during rest, in the left knee,[1].—Violent pressure in right knee, when sitting,[1].—Pressure in the right knee, afterwards in the left, when sitting,[1].—[**230.**] Cutting in the skin above the left knee,[1].—Stitching in the flesh above right knee, on the inner side,[1].—Very painful stitching in left knee,[1].—Stitching in left knee, when sitting,[1].—Stitches in left knee, when walking,[1].—Burning in skin of right calf,[1].—Burning in skin of left calf,[1].—Boring in the tibiæ,[1].—Boring in the lower part of left tibia,[1].—Boring, first in right tibia, then in left,[1].—[**240.**] Boring in left tibia,[1].—Boring in left tibia, when sitting,[1].—Boring in skin of right calf,[1].—Violent boring in left tibia, when sitting,[1].—Constant violent boring in left shin-bone, when sitting,[1].—Drawing in the shins,[1].—Drawing in the right tibia,[1].—Drawing in centre of left tibia, extending into the ankle,[1].—Drawing in lower part of right tibia,[1].—Drawing in lower part of left shin-bone,[1].—[**250.**] Drawing in left tibia, during rest,[1].—Drawing in calves,[1].—Pressure in lower part of left tibia,[1].—Boring pressure in the tibiæ,[1].—Cutting in a small spot of the skin of the right tibia,[1].—Painless crepitus, as from rubbing dry leather, below the inner bone of right ankle, when lying still,[1].—Boring about the right ankle,[1].—Boring in right ankle, when standing,[1].—Much boring in the right ankle,[1].—Drawing in left ankle, when lying down,[1].—[**260.**] Pressure in ankles when sitting,[1].—Pressure in right ankle-joint, during rest,[1].—Pressure in the left ankle, when sitting (several times),[1].—Pressing in the left ankle,[1].—Violent boring in right great toe,[1].—Boring in the bone on right sole,[1].—Violent boring in left heel,[1].—Boring in dorsum of right foot,[1].—Violent boring in both sides of the right tendo Achillis, when sitting,[1].—Violent, long-lasting, and repeated boring in the right os calcis,[1]. —[**270.**] Boring in left os calcis,[1].—Boring in lower part of right shin-bone,[1].—Drawing in left heel,[1].—Drawing in the right foot, from the sole to the tips of the toes, when sitting,[1].—Drawing in inner edge of right foot, then of the left, when sitting, in the evening,[1].—Drawing in the toes,[1].—Pressure on right foot, when sitting,[1].—Violent pressure on dorsum of left foot,[1].—Tearing in the sole of right foot,[1].—Acute stitching and burning in the ball of the right foot,[1].—[**280.**] Stitching in the toes of the left foot,[1].—Violent stitches in the balls of the foot,[1].—Stretching-apart sensation in the right toes,[1].—Violent boring in plantar surface of right great toe, during rest, ceasing on moving the toe, but again felt as soon as the toe is quiet,[1].—Drawing in right toes, when sitting,[1].—Drawing in right toes when walking or sitting,[1].—Deepseated drawing in left great toe,[1].—Cutting and boring in left great toe,[1].—Cutting in tips of right toes, when sitting,[1].—Stitching in the back of right great toe,[1].—[**290.**] Stitching in tip of right great toe,[1].—Stitching in the tips of right toes,[1].—Stitching on the end of left great toe,[1].—Stitching in right toe.[1].—Stitching in the ends of the toes, when sitting,[1].—Stitching in tips of right toes,[1].—Sharp stitches in the usually painless bunions, while sitting in easy shoes,[1].

Generalities.—General increase of secretions from the stomach, intestines, and kidneys,[2].—Great. general, long-lasting erethism,[1].—Accelerated circulation,[3].—[**300.**] Lassitude,[1].—Sensation of general weakness and discomfort, as if sickness were coming on,[1].—Great weakness on rising in the morning, though after resting well, which lasts for an hour,[1].

Fever.—Remarkable coldness in the back,[1].—Remarkable and long-lasting heat of the skin,[1].—Internal warmth,[3].

Conditions.—Aggravation.—(*Bending head to right*), Tension, etc., in muscles to left of nape of neck.—(*When lying down*), Drawing in left ankle.—(*When lying quiet*), Pressure in both forearms; crepitus below right ankle-bone.—(*On slight motion*), Rapid, etc., beats of heart.—(*During rest*), All symptoms remarkably aggravated; pain in left wall of thorax; tension, etc., in muscles to left of nape of neck'; pain in joints of arms, etc.; stitching in right axilla; pressure in both elbow-joints; pressure in left elbow-joint; pressure in right elbow-joint; pain in right forearm; pressure in both wrists; drawing in left tibia.—(*During rest of the part*), Pressure in left forearm; pressure in right wrist; burning in joint of index finger.—(*Contact with salted food*), Pain behind upper incisors.—(*When sitting*), Heaviness of forehead; drawing in frontal bone; cutting pain above forehead; drawing in right cheek; stitches in roots of teeth; pain above left clavicle; pressure in forearm, etc.; pressure in right wrist, etc.; sensation of stretching apart in roots of fingers, etc.; drawing in right fingers; drawing in roots of right fingers; pain in legs; pressing in hip-joint; *boring in right knee;* pressure in right knee; stitching in left knee; *boring in left tibia;* pressure in ankles; pressure in left ankle; boring in both sides of tendo Achillis; drawing in right foot; in evening, drawing in inner edge of right foot, etc.; pressure on right foot; *drawing in right toes;* cutting in right toe-tips; stitching in toe-tips.—(*When sitting or walking*), Tickling in larynx, etc.—(*While standing*), Violent beats of heart, etc.; boring in right ankle.—(*Stooping*), Burning in cheeks; rapid, etc., beats of heart.—(*Touch*), Pain behind upper incisors.—(*On urinating*), Cutting in end of urethra.—(*When walking*), Boring in orbital bone; stitches in wall of thorax; pressure in chest; pressure in left shoulder; pressure in bend of elbow; stretching sensation in right fingers; drawing in roots of right fingers; pain in knee; stitches in left knee; drawing in right toes.—(*Contact with warm food*), Pain behind upper incisors.

Amelioration.—(*While eating*), Dulness of teeth ceases.—(*Motion of arm*), Pressure in right elbow-joint; tearing in left elbow-joint.—(*Moving the part*), Pain in legs.

AURUM SULFURATUM.

Auric sulphide, Au_2S_3.   *Preparation*, Triturations.
Authority.   Molin, Bull. d. l. Soc. Med. Hom. de Paris, 1, 28.

Mind.—Desire for solitude.—Gloomy, anxious, wretched disposition.—Disgust for life.—Vexation.—Rude, disagreeable mood.

Head.—Constant nodding of the head.—Dizziness.—Continual rush of blood to the head.—Great itching of the head, especially at night.—[10.] Lancinations in the occiput.—Burning and smarting of the scalp.—Falling off of the hair.

Eyes.—Beatings in the eyes.—Redness of the lids.—Morning-agglutination of the lids.—Sty near the outer canthus.—Lancinations, itching and pricking of the lids.—Light is painful to the eyes.

Ears.—Burning and lancination in the ears.—[20.] Hardness of hearing.

Nose.—Redness and swelling of the nose.—Crusts in the nose.—Frequent sneezing.—Dry coryza.—Beating and cutting pain in the nose.—Lancination and itching of the nose.—Great sensitiveness of the nose to the least contact.

Face.—Paleness of the face.—Face covered with red blotches.—[30.] Cracked lips.

Mouth.—Numb feeling in the teeth.—Lancinations, drawing, and cutting pains in the teeth.—Dull pains which begin in the upper molars, rise into the whole head, and then go down into the teeth again.—Redness, swelling, and bleeding of the gums.—Discoloration of the tongue and gums.—Aphthæ on the inside of the cheeks only, with smarting and lancinations.

Throat.—Swelling of the thyroid gland.—Pain in the parotids.—Lancination and drawing in the throat.—[40.] Difficult deglutition.

Stomach.—Loss of appetite.—Urgent thirst.—Tasteless, watery eructations.—Watery eructations tasting of the ingesta.—Frequent hiccough.—Nausea.—Inclination to vomit shortly after eating.—Extremely slow digestion.—Heat and lancinations in the stomach.

Abdomen.—[50.] Lancinations in different parts of the abdomen about the waist.—Lancinations and drawings in the right hypochondrium.—Inflation of the abdomen, with tenderness to touch.—Sensation of a ball rolling in the abdomen.—Sensation as if something were tearing in the abdomen.—On standing up, it seems as if something would fall out of the body.—Dull pains in the hypogastrium.—Lancinations in the hypogastrium.

Stool and Anus.—Lancinations, drawings, tearing, itching, and cutting pains at the anus.—Stools like rabbits' dung.—[60.] Constipation.

Urinary Organs.—Nocturnal enuresis.—Thick, yellow, red, and sandy urine.

Sexual Organs.—(*Male.*) Frequent erections, with desire for an embrace, but ceasing immediately.—Impotence.—Heat, smarting, and lancinations in the penis.—Painful swelling of the testicles.—(*Female.*) Redness and swelling of the vulva.—Moisture of the vulva and around the glans.—Heaviness of the genitals in females.—[70.] Heat, lancinations, and itching of the vulva.—Thick, yellowish leucorrhœa, especially in the morning.—Irregular menstruation, sometimes too soon, sometimes retarded.—Suppression of the menses.—Sensitiveness of the uterus to the touch.

Respiratory Apparatus.—Hoarseness.—Dry cough.—Nightly paroxysms of loud cough.—Frequent thick cough, especially in bad weather.—Thick cough, with yellowish expectoration.—[80.] Hard cough, with scanty expectoration of pure blood.—Thick cough, day and night, with insipid yellowish expectoration.—Difficult respiration.—Suffocative attacks at night.

Chest.—Swelling of the breasts; they are painful to touch.—Cracks on the nipple.—Lancinations and pricking under the clavicles.—Smarting and lancinations in the summit of the breasts.

Heart and Pulse.—Palpitations when ascending a height, when running, and after all violent movements.—Dull pains at the heart.—[90.] Lancinations at the heart.

Neck and Back.—Pain when turning the neck.—Cutting pains and burning in the back.—Tearing sensation along the spine.—Lancinations, pricking, and heat in the loins.—Bruised feeling in the loins.

Upper Extremities.—Stiffness of the arms.—Cutting pains in the arms on moving them.—Lancinations and tearing pains in the arm.—Redness and swelling of the back of the hand.

Lower Extremities.—[100.] Difficulty in walking.—Stiffness in the thighs.—Lancinations in the legs.—Swelling of the feet.

Generalities.—Staggering gait.—Painful weariness, stomachache, and nausea before the appearance of the menses.

Skin.—Red pimples on the face.—Pimples on the lips, with heat and short stitches.

Sleep and Dreams.—Sleepiness in daytime, with nocturnal wakefulness.—Nightly restlessness.—[110.] Troublesome, frightful dreams.—Dreams of thieves, assassins, etc.

Conditions. — **Aggravations.** — (*Morning*), Leucorrhœa.—(*Night*), Itching of head; suffocative attacks.—(*When ascending*), Palpitation of heart.—(*After eating*), Inclination to vomit.—(*Before menses*), Painful weariness, etc.—(*After violent movements*), Palpitation of heart.—(*On moving the part*), Pain in arms.—(*When running*), Palpitation of heart.—(*In bad weather*), Cough.

BADIAGA.

Spongilla fluviatilis (Spongia palustris, Linn.). Section Protozoa of the animal kingdom. *Common name*, Fresh-water sponge. *Russian name*, Badiaga. *Preparation*, Trituration of the dried sponge gathered in autumn

Authorities. (Hering's Résumé, Hahn. Monthly, 2, 123.) 1, G. Lingen, effects observed from triturating the drug; 2, L. Bedford, provings with the 30th dil.

Mind.—A moan or shriek, caused by the pain in the side,[2].—In spite of the headache, he is still clear in his mind, and more inclined to mental activity than before,[1].

Head.—Dull, dizzy feeling of head,[2].—Headache, does not affect the mind,[1],—Headache commencing between 1 and 2 P.M., lasting till between 6 and 7 in the evening (seventh and ninth days),[2].—Headache with inflamed eyes,[2].—During the day, more or less headache, *with pain in eyeballs*, worse in the left ; more from 1 o'clock in the afternoon till 7 in the evening (sixth day),[2].—*Headache from 2 P.M. till 7 A.M., with slight aching pains in the posterior portion of both eyeballs*, and in the temples (fifth day),[2].—Headache, coryza, and some other symptoms, better on the fifteenth day, less during the afternoon (twelfth day). Dull during the afternoon, beginning at 1 o'clock (thirteenth day),[2].—[10.] Headache and soreness of the body, aggravated from 7 to 10 in the evening, on a rainy day (fourteenth day) ; slight on the fifteenth day, from 1 to 3 in the afternoon (sixteenth day),[2].—Frontal headache, during the forenoon, worse in the temples, *and extending into the posterior portion of the left eyeball, aggravated by moving the eyes* (tenth day) ; the same on the eleventh day, but worse in the afternoon until late in the evening ; the same the thirteenth day, *extending to both eyeballs, aggravated by moving them in either direction;* worse in the afternoon, with heat in the forehead and dull aching in the temples,[2].—During the afternoon, heat, pain, and congestion in the forehead, worse at 7 in the evening (tenth day),[2].—Congestion in forehead,[2].—In forehead, drawing,[1].—In temples and eyeballs, pain ; to the temples from eyeballs,[2].—A very severe headache on the top of the head, remains the same in all positions, better at night *after sleeping*, and better in the morning, returning violently after breakfast, lasting several days. C. Hg.—Scalp sore to the touch, with tetter-like eruption on the forehead, and dull, dizzy feeling of the head during the forenoon (twelfth day); soreness less on the fifteenth day,[2].—Itching of the scalp, with much dandruff, like tetter, and dryness of the hair, thirteenth day; tetter less on the fifteenth day; all disappeared on the seventeenth day; hair again soft and oily; this whole change taking place last night mostly,[2].—An excess of dandruff or dry tetter-like appearance of the scalp, with slight itching (eleventh day),[2].

Eyes.—[20.] Under the eyes, blue,[2].—Scrofulous inflammation of the eyes, with hardening of the Meibomian glands. N. N.—The right eye is irritated and somewhat inflamed, with headache during the afternoon, same as the seventh and eighth days,[2].—*Bluish-purple margin of the eyelids, and blueness under the eye* (twelfth day),[2].—Twitching of the left eyelid,[1].—*Headache extending to the eyeballs,*[2].—Pain in left eyeball from temples; from forehead,[2].—Pain in the left eyeball and temple, quite severe, extending to the left side of the head and forehead (eleventh day),[2].—Pains in the eyeballs extending into the temples, aggravated by turning them in either direction (ninth day),[2].—At 3 P.M., in the posterior portion of the right eyeball, a severe intermitting pain, more or less severe during the afternoon (third day); same, and in temple (fourth day); in left eye (sixth day),[2].—Slight aching pains in the posterior portion of both eyeballs and in the temples (with headache from 2 P.M. till 7 in the morning), (fifth day),[2].—[30.] *The left eyeball quite sore, even upon closing it tightly* (twelfth day),[2].

Ears.—During the afternoon, very *slight shocks heard in the ear as of very distant artillery* (nineteenth day); the same three or four times *during afternoon and evening* (twentieth day); occasional and momentarily up to the twenty-seventh day,[2].

Nose.—Occasional sneezing, with more profuse coryza, most on the left side, with occasional stoppage of the nose; worse in the afternoon and evening (eighth day),[2].—*Sneezing with coryza* at times during the day, with a cough as from cold, more during the afternoon (fifth day); cough causing sneezing and profuse coryza (seventh day),[2].—Sneezing, fluent coryza, with stoppage at the nose at times (tenth day),[2].—Profuse discharge from the left nostril (twelfth day); thick yellowish mucus, more during the afternoon; it is also hawked up (thirteenth day),[2].—His catarrh lessened perceptibly,[1].—Coryza and cough (ninth day),[2].—Itching of the left wing of the nose,[1].

Face.—*Pale, ashy or lead color of the face* (twelfth day),[2].—[40.] Left cheek and malar bone quite sore to the touch (thirteenth day),[2].—Stiffness in the maxillary joints. C. Hg.

Mouth.—In a decayed back-tooth, drawing,[1].—During the afternoon, *the mouth and breath hot and feverish, with thirst for large quantities of water at a time* (tenth day),[2].—Mouth and tongue as if scalded,[2].—Bad taste in mouth, evening,[2].

Throat.—*Hawked up a viscid solid lump of bloody mucus in the morning* (twelfth day). Next day, when first getting out of bed, *a mass of hard, gluey, bloody mucus, tough and dry* (thirteenth day),[2].—*Throat inflamed and sore,* especially on swallowing, 2 P.M. (eleventh day); increasing same day; quite inflamed and sore, especially on swallowing, while most other symptoms are better or disappearing (twelfth day),[2].—Throat quite sore; tonsils red and inflamed, aggravated much on swallowing; 2 P.M. (thirteenth day); especially upon swallowing solids (fourteenth day); disappeared (fifteenth day),[2].

Stomach.—Good appetite, with less thirst, and with a feeling as if the mouth and tongue had been slightly scalded with hot tea (twelfth day),².—But little appetite; took toast for dinner; at 7 in the evening, for tea, a small piece of toast and cup of tea, with a bad appetite and bad taste in the mouth (eleventh day); better on twelfth day,².—Diminished appetite; bowels costive; urine high-colored (tenth day),².—Thirst for large quantities of water,².—[50.] Less thirst, with a good appetite,².—At 8 A.M., a severe lancinating pain in the pit of the stomach, extending to the vertebra opposite, and to the right scapula, and at times to the right side, resulting there in a pleuritic pain; also, a pleuritic pain on the left side, which, as well as on the right side, is aggravated by contortions of the body, and on full inspiration (tenth day),².

Abdomen.—A lancinating pain, with a bounding movement in the region of the liver, lasting but a few minutes (eighth day),².—(Indurated inguinal glands. Popular remedy,°.)—(Syphilitic bubo in the left groin; a longish swelling as hard as a stone, uneven, ragged, like a scirrhus; at night, violent lancinations, as if with red-hot needles,°.) Rosenstein.— (Buboes originating by consensus or cellular irritation, with shooting pains, if suppuration has not commenced, will disappear in three days completely, if, with rest, low diet, and cold local applications, the tincture of Badiaga is given, one drop in a tablespoonful of water, every three or four hours,°.) Rosenstein.—(Buboes, with decided fluctuation, are scattered and absorbed from six drops of the tincture every day in water,°.) Rosenstein.—(Hæmorrhoids. Popular remedy,°.)

Urinary Organs.—Severe, sharp lancinating pain in and near the orifice of the urethra, lasting but a few minutes, at noon (third day),².— Urine high-colored (tenth day),²; and reddish (twelfth day),².

Respiratory Apparatus—[60.] Breath hot and feverish,².— *Occasional severe paroxysms of spasmodic cough, ejecting viscid mucus from the bronchial tubes, which at times comes flying forcibly out of the mouth*, more during the afternoon, *caused by a tickling in the larynx as if a particle of sugar was being dissolved in the throat* (sixth day). Similar paroxysms during the seventh day, at times causing sneezing, with profuse coryza, most from left nostril; worse after 1 P.M. (seventh day.) During the eighth day quite severe, more in the afternoon (eighth and ninth days),².—Cough with yellowish mucous expectoration (tenth day); not as severe the eleventh day, while other symptoms are about the same, and better in the warm room (eleventh day); less severe and less frequent (twelfth day); much better (fourteenth day),².—Cough causes a sneezing,².—While lying on the right side in bed, and at the moment of becoming unconscious by sleep, severe oppressive suffocative attacks from suspended respiration, causing a quick effort to prevent suffocation, by changing position. This is an old symptom, aggravated during the past week; he often avoided going to sleep in such a position on this account (eighteenth day),².

Chest.—Pleuritic pain on full inspiration,².—Pain in the upper part of the right chest. C. Hg.—Pleuritic pain, also on the left (tenth day); increased, with stitches in both sides, aggravated on motion or full inspiration, afternoon (tenth day); increased, with soreness of the whole body, especially the chest; aggravated during the afternoon and evening (tenth day),².—A severe, sharp, lancinating pain in the right supraclavicular region, in or near the subclavian artery, lasting several minutes during the evening (thirteenth day); lasting but a few minutes and less severe (fourteenth day); severe lancinating drawing from three to five minutes, 9 o'clock, evening (fifteenth day); slight, for a minute at a time, till the twenty-seventh day,[2].—Severe stitches in the sides, especially the right side, from the seventh to the eighth rib, aggravated by the least motion (tenth day); severe, especially in the posterior portion of right side; neither soreness nor stitches remaining in the left side (thirteenth day); the right side also better, and many other symptoms (fourteenth day),[2].—[**70.**] During the afternoon, severe stitches in the sides, especially the posterior portion of the right side, aggravated by the slightest motion, with severe aches and pains in various parts of the body (eleventh day); all gone (sixteenth day),[2].—Pain in the right side only on contortions of the body (fourteenth day),[2].

Heart and Pulse.—Severe, vibrating, tremulous palpitation of the heart, even while sitting or lying quiet, upon the least elating or other emotion of the mind (twelfth day),[2].—While lying in bed, forcible pulsations of the heart felt and heard, extending from the chest up into the neck upon the slightest emotion or thought (twelfth day),[2].—Palpitation of the heart, with a fluttering and vibrating upon the slightest emotion of the mind (thirteenth day),[2].—Occasional spells of severe jerking, fluttering palpitation of the heart, upon a sudden elating thought or emotion of the mind, even while sitting or lying (fifteenth day),[2].—To-night, while lying on the right side, the heart is both heard and felt to pulsate from the chest up to the neck (fifteenth day),[2].—Midnight, while in bed, vibrating palpitation of the heart, lasting but a few minutes, after which, while lying on the right side, a sensation as if the lower lobe of the left lung was settling down or being collapsed; it appeared to have settled from three to four inches, lasting five minutes, and was relieved by changing position (twenty-seventh day),[2].

Neck and Back.—Up into the neck, palpitation,[2].—A very stiff neck, C. Hg.—[**80.**] Occasional severe drawing pains in the nape of the neck, lasting but a few minutes at a time (eighteenth day),[2].—Stitches and stiffness in the nape of the neck, aggravated by flexing the head back and forth, or felt a few minutes at a time, while sitting still (seventeenth day),[2]. —*Soreness and lameness, with stitches in the nape of the neck, aggravated by bending the head back and forth* (thirteenth day),[2].—(Glandular swellings on the left side of the face, throat, and neck, nearly all of the size of a hen's egg, some hard, some suppurating; they disfigured and enlarged the whole region considerably since his early youth, now twenty years; 30th, in often-repeated doses, lessened it very much, more than half the former size,°.) Fielitz.—In the scapula, pain from pit of stomach,[2].—Severe pain in or near the head of the right scapula, lasting but a few minutes (tenth day),[2]. —Painful drawing near the spine to the left, downwards from the shoulder-blade; a similar sensation in the forehead, and slightly in a decayed back tooth,[1].—*Severe lancinating pains and stitches in the posterior right side below the scapula, aggravated very much by throwing the shoulders back and the chest forward, or contortions of the body;* at times eliciting a moan or shriek, caused by the pain (twelfth day),[2].—In vertebra, opposite pit of stomach, pain from front to back,[2].—Pain in the small of the back, hips, and lower limbs (eleventh day),[2].—[**90.**] In the afternoon, sharp pain felt in the right kidney, lasting but a few moments (twenty-seventh day),[2].

Extremities.—Pain in the front of the upper part of the right shoulder, afterwards in the left shoulder and arm, C. Hg.—Palms of the hands hot and dry (tenth day); dry and husky (eleventh day),[2].—Lower limbs pain,[2].—Hips pain,[2].—A pain in the right knee-joint, lasting about twenty minutes, 2 P.M. (ninth day),².—Pain in the left knee-joint on going up or down stairs (twelfth day),².—Several hard, small lumps along the shin bone, C. Hg.—An intermitting pain in the muscles of the lower posterior third of the right leg, with a sore, contracted, clumsy, bruised feeling of the anterior muscles of the lower third of the right leg, which is aggravated by flexing the foot and going up stairs, when the toes have a tendency to drop down, as if the foot was asleep, though without the sensation as if asleep (sixth day),².—The intermitting pain in the *posterior* muscles of the right leg has not been felt since yesterday, but there is an aggravation of all the symptoms in the *anterior* portion of the same leg to-day, especially when going upstairs, walking or flexing the foot, so as to render it quite painful and awkward (seventh day). The sore, numb, clumsy, bruised feeling in the right leg is ameliorated by remaining quiet in the house, aggravated by going up and down stairs several times during the afternoon, rendering it necessary to go up slowly, on account of the uncertainty of step, and tendency of the toes to drop down, which makes it necessary to step higher with the right foot (eighth day),².—[**100.**] A pain running from the anterior of the right leg to the posterior of the right thigh, between 12 o'clock and 1 in the afternoon (ninth day),².—The anterior muscles of the right leg sore as if beaten, and a contracted feeling, sore upon going upstairs or walking, with a numb feeling while sitting or lying (tenth day). The constant sore numb feeling of the muscles of the leg continues to be more or less aggravated at times, especially on going upstairs, or flexing the foot (fifteenth day). Soreness and numbness better, and only slightly troublesome, on going upstairs (sixteenth day),².—Lessened hard cellular swelling of both legs, C. Hg.,°.—Severe crampy pains in metatarsal bones of both feet,².—Sharp, stinging pain in the posterior portion of the right heel, aggravated by the slightest pressure, lasting but a few minutes (eleventh day),².—Bad ulcers on the feet of horses. (Popular remedy,°.)—Hurts of the hoofs of horses. (Popular remedy,°.)—In toes, a tendency to drop down as if asleep,².—Chilblains. (Popular remedy,°.)

Generalities.—During the afternoon, severe aches and pains in various parts of the body, with severe stitches in the sides, especially the posterior portion of the right side, aggravated by the slightest motion (eleventh day); all gone (sixteenth day),².—*A general soreness of the muscles and integuments of the whole body,* especially the integuments, aggravated on motion, and especially by the friction of the clothes (eighth day). *Flesh and integuments feel sore to touch, even of the clothes,* with sensitiveness to cold and cold air (ninth day). *Sore as if it had been beaten, and very sensitive to touch* or the friction of the clothes (tenth day); less during the afternoon (twelfth day); also less sensitive to cold and to cold air, and to touch (thirteenth day); all gone (sixteenth day),².

Skin.—On forehead, tetter-like eruption,².—Itching on scalp,².—[**110.**] Scrofulous diseases, particularly swollen glands. (Popular remedy,°.)—Bruised spots from falls or being beaten. (Popular remedy,°.)—Sensitive to cold and cold air,².—Friction of clothes aggravates soreness of skin,².—Flesh and skin sore to the touch ; cheek and malar bone,².

Sleep and Dreams.—Restless night, could lie a short time only in one position, on account of soreness of the muscles and whole body (eleventh and twelfth days),².—Awoke with frightful dreams, and severe crampy pains in the metatarsal bones of both feet, lasting from fifteen to twenty minutes, at 3 to 4 o'clock (third day),².

Fever.—Heat in forehead,[2].—Feverish hot breath and mouth in afternoon,[2].—Hot and dry palms of hands,[2].

Conditions.—**Aggravation.**—(*Morning*), Hawking bloody mucus; when first getting up, hawking mass of bloody mucus; 8 o'clock, pain in pit of stomach.—(*Forenoon*), Frontal headache; dull, etc., feeling of head.—(*Noon*), Pain in urethra.—(*Afternoon*), Between 1 and 2 o'clock, headache; 1 to 7 o'clock, headache; beginning at 1 o'clock, dull headache; until late in evening, *frontal headache;* heat, etc., in forehead; at 3 o'clock, pain in eyeball; shocks in the ear; sneezing, etc.; discharge of mucus from nostril; mouth, etc., hot and feverish, etc.; 2 o'clock, sore throat; *paroxysms of cough;* same, after 1 o'clock; pain in kidney; 2 o'clock, pain in knee; pains in various parts.—(*Afternoon and evening*), *Shocks heard in ears;* sneezing, etc.; pleuritic stitches.—(*Evening*), 7 to 10 o'clock, on a rainy day, headache, etc.; 7 o'clock, heat, etc., in forehead; bad taste in mouth; pain in supraclavicular region; 9 o'clock, severe drawing in same.—(*Midnight*), In bed, palpitation of the heart.—(2 P.M. *till* 7 A.M), Headache, etc.—(*Ascending stairs*), Pain in right leg; sore feeling in leg; numbness in leg.—(*Bending head back and forth*), Stitches, etc., in nape of neck; soreness, etc., in the same.—(*Bending foot*), Pain in right leg; numbness in same.—(*After breakfast*), Headache on top of head returns.—(*Contortions of body*), Pleuritic pain; *pain in right side.*—(*Friction of clothes*), Soreness of skin.—(*Full inspiration*), *Pleuritic pain;* in afternoon, pleuritic stitches. —(*While lying on right side*), In bed, at moment of becoming unconscious in sleep, suffocative attacks; pulsations of heart heard, etc.; sensation in lung.—(*Mental emotion or thought*), Spells of palpitation.—(*Motion*), *Stitches in sides;* soreness of muscles, etc.; pains in various parts.—(*Moving eyes*), *Frontal headache.*—(*Pressure*), Pain in heel.—(*Going up and down stairs*), Pain in leg; pain in knee-joint.—(*On swallowing*), Throat inflamed, etc.; sore throat.—(*Throwing shoulders back and chest forward*), Pains in side.— (*Turning the parts in either direction*), Pain in eyeballs.—(*Walking*), Pain in right leg.

Amelioration.—(*Morning*), Headache on top of head.—(*Afternoon*), Headache, etc.—(*Night*), *After sleeping,* headache on top of head; pains in the buboes,[∘].—(*Changing position*), Sensation in lungs.—(*Warm room*), Cough.

BALSAMUM PERUVIANUM. ·

Myroxylon Pereiræ, Kl. *Natural order,* Leguminosæ. *Preparation,* Tincture of the balsam that flows from the stems.

Authority. Lembke, N. Z. f. H. Kl., 12, 41, provings with repeated doses of from 15 to 30 drops.

Nose.—Bleeding from the right side of the nose without cause, without coryza, without sneezing, without having blown the nose (eighth day).— Repeated bleeding from the nose without cause, at 7 P.M. Slight blowing of blood from the right side of the nose (ninth day).

Mouth and Throat.—Redness in the arch of the palate, and pain on every touch (thirteenth day).—Redness and pain in the arch of the palate persisted in during the whole time.—The whole arch of the palate and uvula are dark-red, and very painful, especially upon slightest touch; continued for several days.—After every dose, continued scraping of the fauces.

Stool.—The first day, two soft stools.—Profuse fluid stool without pain, at 3 p.m. (fifth day).—A copious liquid stool, painless, at 2 p.m., and again at 7½ p.m. (tenth day).—Hard stool (fourth day).—Passage of blood with the normal stool (does not suffer from hæmorrhoids), (seventh day).

Urinary Organs.—Sticking in the urethra.—Cutting on urinating. —More frequent urinating than usual in the night.—Frequent urinating of much clear yellow urine (sixth and seventh days).—Much clear urine and much urinating (sixth day).—In the third night, more urine than usual.—Urine more scanty and darker (eleventh day).—Red coating on the urinal (fifth day).

Respiratory Apparatus.—Scraping in the larynx in the forenoon.—Severe scraping in the larynx, and cough, a quarter of an hour after taking it.—The same dry cough with scrapings, evenings in bed (fifteenth day).

Upper and Lower Extremities.—Several times, severe oppressive pain in the right wrist (eleventh day).—In the morning, severe pain in the left tibia, several times repeated.—Soon after rising, severe pain in the left tibia.—Violent boring in the right tibia, at 8 a.m., afterwards in the left (twelfth day).—At times, severe boring pain in the tibiæ and ankles; scratching in the throat, and long-continued dry cough at 11 p.m., in bed (fourteenth day).—Drawing in the tibia.—Tearing in the tibiæ, evenings in bed.—Continued boring in the left ankle, afterwards in the right (seventeenth day).

Sleep and Dreams.—Many dreams of various things.—In the night, very many dreams, mostly concerning the duties of the day.

Conditions.—Aggravation.—(*Morning*), Soon after rising, pain in left tibia.—(8 a.m.), Boring in right tibia.—(*Forenoon*), Scraping in larynx. (3 p.m.), Profuse stool.—(7 p.m.), Bleeding from nose.—(2 p.m. and 7.30 p.m.), Copious stool.—(*Evening*), In bed, cough, etc.; pain in tibia; in bed, tearings in tibiæ.—(*Night*), Frequent urination.—(11 p.m.), In bed, scratching in the throat, etc.—(*Touch*), *Pain in arch of palate;* pain in arch of palate and uvula.

BAPTISIA.

Baptisia tinctoria, R. Br.　*Natural order,* Leguminosæ.

Authorities. 1, Dr. Wm. L. Thompson, N. A. J. of Hom., 5, 547 (dose not given); 2, Dr. J. S. Douglass, N. A. J. of Hom., 6, 230 (took repeated doses of 1 to 3 drops of tincture); 3, Dr. S. R. Beckwith (ibid.); 4, W. Rowley, ibid.; 5, L. W. Sapp, ibid.; 6, J. E. Smith, ibid.; 7, T. B. Hoyt, ibid.; 8, Dr. Hadley, Trans. of N. Y. St. Hom. Med. Soc., 3, 325 (took 10 to 25 drops of tinct.); 9, Miss Hadley, ibid. (took 15 drops of tinct.); 10, Dr. Burt, Hale's New Remedies (took 10 to 200 drops of tinct., and 30 grains of bark subcutaneously); 11, Dr. Burt, ibid. (took 4 to 14 grains of Baptisin); 12 Dr. Wallace, Med. Investigator, 1873 (three provings with the one-tenth).

Mind.—The brain a little stimulated,[2].—Febrile excitement of the brain, like a beginning febrile delirium in a greater degree,[9].—A sort of excitement of the brain which is the preliminary, or rather the beginning, of delirium; with him it never fails to take place if the fever continues, and increases to considerable intensity,[2].—Disposition to talk,[2].—Low spirits (third day),[4].—Unhappy (second day),[2].—Felt very gloomy for several days (third day),[11].—*Cannot confine his mind; sort of wild, wandering feeling,[7].—Mind seemed weak, rather than confused (second day),[2].—[10.] Inactive mind,[3].—*Indisposed to think; want of power to think (second day),[2].—Dull, stupid feeling after breakfast,[5].—Very distinct recollection of what he had been reading,[2].—Inability to memorize as usual,[6].

Head.—Confused feeling in the head,[1].—Slightly confused feeling of the brain,[2].—Dulness in the head,[1].—A little dulness of the head (second day),[2].—[20.] Slight dulness in brain all day (second day),[6].—Dull, stupid feeling all over the head, with severe pain at the occiput,[7].—Morning, after rising, dull heavy feeling of head, and headache,[5].—Head feels very heavy,[10].—Head feels heavy, as though he could not sit up,[7].—Head feels very heavy, with pain in occiput (after one hour),[12].—Swimming sensation, very like that experienced before the operation of an emetic,[1].—Slight dizziness and languor,[3].- -**Vertigo,**[7].—*Vertigo, and sensation of weakness in the entire system, especially in the lower limbs, with weak knees,[1].—[30.] Headache day and night, causing a sensation of wildness,[7].—Pain in base of brain, with lameness and drawing pain in cervical muscles (after twenty minutes),[12].—Heavy pain at base of brain (after twenty minutes),[12].—Slight pain of head, with bruised feeling of forehead (third day),[6].—Head felt large,[2].—Head feels large and heavy (after twenty minutes),[12].—Fulness of the external vessels of the head and face,[2].—Head full, and feels heavy (after twenty minutes),[12].—Hard, dull headache, very much worse by moving (30 grains crude bark), (second day),[10].—*Dull, heavy headache (second day),[11].—[40.] *Dull, heavy, pressive headache,[10].—Slight pressive headache and dull pain in loins (from subcutaneous injection of 10 drops),[10].—Soreness of brain, worse when stooping,[5].—Noise increases the headache,[7].—Severe headache in front (third day),[4].—Pain in the whole anterior part of the head and in the **forehead,**[9].—Some headache in front, afterwards passing to the back part,[4].—In morning, headache in front part of brain,[6].—Frontal headache, with feeling of fulness and tightness of the whole head (after twenty minutes),[12].—*Frontal headache, with pressure at root of nose (after twenty minutes),[12].—[50.] Severe frontal headache, with pressure at root of nose (after one hour),[12].—Slight pain in the frontal sinuses, mostly in the right side,[8].—Slight pain in the right frontal sinus,[8].—Severe pain in frontal sinuses, followed by sneezing,[9].—Heat in forehead (second morning),[5].—Skin of forehead feels very much contracted,[10].—Feeling of tightness across forehead, with pain over right eye (after two hours),[10].—Skin of forehead feeling very tight, with sharp pain in temples,[10].—Skin of the forehead feels as if drawn very tightly over the forehead, with sharp pain over right eye (immediately),[10].—Skin of forehead felt as if it would be pulled to the back part of the head, with numb feeling of forehead and face (from subcutaneous injection of 10 drops, after ten minutes),[10].—[60.] Dull pain in front part of head,[7].—Dull pain in forehead,[10].—In the afternoon, dull pain in the anterior lobes of the brain and in the right frontal sinus,[8].—Dull, heavy pain in forehead,[10].—All the evening, dull frontal headache, with smarting of the eyes and a drawing pain down nose,[11].—Constant dull frontal headache, and dull pain in bowels all the evening,[11].—Pressive pain in forehead,[10].—Dull pressive pain in the forehead (after three hours),[10].—Feeling as if the forehead would be pressed in (from subcutaneous injection of 10 drops, after half an hour),[10].—In evening, soreness in the front part of the head on moving the eyes or turning them upward,[5].—[70.] Frequent pains in right **temple,**[11].—Dull pain in both temples, growing more and more intense,[7].—Sharp pains in both temples (after three hours),[10].—Sharp pains in temples, very often (30 grains crude bark), (second day),[10].—*Sharp pains by spells in right and left temples*,[10].—Burning on top of head and soreness of scalp,[12].—Dull feeling, especially in the occiput, where there was slight pain and fulness (after one and a half hours),[2].—Dull pressure in occiput (second morning),[5].—Soreness of scalp (after one hour),[12].

Eyes.—Eyes shining,[2].—[80.] Congestion of the vessels of the eye; they look red and inflamed,[7].—Eyes feel swollen, with burning and slight lachrymation,[7].—Eyes feel as if being pressed into head, with great confusion of sight; cannot place anything until she looks at it a few seconds; everything appears to be moving,[11].—Eyes smart and ache severely,[11].—Frequent pressive pain over right eye,[10].—Sharp pain over right eye, then over left,[7].—Partial paralysis of the eyelids; it is very difficult to keep them open,[11].—Lachrymation on going into the open air (third day),[6].—Walking in open air produced continual and profuse lachrymation (third day),[2].—*Soreness of eyeballs*,[7].—[90.] *Eyeballs feel sore and lame on moving them* (after twenty minutes),[12].

Ears.—Dulness of hearing,[7].

Nose.—Sneezing, and feeling as after taking a severe cold (after twenty minutes),[12].—Catarrh,[7].—Thick mucous discharge from nose,[1].—Dull pain at root of nose,[7].—Severe pressure at root of nose (after twenty minutes),[12].—Soreness extends to posterior nares (after twenty minutes),[12].

Face.—Sallow appearance of countenance,[5].—*Hot and perceptibly flushed face*,[2].—[100.] Face feels flushed and very hot,[7].—Cheeks burn,[7].—Burning and prickling of left side of *face and head*,[12].

Mouth.—Teeth and gums have been very sore for two days; by pressing on them with the finger, large quantities of blood ooze from the gums (third day),[11].—Tongue coated whitish, and slightly congested (second morning),[5].—Slight yellow coat on tongue,[5].—*Tongue coated yellow*,[10 11].—*Tongue coated yellow along the centre* (second day),[10 11].—*Tongue coated at first white, with reddish papillœ here and there, followed by a yellowish-brown coating in the centre, the edges being red and shining*,[7].—Tongue coated yellow, with flat, bitter taste (second day),[11].—[110.] On waking, tongue dry, with the same burnt feeling (second day),[2].—Tongue feels thick and swollen,[7].—Tongue feels as though it had been scraped,[1].—Numb pricking sensation of the tongue,[7].—* Well-developed ulcers in the mouth*,[1].—Long-continued flow of saliva,[1].—*Saliva rather abundant, somewhat viscid and flat tasting*,[2].—Profuse flow of sweetish-bitter saliva, followed by a dryish or glutinous substance; lips stick together,[7].—In the morning, increased flow of saliva of a pleasant taste,[8].—Increased flow of saliva in the evening,[8].—[120.] A most copious flow of saliva, followed by sore throat, with scraping and burning,[1].—In a short time, an increased secretion of saliva, followed by slight pain in the right lung,[8].—Taste of food not quite natural,[2].—Flat taste in mouth (9 A.M., second day),[10].—*Flat, bitter taste in mouth*,[11].—Bad taste in mouth,[7].—Filthy taste, with flow of saliva,[3].

Throat.—In the afternoon, fulness of the throat,[9].—Slight angina; throat feels swollen or full, with oppressed respiration,[7].—* Constrictive feeling in throat, causing frequent efforts at deglutition*,[1].—[130.] Sore throat, extending to the posterior nares (after one hour),[12].—*Throat sore, and feels contracted* (after twenty minutes),[12].—Sore throat, with scraping and burning, preceded by a most copious flow of saliva,[1].—Tickling in the throat, constantly provoking to cough,[1].—*Tonsils and soft palate look very red*, but are not painful (second day),[11].—Tonsils congested,[11].—*Tonsils and soft palate* *congested* (second and third days),[11].—Tonsils very much congested, with frequent inclination to swallow, which produces pain in the root of the tongue,[11].—Fauces and tonsils very much congested,[11].—Scraped sensation extends through the fauces,[1].—[140.] Dryness and roughness of the pharynx, extending to the nares, with a stringent sensation, followed after a little by an increased secretion from the parts, especially the pharynx,[8].—Raw sensation in pharynx, with a large amount of viscid mucus,[1].—Pricking sensation in upper part of pharynx,[1].

Stomach.—*Loss of appetite,*[3 5].—Thirst,[5].—Constant desire for water,[7].—Frequent gulping up of air (from subcutaneous injection of 10 drops),[10].—Frequent eructations of flatus,[1].—*Nausea,*[1 4].—Slight nausea and want of appetite,[7].—[150.] Slight nausea, with increased heat,[3].—Feeling as though it would be a relief to vomit,[1].—Feeling as if he would vomit, but no nausea, with severe shooting pain in the left kidney and left side of the umbilicus (from subcutaneous injection of 10 drops, after fifteen minutes),[10].—Gone, empty feeling at stomach,[2].—Pains in the stomach, and feeling as if there was a hard substance in it,[5].—Severe pain every few minutes in the cardiac portion of stomach (after five hours),[10].—A good deal of pain in epigastric region all night,[10].—Slight pain all day in stomach and right hypochondriac region; pain in right side very severe when walking,[10].—Slight pain in stomach and right hypochondriac region and umbilical (from subcutaneous injection of 10 drops, after half an hour),[10].—Pain in stomach, abdomen, and right hypochondrium, passing down to right iliac region (third day),[4].—[160.] Constant pain in stomach and liver, quite sharp at times,[10].—Constant pain in stomach and right hypochondriac region,[10].—Constant pain, of a drawing character, in the epigastric and right hypochondriac regions, very severe when walking,[10].—Constant pain in stomach and right hypochondrium of a dull, aching character, and extending to the spine; very much worse by motion,[10].—At night, frequent pain in the epigastric region, very much worse by turning over, which he had to do all the time,[10].—Great distress in epigastric and umbilical regions, with great rumbling,[11].—Great distress in stomach and bowels all the forenoon, with desire to vomit,[11].—Constant burning distress in the epigastrium, with severe colicky pains in the umbilical, and especially in the hypogastric region, every few seconds, with rumbling in the bowels and desire to vomit, but no nausea (30 grains crude bark),[10].—In evening, cramp in the stomach,[5].—Heavy aching pain in stomach and liver, with very hot sensation in those parts,[10].—[170.] Constant aching distress in the stomach and umbilical region, with a great deal of pain in region of gall-bladder,[11].—Constant dull aching pain in the stomach and liver,[10].—Dull pain in the epigastric region,[10].—Dull pain at the pit of the stomach, and constriction of the diaphragm,[8].—Pressure at stomach, with belching of large quantities of flatus,[12].—Stitching pain in cardiac extremity of stomach,[6].

Abdomen.—*Pains in liver* (third day),[6].—Dull pain in right hypochondriac region (after three hours),[10].—*The pain in the liver extends from the right lateral ligament to the gall-bladder; it is almost impossible to walk, it makes the pain so severe in the region of the gall-bladder,*[10].—Suffered constantly and severely all day with pain in the *liver* and stomach; the pain caused a numb feeling to pass all over the body,[10].—[180.] Good deal of dull pain in liver, stomach, and umbilical region (second day),[10].—Soreness in region of liver,[5].—*Constant dull pain in region of the gall-bladder; very severe on walking,*[10].—*Severe pain in region of gall-bladder;* lasted one hour,[11].—Good deal of distress in the umbilical region all day (second day),[11].—Constant dull pain in the umbilical region,[11].—Constant aching pains in umbilical region (30 grains crude bark, second day),[10].—Constant slight pain in the umbilical region,[11].—Constant dull pain in the umbilical and hypogastric regions; by spells the pain in hypogastric region very sharp,[11].—Constant dull aching pains in umbilical region, aggravated by a full inspiration (second day),[10].—[190.] All day, constant pain in umbilical region, with slight rumbling of bowels (second day),[10].—*Fulness of abdomen,[7].—*Distension of abdomen,[1].—Flatulence,[7].—Loud borborygmi (third day),[6].—Rumbling in the intestines,[1].—Slight rumbling in the bowels,[10].—Rumbling, with desire for stool,[11].—Slight rumbling in the bowels, with a mushy stool (after three hours),[10].—Dull aching distress in bowels (second day),[11].—[200.] Dull pain in abdomen on pressure,[5].—Quite a number of times there have been sharp shooting pains all through the bowels,[10].—Soreness of abdominal muscles, as if from cold or coughing severely,[7].—Pain in hypogastrium,[7].—Glands of left groin very much swollen, one of them as large as a common-sized hickory-nut; very painful when walking (second day),[11].—Dull drawing pain in right groin,[10].—Severe drawing pains in right groin and testicle and right foot,[10].

Stool and Anus.—Bowels loose next morning (very uncommon),[6].—*Diarrhœa (third day),[6].—*Diarrhœic stools dark,[3].—[210.] Soft stools (first and second days),[10].—Soft mushy stool,[11].—Soft papescent stool (second day),[11].—*Stool papescent, with a large quantity of mucus, but no real pain,[11].—Bowels costive,[2].—Bowels costive for two days,[5].—Constipation (fourth day),[6][7].—Constipation throughout the period of proving (eight days),[2].—Constipation severe, with hæmorrhoids in the afternoon; quite troublesome (fifth day),[6].

Urinary Organs.—*A sort of burning when urinating,[7].—[220.] Urine is of a whitish color, does not change blue litmus, and has no effect on red paper (second day),[11].—Urine high-colored,[5].—*Urine not very copious, but of dark-red color,[7].

Respiratory Apparatus.—In morning, swelling of the epiglottis,[5].—Increased secretion from the bronchial tubes and fauces, with expectoration of mucus,[8].—Hoarseness to such an extent as to require the utmost effort to be understood,[1].—In afternoon, disposition to cough quite troublesome,[9].—Lungs feel easier and stronger than usual (curative reaction),[9].—She was cured by this proving of a troublesome cough of long standing,°[9].—Constant want to take a full breath,[2].—[230.] In the afternoon, difficulty of breathing,[9].—At 6 P.M., oppressed breathing, with cough, soreness of right lung, and sneezing,[8].—*Awoke with great difficulty of breathing; the lungs felt tight and compressed; could not get a full breath; felt obliged to open the window to get his face to fresh air, with the same burning heat of surface, dry tongue, increased pulsations of the heart, and accelerated pulse, and the same peculiar feeling of the brain as on first night. An hour passed before he could breathe easily and felt comfortably cool,[2].—*On lying down, difficulty of breathing, in half an hour becoming so great that he was obliged to rise; afraid to go to sleep from a feeling of certainty that he should immediately have nightmare and suffocations.—This difficulty of breathing is not so much from constriction of the chest as from a feeling of want of power in the respiratory apparatus, such as he had only felt during a fever,[2].

Chest.—Constriction and oppression of the chest,[3].—Tightness of chest and desire to take a deep inspiration (after twenty minutes),[12].—In the afternoon, tightness of the chest,[9].—Oppression of chest and difficult breathing,[12].—Sharp pains in chest when taking a long breath,[7].—Pain through left of chest,[12].—[240.] Pain in the right lung, continuing some time; less pain in the left lung, with some soreness,[8].—Rheumatic pains in right side,[5]. —Dull pain in the sternum,[8].—In the afternoon, sensation of weight and oppression in the præcordial regions, with a feeling of unsatisfied breathing,[8].

Heart and Pulse.—Feeling of greatly increased compass and frequency of the pulsations of the heart; pulsations seem to fill the chest,[2].— Throbbing in heart, so as to be distinctly heard,[6].—Pulse, at first accelerated, afterwards became very low and faint,[7].—Pulse slow and weak (third day),[4].—Slow, round, full pulse,[3].—The pulse (usually but little over 70) I judged to be 90 or over, full and soft,[2].—[250.] Pulse 70, rising, about 2 o'clock P.M., to 100,[5].

Neck and Back.—Neck stiff and lame (after twenty minutes),[12].— *Stiffness and lameness of cervical muscles* (after one hour),[12].—Pain in neck, unbearable on moving head (after twenty minutes),[12].—Soreness of muscles of neck,[5].—Twitching in latissimus dorsi of left side (third day),[6].—Lameness of muscles of back and chest, especially when moving the head (after twenty minutes),[12].—*Back and hips are very stiff, and ache severely* (second day),[11].—Pain in back extending to sacrum,[3].—Slight backache (third day),[11].—[260.] Back aches severely, aggravated by walking (second day),[11].—Dull heavy aching in lumbar region on going to bed at night,[5].— Dull aching pain in lumbar region; very severe when walking (second day),[10].—Dull pain in small of back (after three hours),[10].—*Dull pain of the sacrum, compounded of a feeling as from pressure, and fatigue from long stooping, and soon extending around hips and down right leg*,[2].

Extremities in General.—Wandering pains in all the limbs, with dizziness,[12].—*Aching in limbs*,[3].—*Drawing pains in arms and legs*,[10].—At times, drawing pain in right wrist and left ankle,[11].—Prickling of hands and feet, with numbness; worse on motion,[12].—[270.] Peculiar thrilling sensation through both hands and feet, somewhat like going to sleep or a want of circulation,[2].

Upper Extremities.—Constant twitching in left deltoid muscle (since taking first dose),[6].—Pain in left shoulder and arm (after twenty minutes),[12].—Pain in left shoulder, extending down the arm (after one hour),[12].—Drawing pain in shoulder and arms, more in the left (after twenty minutes),[12].—Feel sore and stiff about shoulders and chest (second day),[12].—*Numbness of left hand* and forearm, with prickling (after one hour),[12].—Numb prickling pain of hand and arm, worse by movement; sharp darting pain through the fingers (after twenty minutes),[12].—The hands felt large and were tremulous,[2].

Lower Extremities.—Lower limbs, on walking, feel weak and vacillating,[2].—[280.] Pain in hips and legs, with numbness (after twenty minutes),[12].—Drawing pains in the left hip (second day),[11].—Drawing pains in right hip and both calves (30 grains crude bark),[10].—Soreness in anterior part of thighs, worse after sitting awhile (third day),[6].—Darting pain in left knee and malleolus of left side (third day),[6].—Drawing pains in legs,[11].—Legs ache,[10].—Cramp in calves of legs whenever he moves them,[11]. —Drawing pain in calves of legs,[10].—Severe drawing pain in both calves,[10]. —[290.] Frequent drawing pain in calves (second day),[11].—Drawing pains in the legs (after three hours),[10].—Foot and leg prickly, and can move but little,[12].—*Left foot numb, and prickles* (after twenty minutes),[12].

Generalities.—*Restless*,[3].—**Restless; does not sleep quietly; wants**

to get up, and yet does not want to,[7],—*During the evening, uneasy, restless; could confine himself to nothing; wanted to be moving from place to place (second day),[2].—No disposition to move,[3].—On going to bed, feeling of inability to make either physical or mental exertion,[2].—*Great languor,[5].—[300.] Feels weary and obliged to lie down (after twenty minutes),[12].—After walking, feeling of rather painful weariness of back and lower limbs, especially the right, and the right shoulder and arm,[2].—Painful weariness of the whole left side of body (after one hour),[12].—*General tired, bruised, sick feeling in all parts of the body, yet does not feel very badly (third day),[6].—Debility,[3].—Muscular debility,[3].—Through the day, rather weak (second day),[2].—*Feel rather weak and tremulous, as though recovering from a fit of sickness, and as yet incapable of vigorous mental or physical exertion (third day),[2].—Feeling very weak, and trembling a good deal,[10].—Very weak and faint,[11].—[310.] *Sensation of weakness in the entire system, especially in the lower limbs, with weak knees and vertigo,[1].—Prostration (third day),[4].—Feeling of great prostration, with flashes of heat from small of back in all directions,[4].—Prostration and increased perspiration upon the least exertion,[9].—Felt stronger on walking in open air (third day),[2].—Very faint and weak; legs tremble and ache,[11].—Paralysis of whole left side; left arm and hand entirely numb and powerless,[12].—General feeling of having slept too long and too hard, with a bloated feeling of the eyes (third day),[2].—Feel as though had taken cold; throat sore, and sneezed several times,[12].—*Indescribable sick feeling all over,[5].—[320.] Rheumatic pains and soreness all over the body,[7].—Stiffness of all the joints, as though strained,[7].—Feel stiff and sore all over; dread to move,[12].—Each time after waking from the nightmare, the parts on which he lay soon became exceedingly painful, especially the sacral region and hips. After lying for not more than ten minutes upon the back, the sacral region became intolerably painful, as though he had lain on the barn-floor all night, and inducing the conviction that a short continuance of the position would produce bedsores. When turning on the other side, the same sensation was produced on the hips, obliging him at last to turn on his face to relieve these parts,[2].—Intolerance of pressure on all parts on which pressure was made; could not rest back against chair without pain from the pressure; obliged to change sitting posture every few minutes from same cause; even the feet became equally painful from resting on the floor,[2].—Slight erratic pains in various parts (fourth day),[6].

Skin.—Livid spots appear all over the body and limbs; size of pea to three-cent piece; thickest on body; without sensation; not elevated, and irregular in shape (after six weeks),[12].

Sleep and Dreams.—Drowsiness; disposition to have eyes half closed (third day),[4].—Feel drowsy, and must sleep (after three hours),[12].—Drowsy, stupid, tired feeling,[3].—[330.] Unusual sound sleep,[5].—Deep sleep till 3 A.M.,[5].—Slept profoundly all night, and was not even waked in the morning by the breakfast-bell, a very unusual occurrence (second day),[2].—Slept well until midnight, then could not sleep any more,[10].—*Slept very well until 2 A.M., then very restless till morning,[10].—Slept until 2 A.M., then could not sleep any more,[10].—*Slept until 3 A.M.; could not sleep any more, but had to toss about constantly (30 grains crude bark, second day),[10].—Slept well until 1 A.M.; awoke with severe cutting pains in hypogastric region, with loud rumbling of the bowels; very restless after (second day),[11].—Slept two or three hours, and waked from a troublesome dream, with difficult breathing, a sort of nightmare; felt on waking as if the room was insufferably hot and close, hindering respiration,[2].—After sleeping about two hours, had nightmare, from which he seemed to be a long time in rousing himself by violent efforts to move and to make a noise. The anxiety continued some time after waking. (Has never had nightmare for many years, except when sleeping on back, or, very rarely, on left side. In all the instances recorded, was sleeping in usual position, on right side),[2].—[**340.**] Lay down and slept an hour, waking from a sort of nightmare with moderate tightness of the chest and correspondingly difficult breathing, which was soon over (after one and a half hours),[2].—Slept well the remainder of the night, after having, for a short time, slight febrile chilly horripilations over the lower limbs and back,[2].—Had a very restless night (second day),[11].— At night, sleepless, disturbed,[6].—*Restless night, with frightful dreams*,[10].— Dreams at night,[5].—When asleep, continual dreaming,[6].—Dreamed all night; in dreams triumphed over all opposition,[6].—Dreams about fighting and disputations, but always comes off best,[7].—*Frightful dreams*,[10 11].—[**350.**] Dreamed of being bound down with a chain across the mouth,[10].—At night, slept two or three hours, and dreamed of laboring hard in deep snow, suffering with heat from the exertion, and finally being smothered in the snow,[2].

Fever.—Surface of body chilly,[1].—Slight chill about 11 o'clock A.M.,[5]. —Forenoon, chill over back while sitting by a hot fire,[5].—In evening, great chilliness on going into open air,[5].—Slight chilliness in the lower limbs and back (very soon after taking),[2].—In evening, chills over back,[5].— Most uncomfortable burning heat of the whole surface, especially the face; it compelled him to move to a cool part of the bed, and finally to rise and open a window and wash his face and hands; with these symptoms there was a peculiar feeling of the head, which is never felt except durir.g the presence of fever,[2].—On waking at 3 A.M., flashes of heat and feeling as if perspiration would break out,[5].—[**360.**] General heat after going to bed,[5]. —Burning sensation over the whole body, followed by perspiration, vomiting, and diarrhœa,[3].—Heat of the face (after a few minutes),[2].—Flashes of heat over face,[5].—At night, heat and burning in lower extremities so intense as to prevent sleep much of the night,[6].—Chill all day, with fever at night,[7].—Whole surface of body feels hot and dry, with occasional chill, principally up and down the back, as if ague were coming on,[7].—Extremities feel hot, except the feet, which are cold,[7].

Conditions.—Aggravation.—(*Morning*), After rising, dull feeling of head, etc.; frontal headache; increased saliva; swelling of epiglottis; on waking, 3 A.M., flashes of heat, etc.—(*Forenoon*), Distress in stomach, etc.; chill over back; about 11 A.M., slight chill.—(*Afternoon*), Pain in anterior lobes of brain, etc.; fulness of throat; disposition to cough; difficulty of breathing; 6 P.M., oppressed breathing, etc.; tightness of chest; sensation of weight, etc., in præcordial regions.—(*Evening*), Frontal headache, etc.; on moving eyes, soreness in front of head; increased saliva; cramp in stomach; uneasy, etc.; chilliness; chills over back.—(*Night*), Pain in epigastric region; difficulty of breathing; on going to bed, pain in lumbar region; heat, etc., in lower extremities.—(*Going into open air*), Lachrymation.— (*Walking in open air*), Lachrymation.—(*After going to bed*), General heat. —(*Beer*), All symptoms.—(*After breakfast*), Dull feeling.—(*Full inspiration*), Pains in umbilical region; sharp pains in chest.—(*Lying down*), Difficulty of breathing.—(*Motion*), Headache; pain in stomach, etc.; prickling of hands, etc.; numb pain of hand, etc.—(*Moving head*), Pain in neck; lameness of muscles of back, etc.—(*On moving legs*), Cramp in calves.— (*Noise*), Headache.—(*After sitting*), Soreness of thighs.—(*Stooping*), Soreness of brain.—(*Turning over*), Pain in epigastric region.—(*On waking*), Tongue dry.—(*Walking*), Pain in right side; pain in epigastric, etc., regions; *pain in gall-bladder;* pain in glands of groin; backache; pain in lumbar region; weakness in lower limbs, etc.—(*After walking*), Weariness of back, etc.

Amelioration.—(*Walking in open air*), Felt stronger.

BARTFELDER (ACID SPRING).

Cold springs in Upper Hungary; temperature from 45° to 50° F.

Analysis (Schultes), 16 ounces furnished 11.59 grains of residue, containing sodium carbonate, 6.07 grains; sodium chloride, 3.03; potassium carbonate, 0.75; potassium chloride, 0.62; ferrum carbonate, 0.40; silica, 0.35; extractive, 0.37.

Authority. Dr. Schreter, Archiv. f. Hom. Heilk., 19, 1, 176; provings by himself (1); his wife (2); and a child (3); from sitz-baths, and from drinking the water.

Mind.—During the whole time there is a kind of slight intoxication, though no special exhilaration; nor is he less active; especially he sees indistinctly, particularly when walking,[1].—Lively and contented,[1].—Disposition rather earnest than lively,[2].—More fretful and sensitive; every trifle vexes him; he is morose, reflective; will not speak nor answer,[1].

Head.—Confusion of the head after drinking, as after intoxication. With this she is not lively, but rather indifferent and in an earnest mood,[2]. —Confusion of the whole head, burning and dry sensation of the eyes, and qualmishness in the stomach,[1].—Headache as if stupefied with pressive heaviness in the brain,[1].—Heaviness in the whole head, especially in the occiput; it draws the head backwards,[1].—Pressive heaviness of the head with drawing in the neck,[1].—Heaviness in the head immediately on waking,[1].— [10.] Plethoric persons suffer on drinking the water with severe congestion of the head,[1].—Boring headache, which concentrates itself in the right eye, at evening in the open air,[1].—Constrictive sensation in the forehead, extending down to the root of the nose, in the evening after smoking,[1].—Drawing tearing headache in the occiput, extending down to the neck, with a waving sensation in the brain after one-half hour,[1].—Drawing tearing headache in the occiput, extending into the neck, even while in the bath,[1]. —After the bath, when he lies in bed to rest, the drawing in the occiput and in the neck repeats itself, with throbbing and pulsation in the occipital vessels,[1].—Pulsating in the occiput and neck, with sticking pains therein,[1]. —Throughout the whole time scurf on the occiput; it itches and, after scratching, becomes covered with a yellowish amber-like scurf, and at the same time exudes a moisture,[1].

Eyes and Ears.—Burning and dryness of the eyes, with confusion of the head, and qualmishness in the stomach,[1].—After coition, pressive pain over the left eye and in the eyeball itself,[1].—[20.] In plethoric persons the eye becomes agglutinated at night from using the water,[1].—In plethoric persons agglutination of the eyes at night, and a violent congestion of the head is caused by the use of the water,[1].—Especially on walking he does not see distinctly, throughout the whole time as if he were slightly intoxicated,[1].—Sticking in the ears,[2].

Nose and Mouth.—The corners of the nose become eroded, as in severe coryza. Constrictive sensation in the upper incisors, as if they were

firmly pressed together, and hence became asleep, a kind of numb sensation,[1].—A hollow tooth becomes ulcerated, with swelling of the cheek,[2].—
After becoming chilled in the night she is attacked with a raging toothache,[2].—Toothache in a hollow tooth, a kind of tearing-drawing, aggravated
by cold water and by touch of the finger,[1].—Grumbling in a hollow tooth,[1].
—Throbbing pain in a hollow tooth,[1].—[30.] Inky taste on the tongue, at
night on waking,[1].—He is obliged to expectorate much frothy saliva,[1].

Throat.—Much hawking and raising of mucus,[1].—Dryness in the
throat,[1].—Scratching in the throat, causing a dry cough,[1].

Stomach.—Appetite increased, especially in the evening,[2].—Sensation
of hunger soon after breakfast, which disappeared after eructations,[1].—
Eructations after the acid water,[2].—Eructations soon after drinking the
acid water in large quantities,[1].—Empty eructations in the evening,[1].—[40.]
Eructations, as of bad eggs, in the morning,[1].—Eructations, with a crawling passage of air through the nose several times (after six minutes),[1].—
Qualmishness in the stomach, with confusion of the head, and a sensation
of dryness of the eyes,[1].—Nausea,[1].—Vomiting at breakfast,[1].

Abdomen.—Distension of the abdomen,[1].—Abdomen distended like
a drum,[1].—Distension of the abdomen with passage of flatulence,[2].—Passage of flatulence,[1].—A kind of colic, pinching-drawing pain in the abdomen, in the morning on waking, immediately after a glass of the water,[1].

Stool and Anus.—[50.] Crawling in the rectum,[1].—The hæmorrhoids protrude very much, and pain when walking,[1].—(The hæmorrhoids
protrude with the stool),[1].—Burning in the hæmorrhoids during the sitz-
bath,[1].—Desire for stool (after ten minutes),[1].—Desire for stool, which is
more firm, though normal in form,[1].—At night desire for stool, but with much
pressure; no stool follows,[1].—Hard stool in the morning,[1].—Stool twice in
the day, consisting of large cohesive masses,[2].—Stool in the morning immediately on waking, and followed by a second, and in two hours by a third;
the last is pasty, dark greenish-brown, with protrusion of the hæmorrhoids,[1].
—[60.] Stool six times in the day, the first normal, the others liquid with
mucus and bright-red blood, with great protrusion of the hæmorrhoids; also,
at other times, frequent desire for stool when only blood passes. On walking, the hæmorrhoids become strangulated and cause a constant desire, tenesmus, and pressure in the rectum,[1].—Stool copious, soft, normal in form and
color,[1].—One hard stool like nuts and sheep dung,[1].—No stool during the
day,[1]. [Secondary action.]

Urinary Organs.—Discharge of a little mucus from the orifice of
the urethra, which leaves a spot as of semen,[1].—Burning in the orifice of
the urethra during a cold bath,[1].—Burning, twinging sensation in the orifice of the urethra during a bath,[1].—Burning when urinating, with a gnawing sensation along the urethra, even when not urinating,[1].—Urging to
urinate, with burning and cutting, which returns later, and even when walking,[1].—Frequent urinating day and night,[2].—[70.] Frequent urinating of
clear white urine,[2].—Frequent urinating, though little at a time,[1].—On urinating in the morning the stream is always interrupted; is obliged to stop
eight times and commence again before the bladder is emptied,[1].

Sexual Organs.—*Male.* Throughout the whole proving, no erections and no sexual desire, though to-day when caressing sudden desire for
coition, which was reciprocal; his wife had until this time complete want
of sexual desire (seventh day),[1].—Strong erections toward morning, and
also in a warm bath; on coition, however, very little sensation, and none
with the ejaculation; the semen is watery (seventeenth day),[1].—Burning

in the genitals and hæmorrhoids during a sitz-bath,[1].—The testicles are heavy, larger, and seem swollen in the evening,[1].—*Female*. Biting and burning internally in the female genitals; feeling well generally after a bath,[2].—Sticking in the female genitals,[2].—Usually after menstruation there was desire for coition, but this time none, and on coition only transient enjoyment,[2].—[**80.**] Menstruation appeared on the thirty-second day (the previous time on the fortieth day), the first day more profuse than usual, the blood passed in clotted masses like liver, is very fetid; the second day no blood only at night; the third day almost none; formerly she had pains, this time none,[2].

Respiratory Apparatus and Chest.—Hoarseness during the whole proving; most severe in the morning,[2].—Hoarseness, even in the bath, and also in the morning on waking,[2].—Hoarseness and a scraping sensation in the throat,[1].—Difficult breathing,[1].—Sticking in the chest, with pressure of breathing, and dryness in the throat in the afternoon,[1].

Heart and Pulse.—After drinking coffee, palpitation of the heart, anxiety, heat, congestion of blood in the head, with confusion, sleepiness, and restlessness in the whole body (after two hours),[1].—Cramp of the heart; it seems as if it were constricted, though only for a moment with a stitch,[1].

Neck and Back.—Oppressive pain in the neck, extending into the occiput,[1].—He feels sore below the shoulder and in the lumbar region, especially on elevating the arms, and on walking,[1].—[**90.**] He feels bruised and lame in the small of the back in the evening,[1].

Upper Extremities.—Trembling of the arms and hands, even when resting them upon anything; if he holds anything in the hands the trembling is worse,[1].—The balls of the little finger of the left hand feel frozen, are red, itch, and burn for several days, most severely in the morning,[1].

Lower Extremities.—Bruised pain in the flesh of the nates and hip-joint,[2].—While walking the knees knock together, and a sensation of fatigue and weakness in the thick flesh of the thigh,[1].—Weakness of the knees, especially on walking; they knock together,[1].—Throughout the whole proving, weakness of the knees and heaviness of the feet,[2].—Weak in the knees, especially when walking, with yawning,[1].—Spasmodic contraction in the left calf,[1].—Throbbing and pulsating in the tendo Achillis of the left foot, as if something were in it, and then it goes to sleep as if it became numb; this disappears on walking, and returns on sitting still (noticed during a walk in the morning),[1].—[**100.**] The right heel feels frozen; this extends as far as the toes,[1].—At night, in bed, sticking in a corn, which wakes him,[1].—The nails of the toes are colored bluish, as if from tan, especially in the corners where they are covered by the neighboring toe,[1].—The skin between the toes is inky black,[1].

Generalities.—So weak that he can scarcely rise for sleepiness, in the forenoon,[1].—General well feeling after a bath,[2].—Transient swarming sensation in the face and on the body,[2].

Skin.—Nettlerash for several days, especially in the morning and evening, with sticking pains, which compel him to scratch, after which it burns,[1]. —A tetter on the forehead and below the right eye, which itches very much, and dries up after a few days,[1].—During the last days of the proving a pustular eruption appeared on the abdomen as large as a half dollar, with itching in the evening; it then became dry, and remained stationary for some time,[2].—[**110.**] On the right nates a small furuncle, which dries up after awhile,[1].—In a cold bath, a pricking sensation, as with needles; the whole body becomes red, with elevated patches like nettlerash; especially are\the hands and feet swollen, so that he cannot extend the hands well for two hours; the legs become red,[1].

Sleep and Dreams.—Yawning,[1].—Much yawning in the forenoon. —Sleepy and weak the whole day,[1].—Very sleepy in the morning; he has no will to rise, and feels chilly,[1].—In the forenoon and afternoon so very sleepy that she is obliged to sleep several hours; at night many dreams and restless sleep,[2].—For three nights he wakes several times, but soon sleeps again,[1].—(Falls asleep late and wakes early, with restless, indistinct dreams),[1].—Vivid dreams of funerals,[1].—Dreams at night of journeyings, with restlessness and anxiety,[1].—[120.] Anxious dreams of being pursued,[1].

Fever.—Dread of a cold bath; he will not remain long in it,[1].—(In the night while asleep he took off his shirt, laid the pillow at the foot of the bed, and finally awoke on account of chilliness. The child has two attacks of fever like quartan fever: chilliness in the evening, alternating with heat without thirst, with pain in the head and abdomen without sweat; it disappears after several loose stools; this followed eating pears,[3].)—After the bath internal shivering and chilliness in the hands, with blue nails and burning heat over the whole skin,[1].—Heat in the face, alternating with shivering in the back (after one and a half hours),[1].—Heat and confusion of the head,[1].—Heat and sweat on the forehead (after half an hour).—Heat and sweat on the forehead, with restlessness after coffee,[1].

Conditions.—**Aggravation.**—(*Morning*), Eructations; on waking, immediately after a glass of water, colic in abdomen; *hoarseness*; itching, etc., in little finger; nettlerash.—(*Forenoon*), Yawning.—(*Afternoon*), Dryness of throat.—(*Evening*), In the open air, headache, etc.; eructations; testicles seem swollen; bruised feeling, etc., in small of back; nettlerash; itching on abdomen; chilliness.—(*Night*), On waking, inky taste on tongue; agglutination of the eye; in bed, sticking in corn.—(*During the sitz-bath*), Burning in the hæmorrhoids.—(*At breakfast*), Vomiting.—(*After being chilled*), In the night, raging toothache.—(*After drinking coffee*), Palpitation of the heart, etc.; heat, etc., on forehead, etc.—(*After coition*), Pain over left eye, etc.—(*During a cold bath*), Burning in orifice of urethra; prickling sensation, etc.—(*Cold water*), Toothache.—(*After drinking*), Confusion of the head.—(*Holding anything in hand*), Trembling of the arms and hands.—(*After scratching*), Nettlerash burns.—(*On sitting still*), Throbbing, etc., in tendo Achillis returns.—(*Touch of the finger*), Toothache.— (*On waking*), Immediately, heaviness in the head.—(*When walking*), Sees indistinctly; hæmorrhoids protrude, etc.; hæmorrhoids become strangulated, etc.; sore feeling below shoulders, etc.; knees knock together; *weakness of the knees.*

Amelioration.—(*Evening*), Appetite increased.—(*After a bath*), General well feeling.—(*After eructations*), Sensation of hunger disappears.— (*On walking*), Throbbing, etc., in left tendo Achillis, etc., disappears.

BARYTA ACETICA.

Barium acetate, $C_2H_3O_2Ba$.   *Preparation,* Triturations.
Authorities. 1, Gross, Hahnemann, Chr. Kr., 2, 245; 2, Adams, ibid.; 3, Stapf, ibid.; 4, Hartmann, ibid.; 5, Hartlaub, ibid.; 6, Rückert, ibid.; 7, Rummel, ibid.; 8, Dr. Demoor, Rev. Hom. Belge, 1, 43 (from Dr. Lagard, Union Med., 1872, 537, a case of poisoning, by taking a solution of Bar. ac. by mistake for Sulphovinate of Soda, as follows: Bar. ac.,

grammes 30; syrup of currants, grammes 60; water, sufficient to dissolve. A portion only of the liquid was taken, but with a fatal result); 9, ibid.; (the physician in the last case took 8–10 grammes of the liquid to test it.)

Mind.—Sudden, excessive, but transient anger and wrath, even to rage from very little cause; easily provoked to action (after many days),[1].—Anthropophobia,[1].—All self-confidence has disappeared,[1].—Sad mood,[1].—Grief at every trifle,[1].—Great solicitude and anxious care,[1].—She is very anxious and careful about very insignificant things, which formerly were perfectly indifferent to her,[1].—Solicitous and fearful. The slightest noise in the street seems to him like a fire alarm, and he is frightened thereat, so that he starts in every limb,[1].—Dread. When walking in the street, she imagines that people are criticizing her, and judging her wrongfully, which makes her anxious, so that she will not look up, will look at no one, and sweats all over,[1].—An evil, fearful suspicion suddenly takes possession of her, as if, for example, a loved friend had been taken suddenly deathly ill,[1].—[10.] Out of humor, fretful,[1].—Fretful, morose, disinclined to work,[2].—Exceedingly obstinate, irritable mood; excited about trifles (very soon),[3].—*He wavers for a long time between opposite resolutions* (after several days),[1].—*During the day she resolves to undertake a certain matter in the evening, but scarcely is the time come when she repents it, and is undecided whether she shall do it or not,*[1].—Extreme irresolution; he proposes a short journey, but as soon as he makes preparation he changes his mind, and is inclined to remain at home,[1].—*Forgetfulness. He forgets the words he was about to speak. In the midst of a speech he is often unable to remember a very common word,*[1].

Head.—Confusion of the head, which extends to the temple and forehead,[2].—Confusion, dulness, and heaviness of the head,[1].—Vertigo on moving the body,[2].—[20.] Dulness in the head,[2].—Dulness in the head, with tensive confusion in the forehead and eyes, especially in the inner canthi,[1].—Light feeling in the head, as if it was empty (after three or four hours),[9].—Violent pressing in the whole head, as though it would burst asunder, especially violent in both frontal eminences, and over the orbits (after four and a half hours),[4].—A burrowing headache in the forehead and temples,[1].—Stupefying, dull pressure in the forehead, just over the root of the nose,[1].—Painful pressure in the forehead, just over the right eye,[5].—Dull pressing pain from within outwards in the whole forehead, especially in the orbits, very much aggravated on raising the head erect, disappearing on stooping (after ten hours),[4].—Small, severe stitch in the right frontal eminence, from within outwards (after nine hours),[4].—Twitching deep, internally in the temple, orbit, and ear of the left side,[1].—[30.] Pressive pain in the left temple (after some days),[1].—A heavy, pressing thrust in the left temple, extending outwardly (for two and a half hours),[1].—A burrowing headache, in the top and front of the head, almost daily in the morning after rising, continued through the forenoon, and disappearing in the afternoon. On shaking, the brain feels loose,[1].—Pressive pain through the right half of the brain, from the neck to the frontal protuberance (after one and a half hours),[4].—A pressing-asunder stitch, beginning in the left side of the head, traversing the whole left occiput, and ending in the cervical vertebræ (after nine hours),[4].—Heavy sensation in the whole occiput, especially close to the neck, with a tension of the same, though without influence upon motion (after four hours),[4].—Sudden sensation as of drawing, extending from the occiput over the right ear and lower jaw,[1].—Dull, pressive pain in the occipital bone, extending from the cervical vertebræ behind the right ear, obliquely to the parietal bone, in the afternoon, at 4 p.m., and afterwards, the following day, at the same hour,[4].—The scalp is painful to every touch,[6].—A creeping over the scalp, as if the hair stood on end, without cold sensation,[1].—[40.] Here and there in the scalp slow, fine stitches, which compel scratching,[1].

Eyes.—Aching and fatigue in the eyes, with pressure in them,[1].—Dull pressure in the left eye after a twinging pain in the left temple and orbit, with a sensation as though the eye would water, and a kind of weakness which compels her to frequently close them. Finally this presses also in the right eye,[1].—Pressure deep in the eyes, which is worse if she looks at one point, or upwards and sidewise, but is relieved by winking or looking downwards (after several days),[1].—Continual pressure on the eyeballs,[1].— Rapid alternation of dilated and contracted pupil, whereby it is not quite round, and seems to have several obtuse angles (after five minutes),[1].— *Everything seems enveloped in a mist for several minutes. If she closes the eye and presses the ball a little with the hand there is a pressive pain in the ball,*[1].

Ears.—A drawing stitch in the left mastoid process, aggravated at intervals in a small spot, which is exceedingly painful afterwards, especially on touching it or turning the head,[1].—Severe stitch, so that she must cry out, several times in the day, below the right ear, near ramus of the lower jaw (after twenty-four hours),[1].

Face.—Cadaverous pallor,[9].—[50.] Pale face, drawn features, eyebrows rather drooping,[8].—*Sensation as if the whole skin of the face were covered with cobwebs,*[3].—Sensation of heat in the face, without redness,[5].— Sensation as if the whole face were exceedingly swollen; it was, however, only very slightly so, although the usual deep furrows in the face had almost entirely disappeared, and the face seemed smooth for some hours (after half an hour),[3].—Tension in the face which draws down the eyelids, with inclination to expectorate saliva,[1].—Tensive sensation in the whole face, with nausea and diarrhœic stool (after one and a half hours),[5].—Exceedingly unpleasant sensation extends over the whole skin of the face and scalp, and especially the temporal region, as if something were drawn tightly over it, with a cold sensation in the face (very soon),[3].—Painful stitch in the face,[7].—Broad wheals on the upper lip under the skin, very painful to touch,[2].—Feeling in the upper lip as if it were swollen, with a sensation on the inner surface and on the palate, as if burnt or numb,[3].

Mouth and Throat.—Swelling of the gum of the right upper back teeth, it looks red, and has a dark-red narrow border around the teeth; from cold drinks the tooth pains, and its vicinity is sensitive,[1].—[60.] Cold tongue, somewhat black,[8].—Pustules in the right corner of the mouth, painful to touch,[2].—Sudden spitting of saliva, without nausea,[1].—Very bitter taste in the mouth with the natural taste of the food,[1].—Detestable taste in the mouth,[8].—Horribly disagreeable styptic taste of the drug, lasting more than twenty-four hours,[9].—Utterance imperfect,[8].—Pungent taste in the throat on smoking tobacco (which he is accustomed to), (after three-quarters of an hour),[4].

Stomach.—Great appetite all day; and if he has eaten so as to be only moderately satisfied he is soon again hungry; if he becomes completely satisfied, he feels great discomfort and heaviness therefrom,[1].—Aversion to eating, and yet a sensation of hunger,[6].—[70.] Very little appetite, with a natural taste of the food; no hunger,[1].—Little appetite; when he attempts to eat it will not go down; food has a natural taste but is repugnant to him, and eating gives discomfort,[1].—Satiety the whole day; whatever she eats is without hunger,[1].—If she eats even a very little she is completely satisfied, and experiences a painful heaviness in the stomach as from a stone, with a sensitive gnawing; the pain is relieved by sitting erect or bending backwards, but only for a short time; it is very much aggravated by sitting bent,[1].—Very urgent thirst for forty-eight hours, only to be allayed by holding a small piece of ice in the mouth,[1].—Empty, tasteless eructations (quarter of an hour),[1].—Empty eructations, with insipid taste and collection of water in the mouth, without nausea,[1].—Eructations of air with a sensation in the epigastric region, as if it would force itself painfully through it, which causes a sore sensation; afterwards, tasteless eructations follow,[1].—Nausea,[8].—Sensation of nausea in the stomach, qualmishness,[2].— [80.] Nauseous sensation; an uncomfortable feeling with a kind of qualmishness,[1].—Nausea in the stomach when walking, aggravated on touching the epigastric region; without collection of saliva,[2].—Nausea, followed by sudden and very copious vomiting of bile, and a brownish substance (consisting, no doubt, of the chocolate taken that morning), (after ten hours),[5].— Retching,[8].—Several attacks of very copious vomiting,[8].—Vomiting almost regularly every hour, for twenty-four hours,[8].—Heaviness in the stomach, with nausea in the morning, and fasting; disappears after breakfast (after many days),[1].—Heaviness in the pit of the stomach as from a load, making respiration difficult, relieved by deep breathing, but aggravated by carrying even a slight weight,[1].—Heartburn after some eructations,[2].—Sudden drawing pain in the pit of the stomach from time to time,[1].—[90.] Pressure in the epigastric region with oppressure of the breath, and sensation as if on deep breathing the breath were arrested there, together with a rough voice, which is only transiently relieved by frequent hawking; the pressive pain is aggravated by the slightest food,[1].—Sensitive, dull sticking just below the pit of the stomach, near the ensiform cartilage, which continues as a simple pain,[1].—*Painful writhing sensation in the stomach when, on eating, the food passes into it, as if it had to force its way through against sore places,*[1].— Even when fasting she feels a sore pain in the stomach for several days together,[1].—*Sore pain in the pit of the stomach,* on external pressure and on breathing (first day),[1].—The pressive, sore sensation and gnawing in the stomach are most severe when standing and walking, as also when sitting bent; when lying on the back, on bending forward, or when pressing on the stomach with the hands, she feels only the painful pressure, not the gnawing,[1].

Abdomen.—Pressive pain on a small spot in the right hypochondriac region only when breathing (especially when breathing deep), the place is painful to pressure (second day),[5].—Borborygmi,[8].—Borborygmi (after two hours),[9].—Rumbling and grumbling in the abdomen,[2].—[100.] Severe rumbling and gurgling in the abdomen,[1].—Gurgling in the abdomen on moving it. Sensation of much fluid, although she had drank nothing (in the afternoon),[1].—Unpleasant sensation in the upper abdomen, as before vomiting,[6].—Sensation in abdomen as if diarrhœa would ensue, with chilliness,[1].—Pinching in the upper portion of the left side of the abdomen, in a small spot just below the left hypochondrium, increased by pressure with the fingers (after quarter of an hour),[4].—Griping pain extending through the whole abdomen from above downward,[2].—Sudden, violent, pinching pain in the region of the transverse colon, as from flatus pressed forcibly through it,[2].—Violent pain as from diarrhœa, drawing, here and there, through the whole abdomen; relieved for a short time by a loud rumbling in the bowels,[2].—Some sudden, sharp stitches in the right side of the abdomen which make her cry out,[1].—Sudden, constrictive pain in the lower abdomen above the pubis, which is worse by paroxysms; it gradually disappears (after five minutes),[1].—Suddenly a violent stitch from the right groin into the abdomen, so that she starts,[1].

Stool.—[110.] Frequent desire for stool, although she goes no more frequently than usually, and the passage then is natural,[1].—Urging to stool, with violent pain in the abdomen, as if the intestines were spread out, then a soft stool followed by renewed urging (after one hour),[5].—*Frequent urging to stool, with painful aching in the lumbar region,* and creeping coldness over the head and along the thighs *as in dysentery, and then a soft stool at short intervals;* continuing pain in the loins with *renewed urging to stool,*[1].—Involuntary stools,[8].—Soft granular stool without any difficulty,[1].—Stool soft, finally becoming like diarrhœa,[2].—Half liquid stool (after two hours), followed by constipation,[9].

Urinary Organs.—Increased discharge of urine,[2].—He is obliged to pass clear, watery urine frequently, though only a little at a time,[3].—Frequent and copious urinating in the morning, fasting, without having drank anything,[1].—[120.] When appetite improved and thirst lessened, the urinary secretion became very considerable,[8].—Almost complete incontinence of urine and fæces,[8].—Clear and abundant urine,[8].—During twenty-four hours the urine held a great deal of mucus in suspension, but no baryta was found on analysis,[8].

Sexual Organs.—Red, eroded, moist, burning, hot spot between the scrotum and the thigh,[2].—Profuse sweat of the scrotum,[2].—A formerly swollen epididymis swells anew very violently,[2].—Diminished sexual desire,[2].—Menstruation is somewhat more profuse, and continues longer than usual, but is not accompanied by the usual pain (curative action),[1].

Respiratory Apparatus.—Pressure just below the larynx, which does not affect swallowing (after three hours),[4].—Voice rough on account of tough mucus, which constantly collects in the fauces and larynx for several days together; on hawking he raises but little, and makes his voice clear for but a short time,[1].—[130.] Voice extinct,[8].—Respiration very slightly affected,[8].—Respiration gradually more and more embarrassed,[8].—Respiration imperfect and very frequent; respiratory sound almost imperceptible,[8].

Chest.—Pressive heaviness across the chest, increased on inspiration, which gives a sticking pain below the end of the sternum (after half an hour),[4].—Itching on the chest,[5].—Transient stitch in the right side of the chest, between the sixth and seventh ribs,[4].

Heart and Pulse.—Dull, deep sounds of the heart,[8].—Pulse 125–130, very small and very frequent,[8].—Pulse slower than normal by sixty-five beats,[8].—[140.] Pulse remained pretty regular, but notably slackened (56 instead of 70). (In similar cases has been observed to fall to 25,[8].)—Marked, but very short-lasting, irregularity of pulse, on one occasion,[8].

Neck and Back.—Pressive, tensive pain of the left side of the neck during rest and motion,[4].—After the first vomiting, the muscular relaxation affected the posterior muscles of the trunk; he was too prostrated to remain in his arm-chair, and had to go to bed,[8].—Sensation of heat in the back,[5].—*Anxious sensation, with discomfort and restlessness in the lumbar region like urging to stool;* relieved transiently by the passage of flatus or eructations of air; at last, several stools follow at short intervals,[1].—A throbbing, grumbling sensation in the small of the back,[1].

Extremities in General.—Scarcely able to sit up in an arm-chair; extreme muscular relaxation in every limb (after fifteen hours).—A transient stitch on the left shoulder-blade, and on the outer side of the right thigh,[5].

Upper Extremities.—Heaviness of the left arm, it is moved with difficulty; the shoulder alone seems to act; the hand and forearm are paralyzed (after seven hours),[8].—[150.] Sensitive drawing in all the bones of the right arm,[1].—A sudden, transient, pinching pain on the left shoulder-blade (after half an hour),[5].—Painful digging in the left shoulder-bone,[1].—In the bones of the right arm a sensitive pain at a small spot,[5].—Pain, as if beaten in the middle of left humerus,[1].—Transient, painful drawing in the left forearm, as if in the bone during rest and motion (after one and a half hours),[5].—Bruised pain, worse by paroxysms, on the back of the forearm, as if in the bone (after many days),[1].—Rhythmical twitching in the external condyle of the wrist,[1].—Twitching in the inner condyle of the wrist in slow, wavelike paroxysms in the morning when lying in bed,[1].—Cramp-like, pressive pain in the right wrist, extending from within outward (after three and a half hours),[4].—[160.] Tearing of the wrist-joint, extending to the tips of the fingers,[1].—Burning-crawling on the back of the hand and fingers during the day, only transiently relieved by scratching,[1].—Violent, small stitches in the lowest joint of the left index finger, during rest and motion (after nine and a half hours),[4].

Lower Extremities.—Giving way of the right leg, then of the left leg (after eight hours),[5].—Tearing extending down the leg, most painful, and lasts longest in the knees, and also in the other joints, the nates, the hips, and the ankles,[1].—Intermitting tearing from above downwards, in the right nates,[1].—Tearing in the external and anterior side of the thigh, extending downward under the skin, as far as the knee when walking (after seven hours),[5].—Painful aching on the inner side of the left knee on rising and putting the leg forward in walking (after many hours),[1].—Pressive pain in the left knee, more towards the inner side when sitting; on extending the foot, it becomes a dull, pressive sensation,[4].—Sharp stitches in the inner side of the left knee, sudden, so that she starts,[1].—[170.] Violent stitches through the left knee on going upstairs, they leave a kind of painful paralysis in it,[4].—A feeling of weariness in the legs; jerks in the foot,[1].—Feeling as of a cold air just along the leg as far as the condyles,[1].—*Drawing pain down the whole left leg,*[1].—Tearing extending from the knee downward under the skin, when walking (after seven hours),[5].—Sensitive drawing in a small place in the left tibia (after three-quarters of an hour),[5].—Drawing pain in the left sole,[5].

Generalities.—Lies on his back in bed, deprived of voluntary motion,[8].—The paralysis extends rapidly from above downwards, affecting first the abdominal muscles, next those which have their insertions in the chest, then those of the neck, and lastly, the sphincters of the bladder and rectum,[8].—Great fatigue; he desires to lie or to sit constantly,[1].—[180.] The muscular relaxation lasted twenty-four hours, then gradually, but quite rapidly diminished, following the same course as when it came on. In less than twenty hours after the first slight movements of feet and hands, he was able to hold himself in a chair, and sit up in bed, and could soon take a few steps on the floor of his room,[8].—General debility (after three or four hours),[9].—Alarming debility (after two hours),[9].—Increased weakness, could scarcely put out his left arm to ring the bell,[8].—Loss of vigor and power; when standing, the knees give way; the spine pains, especially in the lumbar region, as if he had taken a long ride; he feels uncomfortable in the whole body, and desires constantly to sit, or rather lie; would rather walk than stand,[1].—After eating, depressed, weak, uncomfortable, with constant desire for stool, and an anxious sensation in the lumbar region, when at rest,[1].—Inability to cough, to expectorate, to articulate words of more than two syllables (owing to failure in expiration), or to lift the head from the pillow,[8].—The general system remained feeble for more than a month; the discoloration of the tissues and emaciation lasted still longer, and sleep did not become sound and refreshing until eight or ten weeks had elapsed,[8].—Death in about twelve hours after taking the poison, with undisturbed intellect, and without having stirred from his supine posture,[8].—Indescribable malaise (after three or four hours),[9].—[190.] Drawing in the whole body, now here, now there, especially in the joints,[1].—Dull pressure as if bruised, slowly increasing and decreasing, here and there, in a small spot,[1].—The whole body feels bruised, with weariness and heaviness of the limbs,[1].—The symptoms (tearing, drawing, throbbing), in the head and the limbs, appear more on the left side,[1].

Skin.—Eruption of acne pimples on the chest, they disappear in a few days,[8].—Pustules on the left middle finger, with a sore pain on touching,[1].— Fine sensitive stitches here and there in the skin,[8].—Intolerable crawling in the whole body, especially on the back, hips, legs, ankles, the back of the feet and fingers, wakes him at night, keeps him constantly scratching, which, however, only transiently relieves, after three nights in succession,[1]. —*Crawling and burning needle-stitches, here and there,* often sudden in a small spot; she is compelled to scratch and rub, although it *does not relieve,*[1]. —Feeling as if the head and face were covered with parchment,[9].—[200.] Very disagreeable formication and pricking under the skin of the head and face,[9].

Sleep and Dreams.—Frequent yawning, whereby the eyes become suffused,[1].—Yawning, stretching, and sleepiness,[7].—Overpowering sleepiness,[6].—She cannot help falling asleep in the afternoon, and nods continually,[1].—Wearied with sleep in the forenoon,[1].—Although he was very tired and sleepy on going to bed, yet the first sleep was very uneasy and frequently interrupted, he awoke frequently without cause,[2].—She wakes more frequently at night than usual; she seems too hot, throws off the covering; her feet ache as if she had stood for a long time during the day; this disappears after rising and walking about,[1].—In the morning when waking he does not feel refreshed; the limbs are tired as if bruised; he feels better, however, after rising,[2].—Confused dreams, restless sleep, frequent waking, and a great fatigue, so that he soon falls asleep again,[1].—[210.] Confused, commingled dreams,[1].—Vivid, strange dreams,[2].—Dreams of dead persons (i. however does not frighten him), with murmurings in sleep (first night),[5].

Fever.—Skin cool,[8].—Skin cool, even cold and rather moist,[8].—Skin cold and covered with profuse sweat,[8].—Chilliness, especially in the arms with goose-flesh, and yawning, in repeated attacks,[1].—Shivering chilliness in the head, with dull tension in the malar bone as if there would be goose-flesh in the face, as if the hairs stood on end,[1].—Chilliness and freezing extend down through the whole body, in repeated attacks with cold hands (after seven hours),[1].—Chilliness in the forenoon, coldness rising in the pit of the stomach with painful pressure, so that it seems if the hairs were drawn together; it then extends slowly down the arms and legs into the feet,[1].— [220.] Short attacks of shivering, with quick flashes of heat, mostly in the back; the chilliness seems to extend from the face, in which there is a feeling of tension (after one hour),[3].—After repeated chilliness extending from the pit of the stomach, the whole body becomes warm except the feet, which remained cold; after ten minutes, chilliness again,[1].—Flushes of heat over the whole body, followed by exhaustion, so that the hands sink down; the face and hands hot, the rest of the body cold,[1].

Conditions.—Aggravation.—(*Morning*), After rising, headache in top, etc.; when fasting, heaviness in stomach, etc.; when lying in bed, twitching in condyle of wrist.—(*Forenoon*), Chilliness.—(*Afternoon*), At 4 o'clock, pain in occipital bone.—(*On ascending stairs*), Stitches through knee.—(*When breathing*), Pain in right hypochondriac region.—(*Carrying a weight*), Heaviness in pit of stomach, etc.—(*From cold drinks*), Tooth pains.—(*After eating*), Depressed, etc.—(*The slightest food*), Pain in epigastric region.—(*Inspiration*), Heaviness across chest.—(*On moving the body*), Vertigo.—(*Pressure with fingers*), Pinching in upper abdomen.—(*Raising head*), Pain in forehead.—(*On rising and putting leg forward in walking*), Aching in left knee.—(*When sitting*), Pain in left knee.—(*Sitting bent*), Heaviness in the stomach; pressive sensation and gnawing in stomach.—(*On smoking tobacco*), Pungent taste in throat.—(*Standing*), Pressive sensation and gnawing in stomach.—(*Touch*), Stitch in mastoid process.—(*Touching epigastric region*), Nausea in stomach.—(*Turning head*), Stitch in mastoid process.—(*Walking*), Nausea in stomach; pressive sensation and gnawing in stomach; tearing in thigh; tearing from knee downwards.

Amelioration.—(*Morning*) After rising, tired feeling in limbs.—(*Bending backward*), Heaviness in stomach.—(*Bending forward*), Gnawing in stomach.—(*After breakfast*), Heaviness in stomach, etc., disappears.—(*Deep breathing*), Heaviness in pit of stomach.—(*Eructations of air*), Anxious sensation, etc., in lumbar region.—(*Lying on back*), Gnawing in stomach.—(*Passage of flatus*), Anxious sensation, etc., in lumbar region.—(*Pressing with hand*), Gnawing in stomach not felt.—(*After rising and walking about*), Aching in feet disappears.—(*Sitting erect*), Heaviness in stomach.—(*On stooping*), Pain in forehead disappears.

BARYTA CARBONICA.

Barium Carbonate, BaCO₃. *Preparation*, Triturations.

Authorities. 1, Hahnemann, Ch. Kr., 2; 2, Nenning, ibid; 3, Rückert, ibid.; 4, Hartlaub, ibid.; 5, Rummel, ibid.; 6, Gross, ibid.; 7, Neumann, ibid. (Krank. d. Vorst., observed in scrofulous children treated by Bar. c.); 8, Hering, Hom. V. J. S., 10, 95, symptoms from 12th, 24th, and 30th; 9, Effects of taking half a cupful with water, A. H. Z., 8, 26 (Wilson, Coll. Phys., 1834).

Mind.—Emotions. Slight delirium and stupefaction at night, as in fever,[1].—He imagines he walks on his knees (Rust),[8].—Children do not desire to play,[7].—Lachrymose at night,[1].—Sad and fearful; he has all kinds of sad thoughts about his future state, and thinks that he is lost entirely; in the evening (after thirty-five days),[2].—Dejected; he does not wish to speak,[1].—Suddenly becomes dejected in the evening,[8].—Dejection and dread of men,[7]*. [*In scrofulous children treated by Baryta.]—Extremely despondent and depressed; she believes that she must die; cries (seventh to tenth day),[2].—[10.] Despondent and anxious,[7].—Anxious; evenings in bed; she feels obliged to open her clothes,[1].—Great fear and cowardice,[1].—Great ennui and ill-humor,[2].—Peevish and quarrelsome,[2].—

Good humor becomes mischievousness,[1].—*Great irresolution about small things; he wants to drink the cup of coffee, then again not; does not know what he shall do,[8].—**Intellect.** In the morning, on waking he feels stupid,[1]. —Children are inattentive when studying,[7].—Want of memory (after sixteen hours),[1].—[20.] *Great forgetfulness, so that he does not know what he has just spoken (after twenty-seven days),[2].

Head.—Confusion and Vertigo. Confusion in the head when sitting; passes off in the open air (after twenty days),[2].—Confusion and heaviness in the head in the evening, with sleepiness; the head constantly falls forward; at the same time he is fretful and tired (after forty-six days),[2].— Dulness in the head; confusion in the head, in the morning on waking, and in the whole forenoon (after twenty-seven days),[2].—Vertigo,[3].—Vertigo on rising up from stooping,[2].—Vertigo, so that he does not know where he is when walking along a little path,[2].—Vertigo, with headache on stooping (after twenty-five days),[1].—Vertigo, with nausea on stooping,[1].—Vertigo, so that everything seems to turn around suddenly on raising the arm (after twelve days),[2].—[30.] Vertigo in the morning after rising, everything turns around, with a faint, nauseous sensation in the stomach (eighth to eleventh day),[2].—Dizziness in the head, so that he must sit and hold it still, with nausea,[1].—**General Sensations.** Humming in the head, as of boiling water (after twenty-seven days),[2].—When she raises herself, it seems as if her head would tumble about,[8].—Feeling as if the brain were loose; it seems to fall here and there when moving the head (after forty-five days),[2]. —In the morning on waking, first heaviness, then after rising, heat in the head, with coldness in the hands and feet,[1].—Headache from walking,[1].— Headache in the evening, with which every noise, especially the human voice, hurts the brain very much (after five days),[1].—Distending pain in the head and nose,[8].—Headache, as if the head were pinched together,[8]. — Severe sticking in the whole head, increasing and decreasing (after three days),[1].—[40.] Sticking in the head comes on immediately from the warmth of a stove,[2].—Violent stitches in the brain, with heat and crawling in the head (after fifteen days),[2].—On stamping with the feet, a shaking in the brain; great rush of blood to the head; it feels as if the blood stagnated there, and could not circulate (after twenty-seven days),[1].—Itching, creeping here and there in the head, which disappears on scratching,[2].—**Forehead and Temples.** On stooping, a sensation as if everything would fall forward in the forehead (after sixteen days),[2].—Pressive pain in the forehead from within outward (twelfth day),[2].—Pressure, with heaviness in the right side of the forehead,[2].—Violent, dull stitches in the left frontal eminence, on stooping when washing,[2].—Severe throbbing in the forehead, deep in the brain on stooping (after thirty days),[2].—Tensive sensation in the whole skin of the forehead, it seems too tight; after a meal,[2].—[50.] A burning stitch in the right temple,[2].—Dull stitches above the right temple, in the morning when yawning,[2].—Pulsating in temples,[9].—**Vertex and Parietals.** Pressure in the brain beneath the vertex, extending towards the occiput, on waking from sleep, with stiffness of the neck,[1].—Tearing on the vertex,[4].—*Pressive sticking on the vertex, which extends through the whole head, whenever he stands in the sun,[2].—Tension, with burning in a small spot on the left parietal bone (after one hour),[2].—Painful squeezing together of the head from both sides, then tearing in a small spot on the left parietal bone, and afterwards in the left side of the occiput,[2].—Fine tearing in a small spot on the right parietal bone, deep in the bone,[2].—Tearing, with twitching at short intervals, deep in the brain, beneath the right ear, immediately renewed by touching,².—[60.] Sticking in the sides of the head, also after dinner and in the evening, when it is most severe in the left side,².—Dull stitches in the left side of the head, extending from the occiput to the frontal eminence, or alternately here or there,².—Throbbing, with sticking in the left side of the head (after seven days),².—Pain, as if the hairs were pulled up on a small spot on the right parietal bone,².—*Occiput and Exterior.* Rheumatic pain in the occiput, with swelling in the glands of the neck,².—Tearing in the left side of the occiput, relieved by bending the head backwards,².—Throbbing in the occiput, extending to the frontal eminence; in the evening (after five days),².—An old tumor hitherto painless on the scalp becomes larger, and begins to pain as if ulcerating, when touched,¹.—The hairs fall out when combing (after four days),⁵.—Crawling as from ants over the whole scalp; in the evening,².

Eyes.—In General. [70.] The eyes are swollen in the morning,¹.—Redness of the white of the eye and lachrymation,¹.—Redness of the white of the eye, and a white pimple upon the eye near the cornea,⁴.—Weakness of the eyes, especially in the evening by candlelight; during the day, a cloud is before the left eye; by candlelight, a glimmer,⁸.—Violent pains in the left eye, and extending thence over the temple into the ear (after twenty hours),¹.—Burning in the eyes on exerting vision,².—Dry heat, and pressure in the eyes,⁴.—Pressure in both eyes, with itching as from dust,².—*Itching of the eyes,*¹.—Tearing in the eyes,⁴.—[80.] Itching, burning pressure, soreness, and dryness in the eyes,¹.—*Orbit, Brow, and Lids.* Sensation, as if a burning spark passed from the upper margin of the right orbit to the root of the nose,².—Sharp drawing over the left eye, extending from the nose towards the temple; in the evening,⁴.—Swelling of the lids in the morning,¹.—Inflamed redness of the eyelids internally,¹.—Matter externally on the lids, especially in the morning,¹.—Agglutination of the eyes,¹.—The eyes are difficult to open in the morning,¹.—The eyes close in the evening in the twilight,¹.—Twitching tearing in the right upper lid,².—[90.] A stitch through the left upper lid,².—Itching on the border of the upper lid,².—Sties in the left internal angle of the eye,⁸.—Agglutination of the eyes in the external canthi at night,².—Burning in the eyes in the inner canthi, with profuse lachrymation,².—Pressure in the external canthus, as if a grain of sand were in it,².—Twitching-sticking in the external canthus,².—*Balls and Vision.* The eyeballs are painful,⁴.—Frequent obscuration of vision,¹.—After a meal a gauze comes before the eyes,¹.—[100.] *Sensation as of gauze before the eyes, in the morning and after a meal,*¹.—Sparks before the eyes in the dark,¹.—Sparks of fire before the eyes, and tearing in them,⁴.—The candlelight is encircled by a halo with rainbow colors,¹.—Black spot before the eyes (after twenty-four hours),¹.—Double vision,⁹.

Ears.—External and Subjective. *The gland below the right ear is swollen and painful to touch,¹.—Tearing behind the right ear,².—Crawling pain in the bones in front of the right ear,².—Boring in the right ear so violent that she must cry out,².—[110.] *Drawing pain in the ears, a kind of twinging earache,*¹.—At night, frequent drawings in the ears,¹.—Tearing in the left ear, extending outward,².—*Tearing, with boring and drawing in the bones in front of the right ear,*². Sticking deep in the left ear,².—Severe stitches in the ear constantly for two days (after twenty-eight days),¹.—Throbbing and hard pressure after midnight, deep in the right ear, upon which he lay, and, upon turning to the left side, in the left ear,².—Crawling and twitching in the left ear,².—*Itching in the ears (after twenty-four days),[1].—Severe itching in the left ear,[2].—*Hearing.* [120.] Sensation as if hard of hearing,[5].—*Hardness of hearing first days,*[1].—*Severe buzzing in the ears, in the evening, like a ringing of bells and a violent wind,*[1]. —Cracking in both ears when swallowing,[1].—* Crackling in one ear on swallowing, as if it were breaking,*[1].—Cracking in the ear, when walking fast, when swallowing, sneezing, etc.,[1].—Crashings in the ears at night,[1]. —He cannot lie upon the left ear, because there is a crackling in it which extends to the right ear, which prevents his sleeping (after eleven days),[1]. —*A reverberation in the ear in blowing the nose violently,*[1].—Ringing in the ears,[4].—[130.] Ringing in the ears,[9].—Violent, long-continued ringing in the ears,[1].—Roaring and buzzing before the ears (after twenty-eight days),[1]. —Increased roaring of the ears; difficulty of hearing (in several),[5].— Sounding in the ears, even when breathing, like a sounding-board (after two days),[1].—Stunning noise in the ears (after two days),[1].—Throbbing in front of the left ear if he lay upon it,[1].—Throbbing like a pulse in the (left) ear, upon which he lay at night,[2].

Nose.—The nose seems swollen and internally agglutinated,[2].—The nose is stopped,[1].—[140.] *Obstinate dryness* of the nose,[5].—Frequent but transient catarrh, sometimes only for one hour,[1].—Continual catarrh, with stopped sensation in the nose (fifteenth day),[2].—Fluent catarrh, which rapidly appears and soon again disappears,[4].—Fluent catarrh, with a hollow deep voice and dry cough, in the morning and during the day, but not at night,[1]. —Frequent discharge of mucus from the nose,[2].—* Discharge of thick, yellow mucus from the nose,*[4].—Frequent inclination to blow the nose, with discharge of thick mucus, whereupon a constant sensation of dryness remains (eighth day),[2].—Sneezing, so violent the brain is shaken by it; it leaves behind a feeling of dizziness (first day),[2].—Frequent sneezing in rapid succession, in the evening,[4].—[150.] *Frequent nose bleeding,*[1].—Frequent and profuse nose bleeding (after twenty-four hours),[1].—Bleeding of the nose several times a day (after twenty-four days),[1].—Nose bleeding in the morning when in bed, bright red blood,[2].—The nose bleeds easily when blowing it or cleaning it,[1].—Every time when blowing the nose a stream of blood,[2].—The nose pains in the tip and margin,[8].—Burning in a small place on the top of the nose, as from a drop of hot fat.[2].—Crawling on both sides of the nose,[1].— The smell is very sensitive,[4].

Face.—[160.] *Face puffy,*[9].—* Pale face,*[9].—Redness of the face in the evening (after twelve days),[2].—Great redness in the face, with purple-red lips, and severe congestion of blood immediately,[1].—Twitching in the left side of the face,[2].—Sensation of swelling in the face,[2].—Sharp stitches in face,[2].—*Tensive feeling in the whole skin of the face,*[2].—Rough, red spot on the right cheek,[2].—Swelling of the left cheek and the region behind the ear, with pain in the temple (after thirty days),[1].—[170.] Crawling or creeping in the left cheek (first day),[2].—Swelling of the upper lip, with burning pain,[2].—Lower lip cracked,[4].—Vesicles on the lower lip,[2].—In the morning, after rising, the lips are dry,[2].—The upper lip feels swollen,[2].— Burning in a small spot on the red part of the lower lip (after seventeen days),[2].—Dry sensation in the lips and in the gum; drinking does not relieve it,[4].—Burning, smarting in the lower lip,[2].—Painful gnawing in the left side of the lower jaw,[2].—[180.] Tension in the lower jaw extends as far as the os hyoides,[8].—* Cannot close the lower jaw without great pain in the articulation,*[1].—Pressure under the chin, increased by touch and by moving the lower jaw,[2].—Tearing in the lower jaw of the right side,[2].—A stitch in the middle of the lower jaw,[2].—Glands on the under jaw are painful,[1].

Mouth.—Teeth and Gums. (Tooth becomes rapidly hollow,[1].)—A sound tooth becomes loose, and pains when eating and for some time afterwards,[1].—At times, an involuntary chattering of the teeth,[8].—*Frequent and profuse bleeding of the teeth*,[1].—[**190.**] Toothache, evening in bed, not by day (after eight days),[1].—Burning pain, now in the upper, now in the lower teeth of the left side, with accumulation of much saliva in the mouth; he cannot lie upon his side because the side of the head feels as if pressed in, and it throbs in the left ear,[1].—Tensive and sticking pain in all the right teeth,[1].—Boring in the teeth as if they would be rent asunder, if he takes anything cold or warm into the mouth,[1].—Crawling-burning in the lower teeth (after thirty-six days),[2].—A sensitive crawling in the tips of the teeth, in the evening (after six days),[2].—Drawing, jerking, throbbing toothache, as though something were seated under the teeth, extending into the ear and the right temple,[1].—Painful gnawing in the roots and gum of the back teeth,[2].—Grumbling in the back teeth,[2].—Grumbling in a decayed tooth during the day,[8].—[**200.**] Tearing in the back teeth,[2].—A sore, painful toothache; she cannot touch the teeth,[1].—Throbbing pain, with great sensitiveness in the lower back teeth, in the morning after rising,[2].—Gum swollen about a hollow tooth,[8].—The gum bleeds and seems to retract from the teeth,[5].—**Tongue.** A vesicle under the tongue,[2].—Pointed vesicles in the middle of the tongue,[1].—Burning vesicles at the tip of the tongue, of long duration (after six days),[2].—Tongue much coated,[1].—*Tongue coated, as if fuzzy*,[8].—[**210.**] Hardness of a spot in the middle of the tongue, with burning under touch for several days (after eighteen days),[2].—Dryness of the tongue in the morning, with sensation as of swelling in the throat when swallowing,[1].—Pain in the side of the tongue, as from vesicles,[1].—Tearing on the left border of the tongue, which smarts and pains as if sore,[1].—*Smarting, burning pain in the tip of the tongue,* (fourth day),[2].—Rawness on the tongue, in the morning on waking; if it touches the palate it feels as if it were a grating-iron (after thirty-one days),[2].—**Mouth, Saliva, and Taste.** *The whole mouth becomes filled with inflamed vesicles, especially the palate and the inside of the cheeks*,[1].—Much thick mucus in the mouth,[2]. —*Much trouble with tough phlegm, which has no end; from it the mouth becomes very dry, and therefrom a kind of thirst*,[8].—Intolerable odor from the mouth, which he does not perceive himself (after five days),[2].—[**220.**] Dryness in the mouth, in the morning after rising,[2].—Mouth is sticky,[1].—The mouth feels numb in the morning (third and fourth days),[2].—Stitches in the palate, as with needles (after nine days),[2].—Continual spitting of saliva for eight days (after thirty-eight days),[2].—The mouth is constantly full of water which rises from the stomach (after fourteen days),[2].—During the morning sleep, saliva runs out of the mouth,[1].—Taste completely lost for several days,[2].—Sweet taste behind the root of the tongue (after nineteen days),[1].—Mouth bitter and slimy, with coated tongue (sixth day),[2].— [**230.**] Foul, bitter taste and smell in the mouth,[1].—*Foul taste in the mouth every morning,* with very coated tongue,[1].—Salty taste in the mouth and throat in the afternoon,[1].—Sour taste in the mouth, in the morning after rising (after forty-eight days),[1].—Sour taste in the mouth in the evening,[1]. —Sour taste in the mouth before eating, not after it,[1].

Throat.—In General. *Takes cold very easily, and has an inflammation of the throat in consequence,[1].—Dryness and severe painful sticking and pressure, as from swelling, in the back part of the left side of the throat, only when swallowing (after four days),[2].—*After chilliness, and heat, and bruised feeling in all the limbs, an inflammation of the throat, with swelling of the palate and tonsils, which suppurate, and on account of which he cannot open the jaws, neither speak nor swallow, with dark-brown urine and loss of sleep (after eighteen days),[1].—Feeling as if there were much mucus in the throat, and hence much desire to drink in order to relieve the sensation,[1].—[240.] A feeling as though the throat were swollen internally in the morning, when swallowing, with dryness of the tongue,[1].—*Attacks of choking in the throat after dinner, when sitting and writing, with sensation as if the thyroid gland were pressed inward, which thereby impedes respiration (after twenty-eight days),[1].—Choking or constriction in the throat, with arrest of breathing, so that he is obliged to open his clothes during dinner (after twenty-six days),[2].—*Constriction in the throat, with sensation on swallowing as if a plug were in the region of the larynx; worse in the afternoon,[2].—Pressive pain in the throat when swallowing,[1].—Sticking in the throat (after fourteen days),[2].—Sticking pain in the throat on swallowing,[1].—*Sticking in the throat, worse when swallowing, with dryness, in the evening (after six days),[2]. —Pain in the throat from taking cold; a sharp stitching pain when swallowing (seventh day),[1].—*Smarting pain in the throat when swallowing, though most on empty swallowing; therewith the throat is painful externally on both sides to the touch,[1].—[250.] Rawness in the throat, followed by severe paroxysms of cough (after one hour),[2].—*Rawness and smarting in the throat after a night-sweat, more painful on empty swallowing than when swallowing (soft) food (after forty-eight hours),[1].—The throat is scraped and raw, worse after swallowing (after two days),[2].—Tickling in the throat, which causes a constant hawking,[2].—*Pharynx and Tonsils.* When sneezing, a sensation in the pharynx as if a piece of flesh had become loosened in the upper part of the fauces, with burning at that spot (after four days),[2].—A feeling in the pharynx following previous scratching, as if a plug or a morsel had become lodged there,[1].—*A sensation in the pharynx as if a fine leaf lay before the posterior nares, in the morning after waking (second day),[2].—Swelling of the left tonsil,[1].—*Swelling of the submaxillary gland (after thirty-nine days),[1].

Stomach.—Appetite and Thirst. Insatiable,[1].—[260.] Hunger, even on rising in the morning (after two days),[2].—(Desire to nibble,[1].)— *Sensation of hunger in the stomach, but no appetite (after ten days),[2].—Want of appetite,[4].—Appetite slight for several days,[2].—Loss of appetite for three weeks (after twenty-six days),[1].—Indifference to sweet things,[1].—Aversion to fruit, especially to plums,[1].—Thirst almost every evening at 6 o'clock (after sixteen days),[2].—Thirst, with dryness in the mouth,[2].—*Eructations and Hiccough.* [270.] Frequent eructations,[1].—Incessant eructations,[1]. —Many eructations in the afternoon (after twenty-five days),[1].—Eructations from the afternoon until far into the night, which prevent his going to sleep (after forty days),[1].—After dinner, suppressed eructations, followed by spasmodic constrictive pain in the stomach (after seven days),[2].—Forcible eructations, with pressure in the stomach, as if a stone rose and fell down again,[2].—Empty eructations wake him from sleep in the morning (after forty-two days),[1].—After a (natural) stool, much empty eructations (after a few hours),[1].—Frequent eructations of air, with sensation as if a lump of the size of a hazel-nut rose with them, in the morning (after nineteen days),[2].—Eructations sweetish, or of bitter water, after dinner,[2].—[280.] Frequent bitter eructations,[2].— Rancid eructations,[2].—Sour eructations daily, a couple of hours after eating,[1].—Hiccough,[1].—Violent hiccough in the forenoon and after eating,[2].—*Nausea, Vomiting, and Sensations.* Nausea, as from foul stomach, in the morning,[2].—Nausea in the morning, fasting, with palpitation and anxiety,[1].—Frequent vomiting of mucus,[1].— Vomiting fluid, water and chalk, followed by prostration,[9].—*A feeling of weakness in the stomach, which disappears after eating,*[2].—[**290.**] Cold and empty feeling in the stomach,[2].—It seems as if the stomach hung down loose,[8].—Pain in the stomach,[3].—Burning in the region of the stomach in the afternoon,[2].—Feeling of repletion in the stomach,[2].—Fulness of the stomach, after eating, as if he had eaten too much,[4].—Pain in the stomach as if it were too full and tense; urinating difficult,[8].—Sense of tension and heaviness in pit of stomach, as from flatulence and palpitation,[9].—Constrictive pain in the stomach in the afternoon,[2].—*Pressure in the stomach, as from a stone; relieved by eructations,*[2].—[**300.**] Severe pressure in the stomach, with nausea, after eating bread, not after cooked food, even when very little, with collection of saliva in the mouth,[1].—Pressure and choking in the right side of the stomach, extending into the chest, as if a hard body pressed upward with difficulty, from morning to afternoon,[2].—Drawing-tearing in the pit of the stomach, with a feeling as if a heavy body were there, on becoming erect and on stooping (after seventeen days),[2].—Fine stitches through the stomach into the spine,[2].—*Sensitiveness of the pit of the stomach; on stepping hard he feels every step painful in it,*[6].—Ulcerative pain in the stomach when pressing upon it,[1].

Abdomen.—Hypochondria and Umbilicus. Pressive pain in the region of the liver, more when moving, and still more when touching it,[1].—Short sticking below the right hypochondrium, without affecting respiration (after half an hour),[4].—Violent dull stitch in the left hypochondrium,[2].—Pains in the abdomen about and below the navel, which extend downward into the thigh; with violent pain on the left side from the point of the hip, extending forward, and pain in the region of the right groin (after three days),[8].—[**310.**] Pains in the abdomen so violent that the navel is retracted, and he is obliged to crouch; in the evening,[2].—Pinching around the navel, more in sitting than when moving,[2].—Pinching around the navel on the slightest motion made at night when lying down, and by day when sitting; passage of flatus relieves the pain, and it ceases entirely when walking (after twenty-seven days),[2].—Sudden stitches below the navel (after four days),[2].—*In General.* Fulness of the abdomen (after nineteen days),[2].— *Distension of the abdomen,*[1].—*Painful distension of the abdomen,*[1].—*Hard, tense abdomen,*[1].—Offensive flatus,[2].—*(On turning in bed, it seems as if the intestines fell from one side to the other),*[8].—[**320.**] After a customary walk, pain in the abdomen, followed by an exhausting night-sweat (fifth day),[1].—On account of pains in the bowels he cannot sleep at night; whenever he moves a little, the pains return (after twenty-seven days),[2].—Tension of the abdomen, with sensitiveness of the abdominal walls when touched,[2].—A feeling in the abdomen as if something in it were swollen,[1].—Many troubles in the abdomen from flatulence, whereby the hæmorrhoids protrude, with pain when sitting,[1].—Feeling of contraction in a spot of the size of the hand in the left side of the upper abdomen (after two days),[2].—Pinching in the bowels, with nausea,[1].—Pressure in the right side of the abdomen in the morning, after waking, in bed; disappears after rising,[1].—Pressive pain in the forepart of the abdomen, as if external to the intestines, in the muscles, especially at evening, becoming unendurable when walking and on motion; speedily relieved when sitting and lying, but soon returning on walking (after twenty-four hours),[1].—Severe cutting pain in the abdomen wakes him about midnight,[1].—[330.] Painful cutting in the abdomen, especially around the navel, in the evening (after fifteen days),[2].—Cutting colic at night,[1].—Severe drawing-cutting, extending upward in the left side of the upper abdomen,[1].—Stitches in the right side of the abdomen when hiccoughing, when turning the body, when yawning and breathing deeply, not when walking,[1].—A stitch in the right side of the abdomen, and, at the same time, in the small of the back (after two days),[2].—Throbbing here and there in the abdomen,[8].—*Hypogastrium and Iliac Region.* On urinating, pinching in the lower bowels,[2].—Drawing pain deep in the lower abdomen, down along the right groin, as from a string (after two days),[2].—Pressure in the abdomen, above the pubes, in the morning, in bed, when lying on the back,[2].—(Inflammation of a hernial ring (after three days),[1].)—[340.] A pressing outward in the abdominal ring on moving and during stool,[1].—Cutting in the lower portion of the bowels at night, with pressure towards the rectum, with rending pains in the intestines, with a feeling of fulness above the pubes, as though everything were stopped and the abdomen would burst, when lying out straight; afterwards, stool, first hard, knotty, then liquid, with much pressure, with relief of the pain in the bowels, followed by burning in the anus (after two days),[2].—Itching in the hernial ring,[1].

Rectum and Anus.—Sticking in the rectum the whole day, and a hard stool,[1].—In the anus, many hæmorrhoids of the size of a hazel-nut, with smarting and sticking pains,[1].—Not only with the stool, but also with urination, the hæmorrhoids protrude,[5].—After the stool, moist hæmorrhoids,[1].—Passage of blood from the anus frequently, with distension of the abdomen,[1].—Burning in the anus,[5].—With the (natural) stool, burning in the anus,[2].—[350.] Biting in the anus,[1].—Crawling in the anus,[1].—Painful soreness around the anus, as if he had been excoriated (after five days),[5].—Sore pain and burning around the anus towards evening,[5].

Stool.—Very frequent desire for stool,[1].—Urgent desire for stool; she cannot retain the stool because it is forced out rapidly,[1].—Frequent small stools, with feeling of great relief,[8].—Diarrhœic stool (first and thirtieth days),[2].—Diarrhœic stool, mixed with blood (in a child),[1].—Diarrhœa at night, with hæmorrhoidal pains,[8].—[360.] Diarrhœa towards morning, preceded by pain in abdomen; later in the day, suddenly, yellow stool, with mucus and blood,[8].—Soft stool, with very urgent desire (previously there had been a hard one), followed by a burning and a pressing asunder in the rectum (first and second days),[2].—Stool very hard, difficult to pass, with pain in the rectum and bloody mucus,[1].—Tough stool one day; hard stool, with burning in the anus,[2].—Light-colored stool,[1].—*Passage of round worms*,[1].—A passage of round worms in the stool,[2].—Small pin-worms pass with the stool (in an adult),[8].—Blood with the stool,[8].—Stool omits sometimes for one day,[2].

Urinary Organs.—[370.] Increased purulent gleet,[8].—On urinating, burning in the urethra (fifteenth day),[2,8].—After dinner, much desire to urinate,[1].—Urgent desire to urinate; she cannot retain the urine, it passes so rapidly,[1].—After urinating, renewed desire therefor; afterwards, every time when walking, a few drops of urine pass; disappears on sitting,[1].—Frequent passage of urine every other day (after twenty-nine hours),[2].—Increased urine; she rises twice every night to urinate; passes much each time (after nineteen days),[2].—Seldom and scanty urine, with burning in the urethra (eighth and seventeenth days),[2].—The urine, clear on passing, soon becomes cloudy (Bute),[8].—The urine has a yellow sediment,[1].

Sexual Organs.—(*Male.*) [**380.**] Numbness of the genitals, for several minutes (after twenty-eight days),[1].—Slow erection (ninth and fourteenth days),[1].—Erection in the morning before rising, which was seldom the case (after seventeen days),[2].—Erection all night (thirtieth day), (secondary action),[1].—In the evening, sudden erections, more violent than for a year, with shivering and such desire that coition was necessary (after ten hours),[1].—Erections while riding, with impotence,[8].—Twitching in the glans,[8].—Violent itching on the right side of the scrotum, which he cannot sufficiently scratch,[2].—Burning in the left testicle (after thirteen days),[1].—*Much increased sexual desire* (secondary action),[5].—[**390.**] Diminished sexual desire,[6].—Falls asleep during coition, without emission of semen (twenty-first day),[1].—Sexual desire disappears the first day,[1].—(In coition, emission takes place too soon),[8].—Emissions in a man thirty years old, who never before had the like,[8].—Several emissions follow each other in close succession (in a married man), followed by exhaustion (after thirty-five days),[1].—Profuse, nightly emissions shortly after coition (fourth day),[1].—Emissions in an old man followed by a feeling of dryness in the whole body (after ten days),[1].—(*Female.*) Discharge of bloody mucus from the vagina, with anxious palpitation and restlessness of body, pain in the small of the back, weakness amounting to faintness,[1].—Painful drawings like tearings by jerks in the pudenda, so that she must cry out, in the evening (after four days),[1].—[**400.**] Continually increased sexual desire in women (curative action),[1].—Increased desire for coition in women, which is more violent and lasting (curative action),[1].—Menstruation appears two days too early,[2].—Menstruation appears too early and is too profuse,[1].—Menstruation very scanty,[1].—Menstruation very scanty, lasting only one day, usually lasts two or three,[2].—During menstruation, a pressure like a heaviness over the pubes in every position,[2].—During menstruation, cutting and griping in the bowels,[2].

Respiratory Apparatus.—Stitches in the air-passages (second day),[2].—*In the larynx a feeling as if he inspired only smoke* (after twenty-seven days),[2].—[**410.**] Hoarseness (after fourteen days),[1].—Hoarseness, or rather loss of voice (for several weeks),[1].—Cough after midnight,[2].—Suffocative cough,[1].—Cough excited by continued speaking (after thirty-five days),[2].—Dry cough in the morning after rising, followed by a sensation as if a hard body were falling down in the chest (twentieth day),[2].—Dry short cough in the evening,[1].—Dry cough for three days, caused by a tickling in the bronchi and in the præcordial region, which is relieved only at night, sometimes also after dinner,[2].—Violent dry cough in the evening, followed by weakness in the head,[2].—Cough with expectoration of mucus,[1].—[**420.**] Cough, from an incessant irritation, with mucous expectoration,[2].—A loose cough, with salty, starch-like expectoration, having lasted four weeks, disappears (curative action),[2].—Arrest of breathing, either in coughing or not (ninth day),[2].

Chest.—Pains in the chest,[4].—Fulness in the chest, and painfulness as if bruised in the left side,[2].—A fulness in the chest with short breathing, especially on ascending, with stitches in the chest, especially on inspiration,[2].—Pressure and tickling in the chest with dry cough, disappears (curative action),[2].—Stitches extending from the chest to the shoulder,[4].—Sore pain in the chest and on it, externally,[2].—When coughing, a sensation of soreness in the chest,[2].—[**430.**] Sensation of severe palpitation on the forepart of the chest,[2].—Burning externally in the whole breast, with redness of the skin,[2].—Tearing and sticking externally in the breasts (after nineteen days),[2].—Pain in the right ribs, with cold hands and feet, and heat and redness of the cheeks (after two days),[1].—Transient burning in the left side of the chest,[2].—Sudden sticking and burning, so that she cried out on account of it, deep in the left side of the chest, in the afternoon (after four days),[2].—Transient stitches in the right side of the chest caused her to cry out, in the evening (after two days),[2].—Stitches in the left side of the chest (after four hours),[1].—Small stitches in the left side of the chest on every respiration (after nineteen days),[2].—A violent stitch in the left side of the chest on lifting a heavy weight with both hands (after twenty days),[2].—[440.] Throbbing, with sticking pain in the left side of the chest, extending upward from the pit of the stomach,[2].—Dull stitches under the sternum, deep in the chest, followed by a bruised pain at that spot (first day),[2].

Heart and Pulse.—Violent, long-lasting palpitation,[9].—At times violent palpitation (during the first fourteen days),[1].—Palpitation of the heart when lying on the left side,[1].—Palpitation of the heart, which is renewed when thinking of it, for then it makes her anxious, most at midday,[1]. —Pulse full and hard,[9].

Neck and Back.—Swelling in the neck, which, after a time, extends over the whole head, with redness and ulcerative pain in the skin, and *great swelling of all the glands of this region for several days* (seventh day),[2]. —Stiffness in the neck on waking from midday sleep (after twenty-four hours),[1].—Boring bone pain in the neck, which is neither increased nor diminished by motion nor by touching (third day),[1].—[450.] *Several swollen glands in the neck and occiput*,[1].—Dislocating pain in the left shoulder-blade,[1].—Burning in the upper part of the right shoulder-blade,[2]. —Burning stitch on the outer border of the shoulder-blade (second day),[2]. —Dull stitches through the left shoulder-blade to front of the chest (third day),[2].—Bruised pain between the shoulders (fifth and tenth days),[2].—In the morning, on rising, pains between the shoulders, so that he is quite stiff therefrom and cannot turn himself; afterwards, they extend into nape of neck and left shoulder, where they are very violent, then into the vertex and across the pectoral muscles into the left nipple,[8].—Weakness and powerlessness in the spine, it falls together when sitting a long time,[4].— Great pain in the right side of the back on lying down,[1].—Tensive pain extending from the spine forward, under the right ribs when rising from sitting, and when stooping far forward (to lift something up),[1].—[460.] Backache, as if he had lain too hard,[1].—Throbbing in the back and severe pulsation during rest, especially after emotionable excitement (first day),[1]. —Heaviness in the *small of the back* and in the loins, as from taking cold,[1].—Pain in the small of the back (after twelve days),[1].—Painful drawing in the small of the back, as if a heavy body broke down (after six days),[2].—*Tensive pain in the small of the back*, worse in the evening, so that he could not rise from sitting nor bend himself backward,[1].—Sticking in the small of the back, worse when sitting than on motion (after eleven days),[1].—A violent stitch in the small of the back,[2].—A sore pain extends from the small of the back around the abdomen externally,[2].—During menstruation, bruised pain in the small of the back,[2].—[470.] Burning in a small spot on the left side of the lumbar vertebræ, and at the same time in the lower part of the left shoulder-blade, worse when rising from sitting, better when walking; also at night, so that he can lie upon only one side (seventeenth and nineteenth day),[2].—Burning in the loins, which extends across through the abdomen,[1].

Extremities in General.—Excessive weakness in all the limbs in the afternoon, then towards evening; sweat at night; vomiting; this all reappears (according to a three-day type),[4].—The feet, the arms, etc., go to sleep on lying upon them,[5].

Upper Extremities.—Audible cracking in the *shoulder-joint,* on every motion of the arm (after eighteen days),[2].—Throbbing, alternating with tearing, now in the left shoulder, now between the shoulder-blades, also at night (nineteenth day),[2].—*In the axillæ under the arms, frequent pain in the glands,*[1].—Swelling of the right arm with pain of the axillary glands,[1]. —The arms are heavy and trembling,[1].—The arms fall asleep when lying upon the table,[5].—[480.] The left arm falls asleep, she can only bring it to again by much rubbing,[1].—Pain in the bone of the upper arm as if an ulcer would form,[1].—Tension here and there in the arms, always only in a small spot (second day),[2].—Twitching-tearing in the bend of the right *elbow,*[2].— Twitching almost like shuddering in the bend of the left elbow, extending to the middle of the upper and forearm,[2].—Pain as from a blow, above the left elbow,[2].—Pain in the elbow, as if bruised,[1].—Paralytic pain in the *forearm* in the morning, disappearing on motion, and returning during rest,[2].— In the left forearm painful tearings extending from the middle of it to the wrist,[2].—In the wrist and in other parts of the right arm, tension or drawing,[2].—[490.] Drawing in the left wrist, extending to the middle of the upper arm,[2].—Sudden tearing pain in the wrist,[2].—Dull sticking in the left wrist, relieved by motion,[2].—Distended veins in the hands, with redness thereof (twelfth day),[2].—The hands tremble when writing,[2].—Pinching pain in the hand,[5].—Wrenching pain in the back of the hands,[2].—At first crawling in the hands, then they fall asleep,[2].—Cracking in the joints of the thumb and little finger on moving them,[2].—Drawing in the last joint of the thumb and also in the fourth finger, so violent that it seems as if the finger would be torn off,[2].—[500.] Drawing pain in the last joint of the thumb,[2].—Drawing under the thumb-nail,[2].—Drawing in the index-finger as if paralyzed, with a sensation on touching it or bending it as if it were pithy, especially at the tip,[4].—Stitch in the last joint of the thumb, also suddenly in the tip of the thumb, so violent that it frightens him,[2].—Throbbing in the middle joint of the middle finger as of a hammer,[2].—Ulcerated nail on the left fourth finger (second day),[1].

Lower Extremities.—Hip and Thigh. Tension in the legs extending up to the hips, as if all the tendons were too short; most severe when standing, relieved when lying (thirty-seventh day),[2].—Pain in the right hip-joint on walking in the open air,[1].—Pinching pain in the right hip-joint, as if it were stiff or screwed up, it extends downward along the front of the thigh,[2].—Sudden stitches in the hip-joint, as if it would be wrenched out, with pain on walking, as if it would break to pieces,[1].— [510.] Burning in the nates,[1].—Drawing pain in the right nates, as if the flesh were torn off,[2].—Violent stitches in the nates,[2].—Sticking-itching in the nates,[2].—Twitching in the thigh above the right knee,[2].—He drags the legs, especially on ascending steps, on account of a sensation of lameness in the middle of the thigh,[3].—(Neidhard),[8].—She said she had pains in the thigh during sleep,[8].—Burning in the bend of the thigh, as if in the bone when sitting,[7].- Drawing down the front of the thigh as if in the bone, relieved when walking (twenty-seventh day),[2].—A feeling of pressing-inward in the bend of the right thigh,[2].—[520.] Sudden, dull sticking on the inner surface of the thigh which frightened him (fourth day),[2].—Violent sticking in the right thigh, so that he could scarcely walk (fourth day),[1].—Tearing in the right thigh in the morning after rising, relieved by the warmth of the bed (nineteenth day),[2].—From the left foot, internal stitches through the whole thigh into the testes, hinder walking,[8].—Excessive bruised feeling in the thighs,[8].—Violent bruised pain in the middle of the right thigh, which after awhile extends over the whole leg, and lasts from the afternoon till towards midnight,[2].—A blow in the thigh above the right knee when standing, so that he believed he would fall forward,[2].—*Knee, Leg, and Ankle.* Pain in knees and legs,[9].—Tearing on the inside of the knee, extending to the middle of the tibia, relieved when walking, returns when sitting,[2].—Cutting-burning in the right knee-pan,[1].—[530.] In the right knee, at times, a rapid momentary pain, like a cutting with a knife, which makes the leg lame,[1].—*Stitching pain in the knee joints,[1].—(Burning soreness in the knee-pan),[8].—Twitching in the right calf,[2].—Weakness in the legs in the morning, so that he sinks down (tenth day),[2].—In the lower leg, especially in the right tibia, paralytic pain relieved by elevating the leg, as for example, on a sofa,[5].—Tension in the tibia, in going down a mountain (sixteenth day),[2].—Tension in the tendons of the calf as if they were too short (fifteenth day),[2].—Tension and tearing in the legs, relieved by walking (sixteenth day),[2].—Much cramp in the legs,[1].—[540.] Cramp in calves,[9].—Cramp in the calf on stretching out the leg,[1].—Drawing pain as if in the bones of the leg, in the evening when sitting, was obliged to stand and walk about,[1].—Tearing and tension in the bones of the legs, extending downward to the feet, somewhat relieved when walking (fifteenth day),[2].—Crawlings in the left calf as though going to sleep, when sitting,[2].—Pains in the legs at night, as if he had taken a very long walk or danced too much,[1].—Pain as from a sprain in the ankle,[1].—Pain as from a sprain in the ankle, and on the back of the foot, even when at rest, with severe sticking, on motion,[1].—*Feet and Toes.* Trembling in the feet when standing, so that he is obliged to take hold of something to prevent falling (tenth day),[2].—When walking in the open air, the right foot becomes cold, and there is a tension in the calf,[1].—[550.] Uneasiness in the feet,[1].—Uneasiness in the feet when sitting, is constantly obliged to move the leg, in order to relieve the tension in the thigh, and the burning in the pubic region,[2].—Drawing pain in the feet, only when walking,[1].—Tearing in the feet extending to the knee, worse on motion,[2].—Sticking deep in the ball of the right foot,[2].—Ulcerative pain in the ball of the foot on stepping, especially in the morning after rising,[2].—Sticking in the heel,[1].—Burning in the soles of the feet the whole night, yet he cannot endure anything cool on them,[2].—Spasmodic pain in the soles of the feet,[4].—The tough skin on the sole of the foot pains as if sensitive when walking, like a corn,[1].—[560.] Pinching in the toes on stretching out the foot,[1].—Drawing pain in the toes (after five days),[1].—Drawing, violent tearing in the right great toe towards the tip,[2].—Tearing and stitching in the left great toe by the nail, with continued sensitiveness of the place, with great fretfulness (first day),[2].—Corns make their appearance on the toes,[1].—Pinching pain in the corns,[1].—Sticking in a corn,[1].

Generalities.—Trembling through the whole body, in the morning on rising,[1].—After dinner, great indolence and dread of labor,[4].—Walking in the open air is difficult for him; but the farther he walks the easier it becomes,[1].—[570.] A short walk fatigues him very much; he is obliged to sleep soon afterwards,[1].—*Weary, as with sleepy eyes during the whole day,[8].—*After eating, so tired that she cannot raise the hands; she is too weak to masticate,[8].—Great weakness; can scarcely raise herself in bed; if she does, the pulse immediately becomes rapid, jerking, and hard, and after several minutes scarcely perceptible,[8].—Great weakness and lassitude of the body, so that he almost sinks down, in the evening at 8 o'clock,[4].—When lying, a weakness, which generally seems a kind of heaviness; is most insupportable,[2].—Faint feeling at night; she is obliged to vomit profusely on the following day; is still nauseated the second night,[1].—Unusual sensitiveness of all the senses,[4].—Feeling generally sick,[4].—A very unpleasant relaxed condition of the joints,[1].—[580.] The whole upper part of the body feels numb and stiff,[8].—At night everything rocks within him, as in a ship,[8].—Tight and tense feeling in the whole body, with anxiety in the forenoon,[2].—Pinching pressive pain in many places in the body,[5].—Drawing in the whole body, now here, now there (after seven days),[2].—Drawing, alternately in the right shoulder, in the legs, in the arms, in the occiput, and in the eyes, with heaviness of the occiput, great weakness, and sleepiness, causing dizziness,[4].—Sticking as from needles in the whole body,[1].—Sometimes, stitches in the joints,[1].—Feeling bruised over the whole body, and very weak (after twenty-four hours),[1].—Feeling bruised over the whole body, in the morning on waking (eleventh day),[1].—[590.] In the morning at 8, suddenly feels as if the circulation ceased; a tingling in the whole body, extends into the tongue and the ends of the fingers and toes, with anxiety for fifteen minutes; then feels deathly tired,[8].

Skin.—Desquamation of the skin on the back of both hands (twentieth day),[2].—Dryness of the skin of the hands like parchment (fifth day),[4].—The skin on the back of both hands is rough and dry,[2].—The skin on the tips of the fingers becomes chapped and scales off,[2].—Eruption on the right eyebrow, with a sticking pain when touched,[1].—Eruptions on the ears,[1].—*Fatty tumors, especially about the neck,° (St. Cl. S.).—Pimples in various places, for example, on the arms, hips, nose, upper lip, forehead, etc.,[4].—Pimples on the sides of the scalp,[2].—Small pimples in the face like boils, though without sensation,[2].—[600.] A cluster of small, itching pimples, with a red base below the left corner of the mouth,[2].—Itching pimples in the neck close to the scalp (third day),[1].—Itching pimples on the wrist,[2].—Pimples on the feet, which spread like the itch,[8].—(Tetterlike) rash on the upper part of the forehead, with a sensation that is more burning than itching,[1].—Small boils on the forehead,[2].—A very uncomfortable small boil on the right wing of the nose, near the tip,[8].—(Boils on the upper arm),[8].—Small boils on the nates,[2].—A small wound becomes easily unhealthy, for example, having got a splinter in the finger, which was drawn out again, the wound would not heal; it ulcerated and throbbed; the pain prevented her sleeping at night,[1].—[610.] Burning in many places on the skin, now here, now there (seventeenth day),[2].—Severe itching over the whole body, which prevents her sleeping for several hours at night (twenty-ninth day),[1].—Itching here and there, which is only partially relieved by scratching,[2].—*Itching here and there; scratching is followed by a violent pain,[5].—Burning-itching, here and there,[2].—*Itching and biting on the scalp, and on the temples (after third day),[1].—Itching, evenings in bed, now in the face, now in the back, now in the hands,[1].—Itching upon the left shoulder-blade, with small pimples after scratching,[2].—*Severe itching in the thighs, even at night (eleventh day),[1].—Violent itching on the back day and night,[1].—[620.] Much itching, with eruption upon the back,[1].—Itching on the small of the back and between the nates; must scratch it raw,[5].

Sleep and Dreams.—Much yawning, every morning,[1].—Frequent, severe yawning,[2].—Great sleepiness after dinner, every day,[2].—Great sleepiness in the evening, his eyes close involuntarily,[4].—Falls asleep late in the evening, and then the sleep is very restless with dreams,[2].—Frequent waking at night, every hour,[2].—Frequent waking at night; child calls for its parents,[1].—Loss of sleep at night, on account of a sensation of great heat,[2]. —[630.] Evenings in bed the thought which she had had through the whole day that she would sleep very well prevented her sleeping all night,[1]. —Sleepless,[9].—Starting in the evening on falling asleep, as from fright, so that the whole body rises up,[2].—Is not refreshed by afternoon sleep, heavy, feels bruised; the head is painfully confused; constant yawning (after four hours),[1].—Talking during sleep (in an old man),[8].—*Dreams nearly all night*,[1].—Confused dreams for several nights, so that in the morning on rising it is some time before she collects her mind,[4].—*Anxious dreams almost every night*, with restless sleep,[1].—Anxious dreams at night, with heaviness of the head in the morning,[1].—Frightful dreams,[2].—[640.] Frightful dreams, on account of which she wakes in a sweat,[2].—Frightful dreams of fire and the like (after eight days),[1].

Fever.—Coldness. Great sensitiveness to cold (after twelve days),[1].— Constant coldness, as if cold water were dashed over her; worse in the afternoon (seventh to tenth day),[2].—Sudden chill, with gooseflesh; external coldness; bristling of the hairs; in the forenoon,[2].—At 8 o'clock in the evening, coldness of the whole body, with shivering beginning in the feet, with bristling of the hairs (twentieth day),[2].—Chilliness, with thirst in the afternoon (seventh day),[2].—Chilliness on going into a room from the open air,[2].—Shivering in the arms, which disappears by the warmth of a stove, but is aggravated by the least draft of air; in the afternoon,[2].—Coldness of the hands, with itching,[2].—*Heat.* [650.] Skin hot and dry,[9].—Alternations of heat during the day (ninth day),[1].—Transient heat frequently rising in the head (fourth day),[2].—The whole night, restless on account of internal heat (in a child),[8]. —*Heat at night and anxiety*, so that he does not know what to do with himself; lasts till morning on rising (fifth and fourteenth days),[2].—She cannot lie upon the left side, on account of orgasm of blood and violent palpitation, with a feeling of soreness in the heart, and great anxiety,[1].—He is attacked with heat when eating or drinking,[1].—After dinner he becomes very warm and uncomfortable, and feels a pressure in the right side above the stomach,[1].—Violent heat and sweat in the head, then thirst in the evening (eleventh day),[2].—Heat toward evening, with little thirst; violent pulsation extending into the head; on rising, vertigo, even to falling; heat the whole night, with disturbed sleep; next day violent thirst; pours down whole glasses of water, with very thick, white coating on tongue,[8].—[660.] Heat in the head, in the morning on rising, and sticking as with knives (after seventeen days),[2].—Dry heat of the face in the afternoon (twelfth day),[2].—Hot hands; frequently dips them into cold water,[8].—*Coldness and Heat.* Alternation of coldness and heat towards evening,[1].—Chilliness in the forenoon, suddenly in the evening he becomes too warm in the whole body, and the blood pulsates in the head,[1].—Dry heat the whole night, with sleeplessness, and, if she put her hand out of bed, coldness, chilliness, and thirst (twelfth day),[2].—Now heat, now coldness, the whole night,[2].— Cold sensation in the right side of the head, as from ice, and at the same time a burning sensation,[2].—A burning cold sensation in the forehead, in the forenoon (seventh day),[2].—Icy coldness of the feet from afternoon till evening, with heat in the whole body after lying down (seventh day),[2].— [670.] Heat and redness, frequently of one cheek, with coldness of the other,[1].—*Sweat.* Sweat for several nights, after midnight (seventh day),[2].

—Exhausting night-sweat (thirteenth day),[1].—Profuse sweat on the left side, especially on the head,[4].—Sweat on the inner surface of the hands and fingers in the afternoon (eighteenth day),[2].

Conditions.—Aggravation.—(*Morning*), On waking, feels stupid; on waking, confusion in the head; after rising, vertigo; on waking, heaviness, etc., in head; when yawning, stitches above right temple; eyes swollen; swelling of the lids; matter on the lids; eyes difficult to open; *sensation as of gauze before the eyes;* in bed, nose-bleed; after rising, lips dry; after rising, pain in lower back teeth; dryness of tongue; on waking, rawness on the tongue; after rising, dryness in the mouth; mouth feels numb; *foul taste;* after rising, sour taste in mouth; when swallowing, feeling as if throat swollen; after waking, sensation in the pharynx; frequent eructations; nausea; fasting, nausea; after waking, in bed, pressure on right side of abdomen; in bed, when lying on back, pressure in abdomen; after rising, cough; on rising, pain between shoulders; during rest, pain in forearm; after rising, tearing in thigh; weakness in the legs; after rising, pain in ball of foot; on rising, trembling; on waking, bruised feeling all over; at 8 o'clock, suddenly, feeling as if the circulation had ceased, etc.; much yawning; on rising, heat in head.—(*Forenoon*), Confusion in head; hiccough; from morning to afternoon, pressure, etc., in right side of stomach; tight feeling in whole body; sudden chill; chilliness; burning cold sensation in forehead.—(*Noon*), Palpitation of heart.—(*Afternoon*), Salty taste in mouth; constriction in throat; eructations; burning in region of stomach; pain in stomach; sticking, etc., in chest; weakness in the limbs; coldness; chilliness; shiverings in the arms; dry heat of the face; from afternoon till evening, coldness of the feet; sweat on the hands.—(*Towards evening*), Pain, etc., around anus; heat, etc.; alternations of coldness and heat.—(*Evening*), Sad, etc.; suddenly, becomes dejected; in bed, anxious; confusion, etc., in head; headache; sticking in the sides of the head; throbbing in occiput; crawling over scalp; weakness of the eyes; drawing over left eye; in the twilight, eyes close; buzzing in ears; frequent sneezing; redness of the face; in bed, toothache; crawling in tips of teeth; sour taste in mouth; sticking in throat; at 6 o'clock, thirst; from afternoon until far into the night, eructations; pressive pain in forepart of abdomen; cutting in abdomen; sudden erections; drawings in the pudenda; dry cough; dry, short cough; stitches in right side of chest; pain in small of back; when sitting, pain in the bones of the leg; at 8 o'clock, great weakness, etc.; in bed, itching; becomes too warm, etc.; sleepiness; 8 o'clock, coldness all over.—(*Night*), Lachrymose; agglutination of eyes; drawing in ear; crashings in ears; on slightest motion, when lying down, pinching around the navel; cutting colic; cutting in lower bowels; when lying out straight, feeling of fulness above pubes; diarrhœa; burning in left side of lumbar vertebræ; throbbing in left shoulder, etc.; pains in the legs; faint feeling; everything rocks within him; restlessness from heat; *heat with anxiety;* dry heat, etc.; now heat, now coldness.—(*About midnight*), Cutting pain in abdomen.—(*After midnight*), Throbbing, etc., in right ear; cough; for several nights, sweat; exhausting sweat.—(*Towards morning*), Diarrhœa.—(*Least draft of air*), Shivering in arms.—(*Walking in open air*), Pain in right hip; right foot becomes cold, etc.—(*On ascending*), Fulness in the chest.—(*On blowing nose*), Reverberation in ear; *bleeding at the nose.*—(*When breathing deeply*), Stitches in right side of abdomen.—(*When coughing*), Sensation of soreness in chest.—(*On descending a mountain*), Tension in the tibiæ.—(*After dinner*), Sticking in sides of head;

when sitting and writing, attacks of choking in throat; suppressed eructations; eructations sweetish, etc.; desire to urinate; every day, great sleepiness; becomes very warm, etc.—(*Before eating*), Sour taste in mouth.—(*When eating*), And for some time afterwards, sound tooth becomes loose, etc.—(*When eating or drinking*), Heat.—(*After eating*), Daily, in two hours, sour eructations; violent hiccough; feeling of repletion in stomach; tired.—(*After eating bread*), Pressure in stomach.—(*After emotional excitement*), Throbbing in the back, etc.—(*On exerting vision*), Burning in eyes.—(*Passage of flatus*), Pinching around navel.—(*When hiccoughing*), Stitches in right side of abdomen.—(*On inspiration*), Stitches in the chest.—(*On lifting a heavy weight with both hands*), Stitch in left side of chest.—(*When lying*), Weakness.—(*On lying down*), Pain in right side of back.—(*When lying on ear*), Throbbing in front of ear.—(*When lying on left side*), Palpitation of heart.—(*After a meal*), Tensive sensation in skin of forehead.—(*During menstruation*), Pressure over pubes; cutting, etc., in bowels; pain in small of back.—(*Motion*), Pain in region of liver; pains in bowels; pain in abdomen; pressing out in abdominal ring; sticking in ankle, etc.; tearing in the feet.—(*Moving lower jaw*), Pressure under the chin.—(*On raising herself in bed*), Immediately, pulse becomes rapid, etc.—(*On raising the arm*), Suddenly, vertigo.—(*On every respiration*), Stitches in left chest.—(*While riding*), Erections.—(*When rising from sitting*), Pain from the spine forwards; burning on left side of lumbar vertebræ.—(*On rising from stooping*), Vertigo; seems as if his head would tumble about; drawing, etc., in pit of stomach.—(*After scratching*), *Violent pain;* pimples on shoulder-blade.—(*When sitting*), Confusion of head; pinching around navel; sticking in small of back; burning in bend of thigh; tearing on inside of knee returns; crawling in left calf; uneasiness in the feet.—(*When sitting a long time*), Weakness, etc., in spine.—(*During sleep*), Pains in thigh.—(*When sneezing*), Cracking in ear; sensation in pharynx.—(*Continued speaking*), Excites cough.—(*On stamping with the feet*), Shaking in the brain, etc.—(*Standing*), Tension in the legs; trembling in the feet.—(*On standing in the sun*), Sticking on vertex.—(*During stool*), Pressing out in abdominal ring.—(*After stool*), Much empty eructations; moist hæmorrhoids.—(*On stooping*), Vertigo; sensation as if everything would fall forward in the forehead; when washing, stitches in frontal eminence; drawing, etc., in pit of stomach.—(*When stooping far forwards*), Pain from the spine forwards.—(*On stretching out the foot*), Pinching in the toes.—(*On stretching out the leg*), Cramp in the calf.—(*When swallowing*), Cracking in both ears; crackling in one ear; dryness, etc., in back part of throat; sticking in throat worse.—(*Empty swallowing*), Smarting pain in throat; rawness, etc., in throat.—(*After swallowing*), Scraping in throat.—(*On taking anything cold or warm into mouth*), Boring in the teeth.—(*Touch*), Renews tearing in brain; pressure under chin; pain in region of liver; indolence, etc.—(*When turning body*), Stitches in right side of abdomen.—(*On turning in bed*), Intestines seem to fall to one side.—(*On urinating*), Pinching in lower bowels.—(*On waking*), Pressure in the brain; from midday sleep, stiffness in neck.—(*On walking*), Headache; pain in abdomen becomes intolerable; drawing pain in the feet.—(*When walking fast*), *Cracking in ear.*—(*After walking*), Pain in abdomen.—(*On going into warm room from open air*), Chilliness.—(*From warmth of stove*), Immediately, sticking in head comes on.—(*When yawning*), Stitches in side of abdomen.

Amelioration.—(*Morning*), After rising, pressure in side of abdomen.—(*Night*), Fluent catarrh ceases; dry cough.—(*In open air*), Many symptoms disappear; confusion of head passes off.—(*Bending head backwards*), Tearing in occiput.—(*During dinner*), Many symptoms seemed to abate.—(*After dinner*), Dry cough.—(*After eating*), Weak feeling in stomach disappears.—(*Elevating leg*), Pain in lower leg.—(*Eructations*), Pressure in stomach; pains in the chest.—(*Lying*), Pain in abdomen; tension in legs.—(*Motion*), Many symptoms disappear; pain in forearm; sticking in wrist.—(*On scratching*), Itching, etc., in head disappears.—(*Sitting*), Pain in abdomen; desire to urinate ceases.—(*Standing*), Many symptoms.—(*When walking*), Pain around navel ceases; burning on left side of lumbar vertebræ; drawing down thigh; tearing on inside of knee; tension, etc., in legs; tearing, etc., in bones of leg.—(*Warmth of bed*), Tearing in right thigh.—(*Dry, warm applications*), Pains in chest.

BARYTA MURIATICA.

Barium chloride, BaCl$_2$2H$_2$O. *Preparation*, Solution of the crystals in water (1 to 10), for the lower dilutions.

Authorities. 1, S. Hahnemann, Hom. Archiv., 3, 3, 186; 2, Hufeland, ibid.; 3, Dürr (in Hufeland's Journ., 11), ibid.; 4, Bernigan (Dissert.), ibid.; 5, Thuessink (Waarnem, iii), ibid.; 6, Kohl (in Hufeland's Journ.), ibid.; 7, Mother (in Saml., f. p. Aerzte, 17, etc.), ibid.; 8, Gebel (Hufeland's Journ.), ibid.; 9, Crawford (in Med. Presc.), ibid.; 10, Schaeffer (Kuhn's Mag., 1), ibid.; 11, Schönemann (Hufeland's Journ., 20), ibid.; 12, Michaelis, ibid.; 13, Orfila in A. H. Z., 8, 297; 14, Henke's Zeitschrift, in A. H. Z., 8, 350, poisoning of a woman, æt. 42, by half an ounce, taken for gastralgia; 15, Schwelgæ, from Wibmer, general statement of effects of $\frac{1}{5}$ to 3 grains; 16, Walsh, Lancet, 1859, a girl, æt. 22, took a teaspoonful by mistake for epsom salts; 17, Wolf, Casp. Woch., 1850, a student took three teaspoonfuls.

Mind.—Anxiety,[2 10 15].—Great internal anxiety, which bends one together,[14].—Great anxiety, with retching,[2].

Head.—Vertigo,[2].—Vertigo; whatever he looked at seemed to turn around,[1].—The head is affected,[3].—Feels so heavy in the head that he can scarcely sit up,[1].—Headache,[13].

Eyes and Ears.—Eyes deeply sunken (after one and a half hours),[16]. —[10.] Catarrh of eyes, ears, nose,[15].—The eyes become quite stiff, he cannot move them,[1].—Left eyelid paralyzed,[17].—Deafness,[13].

Face.—Face pale, with an anxious expression (after half an hour),[16].— Face red,[15].—Spasmodic drawing of muscles of face,[14].—Sensitive drawing in the muscles of the face,[2].

Mouth and Throat.—Looseness of the teeth,[6].—Toothache, at first fine sticking, then (twitching), throbbing, like the beat of the pulse, especially after sleeping, and after midnight, which compels him to sit up in bed, but which is neither increased nor diminished by touching it, nor by biting, nor by cold water,[1].—[20.] Coated tongue,[2].—Tongue and mouth dry,[15].—Offensive smell from the mouth, as from mercury,[6].—Swelling of the palate,[6].—*Swelling of the salivary glands,*[6].—Profuse salivation,[2].—Bad taste in the mouth, even the food tastes badly,[1].—Swallowing difficult,[15].

Stomach.—Loss of appetite,[2 15].—Nausea,[2 7 14].—[30.] Nausea, immediately,[7].—Nausea (after half an hour),[16].—Retching,[2 14].—Increasing and incessant, tormenting, ineffectual retching; cannot lie,[14].—Inclination to vomiting,[9][10].—Violent vomiting,[13].—Violent vomiting of slimy, watery fluid,[14].—Vomiting of everything taken, with stringy mucus (one and a half hours),[16].—Vomiting of small portions of a nauseous looking and tasting substance, for six hours,[7].—Vomiting in the morning,[6].—[40.] Violent vomiting, with anxiety,[8].--Vomiting and pain in the abdomen,[17].—Troubles with the stomach,[8].—Pain in the stomach,[16].—Warmth in stomach goes to chest and head,[15].—Cramp in the stomach,[10].—Pressure in the stomach,[2].—Pressure in the stomach, and nausea, with great anxiety,[2].

Abdomen.—Pain in the abdomen,[2].—Continual pain in the abdomen,[17].—[50.] Burning pains in the abdomen,[10].—Violent burning in the abdomen,[16].—Slight colic,[15].—Pinching pain in the pelvic cavity,[10].

Stool.—Diarrhœa,[15].—Continued diarrhœa,[2].—Painful diarrhœa,[16].—Profuse diarrhœa, without pain in the bowels, for ten hours,[7].—Liquid stool,[2].—Stool greenish and chopped,[1].—[60.] Stool coated with mucus,[1].

Urinary Organs.—Painful urinating,[6].—Increased desire for urinating,[2].—Constant urinating,[6].—Involuntary urinating,[6].—Increased urine (after twenty-four hours),[15].—Urine has white sediment,[8].

Sexual Organs.—Frequent emissions at night,[3].—Induces menstruation,[10].

Respiratory Apparatus and Chest.—Voice weak,[17].—[70.] Cough,[2].—Dyspnœa,[2].—Oppression,[9].

Heart and Pulse, and Back.—Beating of the heart irregular, pulse scarcely perceptible (after one and a half hours),[16].—Pulse rapid, full,[15].—Pulse soft and irregular,[17].—Pain in the back,[10].

Extremities.—Swelling of the hands and feet,[2].—Trembling of the limbs, faintness, twitchings,[10].—Twitchings in hands and feet,[14].—[80.] Extreme weariness of the muscles of the limbs (after one and a half hours),[16].—(The limbs are cold, paralyzed),[7].—Hands and feet paralyzed,[17].—Painless twitching in the arm, especially at night,[1].—Tension in the legs,[10].—Cramp in the toes,[1].

Generalities.—Trembling,[15].—Convulsions,[13].—Death, with violent convulsions (after seventeen hours),[16].—Immobility of the body,[12].—[90.] General paralysis, for two days,[12].—Weakness,[15].—Laxity of the muscles of the body, and sinking of the strength, so that he was scarcely in a condition to crawl or move the limbs,[7].—The body feels so heavy that he cannot keep up, like loss of power,[1].

Skin.—Skin inflamed,[15].—Small eruptions on the skin,[2].—Itchlike eruptions on the body and throat,[4].—Itching eruption on the neck,[5].—On the side of the tip of the nose, a broad red pimple, with a biting, tickling, sore sensation, with small fine stitches on touching and rubbing it, though these sensations do not cause him to scratch it,[1].—Scurf-like eruption on the abdomen and thighs,[11].—[100.] A kind of scurf; profusely suppurating eruption on the scalp,[5].—Suppurating glands discharge more,[15].—Tearing-burning in denuded spots,[2].—Biting pain in the skin,[1].

Fever.—Surface cold (after one and a half hours),[16].—Ice-cold extremities (after half an hour),[17].—Tertian fever,[10].—Dry heat of the whole body both day and night,[3].—Internal heat in the upper part of the chest,[1].—Fever with thirst,[15].—[110.] Increased perspiration,[2].—Sweat,[15].

Conditions. — **Aggravation.** — (*Morning*), Vomiting. — (*Night*), Twitching in the arm.—(*After midnight*), Toothache.—(*After sleeping*), Toothache.

BELLADONNA.

Atropa Belladonna, L. *Nat. order*, Solanaceæ. *Common names*, Deadly Nightshade. (German) Tollkirsche. *Preparation*, Tincture of the whole plant, when beginning to flower.

Authorities.† (1 to 85 from Hahnemann, R. A. M. L., 1.) 1, Hahnemann; 2, Baehr; 3, Gross; 4, Hbg.; 5, F. H——n; 6, Hartung; 7, Hrn.; 8, Htn.; 9, Kr.; 10, Ln.; 11, Lr.; 12, Mkl.; 13, Rkt. d. j.; 13a, Stf.; 14, W. S.; 15, Ackermann;‡ 16, Albrecht, poisoning of two adults and a boy by the berries; 17, Baldinger, poisoning of four adults;§ 18, Baylie;‡ 19, Boucher, poisoning of five children; 20, Buchave, symptoms observed in hooping-cough patients after the administration of large doses of the extract; 21, Bucholz, effects of two-grain doses of the powdered root given to a boy, as prophylactic of hydrophobia; 22, Buch'oz, poisoning of a young boy; 23, Carl, symptoms produced by a decoction of the root in a chronic sufferer from rheumatic gout; 24, Cullen, effects of the infusion in a sufferer from cancer of the lips; 25, De Launay d'Hermont, poisoning of an adult; 26, De St. Martin, poisoning of a boy of four years; 27, De Meza, effects of a five-grain dose of the powdered leaves in a case of tumor of the breast; 28, Dillenius, poisoning of a mother and six children; 29, Dumoulin, poisoning of two little girls; 30, Eb. Gmelin, poisoning of an old man; 31, El Camerarius, poisoning of four children; 32, Elfes, poisoning, boy of seven years; 33, Erhardt, effect of berries in a boy of seven; 34, Evers, i, case of serous apoplexy, in which Bell. was given; 35, Evers, ii;‖ 36, Faber, general statement of effects of Bell.; 37, Grimm, poisoning of child of three; 38, Gmelin, general statement of poisonous effects; 39, Gœckel, poisoning of child of five; 40, Greding, effects of Bell. administered to epileptics and epilepto-maniacs, and in jaundice; i, man, æt. 29; iii, woman, æt. 35; iv, man, æt. 24; v, woman, æt. 23; vi, woman, æt. 20; vii, man, æt. 35, subject to raving in connection with his epilepsy; viii, man, æt. 20; ix, woman, æt. 25; x, woman, æt. 40; xi, youth of 16; xii, man, æt. 33, an epilepto-maniac; xiii, man, æt. 28, a melancholio-maniac, in whom epilepsy supervened; xiv, woman, æt. 37; xv, woman, æt. 38; xvi, man, æt. 38, epilepto-maniac; xvii, woman, æt. 29, epilepto-maniac; xviii, woman, æt. 32, epilepto-maniac; xix, man, æt. 23; xx, woman, æt. 34; xxi, man, æt. 34, epilepto-maniac; xxii, woman, æt. 42, a violent epilepto-maniac, raging and convulsed throughout; xxiii, a youth of 15; xxiv to xxvi, cases of jaundice; 41, G—ch, effects of an infusion of Bell. leaves given as an injection for incarcerated hernia; 42, Hasenest, poisoning of a young woman; 43, Henning, effects of grain doses of the powdered leaves given for the cure of pemphigus; 44, Hochstetter, effects of an infusion in an adult; 45, Hoffmann, statement of the effects of soporifics in general, including opium; 46, Horst, poisoning of an adult by the inspissated juice; 47, Hoyer, poisoning of an old woman; 48, Hufeland;‖ 49, Juste, effects of a single full dose, in an adult, given as a prophylactic of hydrophobia; 50, Lamberger, a narrative of the five months' treatment of some mammary indurations by an infusion of Bell.; 51, Lentin, effects in a case of mammary scirrhus; 52, Lottinger;‖ 53, Monetti, poisoning of a

---

† All of Hahnemann's authorities are given; others are carefully selected.
‡ Not accessible.
§ By the berries understood always unless differently stated.
‖ Not found.

puppy by the juice of the berries; 54, Mappus, fatal effects of a large
quantity of the juice mixed with wine; 55, Mardorf, poisoning of several
persons; 56, May;† "a baccis in infantibus," Hahnemann in Fragmenta de
Vir.; 57, Med. Ch. Wahrn.;† 58, Moibanus, poisoning of a man; 59, Müller,
effects of Bell. taken for angina faucium in a man of 50; 60, Münch, effects
of 4 to 14 grains of the powdered root given as a prophylactic of hydrophobia; 61, Ollenroth, effects in a case of mammary scirrhus; 62, Porta,
effects of a strong infusion; 63, Rau, poisoning of a man; 64, Remer, effects
of full doses of the powdered root, in a case of melancholia occurring at the
climacteric; 65, Sauter, i, effects when taken in fully developed hydrophobia;
66, Sauter, ii, poisoning of a child; 67, Sauvages;† 68, Schäffer, effects
when given to children for pertussis; 69, Schreck, fatal poisoning of a boy;
70, Sicelius;† 71, Solenander, poisoning in an adult; 72, Timmermann;†
73, Vicat, an account of the general effects of the leaves and berries; 74,
Wagner, poisoning of two old women and some children; 75, Wasserberg,
proving on himself; 76, Weinmann, effects of Bell., cited by Gmelin; 77,
Wetzler;† 78, Weinhold;† 79, Wierus, poisoning of an adult; 80, Wiede-
mann, effects when given freely to children for hooping-cough; 81, Ziegler;†
82, Ray; 83, Ware; 84, Wells; 85, Struve; (86 to 140 from Hencke's
résumé, Hom. v. j. Sch., vol. 16); 86, Burkner, effects of 8 grammes of the
extract; 87, Commaille, took half of an infusion of 3 grammes of herb
Bell.; 88, Frank, proving (from A. H. Z., 32) of the 1st dil., 10 to 50
drops; 89, ibid., proving of a solution of the extract; 90, ibid., proving by a
girl, æt. 23, with 50 drops of the 1st dil.; 91, Kluky, provings by 12 persons, with the extract, $\frac{1}{8}$ grain to 1 dr. doses; 92, Purkinje, proving with
20 drops of an aqueous solution of the extract; 93, Scheidtweiler, took a
piece of the extract; 94, Schlosser, effects of a small dose of the extract;
95, ibid., effects of $\frac{1}{260}$ gr. of the extract applied to the eye; (96 and 97
omitted); 98, Waltl, effects of 4 grains of the dried root; 99, Wasserberg,
effects of pills of Bell. extract; 100, Boulduc, poisoning of several children;
101, Buchner, chronic poisoning of a man; 102, Buchner, poisoning of a
girl, æt. 3; 103, Lipp, Dissert., poisoning of children; 104, Caffarelli, effects
of a clyster of herb. Bell.; 105, Couty, effects of a liniment of Bell. ext. and
a clyster of Bell. ext. for a periodic pain in the bowels; 106, Fink, poisoning by berries, man, æt. 19; 107, Frank, poisoning of an old man; 108,
ibid., poisoning of an old woman; 109, ibid., poisoning of a young man and
woman; 110, Fritze, poisoning of a child; 111, Gerson, poisoning of several persons; 112, ibid.; 113, Goldschmidt, poisoning of a boy; 114, Gaul-
tier de Claubry, poisoning of soldiers; 115, ibid., poisoning of a family by
an infusion of herb. Bell.; 116, Hirschman, poisoning of a child; 117,
Jolly, poisoning of a man by 46 grains of Bell.; 118, Köstler, poisoning of
two boys; 119, Koch, poisoning of a boy; 120, Krämer, poisoning of a
boy; 121, Kurtz, poisoning of two children; 122, Labbe, poisoning of a
man, 20 years old, by an infusion of herb. Bell.; 123, Laurant, poisoning
of a boy by 20 grains of ext.; 124, ibid., poisoning of a child, 1½ years old,
by 10 grains of ext.; 125, Liedbeck, poisoning of a boy; 126, Melion,
poisoning of two children; 127, Pinard, poisoning of several children; 128,
Rosenberg, poisoning of a man; 129, Salzb., Med. Chir. Ztg., poisoning of
a man by a clyster of 3 quarts of a decoction; 130, Seiler, poisoning of a
boy; 131, Teschemacher, poisoning of two women; 132, ibid., poisoning of
two girls; 133, ibid., of a woman; 134, ibid., of two children; 135, Trapen-

---

† Not found.

art, poisoning of a man ; 136, Vosnack, poisoning of a man ; 137, Wenzel Huber, poisoning of a boy ; 138, Gazette d. Santé, poisoning of two children ; 139, ibid., of a man ; 140, Zabri, from Kürner Wurt. Carr. Bl., poisoning of two adults and five children ; (141 *to* 176 *are taken from Roth's résumé j. d. l. Soc. Gal. (Mat. Med.*), 4, 402, *where references are furnished, but no details*). (On subsequent critical research, most of these additional authorities given by Roth have been found to refer to the effects of Bell. when given to patients ; they are therefore omitted, though the subsequent numbering could not be changed without great trouble.) (177 *to* 213 *are taken from Hughes's monograph on Bell., Hahn. Mat. Med., Part III.*) 177, Hughes, case ii, poisoning of a child with 8 to 12 grains of ext.; 178, Hughes, iii, Dr. Gray, effects of 8 to 10 grains of ext. on self; 179, poisoning of an adult by half an ounce of liq. Bell.; 180, poisoning of a boy by ext.; 181, ditto ; 182, ditto ; 183, ditto ; 184, poisoning of a child of four by berries ; 185, poisoning of a lady by a dr. of ext.; 186, poisoning of six persons ; 187, ditto of ten persons ; 188, effects of Bell. plaster to an abraded surface ; 189, poisoning of seven persons by berries ; 190, poisoning of a boy of 14 ; 191, poisoning of a man of 75 by ext.; 192, miscellaneous ; 193, poisoning of a man ; 194, effects, from Harley ; 195, Schneller, provings with $\frac{1}{4}$ to $4\frac{1}{2}$ grains of ext.; 196, Anstie ; 197, Christison ; 198, Hempel ; 199, Höring, poisoning by 25 grains of ext.; 200, Orfila ; 201, Pereira ; 202, Taylor ; 203, Trousseau et Pidoux ; 204, Lancet, 1844, effects of ext. to forehead ; 205, Lancet, 1854, effects of 3 grains of ext.; 206, B. J. of Hom., poisoning of a boy ; 207, Teste, poisoning of girls by decoct. of leaves ; 208, Aldridge ; 209, Fuller, a number of children treated with the ext., for chorea ; 210, Lond. Med. Rec., 1873 ; effects of $\frac{1}{2}$ gr. of ext., three times a day, for 12 days, for diabetes insipidus ; 211, Boecker, Beiträge ; 212, Ley, in Lancet, 1844 ; 213, Schroff; (214 *to* 241, *additional provings, and selected poisoning cases*) ; 214, Hering, symptoms from Archiv, 13, 2, 181 ; 215, Houat, proving of the 15th dil.; 216, L. B. Wells, provings, N. Y. St. Hom. Med. Soc. Trans., 10, 129, Miss F. B., æt. 22, took 4th dil.; 217, ibid., Miss C. E. C., æt. 19. took 4th dil.; 218, Dr. Schenk, ibid., took 10 to 30 drops of tinct., repeated for several days ; 219, Robinson, provings with the 200th and 30th, B. J. of Hom., 25 ; 220, Voigt, in Summarium, 1835, poisoning of a woman by a suppository of the ext.; 221, Goldschmidt, Casp. Woch., 1838, poisoning of a boy ; 222, Vierdier, Journ. de Montpellier, 1844 ; poisoning of a girl by infusion of the leaves ; 223, Evans, Br. Med. Journ., 1861, poisoning of a girl, æt. 9 ; 224, Woodman, Med. Journ. and Gaz., 1864 ; a man, æt. 24, took two oz. of a liniment composed of ext. of Bell., glycerin and water ; 225, Asprea, Lo Sperimentale, 1870, poisoning of a woman by a clyster of ext.; 226, Rollet, Wien. Med. Woch., 1865, poisoning of two boys ; 227, Smith, E. P. K., N. A. J. of Hom., 14, 553 ; poisoning by an infusion of Bell. leaves ; 228, ibid., poisoning by teaspoonful doses of Tilden's ext.; 229, Dufresne, Bib. Hom. d. Geneve, 1, 322 ; 230, Marsh, N. Am. J. of Hom., 4, 122, poisoning by 17 grains of ext.; 231, Hollier, Pharm. J., 16, 549, poisoning by decoction of Bell. roots; 232, N. Am. J. of Hom., 1, 182, poisoning of four women by the herb in brandy ; 233, Journ. Hebdom., 1834, poisoning of two children by 12 and 24 grains of ext.; 234, Hirschel's Zeit. fur Hom., 12, 16, poisoning of a boy ; 235, A. H. Z., 85, 175, poisoning of seven persons by eating beans cooked in a dish that had contained Bell. ext.; 236, Guarda, Quart. Hom. Journ., 1, 482, symptoms after 12 grains of the ext. taken for sleeplessness ; 237, Schleissteher, effects of the root of Bell. mixed with the food, attempt to

poison, Z. f. Hom. Kl., 1, 213 ; 238, Tardieu, Etude sur empois., effects of
Bell. plaster ; 239, ibid., poisoning by infusion of the leaves, three persons ;
240, ibid., poisoning of a man from eating without washing his hands, after
digging Bell. roots ; 241, Macfarlan, proving with the 6ᵐ (Fincke).

Mind.—Emotions, Rage, and Fury. *Anger, proceeding even
to paroxysms of convulsive rage,²¹⁵.—*She tosses about in her bed in a perfect
rage,⁶⁵.—*Rage; the boy does not know his parents.†—[Rage; he injures himself and others, and beats about him],⁴⁰ (Case 12).—*He bit at whatever came
before him,⁶⁰.—**Inclination to bite those around them,**²⁹.—[He tries to bite
those standing about him, at night],⁴⁰ (Case 18).—*Instead of eating what
he had asked for, he bit the wooden spoon in two, gnawed the plate, and
growled and barked like a dog,⁶⁰.—**She attempted to bite and strike her
attendants, broke into fits of laughter, and gnashed her teeth. The head
was hot, the face red, the look wild and fierce,**¹⁸⁶.—[10.] [*Inclination to
bite those about him, and to tear everything about him to pieces],²⁹.—
*Inclination to tear everything about them to pieces,²⁹.—*She tears her
nightdress and bedclothes,⁶⁵.—[He tears everything about him, bites and
spits],⁶⁵.—[He strikes his face with his fists],⁴⁰ (Case 12).—They stammered
out violent language,²⁹.—**Fury,**⁷⁹ ⁶⁷.—**Raging violent fury,**¹.—*Furious
delirium,⁸⁶ ²³¹.—**Fury ; she pulled at the hair of the bystanders,**⁵⁵.—[20.]
The forcible administration of fluid medicine makes her furious,¹⁷.—*[Fury,
with grinding of teeth and convulsions],⁵⁶.—**Such fury (with burning heat of
the body and open, staring, and immovable eyes) that she had to be held
constantly, lest she should attack some one ; and when thus held, so that
she could not move, she spat continually at those about her,**¹⁷.—**Mania.**
Mania, in which the patient was often very merry, sang and shouted ; then
again spit and bit,³².—Madness ; in his exceeding restlessness he jumped on
the table, bed, and stove,¹²⁰.—Violent madness ; the children scratched
themselves with their nails,¹²⁷.—Insanity,⁴⁴.—Insanity, with various gesticulations,⁴⁴.—He is beside himself, raves, talks much about dogs, and his arm
and face swell,⁶⁰.—*Insanity; they stripped themselves, and, clad only in their
shirts, ran out into the streets in broad daylight, gesticulating, dancing, laughing, and uttering and doing many absurd things,²⁸.—[30.] Crazy fits, with
great loquacity or absolute speechlessness, or with absurd buffoonery, fantastic gestures, and improper behavior,²¹⁵.—*Left the house and stripped
themselves naked; one woman went into the fields to work, at night ; another
went into the street before the house to dust and sweep ; another, with excited singing, cut open the pillows, and scattered the feathers about the
yard and street ; another went naked to the neighbors to caress the men,²³².
—*The paroxysms of madness were occasionally interrupted by loud laughing
and grinding of the teeth ; **the head was hot, the face red, the look wild
and staring;** pulse small, and very frequent; **pupils dilated ; the arteries of
the neck and head visibly pulsating;** pulse full, hard, and frequent,¹²⁸.—
She did foolish things, tore her clothes, pulled stones out of the ground and
threw them at the passers-by,⁶⁵.—He took a piece of bread for a stone, and
threw it far away, laughing violently and running about the room,¹¹³.—
Ridiculous gestures ; she feels after those about her ; now she seats herself ;
now she acts as if she were washing or counting money, or as if she were
drinking,⁴².—[He claps the hands, wags the head to either side, while
stringy saliva hangs down from the lips],⁴⁰ (Case 22).—[She claps the
hands together over the head, with a short, very violent cough, which
threatened suffocation at night],⁴⁰ (Case 22).—*He talks like a maniac, with

† Made up of S. 1409 and 42.

staring, protruded eyes,[20].—**Delirium**. *Delirium*,[46].—[40.] Delirium (mother and child, within an hour),[228].—Continued delirium,[234].—Constant delirium,[46].—*Rambling delirium*,[81 56 31 30 21 57].—Idle musing; raving; delirium, with illusions of the senses,[215].—Delirium, returning by paroxysms,[16].†—*Delirium, either continuous or recurring in paroxysms, mirthful at first, but subsequently changing to fury*,[73].—Delirium; she lay upon one side, the head bent forward, and the knees drawn up, gesticulating violently, and murmuring unintelligible words,[225].—*Very delirious; she would persist that there were very horrid monsters all over the room, staring at her*,[185].—Wildly delirious, but quite fantastic, almost hysterical, laughing, crying, and not at all conscious,[183].—[50.] During the delirium, loud screaming, cries, and laughing,[234].—*Delirium; the boy jumped out of bed, talked a great deal, was lively, and often laughed; consciousness was entirely gone; he did not recognize his parents*,[113].—Delirium; the child is very restless, talks confusedly, runs, jumps, laughs convulsively; face purple; pulse accelerated; the look very much changed; he has fever (after one hour),[128].—*In the evening he was seized with such violent delirium that it required three men to confine him. His face was livid; his eyes injected and protruding, the pupils strongly dilated; the carotid arteries pulsating most violently; a full, hard, and frequent pulse, with loss of power to swallow*,[193].—The delirium was of a busy, restless, vivid character, but generally rather pleasing than otherwise. The patients appeared to think they were pursuing their ordinary occupations; one boy appeared eager in flying a kite, another pulled tables and chairs about, thinking he was working in a coalpit, and a woman appeared to be remarkably busy with her household duties. All their movements were of a quick excited character, strikingly resembling delirium tremens,[187].—The delirium was attended with phantasms, and in this respect resembled that caused by alcohol, but the mind did not run on cats, rats, and mice, as in the case of drunkards. Sometimes the phantasms appeared to be in the air, and various attempts were made to catch them or chase them with the hands; at other times they were supposed to be on the bed. One patient (a woman) fancied the sheets were covered with cucumbers,[189].—His delirium would now be of a merry, now of a quarrelsome character; sometimes he would see figures which he tried to catch, etc.,[137].—The slight delirium that followed the action of the narcotic was of a strange, yet not unpleasant, kind. The intellectual operations at times were very vivid. Thoughts came and went, and ludicrous and fantastic spectacles were always uppermost in my mind. I was conscious that my language and gesticulations were extravagant, yet I had neither the power nor will to do otherwise than I did; and, notwithstanding my bodily malaise, my mind was in a state of delightful exhilaration,[178].—She complained first of "a sensation of madness in her brain," then suddenly lost the power of speaking and swallowing, and fell into a comatose state. The head was bent forward on the chest, eyes closed, breathing heavy and stertorous, pupils widely dilated, hands and feet cold, pulse scarcely perceptible, jaws firmly fixed. After rousing, appeared conscious when spoken to, but could not answer. Soporose throughout the day, speech gradually returning. (Second day.) Has passed a restless night, *sleep being much disturbed by frightful dreams; complains of intense pain in the head, and says that it feels enormously large*; **great intolerance of light and noise**. At noon, *very delirious, and would persist that there were horrid monsters all over the room staring at her*. (Third day.) Head much relieved after leeching.

† Not found.

Passed a restless night, her sleep, she says, being disturbed by "miserable phantoms." From this point gradual amendment took place,[185].—Soon after the spasms, delirium (in which, however, the patient knew his doctor),[238].—[60.] Delirium, with fierceness,[47].—*Delirium and heat,[16].—Violent delirium, alternating with lethargy; the boy appeared very much heated,[119].—*Excited and delirious, with violent motion of the arms and legs, increasing to a raging delirium,[235].—At times he is delirious, at times he answers rightly when questioned, and bemoans himself,[31].—She mutters like one asleep,[42].—Senseless talk,[31] [20] [10] (Case 5).—Continual senseless chattering and laughter (after half an hour),[104].—Speech loud, disconnected,[223]. —[70.] [*Delirious talking; obscene],[40] (Case 11).†—She spoke constantly and rapidly, talking nonsense,[66].—Speaks in broken sentences and deliriously,[240]. —*Her mind was disordered, so that speech did not correspond to thought, nor thought to sense, nor sense to the objects present,[37].—Her heightened but deluded fancy conjures up before her a multitude of beautiful images,[9].— The boy's fancy was very active, but he passed quickly from one idea to another; they were mostly of a lively character, relating to his plays,[118].— Hallucinations and confusion of mind,[91].—Hallucinations, with vertigo,[122]. —Hallucinations, with great restlessness; she did not know the bystanders; she laughed out,[222].—*He imagined he saw things not present,[80] [236].—[80.] Groped for things which did not exist,[237].—He imagines he sees birds flying off through the chimney, and wishes to follow them by the same route,[229].—[Delirious talk of dogs, as if they swarmed about him],[48].—Talks of wolves being in the room; with full pulse,[41].—He looked about; he talked about mice and other dark-colored animals which he saw,[233].—Visions of wolves, dogs, giants, and fire,[215].—At the height of the poisoning, the woman was in a state very closely resembling that so often seen in delirium tremens. Excessive terror was painted on her countenance, and she responded to all questions by pointing with a trembling finger to swarms of unclean beasts, which she fancied were scrambling all over the walls, beds, table, etc., of the wards (from 5 grains used as a suppository),[196].—Fancied he saw ghosts and animals in the fire,[237].—He imagines he sees ghosts and various insects,[98].—He imagines he is riding on an ox, or some such thing,[41].—[90.] It seems to her that her nose is transparent, and a spot on the left side of the head transparent and colored brown,[9].—[He raves as in a dream, and cries he must go home, because everything is burning up there],[40] (Case 21).‡—Lying in bed in the evening, it appears to him as if he were floating away with his couch; ten evenings in succession he imagined, immediately after lying down, that he was floating in his bed,[5].—Lively and playful the next morning, apparently well, but completely unconscious, so that when he was offered a piece of bread he thought it was a stone, and threw it from him,[221].—*He sought continually to spring out of bed,[30].—*When put into bed, he sprang out again in delirium, talked constantly, laughed out, and exhibited complete loss of consciousness; did not know his own parents (this lasted the whole night),[221]. —*In his delirium he threw himself down from a height,[21] [22].—She jumped into the water,[66].—*In his delirium he picked at the bedclothes and threw them off, and sought continually to spring out of bed,[30].—Condition resembling constant intoxication,[215].—[100.] Intoxication,[1].—State of joyous intoxication; she danced and jumped about in such a way that the neighbors

---

† See S. 864.
‡ These two symptoms are taken from the following: "On December 6th, raved in his sleep; he cried out, 'All is on fire at home; it is necessary that I should return there.'"

thought she had been drinking,[239].—State of intoxication, with disturbed vision and difficult speech; he imagines that he cannot move his tongue (after five hours),[239].—As if drunk, immediately after a meal,[1].—Directly after a meal, as if intoxicated (after six and a half hours),[11].—Intoxication immediately after drinking the least quantity of beer,[1].—Great excitement; now he sings, now scolds, while the limbs are in constant motion,[137].—Various gesticulations,[41].—[She makes preparations for returning home],[40] (Case 21).—A tailor was poisoned with a Belladonna injection, and for fifteen hours, though speechless and insensible to external objects, went through all the customary operations of his trade with great vivacity, and moved his lips as if in conversation,[197].—[110.] He performs foolish ridiculous tricks (after one to eight hours),[1].—The speech was more incoherent in the evening,[15].—[Nightly delirium, which is absent during the day],[40] (Case 7).—[Incoherent ravings at night; during the day he is in his right mind],[40] (Case 16).—The delirium ceases after a meal,[5].—Talkativeness,[233 235].—Constant unintelligible talking,[238].—*Garrulity; he constantly uses foolish and absurd language, at which he often laughs aloud; when addressed he turns toward the speaker, but does not answer correspondingly (after half an hour),[136].—Great garrulity, with a silly unmeaning smile and laugh,[115].—Garrulity, unlike his usual mood, with squinting and extremely stupid expression,[123].—**Desires and Aversions.** [120.] Takes pleasure only in voluptuous ideas,[215].—Inclination to violent exercise and rapid travelling,[215].—Fondness for games of chance, [215].—Love of solitude, aversion to society, and dislike to conversation,[215].—Dread of solitude, of ghosts and thieves,[215].—Not inclined to talk; he desires solitude and quiet; every noise and the visits of others are disagreeable to him,[7].—She abhorred all liquids, and acted frightfully, bit the jaws tightly together, and raved so that she was obliged to be tied down,[108].—Aversion to all fluids, so that she demeaned herself frightfully at the sight of them,[17].—Abhorrence of all liquids; he would scream violently as soon as a spoon or glass containing liquid was brought to his lips, would convulsively set his teeth together, and, if forced to swallow some, violent general convulsions would immediately occur,[118].—**Moods.** The expression and actions denoted uncommon cheerfulness; with incessant senseless talking,[130].—[130.] Merry craziness,[67].—In the evening, the boy was uncommonly lively and cheerful; he laughed, screamed, sang, and quarrelled in a loud voice, but very soon became sick, and vomited,[137].—Unrestrained and exuberant mirth; inclined to quarrel without cause, and disposed to laugh in an annoying manner,[6].—Very mirthful mood; he is inclined to sing and whistle (in the evening, after thirteen hours),[14].—Great mirthfulness after supper; the vital powers were increased to an extraordinary degree for a quarter of an hour, after which came drowsiness,[12].—Frequent laughter,[40] (Case 5).—Loud laughter,[37 29 44 57].—Constant loud laughter,[23].—Involuntary, almost loud, laughter, without having any laughable thoughts,[13].—Stupid laughter and merry delirium,[236].—[140.] She laughs a long time with herself,[40] (Case 5).—Continual laughter, whereby the subjects jumped high up, from emotions of wild joy, danced, made the most remarkable gesticulations, and performed different motions of the body with the greatest rapidity and dexterity (after one hour),[112].—[She breaks out into loud laughter, sings, and touches things near her],[40] (Case 17).—[Laughing and singing, she touches objects around her the whole day],[46] (Case 22).—Singing,[233].—He sings and warbles,[57].—Singing and loud talking in sleep,[1].—[*Weeping*],[29].—Very excited mood; she is readily brought to weep,[2].—Violent weeping, whimpering, and howling without cause, accompanied with timorousness, usually within twelve hours,[1].—[150.] Weeping and extreme ill-humor on awaking out of sleep,[1].—In the intervals free from spasms, she utters the most violent cries, as if she were suffering great pain,[37].—Dejected, despondent,[19].†—She is so anxious and confused that she fears she is about to die,[72]. —Anxiety and inquietude,[30].—Very anxious and timorous,[12].—*By day, great anxiety ; she has no peace anywhere ; it seemed to her as if she must flee away,*[1].—*Anxiety, anguish, trembling, constant restlessness ; groans, cries, and weeping, especially in the afternoon and at night,*[215].—Anxiety during the menses,[50].—Much anxiety, followed in an hour by perspiration,[43].— [160.] In her momentary lucid intervals she complains of intolerable anguish, so that she wishes to die,[17].—In walking in the open air, she is overwhelmed with tearful anguish ; she is weary of life, and inclines to drown herself,[1].—[She begs the bystanders to kill her],[40] (Case 22).—Tearful timidity,[1].—Timid mistrust,[1].—Cowardice, distrust, suspicion, inclination to run away,[215].—He starts in affright very readily, especially when any one approaches him,[13].—Events which had been previously anticipated with pleasure appeared to him in an anxious light ; he thought them fearful and dreadful,[13].—*Timorous insanity ; he is afraid of an imaginary black dog, of the gallows, etc. ; more in the first twelve hours than afterwards,[1]. —On seeing a drink which was offered him, he became very restless, the gesticulations and rolling of the eyes became more violent, and the face assumed an expression of great fear,[137].—[170.] He feared that death was near,[30].—[She is so anxious and confused that she fears she is about to die],[72]. —[She tries to strangle herself, and begs the bystanders to kill her, because she believes that she will certainly die],[40] (Case 22).—[He tries to escape],[65].—He escaped, under some pretext, into the open field,[60].—*Extreme irritability of temper,*[219].—The merest trifle provokes and irritates him ; he is dissatisfied with everything,[215].—Exceedingly irritable and sensitive humor, with inclination to utter abusive language and to strike,[215].—Fretfulness ; nothing seemed right to him ; he was vexed with himself,[5].—He was fretful about this and that,[1].—[180.] Extremely morose and serious,[4].— Silent ill-humors (after eight hours) ; on the two following days he was in his wonted mood ; the day after that, however, his ill-humor returned,[7].— Whining ill-humor about trifles, with headache as if a stone were pressing the forehead,[1].—Want of cheerfulness, ill-humor, inclined to nothing,[1].— Extreme ill-humor after sleep ; he bites those around him,[20].—He is very easily made angry, even about trifles,[7].—Violent quarrelsomeness, which cannot be appeased,[1].—At times he is delirious, at times he answers rightly when questioned, and bemoans himself,[31].—At one time he utters ridiculous nonsense, at another he talks rationally,[1].—After the talkativeness, dumbness,[20].—[190.] Hourly alternation of weeping and fretful humor,[1].—At first, sad, weeping, which then passed into impatient and vehement howling (with chilliness), (after one hour),[1].—Sighing, alternating with jumping and dancing,[55].—Groaning, alternating with bursts of laughter, songs, and gambols,[215].—[At one time he hurriedly grasps at those standing near, at another he starts back in fear],[65].—Disinclination and indifference to everything ; deficient activity of mind and body,[12].—Apathy ; nothing could make an impression on her ; after some days there succeeds a very sensitive, fretful mood, in which nothing gives her pleasure,[1].—Extreme indifference for hours ; one could have taken her life without affecting her,[9].—*Intellect,*

---

† Not found.

Thought. *Paroxysm of cerebral exaltation, with abundance of ideas and images, generally fantastic and incoherent,*[215].—His uncommon liveliness and readiness of thought, and the absence of his customary hypochondriac moods, seemed remarkable to himself and the physician,[129].—[**200.**] *He spoke rapidly and hastily,*[119].—[*Mental confusion*],[70].—Mental confusion, so that he knew not whether he was dreaming or awake,[58].—Confusion of mind; he imagined himself rich, owner of a large house, etc. (after a quarter of an hour),[86].—Confusion of mind, general trembling, transient heat of face (after half an hour),[104].—Confusion of mind, with flickering before the eyes,[103].—Confusion of the senses; sleepy, yet awake, he imagines he is dreaming,[58].—Thoughts became disturbed and confused,[237].—Talked confusedly,[237].—Speech slow and confused,[123].—[**210.**] Disordered consciousness,[43].—First this occurred to him, and then that, he could not think in an orderly manner, and forgot immediately whatever he thought or read about,[11].—His manner of expression is incomplete; speech very difficult,[115].—He sat lost, as one in a dream,[4].—Heedlessness and frequent absence of mind,[215].—Mental weakness,[79].—Weakness of the mind and memory,[215].—Loss of understanding and memory,[215].—Stupidity,[74].—Irrationality, stupidity,[215].—[**220.**] Loss of the thinking faculty; one is stupid, and like an idiot,[215].—Intellectual obscuration,[238].—Obtuseness of sense,[1].—Impaired understanding for some weeks,[63].—Entire disappearance of intelligence,[20 65].—He does not seem to know where he is,[238].—He paid no attention to those about him, in fact, seemed unconscious of their presence; only now and then, when addressed in a loud voice, he stared at the speaker for an instant, like one suddenly roused from a sound sleep. The face was a little flushed (after eight hours),[188].—Disinclination to all kinds of mental exertion,[4].—Aversion and incapacity for all work, and especially for all efforts of thought,[215].—***Memory.*** Lively memory (after twenty-four hours),[1].—[**230.**] He remembers things long bygone,[80].—He remembers things which happened three years ago,[57].—Temporary return of the lost memory,[40] (Case 5).—Diminished memory,[1].—Loss of memory,[237].—Forgetfulness of what had taken place,[235].—His memory, for two or three days after, was very defective,[188].—Memory very poor for two or three days; he remembered nothing which took place after the doctor came,[238].—Very weak memory; he forgets in a moment what he was about to do, and cannot recollect anything,[1].—Absence of mind; he is apt to do his business wrong, and forgets things which he had just intended to do,[14].—[**240.**] During the headache, disappearance of the thoughts; she forgets what she has just thought, and cannot recollect herself,[2].—He did not know his own relations,[79].—The boy does not recognize his parents,[130].—***Insensibility.*** Insensibility, loss of consciousness,[13a 73 42 37 63 30].—Insensibility to all external objects,[197].—Insensibility, rattling breathing, and convulsive movements in the face and hands,[17].—Entire insensibility, stiffness of the lower limbs, extreme distension of the superficial bloodvessels, with strangely red, swollen countenance, very full and rapid pulse, and excessive sweat,[17].—Complete loss of consciousness,[234].—Consciousness disappears; he no longer recognizes his surroundings, and begins to rave (after half an hour),[136].—Loss of the senses,[42 37 63] (after two hours),[30 44].—[Loss of the senses, with convulsions of the limbs],[29].—[**250.**] [Loss of consciousness and convulsions of the arm, at night],[40] (Case 14).—Senselessness, as in intoxication, and a kind of active delirium,[102].—After a little time, loss of consciousness, with stertorous respiration,[230].—He lay four days without taking any nourishment, motionless, like a dead person; he could not be roused,[62].—Lethargic, apoplectic condition; for a day and a night they lay without any motion of the limbs; if pinched by the by-standers, they opened their eyes, but uttered no sound,[74].—The patient's manner was apoplectic, and severe engorgement of the vessels was present. This state of partial coma was alternated by paroxysms of uncontrollable tendency to motion and rapid automatic movement, attended with convulsive laughter. No well-marked convulsions made their appearance, al-though, during the brief intervals of sleep, a slight subsultus of the muscles of the face and extremities was noted.—A sort of coma, with small, weak, unequal pulse,[19].—*Comatose condition, with rattling in the throat, very red face, dilated pupils, convulsions of the upper extremities, very hot skin, with red spots on neck and chest, and feverish pulse* (after half an hour),[109].— Stupor and loss of consciousness,[215].—[260.] Slight stupor or lethargy,[231].— Persistent stupor (after five and a half hours),[239].—Stupor, with violent convulsions of the extremities,[134].—Stupefaction,[20 61 74 79].—Well-marked state of stupefaction,[239].—Very great stupefaction,[61].—Profound stupefac-tion, which, at times, is interrupted by a shrill scream, betraying great anxiety,[140].—Stupefaction and vertigo, from congestion of the head,[129].—He lies as if stupefied; rattling in the throat; twitchings of face and hands (after half an hour),[107].—Stupefaction; she lost consciousness, became rest-less, and struck about her forcibly (after four hours),[126].

Head.—Confusion and Vertigo. [270.] The whole head is mud-dled for many days,[13a].—Bewildered feeling in the head,[219].—Confused and muddled head (after five minutes),[91].—**Confusion of the head,** *aggravated by movement,*[7].—Confusion of the head on moving it, but still more on walking; even when relieved, it returns immediately on walking (after five min-utes),[88].—In the evening, he complains of confusion of the head; with ex-traordinary garrulity,[129].—Confusion of the head, as in incipient intoxica-tion, with continually increasing dulness,[88].—Confusion of the head, with cloudiness and feeling of intoxication, as from smoking tobacco and drinking spirits,[215].—Head confused, with pain in forehead,[195].—*Vertigo,*[20 30 43 71 81 227 237]. —[280.] Vertigo, he staggers as if drunk,[91].—Vertigo, impossible for her to stand, everything turns around (after three hours),[220].—*Vertigo, as if every-thing turned in a circle* (after one hour),[7].—*Vertigo; it appears to him as if objects around him swayed to and fro,*[14].—*Vertigo, mostly at night on turning over in bed, or when getting up in the morning, also when walking, and on every change of position,*[215].—*Vertigo increased on any movement of the body,*[195]. —The confusion of the head gradually increases to real vertigo, which is aggravated on motion,[18].—*Vertigo, with perceptible pulsation in the head, dilated pupils, with nausea* (after one day),[89].—*Vertigo, with rush of blood to the head, roaring in the ears, and slight mistiness of vision* (after one day),[89]. —Vertigo, with headache and drowsiness, relieved after sleeping (after one hour),[98 131].—[290.] Vertigo, with dimness of vision; he saw snow-flakes, etc., before his eyes, and the pupils were much dilated (after one day),[139].— Immediately after, vertigo and dimness of vision, recurring three days after-wards at the same hour,[207].—Vertigo, and a feeling as if intoxicated; gait was tottering, face red and turgid; he was in good humor and remarkably talkative (after half an hour),[136].—Vertigo, with nausea; dazzling of the eyes, reeling, dulness, trembling, and anxiety,[215].—Vertigo, with lassitude, anguish, and fainting,[215].—Vertigo and pain in all the limbs,[86].—Vertigo, and trembling of the hands,[107].—Vertigo, and trembling of the hands, so that they could not perform any work with them,[17].—Vertigo, with trem-bling of the hands and contraction of the fingers,[215].—Attacks of vertigo during rest and motion,[3 215].—[300.] Attacks of vertigo, with dulness of

sense, lasting a few minutes (after twelve hours),[1].—Vertiginous reeling,[55]. —A vertigo-like sensation of reeling in the whole head while sitting,[8].—He attempted to get out of bed with a reeling, drunken motion; his speech was thick and indistinct,[190].—He reeled in walking, held on by the walls, complained of anguish and vertigo, and often spoke irrationally like a drunken man,[17].—Vertiginous staggering,[55 52 50].—The first effect was vertigo, increasing to such an extent as to render it impossible to walk without staggering,[178].—He staggers when walking like a drunken man,[240].—On rising in the morning, she staggered about as if drunk,[25 40].—She rose early from her bed, and staggered to and fro like one intoxicated,[40] (Case 14),[25]. —[310.] While walking, he staggered and spoke senselessly as if drunk,[107]. —It seems as though everything about him was turning round,[215].—Feeling as if he was turning round like a ball, and as if waltzing from right to left,[215]. —Turning round in the head, vertigo with nausea, as after turning quickly in a circle, or as on waking from the morning sleep after a night of revelling,[4].—Such violent turning in the head that he was unable to distinguish objects, much less be serviceable in his occupation,[237].—Turning in the head, and at the same time a similar turning in the scrobiculus cordis; after rising up it became so bad in walking, that she could no longer distinguish anything; everything vanished from before her eyes,[9].—Swimming of the head, as in a state of intoxication,[227].—Dizziness (after five hours),[217]. —*Dizziness with sensation as if a board were before her forehead,[90].—Sensation sometimes of dizziness, sometimes like the vibration of a pendulum, in the head,[215].—*In General.* [320.] *Swelling of the head,[9 46 60].—*Head swollen to double its size,[46].—*Great swelling of the head and redness over the whole body* (in two boys),[60].—Trembling of the head and limbs,[215].—Unsteadiness of the head and hands,[1].—*Throwing the head hither and thither, even to shaking;* then again, convulsive bending forwards of head and trunk,[119].—[Violent shaking of the head],[40]. (Case 6.)—[Violent shaking of the head, frothing from the mouth and loss of consciousness],[40] (Case 14).— [After hiccough, slight convulsions of head and limbs, followed by nausea and lassitude],[40].—*Her head is drawn backwards; she bores deep into the pillow at night,[2].—Unconsciously, he often scratches his head and rubs his nose,[125].—[330.] A kind of cerebral apoplexy seized one of them, causing her to fall down insensible,[207].—Determination of blood to the head; red cheeks,[20].—*Rush of blood to the head; pulsation of the cerebral arteries, and a throbbing in the interior of the head (after five minutes),[88].—*Strong rush of blood to the head, with beating in the temples, and burning in the eyes,[215].—*Congestion of blood to the head, with danger of apoplexy,[215].—Congestion of blood to the head, with bleeding of the nose and extreme dulness,[215]. —A shepherd died comatose twelve hours after eating the berries. At the autopsy the bloodvessels of the head were gorged,[197].—Ebullition of the blood towards the head, without internal heat of the head; when he leaned the head backwards it appeared to him as if the blood rushed into it,[4].— *Confusion as if intoxicated,[13 44 56 70 16].—Confusion of the head as though from much brandy and tobacco,[4].—[340.] Confused head and intoxication, as from wine-drinking, with bloated, red countenance,[16].—During a sudden rigor, great confusion of the head and sight, red eyes and swollen face, which is covered with very small, irregularly shaped, dark-red spots, especially on the forehead,[40] (Case 19).—Constant confusion of the head and drowsiness (after four hours),[3].—Confusion of the head, with swelling of the glands in the nape of the neck (after six hours),[1].—Dull, uneasy sensation all over the head (after half an hour),[217].—Sense of dulness and turning in the head; she felt better in the open air, worse in a room (after quarter of an hour),[13a].—Dulness of the head, with fatigued, torpid, besotted feeling,[215]. —Weariness of the head; inability to raise the head after stooping,[198].— Head heavy (second day),[218].—Heavy, pressing feeling in whole head (after five and a half hours),[218].—[350.] Head heavy all day (first day),[218].—He feels his whole head heavy, as if from intoxication,[13a].—His whole head feels so heavy that he seems about to fall asleep; he is not disposed to do anything,[1].—Head felt heavy on rising in morning (after eight and a half hours),[218].—On stooping, the blood mounts to the head, which becomes heavy as if giddy,[1].—Feeling of heaviness and fluctuation in the head, as if there was a vessel of water in it,[215].—Heaviness of the head and vertigo,[106]. —Weight in the head as though he would fall,[10].—Weight on the head, with dull shootings (after fourteen hours),[207].—*Inclination to lean the head against something hard and cold,[215].—[360.] Headache,[240].—Headache all day (second day),[217].—Slight headache,[239].—[Violent headache],[40] (in several cases).—*Very intense headache,[239].—Pain in the head shifting to the scapulæ,[40] (Case 8).—The pains in the eyes are correspondingly felt in the head, and often even in the heart,[215].—Violent dull headache (soon after),[237] —Headache as if the brain were numb,[1].—Complains of intense pain in the head, and says that it feels enormously large,[185].—[370.] Headache, with confusion and dulness of the senses,[99].—*Headache, with dizziness, aggravated by stooping, and, if relieved, immediately reproduced on motion,[90].— *Violent headache, chiefly in the orbital region, with redness of the eyes and face (after one hour),[117].—Violent headache, and feeling of pressure in the eyes, which were much injected,[199].—*Pain in the head and eyeballs, which felt as if starting from their sockets,[187].—Headache, with transient blindness,[40]. —Violent pains in the head, with swelling of the lids, heat in the face, and lachrymation (after three-quarters of an hour),[93].—Headache and weariness, the face red,[186].—Headache and great lassitude on awaking,[1].—Stupefying headache, with painful lassitude, bad temper, and inclination to lie down,[215].—[380.] Headache, with burning miliary eruption over the whole body,[215].—The headache is worse after dinner and in the evening,[215].—**The pains in the head are aggravated by noise, motion, when moving the eyes, by shocks; contact,** *the least exertion, and in the open air,*[215].—Continuous distension of the whole brain,[10].—Sensation of swelling and extraordinary expansion in the brain,[215].—*The feeling in the head was that of violent congestion, a full, tense, and throbbing state of the cerebral vessels, identically the same sensation as would be produced by a ligature thrown round the neck, and impeding the return of the venous circulation,[178].—* Violent pressing in the whole head from within outwards, as if it would burst (after three hours).[8].—* Headache as if the sutures of the skull were being torn open, and as if a lever were being applied, whereby the head was forced asunder,[10].— *In the open air, the sensation of bursting in the head is very violent,* **and he is afraid to cough on account of the increase of pain it causes** (after three and a half to four hours),[8].—Headache, as if the head were screwed together on both sides, and thereby rendered narrower,[2].—[390.] Feeling of burning and swelling in the cranial bones,[215].—Burning in the brain, with sensation as if the bones of the head had become soft, and fallen apart,[215].— Burning, pressive, lancinating, painful, or crampy pains in the head, chiefly in the forehead, along the orbital vault, at the nape of the neck, and on the right side of the head,[215].—Boring and pressing headache during the day, in different places; in the evening, shooting,[9].—*Incessant drawing and expansive pain in the head, as if something in it rocked or swayed in a jerking *manner*,[1].—Oppressive pain in the head (mother and child, third day),[228].—Sensation of hard pressure over the whole head,[215].—**Pressure in the head, now here, now there, which occupies each time large areas**,[7].—Drawing-pressive headache,[4].—*Pressive headache, especially in the forehead* (after two days),[7].—[**400.**] *Pressure deep in the brain over the whole head, during and after walking in the open air*,[1].—*Painful pressure in the head, especially in the lower part of the forehead directly above the nose, intolerable on stepping or treading*,[13].—Pressure and pulsation in the head, felt mostly in the forehead and eyebrows,[215].—Lancinating headache, causing vertigo, and extending to the eyes,[215].—Cutting-tearing pain in the head, which moves about from one part to another,[7].—*Stabbing through the head, as if with a double-edged knife, in the evening*,[9].—*Three violent severe stabs through the head, from the forehead to the occiput*, **whereupon all previous headache suddenly disappears**,[13a].—Painful shooting in the whole head, especially in the forehead,[13a].—Terrible headache, made up of dull or pressive shootings, which dart through the brain from all sides,[1].—Throbbings in the head,[239].—[**410.**] Violent throbbing of the brain,[227].—*Violent throbbing in the brain from behind forwards, and towards both sides; the throbbing ends on the surface in painful shootings*,[14].—Throbbing sensation, which for a short time alternated between the head and chest. He compared it to the movement of a pendulum (after half an hour),[239].—Pulsating headache, with pressure at vertex,[219].—*Jerking headache, which becomes extremely violent on walking quickly or on going rapidly upstairs, and where at every step there is a jolt downwards, as if a weight were in the occiput* (after forty-eight hours),[14].—Shocks and balancing sensation in the head, mostly when walking fast and going upstairs,[215].—Feeling in the brain as of the swashing of water,[21].—*Forehead.* Confusion of the head about the forehead, and at times a reminder of vertigo (after half an hour),[95].—Cloudiness in the forehead, as if an oppressive cloud moved to and fro, especially under the frontal bone,[3].—A sensation externally, as of contraction of the muscles of the forehead and eyes,[10].—[**420.**] Cold sensation in the brain, at the middle of the forehead,[1].—*He was frequently obliged to stand still in walking, from the violence of the pain in the forehead; at every step it seemed as if the brain rose and fell in the forehead; the pain was ameliorated by pressing strongly on the part* (after six days),[4].—Dull, frontal headache on the left side,[195].—*Headache above the orbits, as if the brain were compressed, so that he was obliged to close the eyes*,[4].—Violent crampy pain in the frontal eminence, which extends down over the zygoma to the lower jaw,[14].—Early in the morning, headache, as if something in the forehead over the eyebrows sank down and hindered the opening of the eyes (after four hours),[11].—*Boring pain under the right frontal eminence, early in the morning, soon after waking*,[3].—Drawing in the head towards the forehead, as if the brain would dilate,[10].—*Drawing pain in the frontal bone and in the nape of the neck, both when at rest and during motion*,[3].—Gnawing pain externally in the frontal eminences,[14].—[**430.**] Oppressive frontal headache,[91].—*Pain in stooping forwards, as if everything would issue at the forehead*,[13a].—A weight at the top of the forehead, which causes vertigo, and a sense as if intoxicated (after fourteen days),[1].—Pressive pain behind and above the eyebrows in the forehead,[211].—*Headache, as if the brain would be pressed out, in the forehead, just above the orbits, which prevents the eyes being opened, and obliges him to lie down* (with excessive contraction of the pupils and very weak voice), (after five and twenty-four hours),[1].—Violent pressive pain in the left frontal eminence, from within outwards,[8].

—*Tensive pressure in the right side of the forehead,*[7].—Pressive pain below the right frontal eminence, which soon occupies the entire forehead (after ten minutes), decreases at intervals, but only to return with greater violence,[3].—Pressive pain under the frontal eminences, soon after waking, on rising,[3].—Headache above the eyes only, like a weight in the head, early on waking; when touching the eye he feels pain,[1].—[440.] *Headache, as if a stone were pressing the forehead, relieved by laying the head down, and stooping, with dilated pupils, and whining ill-humor about trifles (after three hours),*[1].—*Sensation as if the brain were pressed towards the forehead, which disappeared directly on bending the head a little backwards* (after one and a quarter hours),[8].—**Pressive pain in the forehead, so severe during motion that it caused him to close his eyes;** *easier in sitting; he was obliged to lie down, upon which it disappeared; it returned immediately on rising, for two days, and was not aggravated by eating or drinking; but as soon as he went into the open air, the forehead seemed to be pressed in as if a heavy stone lay on it;* on the third day, the pain disappeared entirely, while he was sitting in the room,[4].—Sharp shootings in both frontal eminences, from within outwards (after two hours),[14].—Tearing shootings in the head over the right orbit,[7].—Fine shooting, burning pain in the left frontal eminence (after a quarter of an hour),[8].—Severe shooting in the right frontal eminence, increased by bending forwards, ameliorated by pressure (after five minutes),[13a].—Tearing in the forehead,[4].—Tearing in the forehead, externally,[1].—Violent pains of a tearing character in the anterior part of the head,[3].—[450.] Burning-tearing pain in the left frontal eminence (after four hours),[8].—Strong pulsation of the bloodvessels in the forehead, and pain as if the bones were lifted up,[4].—*Temples.* Severe pain through temples,[227].—At 3 P.M., slight headache in left temple (second day),[217].—Cramplike compression at the temples and forehead,[215].—Dull, darting pain in right temple, affecting the eye (after five minutes),[218].—*A drawing-down in the temples and in the right orbit,*[1].—Drawing and pressive pains in the right temple, with sensation as if it would burst,[215].—Cutting pressure in the temples, from within outwards, which increases in violence, spreads through the brain, and there passes into a strong throbbing, constant in all positions,[14].—A pressive feeling of weight from the centre of the brain towards the temples, with diminution of hearing in both ears,[12].—[460.] *Pressive pain in the right temporal region, which on supporting the head with the hand increases to a sense of bursting, and extends into the right frontal eminence* (after eight hours),[8].—Tearing pressure in the right temple, and in the vertex, which extends in various directions,[7].—Violent pressure in the left temple, from without inwards, which spreads itself over the entire anterior half of the brain, on that side where the head is supported by the hand (after three-quarters of an hour),[8].—**Stabbing as if with a knife, from one temple to the other,**[2].—Pressive shootings in the temples, from within outwards,[14].—*Violent shooting pain in the right temple, for a quarter of an hour (after twenty-five hours),*[13a].—Dull shooting in the left temple, from within outwards,[11].—Throbbing and beating of temples,[228].—*Vertex and Parietals.* Crampy pain, passing off rapidly, in the right side of the vertex (after eleven hours),[14].—Pressing in the right vertex, shifting to the left and then back again to the right,[12].—[470.] Tensive pressure in the left vertex and in the forehead (after twenty-four hours),[7].—*Headache in the vertex, a kind of twisting, sometimes also digging, sometimes tearing; the pain became much more violent on external pressure; the skull seemed to be quite thin, as if it could be pressed through,*[9].—Tearing pain in the right *vertex*, increased by movement,[8].—Slight lateral headache (third day),[217].—Pain in left parietal bone, extending to the temples (after five hours),[217].—Headache in left parietal bone, increasing and extending to right temple (after forty minutes),[217].—In about three-quarters of an hour after rising, and after stirring around quite briskly, the right side of the head ached, but without that heavy feeling (after nine and a quarter hours),[218].—Drawing pain in the right side of the head, and at the same time in the right arm, when at rest after dinner,[4].—*Incessant, dull, pressive pain on one or other side of the head* (after five and twenty-four hours),[1].—Violent pressure from within outwards, in the whole left half of the brain, especially violent in the forehead (after two and a half hours),[8].—[**480.**] Sensation as if a bar of iron was pressing on the head in the direction of the ears, with hardness of hearing,[215].—Darting pain under left parietal bone (after four hours),[217].—*Sharp cutting pain in the right side of the head, from the frontal to the occipital region, becoming general, and at last settling in left parietal bone,[217].—*Stabbings in the right side of the head, as if with a two-edged knife, which next are felt in the front of the head, then in the vertex, then in the occiput, so that she cannot lie on either side,[9].—Throbbing aches in the parietal region, lasting nearly two hours (after five and a half hours),[218].—Occiput and External.* Occipital headache,[214].—*Sensation of weight, with violent pressing, in the occiput* (after two and a half hours),[8].—Throbbing pressure in the left side of the occiput (after five hours),[8].—A cutting pain in the head to the left of the occipital protuberance,[3].—In the evening, some severe stabs in the occiput, immediately behind the ear, rapid as lightning, so that he could have cried out (after six days),[1].—[**490.**] Some dull shoots in the left side of the occiput,[10].—Nodosities resembling small exostoses, at several places on the head,[215].—Eruption of hard and very sensitive pimples on the scalp,[215].—Crusty herpetic eruptions, scales and ulcers, on the hairy scalp,[215].—Sensation as if the hair on the top of the head were being pulled (after three and a half hours),[217].—Pain externally in the whole head, resembling that which remains in the integument after strong tugging and pulling at the hair,[13].—*The head externally is so sensitive that the least contact, even the pressure of the hair, gives her pain,[9].—Soreness of roots of hair,[227].—Crampy pain on the scalp, with feeling as if the hair was being plucked out,[215].—Raw pain on the scalp, as if it had been burnt,[215].—[**500.**] The hair of the head, which was previously naturally electric, is so no longer (after twenty-four hours),[1].—Falling off of the hair, chiefly around the head,[215].—Hairs which become discolored, break easily and fall off,[215].

Eyes.—In General. Puffy appearance about the eyes,[230].—Black circle around the eyes, as if one had received a blow,[215].—Eyes inflamed, red, and bloodshot, even to the iris,[215].—*The eyes are inflamed, and have a wild expression,[114].—Inflammation of the eyes; the conjunctiva is covered with red vessels, with shooting pain; the eyes water,[4].—Inflammation of the eyes; swelling of the veins of the sclerotica, with a tickling sensation,[1].—Inflammation of the eyes; the cornea is dimmed, and the lids are swollen (after five minutes),[86].—[**510.**] The look is somewhat dim, uncertain, unsteady, as in amaurosis, without his suffering in the least from that disease,[115].—*The eyes are very animated, with fully dilated pupils,[19].—Bold look,[29].—*Had a staring expression (for three days),[230].—*The eyes had a staring look,[29 59 180].—Staring eyes.—Though he is blind, the eyes are open,[31].—Protruding eyes (after one hour),[114].—Eyes protruding,[186].—*The eyes are projecting and sparkling,[37].—[**520.**] *Protruding, sparkling, furious *eyes;* sometimes without expression, dull, and filmy,[215].—*The eyes protruding, glaring, and wholly insensible to light* (after four hours),[126].—*Protruded eyes, with dilated pupils* (after six hours),[12].—*The eyes protruding; pupils dilated; with a staring look,*[132].—*The eyes are protruding, shining, the pupils dilated, and completely insensible to light* (after four hours),[121].—The eyes protruding very much, immovable, sometimes as if swimming in tears, with dilated pupil,[129].—Eyes closed (after six hours),[239].—Eyes half closed, threatening (after one hour),[112].—Eyes were glittering, fixed,[233].—Eyes sparkling, fixed, glittering, and prominent (second day),[227].—Yellowness of the white of the eyes,[1].—[**530.**] In the morning, the white of the eye is streaked with red, with pressive pain,[1].—Yellowish hue of the sclerotica,[215].—Bluish sclerotica (in the sopor),[236].—[The eyes are red, glittering (glassy), and turn about in the head],[65].—Mucous membrane of eyes and lids deeply injected, and much swollen (after six hours),[239].—*Squinting,*[233].—Strabismus,[215].—[The eyes are distorted],[40] (Case 8).—*The eyes become distorted, with redness and swelling of the face,*[20].—*Spasms of the eyes, distorting them,*[69].—[**540.**] Eyes spasmodically turned up, and showing only the whites,[215].—The eyes turn spasmodically round and round,[19].—Rolling of the eyeballs (for three days),[230].—The eyes, which protrude from their sockets, roll around,[103].—*The eyes are in constant motion, the pupils extremely dilated,*[137].—Eyes and hands are in constant spasmodic motion,[19].—Eyes alternately fixed and very movable,[200].—Sometimes the eyes rolled wildly about, at others they were immovable, fixed on one point,[118].—Pressive pain over right eye,[219].—The eyes tire very soon on reading,[94].—[**550.**] *Eye dry; motion attended with a sense of dryness and stiffness,*[178].—*Dryness of the eyes* (the nose, the mouth, and the gullet),[75].†—*Feeling of burning dryness in both eyes,* more violent alternately in the one or the other (after seven hours),[12].—*Pain and burning in the eyes,*[40] (Case 1).—Very frequently repeated sensation of heat in the eyes, and as if the eyes swam in tears,[94].—*Feeling of heat in the eyes; it was as if they were surrounded by a hot vapor,*[1].—While walking in the open air, a sensation of heat blowing against the eyes, and fine sticking pains, afternoons; at the same time drowsiness (after five minutes),[88].—*Burning heat in the eyes,*[215].—Burning in the eyes, coupled with acute itching; both, however, cease when the eyes are pressed upwards,[12].—Intolerable burning and dryness of the eyes,[215].—[**560.**] Sensation of burning and roughness in the eyes, as from sand or pepper,[215].—His eyes seemed to him to be too large,[237].—Aching pain in eyes,[228].—Drawing pain under the left eye from below upwards,[1].—Feeling in the eyes as if they protruded,[13a].—Pressure in the eye, as of a grain of sand,[40] (Case 5).—A general pressure in both eyes, as if hard spring-water had got into them,[10].—Pressive and digging pain in the eyes, felt even in the head,[215].—Shooting in the eyes from within outwards,[9].—Smarting in both eyes,[4].—[**570.**] Crawling, pressive pain in the eyes, as if they were full of sand; she was obliged to rub them (after one hour),[15 11].—Itching of the eyes, with lancinating pains from one canthus to the other,[215].—*Sensitiveness of the eyes,*[91].—**Brow, Orbits, and Lids, Lachrymation.** A pressive pain in the left supraorbital ridge, together with distressing weakness of vision of the right eye on writing, whereby the letters swam; and an oppressive sensation, as if the right eyelid hung down paralyzed,[94].—Pain in the orbits; often it feels as if the eyes were being torn out, sometimes (and more lastingly) as if they were being pressed into the

---

† The observer adds after "eyes," "with burning in these and in the lids."

head; in addition to which there is a pain which presses down from the forehead into the eyes,³.—Darting pain in and near the orbit of the left eye and near the vertebral extremity of the eighth rib (after four hours),²¹⁷. —A confused pressure comes in the right orbit, and alternately shifts into the forehead and back again,³.—Pressing pain in the upper part of the socket of the eyes (after four and one-quarter hours),²¹⁷.—Dilated eyelids; eyes wide open,¹.—*The lids wide open; eyes shining and protruding*,¹³⁵.— [580.] The lids are wide open, the eyes protruding far from their sockets, rolling, squinting, and almost insensible to external impressions,¹⁰⁶.—Both eyelids tumid,¹⁹⁰.—Swollen lids, which are ulcerated and bleared,²¹⁵.—Slight swelling of the lower eyelids (after four and one-quarter hours),²¹⁷.—The palpebræ of the left eye were puffy, and redder than those parts on the right side; and the upper left lid was prolapsed, as in ptosis,¹⁷⁹.—A livid, lead-colored spot upon the eyelids contrasted horribly with the deathlike paleness of the face (in the sopor),²³⁶.—Tarsal edges of lids injected,¹⁹⁵.— Sties on the upper lids,²¹⁵.—Frequent jactitation of the eyelids,²¹⁵.—Twitching and convulsions of the lids,¹⁰².—[590.] An incessant quivering (and blinking) of both eyelids,¹⁰.—Quivering of the left upper lid, and a slight burning in the outer canthus, with dilated pupils,⁸⁹.—An incessant trembling and quivering of the right upper eyelid, continuing the whole day, and at last becoming painful,⁶.—Spasmodic and involuntary closure of the lids, even when the eyes are shut, as if a bright light was shining on them,²¹⁵. —Heaviness of the lids (¹⁹⁵), especially of the right upper lid,¹³.—Heaviness of the lids, with a feeling as if a sticky mass were lying between them and the ball, which compels rubbing; pupils dilated; confusion of the head, and drowsiness (after two and one-half hours),⁸⁸.—Throbbing pain in the lower eyelid towards the inner canthus, with great inflammatory swelling at that point, and much lachrymation, for half an hour (after thirty-two hours),¹².—The internal canthus of the left eye is very painful, even to a slight touch,³.—Itching shoots in the internal canthi, which rubbing only temporarily removes (after one hour),¹⁴.—Swelling and suppurative inflammation of the left caruncula lachrymalis, at first with burning, afterwards with pressing pain, for three days (after four days),¹².—[600.] *In the morning the lids are completely agglutinated*,⁹ ¹².—Trembling mucus before the left eye, so that she must rub it frequently,⁹⁰.—*Lachrymation,*¹².—Flow of tears, which seem to burn the lids,²¹⁵.—Involuntary lachrymation,¹.—*Lachrymation, with great photophobia; all light is intolerable,*²¹⁵.—*Total absence of lachrymation, and motion of the eyes, attended with a sense of dryness and stiffness; the conjunctival vessels fully injected,*¹⁷⁸.—**Conjunctiva and Ball.** Conjunctival sac injected with blood,²³⁵.—Conjunctiva injected, bluish,²¹³.— The conjunctiva of the ball is injected with bluish blood,¹¹⁴ ¹¹².—[610.] The conjunctiva red, the lids heavy, the eyes shining, and as if swimming in tears (after five minutes),⁸⁸.—*The conjunctiva red, the pupil much dilated; look staring,*¹⁰⁵.—*Tunica conjunctiva highly injected, and the whole eye prominent and preternaturally brilliant,*¹⁷⁷.—The vessels of the conjunctiva and the white of the eye are congested with blood, the pupils dilated, and the ball is generally turned upward (after two hours),¹²⁵.—Eyeballs unnaturally prominent (after six hours),²³⁹.—*Eyeballs red and prominent,*¹⁹⁷.—Pimples and ulcers on the cornea,⁷¹⁵.—The eyeball has a constant trembling motion,¹⁴⁰.—*The surface of the ball became quite dry, which caused a very disagreeable and uncomfortable sensation, which could not be relieved by winking or continued closing of the eyes* (after one hour),⁹².—Pain in eyeballs,²²⁷.—

[620.] Pain in the eyeballs, intolerance of light, and conjunctival inflammation, followed by dilated pupils and loss of sight permanently,[204].—When she closed the eyes, a pressive pain deep in the eyeball,[13a].—*Pupils.* *The optic disk greatly deepened in tint, and the retinal arteries and veins much enlarged, the veins most markedly so* (from one drachm of extract), (after an hour and a half),[206].—*Dilated pupils* (nearly every prover).—*Dilatation of the pupils* (after three and one-half hours),[66].—*Next to its influence on the circulation, the most prominent effect of the action of Belladonna consists in dilatation of the pupils,[194].—Pupils partially dilated,[239].—Considerable dilatation of the pupils (after six hours),[239].—Pupils strongly dilated,[240].—Great dilatation of pupils,[230 234].—[630.] *Pupils remarkably dilated,*[231].—The pupils uncommonly dilated, so that the iris becomes almost a line (after seven hours),[112], etc.—Extreme dilatation of the pupils,[19].—Extreme dilatation of the pupils (from the application of a fresh Belladonna leaf to an ulcer below the eye),[82].—The pupils extremely dilated, not at all sensitive to light, while vision seemed to be totally lost (after four hours),[126].—Dilatation of the pupils, especially the right (after five minutes),[86].—The right pupil shows a very large circular dilatation,[94].—Complete dilatation of the pupil of the right eye, and blindness for three weeks (from injecting the juice of the plant into the eye). Dazies.—In the sopor, the pupils paralytically dilated,[236].—*Dilated, immovable pupils,*[56 233].—[640.] *Pupils dilated, insensible,*[220].—*The pupil dilated and immovable,* the eye totally devoid of expression,[115].—Dilatation of the pupil, with weakness of sight (after one hour),[98].—Dilatation of the pupils, with presbyopia,[189].—Pupils strongly dilated, and contracting imperfectly,[238].—Widely dilated and sometimes contracted pupils,[215].—*Contracted pupils* (after ten minutes),[3] (after one and a half hours),[14] (after two and a half hours),[11].—The dilated pupils become somewhat smaller after several hours, but the right was less contracted than the left (after five minutes),[88].—Very contracted pupils the whole day, which first begin to dilate in the evening,[13a].—Excessive contraction of the pupils, with headache,[1].—[650.] *Irides insensible to light,*[231].—Pupils insensible, and extremely dilated (after six hours),[239].—*Vision.* Vision disturbed,[231].—Disturbed vision and hallucinations,[240].—Disturbance of the visual power and presbyopia, with dilated pupils,[83].—Imperfect sight, objects appearing white to him,[180].—Weak or feeble vision,[91].—Eyes were somewhat weak, or objects were seen as if through glass, not obscured,[211].—Weakness of vision increased, without any dilatation of the pupils,[195].—Weakness and transient loss of sight, with widely dilated pupils, as in amaurosis,[215].—[660.] Great failure of sight,[220].—[Great obscuration of sight],[49].—Obscuration of sight from dilated pupils,[20].—On writing, he must close the eye whose pupil is more dilated, in order to see the lines plainly (after a quarter of an hour),[94 95].—Obscuration of sight, with extremely dilated pupils,[40] (Case 26).—Obscuration of vision, so that he could not distinguish surrounding objects; dilated pupils,[105].—Complete obscuration of vision, so that she could not walk alone without running against everything; the eyes look as if quite amaurotic,[114].—Dulness of sight for three hours,[40] (Case 17).—Sight and hearing quite dull; he did not answer to loud calling (after four hours),[121].—Dulness of sight, with trembling of all the limbs,[40] (Case 1).—[670.] Extreme dimness of sight,[61].—Dimness and weakness of sight,[215].—*Dimness of sight or actual blindness,*[21 31 40 42 49 50 66].—Dim sight and blindness, with dizziness, headache, and weakness of the imbs,[215].—Dimness of sight, dryness of the mouth, and pain in the abdomen,[40].†—Dimness of sight alternating with cramps in the hands and feet, cloudiness of the head, and lassitude of the limbs,[40] (Case 18).—Indistinctness of vision was most complained of when the pupils were of their natural size, and were contracting freely under the stimulus of light,[209].—The impaired vision of Belladonna is chiefly or entirely presbyopia. In two cases, magnifying glasses enabled the subject to read with ease,[201].—Longsightedness (presbyopia) as in old age,[52].—Presbyopia; he can only read large type,[215].—[680.] Distant objects appear clearer than near ones, with dilated pupils,[94].—He can see distinctly only quite distant objects and completely parallel rays, as those of a star in the heavens (after injecting the juice of Belladonna into the eyes),[83 84].—A feeling as if he could see nothing, and yet he saw when he tried to see something, and strained his eyes for the purpose,[13].—The visual power appeared almost lost, but if the boy's attention was aroused he recognized the persons about him, but only for a few moments, after which he returned to the land of dreams; he imagined he saw a number of different objects, flies, birds, fishes, horses, soldiers, etc., with which he was constantly busy,[118].—Vision as if through a fog, the lids heavy, and in the eyes a sensation as if they protruded from their sockets,[89].—Darkness before the eyes, while looking, in the morning,[106].—In reading, he can discern nothing in the book but the white margin which surrounds the area of black letter-press,[58].—The sight of the right eye had become rather clearer, but that of the left eye more impaired, the upper lid more tumefied and prolapsed, the conjunctiva more vascular, and raised above the margin of the transparent cornea, which in a few days became opaque, and a small quantity of a puriform fluid had accumulated in the anterior chamber of the eye,[179].—Vision is not present in the left eye, the lid of which is drooping, inflamed, and very painful when touched,[181].—She says, "can see distinctly for a moment only, and then my face becomes horribly distorted" (after twenty-eight hours),[185].—[690.] He sees nothing close at hand; at a distance everything appears double,[13a].—Vision at times lost, at times only obscured, with excessively dilated and quite immovable pupils,[32].—Loss of sight at sunset,[215].—While walking in the open air, and in bright light, vision was weaker than in a room, or in the dark,[94].—Transient blindness, with headache,[40] (Case 17).—Blindness,[42 66].—He awakes blind,[31].—Such notable blindness was observed, that she could not read ordinary print,[50].—Complete blindness,[223].—[700.] He was quite blind, and stared vacantly,[183].—The eyelids did not close when the hand was passed suddenly before them. He had evidently lost the power of vision, although he stared fixedly at objects as if he saw them,[190].—[Blindness; the pupil of the right eye is extremely dilated and incapable of contraction],[40] (Case 11).—The visual power is altogether lost (in a state of stupor), (after four hours),[121].—Vision so completely lost that even the brightest light cannot be distinguished,[197].—Retina quite insensible to the influence of strong daylight,[179].—[Photophobia; he avoids looking at the light],[49].—Her room was darkened (light was unendurable),[228].—She sees objects inverted,[43].—*Diplopia (after six hours),[239].—[710.] *Double vision,[220 222 227].—Objects are seen double,[43 76 185].—Objects appeared double, and they seemed to revolve and run backwards,[190].—*Objects appear double, upside down, or crooked,[215].—*Every object in the room, both real and spectral, had a double, or at least a dim outline, owing to the extreme ditatation of the pupils,[196].—[Objects are seen manifold and dark],[65].—The sight (e. g., of letters) is multiplied, not clear, and irregu-

---

† Not found.

lar (after one hour),[98].—Reading by lamplight was difficult; the lines
jumped hither and thither,[99].—Letters swim while reading,[195].—Evenings,
in bed, on reading as usual, the letters flowed one into the other, so that it
was utterly impossible for him to read,[89].—**[720.**] Objects seem to tremble
and scintillate, as if viewed through a mist,[215].—Illusions of vision; saw
everything confused, as if through a fog or smoke,[236].—After vertigo came
on the affection of the eyesight, every object growing dim, as though a
cloud were between the eye and it; sometimes objects appeared double, and
passed before the eye with an undulating motion. I observed that by a
strong effort of the will a concentration of the nervous power, this paralysis of the retina (?) might for a moment be combated, but only to return
with greater severity when the mental effort had been succeeded by its corresponding relaxation. The pupils were immovably dilated,[178].—Without
glasses he could see the letters larger than usual; he saw sharper with the
left eye than with the right, which was not the case in the normal state,[89].
—On seeing himself in a glass, he asserted that he squinted badly, and
that both eyeballs were turned towards the nose,[239].—On reading, the letters
shone, partly like gold, partly like blue size, and trembled,[21].—***Everything
he looks at seems red,**[215].—***A large halo appears round the flame of the
candle, party-colored, the red predominating; at times the light seems as
if broken up into rays,**[12].—* *The flame of a candle appears encircled by a colored halo,* or stretches out and is lost in long rays,[215].—All colors appear to
him reversed; the black stove seems white, red objects of a pale yellow,
the burning light brilliant in all colors, etc.,[129].—**[730.**] Mist before the
eyes,[21].—***He sees sparks before the eyes,**[81].—* *Large bright sparks before
the eyes,*[1].—[* *He sees sparks, as of electricity, before the eyes, especially on
moving them*],[81].—* *Occasional flashes of light before the eyes,*[190].—When laying her hand upon her swollen cheek she sees flames before her eyes, and
the air seems to her like a fog-mist,[9].—She sees in the ceiling of the room
a white star as large as a plate; and across it, from left to right, light, sil-
very clouds seem passing; oftentimes and in various places,[9].—* *Chromopsia*
(after six hours),[239].—Muscæ volitantes, flames and sparks before the eyes,[215].
—In the morning on going out (about 10½ A.M.), black points and stripes
before the eyes, which soon disappear and soon return (no trace of them
in the afternoon),[211].—**[740.**] Vision confused in a high degree; they constantly endeavored to grasp fancied surrounding objects, as persons, blades
of grass, handles, etc.,[114].—Visions; he sees only dark-colored animals,
black cats, etc.,[125].—He stared now straight before him, now around, and
screamed out that he saw rats, mice, dogs, cats, and large black animals
(always only *dark* objects) on the walls, furniture, etc. These dark visions
lasted four hours. About this time the body, especially the cold extremities, began to grow warm, his face became lively and red, the eyes viva-
cious, bright, expressive of joy and astonishment; the lips dry; speech
was short, but articulation distinct; his answers to questions were hasty,
laconic, and dry. It was very difficult to draw his attention for a moment
from his yet all-brilliant visions; he was enraptured, appeared happy, and
content; his limbs were in constant motion; he groped with his hands after
colored butterflies, shining insects, etc., which he fancied he saw on the
physician's clothes,[123].—Nothing could rid my eyes of the most disgusting
spectral cockroaches, swarming all over the room,[196].

Ears.—In General. *Inflammatory swelling of the ears, and also of
the parotids,*[215].—Wind rushes out of her ears,[40] (Case 9).—Very abundant
secretion of cerumen,[215].—Purulent discharge from the ears,[215].—Purulent

moisture exudes from the ears, for twenty days,[5].—Bleeding from the ears,[215].—[750.] Violent pressure on the mastoid process below the ear,[3].—Incisive thrusts through the mastoid process below the ear (after twelve hours),[14].—Behind the left ear the muscles are painful as far as the throat, as if they were violently pressed upon, and a similar pain also in the muscles of the forehead,[4].—Pressing tearing behind the right ear (after half an hour),[8].—Slight cutting pain behind the ears (after fifty minutes),[217].—Tearing pressure in the lower half of the cartilage of the right ear,[7].—Tearing pain on the posterior side of the cartilage of the left ear,[14].—Drawing pain from the ears into the nape of the neck,[4].—A transient shoot darts from the ear to the chin (after one hour),[14].—Great liability to be cold, and to be affected as from chilblains in the ears,[215].—[760.] Sensation of heat, with drumming in the ears,[215].—Burning in the ears, with deafness,[215].—Pinching in the ears, first in the right, then in the left, immediately after hiccough,[9].—Slight earache (after three and one-third hours),[217].—Earache, accompanied with great headache,[215].—Otalgia in the left ear (after five days),[4].—Boring pain close to the right ear,[9].—A disagreeable pressure in the meatus, as if one were boring in it with the finger,[10].—Feeling in the external meatus, as if some one pressed upon it,[13].—Tearing externally in the right ear, from before backwards,[4].—[770.] *Tearing in the internal and external ear, in a downward direction,[1].—Tearing pain in the right external ear, and the whole of the right side of the face downwards (after twenty-four hours),[1].—A very disagreeable feeling in the right ear, as if it would be forcibly torn out of the head,[3].—Pain in the ears and temples, as if they were being alternately torn out and pressed in, alternating with a similar pain in the orbits,[3].—Shootings in the external meatus,[13].—Shootings in the internal ear, with hardness of hearing on that side,[1].—Shootings in the internal ear, during eructations from the stomach, having the taste of the ingesta (after twelve hours),[1].—*Acute thrusts in the internal ear, with pinching, like earache,[14].—Pulsation in the ears, with increased sharpness of hearing,[215].—

Hearing. [Increased sensitiveness of hearing],[66].—[780.] *Very sensitive to loud tones, he starts every time,[125].—Hardness of hearing,[239].—[Difficult hearing],[40] (Case 23).†—Deafness, as if a skin were drawn over the ears,[1].—Attacks of deafness, from congestion of blood, chiefly in the evening,[215].—He could neither hear nor speak plainly,[180].—Total loss of hearing and speech (after four hours),[126].—What was said to him sounded like a humming noise,[239].—*Noises in the ears,[73].—Ringing in the ears,[195].—[790.] Ringing in the ears (morning after taking),[230].—Occasionally disturbances of hearing, as singing in the ears,[201].—In the morning, immediately after waking, a fluttering and bubbling before the ears,[1].—He fancies he hears distant voices, or the warbling of birds,[215].—Whistling and vocal murmurs in the ears, with pressive distensive pains as if something inside was trying to enlarge the cavity,[215].—Roaring in the ears, vertigo, and dull colic,[40] (Case 9).—*Roaring or ringing in the ears,[91].—*Roaring, tingling, and humming in the ears,[215].—Remarkable roaring in the ears, and at the same time flickering before the eyes, especially the left, so that he was obliged to rub them frequently, with twitching of the left upper lid (after five minutes),[89].

First, a din as of trumpets and kettledrums in the ears, and as of the rushing of wind, immediately; afterwards a humming and buzzing, worse when sitting, better when standing and lying, still better when walking,[1].

Nose.—Objective and Discharges. [800.] *Tip of the nose red,

---

† Immediately after a severe epileptic paroxysm.

swollen, and shining,[215].—**Sudden redness in the tip of the nose, with a burning sensation,*[14].—Redness of the Schneiderian membrane,[91].—[Very cold nose],[40] (Case 12).†—Ulcers, crusts, and fissures in the nostrils and at the border of the nose,[215].—The mucus in the nostrils dried to crusts,[211].—The boy often bores his nose,[118].—Frequent sneezing,[215].—Paroxysms of sneezing,[223].—**Frequent dry sneezing, with tickling, especially in the left nostril,*[195].—[810.] Coryza, with discharge of clear and whitish mucus,[215].—Fluent coryza, on one side of the nose, and from one nostril only,[1].—Coryza with offensive smell in the nose, as if of herring-pickle, especially when blowing the nose,[9].—Now stuffing in the nose, now water flows from it,[2].—Left nostril somewhat moist, followed by sneezing and collection of mucus in the nose, throat, and air-passages (third day),[211].—The right nostril somewhat stopped, followed by sneezing, and afterwards a slight coryza,[211].—**Mucus mixed with blood blown,*[195].—Discharge of clotted blood when blowing the nose,[215].—Bleeding of the nose immediately, the whole night, early in the morning,[1].—Hemorrhage through the nose and mouth (when throwing up the berries, from the operation of an emetic),[74].—[820.] ** Very frequent epistaxis, with pulsative pains in the head, especially at night when in bed, and on waking in the morning,*[215].—**Sensations.** **Dryness of the nose and lips, the latter very red,*[119].—Dryness of nasal cavity, with dull frontal headache,[195].—**Dryness of the Schneiderian membrane, and of the eyes, with a burning sensation in them and in the lids,*[90].—Dryness and obstruction of the nose, for several weeks,[215].—**Sensation of dryness of the Schneiderian membrane* (after one hour),[92].—The left nostril is very painful and closed up by matter in the morning,[13a].—Sensation as if the nose were full of blood, and on the point of bleeding,[215].—Cramp at the root of the nose,[14].—Drawing pains in the nose, with sensation as if it was turned up towards the forehead,[215].—[830.] Painful drawing over the left half of the nose,[4].—Pressing pain in the bones of the nose,[3].—Pressure, stitches, and pulsations in the nose,[215].—Fine stitches in the tip of the nose, the whole night, beginning in the evening,[3].—Fine shootings below the nose (after half an hour),[14].—Bruised pain in the bones and cartilages of the nose,[215].—Above the wing of the nose, pain as if bruised on touching the part,[1].—**Smell.** **Great sensitiveness of smell*; *the faintest odor, especially that of tobacco, is unbearable,*[215].—*Olfaction too sensitive*; *the smell of tobacco and soot is intolerable to him* (after one hour),[1].—Camphor is loathsome,[2].—[840.] Olfactory organs insensible to the strongest stimulants (after six hours),[239].—Bread smells (¹), and tastes sour,[14].—Smell like rotten eggs before the nose, for a quarter of an hour (after four hours),[11].—Smell of rotten eggs, and of fresh fish, before the nose,[215].

Face.—Objective. Stupid expression,[233].—Rather stupefied expression,[238].—The expression of the face is stupid astonishment, the eye is lifeless (after ten hours),[110].—Countenance anxious but vacant,[231].—Expression was lively, denoting joy and astonishment,[233].—Extremely haggard face, expressive of uneasiness and anxiety,[215].—[850.] The face is sunken, and covered with a cold clammy sweat,[129].—The features are disfigured, and on expiration the boy puffs as if hot,[125].—Countenance pale,[230].—Paleness of the face,[70].—[Sudden paleness of the face, lasting some time],[40] (Case 16),‡—Paleness of the face, with increased appetite,[40] (Case 5).—Paleness of the face, with thirst,[40] (Case 5).§—The child was pale, cold, and as if in a

---

† Continuing during seven days of mania.
‡ Such sudden pallor is not uncommon in epileptics.
§ Not found.

fainting condition,[124].—Pale, yellow, earthy complexion,[215].—Jaundiced complexion,[215].—[860.] The habitual coppery face of the old man became violet, and the conjunctiva bulbi was injected with bluish blood,[115].—Bluish redness of face,[228].—Bluish-red face, with great heat of the body, every evening,[86].—The pale face becomes suddenly red,[215].—[Frequent excessive paleness of the face, suddenly changing to redness, with cold cheeks and hot forehead],[40] (Case 11).†—*Unwonted redness of the face,*[10].—*Great redness of the face* (after two hours),[220].—*Remarkable redness of the face* (after one hour),[98].— *Face extremely red,*[235].—Blood-red countenance,[86].—[870.] *Glowing red, hot face (after half an hour),[105].—*Glowing redness in the face, with violent inexpressible pains in the head,[13a].—Face dirty-red,[240]. —Scarlet redness of the face and chest during sleep,[68].—*The face was very red, with a staring look,*[119].—Face red ; eyes shining, and seem to be swimming in tears (after two and a half hours),[90].—*Very red face, with general warmth and great restlessness,* this, however, was soon followed by paleness of the face and lassitude,[123].—*Redness and heat of the face, with great thirst,*[40] (Case 14).—Very red, hot face, with icy coldness of the limbs,[13a].—*Face red and hot, and face, neck, and chest much swollen,*[199].—[880.] *Great redness and heat in the face, without sweat* (after twenty-four to thirty hours),[12].—* The face was red and turgid,*[178].—*Red, swollen face,*[56].—*Red and swollen face* (after two hours),[86].—The face was red and swollen, but the rest of the body pale,[37].—The face red and distended, the look disturbed and threatening,[106 135].—*The face scarlet and swollen,* especially about the eyes,[102].—[Red, swollen face, with staring eyes],[49].—The face of a usually pale and lean man is uncommonly red and swollen ; the heat is general and strong, the pulse full and rapid, with excessive sweat (after half an hour),[107].—Red spots like scarlatina, and purple blotches like bruises on the face,[215].—[890.] There appeared on the face, especially on the left cheek, along with increased heat, red irregular patches of the size of a crown piece, which disappeared and again returned,[195].—Dark-red spots in his face, resembling the rash of scarlet fever ; with full pulse,[80].—[The skin of the face is thickened as if an eruption would break out],[65].—Tense and rough skin of the face,[215].—Face full of wrinkles,[215].—*Swollen face,*[1 60]. —Face swollen (after six hours),[239].—Face greatly swollen (after six hours),[239].—*His face was so much swollen and red as quite to change his usual appearance.* His daughter remarked that the wrinkles of old age had disappeared, and he seemed much fatter than usual,[189].—Swelling of the face, especially of the lips,[50].‡—[900.] Erysipelatous swelling of the face,[215]. Face full and flushed ; amendment was indicated by a diminution of heat and fulness of face, and by returning consciousness,[179].—Puffy, flushed, and mottled face,[215].—*Tumefaction and redness of the face and lips,*[184].—*The face is much swollen and hot,*[20].—* Great swelling of the face, and intense heat, which at times extends over the whole body,*[20].—Face swollen, eyes dim, and pupils dilated (after ten hours),[110].—Hard, large swelling in the face near the nose and eye, with swelling also of the parotid gland on the opposite side, of five days' duration,[40] (Case 19).—The muscles of the face show a remarkable mobility (after one hour),[112].—*Spasms in the face,*[38].—[910.] *Spasmodic action of the muscles of the face,*[198].—Alternating contortion of the muscles of the face,[234].—Convulsions of the facial muscles, with ridiculous motions of every description,[103].—Convulsive motion of the mus-

---

† Occurring during a succession of epileptic paroxysms.
‡ In connection with S. 367.

cles of the left side of the face, especially of the left corner of the mouth,[106]. —*Convulsive movement of the facial muscles, with distortion of the mouth,[215].—Distorted features,[19].†—The face is disfigured by convulsions and swelling,[103].—[She distorts the facial muscles horribly, sticks the tongue far out, clucks with the tongue, and retches even to vomiting, by paroxysms],[40] (Case 13).—Twitchings of face and hands (after half an hour),[107]. —*The muscles of his face, jaws, and limbs were agitated by convulsive twitchings (from the leaves),[202].—[920.] Convulsive play of the facial muscles, with grinding of the teeth, and at times stretching and extending of the limbs,[118].— *Sensations.* Numbness of the face,[201].—It appeared to him as if his face had become swollen (after three hours),[190].—Sharp pains in the facial bones, with sensation as if they were swollen,[215].—Neuralgic pains extending from the temples to the lower jaw, and accompanied with pulsative and pressive pains in the head,[215].—*Cheeks and Lips.* Cheeks very red,[222].—The cheeks purple-red (after one hour),[112].—Redness of the cheeks; the face is turgid, with general heat (after two and a half hours),[130].—On awaking in the morning, a small, bluish-red spot on the left cheek, which gradually increases in size, until the bluish-red swelling occupies the whole cheek, excessively aggravated by movement; after some days the other cheek swelled, and the swelling lasted eight days,[9].—Swelling of the cheek with burning pain,[5].—[930.] Swelling, sometimes of one cheek, sometimes of the other,[215]. —Swelling of the left cheek near the nose and eye, which came on in the night, increased the next day, with heat, and lasted five days,[40] (Case 13).— *Pressing below the right zygoma,[3].—*A tearing and drawing below the right zygoma (after quarter of an hour),[3].—Pinching pressure on the left zygoma,[14]. —The lips, and especially the upper one, crack in the middle, in sneezing and coughing,[1].—Lips enlarged, chapped, full of phlyctenæ,[215].—*Great swelling of the upper lip; it feels tense on opening the mouth,[1].—Abscess of the upper lip, causing painful swelling, with fever, headache, and loss of appetite, ending in free discharge of pus,[50].—Spasmodic movements of the lips,[89].—[940.] *A man suffered with a sardonic laugh for years, after Belladonna poisoning,[101].—*Dry, burning, swollen, and hardened lips,[215].—At the outer edge of the lips, a burning pain, and small vesicles (after twenty-four hours),[13a].—*The lips, mucous membrane of the mouth, fauces, and nose, very hot and dry,[226].—Drawing in the upper lip, with subsequent red swelling,[9].— *Jaws and Chin.* Jaws firmly closed,[42].—Lockjaw,[16].—*The jaws are closed convulsively, and very difficult to open,[135].—She closed her teeth so firmly that it became necessary to break out a tooth in order to pour fluids down her throat,[17].—*On attempting to pour down liquid, tetanic closure of the mouth, and regurgitation of the liquid (after four hours),[121].—[950.] *The lower jaw is pressed convulsively against the upper, with a red face, and a peculiar staring look,[140].—*Convulsive closing of the jaws, and contraction of the muscles of the face and extremities; next day, increase of convulsive movements, with redness of the face, and profuse perspiration; great rigidity down the spine,[184].—*She clenched her teeth together, so that great force could not open them ([42]), with startings in all the limbs and chilliness,[60].—Cramp and compression of the jaws,[215].—She feels as if her lower jaw were drawn backwards; it hurts her much to advance it, and biting causes excessive pain,[14]. —Clucking (as of a hen) along the under edge of the lower jaw,[14].—Fine shootings in the socket of the maxillary joint (after one hour),[14].—*Shootings extending from the superior maxilla into the internal ear,[1].—*Shooting

† Not found.

and tension of the lower jaw, in the direction of the ears,[13]—On masticating, a violent shooting in the right maxillary joint, extending into the ear, which continues for some time after he has finished, though it then rather resembles a drawing or pulling,[13a]—**[960.]** *Fine tearing on the inner surface of the corner of the left lower jaw, in the left tonsil and behind the latter, unaffected by contact; the tearing is more violent during deglutition,*[7]—A nestling, spasmodic sensation in the chin,[1]—Sharp shootings in the chin,[14].

Mouth.—Teeth and Gums. Teeth turn yellow and decay,[215]—Suction of the hollow teeth with the tongue causes blood to flow from them, without pain,[14]—Grinding of the teeth,[134]—Violent grinding of the teeth,[60]—[Grinding of the teeth, with copious saliva running from the mouth],[40] (Case 6).—[Grinding of the teeth and spasm of the right arm],[40] (Case 20).—[Gnashing of the teeth, with much froth from the mouth, smelling like bad eggs],[40] (Case 22).—**[970.]** The front teeth are as if too long,[1]—The child complained of great pain in his teeth (after forty-eight hours),[184]—An indefinite slight pain in both upper middle incisors, rapidly running through them (after five minutes),[88]—Toothache, with drawing in the ear,[1]—Toothache, with swelling of the cheek, especially on the right side,[215]—Cramplike drawing pains in the teeth, as if they were being pulled out,[215]—(A digging toothache, of brief duration),[1]—Toothache rather drawing than shooting,[1]—Unpleasant sensation, as if her teeth would be forced out of her head,[219]—A drawing in the anterior molars of the right upper jaw, remaining unchanged under all circumstances,[3]—**[980.]** **Dull drawing in the upper right row of teeth, through the whole night;** the pain would not permit sleep; the painful part was somewhat swollen (with burning pain), and felt hot to the touch; sometimes, painful jerkings in the teeth,[4]—Toothache, a sharp drawing from the ear down to the hollow tooth of the upper jaw, wherein the pain becomes boring, easier while eating, more violent afterwards, never entirely ceasing during the day, but most violent at night, and completely preventing sleep (after drinking coffee, the pain becomes a dull jerking and boring),[198]—Tearing pain in a lower hollow tooth and in a sound molar adjoining; the pain becomes excessive from contact with air or food (after four hours),[7]—A fine shooting pain in one of the upper hollow molars during the whole day, in consequence of which he can hardly sleep at night, followed by swelling of the cheek,[1]—He wakes up after midnight with violent tearing (?) in the teeth,[1]—On admission of the open air, a steady pain in the teeth, a simple toothache, like a soreness,[1]—Toothache in the evening after lying down, and during mental occupation, a dull pain in the nerve of the fang of the tooth, almost as if it were sore, and, when worse, like a continual cutting,[1]—The teeth are painful in biting anything, as if the roots were ulcerated and would break short off,[1]—Several very painful jerkings or bubblings in the nerves of the fangs of one or more teeth,[1]—Toothache, worse in the evening, at night, after eating, in the open air, and by any contact,[215]—**[990.]** The toothache does not come on during a meal, but in the first few minutes after; it increases gradually to a high degree, and as gradually diminishes; it does not follow drinking,[1]—Constant inclination to pass the tongue over the teeth, in order to relieve the pains,[215]—Frequent bleeding of the gums,[215]—The gum bleeds near to a hollow tooth (after six days),[14]—Vesicle in the gum below one of the front teeth, with pain as if it were burnt,[1]—Extremely painful swelling of the gums on the right side, with fever and sense of chill,[40] (Case 20).—Heat in the gums, with itching and throbbing,[1].—The gum, on being touched, pains as if ulcerated,[1].—Scraping and scratching in the gums, unaffected by external influences,[14].—Pulsation and pain as from an abscess in the gums, which are inflamed and swollen,[215].—[1000.] Itching of the gums (after half an hour),[109].—Extremely troublesome itching in the gums, with pain in the throat,[17].— **Tongue.** The tongue is white-coated (after a quarter of an hour),[91].— Tongue covered with a tenacious white coating, which comes off in shreds,[238]. —The tongue is white-coated; appetite very slight.[89].—Whitish, yellowish, or grayish coating on the tongue,[215].—[The tongue is covered with a quantity of tenacious yellowish-white mucus],[49].—The vessels beneath the tongue are bluish, and injected with blood,[119].—Tongue rather dark, but moist (after twenty-eight hours),[185].—**The tongue and palate dark-red; she complains of dryness of the throat, and of difficult swallowing** (after half an hour),[104].—[1010.] Furred tongue,[140].—The tongue is moist and white-coated,[119].—Tongue rather moist, rosy red,[233].—* *The papillæ on the tongue are of a deep red color, inflamed and much swollen* (after three days),[13a].— Cracked, white-coated tongue, with much flow of saliva,[4].—The tongue is swollen (after six hours),[102 103].—The swollen tongue is pressed close behind the lower incisors,[125].—The swollen tongue projects beyond the lips, and is turned, now here, now there,[116].—Cramps at the base of tongue (after fourteen hours),[217].—* *Trembling of the tongue,*[76].—[1020.] Stammering of the tongue,[63].—Tongue heavy, thick, and as if paralyzed,[215].—Impaired mobility of the tongue; consequent impeded speech and difficult swallowing,[91].— Tongue as if paralyzed; dry and cracked,[129].—Tongue felt paralyzed; difficulty in articulating,[230].—Vesicles and small burning pimples on the tongue,[215].—***Dryness of the tongue,*[134].—* *Tongue parched,*[228].—The tongue dry, as if covered with a crust,[137].—Tongue dry, of a yellow-brown color,[206].— [1030.] * *The tongue hung dry from the child's mouth, and was swollen thick; it was scarcely possible to get some drops of milk into the mouth* (after ten hours),[119].—* *Tongue dry, cracked, difficult to move,*[226].—***Dryness of the tongue and throat, becoming so great as to interfere with speech,**[238].— He noticed that his tongue and throat were extremely dry, and that his tongue was covered with a white clammy fur, which he could pull off in strings. He drank some water, which seemed even to increase the sense of dryness of the tongue,[168].—Tongue, mouth, and fauces devoid of moisture, as if they had been composed of burnt shoe-leather. The secretions of the glands of the mouth, and the saliva, were entirely suspended. A draught of water, instead of giving relief, seemed only to increase the unctuous clammy state of the mucous membrane,[178].—A feeling as if the tongue lay deeper in the mouth than usual, and so the buccal cavity was more spacious,[9].—The tongue feels as if asleep, lifeless, and furred (in the morning),[9].—Feeling of coldness and dryness of the anterior half of the tongue,[9].—The whole tongue is painful, especially to the touch,[13a].—Feeling in the tip of the tongue, as if there were a vesicle on it, which caused a burning pain on being touched, for two days,[4].—[1040.] In the middle of the tongue, which is coated white, a severe smarting pain, as if from a vesicle (after three days),[13a].—**Mouth in General.** Slimy mouth, with the feeling as if a bad smell came from his mouth as when the stomach is disordered,[1].—**Slimy mouth in the morning on waking, with pressive headache, both of short duration,**[1].—Raw places in the buccal cavity and on the palate,[215].—Bad smell from the mouth, especially in the morning and when fasting,[215].—The mouth is drawn on one side by spasms,[26].—[The right corner of the mouth is drawn outward],[40] (Case 11).†—Convulsive chewing and foam from the mouth,[125].—[*Paralytic weakness of the internal parts of the mouth*],[52].—**Dryness in the mouth**,[50 81].—[**1050.**] *Dryness of the mouth* (after a quarter of an hour),[87 122].—*Dryness of mouth* (second day),[228].—*Dryness in the mouth, which is almost beyond relief*,[27].—On chewing dry bread, he could not collect it to a mass,[92].—Constant spitting, without ejecting saliva,[137].—Aridity in the mouth, as if the mucous membrane had been removed by some pungent or corrosive substance,[52].—Sensation of great dryness of the mouth, with very irritable temper; at the same time, the mouth and throat look moist,[1 13a].—Sensation of great dryness in the mouth; there was a very little tenacious mucus on the tongue, and the lips were hot and peeled off,[1].—*Dryness in the mouth, with thirst,*[1 10 101].—*Dry, burning mouth, with great thirst,*[215].—[**1060.**] **Dryness of mouth and throat,**[231].—His mouth and fauces at this time (to use the words of an attendant) were as dry as a chip,[191].—*Dryness of the mouth and pharynx, with a sense of constriction of the throat* (after one hour),[112].—Dryness in the mouth; he sits at table and chews his food, without being able to swallow it; the throat felt as if constricted (after half an hour),[107].—*Dryness of the whole inner lining of the cheek, the tongue, which looks as if burnt, the roof of the mouth, and the pharynx,*[114 115].—*Great dryness of mouth and pharynx, with thirst,*[95].—*Troublesome, continued dryness of the mouth, lips, and throat, with a violent longing for drink, but not satisfied by drink,*[91 98].—*Feeling of dryness in the mouth and throat; especially troublesome on attempting to swallow,*[92].—**Dryness of the mouth and throat, with difficult swallowing,**[235].—*Excessive dryness of the mouth and throat, especially the tongue; patient cannot swallow,*[128].—[**1070.**] Dryness in the mouth and throat, with a scraping sensation in the same, and difficult swallowing,[89].—Dryness of the mouth and throat, with difficulty in swallowing; water did not pass down easily; with frequent expectoration of mucus from the pharynx,[89 140].—*Dryness, burning and scraping in the mouth and throat,*[106].—*Burning in the mouth,*[237].—Sensation as if the whole mouth was burnt and full of phlyctenæ,[215].—Heat and dryness of the mouth and pharynx, with thirst and nausea,[102].—*Sensation of heat and dryness in the mouth and pharynx, extending to the stomach; the epigastric region was painful and swollen, with constant thirst,*[103].—Soreness on the inside of the cheek; the mouth of the salivary duct is as if eroded,[1].—Raw feeling at the corners of the mouth, as if they would ulcerate,[13a].—*Saliva.* Salivation,[1].—[**1080.**] Abundant salivation,[61].—The saliva in her throat was thickened, tenacious, white, and clinging to the tongue like glue, so that she was obliged to put something fluid into her mouth,[70].—Tenacious saliva hangs in long strings from the mouth,[40] (Case 20).—Viscid saliva, which adheres to the tongue and escapes in stringy foam from the mouth,[215].—Tenacious mucus in the mouth ([12]) with sensation of dryness, ([7]) hanging in long strings from the mouth,[40].—Following the pain in the forehead, an increase of saliva in the mouth; mucus also collected in the upper part of the throat, which was raised by hawking,[211].—He has much mucus in the mouth, especially in the morning after rising, sometimes of a putrid taste,[7].—His mouth is full of mucus in the morning; he has to wash it out from time to time; it disappears after a meal,[1].—Accumulation of water in the mouth in the evening for half an hour,[9].—*Thick, whitish mucus accumulates in the mouth and throat, with constant inclination to hawk and swallow,*[215].—[**1090.**] Foam from the mouth,[129].—

---

† See note to S. 175.

Bloody foam issues copiously from the mouth (shortly before death),[16].—
[Bloody foam from the mouth, convulsions of the head, and gnashing of the
teeth, from morning till noon],[40] (Case 22).—*Taste.* Insipid taste in the
mouth,[4].—Slight sweetish taste in the mouth,[4].—Weak, aromatic taste,[91].—
Disgusting taste in the mouth, with clean tongue,[1].—Disagreeable, nauseous
taste in the mouth and empty eructations,[89].—Clammy taste, with white-
coated tongue, and sense of emptiness in stomach,[91].—Slimy taste in the
mouth,[1].—Pappy taste in the mouth, with white furred tongue (three hours
after one-quarter grain),[195].—[1100.] Salt sourish taste in the mouth,[13a].—
He had a taste in the mouth like sour wine,[99].—Bitter taste, or taste
of blood, and sometimes a slimy and nauseous taste in the mouth,[215].—
Spoiled taste in the mouth,[40] (Case 8).—Putrid taste comes up out of the
fauces, even when eating and drinking, although food and drink have
their proper taste,[14].—Putrid taste in the mouth after she has eaten,[1 12].—
Extraordinary taste of the saliva,[73].—At times everything eaten tastes
salt,[215].—Salt taste of food, as if everything had been salted (after twenty-
five hours),[13a].—At the commencement of a meal food has its proper taste,
but all at once everything appears to her to taste too salt or disagreeably
insipid, with a feeling in the throat as if she should vomit what she had
taken,[13a].—[1110.] In the evening the bread and butter, or at least the
last of it, tasted very sour, and he generally experienced more or less heartburn afterwards, which continued for two hours (on eight evenings in
succession) (after four days),[1].—Broth which had been taken appeared sour
and left a scratching sensation in the throat,[92].—(Bitter taste of the bread
and apples in the evening),[1].—Loss of taste,[52].—*Speech.* Speech rapid,
interrupted,[233].—Speech slow, impeded,[243].—Paralytic weakness of the organs
of speech,[1].—Stammering weakness of the organs of speech, with full consciousness,[1].—Stammering speech,[20 63].—He stammers like one intoxicated,[20].
—[1120.] Indistinct speech; stuttering,[215].—They utter badly articulated,
confused sounds,[114].—Difficult articulation,[240].—Speech became more and
more difficult,[239].—Difficult speech, difficult breathing, and great lassitude;
afterwards anxiety,[1].—Speechlessness,[74].—Dumbness,[42].—She suddenly lost
the power of speaking and swallowing and fell into a comatose state (after
one hour),[185].

Throat.—In General. *The mucous membrane, from the posterior
third of the palate as far down as could be seen, was of a deep crimson color,
and the tonsils were much enlarged,*[192].—Redness of the throat, and burning
along the whole alimentary canal,[197].—[1130.] Aphthous inflammation of
the throat,[197].—A great deal of mucus accumulates in the throat, interrupt-
ing respiration, and giving rise to constant hawking,[215].—Some mucus in
the upper part of the throat, with a general sensation as if a catarrh of the
throat and fauces would develop; the arches of the palate, tonsils, and posterior wall of the pharynx were swollen and inflamed (repeated in different
provers), (seventh day),[211].—*As soon as the throat began to feel sore, there
was a great expectoration of light mucus,*[230].—Raising of a quantity of phlegm
from the throat (after three-quarters of an hour),[93].—Spitting of blood from
the throat,[215].—In her unconsciousness, she frequently put her finger deep
into her throat, scratched at her gums, and pressed her throat with both
hands,[17].—The throat is swollen internally,[63].†—*Dryness in the throat,*[78 220]
—Dryness of throat (mother and child, within an hour),[228].—[1140]. *Great
dryness of the throat,*[74 219].—*Excessive dryness of the throat,*[239].—Dryness of

---

† Not found.

the throat, without difficulty in swallowing or speaking (after one hour),[239].
—*Dryness and burning of throat,[228].—Pain in the throat,[17] [40].—At first, he
complained of pain in the throat,[180].—Pain in the throat and colic,[40] (Case
6).—*Sensation of heat and dryness in the throat (after five minutes),[179].—
*His throat became hot and dry,[190].—*Violent burning in the throat (the
mouth at the same time being naturally moist), which is not at all relieved
by drinking, but is by a little sugar, though only for a moment,[2].—*Burning
heat, great dryness, and roughness in the throat,[215].—*Sensation as if a large
tumor was growing in the throat and stopped it up,[215].—[1150.] Sensation of
constriction in throat (after five hours),[131].—His throat and fauces felt constricted on account of the too great dryness of the mouth; there was not
a particle of mucus there, and only moderate thirst, yet he could swallow
the milk he was drinking,[13a].—Constriction of the throat with choking sensation,[215].*—During deglutition, feeling in the throat as if it were too narrow,
or drawn together; as if nothing would pass properly (after two hours),[13a].
—Painful constriction in the throat, which extended to the stomach, with
burning and violent thirst,[106].—A pressive sensation in the throat, in the
region of the tonsils (seventh day),[211].—Something seemed to her to rise up
out of the abdomen and to press on the throat, with retching, but without
sense of nausea or vomiting,[13a].—Shootings in the throat on the left side,
alike between and during the acts of deglutition,[8].—*A violent shooting pain
in the throat on swallowing and breathing,[13a].—Soreness of throat (after five
hours),[227].—[1160.] Throat a little sore (after reading aloud one hour),[218].—
*Soreness extending from throat to ears (morning after taking),[230].—*Felt
great soreness in the throat, which looked very red about the tonsils and palate,[230].
—*He felt great soreness in the throat, which looked very red about the tonsils
and palate. The soreness extended to the ears,[192].—*Sore throat, which increases every hour; heat, scraping, narrowing, and feeling of soreness,[9].—Sore
throat; during deglutition, scraping in the soft palate and sensation as if
the part had been rubbed sore,[1].—For a week afterwards he had sore
throat, difficulty of swallowing to a great degree, with considerable redness
of the mucous membrane of the mouth and fauces; the tonsils slightly
swollen (from one dose of gr. 4½ of the ext.),[195].—Some tickling now and then
in the throat (after ten days),[230].—*Tonsils, Fauces, and Pharynx.*
*Tonsils inflamed,[228].—In the throat, inflammation of the tonsils, which
suppurate after four days, during which time he cannot swallow a drop,[40]
(Case 25).—[1170.] Inflammation and swelling of the tonsils, and of the
entire throat,[215].—Small pimples and abscesses on the tonsils,[215].—Cramp
extending from right tonsil to the top of the pharynx (after fourteen
hours),[217].—Inflammation of the fauces,[63].—Tenacious mucus in the fauces,[40]
(Case 6).—Throwing up of blood, seemingly proceeding from the fauces,[24].†
—*Dryness of the fauces, causing excessive difficulty of swallowing, and al-
teration of the voice,[189].—*About the fauces the sensation of dryness was
most distressing. It induced a constant attempt at deglutition, and finally
excited suffocative spasms of the fauces and glottis, renewed at every attempt to
swallow,[178].—Burning sensation in the fauces ([185]), every time she took a
dose,[43].—Long-lasting burning pain in the fauces; food and drinks burn

---

† It ended in death. Also after death blood flows from the nose, mouth, and
ears of those who have been poisoned by Belladonna; they have a blackish-violet
hue, either in the face only or on one side of the body, or over the whole surface, or
these parts are covered with gangrenous spots; the epidermis peels off easily, the
abdomen becomes inflated, and putrefaction sets in sometimes within twelve hours,
as Eb. Gmelin and Faber have stated.

like brandy,[64].—[1180.] Severe spasm of the pharynx (after six hours),[106].
—Dryness of the pharynx,[24].—Slight burning sensation in the upper part
of the pharynx; must frequently swallow; this was rather more difficult than
usual, as if the pharynx were spasmodically constricted; this lasted for
some time and returned at intervals (sixth day),[211].—Constriction of the
pharynx,[186].—Great constriction of the pharynx,[24].†—Great constriction of
the pharynx from dryness of the part,[24].—Sensation of constriction in
pharynx, at the same time the throat feels very dry, and is actually destitute of moisture,[115].—Painful narrowing and contraction of the pharynx;
when preparing to swallow it feels tense and stretched, even when nothing
is swallowed; during actual deglutition it is not more painful, the feeling of
the fauces being narrowed itself amounts to pain (after sixty hours),[14].—*Sore
throat, shootings in the pharynx, and pain as from an internal swelling, only
felt during deglutition, and upon turning the head round; likewise when feeling the side of the neck, but not when at rest or in speaking,[1].—Œsophagus
and Deglutition. *Contraction of the œsophagus, lasting a short time
but frequently recurring, more during deglutition than between, and followed
each time by a scraping sensation in the region of the epiglottis, as if the
latter were raw and sore,[10].—[1190.] Constant urging and wanting to
swallow; it was as if he would choke if he did not swallow,[1].—The throat
is painful during deglutition and expectoration, a sensation of swelling,
more on the left side,[5].—Swallowing caused a pressive pain in the posterior
portion of the fauces,[211].—*Impeded deglutition,[1], and many others.—*Difficult swallowing,[56 103 129 222 230 234].—*Difficult and painful deglutition,[73].—*Extremely difficult and painful deglutition,[215].—Dysphagia (" on account of want
of moisture of the tissue"),[114].—* Only with difficulty and by constantly taking
liquids is he able to swallow solid food,[89].—*He swallows water with the greatest
difficulty, and can only get the very smallest quantity of it down,[31].—[1200.]
Deglutition very difficult, so that of drink, taken even in the smallest
quantity, only a part could reach the stomach; the rest was thrown out
again forcibly, with general spasms (after one hour),[112].—*At first, he pushed
away a glass of sugared water; when, on being coaxed, he attempted to drink
it, only a few drops passed down, the rest was forced out of the mouth by spasmodic contraction of the muscles of deglutition,[106].—Painless inability to swallow,[1].—His throat was contracted so that he could not swallow,[25].—He
chewed his food without being able to swallow it, because his throat seemed
to him contracted,[17].—He cannot swallow on account of the dryness in the
mouth, the fauces, and the nose,[20].—A constant but unsuccessful attempt at
deglutition was observed, and at every renewal of the attempt the muscles
of the throat and pharynx would be thrown into violent spasmodic action,[177].
—External. Painful swelling of the submaxillary glands, also of those
of the neck and nape of the neck,[215].—Strong pulsations of the carotid,[226].—
*Shootings in the parotid gland,[1].—[1210.] * Violent shooting in the right
parotid, extending into the external ear, where it becomes cramplike, and then
disappears (after two hours); it returns again the following day, also at the
same hour,[1].

Stomach.—Appetite. Unnatural appetite; he wants to eat all the
time and relishes everything,[215].—Violent longing for food, and greedy
swallowing of it,[130].—Decided hunger, but no inclination for any one kind
of food,[1].—He is seized with a desire for this or that, but he has no relish
if he eats it,[1].—Appetite for thin broth, and for bread and butter, but for

† See S. 1140.

nothing else,[9].—Appetite very much diminished,[91 98].—Diminished appetite, animal food is especially disagreeable to him,[14].—Loss of appetite,[237].— Complete loss of appetite,[50].†—[1220.] Loss of appetite in the morning, with disgust for all food, especially meat and acids,[215].—Loss of appetite, with increased thirst,[215].—Loss of appetite, with feeling of emptiness and hunger; if he begins to eat, he relishes the food, and eats as usual,[7].— Want of appetite,[37 52].—Want of appetite, with headache,[40] (Case 10).—He ate without appetite or taste; swallowing was somewhat difficult on account of dryness in mouth and throat, with a feeling of fulness in the abdomen; repeated gripings around the navel, as if he were obliged to go to stool; relieved after passing wind,[89].—All his appetite goes away after smoking tobacco,[1].—No appetite; he loathed everything,[1].—Aversion to food,[37 52].— Aversion to food, lasting a long time,[1].—[1230.] [Entire aversion to all kinds of food and drink, with frequent, weak pulse],[40] (Case 16).—Repugnance to acids,[1].—*Thirst.* *Great thirst,*[227].—*Anxious seeking for drink,*[37]. —*Excessive thirst for cold water* (after four hours),[31].—Excessive thirst, with preference for cold water,[215].—Considerable thirst for cold drinks, without heat (after seven hours),[11].—Desire to drink from large vessels and a great deal at a time,[215].—Extremely troublesome thirst,[56].—Violent thirst,[235]. —[1240.] Violent thirst (after one hour),[112].—Violent thirst, which he is unable to satisfy on account of inability to swallow,[106].—Great thirst and difficult swallowing,[223].—Excessive thirst; repeated vomiting, after she had drunk with large swallows,[102].—[Great thirst, frequent micturition, copious sweat],[40] (Case 22).—Unquenchable thirst, with uncommonly slow pulse (after ten hours),[110].—Desire for beverages, without appetite for drinking; he scarcely put the drinking-vessel to his mouth before setting it down again (after eight hours),[11].—Tormented with burning thirst and heat in all parts; she craved drink from time to time, but repelled it when offered,[37]. —Aversion to milk, which she generally and very readily drinks; it appears to her to have a loathsome, very disagreeable smell, and (bitter, sourish) taste, which disappears, however, after continuing to drink,[13a].— Most astonishing thirst in the evening, with watery taste, though all liquids are loathsome to her,[9].— [1250.] Great thirst during the catamenia,[40].— After a long sleep, violent thirst,[40] (Case 19).—After the sweating at first induced had diminished, the thirst increased, and the appetite fell off,[40] (Case 10).—Thirst very slight, notwithstanding the general heat,[123].—No thirst,[222 233].—No desire for drinks; absence of thirst,[1 7].—*Aversion to all fluids, so that she behaves frightfully at the sight of them. The forcible administration of fluid medicine makes her furious,*[17].—Coffee is disagreeable to her,[2]. —Repugnance to beer,[1].—*Eructations and Hiccough.* *Ineffectual inclination to eructate.* *Half-suppressed, incomplete eructations,*[1].—[1260.] Slight eructation,[118].—Frequent eructations from the stomach,[10].—Sobbing eructations; a spasm composed partly of eructation and partly of hiccough,[1]. —Tasteless eructation and flatulence in the bowels, with transient stitches in the left breast; the following night he awoke at 1 o'clock, on account of distension and griping in the hypogastric zone, with troublesome nausea; passing wind relieved (after five minutes),[89].—Eructations tasting of the ingesta,[1].—Sour eructations,[215].—Burning, sour eructations, during which a corrosive acid moisture came into the mouth, with a kind of strangling,[13a]. —Frequent bitter eructations,[215].—Bitter eructations after a meal,[1].—Putrid eructations,[40] (Case 8).—[1270.] Eructations and vertigo,[40] (Case 15)

Eructations with want of appetite,[40] (Case 17).—Several attacks of violent hiccough,[10].—Violent hiccough, which jerked her up, after which she became deaf until the next attack,[9].—Frequent spasmodic hiccoughs, which go on even to suffocation,[215].—[Hiccough with convulsion, alternately of the left arm and right leg, followed by violent thirst, with redness and heat of the head],[40]. (Case 14).—Violent hiccough about midnight,[40] (Case 6) — [Hiccough at night, with profuse sweat],[40] (Case 14).—*Nausea.* Squeamishness after breakfast,[1].—Nausea,[234].—[1280.] *Feeling of nausea* (after two and a half hours),[217].—**Nausea in the stomach,**[7].—Nausea without vomiting,[114].—Frequent attacks of nausea in the forenoon (after seventy-two hours),·.—Nausea, with sensation of fulness in the throat ; nausea gradually changes to burning (after three and five-sixth hours),[217].—Nausea and eructations, with taste of the ingesta,[215].—Nausea and pain in the stomach.[235]. —The influence of medicinal doses on the intestinal secretions is not very marked, but when given by the mouth and in large doses, Belladonna frequently causes nausea, and in poisonous doses vomiting, and sometimes diarrhœa,[194].—Nausea and inclination to vomit (after six hours),[91 103].— Nausea and disposition to vomit,[219].—[1290.] Nausea and desire to vomit (mother and child within an hour),[228].—Nausea and inclination to vomit, but entire inability to vomit,[228].—Nausea and inclination to vomit, often before eating,[215].—(In coughing, the stomach turns, as if vomiting would come on, even when it is empty),[1].—Disposition to vomit when walking in the open air,[1].—Nausea, inclination to vomit, and such violent thirst that they were obliged to drink an excessive quantity of water,[17].—Nausea and inclination to vomit, in the throat (not in the scrobiculus cordis), with occasional bitter eructations, in the evening,[13a].—Ineffectual disposition to vomit; empty retching,[14].—Inclination to vomit; unsuccessful retching; he cannot vomit; inexcitability of the stomach,[56].—Loathing with inclination to vomit, especially when he would eat,[10].—[1300.] Frequent loathing and retching,[40] (Case 2).—*Vomiting.* Vomiting,[231 234 235].—*Vomiting* (after thirty minutes),[227].—Excessive vomiting,[39].—Vomiting (after six hours), followed immediately by sleep for several hours,[31].—Threw her food up within half an hour after eating (soon after taking),[228].—Vomiting of undigested food, which had been taken twelve hours before,[37].—Vomiting of whitish watery substances,[215].—He often spat out or vomited mucus,[40].—Vomiting of mucus after noon,[40] (Case 5).—[1310.] Vomiting of bile and mucus,[27].—Vomiting of bile, with much straining, trembling of the limbs, cold sweat, etc.,[215].— Vomiting of a large quantity of dark bluish-red fluid (containing the berries), followed by loss of consciousness and delirium,[226].—Vomiting, in the evening,[40] (Case 5).—Vomiting, which often occurs in the evening or at night,[215].—Violent vomiting of food, often without nausea or straining, especially after meals,[215].—Vomiting after drinking milk, followed by slight amelioration,[239].— *Vomiting after eating or drinking* (second day),[241].—Vomiting and profuse sweat,[40].—Vomiting, vertigo, and flushes of heat,[40].— Vomiting, with diarrhœa, vertigo, and cramps,[215].—[1320.] Difficulty in exciting vomiting,[177 178 179].—He did not vomit after fourteen grains of *tartar emetic*, and did not even feel nauseated by it,[17].—*Stomach.* Inflammation of the stomach (post-mortem),[39].—Region of stomach is distended but painless,[137].—The pit of the stomach and hypogastric zone were swollen and tense,[103].—After lying down in the evening in bed, distended epigastrium, with tensive pain in the stomach,[1].—*He lay upon his stomach,* with the head resting on the hands and raised up,[233].—It is as if there were something in the pit of the stomach, which always makes him cough,[1].—Feeling of emptiness in the stomach (three hours, after gr. ¼),[195].—Distress in the stomach (after three-quarters of an hour),[216].—[**1330**.] Pain in the stomach (two cases),[182].—Sharp pain over the stomach (after four and a half hours),[217].—Violent stomachache, lasting a short time,[219].—Severe pain in stomach (mother and child, within an hour),[228].—Pain in stomach, with slight nausea (immediately),[217].—*Excruciating pains about the pit of the stomach,*[74].—*At night, periodical pains at the pit of the stomach, with tremor,*[1].—*Burning in the stomach,*[43 42].—Burning of the stomach, every time she took a dose,[43].†—Sensation as if there were burning hot balls in the stomach, and something acid and corrosive in the pylorus,[215].—[**1340**.] Burning pain at the orifice of the stomach,[99].—Burning in the stomach and œsophagus, with desire to vomit,[215].—Heartburn (when smoking); a scraping, burning, smarting sensation remains long after, at the commencement of the throat and upper part of the larynx (after two hours),[1].—After eating, the stomach and abdomen feel swollen and oppressed,[215].—While walking, frequently a squeezing in the scrobiculus cordis, a sort of crampy sensation, which obliges him to draw a deep breath,[8].—Cramp pains in stomach and bowels (mother and child, within an hour),[228].—After eating a very little food, a peculiar contractive sensation in the stomach,[12].—Spasm in the stomach, like cramp,[31].—Long-lasting spasm of the stomach, always during the midday meal,[1].—Spasmodic pressure on the stomach,[91].—[**1350**.] A pressure in the pit of the stomach, in part gnawing,[1].—*Hard pressure in the stomach after eating*([1]), and also later,[7].—Distress as if caused by indigestion (after twenty minutes),[216].—Violent pressure at the pit of the stomach, felt only in walking; it forces him to move slowly (after forty-eight hours),[14].—Violent pressure in the stomach, with inclination to vomit,[195].—Sensation of a bar pressing on the stomach and præcordial region, with crampy and contractive pains, often with inclination to vomit, headache, epistaxis, trembling of the limbs, and great weakness,[215].—Shootings at the pit of the stomach,[1 4].—*Violent shooting cutting pain in the pit of the stomach, forcing one to bend the body backwards, and to hold one's breath,*[1].—Pinching right across the epigastrium and downwards as if in the colon,[12].—*Region of stomach sensitive to touch,*[106].—[**1360**.] Painfulness of the epigastric zone to touch,[102].—Pulsations, uneasiness, and feeling of inflammation in the stomach,[215].—Painless throbbing and beating at the pit of the stomach,[1].

Abdomen.—Hypochondria. Fulness below the short ribs when stooping; fulness at the pit of the stomach and darkness before the eyes (after four days),[1].—The abdomen is tense round the ribs,[31].—When pressing on the epigastrium, pain as if the hypochondria were being pressed out,[1].—Belladonna increases the secretion of bile,[194].—Swollen, painful liver, presenting swellings like abscesses,[215].—Heaviness and pulsations in the hepatic region, with sensation of swelling in that part, and inclination to lean to the left side and to draw up the right shoulder,[215].—Cramps of the liver, involving the chest and exciting paroxysms of cough and suffocation,[215].—[**1370**.] Pulsative pains, with anxiety at the liver, extending to the epigastrium,[215].—Pinching laterally in the abdomen, in the hepatic region, so that in attempting to rise from his seat, he could not for pain,[4].—Dull shootings in the right side of the abdomen near the false ribs,[14].—Sensation of inflammation and swelling of the spleen,[215].—Sharp pain in the splenic region (after six hours),[217].—Pulsative, crampy, and deepseated pains in the region of the spleen,[215].—*Umbilical Region.* A constriction

---

† See S. 1078.

of the belly in the umbilical region, as if a ball or lump were forming,[10].—*Along with the sensation of distension of the abdomen, constrictive pain below the umbilicus, which comes in jerks, and forces one to lean forward bent double (after four hours),[1].—Soon after a stool, a tensive sensation below the navel for only a few moments (second day),[211].—Squeezing and clawing around the umbilicus, so that he was obliged to bend forwards,[4].—[1380.] A squeezing together in the umbilical region, more in the middle of the day and in the afternoon,[1].—After eating, violent pinching below the umbilicus, immediately under the abdominal walls (after two and a half hours),[8].—Griping about the navel (after quarter of an hour),[139].—Dull stabs, as with a knife, in the left side below the umbilicus,[3].—Violent stabs, as with a blunt knife, between the right hip and the umbilicus (after twelve hours),[3].—From the region of the navel, round the left hip as far as the lumbar vertebræ, a shooting stab, as if in one thrust, which terminated with great painfulness in the latter region (after three-quarters of an hour),[3].—Itching shootings in the umbilicus, which disappear on rubbing it (after one hour),[17].—*In General.* Inflammation of the upper part of the abdomen (postmortem),[39].— Abdomen somewhat distended,[221].— Distended, yet neither hard nor painful abdomen,[19].—Distension of the abdomen, with rolling or grumbling of the intestines on the left side,[10].—After a confined motion, distension of the abdomen and heat of head,[40] (Case 14).—Distension of the abdomen, and transient pains in the abdomen,[91].—The abdomen is meteorically distended, the diaphragm pushed forcibly upwards (after five hours),[136].—Meteorism,[102 113 119 130].—Great meteorismus,[226].—Meteorism of the belly, with constipation, in one case subsiding and recurring with the delirium,[203].—[Distended, hard abdomen],[49].—The abdomen distended and very hard,[134].—Inflammatory swelling of the abdomen,[215].—[1390.] Swelling of abdomen, formation of flatulence, and pinching in umbilical region,[195].—Swelling of the belly, and aphthæ in the throat,[197].—The abdomen swollen, the pulse small and frequent,[184].—*Tumefaction of the abdomen,* which was very tender to the touch, constipation and weak pulse,[184].—(Extraordinary and preternatural inflation of the abdomen, after death),[39].—Inflation of the abdomen, as by a mass of water around the bowels, especially in the umbilical region, which becomes prominent,[215].—A drawing-in of the abdomen, with pressive pain (in lying),[4].—Violent recurring rumbling in the abdomen,[3].—Loud rumbling in the abdomen, as if everything there were jumbled topsy-turvy (after half an hour),[13a].—A rumbling and pinching in the belly,[10].—[1400.] Borborygmi and flatulence, which extend from the abdomen even into the stomach, with burning and pressive pains in the præcordial region,[215].—Discharge of much wind,[89].—Very frequent emission of almost inodorous flatus,[1 10].—Flatulence without smell, and sometimes having a putrid odor,[215].—Wind in the bowels, tasteless eructation, and urgency to stool, but which amounted to little,[59].—With the desire for stool, feeling in the abdomen as if diarrhœa would set in, with internal heat in the abdomen (after one hour),[14].—Pain in the belly,[231].—Violent pain in the abdomen,[221 105].—*Feeling of heat in the abdomen as if from a hot iron,*[215].—Occasional heat in the bowels, chest, and face,[215].—[1410.] *Heat in the belly (with anxiety), in the chest and in the face,* with obstruction of the nose,[14].—*Burning in the abdomen,*[16].†—*Burning, compression, and pinching in the abdomen, obliging him to bend double,*[215].—Sensation of fulness in the abdomen, especially soon after a stool (seventh day),[211].—*Colic, spasmodic*

---

† Not found.

tension from the chest to deep in the abdomen, which does not permit the body to be moved in the least (after half an hour),¹.—The abdomen was rather contracted,¹⁷⁹.—Pinching in the intestines,⁴.—Violent pinching deep in the abdomen, which becomes much more violent on drawing oneself in, and in bending the upper part of the body to the left side (after six hours),⁸.—In the evening, always severe pinchings in the abdomen, followed by a soft motion,¹⁹⁵.—Pinching colic, whereby he is obliged to sit with his body bent double, with ineffectual urging to diarrhœa, and subsequent vomiting,¹.— [1420.] An extremely severe griping in the right side of the belly, also, sharp shootings from thence to the right side of the chest, as far as the axilla,¹⁴.—*Colic, as if a spot in the abdomen were seized with the nails, a griping, clutching, clawing*,¹.—Colic,²³⁵.—Continual colic,⁴⁰ (Case 1).—Colics and cramps in the abdomen and in the loins, with inability to keep still,²¹⁵. —[Colic, constipation, diuresis, with eructations and inclination to vomit],⁴⁰ (Case 12).—Very severe colic, with affection of the head and paralytic weakness of the entire right side of the body,²¹⁵.—[Colic, constipation, diuresis, with eructations and inclination to vomit],⁴⁰.—Colic and leucorrhœa,⁴⁰ (Case 14).—(After drinking milk, colic, a few shoots),¹.—[1430.] Colic as from a heavy weight pressing, only when walking and standing, disappearing every time he sits down,¹.—A dull, irritable drawing in the whole circumference of the pelvis; this pain is alternately felt in the sacrum and the os pubis,³.—Drawing in the abdomen as from flatulence, rumbling and passage of wind,⁸⁸.—Drawing pains in the abdomen, with cold feet,¹²³. —Heavy, dull, bearing-down pain in the abdomen and pelvis; (symptom repeated several times, and very similar to what prover suffered at every period), (after two and three-quarter hours),²¹⁶.—Pressure in the abdomen as from a stone, with pains in the loins,⁴⁰ (Case 18).—Pressure, digging, cutting, and stitching in the abdomen,²¹⁵.—Stitching and burning in the abdomen, as also in the hypochondria and loins,²¹⁵.—Fine sticking, as of countless needles, from within outward, in whole abdominal and thoracic cavities,²¹⁴.—(Cutting in the abdomen in the evening, a few hours before going to bed),¹.—[1440.] In the morning in bed, in the left side of the belly on which he is quietly lying, a pressive cutting, which disappears as soon as he lies on the other side,¹⁴.—11.30 A.M., sharp pricking pain in abdomen (second day),²¹⁷.—*Long-lasting painfulness of the whole abdomen, as if it were all sore and raw** (after one hour),¹³ᵃ.—All showed signs of tenderness when pressed even slightly on the abdomen, particularly over the ovarian region,²⁰⁷.—Raw pains in the bowels, as if they were burnt or scraped,²¹⁵.—*Excessive tenderness of the abdomen, which cannot bear the slightest touch,²¹⁵.—Hypogastrium and Iliac Region.** The hypogastric zone is sunken in, soft, and nowhere painful,¹¹⁸.—In the evening, feeling of fulness in the hypogastric zone, very white-coated tongue, want of appetite, slight griping in the bowels, rumbling, and feeling of accumulation of flatulence, which, however, will not pass off,⁸⁹.—Drawings in the hypogastric region on the right side over the horizontal ramus of the pubis, occasioned by wind, which also passed away,⁸⁸.—[Pressure very low down in the abdomen, as from a heavy weight],⁴⁰ (Case 26).†—[1450.] *Violent cutting pressure in the hypogastrium, now here, now there** (after one hour),⁷. —*(In the morning, a pressing, as if everything would be forced out towards the organs of generation, with distension of the abdomen; after the pressing, the abdomen contracted. and this was followed by a discharge of white mucus from*

---

† Apparently a symptom of the patient's disease.

the vagina),[1].—*In the morning, immediately after getting out of bed, a violent, tensive, pressing pain in the whole of the hypogastrium, but especially in the region of the os pubis; it appears as if the hypogastrium (rarely the epigastrium), were spasmodically constricted, sometimes as if it were distended (although not really so); pains which gradually increase and gradually decrease* (after twenty-four hours),[3].—*In the hypogastrium, immediately below the umbilicus, a feeling as if the intestines pressed outwards, chiefly in standing* (after six days),[14].—Cutting in the whole of the hypogastrium, yet most violent in the left side,[3].—When rising from his seat, he feels a pain in the crests of the ilia, as if a sharp body were protruding there,[14].—Swelling of the inguinal glands,[215].—Fine shootings in the left groin,[12].—Severe shootings in the inguinal glands,[1].—In sitting with the trunk bent forwards, a feeling in the right groin as if a hard body pressed outwards,[13a].—[1460.] In the right groin, at the inguinal ring, in sitting with the trunk bent forwards, a feeling as if a hard body pressed from within outwards, without the part feeling hard to the touch (after six days),[14].

Rectum and Anus.—Hæmorrhoidal flow for several days,[1].—Hæmorrhoidal discharge of decomposed blood, even when not at stool,[215].—Sense of constipation,[219].—*Squeezing, constrictive pain in the lowermost intestines, alternately with dull shoots or jerks in the direction of the perineum* (after thirty-six hours),[1].—Contractive pain in the rectum, then ulcerative pain in the epigastrium; thereupon rapid evacuation of mucous diarrhœa; lastly, tenesmus,[1].—Pressing in the rectum towards the anus,[12].—*A sort of tenesmus, a constant pressing and urging towards the anus and genitals, alternating with painful contractions of the anus* (after twelve hours),[1].—Distinct, rapid, severe shootings in the rectum, during stool (after three hours),[1].—Raw feeling with burning and constrictive pains in the rectum,[215].—[1470.] Voluptuous tickling in the lower part of the rectum,[1].—Itching in the lower part of the rectum,[1].—Violent, sudden, painful itching in the rectum and anus,[1].—Prolapsus ani during stool,[215].—Intolerable itching at the anus,[215].—Violent itching, and at the same time constrictive sensation in the anus,[3].—Itching at the anus externally, when walking in the open air,[1].—Itching and moisture at the anus and perineum,[91].

Stool.—Urgent inclination to go to stool,[215].—Constant desire for stool,[1].—[1480.] *Urging to stool, which is thinner than usual, but passes in proper quantity,*[7].—Urging to stool and colic,[36].—*Frequent urging to stool, without result, or with a very scanty and hard evacuation,*[7].—*Frequent urging to stool, sometimes ineffectual, and with tenesmus,*[215].—Ineffectual urging to stool, followed by vomiting,[1].—*Straining to stool; the evacuation is undoubtedly diarrhœic, but very little is voided, and immediately after follows much-increased straining* (after three hours),[13a].—First, a soft diarrhœic stool; subsequently, however, frequent desire for stool, of which little or nothing comes,[14].—Frequent evacuations,[111].—Diarrhœa,[235].—At times, diarrhœic evacuations,[91].—[1490.] When taken by the mouth in poisonous doses, Belladonna sometimes causes diarrhœa,[194].—Copious and frequent stools,[215].—Very frequent small stool; one evacuation is hardly finished before an urging is felt for another,[215].—Small, loose stools, with sharp, stitching pain above the umbilicus (after one and three-quarter hours),[217].—Stools often with sweats and flow of urine,[215].—Frequent thin stools with tenesmus; frequent desire for stool, obliging him to go every quarter of an hour (after forty-eight hours),[1].—[Several watery stools, immediately after profuse sweat],[49].—Frequent watery stools, studded with small white flocks, with colics, cramps in the stomach and limbs, chills, headache, debility, and restlessness,[215].—An offensive, greenish diarrhœa (after nineteen hours),[233].—Diarrhœa with dark discharges (second night),[230].—[1500.] Diarrhœa, inclination to vomit, and pressure at the stomach,[40] (Case 14).—Diarrhœa, with pressure at the stomach, burning in the abdomen, and inclination to vomit,[215].—[Involuntary passage of fæces],[40] (Case 22).—Small, rapid, involuntary evacuations,[1].—Light-colored, rapid, and involuntary stool,[215].—*Involuntary evacuation, temporary paralysis of the sphincter ani,*[29].—Unusually diminutive stool, only very small evacuations resulted for several days,[4].—Stool somewhat less consistent than usual, and colored greenish; this greenish color of the fæces was observed during the whole time of the proving,[211].—Pappy stools mixed with mucus,[4].—Soft, yellowish, greenish, brownish, or whitish stools,[215].—[1510.] Passage is considerably harder and more scanty than usual,[58].—Stool as white as chalk,[76].†—A copious, fluid, greenish evacuation,[124].—Granular, yellow, somewhat mucous stool,[1].—[Greenish stool],[40] (Case 25).‡—[Green stool, with profuse urine, and also with sweat],[40] (Case 24).§—Green stool, fæces enveloped in reddish mucus (seventh day),[211].—*Slimy and bloody diarrhœic stools,*[215].—Stools have a very sour smell,[1].—Discharge of ascarides and lumbrici, with stool,[215].—[1520.] Torpid state of the bowels,[230].—Evacuation slow and dry (after one hour),[92].—Delayed and difficult, although soft stools,[215].— *The passage is perceptibly retarded,*[89 118 126 129 108 119 137 135].—Suppression of fæces and urine, with profuse sweat,[17].—She discharged neither fæces nor urine, but sweated extraordinarily,[108].—[Constipation],[45].—Constipation,[222].—Constipation, with colic, uneasiness, and burning in the abdomen,[215].

Urinary Organs.— *Bladder, Kidneys, and Urethra.*
The bladder half paralyzed,[203].—[1530.] His bladder was full of urine on admission (after nine hours),[190].—Pain in the region of the bladder; desire to urinate; only a few drops of urine were evacuated by the catheter,[223].—Burning in the bladder, with frequent urination, especially at night,[215].—Sensation of turning and twisting in the bladder, as if from a large worm, without desire to micturate,[1].—*Tenesmus of the bladder,*[238].—*Dull pressing in the vesical region during the night,*[1].—Nephritic colic, often accompanied with vomiting,[215].—Painful sensation on urinating and evacuation, for some time,[109].—Irritation in the urinary passages, especially the neck of the bladder, with strangury, and passage of dark, bloody urine, with great heat; scarlet redness of skin, the whole body, palate, and pharynx (after one hour),[17].—Burning in the urethra and violent urging to urinate, without being able to pass any,[106].—[1540.] A long stitch in the urethra, which commenced in the bulb and extended to the orifice, in walking (after three hours),[8].—Between the acts of micturition, dull shootings in the urethra behind the glans, especially during movement,[1].—Raw pains in the urethra, with discharge of a few drops of thick, yellowish mucus, and sometimes of blood,[215].—Titillation in the urethral canal, with feeling as if a sound was being turned round in it,[215].—*Urination.* No inclination to pass water,[230].—Frequent desire to urinate,[222].—*Very frequent desire to urinate, even if only a few drops had accumulated,*[89].—*Frequent desire to urinate, but the urine voided in remarkably small quantities, although of a natural color,*[3 4 20 40].—Urging to urinate, but can only do so drop by drop,[215].—Frequent call to pass water, which yet could only be done after a great effort

---

† Not found.   ‡ Return of bile to stool; curative effect.
§ See note to last S.

and *guttatim*. The urine was normal, and micturition caused no pain,[195].—[155C.] Violent urgency to urinate, the urine, however, passed only with difficulty, in a small stream,[87].—Two hours later, he was affected with extreme desire to micturate, though he could pass only a few drops of perfectly colorless urine. From this time till he lost consciousness his desire to pass urine was constant; wherever he could retire he did so, but succeeded in expelling from the bladder, with considerable effort, only a few drops of colorless fluid,[188].—Frequent urinating,[123].—Frequent micturition, obscuration of vision, and thirst in the morning,[40] (Case 14).—Much urinating,[89].—Some urine passed (after an enema) for the first time (after thirteen hours); twenty-four hours after this urine excreted copiously,[185].—Urine more copious than the drink taken would warrant,[46].—Diuresis,[40].—(Belladonna is, indeed, in the truest sense of the word, a diuretic, and more powerful, perhaps, than any other we possess.)—One other fact relative to the effects of Belladonna is worthy of note, viz., its tremendous diuretic power. I have observed that it does not seem to reach the kidneys until it has been some time in the stomach, and has exerted its specific influence upon the brain. But its power over the secretion of urine is very great. I am confident I passed, in the course of an hour, three pints of urine, accompanied with a slight strangury at the neck of the bladder,[178].—[1560.] The diuretic effect of the drug now (after two and three hours) began to be experienced, the patient evacuating an enormous quantity of limpid urine,[177].—[Frequent micturition of profuse urine],[65].—Frequent and copious emission of urine (after one hour),[138].—Frequent copious emission of pale, diluted, watery urine,[37].—Frequent, rather scanty, discharge of thick, reddish-brown, iridescent urine,[215].—[Diuresis at night, with profuse sweat],[40].—[Diuresis, with the appearance of menstruation],[34].—Emission of urine increased, and mostly involuntary,[130].—*He cannot retain his urine,[1].—Involuntary micturition (in three children),[19].—[1570.] Involuntary emission of urine (in three children),[118].—[*Involuntary emission of urine; temporary paralysis of the neck of the bladder*],[29].—The urine continued to flow involuntarily without interruption, and was like clear spring-water, without smell. When one attempted to catch the urine in a chamber, the patient took the vessel, and held it off with one hand outside the bed, while with the other he held his penis, and continued to urinate,[129].—Unconscious emission of urine while in a stupor,[140].—*His urine escaped from him during a deep sleep in the daytime,[1].—Involuntary urination, often at night and during sleep,[215].—After urinating, cold sweat all over the body,[215].—The urine became more scanty, and passed with exertion (after one hour),[92].—*Diminished urine,[220].—Remarkable diminution in the urinary excretion,[89 137].—[1580.] *The urine was scanty for the first twenty-four hours,[180].—Anuria in two cases,[210].—Excretion of urine now increased, now diminished,[91].—Difficulty in urinating,[230].—Bladder full and distended; the urine flows slowly and sluggishly through the catheter,[226].—Ischuria for twenty-four hours; for six days after this the secretion did not exceed six ounces in the twenty-four hours, very high-colored, and apparently very thick (on twelfth day of taking one-half a grain of extract three times a day for diabetes insipidus),[210].—Violent strangury towards the close,[197].—Violent strangury, with bloody micturition (case of poisoning by 46 grains of the extract),[197].—Could neither urinate nor discharge stool,[237].—He passed no urine, and the bladder was evacuated by the catheter, the quantity being scanty, and strongly ammoniacal,[181].—[1590.] Retention of urine,[126 119 135].—[*Retention of urine, which only passes drop by drop*],[52].—Retention of urine almost invariably occurs during the action of a full dose of Belladonna, and dysuria very often follows. We may encourage a patient to make prolonged efforts to pass urine when fully under the influence of the drug, and he will either fail altogether, or only pass a few drachms, and this not in little jerks which indicate spasm, but in weak driblets. Indeed, the absence of spasm is readily determined. If a full-sized flexible catheter be passed under these circumstances, it meets with no opposition, but passes readily into the bladder, and the urine flows as sluggishly as from the bladder of a patient afflicted with hemiplegia,[194].—Retention of urine; often he would take the chamber without success; he ran much about, could not lie quiet for a minute, and had twitching of the facial muscles (after a quarter of an hour),[122].—Suppression of urine, sometimes with constipation, sometimes with diarrhœa,[215].—Suppression of urine and stool, for ten hours,[1].—*Urine.* Emission of a quantity of watery urine, with sweat,[18].—Frequent discharge of pale, watery urine, with copious sweat,[215].—Whitish urine,[1].—Bright-yellow, clear urine (after four hours),[1].—[1600.] [Clear, lemon-colored urine],[49].—Golden-yellow urine,[4].—[*Yellow, turbid urine*],[15].—Urine with greenish reflections,[215].—*Water deep red*, with a light sediment,[200].—*Blood-colored urine*,[215].—*Urine dark*, and increased,[91].—Emission of dark, bloody urine (after one hour),[117].—Belladonna increases the vesical mucus in the urine,[211].—Urine with a white, thick sediment (after twelve hours),[1].—[1610.] * *The urine becomes turbid like yeast, with a reddish sediment*,[1].—Thick, yellowish-red, brickdust sediment in the urine,[215].—Discharge of gravel with the urine,[215].

Sexual Organs.—(*Male*), Red pimples and growths like small condylomata on the penis,[215].—A soft, painless tumor on the glans,[1].—Frequent erections,[91].—Frequent involuntary erections and involuntary emissions of urine,[200].—Weakness and relaxation of the genitals (from one and seven-eighths grain),[195].—Irritation of the genital organs, in boys, which was manifested by constant erections, and by seizing the member with the hands,[118].—Immediately after urinating, a smarting pain in the outer edge of the prepuce,[1].—[1620.] Heat and redness of the penis, with constant semi-erection,[215].—In the forepart of the glans, an itching titillation resembling a flea-bite,[4].—Sensation as if caused by an accumulation of serum in the scrotum,[215].—Inflammatory swelling of the testicles,[215].—Drawing and lancinating pains in the spermatic cords and testicles,[215].—During micturition, drawing in the spermatic cord,[1].—Before falling asleep in bed in the evening, a tearing upwards in the left spermatic cord, repeated a few times,[12].—Violent shootings in the testicles, which are drawn upwards (after ten, eighteen, and thirty hours),[11].—Increased sexual desire,[215].—Indifference in the night to the distinction of the sexes; no lascivious, lustful thoughts will enter his head; the sexual desire in the imagination is as if extinct,[11].—[1630.] Entire loss of sexual desire,[215].—Discharge of prostatic juice,[215].—Discharge of prostatic juice from a relaxed penis,[1].—Nocturnal pollutions,[215].—Nocturnal emission of semen, during relaxation of the penis,[1].—Nocturnal emission of semen without lascivious dreams (the first night),[11].—Feeble, but abundant, ejaculation of semen,[215].—(*Female*), * *At every step violent shootings in the genital region, as if in the internal sexual organs* (after sixteen hours),[13a].—**Badly smelling hemorrhage from the uterus**,[35]. — * *Burning, pressure, uneasiness and weight in the uterine region*,[215].—[1640.] Cramps of the womb, with feeling as if it was growing narrow,[215].—Before the menses, uterine colic with weakness of sight,[215].— *Burning in the ovarian region*,[215].—Leucorrhœa and colic,[49] (Case 14).—

Flesh-colored or milky leucorrhœa, with a great deal of colic,[215].—Metrorrhagia of light clotted blood,[215].—*[Metrorrhagia, the blood having a bad smell],[3].—*A violent pressing and urging towards the sexual organs, as if everything would fall out there ; *worse on sitting bent and on walking, better on standing and sitting erect* (after ten hours),[13a].†—Bringing on of the catamenia,[1].—Increased menses (curative effect),[50].—[1650.] *Inordinate menstrual discharge may occur suddenly in females,*[212].—Greater flow of the menses, with retardation till the thirty-second, thirty-sixth, and forty-eighth day,[40].—Catamenia appear four days too soon,[1].—*Menses too soon and very profuse, of thick, decomposed, dark-red blood,[215].—Menses sometimes delayed, or of pale blood,[215].—During the catamenia, great thirst,[40] (Case 14).—During the menses, fever, painful lassitude, colic, pains in the limbs, weakness and inclination to remain lying down,[215].—Increased sexual desire in women, especially before the menses and in the evening ; absence of desire, and even aversion to an embrace, in the morning,[215].

Respiratory Apparatus.—Larynx, Trachea, and Bronchi. Catarrh, or cough with coryza,[1].—Catarrh, with cough, coryza, and the head and eyes severely affected,[215].—[1660.] A great deal of tenacious mucus in the larynx and nasal fossæ,[215].—*The dryness extends into the larynx, rendering the voice husky, and often inducing dry cough,[194 195].*— *Painful dryness in larynx, *yet with an unconquerable aversion to all drinks,[237].*—The sensibility of the larynx was so much impaired and deglutition so imperfectly performed, that, on introducing a warm infusion of coffee into the patient's mouth, the liquid collected about the larynx, and his features became alarmingly turgid in consequence of impeded respiration,[179].—Every inspiration causes irritation with dry cough,[1].—Pain under larynx, with hiccough, after eating (from one and seven-eighths grain),[195].— *Sensation as if the larynx was inflamed and swollen, with snoring breathing, and danger of suffocation,[215].—Secretion of a great deal of watery phlegm,[215].—*Sensation as if some one constricted his larynx,[237].—Sensation as if the larynx was narrowed and torn,[215].—[1670.] Spasmodic movement of the larynx as if it was being tied up,[215].—Sensation of ulceration and bleeding of the larynx,[215].—* *Violent scraping in larynx excites a dry cough,*[90]. —* *Tickling and burning in the larynx with violent paroxysms of cough,*[215].— *In the evening, after lying down in bed, tickling-itching sensation in the back part of the top of the larynx, causing a dry, short cough, which he cannot suppress,*[1].—The upper part of the trachea is affected ; he coughs up a substance resembling old catarrhal mucus, of a purulent appearance (in the morning in bed and after rising), (after sixteen hours),[1].—Noise and rattling in the bronchial tubes, with insensibility,[63].—*Voice.* *Now and then, while speaking, the voice, which had been weak, becomes suddenly loud and clear,*[215].—The voice became so sharp and clear that her own father did not know it (naturally somewhat husky),[223].—*Rough, hoarse voice,[1].—[1680.] * *Voice hoarse and weak,*[188].—*Hoarse, rough voice, *with dryness in the throat, the seat of which she accurately located in the larynx; she had to cough frequently, and swallow often; when swallowing, she complained of pain in the larynx,*[90].—Hoarse, dull, shrill, whistling, nasal voice,[215].—*Hoarseness,[73]. —*Hoarseness (after six hours),[239].—* *Hoarseness amounting to aphonia,*[215].— *Hoarseness, which was especially noticed when crying,[10°].—The voice seems changed, and slightly oppressed,[115].—The voice is changed, soft and hoarse,[118].—Speaking is very difficult for him ; he speaks in a piping tone

---

† Lying, sitting, C. D.

of voice,[1].—[1690.] Voice weak,[226].—Temporary loss of speech (aphonia),[67]. —Almost complete aphonia,[114].—*Aphonia, or confused sounds uttered with pain,[201].—*Cough and Expectoration.* Rawness and dryness in the upper part of the larynx excites a cough,[88].—Cough, hollow and scraping,[1]. —Cough, with loss of breath, noisy inspiration, face red and swollen as in hooping-cough,[215].—Cough, especially in the afternoon, at night in bed, and during sleep,[215].—Croupy cough (two boys),[186].—A sort of croupy cough,[134]. —[1700.] *Cough, with a bloody taste in the mouth,*[1].—Cough, with tearing sensation in the chest, and painful shocks at the nape of the neck and in the abdomen,[215].—Cough, with prickings, as if with needles, in the side under the left ribs (after six hours),[11].—Hard fit of coughing, as if something had "gone the wrong way,"[215].—(Attacks of coughing, which end with sneezing),[1].—Attack of coughing, followed by heat,[9].—*Cough commences in the evening (about 10 o'clock), and occurs every quarter of an hour or oftener in three or four fits at a time,*[1].—Night-cough, which frequently awakes her out of sleep, after which, however, she falls asleep again directly,[9].—Cough after eating and great thirst,[40] (Case 12).—*Violent cough during sleep, with grinding of the teeth,*[1].—[1710.] *Before each attack of coughing the child is quiet, and immediately before the cough comes on, she begins to cry,*[1].—During coughing, the child strains much and is fretful,[1].— *Dry cough, whereby the throat is scraped,*[13a].—*Short, dry, noisy, spasmodic or else hollow and hoarse cough,*[215].—Violent, dry cough as if a foreign body had lodged in the larynx, with coryza (after three hours),[11].—Attack of coughing as if one had inhaled dust; he is awakened by it at night, with mucous expectoration,[4].—[For several days in succession, about noon, violent cough, with expectoration of much tenacious mucus],[40] (Case 22).— Mucus in the air-passages expectorated by coughing and hawking,[211].— Expectoration of viscid and whitish mucus,[215].—Phlegm, especially in the morning,[215].—[1720.] At times expectoration of blackish, thick mucus,[233].— In the morning, when coughing, expectoration of bloody mucus,[1].—Spitting of blood,[215].—Hæmoptysis of clear, bright-red blood, rarely coagulated and black,[215].—*Respiration.* Respiration is often sighing, without apparently being otherwise difficult (after eight hours),[129].—[Sighs],[30].†— Stertorous respiration (after a quarter of an hour),[86].—The breathing heavy and stertorous,[185].—Respiratory murmur vesicular, though without rattling,[226].—The breathing was stertorous, and the respiratory sounds, hastily examined over the anterior part of the chest, were modified by râles,[179].— [1730.] Respiration deep, at times yawning (after seven hours),[112].—The breath is hot; respiration accelerated (after half an hour),[118 136 137].— *Respiration rapid and somewhat oppressed,*[130].—Respiration irregular and very rapid,[30 226].—Respiration by jerks, groaning, accelerated,[140].—Violent, short, hurried, anxious respiration (after eighteen hours),[37].—Respiration retarded, at times whistling,[135].—No difference is observed in the rate of respiration, even during the maximum acceleration of the pulse,[194].—Respiration short and hasty,[105].—Respiration short, hurried, sometimes very oppressed,[203].—[1740.] Shortness of breath, anxiety and suffocative fits, especially at night and in the afternoon,[215].—*Shortness of breath after drinking coffee in the afternoon* (after three days),[4].—Intermittent breathing in the night, in sleeping and waking; inspiration and expiration together last only half as long as the pause before the next inspiration; expiration occurred by fits and starts, and was louder than inspiration; inspiration lasted only a little longer than expiration,[1].—At times he breathed, at

---

† Immediately before death.

times he appeared to have drawn his last breath, such attacks recurring four times in a quarter of an hour,[31].—Respiration anxious, and attended with the brazen stridulous sound of croup,[177].—Respiration laborious and occasionally stertorous (post-mortem; congestion of the lungs),[191].—Difficult respiration,[63].—*Breath hot, respiration difficult,[102].—Very difficult breathing,[25].†

Chest.— In General. Inflammation of the lungs,[213].—[1750.] Engorgement and abscesses of the breasts,[215].—*Erysipelatous swelling of the breasts,[215].—The breasts suddenly become flaccid and flat, or else inflamed and swollen, with increased secretion of milk,[215].—Burning in the chest, with sensation as if the lungs were swelling up and inflating the thorax,[215]. —Burning and drawing pains in the nipples, especially the right,[215].—Violent constriction across the chest, as if it were being pressed inwards from both sides (after eight hours),[8].—In the evening in bed, such a constriction in the chest, which did not pass off on coughing for the purpose, that he could with difficulty draw in his breath, just as if the mucus in the larynx prevented him, accompanied by a burning in the chest (after sixty hours),[1]. —*Tightness of the chest,[73].—*Oppression of the chest,[57].—Oppression of the chest and difficult breathing, especially when walking and in the evening in bed, with sibilant mucous and often crepitant râle,[215].—[1760.] Exceeding weight and oppression of the whole chest,[219].—*Painful pressure in the chest, extending into the back,[215].—*Pressive pain in the chest and between the shoulders,[1].—Pressing pain in the chest with shortness of breath, and at the same time between the scapulæ, in walking and sitting,[4].—Acute pressing in the region of the sixth true rib from within outwards (after a quarter of an hour),[14].—Stitches and pulsations in the chest,[215].—In walking, fine stitches below the clavicle from before backwards (after four days),[14].— 3 P.M., stitches in chest and just below right axilla (second day),[217].—Fine shooting pain in the chest,[40] (Cases 11 and 18).—Shooting, disappearing quickly, like stabs with a blunt knife, below the last two ribs, close to the xiphoid cartilage, and above the false ribs (after eight minutes),[3].—[1770.] Scraping, digging, and often lancinating pains in the chest, with constant inclination to cough, often without the ability,[215].—Great inquietude and beating in the chest,[1].—**Sternum.** Pain at sternal extremity of fifth rib (after less than one hour),[217].—Sharp, cramping pain just below the extremity of the sternum, gradually extending to the pit of the stomach and upward to the sternum, and over the cardiac region (after nine hours),[217]. —An acute pressing pain in the sternum directly above the xiphoid cartilage,[3].—Stitches in the sternum in coughing and yawning,[1].—Shooting, pinching pains in the chest, on both sides of the upper part of the sternum,[14]. —A beating pain under the sternum above the scrobiculus cordis,[3].— **Sides.** Pains more in the left than right side of the chest,[215].—*Burning in the right chest,[4].—[1780.] Pressing in the right chest, which causes anxiety,[1]. —Pressing squeezing pain in the left and right sides of the chest,[4].—A pressing pain below the right nipple,[3].—Intermittent, pressing cutting in the right side of the chest, unaffected by either inspiration or expiration (after three hours),[14].—In the right side of the chest, a deeply penetrating and constant stitch, unaffected by the breathing,[14].—Fine stitches in the left side of the chest from the sternum towards the axilla, more violent during motion, unaffected by the breathing,[14].—In the right side of the chest, stitches here and there below the skin, in some measure external,[1].— Stitches in the side of the chest under the right arm, which hinder the

† Not found.

breathing, towards evening,[1].—(Pressive shooting pain in the left side under the ribs),[1].—Constant pressive shooting in the cartilages of the left ribs, more violent, and changing into an almost burning sensation, during expiration (after three hours),[8].—[1790.] A corroding gnawing pain beneath the cartilages of the last ribs on the right side (after two hours),[3].

Heart and Pulse.—Præcordium and Heart. Great anxiety about the præcordia,[74].—Præcordial anxiety during the catamenia,[40].—After dinner and supper, præcordial anxiety, headache, redness of face, and bitter taste in the mouth,[40] (Case 14).—Anxiety was noticed about the heart, a peculiar troublesome sensation from time to time, like that noticed with an intermitting pulse; in fact the pulse did intermit at times (after one hour),[92].—Pressure in the cardiac region, which arrests the breathing, and causes a sense of anxiety,[1].—Sensation of cardiac oppression in the scrobiculus cordis; she could not breathe properly; thereupon nausea, rising up in the throat as if she would vomit; and so oppression and nausea alternated every seven minutes (after a quarter of an hour),[13a].—The action of the heart was feeble (after two hours),[179].—The action of the heart was feeble, and the pulsations of the radial artery were 116 in the minute, regular, and weak (after two hours),[179].—Weak but frequent beat of the heart (after a quarter of an hour),[86].—[1800.] Beat of heart and pulse smaller and somewhat contracted, but not accelerated,[118].—Starts and trembling of the heart, which feels large and heavy,[215].—When she goes upstairs the heart clucks; a sort of palpitation,[13a].—Violent beating of the heart,[222]. —Beating and palpitation of the heart, with great oppression of the chest,[215]. —Violent palpitation,[219].—Violent palpitation, and active, accelerated pulse,[105].—Palpitation of the heart, with pulsation of the carotid and temporal arteries, heat and redness of face; generally with congestion to the head, and fever (after a quarter of an hour),[91].—(During rest, palpitation, with feeling as if the concussion extended to the throat, more violent during movement, and with difficult, slow respiration),[1].—*Pulse.* Very feeble pulse (after one hour),[184].—[1810.] Pulse very feeble and almost countless,[180].—Pulse scarcely perceptible,[185].—Pulse small, contracted, not to be counted,[102 129].—Pulse full, and slightly accelerated,[239].—*Full, frequent pulse, increased by ten beats*,[2].—*Pulse full and quick* (90 to 100), (after six hours),[239].—*Pulse full, about* 120,[178].—Pulse strong, frequent,[222].—Strong, rapid pulse,[10].—*Pulse much increased in force and frequency,*[177].—[1820.] Very small, quick pulse,[1].—Pulse small, compressed, and very quick (120 to 130), (after six hours),[239].—Pulse regular, small, and 120,[226].—Pulse very feeble, and quick,[181].—Pulse extremely accelerated,[220].—Accelerated pulse, strong or small, sometimes full and slow, or small and slow, or hard and tense,[215].—Pulse 80 (second day),[218].—Pulse 80 to 90, and regular,[238].—Pulse 90 (second day),[228].—Pulse 100,[227].—[1830.] Pulse 110,[223].—Pulse 120 to 130,[231].—Pulse very slow and full,[221].—Large, full, slow pulse,[1].—Very small, slow pulse,[4].—The pulse was soft, and slower than usual,[99].—Pulse weak and slow,[225].—Pulse extremely slow, filiform, and irregular,[236].—Pulse sank from 80 to 75 per minute (after ten minutes),[218].—Pulse 70, feeble, and compressible,[190].—[1840.] Pulse 60 (after five and a half hours),[218].— Pulse 37, radial artery full, hard, and firm to the touch, with entire insensibility; a vein being opened in the arm, the blood, which flowed slowly, was dark and thick,[197].—Pulse irregular; one strong beat is quickly followed by four or five weak ones (after half an hour),[136].—Pulse small and intermitting,[106].—Pulse contracted, very accelerated, often intermitting (after seven hours),[112].

Neck and Back.—Neck. *Swelling of the glands on the left side of the neck*, at which spot he also frequently complains of a burning pain,[118].—*Swelling of the glands in the nape of the neck*, with cloudiness of the head (after six days),[1].—*Inflammation and swelling of the glands of the neck and of the back of the throat*,[215].—*Swelling and stiffness of the neck and nape of the neck*, especially on the left side, with crampy pains at the least movement,[215].—Drawing pains and pressure at the nape of the neck,[215].—[1850.] Pressive pain externally in the neck, when bearing the head backwards and when touching the part,[1].—*In coughing, a violent pressing pain in the nape of the neck, as if it would break* (after three and a half hours),[8].—Sharp pain between the last cervical and first dorsal vertebræ (after four and a half hours),[217].—Sensation as if the nape of the neck was struck with a hammer,[215].—*Back in General.* Weakness of the spine, with heaviness of the head, and stooping walk,[215].—Stiffness of the muscles of the back and lower extremities prevents him from sitting up in bed, or raising himself upright; if supported, he is able to stand on his feet, but is unable to move them or to walk,[136].—Rheumatic pain in the back,[40] (Case 15).—Burning sensation, as if the spinal marrow was on fire,[215].—Cramps in the back and chest,[215].—Cramplike pressive sensation in the middle of the spinal column, which becomes tensive when he attempts to straighten the back (after half an hour),[8].—[1860.] During the menses, a cramplike tearing, now here and there in the back, now in the arms,[1].—Pain as if dislocated in the right side of the back and the spinal column,[1].—*Gnawing in the spinal column, with cough*,[1].—Pressive pain at the left of the spinal column, under the false ribs,[4].—Stabbings as if with a knife from without inwards in the vertebræ,[9].—Shooting and gnawing pain in the spinal column,[1].—*Dorsal.* Painful stiffness between the scapulæ and in the nape of the neck when turning the head and neck to and fro, in the morning (after sixteen hours),[1].—Distensive and rheumatic pains, with feeling of dislocation between the shoulder-blades,[215].—Pain between the scapulæ, as from a strain,[1].—Cramp-pain, almost like pinching, between the right scapula and the spinal column,[14].—[1870.] Violent drawing along the spine between the scapulæ, in the evening,[1].—Drawing, cutting pain behind right shoulder-blade,[217].—Pressive pain under the left scapula, more towards the outer side,[3].—Drawing pressure between the right scapula and the spinal column,[7].—Fine shootings in the right scapula,[14].—Repeated electric shoots from the left scapula to the right (after one hour),[12].—*Lumbar.* Burning and weakness in the loins; he walks with difficulty and bent over,[215].—Spasmodic sensation in the left lumbar region,[3].—Cramps and pressure in the loins, extending into the bladder and groins, with inclination to bend over and squat,[215].—Cramps and pains of dislocation in the loins and back, with painful stiffness of these parts,[215].—[1880.] Sharp slight pain in left loin, just above ischium (after ten minutes),[217].—Cutting pain in right loin, and in lower extremity of the sternum (after fifty minutes),[217].—Intensely painful sensation of cramp in the lumbo-sacral region and the coccyx; he can only sit for a short time, and while sitting becomes quite stiff and unable to rise again for pain; he cannot even lie down well; he often wakes at night because of it, and has to turn on the other side because of the violence of the pain; he cannot lie at all on the back; he is relieved chiefly by standing and walking slowly about, but he cannot walk fast (for eight days),[14].

Extremities in General.—Objective. The bloodvessels of the limbs are distended, especially the arteries in the neck pulsate, so that when the lower jaw is opened it strikes against the upper one at every beat, and thus gives rise to a slight chattering of the teeth ; at the same time warmth and feeling of warmth in the whole body, more especially in the head,[5].— Swelling of the injured arm and foot,[60].—Laxity of all the limbs (after a quarter of an hour),[86].—Trembling of the limbs,[102][106].—Trembling and lassitude of the limbs,[40] (Case 1).—Trembling of the limbs; tottering gait, with raising up of one leg, as if he had to ascend a hill; wherefore he falls down, and is unable to rise again without aid,[123].—The limbs are in a constant tremble; if a limb was lifted it would again fall powerless,[105].—[**1890.**] Trembling in all the limbs, inability to walk, distended veins over the whole body, and disagreeable sense of irritation in the throat, for several days,[17].—[With sudden outcries the hands and feet tremble],[40] (Case 1).— Extremities constantly in motion, especially the hands, for he is constantly busy trying to catch brilliantly colored, glittering, fiery hallucinations,[233].— The limbs are in constant motion, even without interruption, during the whole night,[137].—*He slowly moves the extremities upwards, trembling ; then, with greater force, he throws them downwards,*[125].—The extremities would often involuntarily perform the motions peculiar to the daily duties of the individual,[112].—*Twitchings of the limbs,*[81].—(Painful) twitchings in the arms; more in the right than in the left leg,[13a].—Contortions of the extremities,[236]. —Alternate strange distortions of the limbs, and complete immobility,[31].— [**1900.**] Convulsions of the limbs,[234].—*Convulsive movements of the limbs,*[63]. —All the limbs are in convulsive motion,[135].—*Convulsive momentary extension of the limbs on awaking out of sleep,*[1].—[Spasmodic stretching of the limbs, with contortions of the eyes],[40] (Case 12).—Convulsive twitching, turning, and moving of the upper and lower limbs,[137].—Spasms of all the limbs,[60].—[Spasms of the limbs, with hiccough],[20] (Case 14).—Numerous cramps, spasms, agitation, and contortion of the limbs,[215].—*Sensations.* *Heaviness of the hands and feet,*[2].—[**1910.**] [*Lassitude of the limbs*],[70].— Lassitude of the limbs,[81].—Indolence in all the limbs, and indisposition to work,[3].—In course of time the extremities become so feeble, and almost lame, that he could neither stand upright nor raise his hands,[237].—Paralytic weakness of all the muscles of the upper and lower extremities (after six days),[4].—Paralytic weakness, and feeling of paralysis in the limbs, or on one side of the body,[215].—All the limbs seem paralyzed (after six hours),[239]. —[Paralysis of the right arm and right leg],[40] (Case 11).†—Stiffness of all the limbs, under the semblance of ·a feeling of lassitude,[1].—Frequent stiffness and immobility of the limbs; for instance, he was not able to stir his left foot,[13a].—[**1920.**] Great uneasiness in all the limbs, so that he did not know where to put himself,[1].—Burning, pulsative, lancinating, pressive, crampy, or tearing pains in the limbs,[215].—Like gnawing of many ants internally in the bones of arm and thigh creeping from above downward,[214]. —Pulling, jerks, and shocks in the limbs,[215].

Upper Extremities.—In General. Swelling of the arm,[60].— Red or dark swellings on the arms and hands,[215].—Trembling of the arms on the slightest motion,[129].—[He raises the right arm involuntarily, and without his knowledge, above his head],[40] (Case 22).—She occasionally stretched out her arms and hands, as if she would seize something,[20].—His upper limbs move as if affected with chorea,[240].—[**1930.**] The arms and hands were in continual contortions,[19].—Convulsive shaking of the arm, as from excessive shuddering,[1].—Jerking and nervous trembling of the arms and hands,[215].—[Concussive spasms of the arms],[40] (Case 1).—[Spasm of the right arm, with grinding of the teeth],[40] (Case 20).—Cramps and spasms of the arms and hands,[215].—On eating, he would often put his hand instead of the spoon into his soup; often, also, he was unable to find his mouth with the spoon, and would run it alongside,[139].—Sense of great lassitude in the arms, but still more in the hands, as if she must let them hang down,[13a].—Heaviness in both arms,[1].—A heaviness and paralytic feeling in the upper extremities, especially in the left arm,[10].—Heaviness of the left arm, relieved by venesection,[40] (Case 23).—[1940.] Stiffness, so that she could not bend it, in the right arm, upon which she had not lain, at 3 A.M., with a feeling as if it were shorter than the other, and with a tearing pain therein,[13a].—A (sense of) stretching and twisting in the upper extremities,[10].—Paralytic drawing pressure, with weakness, in the right upper and forearm (after four days),[7].—*Shoulder and Arm.* Painful swelling of one of the left axillary glands (after five hours),[1].—Shooting pressure on the top of the left shoulder (after three hours),[7].—Sharp tearing pain under and in right armpit (third day),[217].—Jerking in the shoulders, with numbness and heaviness of the arms,[215].—[Spasm of the right arm, with grinding of the teeth],[40].—Inclination to work the arms, as if performing gymnastic exercises,[215].—Weakness as of paralysis, first in the right upper arm, afterwards also in the forearm (after eight hours),[12].—[1950.] [Paralysis of the right arm],[40] (Case 11).†—[The arm feels numb and painful],[65].—[Rheumatic pain in the right arm, with sense of formication; on the following day spasm of the same arm],[40] (Case 14).—Spraining and contused pain in the arms,[215].—She complained of a very painful cramp in the left arm and in the back, which in the evening extended to the thigh,[40] (Case 6).—Crampy and tearing pains in the arms, starting from the shoulders and stopping at the elbows,[215].—Drawing pain in the inside of the left upper arm,[4].—A drawing downwards in the muscles of the right upper arm, which, when it had reached the region of the elbow, twitched upwards again to the axilla, and there ceased for awhile,[1].—Drawing pain in left arm near insertion of deltoid muscle, relieved by pressure (after five hours),[217].—Paralytic tearing pressure in the anterior surface of the left upper arm (after five days),[7].—[1960.] Paralytic pressure in the left upper arm, with paralytic feeling and weakness of the whole of the left arm,[7].—A violent stabbing pain, as with a blunt knife, below the head of the humerus, from within outwards,[3].—Tearing pain in the humerus,[1] [4].—Bruised pain in the upper arms (after six hours),[14].—*Elbow, Forearm, and Wrist.* A rumbling in the bend of the left elbow, as if water or some heavy liquid were running through the veins,[4].—(When moving or touching the elbow it pains as if burnt),[1].—Paralytic drawing pain in the elbow, and in the fingers of the left hand,[4].—Cutting pain in the interior of the left elbow-joint when walking,[14].—Sharp shootings externally in the left elbow-joint (after seventy-two hours),[14].—Twitching of the tendons and muscles on the inner side of the forearm (after four hours),[121] [126].—[1970.] Feeling of slight warmth along the back of the right forearm, as of approaching numbness, and a slight paralytic feeling along the anterior tibial nerve (in a few moments),[217].—Dull aching in the muscles of the forearm (after half an hour),[217].—Tearing in the flexor surface of the left forearm, and in the palm of the hand and sole of foot,[88].—Sharp pain shooting from the wrist along the course of the ulnar nerve to the elbow-joint (after half an hour),[217].—Acute and tender pain in the radius of the left arm,

---

† See note to S. 864.

near pronator quadratus muscles. (This pain has been present at intervals for years, though not for a few months), (after half an hour),[218].— Cutting-tearing in the lower muscles of both forearms,[8].—Fine shootings in the left forearm (after twenty-four hours),[14].—Dull shootings in the middle of the inner forearm, which gradually increase, and at length become very violent,[3].—11.30 A.M., dull, throbbing pain along the radial nerve of right arm (second day),[217].—Burning-throbbing in the left forearm, near olecranon ulnæ, and posterior ridge of radius, aggravated by touch and light pressure; this sensation repeated itself often during the day; in the evening a similar pain appeared at the base of the scapula, near the angle; this spot appears to be warmer, and also worse on pressure,[88].—[1980.] He is not able to turn the hand easily and freely on its axis (as when dropping into a glass); he can only turn it by jerks; it is as if there were a deficiency of synovial fluid in the carpus; this impeded motion, however, is painless (after four hours),[1].—Paralytic tearing in the carpal bones,[7].—*Hands and Fingers.* Swelling of the hands,[78].— Great swelling of the hand,[60].—Swelling and stiffness of the joints of the hands,[215].—The hands swell and become dry; he could not take hold of anything without dropping it immediately (after three-quarters of an hour),[93].—Constant motion of hands and fingers,[114].—The hands were in constant motion, the boy played with his fingers, pulled and jerked at the covering, and snatched at various imaginary objects,[116].—Feeling of stiffness in the right hand and the fingers; she cannot bend them,[13a].—Dry sensation in the palms of the hands, which felt uncommonly smooth (after one hour),[92].—[1990.] Pain in the bones of the hands as if they were pounded,[215].—Dislocating pain in the joints of the hands,[215].—Tearing pressure in the metacarpal bones and the first joint of the left index finger,[8].— Shooting-tearing in the metacarpal bones of the left hand,[8].—Sharp shootings in the metacarpal bones of the thumb (after one hour),[14].—Slight soreness of the hands (after ten days),[230].—Soreness of the hands on pressure,[230]. —The anterior joint of the middle finger is as if stiff and painful on bending; a simple pain (? sore),[1].—**Painful drawing in the posterior joint of the left middle finger, as if in the periosteum,**[7].—The tips of the fingers of the left hand are painful, as if they had been jammed,[4].—[2000.] Tearing-cutting in the muscles of the right little finger,[8].—**Paralytic tearing in the middle joint of the right index finger,**[7].—During general chill, shootings in the tips of the fingers from below upwards, especially when grasping,[1].—Pain in the tip of the middle finger, as if some foreign body had lodged in it and produced ulceration; the pain is greater when touching the part,[14].—Pulsative or burning pains on the finger tips, as if they had been forcibly pinched or struck,[215].

Lower Extremities.—In General. Five or six spasms of the muscles of the limbs, trunk, and face,[238].—Trembling in the legs,[233].—A sort of stretching; he is obliged to extend the legs (after eleven days),[1].—Weakness of legs,[231].—His legs fail him,[238].—[2010.] He seemed to exercise very little control over the lower extremities, and to have very little power in them. It was clear he must have fallen to the ground had he been left without support. On being led about both legs dragged, but neither one more than the other (after eight hours),[188].—It was some days before she was able to walk, even with the assistance of a person on each side of her; this inability to walk did not arise from weakness, but she appeared to have lost all power of controlling the action of her legs,[185].—Powerlessness of the lower limbs, so that she must lie down, with nausea, trembling anxiety, and vertigo,[17].—Temporary paralysis of the lower limbs,[29].†—[*Paralysis of the lower extremities, together with the neck of the bladder, and the sphincter ani*],[29].—Stumbling, when walking,[233].—Tottering gait,[186 227].—The gait is insecure, tottering; standing is uncertain (after one hour),[98 115].— Staggering,[231].—A drawing heaviness in the legs,[1].—[**2020.**] Painful sensation of heaviness in the right leg, when laying it over the left (after four hours),[8].—An unpleasant sensation in the joints of the lower extremities, particularly in the knees, as if they would give way, especially when walking, and when going down stairs,[1].—***Hip and Thigh.*** Pain in the left hip, with limping,[40] (Case 20).—When lying upon her right hip, she feels a pain in her left; but when she lies upon the painful hip, all uneasiness subsides (after eight or nine days),[1].—Neuralgic pains in the hips, groins, thighs, and knees, coming on in paroxysms, and aggravated in the afternoon and at night, by contact and exercise,[215].—Crampy pains, with stiffness, in the hip and ham, especially on the left side,[215].—Paralytic tension, while walking, in the hip-joints, as if they were dislocated,[14].—Three or four violent shoots in the right hip, when at rest and in motion,[13a].— Heaviness in the thighs, even while sitting,[4].—Excessive heaviness and stiffness in the thighs while walking,[9].—[**2030.**] In walking, heaviness of the thighs and legs, with stiffness of the knee-joints (after twelve hours),[14]. —[Increased heaviness of the thigh and leg (with discharge of yellow mucus from the nose, with increased thirst)],[40] (Case 25).‡—At night, he felt a pain in a small spot on the left thigh, between the knee and trochanter, which changed to a burning-throbbing next day; on close examination, a slight erysipelatous redness was found, which, however, soon disappeared,[88].—Cramp pain in the glutæi muscles, with tension, on bending the body forwards,[14].—Paralytic drawing in the right thigh and leg,[7].—A pain drawing from within outwards on a small spot on the inner side of the left thigh (after one hour),[3].—A knife-stab in the middle of the thigh, more towards the posterior side, immediately after a meal,[3].—**Cutting shoots in the external muscles of the right thigh, just above the knee, only when sitting** (after two hours and a half),[5].—Cutting twitching-tearing in the posterior muscles of the left thigh when sitting (after three-quarters of an hour),[8].—Sore pain on the inner side of the thigh,[1].—[**2040.**] *Pain in the thighs* and legs, **as if they were bruised all over, and as if they were rotten; fine shooting and gnawing along the shafts of the bones, with violent tearing in the joints; the pain gradually rises from the tarsal joints to the hips, obliges him, while sitting, continually to move and shift the feet, and becomes milder when walking** (after four hours),[14].— The ischia feel sore; it seems to her as if she had no flesh on them; nevertheless she has more comfort in sitting on something hard than on a soft seat,[9].—Hard pressure in the middle of the anterior surface of the right thigh,[8].—A fluctuating throbbing pain in the upper and inner part of the left thigh (after twenty-nine hours),[3].—***Knees.*** A twitching in the bend of the right knee (after a quarter of an hour),[10].—A twitching in the bend of the knee, extending upwards into the muscles of the thigh,[1].—[*Tremor of the knees*],[59].—Violent pain in the knee,[13a].—Cramplike pain in the right knee, near the patella towards the outer side, when sitting,[8].—Cramp pain in both knee-joints, particularly about the patellæ; she could not walk upstairs,[219].—[**2050.**] Squeezing and pressing pain in the bend of the right

---

† See Ss. 1505, 1571.
‡ Only an aggravation of the symptoms she had before beginning Belladonna.

knee,[4].—In walking, the outer hamstring of the left knee-joint feels tight, and as if too short; it alternates with a similar sensation in the inner hamstring, but that in the outer one is more intense,[13].—Pressive shooting in the right patella, while sitting (after three and one-half hours),[5].—Dull shoots in the bend of the left knee (after a quarter of an hour),[3].—Prickings below the left patella, when sitting,[3].—Shooting tearing through the left knee, and a crawling on the left sole; at the same time tearing in left hand, in the upper third of the metacarpal bone of the little finger,[88].—Very rapid bubbling, as of water, in the forepart of the left knee, when sitting (immediately),[14].—Tingling-quivering sensation over the right knee when sitting (after a quarter of an hour),[8].—*Legs.* Nervous feeling in the legs, with inclination to keep them all the time in motion, especially at night in bed,[215].—After lying a short time (a quarter of an hour) felt a singular sensation in the legs, a kind of numbness crawling over the legs; right leg affected first,[230].—[2060.] Great weakness in the legs; lasting a long time (after half an hour),[109].—Paralytic lassitude in both legs below the knee ([14]) in going upstairs,[15a].—Tremulous heaviness of the legs,[4].—Heaviness, trembling, and paralytic weakness of the legs,[215].—Uncommon tension in the muscles of the leg, especially in the calf, where he also feels a sort of crawling,[88].—Sensation like a "growing pain" in the right leg, a feeling of stiffness combined with heaviness,[8].—Cramps in the legs,[215].—An oft-repeated sensation, as though he would be seized with a cramp in the calf,[88].—Drawing on the left tibia near the knee,[96].—Pressure in the forepart of the left tibia, when standing,[4].—[2070.] Tearing pressure in the middle of **the inside of the leg, uninfluenced by motion or contact,**[7].—Sharp shootings in the left calf, coming up from the lower part,[14].—Boring or tearing shoots in the tendo Achillis,[1].—Tearing pain in the tibia,[1].—Tearing in the left calf, frequently recurring,[88].—A burning-tearing in the leg upwards through the inner surface of the patella,[4].—Dull tearing in the legs,[4].—Drawing-tearing pain in the right tibia, with sensation of pressing asunder therein (after four hours),[8].—The slightest contact makes the legs feel as if they were being scratched,[215].—A sensation in the legs, drawing from below upwards, as of crawling externally, but internally as of innumerable shootings,[14].—[2080.] A sensation in the leg as if it were jammed, and a commotion (dull tearing) and stir therein, especially at night, relieved by letting the leg hang down (after ten hours),[1].—*Ankle, Foot, and Toes.* While walking in the open air, tension in the right tarsal joint,[1].—Swelling of the feet,[1].—Swelling of the feet, especially in the evening,[215].—When walking he raises up his feet as if he were stepping over a high obstacle,[233].—In walking, he lifts his feet as if he must step over things lying in his way; like a drunken person,[188 70].—Numbness of feet and legs,[231].—Occasional lassitude of the feet, with drawing pain therein,[1].—Sharp pain at the base of the first metatarsal bone of the right foot (after four hours),[217].—The foot was so painful that she had to keep the limb horizontally extended and immovable,[50].†—[2090.] Cutting-drawing at a small spot in the feet, which extends from below upwards, first through the legs and thighs, afterwards through the small of the back up to the shoulders,[9].—A sort of painless drawing or creeping from the heel to the toes, around the bones (after thirty hours),[1].—While walking or bending the foot together, pain in the metatarsal bones as if dislocated,[1].—Tearing pain in the metatarsal bone of the great toe,[1].—Dull shoots in the dorsum of the left

---

† In connection with S. 2898.

foot when sitting; external pressure does not affect them,[14].—When treading upon the left foot, painful shootings dart up to the knee (after thirty-
eight hours),[14].—Creeping in the feet from below upwards (after twenty
hours),[1].—Pain, as if bruised, in the ball of the heel, when treading on it,[1].
—A bubbling in the foot, as when water is dropped therein (after fifty-four
hours),[1].—Burning in the soles of the feet, as if he was walking on fire,[215].
—[2100.] Burning and digging in the soles of the feet,[9].—Tension in the
sole of the right foot, in the region of the heel, changing into a tensive
pressure; when pressing upon the part this pain disappears for some time
(after a quarter of an hour),[7].—Cramp in the sole of the foot, in the evening when in bed, when drawing up the knees,[1].—Boring, digging pain in
the soles of the feet (after several hours),[1].—Drawing pain in hollow of
right foot (after forty minutes),[217].—(While walking) tearing in the sole of
the left foot, with occasional shootings, for a quarter of an hour,[12].—Shooting pain in the soles of the feet (after half an hour),[1].

Generalities.—Objective. In bed, he lay on his belly, the head
bent backwards and the chin resting on the hand, without seeming to take
any notice of what was done or said in the room,[123].—The whole body was
swollen and red,[66].—Increased turgor of the whole body; burning heat of
the skin; extremely red face; hasty motion of the hands,[111].—[2110.] Death
ensued, and a universal gangrene through the whole body, which in a short
time became black throughout, and so flaccid that the cuticle adhered to
the surgeon's hands,[54].—Distension of the superficial veins of the body, with
insatiable thirst,[17].—[The head and the rest of the body drawn quite over
backwards towards the left side, so that he could not walk],[40] (Case 11)†.—
Sudden inflammations,[55].—Transitory inflammations (phlogoses), and rather
difficult breathing,[40] (Case 4).—Apoplectic condition (after epileptic convulsions),[74].—(After death, rapid septic change occurs),[1 54].—(Belladonna
appears to affect more powerfully the flexor surface and fibrous membranes; the left half of the body more than the right),[88].—All motions
are performed with great haste,[137].—All her motions and actions were unsteady and uncertain,[222].—[2120.] In most of the cases the power of the will
over the muscles was so far disordered that the muscular movements were
somewhat irregular, causing a kind of staggering or jerkings,[189].—The
whole body is in constant movement hither and thither, as in chorea,[19].—
Incessant movements of the body, especially of the arms,[19].—Muscles in
constant motion, partly alternate contractions of single muscles, partly automatic motions, startings of the limbs, biting motion, carphology,[226].—
Tremor,[46 25 30].—Spasmodic twitchings for some days (3 grains extract),[205].—
Subsultus tendinum,[32].—Subsultus tendinum and carphologia,[32].—When
the medicine has been given in gradually increasing doses there is subsultus; when a single large dose has been given convulsions occur,[177].—Five
or six times convulsive catchings of the extremities, face, and trunk, such,
he says, as animals have when bitten by venomous serpents (after five
hours),[188].—[2130.] Occasional jactitation,[83].—Frequent and almost uninterrupted spasmodic jactitations, sometimes so violent as to make it necessary to prevent him from being rolled, or partly thrown, out of bed. The
movements of the limbs were of a changing character, now simulating
chorea, now hysterica, and, after a little while, tetanus, even to opisthotonos,[206].—Convulsions,[30].—Strong convulsions and very loud ravings,[17].—
* *Convulsions; distortions of all the muscles,*[26 30 60 63].—The convulsion spread

over the whole body, and produced various frightful contortions (after six hours),[103].—*Repeated convulsions and horrible spasms, especially of the flexor muscles,[37].—*Violent convulsions; distortion of the limbs and eyes,[102].—Alternate strange distortions of the limbs, and complete immobility,[31].—Convulsions, with most ludicrous gestures, and whistling, singing, and crying, all together,[119].—[2140.] Frequent convulsions, often alternating with a throwing hither and thither of the extremities,[125].—The convulsions did not always appear in the same degree; they would alternately slacken, even stop for a time, and return again (after one hour),[112].—[After hiccough, slight convulsions of head and limbs, followed by nausea and lassitude],[40] (Case 14).—Excessive spasms, simulating true epilepsy,[37].—*Epileptic convulsions,[74].—Epileptiform spasms, without clenching of the thumbs,[215].—*Epileptic convulsions, followed by an apoplectic condition,[74].—Repeated convulsions and horrible spasms, especially of the flexor muscles,[37].—Tetanus, with curvature of the body backward or forward, and sometimes to one side,[215].—Inquietude,[19].—[2150.] *Great inquietude; she cannot remain seated long in one place; it drives her about,[9].—*Bodily inquietude; he was obliged constantly to move the whole body to and fro, and especially the hands and feet; he cannot stay long in any position; now he lies, now he sits, now he stands, so that he is always changing his posture in one way or another,[7].—Incessant movement of the body, especially of the arms, with unaltered pulse,[19].—Restless mien,[19].—[He walked round and round in a circle].—Extraordinary restlessness,[223].—Restlessness is a marked result of the action of Belladonna in massive doses,[194].—Great restlessness; the body is thrown now to one side, now to the other; now the chest is raised, and now the abdomen,[137].—Great restlessness, especially of the hands,[238].—Great restlessness; he throws his hands about; pulls at the covering, and searches with his fingers, as after insects (after five hours),[136].—[2160.] *Great restlessness; she beat about her with hands and feet, so that force had to be used to restrain her,[126].—Restlessness; every moment he wished to get out of bed, but would then fall back in great prostration,[105].—*Restlessness at night; grinding of the teeth, and now and then convulsions (after ten hours),[110].—Active movement here and there in bed,[19].—*Restless tossing about in bed,[140].—The boy throws himself about the bed, unconscious,[125].—Great restlessness; the girl threw herself about on the bed, with a sardonic smile,[102].—*Great restlessness; the boy wished to escape, and had to be kept on his couch by force; at the same time he developed a vigor and strength far beyond his age,[118].—Constant uneasiness and agitation; inability to sustain a conversation, or to stay in one place,[215].—Was generally restless and unmanageable, refusing to answer, or to swallow, or to be examined; appeared profoundly intoxicated (after one hour),[194].—[2170.] Restlessness, weariness, hypochondriac moroseness,[215].—He was restless in the extreme, and would not lie down for an instant; his hands were in constant motion; he seemed as if busy moving some light objects. Occasionally he raised his feet alternately some distance from the ground, as if ascending stairs. He moved his mouth incessantly, evidently with the idea that he was talking; but the sounds he uttered were inarticulate and altogether unintelligible,[186].—*Stiffness and Paralysis.* Stiffness of the whole body,[33].—General or partial spasmodic rigidity of the body,[215].—Stiffness of body, whereby the head is drawn backwards, and the body agitated by single jerks, like electric shocks,[140].—On getting up and attempting to stand, felt paralyzed; could walk with difficulty,[230].—[Paralysis, now in one, now in another part],[4]

(Case 11).†—[The left side, especially the arm, is completely paralyzed],"
(Case 11).†—One hour after he had lost the power of articulation, and
presented the general appearance of a person seized with slight paralysis.
He was quite unable to stand or walk, and his limbs were in a state of
tremor and agitation. He became cold, and nearly approaching a state of
insensibility; the eyes had a wild, vacant appearance; the respiration was
laborious and occasionally stertorous. After three hours more the temperature of the body had increased, face swollen, and insensibility more complete.
No active delirium was manifested, but from the general appearance of the
eye and features, no doubt that peculiar derangement existed, subdued
partially by the pressure on-the cerebral organ, so as more nearly to approach the character of apoplexy. He died seventeen hours after taking
the poison. The post-mortem examination showed the presence of great
congestion of the brain, particularly at the base, and of the medulla ob-
longata, together with considerable (serous?) effusion,[191].—*Debility and
Faintness.* Languor and apathy,[215].—[2180.] Lassitude of mind and
body,[7].—Lassitude, indolence, aversion to all exercise and occupation,[215].—
Previous to the catamenia, lassitude, colic, want of appetite, and dimness
of sight,[60] (Case 17).—Feeling of weariness for an hour or two in the afternoon (first day),[218].—Failure of strength,[74].—Failure of strength; great
weakness,[1 74 79].—He falls down without being able to raise himself,[233].—All
her strength goes in an instant,[219].—Weakness,[240].—General debility,[236].—
[2190.] Weakness of the body,[79].—Muscular weakness, almost bordering
on paralysis,[91].—Paralytic weakness of all the muscles, especially of the
feet,[1].—So weak that he could not walk in a room without leaning against
the wall,[237].—General weakness, and such prostration that the girl could
scarcely stand,[102].—Frequently recurring short attacks of great weakness;
she feels as if too heavy, and as if drawn down, so that she would sink together,[2].—Great weakness of the left side, numbness of the left face and
arm, and a prickling sensation in the same parts (from application of the
extract to the forehead),[204].—Weakness, with tottering gait; the knees feel
as if they would give way; he cannot walk,[1].—General feeling of weakness, like a threatening faint, and inability to stand upright,[124].—General
weakness, sick feeling, and apathy,[91].—[2200.] State of prostration (after
six hours),[239].—Great prostration,[25].—Great prostration, with internal burn-
ings,[23].—Prostration of strength, with nervousness,[215].—Fainting fits,[215].—
Attacks of faintness,[40].‡—Attacks of syncope,[224].—*General Sensibility.* Exaltation of the general sensibility, with cheerfulness and agree-
ableness,[91].—*Great irritability and impressionableness of the senses; he
tastes and smells everything more acutely; the sense of taste, of sight,
and of hearing is keener, and the mind is more easily moved, and the
thoughts more active* (after three hours),[1 194].—*Excessive nervous excitability, with exalted sensibility of all the organs; the least noise, the
least light is annoying,*[215].—[2210.] If touched by any person, she jumped
as if in great alarm. This I observed to occur whenever her hair was removed from her face, or when I felt her pulse (after eleven hours),[185].—
Painful sensitiveness of the skin to all contact,[9].—[Excessive sensitiveness to
the cold air],[66] —Complete anæsthesia of the whole body for several days
(after a quarter of an hour),[86].—Upon recovering perfect consciousness
(after thirty hours), a remarkable numbness, extending over all parts of
the trunk and extremities, attracted attention, and persisted for several

days. No pain could be excited while this condition continued, by forcibly pinching the skin of the forehead, or of other parts; and although an unusual sensation was perceived by the patient at the moment, he could not with his eyes averted from the operation point out the precise spot subjected to compression,[185].—*General Sensations. His senses deceive him*,[15].—Pains in all the joints, and a peculiar feeling as if these pains, with a cold sensation, continued to gnaw as far as the tips of the fingers and toes,[119].—In the evening she attempted to stretch herself, but was unable to do so for pain,[9].—On turning in bed, whole system began to feel bad,[230].—Ordinarily, when a pain had reached its highest degree, it disappeared suddenly, and instantly there arose in its stead a pain in some other place,[x].—[2220,] Frequent cramps on the right side of the body, from the clavicle to the region of the spleen,[215].—Cramps and weakness, with ebullition of blood in the. head,[215].—Boring pain in the glands,[1].—Digging pains in the joints, and burning pains in the bones, with great weakness,[215].—(The parts where the shooting pain had been were extremely tender to touch),[x].—Palpitation and tickling in the muscles,[215].—*A beating of the arteries of the head and of all parts of the body, in the morning on waking*,[9].—She was much annoyed by a constant sensation of trembling in all the muscles of the body,[46 185].

Skin.—General Appearance. Cold, painful, long-lasting nodosities and swellings (seemingly a secondary effect),[1].—Distension of the cutaneous veins,[4].—[2230.] Skin appeared white like a statue (unnatural),[230].—Yellowish color of the skin,[215].—*Swelling, heat, and redness of the skin*,[215].—Inflammation of the surface of the whole body,[67].—The affected parts are much disposed to take on a phlegmonous, erysipelatous, and gangrenous character,[215].—Erysipelatous inflammation, which appears, disappears and returns frequently on the face, and sometimes on the chest and nipples,[215].—*Redness of the whole body* ([90]), *with quick pulse*,[20].—*Redness of the whole body, with quick pulse*,[20].—The skin red; superficial veins swollen,[135].—Skin red, with only slight fever,[190].—[2240.] Face, chest, and extremities extremely red,[125].—[Redness and swelling of the affected portions],[65].—In the girl, general scarlet redness,[233].—*Redness, like scarlatina, of the entire surface of the body* (after six hours),[239].—*Scarlet redness of the surface of the whole body, especially of the face, with marked action of the brain*,[71].—*A scarlet redness suddenly spread over the body, especially the face and limbs, with which appeared heat and exaltation of all the faculties;* still without thirst,[134].—Scarlet suffusion of the skin in young children and those who have a delicate skin. Generally, nothing more than a temporary blush, but in rare cases, and in persons who are liable to vascular irritation of the skin, the redness remains, and its disappearance is attended with slight roughness and desquamation,[8].—*Scarlet redness of skin of face and neck, followed, on the second day, by peeling off of the cuticle*,[202].—Scarlet redness of the face and chest during sleep,[65].—Blotches and growths on the skin, like sugillations, ecchymoses, and boils,[215].—[2250.] *Inflamed red patches of the skin, and irregularly-shaped scarlet spots over the body* (after sixteen hours),[1].—Spots and red pimples at the nape of the neck and back,[215].—[Blood-red spots over the whole body, especially in the face, on the throat, and chest],[65].—The skin of the whole body, especially the chest. is spotted scarlet, without heat of the head, or increased temperature of the body,[106].—Dark-red scarlet spots over the whole body, with small, quick pulse, tightness of the chest, an existing cough much increased in violence, delirium, excited memory, rubbing of the nose, and dilated pupils,[90].—Chest and belly are covered with small, red, somewhat elevated, painless spots, frequently disappearing, and then suddenly reappearing, with general redness of the skin,[14].—The chest and thighs are sprinkled over with very small dark-red spots, of irregular shape and size,[40] (Case 19).—The backs of both hands are covered with small red spots, which disappear again speedily,[14].—Dark-red spots on the face, resembling those of scarlet fever, with full pulse,[80].—The skin is rough, and chaps easily,[215].—[2260.] Skin very easily wounded; it seems to be burned and excoriated by contact with the lightest garment,[215].—*Eruptions, Dry.* Small, hard, subcutaneous tumors,[215].—A great many comedones or black pores in the skin,[215].— *Erythema of skin,*[140].—Erythema and burning itching of the vulva,[215].— [*Red, scaly eruption on the lower parts of the body as far as the abdomen*],[81]. —*Scarlet eruption* (first day),[85].—*Eruption like scarlatina all over face and body* (after six hours),[239].—*The eruption, which recalls closely enough that which characterizes scarlatina, has been noticed by numerous observers,*[203].— * The face, upper extremities, and trunk exhibited a diffuse scarlet efflorescence, studded with innumerable papillæ, very closely resembling the rash of scarlatina. The eruption terminated abruptly at the wrists and flexure of the thighs, the rest of the body retaining the natural color. The skin was hot and dry,*[177]. —[2270.] Scarlatina-like eruption on the face and neck, not on the trunk or extremities,[224].—Scarlet eruption on the arms and legs (in several cases),[189]. —Cutaneous eruption resembling measles,[20].—*Eruptions like roseola and scarlatina, with fever, sore throat, cough, headache, etc.,*[215].—Red or whitish miliary eruptions, like nettle-rash, with burning itching,[215].—Miliary and measly eruptions, as also pustules, as of small-pox, on the face,[215].—Papular eruption resembling *lichen agrius*, especially on the hands,[215].—Papular eruption on face, and furuncles,[91].—Small, pale-red papules in the corners of the mouth, with sensibility; they soon disappear without suppurating,[7]. —Red, burning, and very obstinate pimples, especially on the forehead,[215]. —[2280.] Pimples and ulcers on the lips,[215].—A white-tipped pimple under the left wing of the nose, without pain,[1].—Small, red, and very burning pimples on the tip of the nose,[215].—Small, intensely itching pimples on the legs,[215].—At the root of the nose, two small red elevations, which feel painful, as if subcutaneously ulcerated, only when touched (after sixteen days),[14]. —*Moist, Pustular, and Ulcerated.* Blisters, as from burns, on various parts of the body,[215].—Blister on the finger, with painful inflammations,[50].—Eruption on the skin of bullæ, which emit a quantity of limpid or creamy lymph; and therewith such intense pain that the patient, though unaccustomed to suffering, cannot refrain from lamentations and tears. When on the foot, it is so painful that she has to keep the limb horizontally extended and motionless,[50].—Bullæ, which easily burst open, on the palmar surface of the foot, and on the tibia,[50].—[Painful boils on the sternum],[50].† —[2290.] Boil upon the shoulder,[1].—Boils on the calves and thighs,[215].— Pustules and some small ulcers,[238].—Pustulous pimples, with swelling and redness of the surrounding parts,[215].—Small, red, painless pustules appear on the temple, at the right corner of the mouth, and on the chin; when scratched, bloody serum exudes (after thirteen hours),[11].—On the skin of the face a slight pimply exanthema broke out, which suppurated slowly, and dried up in a few days,[195].—Pustules at the borders of the lips, with smarting pain,[14].—A small pustule on the upper lip, with creeping sensation while untouched, but contact produces an itching shooting therein,[1]—

---

† Probably the effect of long-continued wet dressings on the mamma.

Pustules break out on the cheek and nose, which rapidly fill with pus become covered with a crust,[1].—Pustules appear on the nape of the neck and on the arms, quickly fill with pus, and become covered with a crust,[1]. —[2300.] The back, especially in the scapular region, is covered with large red pustules; the whole skin looks red, and smarts as if sore when touched, but in the tips of the pustules there is fine shooting (after ten days),[14].—[A pustule breaking out close to the nail of the right index finger, and emitting a quantity of humor],[40] (Case 15).—Eruption like small-pox, with tendency to invade the brain and mucous membranes,[215].—Herpes and pustules, especially on the face, ulcerating and bleeding easily,[215].—Burning ulcers, which bleed very easily,[215].—Ulcers and crusts on the pinnæ of the ears,[215].—Painful ulceration on the side of the nostrils where the latter unite with the upper lip,[1].—The nostrils and the corners of the lips are ulcerated, but neither itch nor pain,[1].—In the corner of the mouth an ulcer with red edges and corrosive itching,[1].—Corners of the mouth ulcerate, just at the commissure of the lips, with uncommonly severe tearing pains roundabout, even when unmoved and untouched,[1].—**Sensations.** [2310.] Sensation of pinching in a great many places on the skin,[215].—[Prickling biting sensation in the whole skin, especially on the soles of the feet],[65].— Pleasant prickling, as of worms, in all the pores of the skin,[214].—In the evening in bed, itching prickings, like flea-bites, here and there on the skin,[1].—Itching stinging on the scapulæ, inducing him to scratch, whereby it is relieved,[14].—Sensations of formication,[40] (Case 14).—Intolerable itching of the whole body,[215].—[Itching in the whole body, and an eruption of red spots like flea-bites] (after four hours),[65].—Crawling itching over the whole body, fugitive, now here, now there,[14].—Tearing itching here and there, especially after lying down at night in bed; after rubbing, there only remains tearing pain, but this in a greater degree,[1].—[2320.] Frequent scratching of various parts of the body, especially the neck and chest,[226].— Scraping itching of the forehead (after one hour),[14].—(A titillating itching on the left scapula),[10].—During the first few days, occasional creeping-itching of the skin of the legs and back,[230].—Violent itching of the feet,[1].—Biting itching in the feet and their dorsa,[4].—A creeping upwards in the left arm, as when a fly walks along the skin, which frequent rubbing does not remove,[1].

Sleep and Dreams.—Sleepiness. Frequent yawning,[30].—Frequent yawning, as if he had not slept enough (after two hours and a half),[11]. —Frequent yawning, and then shiverings over the body, but which only course along the external surface of the skin, in the evening,[2].—[2330.] Continual yawning,[102].—Yawning like that of an intoxicated person,[55].— [He yawned and retched until the face was blue; while one hand was stretched above the head, the other, unmanageable, kept striking the abdomen],[40] (Case 13).—During the catamenia, yawning and chills coursing along the back,[40] (Case 14).—*Great inclination to sleep,*[114] [130].—Drowsiness (after half an hour),[1].—Drowsiness (after about four hours and a half),[239]. —Great drowsiness,[230].—Notable drowsiness immediately on waking,[3].— Invincible drowsiness, especially towards evening; he falls asleep in spite of himself, wherever he happens to be,[215].—[2340.] Towards evening, even at twilight, drowsiness with yawning; but in the morning he feels as if he had not slept enough,[1].—Uncommon drowsiness and dulness of intellect,[195]. —Drowsiness, often with vertigo and yawning,[215].—Continued drowsiness, with desire to stretch the limbs, from 5 to 11 P.M. (after eleven hours),[12].— Drowsiness full of inquietude,[55].—Drowsiness or comatose sleep, with starting awake full of terror,[215].—Sleepiness; the girl closed her eyes for several seconds, then slowly half-opened them again, as if forcibly resisting sleep (after four hours),[124].—In the morning after rising, uncommon sleepiness, although he had slept well during the night; also, on attempting to read, the letters run together,[89].—Somnolent condition,[42].—Great somnolence,[70]. —[2350.] [*Quite profound somnolency, with subsultus tendinum, pale, cold face and cold hands, and hard, small, rapid pulse*],[56].—Slumber,[67].—Lethargic slumber,[215].—Fit of profound lethargic slumber, with cold face and hands,[215]. —The night sleep was quiet and unbroken, with pleasant dreams,[129].—In the morning he is unable to rouse himself from sleep; on awaking he is very much out of humor,[14].—In some of the patients the delirium subsided into a sort of sleep, attended with pleasant dreams, which provoked laughter,[189].—Sleep at night, with dreams which he cannot remember; he fell asleep earlier than usual, and awoke earlier not unrefreshed, but soon relapsed into the lassitude of the limbs continually present at other times,[3]. —Profound sleep,[28].—Deep sleep for twenty-four hours,[79].—[2360.] Very deep sleep,[1].—Very sound sleep with much dreaming, until towards morning (after five days),[4].—She sleeps much, and if the cough awake her she falls asleep again directly, and yet in the morning she is giddy and tired,[9]. —Heavy sleep, with starts and jerks of the limbs, cries, singing, complaints, etc.,[215].—Soporose condition,[42].—Soporose, stupid condition, from which the child could not be wakened, with convulsions of the facial muscles,[110].— Sopor (after the convulsions),[236].—They lay in a soporose condition, with violent convulsions of the extremities; the head was very hot, the face red, the eyes protruding,[186].—Sopor, coma, or lethargy usually follows the delirium; and sometimes the delirium returns as the sopor goes off,[197].—It is only after moderate medicinal doses that we witness soporific effects; after larger doses, insomnia and delirium occur,[5].—[2370.] Croaking and moaning in sleep,[1].—During his stupefied sleep, he opens his eyes, looks about him wildly, and relapses into stertorous slumber,[17].—During sleep, tendency to bury the head in the pillow, and draw up the legs,[215].—After a good night's sleep, the boy awoke early, looked wild and staring, and his lower extremities were as if paralyzed, so that he could neither stand nor walk,[116].—On waking, fatigue, headache, and aggravation of all the pains,[215]. —*Sleeplessness.* *He starts up as in affright, and awakes,[4].—*He starts as in affright and awakes, when he is just falling asleep,[1].—*In the evening, frequent starting as in affright, when just on the point of falling asleep; *the feet were jerked upwards and the head forwards*,[14].—*She started as in affright, in otherwise quiet sleep, feeling as if she were falling deep down, which caused her to shudder violently,[13a].—Heavy, disturbed sleep, with stertorous respiration,[230].—[2380.] Sleep very light,[10].—*Sleep restless,[218].—*Very restless sleep,[89].—Wakeful from restlessness,[240].—*At night, the boys became restless, spoke irrationally, and could with difficulty be kept in bed,[118].—With restlessness, he woke from the noon sleep, screamed, and stamped his feet,[125].—*Restless sleep, with active dreams,[91].— *Sleep restless, disturbed by dreams and irrational talking,[130].—Uneasy sleep before midnight; the child tosses about, kicks, and quarrels in its sleep,[1]. —[He rises at night, and walks up and down in deep thought],[40] (Case 18). —[2390.] Frequent awaking at night out of sleep, as if he had slept enough (first night),[11].—Frequent awaking out of sleep, and though he turns now on this side and now on that, still he finds no rest, and cannot fall asleep again,[11].—Waking up too early, often with inability to go to sleep again,[215].—*She awakes in the night full of fright and fear; it appeared to her as if there was something under the bed which made a noise; she felt *dry heat on awaking*,[1].—Waking directly after midnight in a sweat, he cannot go to sleep again; and the sweat continues during the waking hours,[1]. —He wakes out of sleep three times about midnight; he raises himself three times to vomit, with cold sweat as from anguish, but in vain,[1].—*Continual but ineffectual efforts to obtain sleep*,[37].—*Sleeplessness*,[1.47.188].—Sleeplessness for several days,[47].—Sleeplessness for several nights,[238].—[2400.] Sleepless until 1 o'clock, not restless; then slept till 6.30 A.M.; rose unrefreshed,[218]. —Nightly sleeplessness, with restlessness and agitation,[215].—Sleep prevented by anguish,[1].—Nightly sleeplessness owing to anguish, with drawing pains in all the limbs,[1].—He cannot sleep at night; a fancy that he has some pressing business hinders him from sleeping,[1].—*Dreams.* He dreams immediately on falling asleep,[1].—Slept well, except dreaming,[218].—She dreams more than usual, but peacefully, and about household affairs,[13a].— Vivid dreams, which, however, he could not remember,[11].—Sleep full of dreams; she was occupied with a great number of people; she wished to get away, but could not,[9].—[2410.] Dreams of performing gymnastic exercises, of walking, running, and riding in a carriage,[215].—He had every night dreams which much fatigued his mind, and was prostrated in the morning when he ought to have got up,[13].—*Anxious and frightful dreams*,[215]. —[*He is constantly awaked out of sleep by fearful dreams and convulsions*],[81]. —He is disturbed by frightful visions when falling asleep,[215].—Frightful dreams vividly remembered,[1].—Fright in dreaming, in consequence of which he awakes with sweat on the forehead and at the pit of the stomach,[1]. —He was constantly awaked out of sleep by frightful dreams and convulsions,[81].—Sleep intolerable, on account of greatly increased pains and frightful dreams,[1].—He dreams of danger from fire, and awakes in consequence,[1].—[2420.] Dreams of battles, fires, and of being pursued by giants,[215].—At night, very stupefied sleep, anxious dreams about murderers and street-robbers; he heard himself shouting loudly once, but did not thereupon come to his senses,[12].—Sleep disturbed by miserable phantoms,[185].

Fever.—Chilliness. Temperature of the skin very low,[225].—Skin at first natural, afterwards cold,[230].—On the emission of a great quantity of urine, and during increased appetite, he was quite cold to the touch,[40].— Coldness of the whole body,[236].—General intense cold, or cold accompanied with partial heat, often with nausea, flow of urine, dimness of sight, drawing and pains in the limbs,[215].—Immediately after meals, excessive coldness, with gnashing of the teeth, and trembling of the limbs while lying. He soon fell asleep; on waking, was moderately warm, had dilated pupils, and eyes shining, protruding, as if swimming in tears; redness of the face,[89].— Hands and feet cold,[235].—[2430.] Hands and feet become very cold,[219].— At times, coldness of the hands, with otherwise normal temperature of the skin,[118].—Quickly passing feeling of coldness in the right hip-joint (after one hour),[14].—The lower extremities are cold and rigid, without being lame,[129]. —*Feet ice-cold; can scarcely be warmed* (after one hour),[98].—Cold feet, with bloated, red face, and flow of blood to the head,[1].—Chilliness,[60].—Chilliness and shuddering, with goose-skin, even near to the warm stove (after one hour),[12].—Chilliness, especially in the arms, with goose-flesh, in undressing; at the same time, redness and heat of the ears and nose,[1].—Febrile chilliness, with fine shooting pains in the chest,[40] (Case 11).†—[2440.] A violent chill seizes her in the back or scrobiculus cordis, or in both arms at the same time, and spreads itself from thence all over the body,[2].—Unusual chill after bathing,[214].—Shuddering during stool,[1].—Slight shuddering, with obscuration of vision, immediately after noon,[40] (Case 1).—The body, at first cold, became warm (after four hours),[233].—Heat of the skin alternating with chills, but without fever,[215].—Fever, with alternate coldness and heat, or shivering followed by heat, especially in the afternoon and at night, once or twice a day, or every two days,[215].—Fever; febrile chill in the morning, followed by slight heat,[40].—Fever; shivering over the body in the afternoon, flushes of heat,[4].—Fever; sudden alternations of heat and chill both without thirst, with sleepiness in the daytime (after twelve hours),[14].— [2450.] Attacks of fever *frequently recurring during the day;* the shaking chills are followed by general heat and sweat over the whole body, without thirst either in the cold or the hot stage,[1].—*Several attacks of fever in one day, during which the hot stage followed the cold within a few minutes to half an hour a^er, always without thirst in either stage, and mostly with confusion of the head,*[7].—Towards evening, fever; convulsive shuddering lifts him up in his bed; two hours after, heat and general sweat, without thirst either during the shuddering or the heat,[1].—Fever; thrills of chilliness running over the whole body (after one hour); four hours after, feeling of heat, and actual heat, especially in the face,[7].—Fever; at night febrile chill, succeeded quickly by heat of body, with frequent micturition and lassitude of the limbs; on the following night two attacks of the same kind, with vertigo and thirst,[40] (Case 1).—Fever; chill in the evening in bed, then heat; the chill commenced in the sacrum, spread itself over the back, and down again over the thighs,[9].—Fever; in the evening while she was undressing, slight chilliness over the body, then heat in the whole of the left side of the body,[1].—Fever; during the external coldness of the body, an internal burning heat,[1].—Head sometimes ice cold, sometimes burning hot,[215].— *Temperature of the head very much increased, *of the rest of the body diminished,*[220].—[2460.] Face hot, extremities cold,[224].—**Heat.** Skin hot,[223]. —Burning skin,[222].—*The body burning hot like fire,* with bluish redness of skin,[127].—*The skin hot, dry, scarlet, especially intense on the face and ears,*[137].—*Temperature of skin very much raised; skin scarlet,* especially on the face and anterior half of trunk (after half an hour),[136].—*Temperature of skin increased, face red, pulse accelerated, with senseless talking, and tottering about as if drunk,*[105 132].—Febrile disturbances,[67 81].—[Febrile symptoms every other day],[65].—Fever after each dose,[51].—[2470.] Morning after taking, had fever without thirst,[230].—[*Burning fever (synocha),* (after twelve hours)],[26].—Evening fever,[41].†—Fever, with phantasies; the boy talked about criminals whom he seemed to see; hearing seemed dull,[125].—Intense, erysipelatous fever, accompanied with inflamed swellings, passing even into gangrene,[1].—(Fever; first putrid taste in the mouth, then heat of the face and hands; the pain increases after the disappearance of the heat),[1].— *Violent heat,*[63].—*Burning heat,*[31].—**Burning heat within and without,**[73]. —*Internal burning,*[23].—[2480.] Burning heat; the distended veins lie like cords on the skin, with loud delirium and violent twitchings (after half an hour),[108].—*Burning heat of the body, with extreme distension of the superficial bloodvessels, and furious delirium,*[17].—*Burning heat over the whole body; skin universally red; pulse full, quick, and extremely frequent,*[119].—Dry, burning heat, generally with swelling of the veins, strong pulsations of the arteries, redness and puffiness of the face, intense thirst, especially for cold water, restlessness, delirium, foolish behavior, frenzy, impulse to beat and

---

† Not found.

kill,[215].—Burning heat in the brain, and simultaneously in the soles of the feet,[215].—Burning in head, palate, and fauces; feet ice-cold,[195].—Burning heat over the face, without thirst (after ten hours),[11].—Sensation of burning heat in the whole face, without redness of cheeks or thirst, with moderately warm body and cold feet (after four hours),[8].—[Every day, after the midday meal, great heat of the body, especially of the head, so that the face from time to time is very red],[40] (Case 12).—After drinking beer, internal heat,[14].—[2490.] Great heat and redness of the cheeks,[20].—Heat all over the body, with bluish redness of the whole surface,[80].—*Great heat, distension of the superficial veins of the body, and insatiable thirst,[17].—*Excessive heat, distended veins, insatiable thirst, with anxiety and trembling (after half an hour),[109].—Heat in the head, externally perceptible (after a quarter of an hour),[13a].—*Heat and redness of the head only,[1].—*Heat and pulsation in the head, with burning of the eyes,[215].—*The head and face hot, the latter somewhat puffy,[238].—*Head hot; face red; eyes protruding; pupils dilated, look staring,[134].—Every day, for twelve days, about noon, sudden heat of head and redness of face, with considerable obstruction of vision and great thirst, lasting an hour,[40] (Case 14).—[2500.] Heat of the head alternating with diarrhœa,[40] (Case 14).—Sensation of creeping heat in the face under the skin (after a quarter of an hour),[14].—Sensation of heat in the face without external redness,[14].—Heat in the face the whole day, as if wine had driven the blood to the head (after twelve hours),[1].—On the face, such an increase of heat that it actually glowed, became brownish-red, and turgid,[195].—Heat and throbbing in the face, with congestion to the head,[215].—Great internal heat about the region of the stomach,[42].—General dry heat in the extremities of the feet and hands, with thirstlessness and paleness of the face, lasting twelve hours,[1].—(In the evening, heat in the hands and feet, but not in the arms and thighs),[1].—Heat, especially in the feet,[1].—[2510.] Great heat (immediately), followed by very profuse sweat,[40] (Case 25).—Great heat of the body; exceedingly violent and rapid pulsations of the arteries, especially in the temporal region, with confusion of the head and subsequent profuse sweat,[40] (Case 24). —Heat from below upwards; a sweat as of anguish breaking out upon her, followed by nausea, with terrible anxiety, the sense of nausea descending lower and lower,[9].—The skin is burning hot, and partially covered with sweat (after one hour),[112].—*Sensation of heat, with actual heat in the whole body, but particularly in the face, which was red and covered with sweat, with confusion of the head (after four hours),[7].—*Sweat*. The general effects of Belladonna on the circulation predispose to sweating,[194]. —Increased transpiration,[91].—Sweat (after some hours),[15].—General sweat, suddenly occurring and as quickly disappearing,[13].—Perspiration which stains the linen yellow,[215].—[2520.] Copious sweat,[219].—Profuse sweat,[40] (Case 6).—[Very profuse, long-continued sweat, staining the linen dark],[40] (Case 13).—Profuse sweat, especially at night,[40].—Profuse night-sweat which does not weaken,[15].—Profuse sweat at night, sometimes only on covered parts,[215].—Profuse sweat, with diuresis,[81 40] (Cases 21 and 22).—Profuse cold sweat of the hands,[1].—Violent sweating every night,[40].—Sweat in the morning,[81].—[2530.] [Sweat all over from four in the afternoon till midnight, then sleep while sweating],[65].—Night-sweat ([4]), which smells like something burnt,[1].—He sweats over the whole body at the least exercise, mostly on the face, down the nose. While walking in a strong wind, and so sweating, colic is induced,[1].—Sweat during the sleep,[20].—[Sweat over the whole body during sleep],[65].—The hair is very often moist with perspiration,[215].—Frequent and profuse perspiration of the face,[215].—Cold sweat on the face, especially after eating,[215].—(Fever; after the chill felt quite well for a few hours, then sweating in the face, hands (?), and feet (?) before the heat came on; no sleep during the hot stage; slight headache with the sweat in the face, but none in the cold stage or in the hot),[1].—Sweat of the feet, without warmth, in sitting,[4].—[2540.] Sweating of the genital organs in the night,[1].—Skin of the whole body remarkably dry,[226].—Skin dry and insensible (after six hours),[239].—Skin dry and burning (after six hours),[239]. —The skin was dry and burning, and the pulse small, wiry, hard, and extremely frequent,[25].

Conditions.—**Aggravation.**—(*Morning*), When getting up, vertigo; on rising, head heavy; early, headache; early, soon after waking, pain under frontal eminences; soon after waking, on rising, pain under frontal eminences; early, on waking, headache above eyes; in about a quarter of an hour after rising, and after stirring about, side of head ached; white of eye streaked with red, etc.; darkness before eyes; on going out, black points, etc., before eyes; immediately after waking, fluttering, etc., before the ears; bleeding of the nose; on waking, epistaxis, etc.; tongue feels asleep, etc.; **on waking, slimy mouth**; bad smell from mouth; after rising, *mucus in mouth;* loss of appetite, etc.; in bed, cutting in belly; pressing towards generative organs, etc.; immediately after getting out of bed, pain in hypogastrium; frequent micturition, etc.; in bed and after rising, phlegm; when coughing, expectoration of bloody mucus; when turning head to and fro, stiffness between scapulæ, etc.; beating of arteries of head, etc.; after rising, sleepiness, etc.; febrile chill; sweat.—(*Forenoon*), Attacks of nausea.—(*About noon*), Cough, etc.—(*Noon*), Squeezing together in umbilical region.—(*Afternoon*), Pains in general; anxiety, etc.; while walking in open air, sensation of heat blowing against eyes; vomiting of mucus; squeezing together in umbilical region; cough; shortness of breath; after drinking coffee, shortness of breath; pains in hips, etc.; feeling of weariness; shuddering, etc.; fever; shivering.—(*Towards evening*), Stitches in chest; drowsiness, etc.; fever, etc.—(*Evening*), Violent delirium; speech incoherent; lively, etc.; mirthful mood; headache; stitches through head; stitches in occiput; in bed, on reading, letters run together; attacks of deafness; face bluish-red, etc.; after lying down, toothache; toothache; accumulation of water in the mouth; sour taste of bread, etc.; astonishing thirst; nausea, etc.; vomiting; pinching in abdomen, etc.; a few hours before going to bed, cutting in abdomen; feeling of fulness in hypogastric zone, etc.; before falling asleep in bed, tearing in spermatic cord; sexual desire; after lying down in bed, tickling, etc., in larynx; about 10 o'clock, cough commences; in bed, constriction, etc., in chest; in bed, oppression of chest, etc.; drawing along the spine; swelling of feet; in bed, when drawing up knees, cramp in sole of foot; in bed, itching pricking on the skin; yawning, etc.; in bed, chill, etc.; while undressing, slight chilliness, etc.; heat in hands.—(*Night*), Pains in general; tries to bite those about him; claps hands together over the head, etc.; delirium; ravings; anxiety, etc.; loss of consciousness, etc.; on turning in bed, vertigo; in bed, epistaxis, etc.; toothache; **drawing in upper teeth**; toothache; hiccough, etc.; vomiting; burning in bladder, etc.; pressing in vesical region; diuresis; in bed, *cough;* shortness of breath, etc.; intermittent breathing; pains in hips, etc.; pain in thigh; in bed, nervous feeling in legs; sensation in leg as if jammed; *restlessness,* etc.; in bed, after lying down, itching; fever; febrile chill, etc.; *profuse sweat;* sweat of the genitals; 5 to

11 P.M., drowsiness, etc.; 4 P.M. till midnight, sweat all over.—(*Before midnight*), Uneasy sleep.—(*About midnight*), Hiccough ; wakes three times, etc. —(*After midnight*), Tearing in the teeth.—(*Every other day*), Febrile symptoms.—(*In open air*), Pains in head ; bursting sensation in head ; pain in forehead ; toothache.—(*On admission of open air*), Pain in teeth.—(*Walking in open air*), Anguish, etc.; pressure in brain ; weakness of vision ; disposition to vomit ; itching at the anus ; tension in tarsal joints.—(*On ascending stairs*), Shocks, etc., in head ; heart clucks ; lassitude in legs.—(*On ascending stairs rapidly*), **Jerking headache.**—(*After bathing*), Unusual chill.—(*After drinking beer*), Internal heat.—(*Bending forwards*), Shooting in frontal eminence.—(*Bending head backwards*), Pain in neck.—(*Bending upper part of body to left side*), Pinching in abdomen.—(*When bending feet together*), Pain in metatarsal bones.—(*In biting anything*), Teeth painful.— (*Blowing nose*), Offensive smell in nose.—(*After breakfast*), Squeamishness. —(*Cold air*), Pains in face.—(*Cold bathing*), Pains in general.—(*Contact*), Pains in general ; pains in head ; toothache ; pains in hips, etc.; itching-shooting in pustule on lip.—(*Contact with air or food*), Pain in lower teeth, etc. —(*Contradiction*), Pains in general.—(*Coughing*), Pain in head ; stitches in sternum ; much straining, etc.—(*When crying*), Hoarseness.—(*During deglutition*), **Tearing in corner of jaw** ; shootings in pharynx, etc.—(*Descending a hill*), Sensation in joints of lower extremities.—(*After dinner*), Headache ; when at rest, pain in side of head ; præcordial anxiety.—(*Drawing oneself in*), Pinching in abdomen.—(*After eating*), Toothache ; putrid taste in mouth ; pinching below umbilicus ; pain under larynx ; cough, etc.; cold sweat on face.—(*Exercise*), Pains in hips, etc.—(*Exertion*), Pains in general ; pains in head.—(*During expiration*), Shooting in cartilages of ribs.—(*When feeling side of neck*), Shootings in pharynx, etc.—(*When grasping*), During chill, shootings in finger-tips.—(*Great heat*), Pains in general.—(*In bright light*), Weakness of vision.—(*After a meal*), As if drunk ; in a few minutes, toothache ; bitter eructations ; vomiting of food ; immediately, stab in the thigh ; coldness, etc.—(*During midday meal*), Spasm of the stomach. —(*After midday meal*), Every day, heat of body.—(*Before menses*), Uterine colic, etc.; sexual desire ; lassitude, etc.—(*During menses*), Anxiety ; thirst ; fever, etc.; præcordial anxiety ; tearing in back, etc.; yawning, etc. —(*During mental occupation*), Toothache.—(*After drinking milk*), Vomiting; colic.—(*Motion*), **Confusion of head** ; vertigo ; headache ; pains in head ; **pain in forehead** ; *pain in right vertex ;* swelling on cheek ; between acts of micturition, shootings in urethra ; stitches in chest ; palpitation, etc.; trembling of arms.—(*After a confined motion*), Distension of the abdomen, etc.—(*Moving eyes*), Pains in head ; *sparks before eyes.*—(*Noise*), Pains in head.—(*Change of position*), Vertigo,—(*Pressure*), Headache in vertex.—(*Light pressure*), Throbbing in forearm, etc.—(*Pressure on epigastrium*), Pain as if hypochondria were being pressed out.—(*Too prolonged repose*), Pains in general.—(*On rising*), Pain in forehead returns.—(*Rising from seat*), Pain in crests of ilia.—(*Sitting*), Reeling sensation in head ; humming, etc., in ears ; stiffness in back ; **shoots in muscles of thigh** ; pain in knee ; shooting in patella ; prickings below patella ; bubbling in knee. —(*Sitting bent*), *Pressing-out feeling in groin ;* pressing towards sexual organs ; shoots in dorsum of foot.—(*During sleep*), Cough ; violent cough, etc.; scarlet redness of face, etc.; sweat.—(*After sleep*), Pains in general ; ill-humor.—(*After a long sleep*), Thirst.—(*Standing*), Colic ; pressure in forepart of tibia.—(*Stepping*), Pressure in head ; shootings in genital region. —(*During stool*), Shootings in rectum.—(*After stool*), Tensive sensation

below navel; sense of fulness in abdomen.—(*When stooping*), Blood mounts to head; fulness below short ribs, etc.; pain in glutei muscles.—(*After supper*), Mirthfulness; præcordial anxiety, etc.—(*Supporting head with hand*), Pain in temporal region.—(*Change of temperature*), Pains in face.—(*After smoking tobacco*), Loss of appetite.—(*Touch*), Pain in neck; throbbing in forearm, etc,; pain in middle finger-tip.—(*Treading*), Pressure in head.—(*When treading on left foot*), Shootings up to the knee.—(*When treading on heel*), Pain in ball of heel.—(*On turning in bed*), Whole system began to feel bad).—(*On turning head round*), Shootings in pharynx, etc.—(*After diminution of sweat*), Thirst; appetite fell off.—(*While urinating*), Drawing in spermatic cords.—(*After urinating*), Cold sweat all over; immediately, pain in edge of prepuce.—(*On waking*), Weeping, etc.; convulsive extension of the limbs; fatigue, etc.—(*Walking*), Confusion of head; vertigo; colic; stitch in urethra; pressing towards sexual organs; oppression of chest, etc.; stitches below clavicle; sensation in joints of lower extremities; tension in hip-joints; heaviness, etc., in thighs; hamstring feels tight, etc.; pain in metatarsal bones; tearing in left sole.—(*Walking quickly*), **Jerking headache.**—(*While walking in a strong wind and sweating*), Colic. —(*Change of weather*), Pains in general.—(*In a wind*), Pains in general; pains in face.—(*Yawning*), Stitches in sternum.

Amelioration.—(*On bending head backwards*), Sensation in brain disappears.—(*After continuing to drink*), Bad smell, etc., of milk disappears.—(*On beginning to eat*), Return of appetite.—(*While eating*), Toothache.—(*Passing flatulence*), Distension of hypogastrium, etc.—(*Letting leg hang down*), Jammed sensation in legs.—(*Laying head down*), Headache.— (*On lying down*), Pain in forehead disappears; humming, etc., in ears.— (*On lying on right side*), Cutting in belly disappears.—(*After a meal*), Delirium ceases.—(*Passing tongue over teeth*), Toothache.—(*Pressure*), Shooting in frontal eminences; pain in left arm; tension in sole of foot.—(*Strong pressure*), **Pain in forehead.**—(*Pressing eyes upward*), Burning in eyes, etc. —(*On rubbing*), Itching shootings in umbilicus disappear.—(*Sitting*), **Pain in forehead.**—(*On sitting down*), Colic disappears.—(*Sitting erect*), Pressing towards sexual organs.—(*Standing*), Humming, etc., in ears; pressing-out feeling in hypogastrium; pressing towards sexual organs; cramp in lumbo-sacral region, etc.—(*Stooping*), Headache.—(*Sugar*), Burning in throat (for a moment).—(*Walking*), Humming, etc., in ears; cramp in lumbo-sacral region, etc.; **bruised pain in thighs, etc.**

BELLIS PERENNIS.

B. perennis, L. *Nat. order*, Compositæ. *Preparation*, Tincture of the whole plant when in flower.

Authority. Dr. Thomas, Br. Journ. of Hom., 16, 325; proving of the tincture, 20-drop doses repeated for fourteen days; of the 3d dilution; effects of external application of the tincture, and of chewing the flowers.

Head.—A little giddiness in the head at times (after two weeks), (from the tincture).—Headache extending from occiput to sinciput (after two weeks), (from the tincture).—Brain feels as though contracted in the frontal region (after two weeks), (from the tincture).

Stomach.—Want of appetite (after two weeks), (from the tincture). —Slight nausea (after two weeks), (from the tincture).

Upper Extremities.—Pain in inner side of right forearm, as of a boil developing (after two weeks), (from the tincture).—Pain in inner side of left forearm, as of a boil developing (after two weeks), (from the tincture).—Pain in middle finger of left hand, as of a gathering, for a short time only (after two weeks), (from the tincture).

Skin.—Development of a small boil (after five hours), (from external application of tincture).—Small boil at the angle of the inferior maxilla, right side (after chewing the flowers).—Painful pimple a little behind the angle of left inferior maxilla (3d dilution), (after third day).—Large boil on back of neck, commencing with a dull, aching pain, some difficulty and bruised pain in keeping the head erect; began as a slight pimple, with burning pain in the skin, increasing until, in six days' time, it was very large, of a dark, fiery, purple color, and very sore, burning and aching pain in it; accompanied with headache extending from occiput to sinciput, of a cold, aching character; brain as though contracted in frontal region, dizziness, etc. (after two weeks), (from the tincture).

BENZINUM.

A product of distillation from Petroleum.   *Formula,* C_6H_6.   *Preparation,* Tincture with alcohol.

Authority.   Dr. J. Heber Smith, N. E. Med. Gaz., 1870.   (Symptoms from a workman in a rubber factory, who for weeks had his hands and arms daily bathed in benzine, and drank water impregnated with it.)

Mind.—Weeping at trifles, and despairing of recovery.—Extremely irritable and faultfinding.

Head.—Severe darting pains in occiput, from below upward, recurring in paroxysms, aggravated by motion, and especially by rising after sitting.

Eyes.—Could not turn eyes upward or to one side without severe aching and throbbing.—Conjunctiva appeared somewhat congested.—A great white hand seemed to appear to him, in the darkness, coming outspread toward his face, causing him in terror to scream for the watcher.

Face.—Occasional sudden puffing up of the left cheek and of the calf of the left leg, as though the parts were filled with air, going off in a few hours, and returning again.

Mouth.—Teeth covered with sordes (during typhoid condition).—Soreness, and sensation of looseness in the upper incisors.—[10.] Tongue parched and brown (during typhoid condition).—Painful, round, white ulcers in the mouth, especially on the inside of the cheeks.—Hot and very offensive breath.

Stomach.—Entire loss of appetite.—Craving for lemons and cider.—Terrible thirst (during typhoid condition).—Extreme thirst for ice-water, satisfied with a sip, but wanting it again directly.

Abdomen.—Continual soreness to pressure in the abdominal walls.—Heat, and grinding, wearing pains in the lower part of the bowels, worse just before stools.

Stool and Anus.—Several times an hour, a stool, smelling of benzine, of lead-colored mucus mixed with bright blood, accompanied by some tenesmus, and followed by throbbing in the anus and rectum, and lancinating pains from below upwards, continuing about five minutes.   These stools followed him with diminishing severity about ten days, preserving their characteristics to the last.

Urinary Organs.—[20.] Pressing pain in the bladder.—After

passing urine, throbbing and smarting in the neck of the bladder and in the urethra for several minutes.—Dark, offensive urine.—Sediment in the urine like red sand.

Respiratory Apparatus, Chest, and Pulse.—Every few days, continual dry, hacking cough.—Continual soreness and aching in the clavicular regions.—Pulse wiry, averaging 96 per minute.

Back and Extremities.—Continual aching and throbbing in the lumbar region, made worse by a full inspiration.—Extreme irritation of the kidneys.—Continual soreness and aching in the muscles of the upper arms.

Generalities.—[30.] Wasted, pallid, and exhausted.—General prostration.—At one time he sank very low, approaching a typhoid condition. —Complained of a sensation of falling through the bed and floor (during typhoid condition).

Sleep and Dreams.—For three nights, before the sweating began, complete insomnia, with unpleasant thoughts crowding the mind, and wide-open eyes, before which photopsic illusions floated continually.

Fever.—Chills seized remote parts and passed toward the head, from the thumbs to the elbows and from them to the shoulders, and from the small of the back to the shoulders and vertex.—Cold compresses came off steaming in a few minutes, smelling of benzine, and stained a deep yellow, which could only be removed by long exposure to the sun.—For seven nights, copious, general, warm sweat, toward morning, very exhausting, followed on several succeeding mornings by perspiration only on the breast, on the side not lain upon, and in the axillæ.

Conditions.—**Aggravation.**—(*Toward morning*), Sweat.—(*Full inspiration*), Aching, etc., in lumbar region.—(*Motion*), Pains in occiput.— (*Rising after sitting*), Pains in occiput.—(*Before stool*), Heat, etc., in lower bowels.—(*Turning eyes upward or to one side*), Aching, etc., in eyes.— (*After urinating*), Throbbing, etc., in neck of bladder.

BENZINUM NITRICUM.

Nitro-benzine ("essence of mirbane," or "artificial" oil of bitter almonds). *Formula*, $C_{12}H_5NO_4$. Prepared by heating Benzol with Nitric acid; the oily fluid formed is washed and rectified; it is miscible with Alcohol, has an odor of bitter almonds, and is very poisonous.

Authorities. 1, Treulich, Wien Med. Presse, 11, 13, two cases poisoned by taking about half a thimbleful; 2, Bahrdt, Archiv f. Deutsch. Heilk., 1871, poisoned by drinking about six drops in some liquor; 3, Letheby, London Hosp. Rep., 1865, J. E. spattered some on his clothes, so that he inhaled the fumes; 4, Ibid., G. G. took a little in his mouth by mistake; he immediately spit it out and rinsed his mouth with water; 5, Ibid., H. A. took a little in his mouth to remove the smell of tobacco; 6, Ibid., a woman cooked some food in a cup which had contained Nitro-benzol; 7, Kreuser, Wurt. corr. Bl., 37 (A. H. Z., M. B., 16, 48); 8, Riefkhol, Deutsch. Kl., 1868; 9, Schenk, Zeit. f. Ger. Med., 1866, a pregnant girl poisoned herself; 10, Muller, ibid., a young man took a teaspoonful in water; 11, Helbig, Deutsche. Mil. Arz., 3, 1873, several soldiers drank some from a flask.

Mind.—Extreme mental excitement (after two hours),[5].—Inability to think connectedly,[5].—Unconscious (after a quarter of an hour),[10].—Unconscious, with leaden color, livid lips, moderately warm skin, and weak, irregular pulse,[6].—Unconscious, with livid face, purple lips, dilated pupils, slow, difficult, and scarcely perceptible respiration, and death,[4].—Loss of consciousness,[2].—Loss of consciousness, fell from her chair (after half an hour),[6].—Loss of consciousness for twenty-four hours,[2].—Comatose some hours,[1].—[10.] Complete coma, which appeared suddenly,[3].—Profound coma, with livid, purple face, closed eyes, moderately dilated pupils, cold skin, difficult, slow respiration, pulse small, slow or accelerated, irregular,[8].

Head.—*Vertigo,*[4][11].—Vertigo and headache,[1].—Headache,[7].—Sensation of formication under the scalp, or as if the hair was bristling up,[1].

Eyes and Ears.—The white of the eye had a livid look, vessels greatly enlarged, pupils much dilated, insensible to the light,[9].—Strabismus,[11].—Staring eyes,[7].—Lids closed,[2].—[20.] Great injection of the conjunctiva bulbi,[11].—Eyeballs roll from right to left constantly,[7].—Eyeballs constantly roll on their vertical axis,[2].—The eyeballs showed a constant turning inward and outward in a slow regular motion, with the visual axes perfectly parallel,[2].—Eyeballs seemed enlarged,[9].— *Pupils dilated,*[1][3], etc.— Pupils dilated, sluggish,[2].—Violent roaring in the ears, and sounds,[1].

Face.—Expression stupid,[3].—Stupid expression of face (after four hours),[4].—[30.] He looked stupid and sick (after four hours),[3].—Face puffy, swollen, and had a relaxed look,[9].—Cyanotic face,[1].—Face cyanotic (fourth hour),[4].—Face blue,[2].—Blue color in the face (after twenty minutes),[11].—Face blue and pale,[7].—Face bluish-gray, sunken,[11].—Face red,[3]. —Face red, with purple lips and cold skin (after two hours),[5].—[40.] Trismus,[2].—Trismus and tetanus,[11].—Lips of a dark blue color,[11].

Mouth.—Tongue white, somewhat swollen,[3].—Tongue thick and soft,[9]. —Mouth clenched,[10].—Mucous membrane of lips and mouth livid and swollen,[9].—Stammering speech,[7].

Stomach and Abdomen.—Burning in throat and stomach,[1].— Nausea (after four hours),[3].—[50.] Inclined to vomit,[1].—Vomiting,[2].—Vomiting (after half an hour),[2].—Vomiting while unconscious,[1].—Vomited what he had eaten (after four hours),[4].—Pains in the abdomen,[2].

Respiratory Apparatus.—Sighing respiration,[1].—Respiration rattling, frequently interrupted,[11].—Respiration regular, somewhat difficult; on auscultation, mucous râles in the large bronchi,[9].—Respiration short and rapid (after three hours),[5].—[60.] Respiration exceedingly slow, so that it frequently seems to cease,[3].—Respiration and pulse continued to become slower until the patient died,[3].—Respiration very superficial and slow,[2].— Dyspnœa (after two hours),[5].—Respiration difficult, catching, and accelerated,[10].

Chest.—Oppression of the chest,[5].—Severe oppression of chest,[1].

Heart and Pulse.—Heart exceedingly irregular (after two hours),[5]. —Palpitation (after half an hour),[6].—The heart beat 120 a minute; carotid and temporal arteries pulsating,[9].—[70.] Pulse small, rapid,[1].—Pulse 100, very weak, and irregular,[2].—Pulse 130, weak, and intermitting (after two hours),[5].—Pulse full and slow,[3].—Pulse scarcely perceptible,[11].

Neck.—Stiff neck,[2].—Stiffness of the neck, trismus, and fibrillar twitchings in the masseter muscles,[2].

Extremities.—Twitchings in the hands and feet,[2].—Twitchings in arms,[2].—Arms spasmodically flexed,[2].—[80.] Arms spasmodically flexed, sometimes extended,[2].—Arms spasmodically flexed at first, afterwards relaxed,[10].—Finger nails colored blue,[11].

Generalities.—Gait tottering and uncertain, as if intoxicated,[3].— Tottering gait, and tendency to fall,[11].—He walked like a drunken man, staggering here and there,[3].—Violent convulsions,[7].—Convulsions paroxysmal,[1].—Convulsions and loss of consciousness; the head sunk upon the shoulder; purple lips, and clenched teeth; the eyes closed (sixth hour),[3].—Chronic cramps and tetanus,[11].—[90.] Tetanic convulsions, relieved for a few minutes by dashes of cold water, and followed by deep coma,[5].—Tetanic spasms of the flexor muscles, especially of the upper extremities and of the masticators,[9].—Faintness,[2].—Sinking,[2].—Was obliged to lie down on account of exhaustion (after half an hour),[5].—Symptoms come suddenly, several hours after taking,[3].

Skin.—The skin, especially the face and neck, also of the extremities, was livid,[9].—Skin bluish-gray,[2].—Skin dry and cyanotic, lips blue,[10].—Irritability of the skin completely lost,[5].

Sleep and Dreams.—[100.] Sleepiness,[3].—Complains of sleepiness (after four hours),[4].

Fever.—Skin cold,[11].—Sweat on the forehead and face,[11].

Condition. — Amelioration. — (*Dashing cold water*), Tetanic spasms.

BENZOIC ACID.

Benzoic acid, C_6H_5,CO,OH. Obtained, by sublimation, from Gum benzoin, or artificially from several aromatic hydrocarbons. *Preparation for use,* Tincture or trituration.

Authorities. 1, Dr. Jeanes, Trans. Am. Inst., vol. i (symptoms obtained from himself and others, sick and well), with the 1st to the 15th potency; 2, Dr. Lingen, ibid. (took of an alcoholic solution $\frac{1}{2}$ gr. to 1 oz., five drops every morning and evening for several days); 3, Keiler, Am. Arzn. Pruf'n, p. 705 (examined the effect of crude doses upon the urine); 4, Nusser, ibid. (took 80 grs. of the 2d trit. at one dose); 5, Petroz, Bull. d. l. soc. med. hom. de Paris, 5, 60 (the original proving); 6, Hauff, from Hering, Am. Arzn. Pruf'n (effects of a drachm daily, an hour after dinner, on a person having arthritic nodes on the fingers, etc.).†

Mind.—The mind is inclined to dwell upon unpleasant things. If he saw any one who was deformed it made him shudder,° [1].—Sadness,[5].—Sense of anxiety,° [2].—Sense of anxiety while sweating,[5].—Activity of mind while at work, afterwards anxiety,[5].—He was much surprised that, while writing, he omitted words every moment, which never was the case before (sixth and seventh days),[4].—Comatose condition. (Ilisch, Med. Zeit. Russl.)

Head.—Confusion of the head,[5].—Confusion of the head, and sleepiness,[2].—[10.] Vertigo, making him fearful of falling sidewise, usually in the afternoon,[5].—Excitement and lightness of the head, when sneezing in the morning,[2].—Sensation as if there were air in the head,[5].—Tired feeling in the head, as from night-watching,[5].—Sensation of coldness in the head,[5].—Sensation of shaking in the head,[5].—The head-symptoms are generally accompanied with depression, lassitude, and loss of appetite,[5].—After mental emotions, headache,[5].—The head-symptoms are worse during rest, return periodically, and are often accompanied with pains in the stomach, nausea, gagging, and cold hands,[5].—Pain and heat in the organs of reverence and firmness,[1].—[20.] Pressure upon the whole upper part of the head and on the spinal column, as if it were pressed together like an elastic body, so

---

† Other authorities taken from Hering, A. A. Pruf'n, are given with the symptoms.

that he stretched himself involuntarily and bent forward. This sensation, without being painful, produces extreme anxiety, two days in succession in the forenoon, while sitting,[2].—Rheumatic pain on the outside of the head,[5].—Formication in the forehead,[5].—Hard throbbing of the temporal arteries,[2].—Pain in the temples, in the region of the organ of constructiveness,[1].—Pain in the left temple,[1].—Hammering pain in the temples, obliging him to lie down,[5].—Tearing pain in the vertex,[5].—Internal pain and bruised feeling in the sides of the head,[5].—Itching of the hairy scalp,[1].

Eyes.—[30.] Distress in the eyes, as from want of sleep,[5].—Burning heat in the eyes,[5].—Burning heat in the lids,[5].—Itching in the outer, and then in the inner, angle of the right eye,[1].—Throbbing in the eyeballs,[5].

Ears.—Swelling behind the ears, which seems to reach the periosteum,[5].—Starting in the ear,[5].—Itching in the left ear,[1].—Puffing in the ears from pulsation of the temporal arteries,[2].—When swallowing, noise in the ears,[2].—[40.] Sensation in the ears like a sound of confused voices, especially when swallowing or when walking in the open air,[5].

Nose.—Redness at the angles of the nose,[5].—Pain in the nasal bones,[5].—Irritation in the left nostril, such as precedes sneezing, yet without being able to sneeze,[1].—Sneezing and hoarseness,[2].—A cold in the head readily occurs from exposure to cold; is renewed every day,[5].—Epistaxis,[5].—Pressure at the root of the nose,[5].—Sensitiveness of the nose,[5].—Itching of the septum of the nose,[1].—[50.] Diminution of the sense of smell,[5].—It seemed to him that he smelled dust, cabbage, or something stinking,[5].

Face.—Circumscribed redness of the face,[5].—Numb feeling in the face,[5].—Burning heat of the face,[5].—Burning heat on only one-half of the face,[5].—Tension in one side of the face,[5].—Pressive sensation in the face,[5].—Trembling of the lips,[5].—Itching of the chin,[5].

Mouth.—[60.] Involuntary biting of the lower lip at dinner, on two successive days,[2].—Stitches in a right lower hollow molar,[1].—Slight cutting pain in the teeth,[1].—Slow jerking in a right upper molar,[1].—The Benzoic oil has been given for toothache,° (A.)—The resin has been used as a chewing-gum in toothache,° (Schrœder.)—Extensive ulcerations of the tongue, with deeply-chapped or fungoid surfaces,[1].—Velvety coating on the tongue,[5].†—Tongue with a white mucous coat in the morning,[2].—Tongue of a slightly bluish color,[5].—[70.] Soreness on the back part of the tongue,[1].—Soreness of the back part of the tongue, felt most while swallowing,[1].—Sensation of soreness and rawness at the root of the tongue and on the palate,[1].—An ulcerated tumor in the left side of the mouth, upon the soft commissure of the jaws, behind the last molar teeth,° [1].—Heat around the mouth,[5].—After-taste of the food,[5].—Slightly acid mucus,[5].—Taste of blood,[5].—The bread tastes smoky,[5].—Flat, soapy taste after drinking water,[5].—[80.] Salty taste of food,[5].—Bitter taste, with pressure at the stomach and eructation,[6].—Bitter taste on drinking coffee or milk,[5].

Throat.—Collection of mucus in the throat,[5].—The thyroid gland feels swollen,[5].—Sensation of swelling or of contraction in the throat,[5].—It feels as if there were little lumps in the pit of the throat, as if food were sticking there. (Fr. Husmann.)—Angina faucium and angina tonsillaris, with the characteristic urine,° [1].—Heat in the œsophagus, as from acid eructations,[1].—Sensation of heat and scratching in the œsophagus and throat. (Pereira.)—[90.] Extremely unpleasant scratching in the throat. (Leh

---

† In both cases there was not the least suspicion of syphilitic affection; in both cases high-colored, strong-smelling urine,[1].

mann, Phys. Chimie.)—Difficulty in swallowing,[5].—Incomplete swallowing,[5].

Stomach.—Increased appetite in the evening,[5].—Loss of appetite, mornings,[2].—In the evening, thirst with sleepiness,[5].—Singultus,[1].—Nausea, mornings,[2].—Nausea, with gagging; with disturbances about the head,[5].—Nausea, with loathing, and constant malaise,[5].—[100.] Vomiting of a salty substance,[5].—Bitter vomiting,[5].—With pregnant women, gastric derangements when ascending a height,[5].—Sensation of warmth in the stomach,[5].—Burning in the stomach. (Honigberger.)—Pressure in the stomach and eructations,[6].—Fatigued by the pressure of the clothes on the epigastrium,[5].

Abdomen.—In the region of the liver, constant, fine, but violent stitching, midway in the upper portion thereof; it seems to be superficial, and is not increased by pressure (seventh day),[4].—Obstruction of the liver,[°]. (Honigberger.)—Cutting about the navel, relieved by stool,[5].—[110.] Uncommon discharge of wind downward in the afternoon and evening of first day,[4].—Pain in the left side of the abdomen, immediately below the short ribs,[1].—Sensation of heat throughout the abdomen,[1].—Tearing bellyache,[5].—Tensive pain in the groins,[5].

Stool and Anus.—Contraction of the extremity of the rectum,[5].—Stitching in the rectum,[5].—Slightly elevated, round surfaces, of a wartlike appearance, and circular form, varying in diameter from half an inch to an inch and a half, at places running into each other, nearly covered both sides and the bottom of the sulcus ani, and causes much smarting and soreness of the part, with strong-scented and highly-colored urine[°] (after previous use of Copaiva for chancre),[1].—Fine stitching in the anus, on the evening of first day,[4].—Formication at the anus,[5].—[120.] Urging to stool, with ineffectual straining,[5].—Bowels freely open, with extraordinary pressure to stool,[1].—*Diarrhœa of children; the discharge is copious, watery, clear-colored, very fetid; the urine at the same time is uncommonly deep-red, and the urinous odor very strong (in very many cases curative, or at least relieving)[° 1].—*Frothy stool,[5].—*Fetid, watery, white stools, very copious and exhausting, in infants, the urine being of very deep-red color,[° 1].—Putrid, bloody stool,[5].—Insufficient stool,[5].

Urinary Organs.—Vesical catarrh,[°]. (G. Bird.)—Irritability of the bladder. Too frequent desire to evacuate the bladder, the urine normal in appearance,[° 1].—Gleet,[°]. (Honigberger.)—[130.] Urine at first increased in quantity only, and not in frequency. In a few days urination became exceedingly frequent, with strong pressing and discharge of a clear urine. Urine of an aromatic odor and saline taste, the odor long retained; most in the forenoon,[2].—Urine more copious, somewhat turbid, otherwise of a natural color and odor. After the daily use of a drachm after dinner, no Benzoic acid was found in the urine, traces of urea, and only mere traces of Hippuric acid,[6].—Enuresis nocturna of children, where Nitrum failed,[°]. (Young.)—Decrease of the quantity of urine,[5].—Urine aromatic,[2].—*Fetid urine, with prolapsus uteri. (C. Hg.)—Urine of a very repulsive odor, of a changeable color, brownish, cloudy, of an alkaline reaction; effervescing with hydrochloric acid; white, flocculent sediment in the urine immediately after its passage, consisting of the phosphate and carbonate of lime, without uric acid. The patient was pale, languid, with a sense of weakness in the loins. (Farquhar.)—Thick urine,[5].—Bloody urine,[5].—Hot, scalding urine, of a deep-red color, and strong odor, causing so much suffering in its passage that this was performed but once a day,[° 1].—Morbid condition of the urine, as in persons with calculus or gouty diathesis,[°] (Ure), with concretions of urate of ammonia,°. (Neidhard.)—[**140.**] *Urine highly colored, *sometimes of the color of brandy;.* the urinous odor exceedingly strong,° [1].—Urine of the above character, of a specific gravity greater than that of healthy urine; passed into the same vessel, it retains its place below the healthy urine without admixture, and, though of a very deep-red color, deposits no sediment,° [1].—*Dark reddish-brown urine,* of greater specific gravity than normal, with an acid reaction, even after some weeks; at the same time many fleeting pains deep in the region of the bladder, not when urinating, but at other times; also with deposit of mucous granules, and, when standing, becoming, in a few days, covered with a thick, filmy crust,° (one-twentieth grain of the undiluted acid). (C. Hg.)—A granular kind of mucus, mixed with phosphates, in the sediment of the urine,°. (Garrod.)— Affords no relief where there are phosphates in the sediment. (G. Bird.)— After thirty-two grains of pure Benzoic acid, taken in the evening before going to sleep, the morning urine reacted uncommonly acid, even after being evaporated, and standing twelve hours, whereupon only the usual sediment of earthy salts presented itself. The Uric acid and urea were both contained therein, apparently in normal quantity,[3].—A scruple, taken an hour after a meal, was followed, in some hours, by five or six ounces of urine; on adding Hydrochloric acid to this an abundant precipitate of Hippuric acid appeared, but no trace of Uric acid. (Ure.)—One of the few acids which manifestly increase the acidity of the urine. (Lehmann.)— Increases the acid of the urine and makes it slightly irritant. (Garrod.)— Not the uric acid but the urea disappears. (Garrod.)—[**150.**] Dark or highly colored offensive urine, quite peculiar (after suppressed syphilis and gonorrhœa. In many cases),° [1].†—In cases with an excess of uric acid in the urine, the urine becomes normal after the use of Benzoic acid,°. (G. Bird.)—Never saw anything so effectual; the urine was clear after the first dose, and in two days was entirely free from mucous deposits; the irritability of the bladder was diminished, and in four days the patient could be left to himself,°. (Soden.)

Sexual Organs.—Male. Painfulness of the genitals,[5].—Pressure at the genitals.—Raw pain of the genitals,[5].—Smarting of the frænum præputii,[1].—A thrilling, almost painful sensation on the left side of the glans penis, extending into the urethra, so severe as to occasion starting, ending in a sensation of tickling and itching,[1].—Itching on the glans,[1].— Itching in the sulcus behind the corona glandis,[1].—*Female.* [**160.**] Menstruation too early,[5].—Retarded menstruation,[5].—Weakness after the menses,[5].—Too long-lasting lochia,[5].

Respiratory Apparatus.—Copious secretion of mucus in the bronchi,[5].—Slight transitory hoarseness and thrice-repeated sneezing, in the morning, with a pleasant excitement and lightness (Leichtigkeit) of the head, which, together with its more rapid disappearance, distinguished it from the more ordinary symptoms of taking cold, of the prover,[2].—Rather increased than diminished the cough. (Pereira.)—When the fumes of Benzoin alone are produced they occasion a cough. (Schrœder, Arneischatz.) —Violent cough from inhaling the fumes. (Pereira.)—Produced an exhausting cough in healthy persons (the flowers). (Med. Zeit. Russlands.)— [**170.**] Given for a tormenting, tight cough, every powder produced a violent cough, then extraordinary weakness, sweat, and a state of coma lasting an hour; at the same time the skin is paler and cooler; the pulse weaker

---

† The gonorrhœa was, in most cases, suppressed by Bals. copaiv.

and less frequent; respiration normal (*from the sublimated but not purified flowers*). (Ilisch, in Med. Zeit. Russl., 15, 1852.)—Cough seems produced by something acrid or dry in the chest,[5].—Cough after a slight cold,[5].—Slight hacking cough, directly after rising (second day),[4].—Cough excited by inspiration,[5].—Troublesome, constant, dry, hacking cough, after suppressed gonorrhœa,[1].—Cough, followed by expectoration of greenish mucus,[5].—The respiration at times somewhat whistling (second day),[4].—Difficulty of breathing on awaking,[5].—Asthma, with inflammatory rheumatic complaints,[0] [1].

Chest.—[180.] Burning in the nipples,[5].—Sensation of swelling in the mammary glands, also in the thyroid gland,[5].—Morbid agitation in the chest,[5].—Sense of roughness in the chest,[5].—Painful starting in the chest,[5].—Sensation of swelling in the chest,[5].—Can scarcely bear the pressure of clothing on the chest,[5].—A cutting sensation in the chest,[5].—Fine, slight stitches in the middle of the chest (evening of the first day),[4].—Pain sometimes in the middle of the breast; a kind of stitching (second day),[4].—[190.] In the evening in bed, somewhat of stitching in the chest, especially on breathing deeply (first day),[4].—It is said to furnish the greatest relief in diseases of the chest; reduces the obstruction of the pulmonary vessels, and promotes expectoration,[0]. (Lewis's Mat. Med.)—In the last period of simple pneumonia, where great weakness prevails,[0]. (Schregar.)—Typhus pneumonia; asthenic affections of the chest. (Schregar.)—Asthenic pneumonia of a young man; after the strength had sunk daily, the difficulty of breathing increased every hour till it attained a fearful degree,[0]. (Goldschmidt.)—Pain in the left side. (Honigberger.)—Pain about the third rib on the right side, midway between the sternum and the side; increased by respiration,[1].—Deep penetrating pain in the posterior part of the left side about the sixth rib (second day),[1].—Pain in the left side about the sixth rib, increased by deep inspiration, and by bending the body to either side,[1].—Pressure on the ribs,[5].—[200.] Stitching in the right side of the chest,[5].—Weak feeling in the præcordial region,[5].

Heart and Pulse.—Undulating beating of the heart,[5].—Intermittent beats of the heart,[5].—Palpitation of the heart with trembling,[5].—Palpitation of the heart while sitting, also after drinking,[5].—Awakes after midnight, with palpitation of the heart; every morning at 2 o'clock, with heat and hard pulse. Throbbing of the temporal arteries prevents his getting to sleep again,[2].—Wakes after midnight, with violent pulsation of the heart and temporal arteries (pulsation 110 in the minute), without external heat, and cannot fall asleep again. In the morning, the tongue covered with a white mucous coat; some nausea and total loss of appetite. Had eaten peaches in the evening. In the afternoon, at four o'clock, all these symptoms had vanished (fourth day),[2].—*Pain in the region of the heart*,[1].—The pains change their place incessantly and suddenly, but are the most constant in the region of the heart,[1].—[210.] Pulse full,[5].—*He wakes every morning about 2 o'clock from strong internal heat, and a hard, bounding,* but not quickened pulse, so that he must lie awake upon his back, because the pulsation of the temporal arteries sounds like puffing in his ears, and prevents him from going to sleep again (lasting eight weeks),[2].—Accelerated pulse (first, second, and third days),[2].—Pulse slow,[5].—Pulse slower and weaker (*from the sublimated but not purified flowers*). (Ilisch, in Med. Zeit. Russl.)

Neck and Back.—Stiffness of the neck, but only on one side,[5].—Pressure in the nape of the neck,[5].—Violent itching in the nape of the neck,[5].—Pain in the right side of the back, between the tenth dorsal vertebra and the side,[1].—Pressure upon the spinal column,[2].—[220.] Hot burning pain in left kidney, with drawing when stooping,[0]. (Neidhard.)—Dull pain in the region of the kidneys,[1].—Sore pain in region of left kidney,[0]. (Neidhard.)—Nephritic colic,[0]. (Williamson.)—Sense of coldness at the sacrum,[5].—Starting in the loins,[5].—Stiffness in the loins, with pains in the kidneys,[0]. (Neidhard.)

Extremities in General.—Nodes on the joints of the upper and lower extremities, knicking and cracking on motion,[1].—In both wrists, between the metacarpal bones, abundant gouty deposits, and swelling of the elbow-joints. The ankle, also, is not free (1 drachm daily for six months),[0][6].—Old, gouty concretions,[0]. (Neidhard.)—[230.] Tearing and fine stitching in various parts of the limbs,[4].

Upper Extremities.—Sensation of swelling under the axillæ,[5].—Tearing pains, apparently in the bones of the arm,[5].—Fine or severe stitching on the outer surface of the right arm; afterwards on the left arm, inner surface (evening of first day),[4].—Tearing below, in the right radius,[4].—Tearing at the outer surface of both wrists, as if in the bones (third day),[4].—Cold hands,[5].—Cold hands with head symptoms,[5].—A kind of itching in the palm of the right hand, with slight but deep tearing in the upper metacarpal joints of the little and ring fingers (evening of first day),[4].—The fingers are as if swollen; a ring became too small (second day),[4].—[240.] The fingers remain somewhat swollen; therewith tearing and fine stitching in various parts of the limbs, especially in front at the metatarsal joint of the right great toe (fourth to seventh days),[4].—Pain in the finger joints of the right hand,[1].—Paralytic pain of the fingers,[5].—Tearing in the metacarpal joint of the left thumb,[4].—Tearing deep in the upper joints of the left index finger (second day),[4].

Lower Extremities.—Lassitude in the lower extremities,[5].—Sensation as if the lower limbs were tightly bandaged,[5].—Pain in the right hip,[1].—Gnawing pain in the left hip, then in the thigh, next in the knees, then in the toes,[1].—Pain in the left hip, in the knee, and the toes at the same time; the worst in the toes; leaving the toes, it seats itself in the muscles of the calf, and then in the knee. After leaving these parts it appears in the right thigh and ankle,[1].—[250.] Tearing pain in the anterior surface of the thigh,[5].—*Swelling of the right knee, with pain as of ulceration of the whole leg, with pains in the kidneys,*[0]. (Neidhard.)—*Cracking in the knee-joint,*[5].—*Sense of dryness in the knee-joint,*[5].—Pain in the right knee,[1][4].—Pain in the left knee,[1].—*Pain in both knees,*[1].—Drawing pain in the knees after drinking wine,[5].—Pain in the gastrocnemii,[1].—Sharp pain in the left ankle during the time it supports the weight of the body while walking,[1].—[260.] When supporting a slight part of the weight of the body upon the left foot, severe pain in the tendo Achillis, close to the os calcis,[1].—Pain in the right tendo Achillis and in the region of the heart at the same time. After leaving the right, the pain appears in the left tendo Achillis,[1].—Numbness in the toes,[5].—Pain in the toes,[1].—Pain in the large joints of the great toe, with slight tumefaction and redness,[1].—In the small toes of the right foot, especially in the middle joints, a kind of deep sensitive tearing; subsequently, in the right knee, the last joint of the metacarpal bone and of the left thumb, and in the radius of the right forearm, etc. (second day),[4].—Deep, persistent tearing in the lowest joint of the great toe (second day),[4].—*Tearing and stitching, especially in the metatarsal joints of the right great toe,*[4].—Stitch passing perpendicularly upward through the right great toe, followed by a burning, which increases gradually to a stitch; appearing afterwards in the left great toe, from which it vanishes with a thrilling sensation, in the morning while lying down (eighth day),[2].

Generalities.—Emaciates (the resin). (Schrœder.)—[**270.**] Trembling, with palpitation of the heart,[5].—* *Weariness and lassitude*,[5].—Extreme weakness, sweat, and comatose condition. (Ilisch., in Med. Zeit. Russl.)—A pain passes from the right hand, and appears in the left arm, extends downwards into the elbow, and next appears in the region of the heart; later in the right thigh and ankle,[1].—Purifies the blood, and is used in vulnerary potions,° (tincture of the flowers). (Schrœder.)—Syphilitic rheumatism,° [1].

Skin.—Eruption of red spots on the fingers,[5].—Itching on various parts of the body and extremities, yielding rather an agreeable feeling on being scratched, but leaving a burning,[1].

Sleep and Dreams.—Sleepiness, with dulness of the head,[1].—Sleep tolerably sound; somewhat disturbed by dreams the first day; the following day good,[4].—[**280.**] Deep sleep,[5].—Starting up from sleep,[5].

Fever.—Horripilation before stool,[5].—Cool, pale skin, with sweat, weakness, and coma. (Ilisch., in Med. Zeit. Russl.)—Coldness of the back,[5].—Coldness in the knees,[1].—Feeling of coldness in the knees, as if blown upon by a cold wind (ninth day),[1].—Cold feet,[5].—Violent internal heat on waking,[2].—Heat during the coryza,[5].—[**290.**] Sense of heat in the œsophagus,[1]; in the stomach,[5]; in the belly,[1].—Heat, with sweat,[5]; heat, with cold in the head,[5]; with nightly palpitation of the heart,[2].—Coldness, with feeling of heat,[5].—Coldness, then heat and sweat,[5].—Gentle, universal exhalation from the skin (evening of the first day),[4].—Slight sweat after the disappearance of the other symptoms,[5].—Subsequently a very copious perspiration. (Lehmann.)—The crystals produce sweat in syphilis, with very great benefit, especially when mixed with Guaiacum. (Schrœder.)—Copious night-sweat, after taking 32 grains, in the evening; the first night, not the following, from repeated doses,[3].—Sweat, with anxiety,[5].—[**300.**] Sweat, with itching,[5].—Sweat while eating; while walking,[5].—Sweat of the feet,[5].—Sweat, with aromatic odor,[5].—Cold sweat on the head,[5].—Cold sweat on the face,[5].—Cold sweat on the face, with heat,[4].—Cold sweat on the feet,[5].—Exhalation from the skin less active than before, while a drachm was taken every day for six months,[6].

Conditions.—Aggravation.—(*Morning*), On waking, head symptoms occur; when sneezing, excitement, etc., of head; white coat on tongue; loss of appetite; nausea; directly after rising, cough; on waking, difficulty of breathing; while lying down, stitch through great toe, etc.; on waking, heat.—(*Forenoon*), While sitting, pressure on head, etc.; urinary symptoms. —(*Afternoon*), Vertigo.—(*Evening*), Symptoms of nose; thirst, etc.; in bed, especially on breathing deeply, stitch in chest.—(*After midnight*), 2 A.M., wakes, with palpitation; wakes, with heat, etc.—(*Every day*), Cold in head renewed.—(*Open air*), Eye symptoms.—(*When walking in open air*), Sensation of voices in ear.—(*Exposure to draught of air*), Head symptoms.— (*When ascending a height*), In pregnant women, gastric disturbances.— (*Bending body to either side*), Pain in left side.—(*When blowing nose*), Trunk-symptoms.—(*On drinking coffee*), Bitter taste.—(*During coryza*), Heat.—(*After drinking*), Palpitation.—(*While eating*), Sweat.—(*After mental emotion*), Head-symptoms occur.—(*Inspiration*), Excites cough.— (*On drinking milk*), Bitter taste.—(*On moving after long sitting*), Trunk-symptoms.—(*Periodic*), Head-symptoms.—(*Reading by artificial light*), Eye-symptoms.—(*Respiration*), Pain in side.—(*Rest*), Head-symptoms.—(*While* *sitting*), Palpitation.—(*Before stool*), Horripilation.—(*When swallowing*), Noise in ears; sensation of voices in ear; soreness of tongue.—(*On turning in bed at night*), Trunk-symptoms.—(*Uncovering oneself*), Head-symptoms.—(*When walking*), Stomach-symptoms; eye-symptoms; sweat.—(*After drinking water*), Flat taste.—(*After drinking wine*), Pain in knees.

Amelioration.—(*Evening*), Increased appetite.—(*After eating*), Mouth and throat symptoms.—(*Friction*), Symptoms of the face.—(*External heat*), Symptoms of the face.—(*Pressure*), Symptoms of the face.—(*After stool*), Cutting about the navel.

BERBERINUM.

Alkaloid, derived from the roots of Berberis vulg. and Columbo (Cocculus palmatus); $C_{21}H_{19}NO_5$. *Preparation*, Trituration.

Authority. Herberger, Buchner's Repert. f. d. Pharm. (from Wibmer); took four grains in the morning.

Stomach and Abdomen.—Eructations.—Cuttings and rumblings in abdomen.

Stool and Anus.—Painless desire for stool.—Copious fluid stool, with pains in abdomen.—Thin evacuation, without pain.

Generalities.—Weak, sick feeling.

BERBERIS.

Berberis vulgaris, Linn. *Nat. order*, Berberidaceæ. *Common names*, Barberry. (German) Sauerdorn. (French) Le Vinettier. *Preparation.* Tincture of the bark of the root.

Authorities. Symptoms not designated are from Hesse (Journ. f. hom. Arznium, 1, 1834), obtained as follows: took, himself, an infusion of half an ounce of the root, after four days a third infusion of the same evaporated from six to two ounces; the second prover, a stout unmarried woman, æt. 26, took infusions of six drachms of the root; the third, a married woman, æt. 35, took infusions and powdered bark of the root; the fourth prover, a male teacher, lean and phlegmatic, took similar infusions; the fifth, a servant girl, æt. 19, took the same.† Dr. Hesse, in his introduction, says: "I have also made some experiments with potencies, and will give a short account of them here because I *did not* include in the résumé all of the symptoms, especially those which did not coincide with those obtained from large doses." These provings are now for the first time incorporated in the résumé as follows: 6, The fourth prover took a drop of the 5th potency; 7, A servant girl, æt. 18, took repeated doses of the 6th; 8, A girl, æt. 14 (never menstruated), took the same; 9, A servant girl, æt. 19, took the same; 10, An old woman, æt. 60, healthy, took one dose of the 30th.

Mind.—Mental dejection, with difficult thinking and weakness of memory.—Anxious sensation if she moves, stands a long time, rises from sitting, even in the morning when rising, and while in bed and rising from it.—Anxious mood, with great fear and fright from 4 o'clock in the afternoon till going to sleep; in the twilight some dogs and children appeared as large again as natural.—Out of humor; he is satisfied with nothing.—

---

† These five provings are not designated in any way by Hesse.

She experiences a certain ill-will, a spirit of intrepidity.—Very fretful, peevish mood, even becoming a loathing of life. Remarkable melancholy and disinclination to speak, which she can in no way overcome, with quiet, not thoughtful, sensual longing (second and third days).—Indifferent, depressed mood, with slight interest in the outer world, disinclination to work, confusion.—Indifferent, quiet, even apathetic mood at times.—Contemplation of necessary mental work becomes difficult, and affects the head very much, especially in the morning.—[10.] During mental work, external occurrences easily cause disturbance, usually unnoticed; he easily loses the connection, becomes fretful, and must cease work.

Head.—Confusion and Vertigo.

Confusion of the head, as if coryza would follow.—Tensive-pressive confusion of the whole head, as if a cap were drawn over it, and as if it would be drawn downward from behind (several times).—Confusion and dizziness in the head (after two hours). —Confusion, heaviness of the head, often also with pressure in the forehead, and great prostration and fretfulness; chilliness, sometimes with slight heat between the attacks of chilliness; this commences in the morning after waking, continues till after midday, when it is followed by an increased warmth, especially in the head, with symptoms of an impending coryza, especially moisture of the nose and sneezing, which, however, goes no farther; these attacks are repeated during the long proving, and aggravations always begin with them.—Feeling of intoxication in the head (after two to three hours).—*Vertigo and dizziness in the head (after half an hour). Vertigo on stooping (first day).—Vertigo on walking, so that she almost fell, with faintish weakness (eighteenth day).—Vertigo and sensation of fainting, with great weakness (tenth day).—[20.] During rather hard work, with frequent stooping and exertion of the arms, a whirling vertigo on rising up, so that she must turn from left to right and forward, and with difficulty keeps erect; with attacks of faintness, pressive frontal headache; followed by chilliness in the back and in the occiput, as in the coldest winter; for half an hour (forty-fourth day).—*Dizziness in the head (first day).—Head in General. Feeling of emptiness, and gloominess in the head repeatedly.—Feeling of heaviness in the head.—Heavy, pressive headache, with great weariness and prostration (third day),[8].—*A feeling in the head as if it were becoming larger (after an hour and a half).—Feeling of fulness in the head, especially in the forehead (after two to three hours).—*A puffy sensation in the whole head (after nine hours).—Tensive sensation in the head (after nine hours).—Headache as if the skull would burst; on stooping, a sensation as if something shook in the head, and as if everything would come out at the forehead (first day),[9].—[30.] Dull, pressive, sticking headache (after nine hours).—Pressive pain in the whole head (after an hour and a half).—Pressive headache, especially in the forehead, but also extending towards the vertex (after three hours).—Pressive headache, especially in the forehead, as if it would bruise the head, or also as if it would be pressed down by a heavy weight (second day),[7].—Pressive headache, with heaviness and confusion of the head, especially in the morning hours during the first days, and returning afterwards at times.—*Tearing pain in the whole head, now here, now there, in the forehead, in the temples (frequently returning the first weeks).—Forehead. Stupid sensation in the forehead (after half an hour, and after ten hours).—On stooping, a painful sensation in the forehead and in the eyes, as if the brain were heavy and fell forward (after ten hours).—Pressive headache, as if the forehead would press out (first day),[9].—Pressure in the forehead for several days together.—[40.] An outward-pressing headache in the forehead and temples (ninth day).—Pressive-tensive headache in the forehead, temples, and eyes (after three hours, and frequently later).—Pressive headache, now over the eyes, now in the frontal eminences, now in the temples, now in other places in the forehead (seventeenth day).—A pressure in the upper part of the right frontal region (seventh day).—Pressive-twinging tensive pain in the forehead several times repeated during the first days, caused and increased by stooping, better in the open air (as most of the head symptoms are generally).—Sticking headache internally in the forehead (after nine hours).—Sticking tearing headache in the forehead and temples, sometimes lasting only half a minute, sometimes several minutes, rarely longer.—Sticking pain in the forehead and in the temples, now very fine, now very severe; seldom continuous, but rather coming and going in paroxysms, generally ceasing suddenly.—Headache in the forehead, sticking, paroxysmal, lasting one-half to three minutes, especially shooting suddenly through the supra-orbital region (after half an hour and ten hours, and frequently).—Sticking, shooting, or also twitching or rolling pain, at several points in the left frontal region, about an inch above the margin of the orbit, extending outward and upward (after three hours).—[50.] Violent stitches in the right forehead extending outward to the side (fifth day).—Stitching pain and jerking in the forehead, also in the upper part of the head when stooping (after nine hours).—*Temples.* *A peculiar cold sensation in the right temple* (one hundred and eighth day).—Tensive pressive pain in the left temple.—Pressive pain in the right temple extending forward to the eye, as if in the bone, with stitches shooting into the forehead (third and fifth days).—Pressive pain in the right temple, as if it were thick, or would be pressed out, increased by touch (after half an hour).—Dull stitches in the right temples (after two hours and a half).—Piercing stitches in the left temple (second day).—A stitch from without inward in the right temple (after two hours).—Jerking stitches in the right temple extending into the right eye. then shooting into the vertex (after four hours).—[60.] Twitching, tearing pains at times in the temples (first day),[9].—Slight tearing in the temples and forehead (seventh day).—Slight transient tearing in the right temple and the right cheek (after twelve hours, and frequently also afterwards).—*Parietals, Occiput, and External.* Single stitches in the left parietal region.—Tearing pain in the left parietal eminence; it pains somewhat on touch.—Pressive-tensive pain in the occiput, as if the scalp were too small and the brain too large (second day).—Tearing in the left occipital region.—Tearing pain in the left occipital region for two days in succession, lasting several hours; and returning it extends upward from the throat and neck to this place (twenty-sixth day).—The integuments of the head and face feel puffy and tense (after two hours and a half).—Tensive sensation in the scalp and the skin of the face, as if the head were swollen; the scalp is difficult to move (first and second day).—[70.] A tensive numb sensation of the skin of the head and face (after three and four hours).—Smarting or corrosive sensation in the skin of the head and face, now here, now there, aggravated by rubbing; sometimes, afterwards a red spot appears.—Corrosive itching or sticking in the skin of the head and face, in various places, repeatedly.—Itching below the hair, chiefly in the occipital region, either simple or biting or burning, associated with fine stitches, frequently with a sensation of warmth in the skin, mostly in the evening, causing scratching, by which it disappeared for a moment, but soon reappeared in other places, sometimes lasting only a few minutes, sometimes several hours (thirty-sixth, seventy-fifth, ninety-third, and one hundred and seventh days, etc.).

Eyes.—In General. In most of the provers the eyes seemed to lie deep, encircled by blue or dirty-gray rings for a long time.—The eye was excessively and uniformly red (second day),[7].—Inflammation of the eyes became so much worse in the afternoon that it is like what I have experienced from large doses (second day),[7].—The eyes feel very dry (second day),[7].—Dryness in the eyes almost constantly.—Dryness and biting or burning, also sometimes an itching sensation in the eyes, frequently also with a feeling as if sand were between the lids and the eye, at times with a slight redness of the conjunctiva of the lid and even of the ball; this symptom did not only appear very early, on the first or one of the first days, but also lasted throughout nearly the whole proving, with intermissions.—[80.] A feeling of stiffness in the eyes, with dragging (first and second days).—Bubbling sensation in the right eye lasting a quarter of an hour (eleventh day).—A bubbling sensation in the left eye, transient (after four hours, and also in the evening of third day).—Painfulness of the eyes (second day).†—Pain in the eyes, as after crying.—A somewhat painful sensation on beginning to read or write (seventh day).—A sensation in the eyes as if they were cold, as when one goes into the cold air, with some lachrymation on closing them (seventieth day).—Burning in the eyes, from 12 o'clock (first day),[9].—Burning sensation with dryness and redness in the eyes, with some matter in the canthi (seventeenth day).—Violent burning in the eyes which were very painful, especially on moving them (second day),[7].—[90.] Burning in the eyes at 3 o'clock in the afternoon, and at the same time a sensation as if sand were in them; they continued to get worse until she went to sleep; the left eye was worse than the right (first day),[10].—Violent burning and dryness in the eyes with a dim look to them; great redness of the conjunctiva of the lids, and a dim, indistinct look, as if there were a mist before the eyes, in the morning after rising, for several hours (sixty-third day).—Troubles with the eyes increased towards afternoon, and especially in the evening; the eyes burn like fire and are very dry (third day),[9].—Pressure in the eyes (after seven hours). —Pressure in the eyes, as if he had cried a long time.—Pressure and burning in the eyes (after two hours).—Pressure in both eyes, and pain on moving them, less during rest, accompanied by heat and burning in them (second day),[7].—Sensation in the eyes as if they were forced out (second to fourth day).—Sticking in the eye, mostly coming from other parts, as drawing from the forehead or from the temples into the eyes, or rising in the eyes, and spreading hence to the forehead; usually sudden shooting stitches.— A digging-sticking pain lasting several minutes, beginning deep in the eye and extending obliquely across the middle of the upper orbital margin upward and outward into the forehead, first in the right, and soon after in the left eye (seventeenth day).—[100.] Several piercing stitches in the eyes. —Four stitches shoot from the eye outward into the forehead, so violent that she is frightened (seventeenth day).—A slight, sometimes sensitive tearing in the eyes.—Throbbing in the left eye, for a short time (after three hours).—*External Parts.* Itching in the eyebrows, burning, biting or sticking, frequently returning, sometimes with fine burning, or burning-itching sticking.—Tensive sticking pain over the right orbit (ninth day).—

---

† Most of the eye troubles seem to be aggravated in the open air; motion of the eyes aggravates the pain.

Biting, fine sticking, and itching pain in the margins of the orbits, in the skin, especially in the inner canthus.—Tearing pain in the upper margin of the left orbit, extending towards the forehead (third day).—Tearing pain in the inner angle of the right orbit, extending towards the nose and forehead (fifteenth day).—Tearing in the bone in the margin of the orbits, especially the lower margin, frequently extending into the orbital cavity; sometimes it only begins to pain when touched (twenty-ninth day, *et seq.*) —[110.] Tearing in the outer side of the left orbit, with tendency to lachrymation.—Several stitches from the left orbital margin shoot quickly to the right frontal eminence (after half an hour and ten hours).—Twitching in the region of the right upper orbital margin (second day).—The eyelids became much inflamed and swollen, especially the left (fourth and fifth days),[9].—The eyelids are red on the inner surface, and the margin covered with a white frothy fluid (first day),[9].—In the morning after rising, a fine white crusty substance on the dry margins of the lids.—The left eye was agglutinated in the morning (second day),[10].—Twitching in the lids when reading by lamplight, seldom by daylight.—Heaviness in the lids on motion.—A feeling in the eyes as if there were two drops of cold water between the margins of the lids, or between the lids and the eyeballs.—[120.] In the inner angle of the left eye a feeling as if a foreign body were in it; the lachrymal caruncle seemed somewhat inflamed; the conjunctiva in the inner canthus was very dry.—In the morning, after rising, a sticky sensation in the margin of the lids.—Sensation of dryness in the lids if they are closed (after two hours).—Fine burning or biting at different small spots on the lid.—Pinching-tearing pain in the eyelids (sixty-third day).—Tearing drawings and twinges in the lids.—Fine sticking, a very sensitive pain on the border of the left upper lid rather towards the outer part, as from a needle, lasting one-half minute twice in succession; it then becomes a burning.—Biting pain beneath the right lower lid.—Tearing in the upper lids.—Tearing in the lower lid of the left eye.—[130.] Crawling-biting sensation on the margin of the right lower lid repeatedly, becoming a twitching, bubbling sensation in the lid, several times repeated in a quarter of an hour.—Itching in the lids, at times burning, biting or fine sticking, seldom smarting.—Itching in the canthi; at times biting or sticking.—The conjunctiva of the margin of the lids is very red, and also the sclerotic (second day),[7].—*Ball and Vision.* Painful tearing in the left eyeball, intermittent, extending obliquely from above downward and outward, lasting two minutes.—At times the vision is somewhat dim; it seems better near than far.—The eyes become dim and felt as though she should soon go to sleep (first day),[10].—Sensitiveness of the eyes to bright sunlight at times, though not very great.—Daylight blinded her more than lamplight (second day),[7].—If she wishes to look at anything fine, she is obliged to hold her hand before her eyes to shield them from the daylight, and still more from the lamplight, which blinds her (third day),[9].—[140.] If she exert the eyes in sewing, it becomes black before them (third day),[9].—She was not able to sew, because everything seemed to run together (second day),[7].

Ears.—Below and behind the right ear, a small swelling of the size of a hazel-nut, not very painful, apparently a swollen cutaneous gland (fourth to eleventh day).—On the left external ear, near the head in the skin, a pimple of the size of a millet-seed, painful to touch; it disappears after six or seven days (fortieth day).—Great heat in the left outer ear, then after one and a half hours great coldness of the same and of the temples (after eight hours).—Tensive, violent stitching-pressing pain, with sticking in the right ear, as if something were digging in the ear, lasts half a minute in the evening (seventeenth day).—Drawing pain in the ears, ending in several stitches lasting several minutes, frequently during the day (eighteenth day).—Pressive pain with stitches in the right ear, as if something were digging in it, lasting half a minute in the evening (seventeenth day).—Pressing-sticking pain starts from the side of the throat below the jaw, quickly passes out of the ear with a slight or severe stitch, especially upon the left side (eleventh day).—A piercing-sticking pain in the right ear, in slow stitches, as if a powerful animal were in the ear and stung with a thick sting, in the afternoon at 5 o'clock for a quarter of an hour (seventeenth day).—[150.] A long jerklike stitch in the right ear, as if it came out through the drum, when at work, while sitting, as if a nail were forced through, or as if a living, stinging animal were in the ear, so violent and surprising that she starts up and involuntarily grasps the ear, with fine digging stitches between the pains, with a sensation as if the ear were full and dragged downward, lasting from ten minutes to a quarter of an hour (seventh and fifteenth days, as also at other times).—Tearing-sticking in the internal ears, alternating with the same symptoms in other parts of the head (eleventh day, and frequently).—Drawing stitches deep in the right ear from below upward, lasting about twenty seconds.—Tensive violent stitches in the right ear from without inward.—Several stitches in the right ear (second day).—Moderate pressive stitches in slow sensitive jerks deep in the right ear for a minute, repeated after a quarter of an hour; then, after half an hour, tearing in the antitragus for half a minute (twenty-fifth day).—About fifteen bubbling stitches in the left ear from without inward, at last a continued stitching, then changing to pressure, then a stopped sensation for half a minute (sixty-fifth day).—Two stitches, as with fine thorns, in the left ear (after three hours).—Pressive, painless throbbing and whizzing in the left, seldom in the right ear, in quickly following shocks, two to fifteen in number, as if the air or the wing of a bird struck against the drum, with a feeling of dryness and coldness in the ear, very frequently repeated (thirtieth, thirty-second, fortieth, and one hundred and first days).—Tearing in the bone behind the left ear.—[160.] A slight tearing in the external ears.—Tearing in one or the other internal ear, mostly only for a short time, now severe, now slight.—Itching in the outer ears, now simple, now biting, or burning, or sticking, with fine stitches and increased sensation of warmth; at times also several pimples on the outer ear.—Ringing in the right ear, long continued, beginning deep, then becoming higher, several times during the day, and for several days together (thirtieth and thirty-second day).

Nose.—The nose and eyes are moist, as if a coryza would come on (after eight hours).—Profuse fluent catarrh (seventeenth day).—*The mucous membrane of the nose seemed in most of the provers dry, with little discharge;* in one prover, however, at a later time, a coryza, which lasted several minutes, appeared in the left nostril, and apparently involved also the frontal and maxillary sinuses; in the beginning, a yellow, burnt-smelling water, afterward purulent, sometimes whitish, at times yellowish or greenish mucus, also of a burnt smell and taste, was blown from the nose and hawked up, especially in the morning, though not a large quantity.—In the morning, on rising, she loses a few drops of clear blood from the left nostril, which had never before been noticed (ninth day).—At about 6 o'clock in the morning some drops of clear blood are discharged from the left nostril, followed by a pressing pain in the left temple extending forward to the eye (ninth day).—*Dryness of the nose*, and a sensation as if she would have a catarrh, with frequent sneezing (second day),[7].—[**170.**] Biting gnawing sensation at the tip of the nose.—Crawling in the left nostril very sensitive, as if she would sneeze, which she did not do (first day).—Frequent crawling, biting, or itching in the nostrils.—Itching in the skin of the nose, at times burning, biting, or fine sticking; also fine burning or itching stitches, at times some pimples arise upon it.

Face.—In General, and Cheeks.
Pale expression of the face (in persons much affected by the drug), *a dirty grayish look, sunken cheeks, deeply seated eyes, surrounded by bluish or blackish-gray circles; very sickly expression for a long time.*—A dark red, very painful, small spot appears, following a transient sensation of coldness; it soon enlarges, and by and by extends over the whole face, with a sensation of great heat; this symptom repeated several times in one afternoon (fifth day).—A feeling as if cold drops of rain spattered in the face on going from the house into the open air, several times (seventieth day, *et seq.*).—A chilly, tearing pain in a small spot on the left cheek.—Pressive pain, sometimes alternating with tearing, in the left upper jaw.—Sticking cold sensation in a small spot on the left cheek.—[**180.**] Tearing, pressive pain in the left cheek-bone, especially in the malar fossa (tenth day).—Tearing, sticking pains in both cheek-bones (fifteenth day, *et seq.*).—Tearing, sticking pain in the right cheek, shooting by jerks into the temples, lasting for several minutes (after two and a half hours).—Severe tearing in the posterior portion of the left cheek-bone in three violent jerks from below upwards.—Tearing pains in the right upper jaw, extending from the angle in front of the ear into the temple.—Aching pressing jerk in the right cheek, as if one had received a box on the ear (thirty-third day).—*Lips and Chin.* A bluish-red color on the inner side of the lower lip.—On the inner side of the lower lip towards the angle, a dull red, somewhat bluish spot about the size of a small bean.—*Dryness of the lips.*—In the morning after rising and also during the day, a sticky feeling on the margin of the lips.—[**190.**] Fine burning in several small places in the upper lip.—Burning in the outer margins of the lips for half a minute, frequently also longer, as if they had been covered with pepper-water, or were swollen, several times.—Burning sensation in the upper lip, in the right corner of the mouth, as from pepper, with a bubbling sensation and a drawing-downward feeling in it (twenty-second day).—In the right half of the lower lip a pressive-pinching pain, as if it were pinched with the fingers for several minutes.—Fine stitches in the margin of the lips; sometimes itching, sometimes burning.—On the left side of the upper lip a twitching, bubbling sensation, as if something were jumping on it for several minutes.—Slight tearing in the left side of the upper lip, with some burning and tingling.—Fine, painless, quick throbbing in the upper lip just over the right corner of the mouth, for half a minute.—Itching in the lips, which disappears on rubbing, but soon returns; sometimes biting or burning.—Cold burning sensation on the left side of the chin.—[**200.**] On the margin of the horizontal ramus of the right lower jaw, about the middle, a pressive pain in the bone, as if the place were squeezed together with two fingers (fifty-fourth day).—A burning stitch in the left side of the chin.—Pain in the lower margin of the left lower jaw, near and just in front of the angle for half an inch, only noticed when touching it, feeling as if one had received a blow on this spot, for several days in succession (forty-sixth to fifty-second day).—Pressive-sticking pain in the jaws, especially in the

lower, during the day and also in the night (thirteenth day).—Jerking stitches in the angle of the left lower jaw, digging-biting extending in the row of teeth on the lower jaw and the back teeth for half a minute, as if the gum were loosened from the teeth, or as if they were raised up..

Mouth.—Teeth and Gums. Dull aching in the back teeth of the left upper jaw, as if they were too long.—Slow digging pain in a right upper incisor in the root, as if it were denuded from the gum, for several minutes (eighteenth day).—A drawing, bubbling pain presses downwards in the first upper incisors of the left side, with a sensation as if the teeth were exceedingly sensitive to the touch, were too long or blunt, and as if something heavy hung upon them; after a few days a small boil in the gum over them.—Tearing in the left upper incisors, extending to the superior maxillary bone (for a quarter of an hour).—Frequent piercing stitches in the teeth of the right side of the lower jaw, as if one of them were carious, with a sensation as if the teeth were too large or blunt, with great sensitiveness to the cold air, especially with tearing and sticking in the lower jaw, in the afternoon and at night for several hours in succession (tenth day).—[210.] Several stitches in the two anterior lower back teeth of the right side, followed by a sensation as if they were too long (after two hours).—Tearing pain in the back teeth of the left upper jaw (tenth day).—Tearing in the two back teeth of the left upper jaw for half an hour, then extending to other parts of the face.—A scraping-gnawing pain in the whole row of the back teeth of the lower jaw of the left side, as if in the roots or necks of the teeth (eighteenth day).—Dirty red scum on the gum of several of the front teeth of the upper jaw, less on the lower jaw and on the back teeth.—On the gum of the upper row several small white pimples; the smallest is of the size of a grape-seed, the largest of a flax-seed, either round or flattened, painless, lasts several weeks.—Above the two upper back teeth of the left side a few small pustules, which become ulcers and continue for a long time.—Slight though noticed bleeding of the gum several times.—***Mouth in General, Saliva, and Taste.*** A painful white vesicle in the forepart of the right side of the tip of the tongue.—On the right side of the tip of the tongue two red pimples as large as a poppy-seed stung violently, especially on touch; the forepart of the tongue seemed stiff and thick (forty-second and forty-third days).— [220.] Sticking-burning sensation in several small points on the left side of the tongue, as from fine needle-points; painfulness of the tongue to touch and motion; no vesicles visible (eighth, ninth, thirty-eighth, and thirty-ninth days).—Some fine stitches in the tongue, especially in the right side (second day).—Nauseous metallic smell from the mouth for a long time.—Dryness and sticky sensation in the mouth of all the provers.—Dryness in the mouth, but still more in the fauces, worse in the morning after rising, with a peculiar sticky sensation, rawness of the mucous membrane, white tongue, diminished secretion of saliva, *or a sticky frothy saliva like cotton;* seldom with thirst and heat; loss of taste or not quite perfect taste; this condition is somewhat relieved by eating and drinking, but it returns; after eating, the taste is somewhat sour.—The mouth and throat feel sticky, pasty, and as if burnt (third day),⁹.—A cold sensation in the left corner of the mouth.—Smarting-burning on the mouth and on the chin, sometimes like a formication.—Sticky saliva.—Insipid, nauseous taste arises from the stomach like heartburn (after one to three hours).—[230.] A scraping-burning taste in the mouth and throat like heartburn (first day).—Long-continued bitter scraping-burning taste of the Berberis root, especially in the palate, of three persons; in one person it seemed as if it came up into the throat;

she could not get free from it nearly the whole of the first day.—Taste as bitter as gall (fifth day).—Bitter taste in the mouth at 8 o'clock in the morning (second day),[8].—Taste as bitter as gall for half an hour, every time after eating (eighth day).—Bitter and sour taste for three hours after taking, and the whole day.—Frequent taste of blood, especially in the morning, sometimes also in the afternoon.

Throat.—Arches of the palate, uvula, tonsils, and pharynx are somewhat red (second and third days).—Dryness in the throat, and pressure in the back part of the palate and pharynx (after eleven hours).—In the upper part of the right side of the throat, just below the angle of the jaw, a digging-sticking pain extends into the ear and out again (seventh day).—Smarting pain on the throat, especially on the right side; scratching increased it, and caused a large, red, hot spot (ninety-fifth day).—[240.] Scraping in the throat (after four hours).—Scraping sensation in the throat as if it were somewhat raw, as if he would be attacked with catarrh (twelfth day).—Scraping sensation in the throat as in commencing angina, so that she is obliged to hawk and raise frequently, without any difficulty in swallowing, for several hours (after four hours).—Scraping sensation in the throat in the morning (second day).—Scraping sensation in the throat in the morning on waking, as if the throat would become sore, which continues until the throat becomes moistened.—Scraping sensation in the throat in the evening, it extends into the pharynx, stomach, and air-passages (third day).—Scraping in throat greatly relieved by drinking water,[7].—Scraping sensation in the throat, especially in the morning after rising, nearly every day for several weeks, sometimes with pain in one side of it.—Pain in the left tonsil caused and increased by speaking, and also by swallowing, with a sensation as if the seed of a fruit were sticking in the throat; the tonsils and the arch of the palate of this side are somewhat red and rather sensitive to pressure, as are also the neighboring parts of the throat to motion (fifth to seventh and seventeenth days).—(Completely developed inflammation of the tonsils, arch of the palate, uvula, pharynx, with bright, fiery redness, and swelling; sensation as if there were a lump in one side of the throat) painful stiffness of the neck as from a blister; great hoarseness, in the morning a discharge of much thick, yellow, gelatinous mucus; violent pains, more on empty swallowing; dryness, scraping, rawness, and burning in the throat, without thirst, extending down into the pharynx and air-passages; tongue white, sticky; *saliva sticky like soapsuds;* the troubles last violently only two days, but for eight days there remains a sensation as of a plug in the throat, and for several weeks rawness, dryness, and scraping in the throat; at last catarrh (eleventh and eighteenth days in two persons).[†]

Stomach.—[250.] Increased appetite (second day).—Increased appetite (after a long-continued use of the tincture of the Berberis root, by a girl suffering from weakness of the stomach, and loss of appetite),[°].—Great appetite (first day).—Very good appetite, almost canine hunger (fourth day).—Very good appetite (after five to six hours); increased appetite in the evening (first day).—Hunger without appetite (third day).—Loss of appetite, with a bilious, bitter taste (eleventh day).—Almost complete want

---

[†] This condition appeared in two women just at the time when an influenza was raging here, which I did not consider associated with this angina. It may be, however, that this attack was dependent in its peculiar development upon this circumstance.

of hunger and appetite; food has almost no taste (seventeenth and twenty-first days).—No real hunger, appetite, or taste (first day).—Severe thirst wakes her several times at night (first night),[7].—[**260.**] Increased thirst with dry mouth, especially in the afternoon, seldom in the morning, in several persons.—*Eructations* (soon after taking the drug).—Eructations frequently alternating with yawning (after an hour and a half).—*Eructations without bad taste or smell* (an hour after taking the drug, and also several times afterwards during first day).—Two hours after taking frequent bilious eructations (lasting nearly half an hour).—Frequent eructations and gripings in the abdomen, as of wind, without passing any (first day),[10].—Hiccough for nearly a quarter of an hour (seventeenth day).—Transient nausea (after one hour).—Nausea lasting one hour (after half an hour).—Nausea and qualmishness before breakfast, disappearing afterwards (second day).—[**270.**] Nausea after dinner; she thought she would be obliged to vomit (first day),[10].—Feeling of discomfort and nausea (after three hours).—*Heartburn* (soon after taking it).—After eating, a pressive sensation in the epigastric region as if it were distended, evenings till 9 o'clock (sixty-first day),[7].—Pressure in the region of the stomach five hours after eating (seventh day).—A sticking pain in the region of the stomach for half an hour and at times afterwards, though returning slighter (seventh day).—A violent sticking, burning, peculiar pain in the stomach, like heartburn, though much more violent, it also extends upward into the pharynx (eighth and twenty-first day).

Abdomen.—Hypochondria. Twice, a bubbling sensation below the tip of the false ribs, in the forepart on the right side, in quick succession; severe bubbling sensation, as if one shook a bottle of water, or as if one forced air into the flesh, on the external border of the right shoulder-blade near the axilla (ninety-seventh day).—*In the hypochondriac region, near the border of the false ribs, about three inches from the linea alba, violent sticking pain for a quarter of an hour, increased by pressure, extending across into the region of the stomach;* it appeared first when walking; walking slowly did not relieve it (after a quarter of an hour), (also noticed from the 5th dilution).—Pressure in the forepart of the right hypochondrium, extending inward into the border of the false ribs (forty-sixth day).—[**280.**] Pressure in the region of the liver, on the margin of the false ribs, about three inches from the linea alba, lasts a quarter of an hour (third day).—On the border of the false ribs of the right side, about two and a half inches from the linea alba, thirty-six to forty successive burning stitches at intervals of four to eight seconds (nineteenth day).—*Sticking-pressive pain in the region of the liver, increased by pressure, corresponding to the region of the gall-bladder, on a small spot;* lasts three hours, though not continuous (second hour and frequently afterwards, even until forty-sixth day).—*Sticking pain, not very penetrating, in the region of the gall-bladder, for several minutes* (after nine hours).—*Sticking pain in the region of the gall-bladder* for a short time, increased by pressure (after an hour and a half).—Drawing-tearing pain below the tips of the false ribs in the left hypochondrium on inspiration; it feels as if something were torn loose at the affected spot.—Pressive pain in the left hypochondrium extends backward or downward.—Tearing-sticking pain in the region of the left hypochondrium, in front (forty-sixth and forty-eight days).—*Umbilicus.* Slight gripings around the navel (after eight hours).—Intermittent pain pressing from within outward in the left side of the abdomen, about an inch from the navel, as if something living were in the spot, about the size of a half dollar, lasting from two to three minutes (twenty-second day).—[**290.**] Cutting-drawing pain in the left side of the navel in a spot of the size of a quarter of a dollar, extending deep inward, for a minute violent, then continuing dull for about two minutes. —*Pain in the region about three inches to the side of the navel, corresponding to a place in front of the kidneys, and rather to the side, mostly sticking,* sometimes dull, sometimes fine, or also burning or gnawing, usually only in one side, seldom in both sides; usually confined to a small place or a point, sometimes pressive when it is more diffused, for the most part aggravated only by deep pressure, seldom, then violent, but returning nearly every day, frequently continuing for hours, with momentary intermissions, often continuing only a short time, *often extending to the lumbar region or to the groins, the liver, the spleen, or the stomach.*—Superficial tearing-sticking pain in the left side of the navel.—Twisting pain in the region of the navel, in a place as large as the palm of the hand, for a few minutes (after nine hours).—A few fine, sharp, deep stitches at the left side of the navel.— Fine stitches in the right side of the abdomen, at the side of the navel but somewhat above it, for a minute.—At times, twinging around and above the navel, in the left side of the abdomen (first day).—***In General.*** Fermentation in the abdomen, especially in the region of the colon, with perceptible motion of the intestines, and moving of wind (first day).—Loud rumblings (after nine hours).—Frequent rumblings in the abdomen, so that they can be heard externally (fifth day).—[**300.**] Great rumbling in the bowels followed by the passage of flatus (after two hours).—Slight rumblings and movings in the abdomen, followed by the passage of some flatus (after eight hours).—Frequent passage of copious, seldom offensive, flatus, usually preceded by painless gripings, at times with a sensation of warmth in the anus; all the provers (first, second, and third days).—Movings in the abdomen, as though a stool would come soon; it does not take place (second day).—Feeling of movings in the intestines, not painful, soon after taking it. Writhings in the region of the stomach (after half an hour).— Slight pain in the abdomen, lasting five minutes (after half an hour).— Pain in the abdomen, in the morning, in bed (second day),[8].—Violent burning pain under the skin, and extending into it, in the left side of the abdomen, about four inches from the navel, in a spot about an inch and a half in diameter, lasting half an hour (ninety-fourth day).—Twinging, constricting sensation in the walls of the abdomen, lasting five to eight minutes.—Twinging, constrictive sensation in the upper part of the left side of the abdomen, especially in the left hypochondrium across towards the navel, for a few minutes.—[**310.**] Colic-like pain in the region below the navel, of short duration (third and sixth days).—Transient colicky pain in the abdomen (first day).—At times, gripings in the abdomen (second day).—Slight griping and constrictions in the intestines (sixty-seventh hour).—Painless gripings in the abdomen, followed by the passage of flatus (after two hours).—Aching, pressing sensation in the region of the left descending colon (after eight hours).—Urging and moving in the abdomen before the stool (second and third days).—Writhings in the abdomen (after one hour).— Violent cuttings in the abdomen, lasting for two or three minutes, repeated two or three times (seventh day).—Cutting pain in the abdomen several times in the afternoon, as if diarrhœa would come on; it lasted till the next day, when there was diarrhœa once in the morning and afternoon (fourth day),[8].—[**320.**] Cutting-sticking pain in the abdomen, at times, for several minutes (tenth day).—Cutting-jerking pain about an inch and a half from the linea alba, an inch above the navel, extending in slow drawings outward across the left lumbar region (nineteenth day).—Tearings in the abdomen (after a half hour to one hour).—At 10 o'clock in the evening, on going to sleep, violent, sticking, tearing, colicky pain in the upper part of the abdomen, lasting about an hour, extending into the stomach and in the left side to the left hypochondrium, mostly corresponding to a place in front of the kidneys, very much increased by breathing, motion, and touch; respiration short; the abdomen somewhat distended and hard; the pains return the next morning on becoming erect when rising, though they last only for a few minutes, and return again afterward, though less severe (fourth and fifth days).—Some stitches extend across the abdomen in the region of the stomach (twenty-third day).—A tearing or sticking pain extends around the body in the abdominal muscles.—*Hypogastrium and Iliac Region.* *In the right inguinal region, near the abdominal ring, some varicose veins,* the longest about an inch and a half long; they extend downward to the thigh, preceded by pressing in this region (third day).—Peculiar cold sensation in the region of the right abdominal ring, becoming more like a burning.—Twinging pain in both Poupart's ligaments, also especially above them, extending outward and into the inguinal rings, for a few minutes (third day).—Cutting pain extending inward in the left inguinal ring, as if it were depressed (forty-ninth day).—[**330.**]— Drawing pain above one or the other Poupart's ligament, extending towards the thigh.—In the inguinal region of one side, and above and in Poupart's ligament, especially in the region of the inguinal ring as the chief point, a dragging, sticking pain, with pulselike stitches, sometimes also a painless bubbling sensation, mostly appearing when walking and standing, and thereby aggravated; they extend downward into the testicles and the upper anterior portion of the thigh, outward into the region of the kidneys, at times also beginning in this last place, together with fine stitches in the abdomen in front of the region which corresponds to the kidneys posteriorly, several times.—Just above the middle of the right Poupart's ligament, ten sensitive stitches, extending from without inward, returning after five minutes, and becoming a twinging pain.—Throbbing stitches in the right inguinal region, by paroxysms, shoot suddenly, for a few minutes in succession, down into the thigh, as with needles (seventh day).—A tensive sensation in one or the other inguinal ring, as if a hernia would appear, frequent, especially on standing and walking.—Itching-burning pain in the region of the left inguinal glands.—Pressive pain in the region of the right inguinal glands, which are painful when touched, as if they would become swollen (third day).—Pressure in the left inguinal region (first day).—Pressive sensation in the right groin near the inguinal ring, above and to the outer side of it, as if something would protrude at this place, extending down to the thigh.—Pressive sensation in the region of the inguinal ring, frequently.—[**340.**] Tensive-sticking pain above the right Poupart's ligament, about the middle of it.—Dragging-sticking pain above the left Poupart's ligament, extending outward and upward.—Several stitches in one or the other inguinal region, and above Poupart's ligament.—*Burning-smarting pain in the right inguinal fold, with tension on motion.*—Itching sensation in the region of one or the other inguinal rings.—Above the anterior border of the left ilium, along down Poupart's ligament, five slow drawing or cutting severe stitches, so that she had to cry out.—Dragging-sticking pain extends from the anterior inferior spinous process of the left ilium, and a little above it, towards the inguinal region and the thigh (eleventh day).— Tearing-sticking pain in the anterior region of one or another iliac crest, extending up towards the abdomen.—Tearing-sticking pain across from the spine into the crest of the ilium, at times remaining at this place, at times extending downward into the pelvis, or upward into the muscles.—Tearing-sticking pain in the crest of the ilium to the region of the anterior spinous process, and also farther backward, sometimes at this place only, sometimes extending inward and upward into the walls of the abdomen, mostly towards Poupart's ligament and the region above it, at times downward into the thigh.—[350.] *Deepseated, sensitive, sticking pain in the ilium of one or the other side, an inch to an inch and a half from the spine, extending obliquely inward towards the sacrum, sometimes with bubbling-like, deeply penetrating stitches.—*Five or six sharp stitches, from the origin of the left Poupart's ligament at the ilium, extending along down it; a quarter of an hour afterwards, a stitch shooting outwardly into the left side of the female urethra.—Tearing-sticking pain above the crest of the left ilium, in the morning when waking.—*Tearing pain in the posterior portion of the iliac crest, usually only on one side, extending downward into the gluteal muscles, or into the bones.—Dragging-tearing pain in the anterior portion of the iliac crest, extending into the abdomen to one or the other side.—Gnawing, tearing, ulcerative pain in the same place in the ilium.—Sticking-tearing pain about the middle of the outer posterior surface of the left ilium, severe and deep in the bone, extending from without inward for several minutes, in the morning on waking, when in bed.—Smarting pain in the region of the crest of the right ilium, extending down into the hip (ninety-third day).

Rectum and Anus.—* Constant feeling as though she must go to stool (third day).—In the anus, hæmorrhoids appeared frequently, with a burning pain after a stool; the evacuation is frequently hard and of a dirty blood color externally (second and third weeks, and frequently).—[360.] Irritation in the anus, frequently returning (first and second days).—Sensation of warmth in the region of the anus (first to third day, afterwards frequently).—*Violent burning pain in the anus, as if the parts around it were sore, frequently returning, and continuing a long time (nineteenth, thirty-seventh, fortieth, and fifty-first days, etc.).—Feeling of fulness in the anus after one hour.—Pressing in the anus (seventh day).—*Slight sticking sensation in the anus (fifth day).—Transient stitching in the anus (second day). —Transient slight stitches in the anus (after three hours).—*Burning stitching pain during, before, and after stool (fourth day).—*Tearings extending around the anus.—[370.] *Smarting pain in the anus (third day).—A feeling of soreness and burning in the vicinity of the anus; there arose hæmorrhoids, which lasted several weeks, as large as an acorn, and frequently caused itching and burning (ninetieth day).—* The skin for some distance around the anus feels completely raw, with severe burning for some days; violent pain on touching the sore place, and great sensitiveness when sitting; finally a thin scurf appears on the border of the anus; this condition returns several times, though later in a less degree (sixty-third day).—Throbbing pain in the anus for a minute (in three hours and a half).—Crawling in the anus, as from ascarides (after two and six hours).—Itching in the anus (second day).—Pressive pain in the perineum in front of the anus (for half a minute).—Digging-sticking pain, with short jerking stitches, as if she had been pierced by a thorn and the perineum were pressed upon it, extending deep into the left side of the womb (seventy-second day).—* Crawling, burning, itching in the anus and about it.

Stool.—* Urging to stool (second day).—[380.] Urging before the stool, especially in the colon, and extending into the small of the back (first and

second days).—Tensive urging to stool in the small of the back and anus
(first day).—Stool in the morning, with pressure and pain (third day).—
Stool passes easily (first, second, and third days).—A satisfactory soft stool
passes easily (after a warm infusion of half an ounce of the Berberis root)
(the next morning). Stool at first somewhat hard, then soft (twenty hours
after a second warm infusion of the same root). In the morning of the
second day a similar stool (after a third infusion of the same).—Easy, copious, natural, not hard stool in the evening, which is not usually the case
(first day).—Easy, soft, profuse stool in the morning (second and third days,
in two persons).—Copious, soft stool in the evening, at an unusual time,
(nine hours after taking an infusion of the root, followed in twenty hours
by another similar one.)—Copious, soft stool, followed for half an hour by
a pressive-tensive sensation in the small of the back and rectum (twenty-
four hours after taking one-half drachm of the powdered bark of the root).
—Copious, soft stool at an unusual time in the afternoon; the next morning there followed the ordinary evacuation, preceded by much pressure in
the small of the back and anus (eight hours after two scruples of the root).
—A loose movement three or four times a day, with cutting pains (eighth
to tenth days),[9].—[390.] Three soft stools, usually she had only one or two,
with great urging (third day).—Three copious, thick, pasty evacuations
(six, thirteen, and twenty-six hours after one-half drachm of the powdered
bark of the root). Hard stool (third day).—Diarrhœic stool without cutting pain (second day),[10].—Diarrhœa twice (first day),[9].—Fully developed
diarrhœa, consisting of four pasty, yellowish evacuations, the first six, the
last ten hours, after taking the drug, with rumbling without cuttings, much
passage of wind, at times some nausea, much thirst, heat in the face and
confusion of the head, with increased appetite in the evening (after a decoction of three and one-half drachms of the root).—Stool scanty, thin-
formed, but not hard (fifth day).—Stool scanty and rather hard (seventh
day).—Stool scanty, hard, or also soft, thin-formed, delayed (after three
days, frequently afterwards, in several people).†—The next morning the
usual evacuation seemed harder, not copious (sixth hour), then a more copious, softer stool (after ten hours), afterwards a profuse, pasty evacuation
(after twenty-four hours), again (after twenty-five hours), and again (after
twenty-eight hours), preceded by severe pressure, especially with the first
evacuations (after ten grains of Berberis).—Stool hardish and in small
quantity (fourth day).—[400.] Stool firm, hard like sheep dung, with
much, frequently ineffectual, urging (ninth day).—After the stool a comfortable sensation of relief.—*A long-continued sensation after the stool, as
if one had just been to stool, or as if one had just recovered from a pain in
the anus (first to third day).—Sensation after the stool as if one must soon
go again, with perceptible movement of the intestines (first and second day).
—*Constipation (ninth day).—No stool (second day),[7].

Urinary Organs.—Kidneys and Bladder. *A sticking-
digging, or digging-tearing pain in one or the other kidney regions, *as if
it were suppurating, aggravated by deep pressure.*—Drawing pain in the left
kidney region.—*Tearing, pulsating pain in the right kidney.*—*Tearing

† From small doses the stool seems to be retarded. I leave to others to judge
whether retarded or increased diarrhœa-like stool is the secondary action. The dis-
tinctions seem to me not so easy, because the potencies also produced diarrhœa.
How then will we account for the purging effect of large doses, followed by an inclination to constipation and retention of stool?

pain in the region of both kidneys soon after rising in the morning, which extends sideways and forward, both upward and downward, so that the whole region of the back between the thorax and the pelvis is affected. If she stooped the lower part of the back felt stiff, and it was with difficulty that she could stand up on account of this painful stiffness. This tearing was noticed even when sitting, more severe than when standing; was relieved in the afternoon (second day),[7].—[410.] Bubbling sensation in the left kidney region, extending across into the abdomen and into the bladder (tenth day).†—Burning-itching, biting-smarting pain in the region of the bladder.—**Burning pain in the bladder,** *sometimes when it is full, sometimes when empty, even after urinating, for several times, frequently also in the morning before urinating for the first time.*—**After urinating, a sensation in the bladder as if one must go again soon, or as if some urine remained behind.*—Pinching constrictive pain in the region of the bladder.—Pressive pinching pain in one or the other side of the region of the bladder; on pressure upon it there sometimes arises burning in the whole urethra.—*Drawing-sticking pain in one or the other side of the bladder, extending down into the female urethra, often arising in the lumbar region, and extending along the course of the ureters.—Pressive pain in the region of the bladder when filled, and also when empty, and after urinating, very frequently and continuous in three provers.—* *Violent cutting-tensive pain deeply seated in the left side of the bladder, at last becoming a sticking obliquely in the female urethra, as if in its orifice, lasting a few minutes* (twenty-fifth day).—*Painful cuttings in the left side of the region of the bladder extend into the urethra, coming from the left kidney along the course of the ureter* (nineteenth day). —[420.] * *Cutting constrictive pain in the bladder,* sometimes when full, sometimes when not full, sometimes immediately after evacuating it.—*Violent sticking pain in the bladder extending from the kidneys, only increased by severe pressure after half an hour, without desire to urinate (seventh day).—Tearing-sticking pain in the region of the bladder, especially on the left side, just above the symphysis and extending into it, then passing into the left side of the penis, or also returning higher up.—Violent stitches in the bladder, which compel one to urinate.—Several stitches in the region of the bladder, either when the bladder is full or after urinating, and also at other times (forty-eighth day).—As many as forty stitches in the bladder, pulselike, above the symphysis, at last becoming a slight sticking pain, lasting a short time; returning in a less degree during the next day, when the bladder is not very full (fifty-ninth and sixtieth days).—*Urethra.* **Burning in the urethra.—*Burning pain in the female urethra during and after urinating,* though more at other times (seventh day, and very often at other times).—**Burning in the urethra, usually more towards the anterior, sometimes also more posteriorly, or *along the whole length of it,* often continuing for several hours, for the most part more on one side, usually when not urinating, but sometimes also when urinating and soon afterwards.— The morbid urine seems warmer than usual when urinating.—[430.] Smarting-burning sensation in the left side of the urethra, with intercurrent bubbling-like shocks.—Momentary constrictive pain in the posterior portion of the urethra.—Pressure when urinating (after two hours).—Cutting pain in the urethra, frequently more upon one side.—* *Cutting pain in the urethra,*

---

† The symptoms in the region of the kidney were worse when stooping and when becoming erect, in sitting, and also in lying than when standing, though not always.

after urinating and also at other times (after two hours, and frequently).—Slight sticking in the urethra (after eight hours, and frequently).—*Sticking pain in the female urethra beginning in the bladder*, sometimes in the middle, sometimes on one side.—Sticking pain in the female urethra, as if a thorn were sticking into it.—Sensitive sticking pain in the urethra, extending into the bladder (third day).—Jerking sticking sensation in the female urethra, with a spasmodic constrictive sensation for several seconds.—[**440.**] Several stitches in the urethra.—Smarting constrictive pain in the urethra.—Smarting in the urethra after coition, once even a sensitive pain in it during ejaculation of semen.—Smarting pain in the urethra and the glans, chiefly towards the forepart and upon one side, or extending into the bladder, returning frequently and continuing a long time; either the urethra pains are caused or aggravated by motion.—Smarting-biting pain in the urethra, frequently with a sensation of soreness, more when not urinating, sometimes transient, sometimes continuous, chiefly in the forepart, but sometimes also extending backwards into the bladder or rectum, frequently more pain on one side.—Bubbling sensation in the posterior portion of the urethra when sitting.—Crawling sensation in the posterior portion of the male urethra (for two minutes).—Itching along the urethra.—Crawling-itching pain in the urethra a few times when not urinating, when the bladder is not full.—**Micturition and Urine.** Pressure to urinate (after three hours).—[**450.**] Excessive desire to urinate, especially in the morning immediately after rising.—Sometimes diminished, sometimes increased discharge of urine; when increased the urine is commonly a clear, light water, or slightly tinged, deposits only a slight sediment of mucus, when scanty it usually deposits a sediment; the former is the case in the beginning and during the aggravations, the latter during the reaction of the medicine; at times, however, intercurrent conditions arise (in all provers.)—*Pale, yellow urine, either* **with a slight transparent gelatinous sediment which does not deposit, or a turbid, flocculent, claylike, copious, mucous sediment mixed with a white, or whitish-gray, and later a reddish mealy sediment.** —The clear, saturated, yellowish, thick urine has a decided appearance of the yellow of the Berberis root, seldom remaining clear, but depositing a mucous sediment during the aggravations of the proving, and usually in the beginning; generally very soon or sometimes later becoming separated, flocculent, or like mealy water, *and depositing a copious mucous and mealylike sediment, with white-grayish, white, or dirty-reddish, or red granular sediment*, with yellowish-red crystals upon the bottom and sides of the glass.—*Urine bright-yellow, with a profuse mucous sediment*, but was not cloudy (second day).—Dark, dirty, wine-yellow urine, which commonly separates and deposits a copious sediment, as in the previous case, or only gelatinous flakes.—Greenish urine, clear, or just tinged, in the beginning somewhat turbid, depositing only some mucus, but becoming cloudy, but only seldom settles.—*Inflammatory red urine*, which like the last separates and deposits a thick sediment, seldom remaining unchanged and becoming merely thick.—*Blood-red urine*, **which speedily becomes turbid and deposits a thick mucous and bright red mealy sediment**, *slowly becoming clear, but always retaining its blood-red color, with violent pains in the kidneys* (in one prover).—During convalescence from the drug-disease the urine has for a long time *a clear mucous sediment.*—[**460.**] The changes in the urine vary, increasing and diminishing with the medicinal disease; even on the same day it changes in various ways, it may be even normal; pains in the loins and kidneys frequently accompany the morbid urine, though not always; usually the urine passed first in the morning after rising is cloudy.

Sexual Organs.—Male—Penis. Decided feeling of weakness in the genitals after coition.—A sense of weakness and loss of irritability of the external male genitals after urinating, and also at other times.—The penis seems somewhat shrivelled and retracted.—Frequent erections (first day).—The mucous membrane of the penis seems to be dry.—Cold sensation in the prepuce and glans at times, also with a somewhat numb sensation.—A pinching constrictive pain extends downwards from the mons veneris along the dorsum of the penis.—Several stitches in the glans.—Fine stitching pain in the penis (for half a minute).—[470.] Fine stitching in the penis in the forepart.—Smarting pains in the anterior portion of the left side of the penis coming from the urethra.—Smarting pain in the left side of the penis, more externally, chiefly in the forepart of the mucous membrane of the glans, and in the part behind this spot, when walking and afterwards, also after coition (one hundred and eighth, one hundred and twelfth, and one hundred and twenty-second days, etc.).—Smarting-burning pain in the corona glandis.—Smarting-burning pain in the left side of the penis, especially in the corona glandis.—Smarting-burning pain in the upper part of the right side of the penis.—Smarting-burning itching pain in the prepuce.—*Scrotum and Testicles, Sexual Desires.* Sensation of coldness, light tearings in the left side of the scrotum.—Smarting, constricting pain in the left lower portion of the scrotum, lasting six to eight minutes when walking.—Sore pain in the scrotum, especially in the sides, most frequently on the left.—[480.] Itching in the scrotum, either simple, or burning, or with fine stitches, at times smarting or crawling.—Burning pain in one or the other testicle, seldom in both, as if they would swell.—Constrictive pain in the testicles and in the spermatic cord, with contraction of the scrotum, as if it would be drawn up against the abdomen; the scrotum is shrivelled and cold, with pressive pain in the testicles.—Drawing-pressive pain in one or the other testicle, seldom in both at the same time, sometimes extending up the spermatic cord.—Pressive pain in both testicles, sometimes in only one, sometimes for only a short time, or for several hours.—Cutting-sticking pain, at times very sensitive, in the testicles, at times in only one, at times in both together.—Single or several stitches in one or the other testicle (fortieth, sixty-third, and ninety-first days, etc.).—Smarting or smarting-burning pain in the testicles, at times in only one, at times in both.—Crawling pain in the testicles, usually in only one (most of the pains in the external genitals are caused and aggravated by motion).—*Soft pulpy swelling of the left spermatic cord, especially in the lower portion, several times when walking, with at times drawing, burning, or smarting, or tearing pains, at times also when sitting, with pain extending down into the testicles, especially the epididymis.*—[490.] *Drawing pain in the spermatic cord of the right, frequently of the left side, extending down into the testicles, or up into the abdominal ring.*—Stitching pain in the spermatic cord of one or the other side.—Several fine stitches in the spermatic cord.—Smarting pain in one or the other spermatic cord, at one time in the region of the abdominal ring, at another behind it, at another more beneath it, often extending into the testicles. —*Smarting-burning pain in the spermatic cord, with several stitches, now on one, now on the other side.*—Twinging pain in one or the other spermatic cord, only at the abdominal ring, or also extending down to the testicles.—Diminished sexual desire in both sexes; the ejaculation of semen during coition is usually too soon, and the desire is weak and passes soon away; in women orgasm is delayed, sometimes associated with cutting or sticking pain.—Emission at night, which is usually very seldom.—*Female.* Pinching constrictive pain in the region of the mons veneris and the bladder, sometimes only on one side, sometimes when full, sometimes after emptying the bladder, immediately, or a long time afterwards.—Tearing pain in the mons veneris coming from the inguinal region.—[500.] Twinging-tearing in one or the other side of the mons veneris, sometimes also in this whole region, very frequently.—Burning, itching, or biting, also smarting sensation in the mons veneris.—Smarting-itching pain in the mons veneris. —*Sensation of burning and soreness in the vagina, frequently very sensitive, *especially in the anterior portion, even extending to the labiæ,* sometimes only on one side, but frequently also in the upper part in the region of the orifice of the urethra, often continuing a long time (twenty-eighth and thirty-sixth days, etc.).—In one side of the vagina, especially in the left, fine, or weak, or sharp, or dull, or violent stitches, sometimes like needles, ten to twenty in succession, twinging, or burning, twisting or long drawn out, and leaving the part painful, extending from within outward, at times ending in the urethra, often appearing so suddenly and violently that she is frightened; the vagina, during an examination, is very sensitive when touched with the finger (thirtieth, forty-first, forty-third, fifty-ninth, and sixty-first days, etc.).—Smarting pain in the vagina, usually only upon one side, sometimes continuous.—Menstruation appears as usual two days too soon, but lasts only two days; with it and afterwards violent pain in the back and loins. The second time it appears two days too soon, with pains in the back, and lasts only one day and a half.—In the fourth return menstruation appeared one day too soon, *the discharge was grayish mucus, then bloody, scanty.* The fifth period omitted entirely; on the sixth some watery blood passed; *then until the eighth again grayish mucus; for some days previous to it violent tearing in the limbs, with severe pain in the back;* at times on only one side, with a feeling as if bruised, as if suppurating, almost like labor pains, so that at times she could not lie upon it, especially at night, sometimes also pain in one hip-bone; dragging pain in the thighs, extending into the calves, especially in the veins of the leg, which are injected with blood; also pain in the lumbar region; once in the evening in bed, *violent sticking on the left side of the abdomen two fingers' breadth from the navel, extending in long stitches into the left side of the vagina;* fretful, tired of life mood; great dejection; **smarting pain in the vagina, burning, violent pain and soreness in the anus;** pressive tensive pain in the upper arm and shoulder, extending up into the neck.—Menstruation appears at the customary time and normally, but on the third day it ceases, and reappears on the fifth day, but more like bloody water; accompanied with great weakness and violent drawing, sticking headache.—Menstruation appears at the right time; the second day it is more like bloody water; on the third some drops of dark blood pass; on the fourth a passage of discolored mucus, then nothing more; during the first days dragging pain in the genitals, severe pain in the small of the back, and violent, dragging, pressing, splitting headache on the right side, with a feeling of faintness.— [510.] Menstruation appears at the right time, *but is very scanty,* does not appear in the usual way; at first is pale, expedited by a foot-bath; it never lasts beyond the fifth day, while it usually continues seven days; scarcely half the usual amount passes, and the discharge is more like bloody water. At the beginning much chilliness and pain in the small of the back; violent tearing in the whole body, especially on the left side; painful distension of the abdomen (fourth and fifth days), *violent pain in the kidneys*, also stitches in the chest; very sickly look; violent, bursting headache only during the first days.

Respiratory Apparatus and Chest.—Voice, and Chest in General. Hoarseness, with pain or inflammation of the tonsils.—Oppression of the chest, appearing several times, especially at night with violent fluent coryza.—Tearing in the left pectoral muscles extending towards their insertion in the arm.—Drawing, tearing pain in the walls of the chest, sometimes relieved by stretching or by exerting the muscles.—Violent, sudden, cutting, constrictive pain in front of the middle portion of the chest, extending down to the abdomen, so that she is obliged to bend double for half a minute (twenty-first day).—Single slow stitches here and there in the chest extending inward.—Sticking pain in the anterior middle region of the chest aggravated by deep breathing, together with a short dry cough (twenty-first day).—It seems raw in the chest as in catarrh, and an habitual occasional expectoration from the chest is increased (second to sixth day). —Scraping sensation in the chest (second day).—[520.] Scraping, scratching sensation of rawness and soreness in the chest.—*Sides of Chest.* Pain near the left mammary gland, deep, internally, extending outward and downward through the mammary gland in about ten stitches (eighth day).—A peculiar sensation of coldness in the right side of the chest for a short time (one hundred and ninth day).—Tearing, burning pain in the lower border of the left pectoralis major extending towards the arm.—Tensive drawing pain in the left side of the chest more towards the back (thirty-eighth day).—Sticking, drawing in the left side of the chest on the lower and outer part, extending from the left hypochondrium towards the back and shooting back and forth (seventeenth day).—Pressive pain in the left side of the chest as if between the mammary gland and the wall of the chest, most severe behind the nipple, extending from within outward into the mammary glands so that the middle of the sensation is in the nipple, with a feeling as if the gland were swollen (sixty-fifth and eighty-eighth days).—A bubbling pressive pain in the region of the left pectoralis major for half a minute in the evening in bed, coming from deep in the chest, with tension in this region and somewhat impeded respiration (forty-third day).—Sticking pain in the left mammary gland (ninth day).—Sticking below the left mammary gland towards the heart.—[530.] Tearing, sticking pain extending around the right side of the chest in the forepart (forty-sixth day).—Tearing, sticking pain, extending from the right side of the chest near the shoulder-blade up to the arm and seating itself in the muscles of the inner side of the upper arm for two minutes (seventeenth day).—A stitch in the right clavicle (fiftieth day).—A penetrating stitch in the right clavicle (seventy-third day).—Pulselike stitching in the right clavicle one-third of a minute (fifty-first day).—Single stitches in the right side of the chest from without inward (forty-fifth day).—Several burning stitches as from wasps in the region of the right clavicle (eighty-eighth day).—Some burning stitches in the left side of the chest near the nipple.—Three deep, violent burning stitches below the right clavicle crossing horizontally into the first ribs (seventy-seventh day).—Long drawing stitches, leaving pain in the region of the false ribs of the left side from below.—[540.] Tearing pain in the dorsal side of the left wall of the chest, somewhat below the shoulder-blade.—Tearing in the right side of the chest chiefly in the forepart, sometimes also in the shoulder-blade between it and the spine, two days in succession with oppression of the chest.—Drawing tearing pains in the sides of the chest chiefly in the left more towards the back, also in the shoulder-blades (forty-second day).—Pulsating at last more pressive and tensive, tearing in the left side of the chest below the axilla extending to the ribs for two minutes.—Several rather sensitive stitches in the left side of the chest externally and in the lower portion (after ten hours).—Jerking, intermitting, not severe stitches in the left side of the chest, almost as if she received electric shocks (eleventh day).—Sticking, jerking pain like electric shocks extends downwards from the left breast into the forepart of the left hypochondrium and then extends backwards; the whole lower part of the left side of the chest and of the abdomen is painful (eighth and twelfth days).—Sometimes a bubbling sensation in the right side of the chest somewhat below the middle (twenty-third day).

Heart and Pulse.—Frequent palpitation (twenty-first day).—Painful twinging stitches in the region of the heart extending outward and downward (twentieth day).—[550.] Pulse slow and weak in several persons.

Neck and Back.—Neck. Cold sensation in the left side of the neck in a place of the size of a quarter of a dollar, becoming a slight burning.—Tensive, burning sensation in the upper part of the left side of the neck with stiffness.—Tensive, not very sensitive, pain in the neck with stiffness, lasting for several minutes, several times.—Tensive feeling of stiffness in one or another place on the back or side of the neck.—On stooping, a drawing pain in the neck as if the muscles were tense (after half an hour).—Tearing, pressive pain in the cords of the neck, worse on the left side.—Burning, sticking pain between the shoulders (for ten minutes).—Tearing, sticking pain in the left side of the neck and posteriorly in slow jerks extending upward to the occiput (seventh and eighth days).—Sudden stitches shoot rapidly from the left side of the neck to the muscles on the inner side of the upper arm, so that she is startled by them (twenty-first day).—[560.] Lightning-like stitches shoot from the right clavicle upward on that side of the neck in six to eight jumping-like, long stitches, as if one were pierced with a sharp needle (fourth day).—Shooting, violent, cutting tearings on the left side of the neck in the muscles near the axis, lasting several minutes, with painful stiffness of the neck, so that she is not able to move the head (third day).—Tearing in the left side of the neck for half a minute (fifty-first day).—Slight tearing in the upper part of the left side of the neck.—Rheumatic tearing in the left side of the neck.—Tearing in the right side of the neck several times for half a minute, once also with pain on external pressure (forty-sixth day).—Superficial tensive tearing on the right side of the neck.—*Back.—Dorsal Region.* Just below the left shoulder-blade rheumatic pain extending into the lumbar region.—On the outer lower margin of the right-shoulder-blade and in the ribs externally, she noticed at times when grasping it a violent continued pain, as if the region were swollen, or injected with blood, suppurating (fifty-fifth to sixtieth days).—Drawing in the shoulder-blades and sides of the chest in the region of the pectoral muscles.—[570.] Tearing, sticking pain in the right shoulder-blade across the back, as if the region were ulcerated (forty-second day).—Digging, pulsating stitches in the region of the tip of the left shoulder-blade, extending upward and outward below the shoulder, chiefly along its inner margin (one hundred and tenth day).—Tearing in the tip of the right shoulder-blade (forty-eighth day).—Pressive tearing in the left shoulder-blade extending to the shoulder, the left upper and anterior pectoral region along the expansion of the pectoral muscles.

and also over the forearm and hand (for two days).—Digging, sticking tearing in the tip of the left shoulder-blade.—Tearing pain just below the spine of the right scapula, extending outward to a place as large as half a dollar, first noticed on touch, at ten o'clock in the evening, and continuing the next day (twenty-eighth day).—Pressive-tensive tearing pain in the right shoulder-blade externally, or rather superiorly, towards the shoulder, extending upward into the flesh of the upper arm and into the left clavicle and pectoral muscles; in the latter it is irritating, as if some muscular fibres were torn; movement of the arm is painful and difficult, continuing for a whole day (twenty-fourth day).—Suddenly when leaning against the arm of a chair a violent deepseated pain at the tip and along the outer border of the right shoulder-blade, also extending towards the axilla in the lower portion of the shoulder-joint, involving the whole joint, and extending down along the inner side of the arm to the elbow; the parts seem bruised, swollen or suppurating; the shoulder-joint seems sprained. On raising the arm the sensation extends into the chest and arrests the breathing. The pain often extends from the right side of the neck; it is relieved during rest; pressure and motion increase or excite it anew; the upper arm is painful, deep in the bone, as if there were something living in it; the second day chilliness in the affected part, extending down into the region of the kidneys, with goose-flesh (third to eighth day).—Sticking pain between the shoulder-blades increased by inspiration (eleventh day).—Tearing pain between the shoulders (tenth day).—[580.] Tearing pain in the spine between the shoulders.—Tearing pain in the back between the shoulder-blades, extending towards the lumbar region (after six hours).—Feeling of coldness with a kind of painless tearing in the upper part of the right side of the back (one hundredth day).—Tensive, sticking pain in the region of the lower dorsal vertebra extending toward the lumbar region (second day).— A stitch from the lower portion of the dorsal vertebra extending through the chest, so that it took away her breath; it pains some time afterwards; breathing is on that account more difficult (forty-fifth day).—Frequent tearing on both sides of the dorsal spine.—*Lumbar Region.* A burning-tensive pain in the lumbar and sacral regions.—Burning, burning-itching, or burning-digging in one or the other lumbar region, seldom in both, sometimes also in the sacral region, generally superficial or at times deeper, but then also sticking or gnawing, *frequently extending around the abdomen.* —Tensive stiff feeling in the lumbar region, with a kind of numb sensation, sometimes in the morning, on waking, when lying upon the back, with a decided lameness of the body.—Pressive-digging or gnawing pain in one or the other lumbar regions, as if an ulcer would appear.—[590.] Tearing, dragging pain in the sacrum, with dragging pain in the anus.—*Pressive or tensive pain in the region of the loins and kidneys, sometimes on one side only, sometimes on both, or frequently across the small of the back, at times extending downwards into the posterior portion of the pelvis, of the thighs, and even to the calves, with a feeling of stiffness and lameness or swelling in the back and lower extremities, and a warm sensation in the affected parts, at times also a kind of numbness in them; the sensations alternate often in the lumbar and sacral regions, continuing a long time and frequently returning.—*Sticking or sticking pressing pain, at times slight, at times very sensitive, in one or the other lumbar region, now in a small spot when it is a simple sticking, now in a larger place, when it is chiefly pressing, either exactly in the region of the kidneys, or at times extending above or below, but especially outward, so that it extends around the side of the abdomen in front, or to the region of the hips, *sometimes also in the spine and exte'ding down to the small of the back,* and the region of the bladder and groins; *sometimes fine, sometimes dull; the sticking sometimes extends from the region of the kidneys straight forward into the abdomen, at times with a numb paralyzed, bruised sensation; frequently returning and lasting a long time.* —A violent stitch beginning in the lumbar portion of the spine and extending outward across the left lumbar region (forty-seventh day).—*Some stitches in one or the other lumbar region, especially in the region of the kidneys, at times fine, at times dull, at times as if a nail were sticking in, and so violent and sudden that it stops the breath; from without inward.—*Burning stitches, single or several in succession, in the region of the loins and kidneys.—* Pulselike stitches at short or long intervals from without inward in one or the other lumbar and kidney region.—Slight superficial tearing in one or the other lumbar region.—*Tearing or tearing-sticking pain in the region of the loins and kidneys, usually more upon one side, frequently at the same time in the small of the back,* as if the region were crushed or bruised, with a feeling of stiffness, so that it was difficult for her to rise from sitting, *so that the hands must assist rising; sometimes also involving the hip, the nates, and the upper and posterior portion of the extremities,* at times also with a sensation of numbness.—Bubbling sensation in the lumbar region usually on only one side, sometimes lasting a short time, sometimes several minutes, more when lying and when rising from sitting.—[600.] *A feeling of warmth in the lower part of the back and in the small of the back, as if the lumbar region were asleep, extending down into the sacrum, the hips, and the posterior portion of the thighs.*—Burning-itching in the lower portion of the back.—**Sacral Region.** Burning pain in the sacrum, mostly with tension and pressure.—Drawing pain in the sacrum, usually one-sided, or pressing, or tearing, or alternating therewith.—*Pressive-tensive or pressing sensation in the sacrum, deep, internal, when severe, with a feeling as if the bone would be forced asunder,* frequently with a feeling of heaviness, warmth, or numbness, or buzzing, usually more noticed in the morning in bed immediately on waking, worse when sitting and lying, generally continuing a long time, frequently returning, sometimes relieved or removed by a stool or passage of flatus; sometimes upon only one side, increased by stooping.— Digging pressure, or tearing-sticking pain in the sacrum.—A dull twinging stitch obliquely from without inward and downward, in the left side of the sacrum, in the morning, in bed, on waking, accompanied by pressure.— Twinging pain in the sacrum with desire for stool (on the first days).— Superficial tearing pain in the sacrum, frequently upon only one side.— Tearing or tearing-sticking pain in the sacrum, at times only on one side.— [610.] Bruised and paralyzed feeling in the sacrum, as after unaccustomed long stooping, often in the morning, immediately on waking, mostly worse when sitting and lying than when walking, very frequent and lasting.— Itching in the sacrum, burning, biting, or with fine stitches.—Tearing pain in the region of the left tuber ischii.—Tearing pain in the right tuber ischii, extending forward to the right side of the uterus, for several minutes when sitting.—Bubbling sensation below the tuber ischii, extending inward and downward, as if a worm as large as the finger were forcing its way downward.

Upper Extremities.—Shoulder. Pain in the left shoulder, especially deep in the joint in front, as if in the head of the humerus, as if the parts were swollen, chiefly when moving the arms backward, always noticed on pressure for several hours (fifth day). Pain in the left shoulder externally and posteriorly, as if the arm had been strained or wrenched (thirty-second day).—*A rheumatic, paralytic-like pain in the right shoulder and some stitches over the left eye,*[6]—Superficial tensive drawings in the shoulders.—Tearing-sticking pain in the shoulders.—Burning-sticking in the region of the right acromion, extending into it (one hundred and seventh day).—[620.] Bubbling-like digging pain and a living movement in the forepart of the right shoulder-joint, external to and somewhat below the head of the humerus.—Tearing-sticking pain along the border of the right shoulder, and then extending quickly down the outer side of the arm and ending in a fine stitch in the tip of the little finger.—Tearing pain in the shoulder-joint, especially in the forepart.—Tearing in the left shoulder extending across the whole shoulder-blade and down the back, especially on motion ; it continued several days (sixth day),[9]—Tearings, beginning along the border of the left shoulder, extending up on the side of the neck and throat as far as the left side of the occipital region, where it becomes seated (forty-sixth and forty-seventh day).—Corrosive smarting sensation on the left shoulder.—Pain in the right shoulder as if it would suppurate.—Bubbling-like sensation in the right shoulder, chiefly in the forepart, not painful, as if something living were in it and would bore its way out, severe a few minutes (seventh and fifteenth days).—*Arm.* Weakness and a paralyzed feeling in the arms, becoming painful on exertion after some violent exercise of the arms, and a painful sensation in the muscles for several days, especially on motion, though also at other times, caused or increased by pressure.—Burning pain on the inner side of the left upper arm two inches below the joint, superficial in the skin or just under it, with some pressure at intervals of two or three seconds, whereby the pain becomes worse (twenty-sixth day).—[630.] Tensive pain in the muscles of the right upper arm.—Pressive pain in the arms, especially in the thick muscles of the shoulders, in the inner muscles, and also on the inner side of the upper arm, less of the forearm.—Drawing tensive sensation in the arms at times with slight tearing, often with a feeling of heaviness and loss of power in them.—Violent pressive-tensive pain in the left upper arm, about the middle of the forepart and somewhat inward on the bone, as if something would be torn loose, so that it is sore as far as the bone, for two minutes (fifty-seventh day).—Drawing pain in the outer side of the left upper arm. —Drawing pain in the outer part of the upper arm extending down to the elbow-joint (thirty-fifth day).—Forcible pressive pain in the middle and on the outer anterior side of the left upper arm in the vicinity of the bone, with a heavy sensation, so that she must let the arm hang down for a minute, followed by heaviness, which continues a long time.—Sticking pain in the thick flesh of the left upper arm in front, three inches below the joint.—Five stitches in quick succession on the inner side of the right upper arm, just below the axilla, with burning between the stitches and afterwards.—Six sharp stitches on the inner side of the left upper arm, just below the axilla, as if a fine splinter were thrust deep into the bone, ending in a long-drawn stitch.—A burning stitch, external in the middle of the right upper arm.—[640.] Burning stitch in the thick flesh of the right upper arm.—Tearing on the anterior portion of the left upper arm.—Tearing pain in the muscles of the inner side of the right upper arm for half a minute.—Slight tearing as if under the skin in the outer side of the left upper arm to the middle (for quarter of a minute).—Tearing in the upper and inner portion of the left upper arm for half a minute, with burning.—Tearing pain for a minute deep in the bone, extending from the middle of the inner and anterior portion of the left upper arm down over the elbow-joint, in the radius to the wrist and the inner side of the back of the metacarpus, so that she, being attacked during a somewhat arduous work, is obliged to allow the arm to hang down and incline towards the left side, with a feeling of heaviness and swelling in the arm (forty-fourth day).—Drawing-tearing pain in the left arm at the insertion of the pectoral muscles.—Drawing sticking-tearing below the right shoulder-joint, on the inner and posterior side of the upper arm, in a place in the flesh about two inches long, for a quarter of an hour (twenty-ninth day).—Two pressive tearings in the outer middle portion of the right upper arm, extending to the bone.—Pressive and digging tearing in the bone of the left upper arm, behind the belly of the biceps, from without inward, for an inch in length, lasting twelve seconds.—[650.] In the anterior region of the right upper arm, just below the shoulder-joint, several painful, jerking-like, digging tearings deep in the bone, on a surface of about an inch and a half (ninety-first day).—Four bubbling-like tearings in the muscles of the inner side of the left upper arm, extending from within outward, at intervals of a few seconds (one hundred and twenty-first day).— Bubbling sensation in the muscles in the middle of the right upper arm extending outward (nineteenth day).—Bubbling in the forepart of the right upper arm, two inches below the shoulder-joint, in about twenty pulsations.—Bubbling sensation in the right upper arm, three inches below the joint, external between the muscles and the bone (twenty-second day).— Bubbling sensation in the thick flesh of the right upper arm, on going to bed, as if the muscles were alive, three times in succession (one hundred and fifth day).—*Elbow.* A violent pain in the tendon of the biceps at the bend of the elbow, suddenly after lifting or moving the arm, especially on extending it, and reaching deep into the joint and forward for a way along the radial side of the forearm, as also upward along the outer and posterior surface of the upper arm.—Burning pain in the outer anterior part of the left elbow (one hundred and third day).—Burning in the outer anterior portion of the left elbow, not only in the skin but also deep in the flesh and extending outward, for a minute.—Burning pain as from nettles in the right elbow, between the olecranon to the inner condyle of the humerus (ten seconds).—[660.] Tensive sensation in the flexor surface of the left elbow, a few inches on the forearm, extending forward, especially on extending the arm, for a minute.—A drawing-tensive pain in the outer portion of the left elbow-joint.—Twitching-sticking pain above the right elbow extending upward a few inches.—Crawling-sticking pain in the left elbow. —Tearing-sticking pain in the forepart of the right elbow-joint, especially in the tendons of the muscles, caused and increased by motion, for eight minutes (twenty-seventh day).—Tearing pain in the right elbow extending outward.—Violent tearing in the right elbow, extending slowly along the outer border of the ulna, as if something scraped the bone, and as if it were distended at the same time, with a feeling of lameness and heaviness of the forearm, several times in the day (seventy-fourth day).—Drawing-tearing pain in the right elbow down to the lower portion of the forearm.—Smarting pain in the elbow-joint.—Corrosive pain in the right elbow.—*Forearm.* [670.] A lymphatic swelling in the flexor tendons of the left forearm on the lower and inner border of the ulna, two inches from the wrist, moderately hard, not very painful to touch, almost not at all on motion, not red, only covered with two petechial-like spots an inch long, not very hot, with burning pain in the skin, lasting several days, then slowly disappearing (tenth week).—Numb paralyzed pain in the extensor surface of the left forearm about two inches from the wrist, extending into it, and on motion to the elbow, deep internally; she is obliged to lay the arm out straight; if the hand hangs down the pain becomes more violent, and then the forearm feels as if asleep (twenty-second day).—A cold sensation like tearing in the right forearm on the anterior margin of the radius.—Burning pain in the outer side of the left forearm.—Burning in the styloid process of the right radius; a red spot appears which becomes larger on rubbing (one hundred and first day).—Slight burning pain on the outer side of the radius of the left forearm, some inches below the elbow (one hundred and fourth day).—Biting-burning pain in the middle of the outer side of the left forearm for about five minutes, then becoming a pressive numb sensation.—Biting tearing-burning pain in the ulnar side of the right forearm.—Pinching constrictive pain in the lower external portion of the left forearm.—Pressive-pinching painlike cramp, in the flexor surface of the right forearm, two inches from the wrist-joint, for about ten seconds, soon again for a longer time.—[**680.**] Drawing pain in the left forearm outward external in the flexor surface after exerting it. On long-continued grasping with the right hand, pain in the flexor muscles and heaviness of the hand and forearm.—Pressive pain in the extensor surface of the right forearm (one hundred and sixth day).—Pressure in the flexor surface of the right forearm, two or three inches from the wrist, in a place of the size of a quarter of a dollar, as if it extended into the bones.—Stitching pain in the muscles of the left forearm below the middle of the ulna.—A stitch in the muscles of the left forearm, slowly penetrating inward along the radius for about ten seconds (seventeenth day).—Four stitches in quick succession along the inner side of the right forearm, in the muscles and tendons of the ulna, from about the middle straight downward.—A burning stitch on the dorsal side of the forearm, about two inches from the wrist.—A burning stitch in the right radius, two inches from the wrist, extending from without inward to the bone.—A violent pressive boring stitch in the inner side of the right forearm, four inches from the wrist, as if a nail were forced into the bone for a minute, not increased by pressure.—Tearing in the left forearm, from without inward.—[**690.**] Fine tearing as if under the skin in the flexor surface of the forearm.—Tearing in the right forearm along the inner side of the radius, for half a minute.—Tearing in the muscles in the flexor surface of the radius, extending from the elbow-joint downward, for a minute.—Violent tearing pain in the right forearm, chiefly in the ulnar portion, extending from the elbow into the wrist, and back again, at the same time extending into the posterior lower portion of the muscles of the upper arm, with a sensation of heaviness and powerlessness of the arm, lasting nearly the whole night and even continuing the next morning (sixty-ninth to seventieth days).—Pressive-tensive, exceedingly painful tearing, aggravated by paroxysms, in the left forearm from the elbow-joint into the ulna, especially in its lower portion, deep as if in the bone, extending to the back of the hand and the middle joint of the fingers, with heaviness and powerlessness of the arm, as if she could not raise it, as if it were swollen, returning several hours in succession and lasting each time from one-half to one minute, in the evening, and also again the next morning (forty-fourth day).—Smarting pain on the back of the forearm, just behind the left wrist, aggravated by rubbing.—Smarting or smarting-burning pain in various places on the forearm, several times, especially on the outer side, aggravated by rubbing; at times a red spot appears after it.—*Wrist.* Pain in the wrist after exerting the hand.—Transient burning pain in the wrists.—

Burning pain as from nettles on the back of the left wrist, **aggravated** by rubbing, several times, once extending down between the metacarpal bones of the little and ring fingers.—[700.] Some itching-burning or biting stitches in the wrists.—Gnawing pain in the right wrist, sometimes for only a minute, sometimes for two hours (one hundred and third day).—Pressive pain in the right wrist, chiefly on the outer side, as after a bruise, extending into the hand.—Violent sticking in the right wrist, beginning in the forearm somewhat above it, extending down deep through the joint into the middle of the hand, lasting nearly half an hour, and returning.—A burning stitch in the left external wrist bone, followed by a slight burning. —Slight transient or continued tearing in the wrist-joint.—Tearing in the inner side of the left wrist extending to the flexor surface of the ring finger, penetrating deep into the joint of the hand, and then continuing a jerking-sticking.—Tearing in the wrist, alternating with tearing in the hands and fingers.—Corrosive tearing on the back of the right wrist, extending from the metacarpal bone of the index finger to its last joint.—*Hands.* A sensation as if cold drops of rain fell upon the back of the hand when she went from the house into the open air (seventh day).—[710.] An increased sensation of warmth in the palms of the hands, frequently with itching or crawling, as in chilblains.—Burning pain in the back of the right hand.— Smarting-burning pain in the region between the fourth and fifth metacarpal bones of the right hand, aggravated even by a slight touch (seventy-third day).—Violent pressing digging and humming pain on the back of the whole of the right hand, arising in the region of the first joint of the fingers, with a sensation of heaviness in them, so that she must let them hang down, at 9 o'clock in the evening, little noticed the next morning (forty-fifth day). —Sticking pain in the outer border of the right hand.—Tearing tensive-sticking in the right palm in the region of the metacarpal bone of the little finger, extending deep toward the little finger (for quarter of a minute).— A severe stitch in the palm of the left hand, beginning in the middle of the wrist and extending deep to the middle of the palm, after exerting the hand (forty-fourth day).—Sudden stitches in the left palm, cutting into it from the outer side, shooting back and forth, so that she involuntarily seizes the hand.—A burning stitch on the back of the left hand between the metacarpal bones of the index and middle fingers, from without inward, continuing to burn afterward.—Tearing in the outer balls of the left palm. —720.] Tearing in the middle metacarpal bones of the right hand, with quick pulsations therein, frequently returning in single tearings.—Tearing pain in the outer portion of the back of the left hand, in the region of the fourth and fifth metacarpal bone, soon changing to a gnawing.—Tearing in the left hand along the metacarpal bone of the little finger.—Sensitive tearing on the external margin of the right hand, for a minute, extending forward to the little finger, so that the whole hand is affected.—Wandering tearing in the back of the hand, frequently extending into the extensor surface of the finger, frequently ending in stitches in the tips of the fingers.— Gnawing-smarting pain on the back of the left hand, aggravated by rubbing.—Tearing pulsating pain deep in the left palm in the region of the metacarpal bone of the middle finger, for some minutes (one hundred and second day).—*Fingers.* Slight redness of the tip of the finger and of the back of the first two phalanges, with frequent itching in them, as after slight freezing, several times.—Slight pain, with stiffness in the second joint of the left index finger, chiefly on bending it (ninety-third day).—In the metacarpal bone of the little finger of the right hand, the same pain on motion and pressure, also extending to the neighboring extensor tendons; the joint of the first phalanx is visibly swollen; the pain is sometimes very severe, sometimes less (fifty-first to sixty-third days).—[730.] A peculiar, extremely painful sensation in the tip of the left index finger, something like a panaritium, as if it would suppurate, most severe under the nail, where it seems as if the flesh around it would be torn loose; she cannot rub the skin without causing a most violent pain, and has a severe sensation of heat in it, which, however, is not noticed on examination, also some pain in the second joint of the same finger (fifty-first day).—Burning pain between the metacarpal bones of the second and third fingers of the right hand.—Burning pain in the inner side of the dorsal surface of the right index finger.—Burning pain on the back of the right index finger.—Burning between the thumb and the index finger of the left hand; on rubbing, a red spot appears.—Burning as from nettles on the back of the second joint of the right index finger.—Burning as from nettles in the second joint of the left index finger, with stiffness, especially when bending it (ninety-third day).—Gnawing-burning pain as from nettles in the first joint of the left middle finger, aggravated by rubbing, for several minutes.—Burning pain in the first joint of the left index finger for several days together, aggravated by rubbing; after a time red pimples appear, which do not maturate (one hundred and sixth day).—Burning pain with fine stitches as from insects, along the metacarpal bone of the right middle finger; on rubbing, the pain scatters (ninety-seventh day).—[740.] Jerking-burning pain in the outer surface of the right middle finger from the second joint into the nail, as if in the bone.—Drawing in the second and third joints of the right index finger, for one minute.—A humming pain in the outer side of the third phalanx of the right middle finger (ninety-ninth day).—A humming pain in the tip of the left index finger, as if it would suppurate (seventy-second day).— Pressive pain in the region of the first joint of the left thumb, in the bone, extending into the second joint (ninety-first day).—Biting-sticking pain in the ulnar side of the second phalanx of the right middle finger, for a few minutes.—Fine stitching sticking pain in the flexor surface of the first joint of the left index finger.—A stitch in the ball of the right thumb.—A stitch in the ball of the first joint of the left little finger.—Some stitches in the flexor surface in the first portion of the index finger, changing to slight sticking.—[750.] Two stitches on the back of the first phalanx of the index finger, changing to slight stitches, which last a quarter of a minute.—Six itching stitches in the region of the first joint of the left index finger, on the inner side.—Ten to fifteen stitches as with fine needles from without inward in the middle of the flexor surface of the first phalanx of the left index finger, at last changing to fine continued stitches.—Several violent stitches, at times lasting only a few seconds, at times a quarter of a minute, in the tip of the index or ring finger, at times also involving the other fingers, frequently.—Stitching pain in the inner surface of the right thumb, sometimes caused by pressure upon it.—Burning stitch in the inner side of the metacarpal bone of the right index finger, for ten to fifteen seconds.—A burning stitch on the inner side of the third joint of the left index finger.— A burning stitch on the inner side of the second joint of the left index finger.—Burning stitches on the outer side of the second joint of the right index finger.—Burning stitches in the inner side of the metacarpal bone of the left little finger.—[760.] Fine burning stitches in the second and third joints of the left little finger, for half a minute.—A twitching-cutting stitch extending across from the first joint of the little finger of the left hand into the palm.—Fine pulselike stitches in the tip of the right index finger. Pain with stiffness in the second joint of the right middle finger, in the morning on waking, at first aggravated by pressure, for a few minutes.—Bubbling stitches in the inner side of the tip of the right thumb, deep under the nail, as if shooting out from the bone, for a few seconds (seventy-first day).—Tearing in the balls of the thumbs.—Tearing along the inner surface of the right thumb.—Some tearings in the finger joints.—Tearing in the tips of the fingers, especially of the index finger.—Tearing on the back of the finger, now here, now there, chiefly in the joints.—Tearing under the nail of the left thumb, from without inward.—[770.] Tearing in the inner side of the joint of the left index finger several times during the day, lasting several minutes.—Tearing on the inner surface of the first joint of the right index finger (ninety-seventh day).—Tearing in the metacarpal bone of the right thumb backward toward the wrist, changing to eight penetrating stitches in the same place.—Tearing in the metacarpal bone of the ring finger, somewhat aggravated by pressure, for twelve to fifteen minutes.—Violent tearing on the right side of the index finger, so that she almost trembled, as if the flesh were torn loose from the bone, for a minute (seventy-fourth day).—Tearing from the second joint of the middle finger of the right hand backward along the tendons to the wrist, for half a minute.—In the first portion of the right middle finger, a tearing pain as if sprained, chiefly in the first joint, especially on motion and touch, with swelling of the parts about the joints, mostly on the back and in the sides, also of the phalanx itself, with cracking of the joints on motion (twenty-second to sixtieth day).—Tearing, now slight, now violent, in several fingers, especially on the back, frequently with some stiffness of them, especially in the index and ring fingers, frequently changing into outward shooting stitches in the tips of the fingers, sometimes lasting only a few seconds, sometimes for several minutes.—Tearing along the metacarpal bone of the left index finger, with pulselike stitches extending inward in the bone.—Tearing in the outer side of the left thumb, as deep as the bone, increased by pressure, with some pulselike stitches from without inward, near the joint (seventy-second day).—[780.] Tearing in the ulnar side of the left thumb as deep as the bone, increased by pressure, with a few intermitting pulselike stitches from without inward near the joint.—Tearing along the side of the metacarpal bone of the right little finger, for half a minute, with a sensation of heaviness and powerlessness in the outer portion of the hand.—Burning-tearing in the volar surface of the first joint of the right thumb.—Drawing-tearing in the second joint of the right index finger and near it, on the back.—A humming-tearing in the left thumb, with a feeling as if it were distended and heavy, for a few minutes, several times in the day (sixty-fourth day). —Smarting-tearing pain in the outer surface of the left index finger, aggravated by rubbing, and changing into a burning pain.—Smarting pain on the back of the fingers.—Bubbling sensation in the ball of the right thumb (nineteenth day).

Lower Extremities.—In General. Great weakness of the lower extremities during a walk, so that he scarcely felt them, as if numb (fiftieth day).—Sensation of weakness, and as if bruised, in the lower extremities, sometimes with heaviness and stiffness, and a paralyzed feeling, as after a long march, or as if the parts were strained, as if the muscles were too thick, usually in the soft parts, though not seldom also in the bones, with pain, which is easily excited by motion, though not always aggravated, through nearly the whole period of the proving, sometimes worse, sometimes better.—[**790**.] A feeling in the lower extremities, as if they were becoming emaciated, which really seemed to be the case.—Great heaviness, bruised sensation, and lassitude in the lower limbs, especially in the thighs, mostly in ascending stairs, with great weakness (fifty-first day),'. —Drawing-tensive sensation in the lower extremities over a large surface, sometimes also with slight, rather superficial tearings, and a heavy or stiff paralyzed feeling, especially when rising after sitting a long time.—Violent bruised pain in the whole of the lower extremities, so that he cannot rise from his seat without assistance from his hands; the knees feel used up and appear paralyzed; he suffers especially along the posterior surface, from the loins and sacral region downward; the calves feel as if bruised sore; pressure and motion increase the pains, especially stooping, for six-teen hours; at last the pain extends downward more into the feet (third and fourth days).—*Hip and Thigh.* Burning pain in the region of the left trochanter.—Pulselike burning stitches, extending from the right trochanter downward deep inwardly, lasting half a minute.—Slight draw-ing pain in the region of the right trochanter.—Tearing pain in the region below the trochanter.—Tearing pain in the hip bones of one side near the spine.—Tearing from the posterior border of the hip bones downward and inward.—[**800**.] Creeping cold sensation on the outer side of the thigh, as if quicksilver were running on or beneath the skin, sometimes accompa-nied by tension in the muscles, or a sticking sensation, though painless, mostly when standing, seldom when sitting, at times ending in burning.— On the posterior portion of the left thigh, about five inches from the joint, in the morning after rising, in a spot of the size of a ten-cent piece, a sen-sation as if it were touched by a cold substance, as by a piece of cold metal, or by a cold animal, so that she grasps hold of it in fright; repeated the next day at noon (forty-third day).—Transient sensation of warmth on the outer portion of the left thigh (one hundred and fifth day).—Transient sensation of warmth on the posterior lower portion of the left thigh, ex-tending down into the upper part of the calf (one hundred and fourth day). —Feeling of warmth on the posterior upper portion of the thigh for a short time.—Burning pain in the left nates.—Burning pain on the inner side of the lower portion of the left thigh, aggravated by even slight touch (one hundred and sixth day).—Burning pain in the inner anterior side of the upper part of the right thigh.—Tension in the muscles in the upper and anterior part of the thigh, when walking, frequently changing into a pain.—Tension in the thighs and nates from the hips downward, with numb-ness, and at times increased warmth.—[**810**.] Tensive pain in one or the other bend of the thighs, as if the tendons were too short, when walking. —Drawing-tensive sensation in the posterior muscles of the thigh.—Draw-ing-tensive pain in the muscles of the outer side of the right thigh, out-ward and backward, as if a cramp would come.—Drawing-tensive pain in the tendons of the thigh, extending downward over the knee-cap, when walking, for some minutes.—A pinching sensation in the muscles of the thigh, especially the flexors, and in the calves.—On more violent motion than usual pinching in the muscles of the thighs.—Tensive contraction of the muscles of the thigh, especially on the posterior surface and in the calves, chiefly when walking.—Drawing pain in the nates.—Drawing from the small of the back on one or the other side from the nates down into the thigh.—Drawing pain in the anterior region of the pelvic bone straight outward into the muscles of the thigh.—[**820**.] Drawing pain in the mus-cles of the right thigh, two inches above the knee.—Drawing pain from the region of the trochanter downward into the thigh.—Drawing or drawing-tensive sensation or pain on the inner side of the thigh.—At night when falling to sleep, slight workings, like crawlings or drawings, on the outer side of the left thigh, extending downward over the knee, followed by a cramplike sensation in the calf, with tingling in it and the outstretched foot (forty-seventh day).—Dragging sensation in the nates and the upper posterior portion of the thigh, starting from the sacrum.—Gnawing on the outer upper portion of the left thigh.—Gnawing pain on the posterior surface of the left thigh above the hollow of the knee (one hundred and twenty-second day).—Gnawing sensation on the outer lower region of the right thigh, especially when walking; is caused and aggravated by rubbing (one hundred and eighth day).—Biting-gnawing in the outer lower side of the left thigh above the knee (eighty-eighth day).—Tensive-pressive pain in the thighs, calves, and knees, as if the muscles were too short.—[**830.**] Sticking pain, mostly transient, in the nates.—Sticking pain, often violent, from without inward, in the middle of the posterior or anterior region of the thigh, very frequent in rest and also after motion, confined to a small spot. —Burning-sticking pain in the outer anterior portion of the right thigh below the middle, for a few minutes.—Tearing-sticking pain penetrating deep into the bone, in the outer middle region of the right thigh, several times in succession.—Pulselike sticking pain in the posterior lower portion of the right thigh, for two-thirds of a minute, whereby he imagines that by the finger he noticed a pulsation in the affected part (sixty-fourth day). —Bubbling sticking pain in the middle of the posterior portion of the left thigh.—A stitch in the inner posterior and middle portion of the thigh in the flesh from without inward, long drawn out, when walking.—A stitch through the left thigh, in the forepart somewhat above the middle, from within outward (twenty-first day).—A stitch in the left nates when standing, extending deep into the muscles.—Three violent stitches in the forepart of the left thigh, about five inches from the knee, extending into the flesh, as with a needle, or as if an animal stung one, so that, thinking this, one grasps the part in order to find the animal; quarter of an hour afterwards, two stitches near the knee.—[**840.**] In the posterior and inner side of the left thigh, six inches above the knee, four stitches from without inward, like severe stings from insects.—About thirty bubbling stitches, at intervals of one or several seconds, in the middle of the left thigh, whereby he thinks he can feel a throbbing with the fingers; mostly a touch causes continued pain.—Some stitches in the middle of the left thigh, external, extending upward along it.—Some burning stitches in the outer upper side of the right thigh.—A biting stitch in the inner and lower portion of the left thigh.—A long-drawn stitch in the inner posterior side of the middle of the left thigh, when walking (seventy-fifth day).—Deep violent stitches on the inner side of the right thigh, two inches from the knee, extending obliquely downward in this place to the opposite side, chiefly when stepping upon it; when sitting at rest, rather paroxysmal, less sensitive stitches (one hundred and eighth day).—Pulsating stitches in the muscles of the posterior portion of the left thigh, deep from without inward, lasting a quarter of an hour, when walking and sitting (ninety-third day).—Biting pain in the skin, in a small spot on the inner and upper side of the left thigh.—Gnawing-biting sensation on the outer anterior side of the left thigh about the middle.—[**850.**] Tearing pain in the thick flesh of the left thigh, about the middle of the forepart.—Tearing pain in the forepart of the thigh and downward over the knee.—Tearing pain on the inner side of the thigh.—On the outer side of the left thigh tearing pain, as if under the skin.—A tearing pain in the lower outer side of the right thigh above the knee, extending down into the outer part of the leg and calf.—Tearing or tearing-drawing pain on the outer or inner side of the thigh.—Tearing, or tearing-sticking, or drawing-tearing pain, in the muscles of the posterior portion of the thigh, chiefly about the middle.—Tearing or tearing-sticking pain in the extensor muscles of the thigh, often arising after motion.—Tearing pain in the outer side of the thigh, sometimes only in one side, sometimes spread over the whole thigh, remitting and recurring, chiefly after motion.—Severe tearing pain in the left or right nates, when walking, extending deep into the ischium, for nearly a minute, also of a less severe kind.—[860.] Severe tearing in the left femur, from the trochanter down to the knee-joint, aggravated by paroxysms, for quarter of an hour, when sitting.—Tearing pain in the lower external and anterior portion of the right thigh, sometimes also of the left, when walking, at last changing to a tension.—Biting-tearing pain in the inner, upper, and anterior region of the left thigh, when walking (ninety-third day).—Sore pain in the outer anterior side of the right thigh (eighty-second day).—Sore pain in the bend of the thigh (ninety-first day).—Smarting pain in the outer side of the right thigh, soon after, in the middle of the forepart.—Pressive pinching-throbbing pain in the upper anterior portion of the right thigh, when standing and walking.—Painless bubbling in the lower portion of the right thigh, as if a stream of air as large as a finger, or a worm of the same size, forced itself through the flesh, lasting several minutes (seventieth day).—Bubbling twice in the lower and anterior portion of the right thigh, not far from the knee.—Bubbling sensation in the muscles of the right thigh in the forepart, moving here and there, as if something living were crawling therein.—[870.] Bubbling sensation in the posterior and upper portion of the left thigh, just below the nates, for one minute, slowly digging and working in a spot as large as two hands.—Bubbling sensation in the forepart of the right thigh, evenings in bed, extending along the thigh, with fine interruptions, as if a stream of water or blood forced its way through the flesh (forty-first day).—*Knee.* Great swelling of the veins near the knee-joints, in the lower and posterior portion of the upper part of the calves.—A sensation as if weak, bruised, and paralyzed in the knees, during and after walking, and on rising after sitting a long time, very frequently.—Biting-burning sensation on the inner side of the right knee, for several seconds, returning slightly soon afterwards.—Drawing-burning pain in the right hollow of the knee.—Tension in the knee-joint, now in one side, now in the forepart, especially in the region of the patella, now posteriorly, chiefly in the tendons, as if they were too short, frequently accompanied by a sensation of heaviness or paralysis, especially noticed when moving, particularly when stretching, often caused for the first time thereby. —Violent pinching pain in the right popliteal space and calf, when sitting down in the evening, when lying in bed, lasting an hour, after a moderate walk (eighty-sixth day).—Violent cramp in the left popliteal space, when stepping or stamping, extending downward into the middle of the calf and upward into the thigh, while standing; when she does not step hard it is less, accompanied by tingling and heaviness in the affected parts, as if they were enlarged, for two days in succession (fifty-ninth and sixtieth days).—Drawing pain in the patella, extending downward into the anterior upper portion of the leg, caused by walking, and also arising of itself.— [880.] Gnawing pain on the outer side of the left knee-pan (one hundred and third day).—Pressive pain in the left hollow of the knee, extending through the joint to the patella, with a feeling as if the knee were stiff and swollen; bending, and especially extending the knee, aggravates it; the tendons seem too short (ninety-first day).—Tensive pressive pain in the right patella, and in the ligaments and tendons behind it, after walking.— At night, a sticking-pressive pain across the left knee (thirty-first day).— Tearing-pressive pain in the right patella and in the ligaments behind it, caused by motion.—Sticking, then burning pain below the margin of the left patella, extending inward into the joint, when walking, lasting more than a minute.—Sticking pain in the inner side of the right knee, extending outward into the tendons of this region.—Sticking pain above the margin of the patella, when going upstairs.—Sticking pain through the right knee-joint, from before backward beneath the patella, when walking, so that stepping she starts up and is obliged to favor the foot, four times in succession, returning afterward twice (forty-ninth day).—In the morning, when she goes down stairs, after rising from bed, when bending the knee, a violent sticking pain just above the patella, as from a nail deep inwardly, so severe for several hours in succession that she is lame; afterwards it changes to a pressure (aching), (fifty-second day).—[890.] Slow sticking pain, as if a large nail were forced inward in a small spot in the right knee, in the forepart near the lower margin of the patella, deeply penetrating, disappears during rest, caused by motion, and lasts nearly three hours, with heaviness in the calves.—Drawing-sticking pain in the left hollow of the knee, extending downward into the upper part of the leg, for a minute and a half; the same pain in the inner side of the right knee, rather superficial.—Some stitches shoot through the knee-joint.—Stitches in the knee-joint, now in one, now in another place, especially on the inner side. —Four stitches below the right knee-joint shooting into the knee obliquely from below upward beneath the patella, when walking.—Burning stitches in front above the left knee-joint, so that he is frightened.—Bubbling stitches in the region above the left knee (ninety-fourth day).—Bubbling long-drawn stitches in the tendons of the outer side of the left popliteal space, for a few minutes, when walking and standing (seventy-first day).—On the inner side of the left knee-joint near the patella, violent pain shooting backward into the knee-joint, and through the joint beneath the patella, as if it were swollen and inflamed, when bending the knee, from 4 till 11 in the morning; the pain disappears during rest in an extended position. —Several tearings in the knee-joints more or less severe —[900.] Tearing or tearing-sticking pain in the knee-joint, most frequently in the inner side, though also in the outer anterior and posterior portion, also frequently extending into the neighboring parts.—Tearing in the tendons of the knee, especially the posterior muscles, when walking or standing.—Smarting pain in the forepart of the left knee near the patella, twice in succession.—**Legs.** Sticking pain in the right leg near the lower part of the tibia, when walking.—Sensitive tearing-sticking pain in the left leg, on the side between the tibia and fibula, in the extensor muscles, especially in their tendons, two inches above the joint, extending down into the external malleolus and the outer side of the back of the foot, lasting more than half an hour.— Burning-sticking pain in the middle of the left leg, on the outer side near the tibia about the middle, for about three minutes, several times returning. —Tearing pain along the whole outer side of the right leg, into the external malleolus and down over the outer side of the back of the foot, then also extending upward along the outer side of the thigh.—Tensive pressive-tearing in the outer portion of the left leg, a few inches above the external

malleolus between the tibia and fibula, with intermissions, nearly half an
hour.—Biting-stinging pain in the middle of the outer portion of the right
leg, chiefly when walking and standing.—Corrosive pain on the outer side
of the left leg.—[**910.**] Sensation of coldness, almost tearing, on the front
of the right tibia.—Tearing-tensive pain in the middle of the tibia, extending upward to the knee.—Tensive aching or pressing pain, sometimes accompanied by burning, or warm feeling, or numb sensation, in the tibia, as
if the bone would become distended, with a bruised and heavy sensation
in the leg, sometimes lasting only a short time, sometimes several hours, a
few times with a bubbling sensation, also sometimes alternating with tearing or sticking, or associated with them, when walking and standing, though
also arising spontaneously at times, even in the morning on waking in bed ;
rubbing causes at times burning in the skin of the tibia.—Burning-gnaw-
ing pain on the inner anterior side of the right tibia below the knee, when
walking, aggravated by rubbing.—Sticking pain in the tibia, especially in
the middle, from without inward, mostly in a small spot, when walking and
standing, seldom when sitting.—Tearing-sticking pain near the middle of
the left tibia, extending outward.—Tearing-sticking pain in the middle of
the tibia, in the bone, in intermitting, twinging jerks, for more than a minute, as if the periosteum would be torn loose.—Corrosive sticking pain in
a small spot in the middle of the crest of the tibia.—A single stitch in the
right tibia.—Three stitches in the inner side of the left tibia, about the
middle.—[**920.**] A severe burning stitch in the lower portion of the left
tibia, in the skin on the outer side close to the ridge of the bone, as if it
pierced the bone, so that she starts.—Three fine burning stitches from without inward, externally near the left tibia, a few inches above the ankle.—
Three sudden burning stitches, penetrating inward, in the outer side of the
left tibia, as if she were painfully stung by an insect, so that she starts (one
hundredth day).—Several fine burning-itching stitches on the outer side
near the middle of the right tibia.—Superficial tearing on the tibia, at the
side of it.—Single transient tearings in the tibia.—Tearing pain in various
places in the tibia, most frequent in the middle, frequently extending upward into the knee and downward into the ankle.—Tearing in the sides of
the tibia, sometimes superficial and slight, sometimes deep and violent.—
Tearing, at times tearing-sticking pain in the tibia, down along its inner
surface, with pressive, or bruised, or warm sensation, or burning, as if the
bone would be pressed asunder, when walking and standing, and also when
sitting.—Tingling, very painful tearing in the right tibia, a few inches from
the joint, extending upward, greatly aggravated by pressure, lasting a few
minutes.—[**930.**] Biting-smarting pain in the middle of the right tibia,
aggravated by rubbing and motion, and changing to a sore pain.—Violent
scraping pain in the inner side of the right tibia, from the inner malleolus
upward.—Smarting-burning pain in the upper part of the right calf, externally below the knee, extending backward and downward over the calf,
with a bruised sensation.—Cramplike pain in the left calf, when sitting,
for a few minutes, as if the muscles were bruised (ninety-first day).—Tensive pain in the calves, when walking, especially when rising after sitting
a long time.—Cramplike pain in the upper part of the left calf, evenings
in going upstairs.—Cramplike pain in the left calf, in the evening when
going to sleep, for quarter of an hour.—Cramplike pain in the right calf,
with several stitches, for half a minute, when walking.—Drawing or drawing pain in the calves, now here, now there, usually only in isolated spots,
sometimes with a feeling of being asleep, heaviness, or stiffness.—Sticking

in the upper inner portion of the left calf, soon changing to a bubbling sensation, as if a bloodvessel were throbbing under the skin.—[**940.**]
Sticking pain from within outward in the right calf, somewhat above the
middle, for forty seconds, returning after about ten minutes, and continuing a long time, but moderately.—Sticking pain in the calves, now slight,
now severe, chiefly in the middle, during and after motion, continuing during rest, even arising without motion, though seldom, often penetrating
deeply.—Drawing-sticking pain, extending outward to the middle of the
right calf, for ten minutes.—In the outer portion of the right calf, near the
tibia, a slow, cutting, sticking pain, for a few minutes.—Burning corrosive
sticking on the outer and posterior portion of the middle of the right
calf.—Tearing-sticking pain in the calves, especially in the middle.—A few
or several stitches in succession in the calves.—Burning stitches in the
middle of the left calf.—Biting pain on the outer and anterior portion of
the left calf, when walking.—Tingling sensation in the calves, as of being
asleep.—[**950.**] Tearing pain in the calves in various places, especially in
the middle, sometimes extending into the tendo Achillis or the knee.—
Superficial tearing pain on the outer side of the left calf, extending downward from the knee.—Tensive cramplike tearing in the upper and inner
portion of the right calf, especially when walking and standing (one hundred and third day).—Pressive tearing pain in the left calf, extending as
far as the bones, for several seconds.—Dull, pressive, bruised pain in the
calves.—Bubbling in the left calf, deep in the muscles.—In the outer portion of the middle of the left calf, bubblings, mornings in bed (one hundred and ninth day).—A lymphatic swelling of the left tendo Achillis,
which for some time feels uneven, still more, however, in the depressions
near it, which are almost filled up, only at first dusky, pale-red, afterwards
dusky-red spots along the tendons; at first violent pain on raising the foot,
less when stepping upon it, which after a time is relieved, and only returns
periodically, with a sensation as if a heavy weight hung upon the foot,
disappearing in a horizontal position; when stretching out the foot extending upward into the calf and hollow of the knee, with a sensation as if the
parts were bruised; frequently with pressive or grumbling pain; cramp in
the sole of the foot if the foot hangs down; at first flexion is almost impossible on account of the severity of the pain; sometimes pressive bubbling,
or tearing, or frightful itching aggravated by rubbing, also burning in the
affected parts; at one time desquamation of the skin; chilliness in the
evening of the fourth day; swelling of the affected portion of the foot
after motion, and swelling of the heel, so that the accustomed shoe is
too tight, with burning in it, and cramp in the foot (thirtieth to seventieth
days); decided traces of the swelling last till the two hundred and fifty-
ninth day, only somewhat painful to pressure.—At times severe, at times
slight pain in the tendines Achillis, as if they had been excessively strained.
—Pressive-tensive pain in the tendines Achillis, when standing and walking, and afterwards; seldom when at rest.—[**960.**] Drawing pain or drawing-tearing in the tendines Achillis in the same conditions.—Sticking or
drawing pain in one or the other tendo Achillis.—Sticking pain in the left
tendo Achillis, when walking; more in the posterior portion, in a few paroxysms.—A few stitches in the tendines Achillis.—Burning stitch in the
left tendo Achillis (seventy-third day).—Intermitting stitches in the left
tendo Achillis, when sitting and hanging the foot.—Tearing pain in the
tendines Achillis, sometimes extending up into the calf, usually continuing
nearly all day, when standing and walking, and also when sitting.—Smart-

ing pain on the inner side of the tendines Achillis, extending upward to the calf, while sitting.—*Ankle.* Violent pain below the left internal malleolus, when walking, with swelling of the ligaments and tendons in this region, extending to the inner portion of the foot as far as the great toe (ninety-first day).—Cold sensation, with a kind of painless tearing behind the left external malleolus (one hundred and fifth day).—[**970.**] Burning pain just above the left external malleolus.—Burning pain on the left external malleolus.—Gnawing on the forepart of the right ankle, for twenty seconds.—Gnawing pain on the external malleolus of the right foot, sometimes lasting only a few seconds, sometimes hours.—Gnawing and sticking in the region above and behind the left external malleolus (ninety-eighth day).—Violent pressive pain in the inner right malleolus, for half a minute.—Sudden sticking pain in the left ankle, when running, for twenty seconds, so that he became lame (sixty-third day).—Sticking in the inner malleolus of the right foot, changing to two violent stitches when stepping. —Sticking in the inner side of the left ankle on bending the joint outward, for half a minute.—Biting sticking on the anterior and outer side of the left malleolus.—[**980.**] Pullselike sticking in the left external malleolus from without inward, for six minutes, in the morning when waking, returning after a quarter of an hour as single stitches.—Bubbling-sticking pain in the left internal malleolus, for five minutes, preceded for ten minutes by simple sticking, at last changing to a dull, diffused, bruised, or numb pain, with increased sensation of warmth on the inner side of the leg.—Five violent stitches on the inner malleolus of the right foot, extending across from before backward (fortieth day).—A stitching in the right ankle from without inward, when standing.—Two piercing, very severe stitches in the anterior region of the right ankle, when walking.—Two sharp stitches on the right external malleolus, extending into the joint, when walking.—A burning stitch on the outer left malleolus, changing to a burning-sticking.—A burning stitch in the outer anterior portion of the right ankle, followed by itching.—Two burning stitches below and in front of the internal malleolus of the left foot.—Tearing in the ankles extending, now downward, now upward.—[**990.**] Tearing in the inner malleolus of the left foot down into the heel.—Fine tearing in the forepart of the left ankle across to the inner malleolus and down to the sole of the foot.—Violent tearing in the left external malleolus, extending upward into the tendons, for half a minute. —Tearing in the outer anterior portion of the left ankle, extending upward into the leg and downward into the back of the foot.—Severe tearing, almost sticking, from the left external malleolus upward into the neighboring tendons, for forty seconds.—Tearing in the inner malleolus of the left foot, changing to a burning.—Tearing in the left inner malleolus for half an hour, with a sharp stitch extending inward.—Tensive-tearing pain upon the forepart of the left ankle.—Drawing-tearing pain in the left external malleolus, extending forward and downward.—Tearing, or tearing-tensive, or sticking pain in the malleoli, seldom lasting; very frequently.—[**1000.**] Violent tearing and digging pain in the left external malleolus, extending into the little toe, so that he is not able to move the foot, in the evening when going to sleep, lasting several minutes; afterward several slighter attacks.—Severe pain when touched, in the tendons and neighboring portions of the bone, in the region in front, and somewhat above both malleoli, especially of the left foot, discovered accidentally on motion (fifty-ninth to sixty-sixth days).—Smarting pain in the ankles.—Bubbling twitches from the left internal malleolus across over the joint, as if something living were moving in this place.—Smarting-itching pain on the forepart and sides of the left ankle.—**Foot.** On stretching out the left foot, pain in the forepart of it.—Pain in the feet, especially in the toes, as from chilblains.—Burning pain, as from nettles, on the outer border of the left foot.—Sensation in the left hollow of the foot, as if the tendons were too short, like a cramp, when walking and sitting.—Two sharp stitches in the whole of the outer border of the right foot from without inward, then, on stepping, three more.—[**1010.**] Five violent stitches in the outer and middle portion of the left foot, penetrating from above to the under side, as if the foot would be nailed down, after a few minutes.—Three frightful stitches between the metatarsal bones of the fourth and fifth toes of the left foot, as if a nail were forced from above through the foot, when standing (forty-fourth day). —A tearing in the inner border of the left foot.—Jerklike tearings in the outer border of the right foot, involving the whole extent of the metatarsal bone of the little toe, lasting several minutes, while sitting after a walk.—Corrosive pain on the inner border of the left foot.—Burning pain on the outer portion of the back of the right foot.—Corrosive burning on the outer anterior side of the back of the left foot.—On the back of the right foot across behind the first joint of the four outer toes, tensive pain, becoming sticking on stepping, for a quarter of an hour, in the morning on rising.—Four stitches on the outer side of the back of the right foot, when sitting, leaving a pain after them (fifty-first day).—Tearing pain on the back of the right foot in the middle, extending to the middle toes, when sitting.—[**1020.**] At one time drawing, at another tensive, at another sticking-tearing on the back of the foot, drawing back and forth, at one time less, at another more severe, frequently ending as a stitch in the tips of the toes.—Corrosive pain on the outer side of the back of the left foot.—Bubbling sensation on the back of the left foot, extending towards the little toe.—Pain in a corn in the right sole frequently.—Tingling, at times crawling sensation of warmth in the soles, often at the same time in the toes, and on the back of the foot, as in frozen feet.—Burning in the soles of the feet, especially in the evening.—Sticking-burning pain in the soles of the feet. —A stitch in the left sole just behind the second toe, changing to a slight, frequent, bubbling sensation.—Ten or fifteen sensitive stitches in the sole of the right foot, at the first joint of the middle toe, when standing, from without inward.—A piercing stitch on the inner side of the right sole.—[**1030.**] Two burning stitches penetrating inward in the right sole behind the joint of the first toe.—Crawling-stitching in the sole of the foot and on the back of the first joint of the left middle toes.—Violent pulsating stitches, deep in the left sole not far from the heel, for several minutes, from without inward (twenty-sixth day).—Tearing on the outer border of the right sole.—Tearing pain in the sole of the left foot and in the metatarsal joints of the toes.—Tearing pain in the soles of the feet, now here, now there, frequently with crawling motions, and a sensation of increased warmth therein.—In the middle of the sole of the left foot, rather externally, a pain, as after bruising the foot.—A burning sore pain in the inner side of the left sole.—Stitches in the balls of the feet, seldom lasting more than a few minutes, frequently only half a minute.—Pulselike stitches in the right balls of the feet.—Tearing in the balls of the feet, mostly of the great toe, sometimes only for half a minute, at times lasting for hours, when walking and afterwards, or also when sitting; very frequently, chiefly when stepping, when it is first noticed.—[**1040.**] Sticking pain in the heel, mostly in the lower surface, extending deep into the bones, most frequent on motion and when stepping, often only noticed when stepping.—Tearing-sticking pain in the heel, when walking, especially on stepping, extending deep into the bones, seldom when sitting.—Tingling tearing-sticking in the right heel, extending deep into the bones, lasting a few minutes, as if there were something living in it.—Pulselike sticking pain, especially on the lower surface of the heel, in two to twenty stitches, at times fine, at times violent, from without inward, often changing into stitches lasting a few minutes.—Single stitches in the heel, especially in the lower portion.—Three piercing stitches across through the right heel from without inward, when standing (thirty-third day).—Seven severe stitches from the anterior outer portion of the margin of the left heel at intervals within five minutes, as if a sharp instrument were thrust deep through the skin, when walking, on stepping, so violent that he must sink down (ninety-third day).—Burning-stitching in the inner side of the left heel.—A sensitive cutting stitch in the left heel, slow, occupying half a minute in passing through (seventeenth day).—Tearing pain in the heels, especially when walking and stepping, sometimes also in single tearings, very frequently, seldom when at rest.—[1050.] Sensation of suppuration in the heels, especially after long standing.—*Toes.* A pain, as if sprained, in the metatarsal joints of the toes of the right foot, and away backwards into the middle portion of the foot, with a sensation as if the parts were swollen, for two days, increased by taking hold of it (ninth day).—Burning pain in the tip of the left great toe.—Transient burning on the back of the first joint of the left great toe, while sitting.—Digging pain in the right great toe, as if it would become inflamed.—Tingling-digging pain in the right great toe, for a minute (eighty-seventh day).—Tearing sticking-digging pain in the whole tip of the right great toe, for a minute.—Severe sticking pain in a corn in the left second toe.—Severe sticking from without inward and backward in the great toe, lasting at times only a few minutes, at times for several hours; it comes on while walking, and continues while at rest; with every step there is a stitch (sixtieth, seventy-third, and eighty-fifth days, etc.).—Burning or smarting-sticking on the back of the second joint of the right second toe (seventy-first day).—[1060.] Jerklike sticking in single toes.—Crawling-sticking in the right great toe.—Twinging drawing-sticking in the right fourth toe, extending backwards along the back of the toe into the foot.—Sensitive jerking-sticking in the right great toe from without inward, several hours in succession, worse when walking.—Pulselike sticking pain in the great toes, at times penetrating inward, at times outward.—Stitches in the tips of the toes, especially of the great toes.—Several stitches in the ball of the left great toe, extending forward into the toe (one hundred and second day).—In the ball of the right great toe, frightful stitches, penetrating inward as from a pointed nail (one hundred and first day).—Three stitches through the metatarsal joint of the little toe from above downward (forty-fifth day).—Eight or ten deeply penetrating stitches in the first joint of the left fourth toe (eighty-eighth day).—[1070.] Stitches, frequently sharp, in the tips of the toes, chiefly of the great toes, sometimes penetrating inward, sometimes outward.—Fine burning stitches on the left great toe, as from needles, extending from the ball.—Jerklike severe stitches in the metatarsal joint of the right great toe.—Pulselike stitches in the region of the first joint of the third toe of the left foot, from below upward, when sitting, for twenty seconds.—A stitch on the back of the metatarsal joint of the left fourth toe, extending forward into the toes, while standing (forty-fourth day).—Violent stitches in the under surface of the right great toe, when walking, for five or six minutes.—Tingling pain in the whole of the right great toe, as if it would swell (one hundred and third day).—Crawling and burning in the toes, sometimes with fine stitches.—Crawling in the first phalanges of the four outer left toes.—Tearing in the metatarsal joint of the second toes.—[1080.] A tearing in the ball of the fourth toe of the right foot.—Single tearings in the toes, especially in the joints.—Tearing in the toes, sometimes drawing, sometimes sticking, sometimes burning in the joints, on the surface, and in the tips, sometimes slight, sometimes severe.—Tearing-wrenching pain in the third and fourth toes of the right foot, sometimes with single stitches, lasting nearly the whole day.—Tearing in all the toes of the right foot, while sitting.—Burning-tearing pain in the ball of the little toe.—Violent sticking tearing in the right great toe, from the second joint to the tip, for one and a half minutes, while sitting after walking (forty-third day).—Jerklike tearings in the first joint of the right fourth toe.—Violent pain in the second toe of the left foot, as if it would suppurate, for ten minutes.—A sensation in the tips of the great toes, as if they had been painfully bruised, at times only by a pressure upon them.—[1090.] In the second and third toes of the right foot an ulcerative or bruised pain, for two days, with intermissions (sixth to seventh days).—Burning, corrosive, or sore pain in the toes, especially in the two last and the great toe, sometimes also in the second and third toes, even after a short walk, with pale redness of the toes, as after superficial freezing; tight boots are unendurable; the outer border of the foot frequently suffers also; the skin between the toes is very painful to touch; sometimes with itching-tearing between the toes.

Generalities.—Attacks of faintness with sudden orgasms of blood after a walk; sweat and heat in the upper half of the body, coldness, paleness and sunkenness of the face, oppression of the chest, shortly before going to sleep; on lying down in bed she shivers; she sleeps heavily, tosses about uneasily and has heavy dreams (fifty-first day).—Continued, even slight, occupation fatigues her very much, and sweat breaks out easily.—In the evening frequently great fatigue, so that she cannot keep awake.—In the evening and after supper she was very soon tired, and she was obliged to go to bed very early (first day),[10].—Great fatigue in the evening; he goes to bed two hours sooner than usual, and falls asleep sooner than usual (first day).—Faintlike weakness when walking, standing, or if she rises up, with vertigo (twelfth and thirteenth days).—Great weakness in the limbs, and in the whole body, increased by walking or long standing, even slight exertions affect her very much.—Exhaustion even to trembling, so that she feared that her knees would break down; vertigo on rising up when she stooped (thirteenth day).—[1100.] General prostration, so that she has no desire to do anything, after six to ten hours.—A condition near to faintness, after riding, followed by a short walk, so that she must lie down.—General bruised sensation in the whole body, especially in the lower limbs, as after great fatigue.—After long stooping, she feels as if bruised and unable to do anything (twelfth day).

Skin.—*General Appearance.* The skin frequently becomes sticky and scales off, and a thin, brownish, superficial scurf appears on its inner margin.—Two small red spots on each side of the forehead (sixty-fifth day).—On the forepart of the left shoulder, three small, punctiform, mottled, dusky-red spots, at times smarting slightly (seventy-fourth day).—On the forepart of the right shoulder, two dusky-red mottled spots nearly confluent, one about a quarter of an inch, the other about five-fourths of an inch long, somewhat painful upon grasping it, as after a bruise of the skin or like " vibices" (forty-fourth day).—A pale dusky-red, mottled spot as large as a half-dollar near the external condyle of the left humerus, at times burning and itching as if congested, in the middle of an elevated nettle-rash-like welt.—Small dusky-red, petechial-like, at times slightly itching or burning spots, on the forearm, also at times on the back of the hand, chiefly near the wrist and a few inches from it.—[1110.] A severely smarting spot an inch and a half long, bright red, on the inner side of the left thigh, about five inches from the knee, lasting more than half an hour; rubbing aggravates the pain; the spot disappears the next day.—*Eruptions.* Single, seldom grouped, sticking, red, burning-itching or sticking, or gnawing pimples on the skin, sensitive to pressure, usually surrounded by a red areola, with small tips containing pus, at last changing to brown spots like liver spots.—Several pimples on the lips.—Pimples at times on the chin.—Several pimples on the throat.—Some pimples in the skin of the chest, most numerous on the shoulder-blades.—Pimples on the neck, sometimes isolated, frequently in groups, especially near the hair.—Some pimples on the back.—Some pimples upon the shoulders.—A pimple on the tip of the right elbow, which became much inflamed by rubbing.—[1120.] Isolated pimples on the back of the fingers, at one time one on the radial side of the right ring finger.—On the back of the first phalanx of the right index finger a small superficial pimple as if a wart would form.—Some pimples on the nates.—A few pimples on the thigh.—On the left upper arm just beneath and behind the shoulder a patch of nettle-rash, two-thirds of an inch long, itching somewhat, afterwards desquamating (fifty-fifth day).—An itching spot of nettle-rash on the left upper arm, a few inches above the elbow.—A nettle-rash-like itching spot on the back of the left hand, in the forepart, between the second and third metacarpal bones.—In the ball of the right hand, three superficial semi-transparent small warts, disappearing after some time (one hundred and first day).—Superficially, or rather just under the skin, a wart as large as a millet-seed, on the outer surface of the third phalanx of the right middle finger, slightly itching (one hundred and fifth day).—On the inner right side of the lower lip, a vesicle as large as a small pea, becomes flattened; the next day two smaller ones arise.—[1130.] On the mucous membrane of the lips and cheeks, several very painful and very red inflamed pimples, with deep though not broad suppurating points in the centre.—*Sensations.* Simple pain in the skin in a small spot in the middle of the outer and anterior side of the right thigh, for a minute; after ten minutes some biting stitches in the same place.—Cold sensation in the skin in a small spot below the right nates.—Momentary cold sensation in the skin on the inner anterior portion of the left thigh, as if a few drops of ice-cold water had been spattered on the skin (seventy-sixth day).—In the upper and forepart of the right thigh, a sudden sensation, as if a cold animal a few inches long, about the size of a lizard, lay on the skin, so that she hurriedly shook the clothes in order to get rid of it (sixty-ninth day). —On the posterior lower portion of the right thigh, in a small spot, a sensation as if the skin touched some cold metal or ice, or as if a drop of ice-cold water were spattered upon it, lasting a few minutes while walking (ninety-fourth day).—Momentary cold sensation, as if ice-cold water touched the skin on the outer side of the left leg not far from the knee (seventy-fourth day).—A sensation as if cold water were spattered on the skin at a small spot below the left calf, for a few minutes.—Cold sensation in a small spot in the skin on the upper outer portion of the left leg.—Cold sensation above

the left internal malleolus in a spot in the skin of the size of a penny.—
[1140.] Burning pain in front above the middle of the right upper arm in
the skin (one hundred and third day).—Burning pain in the skin of the right
thumb-inward.—Violent burning pain in the skin on and near the metacarpal bone of the middle finger of the left hand, for a few minutes (seventy-
first day).—A violent burning several times, with itching, that compels her
to scratch, in the right cheek in front of the ear down to the lower jaw
(fourth day),[7].—Sticking, burning pain in the skin an inch from the right
side of the navel and somewhat above it, lasting for half a minute.—
Gnawing pain in the skin in the upper part of the right side of the chest.
—Gnawing pain in the skin of the wrists, aggravated by rubbing.—Gnawing pain in the skin in the upper anterior portion of the right thigh (one
hundred and sixth day).—Gnawing pain in the skin in a small spot in the
left thigh above the middle of the forepart, for a few seconds.—Gnawing
pain in the skin of the calves, mostly caused and aggravated by walking.
—[1150.] Itching burning-sticking woke her frequently in the night, now
here, now there, on the extremities and on the trunk, and which often compelled her to scratch (one and two nights),[10].—A fine stitch in the skin as
from an insect, on the posterior external and upper portion of the left upper
arm (one hundred and fourth day).—Fine stitches in the skin in the inner
surface of the last joint of the left index finger.—A burning stitch in the
skin about two inches to the left of the navel.—Burning stitches in the skin
of the left side of the abdomen, two inches from the navel, followed by itching.—Burning stitch in the skin in the middle of the right thigh externally
and posteriorly.—Fine burning-itching stitches in the skin of the left
heel.—Two sudden biting stitches in the skin of the flexor surface of the
left forearm, two inches from the wrist.—Two biting-itching stitches in the
skin in the middle of the flexor surface of the right forearm on the radius,
lasting for one minute, becoming a biting-itching (eighty-seventh day).—
Smarting here and there in the skin of the chest.—[1160.] Smarting
pain in the skin in the posterior portion of the lower and outer side
of the right thigh, lasting some minutes.—Gnawing, burning, sore pain
in the skin of the right popliteal space, when walking, for a few minutes
(ninety-seventh day).—Corrosive sensation in the skin in the region of the
left lower orbital margin.—A feeling of formication on the right side of the
upper lip.—Violent itching on the external surface of the lids and the skin
of the temples and of the forehead, which compels her to scratch, which
only momentarily relieves her; the region about the eye becomes quite red
in consequence (first day),[10].—Itching on the chin.—Itching in various
places of the skin of the chest, now in front, now in the sides or in the
axilla, chiefly in the skin of the shoulder-blades, obliges scratching, but
thereupon soon disappearing, but readily returning, sometimes biting, or
with fine stitches or burning.—Itching in the skin of the neck, though not
so often as in other places.—Itching on the neck, frequently burning or
biting, also corrosive, with fine stitches, which compel scratching and are
relieved by it, but soon return again.—Itching in the fossa above the left
clavicle.—[1170.] Itching in the lumbar region, at times burning or biting
or sticking, as from hairs or fleas.—Itching in the region of the shoulder,
chiefly on the anterior or posterior border of the axilla, causing scratching,
sometimes burning, biting, crawling, or fine sticking, also in the axilla.—
Itching in the right upper arm externally above the elbow.—Itching, at
times simple, at times burning, or also with fine stitches, in and around the
elbow, more on its outer than on its inner side.—Itching in the flexor surface

of the left forearm.—Itching in the flexor surface of the right forearm, from the elbow-to the middle of the forearm.—Simple or biting-itching in the wrists.—Itching on the back of the hand or in the palms, at one time simple, at another burning or biting or fine sticking or crawling, relieved by rubbing, but soon returning in the same or another place.—Itching in the fingers, a simple burning fine sticking, or stitch-like.—Itching in various places on the thigh, simple or burning or with fine stitches, or biting or fine sticking, causing scratching, by which it disappears but easily returns.—[1180.] Itching on the knee-joint, now in front, now behind, now on one side, simply burning or accompanied by fine stitches.—Violent itching in the skin of the knee and thigh in the afternoon, which causes her to scratch them, after which it soon disappears, but returns again (second day),[7].—Violent itching in the legs, rapidly changing places, sometimes widely extended, often with burning or fine sticking, or a sensation of increased warmth.—Itching in the calves, sometimes burning, biting or with fine stitches.—Itching in the region of the tendines Achillis, sometimes burning.—Itching on the ankles and malleoli, simply burning or fine sticking, sometimes extending to the backs and sides of the feet, also biting.—Itching on the backs of the feet, simple burning, biting, or sticking.—Itching in the soles, now simple, now biting, now burning or fine sticking.—Itching in the heels.—Itching in the toes, especially on the backs, simple burning, crawling, biting or burning, also with fine stitches or fine sticking in them.—Burning itching pain about the middle of the right upper arm, in the forepart and externally, for a few minutes.—[1190.] Violent, smarting burning itching on the back of the left foot, twice in bed before going to sleep, once also in the day when sitting, aggravated by scratching, which she is obliged to do; she is obliged to change the position of the feet in bed constantly and to seek cold places (sixtieth to sixty-second days).—Stitching-like itching on and behind the left external wrist, in the skin.—Biting-itching in the region of the elbow externally, especially somewhat above it, relieved by scratching, which causes a slight redness of the skin.—A biting or burning itching in the flexor surface of the left forearm not far from the wrist.—Biting-itching in the middle of the right leg externally, near the crest of the tibia, aggravated and caused by walking.—Biting-itching pain on the inner anterior portion of the left tibia.—Smarting itching pain in the skin of the right upper arm in the middle of the outer portion, aggravated by rubbing.

Sleep and Dreams.—Yawning, alternating with eructations (after one and a half hours).—Tearing in the left side of the chest (after nine hours).—Repeated sleepiness during the day, especially in the morning, also after eating, so that he is obliged to lie down.—Sleep unusually long, till 7 o'clock in the morning, with a weary and bruised sensation and a pressive pain in the head, back and loins (forty-sixth day).—[1200.] Difficult waking in the morning, when she cannot rightly recollect, cannot collect her thoughts, and must exert all her power to get awake (seventh day).—She is unable to fall asleep before 2 o'clock in the night (twelfth day).—He wakes frequently and very easily about 2 to 4 o'clock, cannot sleep again in spite of the fact that he is still very tired, or he falls asleep again, but also wakes again; with tension in the head, rush of blood to it and excitement.—Frequent waking from sleep in an unusual position on the left side.—Frequently restless sleep disturbed by itching-burning or by anxious dreams.—Restless sleep full of dreams, which is quite unusual.—In the morning when walking he often does not feel refreshed, but weary in body and mind.—At night a condition between sleeping and waking;

in which she is tormented with a system of education, which at times assumes the form of a tree, at another some other wonderful form; she tries in vain to get rid of the image, arouses from slumber and opens the eyes and becomes very fretful about it (ninth and tenth days).

Fever.—Chilliness.—Creeping chilliness at times, especially on going into the cold air (third day),[9].—Slight chilliness before dinner better afterwards (first day).—[1210.] Chilliness, especially during the hours before dinner, at times also afterwards, with ice-cold feet, dryness and stickiness of the mouth, without thirst; pain in the region of the left tonsil. —Slight chilliness in the region of the stomach (after nine hours).—Slight chilliness in the back for about a quarter of an hour, at seven and a half in the evening (seventh day).—Sensation of chilliness in the back and on the posterior portion of the arms, extending down to the hips, in the evening shortly before going to sleep, several times, as if she were wrapped in cloth dipped in ice-cold water, for twenty minutes, after which she became warm; after the second attack, swelling of the left tendo Achillis (twenty-second to thirty-first day).—Chilly sensation in the morning, from 11 o'clock, for a few hours (third day).—Frequent sensation of chilliness in the head, with cold feet, confusion of the head, even pressive headache, as if he would be attacked with coryza, in the morning; the head is often hot therewith; the hands are rather cool than warm.—In the afternoon the warmth extends over the whole body, with tendency to sweat.—In the forenoon, alternating chilliness on the back, on the outer side of the arms and in the calves; in the afternoon, burning stitches, increasing at night, without thirst, without dry mouth; dizziness and violent sticking pain in the head, with angina; on the third and following days, sweat of a somewhat urinous odor.—Chilliness in the hands and feet and in the whole body, with heat in the face, from 11 o'clock on, with ice-cold feet; the hands feel warm.—Chilliness over the whole body, so that she shivers, followed by heat, for a few minutes (second day).—Rapidly-creeping chills, even shiverings in various parts, especially beginning in the face and arms and extending over the back and chest, followed by heat, with anxiety and oppression of the chest, especially in the forenoons and evenings; the heat was so violent that she was obliged to jump into water (third day).—[1220.] Coldness in the whole body in the evening, followed by heat, with increased thirst.—*Heat and Sweat.* —Increased sensation of warmth over the whole body (after eight to nine hours).—Sensation of heat through the whole day (thirteenth day).—Sensation of heat over the whole body, at 6 o'clock in the evening, for about a quarter of an hour, followed by a cool sensation (fourth day).—Increased warmth in the head (from two to three hours).—Heat in the head (second day),[7].—Feeling of great heat in the head; also excited by touch (after nine hours).—Heat in the temples and coolness in the cheeks (after eight hours). —Increased heat in the face (after five hours).—A slight, burning, warm sensation in the face.—[1230.] Burning heat in the face, more subjective than objective, with redness of the cheeks (after three hours).—Transient heat in the face, with redness frequently returning (after ten hours).— Some heat in the face, with a sensation of coldness in other parts; after a few hours the heat extends over the whole body; the hands and feet become warm; without thirst.—Painful burning in the cheeks, with redness (after four hours).—Heat in the hands and in the head, in the afternoon, for several days.—Tingling sensation of warmth in the legs, especially when sitting, as if they had been rubbed with woollen clothes.—Tingling sensation of warmth in the feet.—In the evening and at night the heat increases, with tendency to sweat (tenth to eleventh day).—Sensation of heat in the body, with sweat breaking out easily on motion, standing, etc.; in the evening, about 6 o'clock, slight chilliness.—Heat in the head after eating and in the afternoon of the first day and on many following days; the head sweats easily on exertion, stooping, standing, etc.—[1240.] She sweat several times very profusely after midnight and woke several times on this account (one, two, and three nights),[10].—Inclined to sweat on the slightest exertion, especially in the afternoon, with a feeling of anxiety (eighth to eighteenth day).—At times cold sweat covered the face (first day),[10].

Conditions.—**Aggravation.**—(*Morning*), When rising, anxious sensation; while in bed, anxious sensation; contemplation of mental work becomes difficult, etc.; chilliness, etc.; pressive headache, etc.; after rising, burning, etc., in eyes; after rising, crusty substance in lids; after rising, sticky sensation in margin of lids; drops of blood from nostril; about 6 o'clock, drops of blood; after rising, sticky feeling on margin of lips; after rising, dryness in the mouth; 8 o'clock, bitter taste in mouth; taste of blood; scraping in throat; on waking, scraping in throat; after rising, scraping in throat; in bed, pain in abdomen; on becoming erect when rising, pain in upper abdomen returns; when waking, pain above crest of left ilium; on waking, when in bed, pain in left ilium; soon after rising, pain in region of both kidneys; before urinating for first time, pain in bladder; immediately after rising, desire to urinate; after rising, urine cloudy; in bed, immediately on waking, sensation in sacrum; in bed, on waking, stitch in left side of sacrum; on waking, pain in middle finger; after rising, sensation on left thigh; when going down stairs, after rising from bed, on bending the knee, pain above patella; from 4 till 11 o'clock, when bending knee, pain in knee-joint; bubbling in middle of left calf; when waking, sticking in left malleolus; on rising, pain on back of right foot; sleepiness; chilly sensation; chilliness in head, etc.—(*Forenoon*), Chilliness on back; from 11 o'clock, on, chilliness in hands, etc.; creeping chills, etc.—(*Towards afternoon*), Troubles with the eyes.—(*Afternoon*), Symptoms in general; 4 P.M., till going to sleep, anxious mood, etc.; inflammation of eyes; from 12 o'clock, burning in eyes; 3 o'clock, burning in eyes, etc.; red spot on face, etc.; thirst; pain in abdomen; itching in skin of knee, etc.; heat in hands, etc.; heat in head; inclination to sleep.—(*Evening*), Itching below hair; troubles with the eyes; pain in right ear; scraping sensation in throat; till 9 o'clock, after eating, sensation in epigastric region; at 10 o'clock, on going to sleep, pain in upper abdomen; in bed, pain in region of pectoralis major; at 9 o'clock, pain in back of hand; in bed, sensation in right thigh; when lying in bed, pain in popliteal space, etc.; when going to sleep, pain in left calf; when going to sleep, pain in left malleolus; burning in soles; *great fatigue;* 7.30 o'clock, chilliness in back; shortly before going to sleep, chilliness in back, etc.; creeping chills, etc.; 6 o'clock, sensation of heat through whole body; heat; 6 o'clock, slight chilliness.—(*Night*), Oppression of chest; on going to bed, bubbling sensation in arm; when falling asleep, workings on left thigh; pain across left knee; heat.—(*After midnight*), Very profuse sweat.—(*Open air*), Most of the eye troubles.—(*Going from house into open air*), Feeling as if rain dropped on face.—(*Bending finger*), Pain in joint of finger; burning in joint of finger.—(*Before breakfast*), Nausea, etc.—(*Breathing*), Pain in upper abdomen.—(*Deep breathing*), Pain in middle of chest.—(*After coition*), Smarting in urethra; feeling of weakness in genitals; pain in left side of penis.—(*Going into cold air*), Creeping chilliness.—(*Before dinner*),

Chilliness, etc.—(*After dinner*), Nausea.—(*After eating*), Sour taste; bitter taste; sleepiness; heat in head.—(*During ejaculation of semen*), Pain in urethra.—(*After exerting arm*), Pain in left forearm.—(*After exerting hand*), Pain in wrist; stitch in left palm.—(*Extending arm*), Pain in tendon of biceps; sensation in surface of elbow.—(*On long-continued grasping with right hand*), Pain in flexor muscles, etc.—(*Taking hold of foot*), Pain in right toe joints.—(*Hanging down the hand*), Pain in surface of forearm.—(*Inspiration*), Pain below false ribs; pain between shoulder-blades.—(*Lifting arm*), Pain in tendon of biceps.—(*Lying*), Symptoms in region of kidneys; bubbling sensation in lumbar region; sensation in sacrum; bruised, etc., feeling in sacrum.—(*Lying down in bed*), Shivering.—(*Motion*), Anxious sensation; pain in upper abdomen; tension in inguinal fold; most of pains in external genitals; pain in right shoulder-blade; tearing in left shoulder; bubbling sensation in muscles of arms; pain in elbow-joint; pain in middle finger; pains in lower extremities; pinching in muscles of thighs; tearing in muscles of thighs; tearing in thigh; tension in knee-joint; pain in right patella, etc.; pain in right knee; pain in middle of tibia.—(*Moving eyes*), *Pain in eyes.*—(*Moving arms backward*), Pain in left shoulder.—(*Pressure*), Pain in region of gall-bladder; pain in right shoulder-blade; pain in left shoulder; bubbling sensation in muscles of arm; pain in right middle finger-joint; tearing in ring finger; tearing in left index finger; *tearing in left thumb;* tearing in right tibia.—(*Deep pressure*), Pain in region on side of navel; pain in kidney region; pain in bladder.—(*On raising foot*), Violent pain.—(*On beginning to read or write*), Painful sensation.—(*When reading by lamplight*), Twitching in lids.—(*On rising from sitting*), Anxious sensation; bubbling sensation in lumbar region; sensation in lower extremities; sensation in knees; pain in calves.—(*On rising from stooping*), Whirling vertigo, etc.; kidney symptoms in general.—(*Rubbing*), Smarting in skin of head, etc.; pain in back of forearm; pain in various places on forearm; pain on back of left wrist; pain on back of left hand; pain in tip of fore finger; pain in finger-joint; pain in joint of fore finger; pain in index finger; gnawing sensation on thigh; pain on right tibia; pain in middle of tibia; pain in skin of wrists; pain in skin of upper arm.—(*When running*), Pain in left ankle.—(*Scratching*), Itching on back of foot.—(*Sitting*), Bubbling sensation in urethra; sensation in sacrum; bruised, etc., feeling in sacrum; pain in tuber ischii; tearing in femur; pain in left calf; pain in tendines Achillis; after a walk, tearing in border of foot; stitches on back of foot; pain on back of foot; burning in great toe; stitches in left third toe; tingling warmth in legs.—(*When sitting down*), Pain in right popliteal space, etc.—(*When sitting and hanging the foot*), Stitches in left tendo Achillis.—(*Speaking*), Pain in left tonsil.—(*When stamping*), Cramp in left popliteal space.—(*Standing*), Cold sensation on thigh; stitching in left nates; pain in upper right thigh; stitches in left popliteal space; tearing in tendons of knee; pain in middle of leg; pain in tibia; pain in spot on tibia; tearing in right calf; pain in tendines Achillis; stitching in ankle; stitches in right sole; stitches through heel; stitches in left fourth toe.—(*On standing a long time*), Anxious sensation; sensation of suppuration in the heels.—(*When stepping*), Cramp in left popliteal space; stitch in right malleolus; tearing in balls of feet; *pains in heel.*—(*After stool*), Sensation as if one must soon go again, etc.—(*Stooping*), Vertigo; sensation as if something shook in head, etc.; painful sensation in forehead, etc.; pain in forehead; pain in forehead, etc.; lower part of back felt stiff; symptoms in region of kidney; drawing pain in neck; sensation in sacrum; pain in lower extremities; pain in right leg; feel as if bruised, etc.—(*Stretching*), Tension in knee-joint; stitches between metatarsal bones.—(*Swallowing*), Pain in left tonsil.—(*Empty swallowing*), Pains in throat.—(*Touch*), Pain in right temple; pain in upper abdomen; pain between metacarpal bones; pain in middle finger; pain in left thigh.—(*After urinating*), Sensation in bladder as if one must go again soon.—(*Walking*), Vertigo, etc.; pain in side of penis; pain in lower portion of scrotum; swelling of spermatic cord; gnawing on right thigh; stitch on left thigh; pain in right thigh; pain in left thigh; pain in upper right thigh; tension in muscles of thigh; pain in bend of thighs; pain in tendons of thigh; contraction of muscles of thigh; stitch in thigh; sensation in knees; pain in patella; pain in right patella; pain through knee-joint; stitches below knee-joint; stitches in left popliteal space; pain below margin of left patella; tearing in tendons of knee; pain in right leg; pain in tibia; pain in right tibia; pain in spot on tibia; pain in calves; pain in right calf; pain in left calf; tearing in right calf; pain in tendines Achillis; pain in left tendo Achillis; stitches in right ankle; stitches in right malleolus; pain below malleolus; stitches in left heel; tearing in heels; sticking in right great toe; cold sensation on thigh; pain in skin of calf.—(*After a walk*), Attacks of faintness.

Amelioration.—(*Afternoon*), Tearing in kidney region.—(*Evening*), Increased appetite.—(*Open air*), Head symptoms generally; pain in forehead.—(*Drinking water*), Scraping in throat.—(*Eating and drinking*), Dryness in mouth, etc.—(*Rest*), Pressure in eyes, etc.; pain in right shoulderblade; pain in right knee; pain in left knee-joint.—(*Stretching or exerting muscles*), Pain in walls of chest.

BISMUTHUM OXIDUM.

Hydrated oxide of Bismuth, $Bi_2O_3OH_2$. *Preparation,* Trituration of the oxide prepared according to Hahnemann's instructions.

Authorities. 1, Hahnemann, R. A. M. L., 6, 250; 2, Hermann, ibid.; 3, Hartmann, ibid.; 4, Laughammer, ibid.

Mind.—Solitude is unendurable,[2].—Ill-humor the whole day; he was very quiet and would not talk; in the evenings more cheerful,[4].—*He is morose and discontented with his condition and complains about it* (after twenty-four hours),[2].—Restless peevishness; he is discontented with everything; at times he sits, he lies down; at times he walks around, and remains only a short time in one position, because it becomes very irksome to him,[2].—He commences one thing and then another, but keeps to one thing only a short time.[2].

Head.—*Confusion of the head,*[2].—Vertigo; a sensation as if the head was turning in a circle (after one hour),[2].—*Vertigo; a sensation as if the anterior half of the brain were turning in a circle, several times during the day, lasting several minutes,*[2].—In the morning, long-continued dizziness,[1].— [10.] The head seems as heavy as a hundred-weight (after one hour),[2].— A burning contractive pain in the head, especially in the forehead and eyes,[1].—*Dull cutting pain in the brain, which begins above the right orbit and extends to the occiput* (after three days),[2].—Dull pressive-drawing in the head, now here, now there,[2].—*Dull pressive-drawing in the head, now here, now there,* more violent on motion,[2].—Boring pain from within outward, at times in the right, at times in the left frontal eminence, sometimes in both at the same time (after nine hours),[3].—Sudden digging and boring in the forehead, the eyes, and the nose down to the tip, as with a dull instrument; an alternately contracting and distending sensation,[1].—*Pressure and sensation of heaviness in the forehead, more violent on motion,[2].—*Violent pressive heavy pain in the forehead, especially above the root of the nose and in both temples when sitting (after three and a half hours),[3].—Tearing pain in the forehead above the right inner canthus and in the back part of the orbit (after twenty-four hours),[2].—[20.] Severe pressure in both temples from within outward, not affected by motion or touch (after two and a half hours),[2].—Tearing pressure internally in the right temple, still more externally, increased by pressure,[2].—Pressure and sensation of heaviness in the occiput, more violent on motion,[2].—Twitching-tearing pain in the whole left side of the occipital bone, more violent close to the parietal bone (after two and a half hours),[3].

Eyes.—Mucus in both canthi (after eight and a half and ten hours),[4].—Pressure on the right eyeball, from before backward and from below upward (after ten hours),[2].

Ears.—Tearing pressure in the external cartilage of the ear, which disappears on pressure (after four days),[2].—Drawing pressure in the external meatus in the left ear (after twenty-four hours),[2].

Face.—Earthy-colored face, blue rings around the eyes; the features are quite changed, as if he had been sick,[2].—Pressure regularly recurring at short intervals in the right malar bone, unchanged by touch,[2].

Mouth.—[30.] Drawing pressure in the back teeth, extending from the back teeth into the front, with drawing pain in the cheeks,[1].—The gums are swollen, sore and painful; the whole of the interior of the mouth is just as sore and sensitive,[1].—In the evening, white-coated tongue, without heat or thirst (seventh and twelfth hours),[4].—In the morning a taste of blood; the mucus hawked up is colored with blood,[1].

Stomach.—*Nausea in the stomach; he feels as if he would vomit, especially violent after eating,[2].—*Pressure in the stomach, especially after eating,[2].

Abdomen.—Rumbling in the lower part of the bowels, without sensation,[2].—Loud rumbling in the right side of the abdomen, when standing (after two hours),[4].—Frequent passage of flatus,[2].—Painless rumbling in the lower part of the abdomen,[2].—[40.] Discomfort in the lower abdomen, with pressure, now here, now there (after eight hours),[2].—Pinching pain in the lower abdomen, now here, now there (after seven hours),[2].—Pinching pressure, now here, now there, in the lower abdomen, with rumbling and grumbling,[2].—Pinching pressure in the lower abdomen, and rumbling with desire; a sensation as if he must go to stool,[2].

Stool and Urinary Organs.—In the evening, desire for stool without effect (after thirteen hours),[4].—*He is obliged to urinate frequently, every time profusely; the urine is watery (after twelve hours),[2].

Sexual Organs.—Pressive pain in the right testicle, more severe when touched (after two hours),[2].—At night an emission of semen, without voluptuous dreams,[4].

Respiratory Apparatus, Chest and Heart.—A cough which wakes him at night from sleep, with profuse expectoration, also just as much cough by day,[1].—Oppression of the chest,[1].—[50.] *Pain in the chest and back, with burning and boring,[1].—A hot burning contraction of the chest, so that it is difficult to breathe or to speak,[1].—*Pinching-pressive pain in the region of the diaphragm, extending transversely through the chest, when walking (after two hours),[3].—(Pinching stitches in the region of both nipples unaltered by inspiration or expiration),[2].—Fine tearing stitches in the region of both nipples (apparently superficial in the lungs, and at the same time in the pectoral muscles), at times more severe when inspiring or expiring,[2].—Dull sticking-tearing in the region of the last ribs,[2].—Pressive pain, now more, now less severe, in the right side of the chest, near the sternum in a small spot, unaffected by inspiration and expiration (after four hours),[3].—Severe pressure near the left nipple, extending inward toward the sternum,[2].—Tearing around and near the left nipple (after two days),[2]. —Intermitting stitches in the lowest false ribs of the left side at their union with the dorsal vertebræ,[2].—[60.] Fine stitching in the sternum in the middle, not affected by inspiration or expiration (after eight hours),[3].— Beating of the heart,[2].

Neck and Back.—Sensation of twitching in the muscles of the right side of the neck,[2].—Tensive pressure on the right side of the neck in the cervical vertebræ, during motion and rest (after three hours),[2].—Sharp pressure on the upper border of the right scapula and the clavicle,[2].—Pain in the left side of the back when sitting, as if one had stooped too long (after eight hours),[4].

Upper Extremities.—Pressive tearing in the right shoulder-joint,[2]. —*Paralytic weakness and weariness in the right arm*,[2].—(Spasmodic) contractive tearing in the muscles of the right arm (after fourteen hours),[4].— Spasmodic contractive pain in the anterior muscles of the left upper arm during complete rest of the body (after twenty-four hours),[4].—[70.] Paralytic pressure in the forepart of the right upper arm,[2].—Hard pressure in the left forearm, more in the lower and outer part,[2].—*Paralytic tearing pressure in the right forearm, especially in the bones of the wrist* (after one hour),[2].—*Paralytic tearing pressure in the right forearm, toward the outer side, at times more in the upper part*, at times more in the lower part, which disappears on motion and touch,[2].—Cutting tearing in the muscles of the lower part of the right forearm (after twelve hours),[3].—A grumbling pain in both bones of the left forearm, as if bruised (after thirteen hours),[3].— Violent tearing in the bones of the left wrist (after one and a half hours),[3]. —Tearing in the bones of the right wrist, which disappears on motion,[2].— Sensitive tearing upon and around the right styloid process, extending into the muscles of the hands, less violent in the process itself (after eleven hours),[3].—Trembling of the hands, noticed when eating,[1].—[80.] Feeling of weakness in the hands as though he could not hold a pen, with trembling (after eight hours),[3].—Itching, tearing pressure in the inner processes of both hands, which causes scratching,[2].—*Tearing in the metacarpal bones of the right index and middle fingers* (after eleven hours),[2].—Intermitting fine tearing in the ball of the left thumb (after two hours),[2].—Fine tearing in the last joints of the left fingers,[2].—*Fine tearing in the tips of the fingers of the right hand, especially under the nails* (after three days).[2].—Pressive tearing in the tips of the fourth and fifth fingers of the right hand,[2].

Lower Extremities.—Intermitting hard pressure above the left knee-joint, in the lower part of the thigh, towards the outer side, unchanged by touch or motion,[2].—Drawing in the middle of the calf and the anterior portion of the left leg down into the foot,[2].—Drawing in the right external malleolus, which disappears on motion,[2].—[90.] Tearing pain below the right external malleolus, which every time terminates behind in the tendo Achillis (after nine hours),[2].—Tearing pain in the right heel near and from the tendo Achillis (after five hours),[2].—Fine tearing in the left heel,[2].— Pressive tearing between the two last left metatarsal bones, close to the toes, while sitting (after ten hours),[3].—Fine tearing in the last phalanges of the left toes,[2].—Pressive tearing in the tip of the left great toe,[2].

Generalities and Skin.—*Weakness and exhaustion*,[2].—*Corrosive itching near the tibia and the backs of both feet near the joints, which becomes much worse on scratching; is obliged to scratch himself until it bleeds*,[2].

Sleep and Dreams, Fever.—*In the morning, a few hours after rising, an excessive sleepiness, but after eating he was unable to take his accustomed nap for several days*,[2].—During work he is overpowered by excessive inclination to sleep; he reads without knowing what; he immediately falls asleep and has vivid and confused dreams,[2].—[100.] He lies upon the back at night,[4].—In the evening while slumbering, violent startings, as if he fell (after fourteen and a half hours),[4].—*At night, frequent waking in sleep as from fright*,[4].—*At night, frequent wakings with weariness*,[4].—*Restless sleep at night, on account of voluptuous dreams, without, or frequently with, emission of semen*,[4].—At night, vivid anxious dreams,[4].—Flushes of heat through the whole body, especially in the head and over the chest, without chill preceding or following, in the morning soon after rising (after twenty-four hours),[2].

Conditions.—**Aggravation.**—(*Morning*), Dizziness; taste of blood; flushes of heat.—(*Evening*), White-coated tongue; desire for stool; while slumbering, violent startings.—(*When eating*), Trembling of the hands.—(*After eating*), Nausea; pressure in stomach.—(*When inspiring or expiring*), Stitches in region of nipples.—(*Motion*), Drawing in the head; pressure, etc., in forehead; pressure, etc., in occiput.—(*Pressure*), Pressure in right temple,—(*Scratching*), Itching near tibia, etc.—(*When sitting*), Pain in forehead; pain in side of back; tearing between metatarsal bones.—(*When standing*), Rumbling in abdomen.—(*Touch*), Pain in right testicle.—(*When walking*), Pain in region of diaphragm.

Amelioration.—(*Evening*), More cheerful.—(*On motion*), Pressure in forearm disappears; tearing in bones of wrist; drawing in right malleolus disappears.—(*On pressure*), Pressure in cartilage of ear disappears.—(*On touch*), Pressure in forearm disappears.

BISMUTHUM SUBNITRICUM.

Formula, $Bi_2O_3, N_2O_5, 2OH_2$.   (Magisterium bismuthi.)   *Preparation*, Triturations.

Authorities.   1, Kerner, Heidlbg. Kl. Annal., 1829 (from Wibmer), took 2 drops for heartburn; 2, Wernek, ibid., two girls, about 18 years old, took 6 grains in the morning, fasting; 3, ibid., a boy, 6 years old, took 6 grains after supper; 4, ibid., some men took from 6 to 12 grains at a dose; 5, ibid., a man took 15 grains, and the next day 20 grains; 6, ibid., a man took 15 grains; 7, a man took 40 grains at one dose; 8, Wernek, ibid., took 20 grains immediately after a meal.

Head.—Head somewhat confused on rising,[8].—Vertigo,[7].—Vertigo (after two hours),[8].—Vertigo on violent motion (after one hour),[2].—Slight, transient headache,[6].—Headache, especially in the frontal region,[7].—Headache and vertigo (after first dose),[4].—Headache and vertigo (after one and a half hours),[5].—Heat and confusion of the head (after one hour),[2].—[10.] Slight transient pain in the forehead (after half an hour),[8].—*Pressure in the frontal region*,[5].—*Pressive pain in the frontal region* (after one hour),[2].

Eyes.—Eyes red, sight somewhat dim,[7].—Conjunctiva red,[5].—Redness of the conjunctiva.

Ears and Nose.—Dry nose,[1].—Roaring in the ears,[8].

Mouth and Throat.—Tongue coated,[7].—Tongue furred,[5].—[20.] Tongue coated white,[8].—Offensive taste in the mouth,[1].—Taste bitter,[7].—The fauces and uvula were inflamed, with burning in the throat, difficult swallowing, and thirst,[1].

Stomach.—Appetite completely lost,[7].—Thirst increased,[7].—Much thirst and no appetite,[5].—*Eructations of wind after drinking a glass of water,*[8].—Frequent empty eructations and feeling of discomfort in the stomach, soon followed by a liquid stool, but not bilious (after three hours),[2].—Violent eructations, gripings in the bowels, and sudden slight bilious vomiting (after one and a half hours),[7].—[30.] Nausea and slight bilious vomiting,[8].—*Nausea, with pressure in the stomach* (after one and a half hours),[5].—Vomiting and diarrhœa, with retching and burning in the throat (immediately),[1].—Passage of much flatus from the stomach (after four hours),[5].—Passage of odorless flatus from the stomach,[3].—*Uncomfortable feeling in the stomach* (after half an hour),[8].—*The pressure in the stomach changes to a burning* (after one hour),[7].—*Pressure in the region of the stomach* (after half an hour),[7].—*Pressure in the stomach* (after one hour),[6 8].—*Distressing pressure and burning in the region of the stomach* (after three and a half hours),[5].—[40.] *Some pressure in the region of the stomach, and empty eructations,*[4].

Abdomen.—Rumbling in the intestines, and eructations (after one hour),[8].—Passage of much flatus, followed by a thin bilious evacuation,[6].—Colicky pains in the bowels,[6].—Gripings in the abdomen, followed by two liquid bilious evacuations (second day),[2].

Stool and Urinary Organs.—A liquid bilious stool (after three hours),[7].—Two loose movements in the bowels, with gripings, at 6 P.M. (second day),[8].—Two liquid stools, with gripings, at 4 P.M. (third day),[8].—During the poisoning he passed no urine, and the region of the bladder was not distended,[1].

Respiratory Apparatus and Pulse.—Difficult breathing,[8].—[50.] Pulse spasmodic,[4].—Pulse tense, spasmodic,[5].—Pulse small,[1].—Pulse small, tense, and spasmodic,[7].—Pulse accelerated, contracted,[2].—Pulse somewhat accelerated, small and tense,[2].—Pulse rapid, hard, small, 97,[8].—Pulse, at midnight, 95 and spasmodic,[8].

Extremities and Sleep.—Cramps in the hands and feet,[1].—Night very restless,[8].

Fever.—[60.] Extremities cold,[1].—Temperature somewhat increased,[8].—Heat over the whole body,[8].—Heat in the whole body (after two hours),[2].—A feeling of heat over the whole body,[5].

Conditions.—Aggravation.—(*After drinking water*), Eructations.—(*On violent motion*), Vertigo.—(*On rising*), Head confused.

BLATTA AMERICANA.

"The great American Cockroach," probably *kakerlae insignis.*

Nat. order, Insecta (common in Brazil). *Preparation*, Triturate the live insect with sugar of milk.

Authority. Pathogenesie Bresilienne (Mure).

Head.—Numbness and heaviness of the head.—Pain in the temple, with lancinations now and then (second day).—Aching pain in the temples.—Acute pain in the temples, every now and then, at 4 P.M.

Eyes.—Pricking, as by a fly, in the corner of the left eye, at 10 A.M.—Lachrymation.—Yellowness of the sclerotica. (When the prover had the jaundice, for which the Blatta is considered empirically as a specific, he felt a number of pains which have been reproduced in this proving, such as general prostration, weariness, etc.)

Nose, Face, and Mouth.—Watery discharge from nose.—Yellowness of face.—[10.] Very salt saliva.

Stomach and Abdomen.—Transient bloating at pit of stomach.—Slight colic.—Pain in transverse colon, duodenum, and pit of stomach.

Urinary Organs.—Much heat in urethra, when urinating.—Yellow color of urine, increasing more and more.—Urine of a bright yellow, albuminous (second day).

Chest.—Acute pain in chest, afternoon (second day).—Violent pain in chest, with want of breath (second day).—Pain in right side of chest.

Neck and Back.—[20.] Prickings in right side of neck.—Pain in back, right side.—Pain shifting from back to shoulder-blade.

Lower Extremities.—Sense of weariness in the hams.—Cramp in right leg (second day).—Pain in right leg, from toes to knees.—Pain in feet, here and there, sometimes in the sole (second day).—Pain at left little toe.

Generalities.—Lazy.—Extreme weariness when going upstairs.

Sleep and Fever.—[30.] Frequent yawning.—Chill and shuddering, for half an hour.—Shuddering, with sense of heat and moisture all over.

The proving was interrupted by an accident.

BOLETUS LARICIS.

Boletus purgans, Pers. (Boletus laricis, L.; B. laricinus, Berk.)
Nat. order, Fungi. *Preparation*, Trituration.
Authority. W. H. Burt, W. Hom. Obs., 2, 154, provings with the 3d trit. and the crude substance.

Mind.—Very gloomy and despondent.—Irritated at the least trifle.—Absence of mind.

Head and Eyes.—Head feeling very light and hollow, with deep frontal headache and great faintness.—Dull frontal headache.—Dull frontal headache, aggravated by motion.—Deep drawing pains in forehead.—Neuralgic pains in the temples.—Agglutination of the eyelids every morning, with dull aching pains in the eyeballs.

Mouth.—[10.] Teeth and gums very sore.—White coating on the tongue.—Thick yellow coating on the tongue, so that the marks of teeth are shown.—Flat taste in the mouth.—Flat, bitter taste.—Strong coppery taste for several days.—All kinds of food taste unnatural.—Loss of taste.

Stomach.—Loss of appetite.—Feeling in the fauces as if I would vomit.—[20.] Nausea, lasting but a moment.—Constant nausea, with distress in the stomach.—Nausea and vomiting.—Great faintness at the epigastrium.—Distress in the epigastric and umbilical regions.—Distress in the stomach and umbilicus, with frequent nausea.—Cutting pains in the stomach all night.—Severe sharp cutting pains in the stomach every few minutes, with dull aching distress in the umbilicus, and loud rumbling of the bowels all night.

Abdomen.—Heavy dragging pains in the liver more in the right lobe.—Dull burning distress in the right lobe of the liver and epigastrium, with dull drawing pains in the right lobe of the liver and whole dorsal region.—[**30**.] Dull aching pains in the right lobe of the liver, with dull frontal headache.—Full inspiration produces sharp cutting pains in the right lobe of the liver and whole dorsal region.—Sharp cutting pain near the gall-bladder.—Burning distress in the region of the gall-bladder all the afternoon, with sharp pains in the stomach, and heavy aching distress in the whole liver, especially the right lobe.—Stools preceded by severe pain and distress in the umbilical region, and followed by the same symptoms.—Sharp cutting pains in the umbilical and hypogastric regions before stool.—Sharp cutting pains in the umbilical and hypogastric regions, before stool, and followed by the same symptoms.—Constant rumbling in the abdomen before stool.—Severe dull aching distress just below the stomach, all day, that produces great faintness; it was terrible to endure.—Great distress in the bowels before stool.—[**40**.] Great distress and pain in the bowels after stool.

Stool.—Great disposition to strain after stool.—Twenty grains acted as a cathartic in eight hours.—Forty grains, taken before breakfast, acted as a most violent cathartic in two hours.—Papescent stools, with pain.—Papescent stool, with high fever.—Thin, yellow, papescent stools.—Yellow, papescent stools, mixed with something that looks like oil, in drops the size of a cent down to small drops.—Soft papescent stool, followed by dull, heavy, aching pains in the liver and umbilicus.—Thin, very dark-colored, papescent stools.—[**50**.] Dark, lumpy, dry stools.—Black, lumpy, dry stools, mixed with bile and mucus.—Stools of pure mucus.—Stools of natural consistence, of a dark color, and mixed with bile and mucus.—Stools of bile, mucus, and blood.—Fifty grains produced bloody stools, with high fever.—Stools that run from the bowels a stream of bile, mucus, and black fecal matter, preceded by great burning distress in the epigastrium, right lobe of liver, and umbilicus, and followed by the same symptoms.—Stools of undigested food.

Urinary Organs.—Urine at first diminished, and then slightly increased.—Urine high-colored and scanty.

Pulse and Back.—[**60**.] Pulse 100, soft and full.—Dull heavy pains in the dorsal and lumbar regions.—Severe dull aching pains in the whole dorsal region, that seem to proceed from the liver.—Great weakness of the small of the back.—Severe dull pain in the lumbar region, greatly aggravated by rising up.—Dull aching distress in back and legs.

Upper Extremities.—Great weakness of the arms.—Severe aching distress in the shoulders, elbows, and wrists.

Lower Extremities.—Great weakness of the legs.—Severe aching distress in the hips, knees, and ankles, during the chills and fever.

Generalities.—[**70**.] Great restlessness after midnight.—Very weak and languid.—Great faintness after stool.—Great aching distress in all the joints.

Fever.—Chilliness along the spine, with frequent hot flashes of fever. —Disposition to yawn and stretch when chilly.—Fever all one afternoon and night.—Skin hot and dry, especially the palms of the hands.—Face hot and flushed, with severe frontal headache.—Hands hot and dry. [**80**.] Waking at midnight, two different nights, in a profuse perspiration.

Conditions.—**Aggravation.**—(*Morning*), Agglutination of lids.— (*Night*), Pain in stomach, etc.—(*Midnight*), Perspiration.—(*On full inspiration*), Pains in liver.—(*Motion*), Headache.—(*Rising up*), Pain in lumbar region.—(*Before stool*), Pain in umbilical, etc., regions; rumbling in abdomen; distress in bowels.—(*After stool*), Distress in bowels.

BOLETUS LURIDUS.

B. luridus, Fries.   (B. nigrescens, Pall., etc.)
Nat. order, Fungi.   *Common names*, German, Hexenpilz, Feuerpilz, etc.; French, Fauxceps, or Oignon de loup.   *Preparation*, Triturations.
Authority.   Delle Chiaje, Tossicologia, p. 143 (from Boudier, by Husemann, p. 158), effects of eating the roasted fungi.
Delirium, followed by death (fourth day).—Headache.—Sunken features (second day).—A violet color of the nose and lips (third day).—Intense thirst.—Violent pain in the epigastrium (after two hours).—Meteorismus (third day).—Exceedingly fetid stool (third day).—Pulse small, irregular (second day).—Subsultus tendinum (fourth day).—Urticaria tuberosa (speedily followed by death), (third day).—Cold sweat (second day).

BOLETUS SATANAS.

B. satanas, Lenz.
Nat. order, Fungi.   *Preparation*, Triturations.
Authorities.   1, Lenz, Boudier on Fungi, translated from the French by Husemann, tasted a piece of the fresh fungus, but spit it out soon; 2, Salzmann, ibid., ate some cooked in salt and water, and roasted; 3, six persons poisoned by eating the roasted mushrooms (Wien. Med. Presse), from N. Z. f. H. Kl., 13, 55.

Mind.—Fear and restlessness,[3].—Intellect undisturbed,[3].

Eyes and Ears.—Sparks before the eyes, alternating with obscuration of vision,[3].—Noises in the ears,[3].

Mouth and Throat.—Troublesome dryness in the mouth and throat,[3].—Violent burning and scraping in the throat,[3].

Stomach.—Unquenchable thirst,[3].—Nausea,[3].—Sudden nausea (after two hours),[2].—[10.] Retching and vomiting,[1].—A desire to vomit came very suddenly; between the attacks there was very little nausea, and no pain when vomiting the last time; after about three hours he noticed a slight trace of blood,[1].—He was obliged to vomit (after two hours and three hours, and repeated twenty times within three hours),[1].—Vomiting repeated thirty times within two hours,[2].—He vomited everything that he took,[2].—Salzmann continued to vomit (after the contents of the stomach) a bitter fluid, which was finally mixed with blood; olive oil did not entirely relieve the vomiting, nor when mixed with charcoal,[2].—Epigastric region distended,[3].—Perceptible pulsation in the epigastric region,[3].—Frightful pain in the stomach,[3].

Abdomen.—Abdomen sunken and frightfully painful,[2].—[20.] Obstinate tension of the abdomen,[3].

Stool.—A profuse diarrhœa of blood and of the mucous membranes of the intestines,[2].—Watery evacuations,[3].

Chest and Pulse.—Oppression of the chest,[3].—Pulse scarcely perceptible.[3]

Extremities.—A sudden sensation through all his limbs as though he would be attacked with apoplexy after two hours),[1].—Violent, extremely painful cramps in the muscles of the limbs and of the face,[2].

Generalities.—Loss of all strength,[2].—A great weakness suddenly (after two hours),[1].—So weak that he could scarcely stand or walk (after two to eight hours),[1].—[30.] Excessive weakness, amounting to faintness, whilst the vomiting continued ; repeated ten or twelve times in an hour,[3].—Great discomfort in the whole body,[3].

Fever.—Limbs cold,[2].—Cold sweat over the whole body,[3].

BOMBYX CHRYSORRHŒA.

Lipparis chrysorrhœa. *Class*, Lepidoptera.
Common name, Brown-tailed moth (common on apple and pear trees in Europe). *Preparation*, Tincture of the living caterpillar.
Authority. Calmeil (as in next), effects of handling a cocoon.

In a few hours, painful pricking in the conjunctiva; unendurable heat and burning in the lids, on the neck, and on the sides, especially on the chest. Soon after, redness of these parts, and an eruption of small blisters, with itching and heat.

BOMBYX PROCESSIONEA.

An insect belonging to the class Lepidoptera.
Common name, Procession moth (common in Europe, on oak trees).†
Preparation, Tincture of the live caterpillars.
Authorities. 1, Calmeil, N. Journ. de Med., vol. 9, effects of disturbing a nest; 2, Galignani's Messenger (Pharm. J., 22, 136), a boy shook from a tree an immense number of the caterpillars into his naked breast.

Eyes.—Painful swelling of the lids,[1].—Lachrymation,[1].

Stomach and Extremities.—Nausea,[1].—In the morning, swelling of the hands and finger-joints,[1].

Skin.—Skin covered with large red spots, which were soon followed by a general swelling,[2].—Dr. C. preserved a nest of the caterpillars in a large glass vial, which was not opened for ten years. At length it was opened in the presence of several persons, all of whom caught the eruption,[1].—If a nest of the insects is touched or stirred up, persons within reach of the emanations arising therefrom will be attacked with a papulous eruption, more or less confluent, which will last several days and be attended with violent itching,[1].—The arms are covered with hard, large, uneven, areola-formed tubercles, with a red areola, so thick as to leave hardly any space between,[1].—Eruption of a wonderful number of linear-formed tubercles over the whole arm, and even over the chest and abdomen ; most marked near all the joints,[1].—[10.] Sensation as if a foreign body were under the skin,[1].—Itching of whole body,[1].—A severe itching sensation, so that he was compelled to run home for assistance,[2].—Itching, evenings, not relieved by anything,[1].—Itching of both hands, increasing to a pain,[1].

Sleep and Dreams.—Frequent waking, nights,[1].—Dreams that the arm is being cauterized, and arrows thrust into the muscles,[1].

Fever.—Burning heat ; great desire to scrape the skin,[1].—Violent heat of arms and face,[1].—Fever, somnolency, and delirium, followed by death,[2].

---

† Avenues in the Bois de Boulogne are sometimes closed, to protect the public from the irritation of the skin that the hairs of this caterpillar cause.

BONDONNEAU.

Bondonneau Mineral Water.　(Saintes-Fontaines.)

Chemical Analysis.

In one litre, there was contained

Free Sulphuric Acid, a trace, but it is very perceptible at the spring.
Free Carbonic-Acid, ...　$\frac{2}{3}$ the volume of water.
Bicarbonate of Lime, ... }
　　do.　　Magnesia, ... } 0.390 grammes.
　　do.　　Soda, ...　0.006　"
Potash, salts, ...　a trace.
Sulphates (probably anhydrous) of { Soda, Lime, Magnesia, }　0.043　"
Chloride of Sodium, ...　0 030.
Alkaline, Iodides and Bromides, . . .　0.008.
Arseniates, ...　a trace.
Sesquioxide of Iron with Manganese, . .　0.002.
Silica and Alumina, ...　0.128.
Earthy Phosphates, ...　a trace.
Nitrogenized organic matters, ...　an uncertain amount.

Authority, Dr. Espanet, Journ. de la Soc. Gallicane, 2d Series, vol. 4, p. 65.

Mind.—Gloomy thoughts; painful anxiety.—Irritability, bad humor (from the first).

Head.—Slight vertigo, sometimes followed by obnubilation (during the first days).—Dulness, heaviness and uneasiness in the head, with bad humor.—Compressive headache (continuing after leaving off the water).—The head seems too full, with internal pulsation at the base of the brain, nearly all the time in the evening.—Throbbing in the head, with pricking in the throat.—On moving the head, bruised pain internally, with vertigo (at the beginning).—Feeling of constriction at the forehead, with irascibility.—[10.] Swelling of the temporal veins and of the hands, with throbbing, but without redness (after fifteen days).—Slight lancinating pain, with heat, at the temples.—Drawing and itching in the hairy scalp.

Eyes.—Lancinations in the orbits and in the head, with evening chilliness.—Red, painless swelling of the puncta lachrymalia (in an old man).—A succession of sties for a month after leaving off the water.—The lids feel swollen and tense, especially in the morning.—Drawing in the eyelids from time to time; they are opened with difficulty during the first fortnight.—Itching of the lids and sensitiveness of the eyes to light (after one month).—Yellow tinge of the albuginea, with paleness of the conjunctiva and of the mucous membrane of the palate and lips (after five weeks).—[20.] Redness of the conjunctiva, without pain (after three weeks).—The eyeball feels as if compressed, during the first week.—Sparks before the eyes (during the first fortnight, in a patient laboring under hepatic obstruction).

Ears.—Increased discharge of a clearer mucus (after three weeks).—Dryness with heat in the ears (in the beginning).—Heat and throbbing in the ears (at the beginning).—Sensation of fulness in the ears, with deafness.

Nose.—In the morning, several times, a slight discharge of black blood from the nose (after fifteen days).—Chronic stoppage of the nose, in a gouty subject.—Repeated, short-lasting stoppage of the nose.—[**30**.] Dryness of the nose, with pricking.—Throbbing at the root of the nose, with redness of the nose (after two weeks).

Face.—Paleness and varying color of the face, towards evening.— Chapping of the lips, as from winter weather (just before leaving off the water).

Mouth.—Discolored and denuded teeth, with small ulcers on the gums.—Grinding of the teeth at night (at the close of the season).—Several molar teeth feel too long, and are painful every night.—Tongue pointed, yellow, with bright-red tip.—Tongue coated white, with red papillæ.— Clammy mouth, with sour taste (at the last).—[**40**.] Dry mouth without thirst (unusual).—Sensation of heat and swelling in the mouth (after a repetition of the water).—Abundant saliva (after one month).

Throat.—The bottom of the throat is bright-red.—Dryness of the throat.—Heat with pricking and lancinations in the tonsils (the first days). —Uneasy feeling, as if from congestion of the tonsils (after three weeks).

Stomach.—Great and continual hunger (while taking the waters, and afterwards).—Thirst during the first days; afterwards, entire absence of thirst.—Insipid, mucous eructations, after taking the water.—[**50**.] Epigastric swelling, with habitual heat.—Liquid gurgling in the stomach when lying down in the evening (at the last).—Burning heat, with uneasiness at the stomach after a meal (after two weeks).—Painful heat at the epigastrium, as from flatulence. It shifts about, often becoming seated at the hypochondria, towards the last.—Sensation of fulness, which takes away the appetite (at first).—The epigastrium and hypochondria are sensitive to touch, after the first week.

Abdomen.—Inflation of the abdomen.—Sensation of heaviness in the abdomen.—Tension and heat of the abdomen (towards the last).—Colic, followed by a diarrhœic stool, with tenesmus, after the first days.—[**60**.] Lancinating pains here and there in the abdomen.

Rectum and Anus.—Protrusion of the anus, after every stool, in a child troubled with worms. In a week, this symptom disappeared permanently.—Heat and pricking at the anus (after one month).—Itching at the anus (after fifteen days).—Profuse sweat of the perinæum (after the season).

Stool.—Towards the last, the evacuations become easier and more regular.—Watery and mucous stools (in the beginning).—Stools yellow, afterwards green (in a patient who had had jaundice).—Hard, curled, dark-green evacuations (after one month).—In the beginning, difficult stools at long intervals (in a cachectic patient, previously dyspeptic).

Urinary Organs.—[**70**.] A former discharge from the urethra reappears at the end of the season.—Pricking in the urethra.—Frequent and abundant discharge of urine, which becomes turbid after passing.—The urine is very abundant and clear (in the beginning).—In the beginning, reddish urine, having a strong odor.

Sexual Organs.—Mucous discharge from the prepuce, with itching.—More frequent erections in the morning.—Dry heat of the vagina (in the first fortnight).—Mucous or serous discharge (after three weeks).—The menses appear for the first time (after three weeks).—[**80**.] Regular return of the menses after a five months' suppression.—Menses too early (in a very lymphatic young woman).—The menses, usually regular, are retarded for one week (after fifteen days).

Respiratory Apparatus.—Constant snorting, as if there was a foreign body in the larynx.—In the beginning, irritation and dry cough, with headache.—From time to time, short-lasting hoarseness (towards the end).—Slight dry cough (in a patient with gastritis).—Blood-streaked expectoration (in chronic bronchitis).

Chest.—Paroxysm of spasmodic oppression, with hiccough.—Habitual oppression, with sensation of heat under the sternum, after the first days.— [90.] Sensation of heat, fulness and oppression of the chest (towards the last).—Stitchlike pain in the right lower portion of the chest.

Heart.—Palpitation, the first days.—Tumultuous action of the heart after a meal (after three weeks).—Sense of tension and fulness at the region of the heart (after one month).

Neck and Back.—Drawing and stiffness in the cervical muscles.— Slight pain in the back, shifting about rapidly.—Pains in the kidneys, extending towards the bladder, after every meal.—Slight lancinations, with heat, in the region of the kidneys (after one month).—Compressive pain in the loins (at the last).

Extremities in General.—[100.] The veins on the limbs are more prominent (after the season).—Heaviness of the limbs, with difficulty in moving them (after the season).—Nervous tension and greater agility in the limbs (after one week).

Upper Extremities.—Extreme sensitiveness, with scarcely any swelling, of the axillary glands.—A previous induration of a mammary gland continues.—Constant heat in the palms of the hands.—Stiffness and sensitiveness of the finger-joints.

Lower Extremities.—Dull and deepseated pain in the inside of the thighs (at the last).—Pains, when in bed, in the long bones of the lower extremities.

Generalities.—Increased sensitiveness of the whole cutaneous surface (in the first fortnight).—Cachexiæ, the results of antisyphilitic and febrifuge treatment.—[110.] Convalescences which left the patients in a confirmed cachectic condition.—Various symptoms of former syphilis.

Skin.—Mottled skin, as in cold weather.—Sensitive, colorless pimples, like tubercles, appear in succession, on the scalp, for several days (after six weeks).—Eruption, here and there, of large, red and very sensitive pimples (after the first week).—Small, red, acuminated pimples on the face (after six weeks).—A very itching kind of eruption, like nettle-rash, appears, on the same patient, every time after leaving off the water.—General eruption of furfuraceous blotches (after the fifth day and fifth bath, and lasting until a week after leaving off the water).—A furfuraceous tetter on the nose extends to the external ear, and causes a discharge from the fold of the latter, which disappears with the eruption, in fifteen days, and after taking the water for six weeks.—Eruption of very painful boils, which succeed each other for five weeks.—[120.] Ulcers cease suppurating while taking the waters and for a long while after, with general improvement of the health. —A profusely suppurating fistulous ulcer on the tibia leaves off suppurating.—General itching, especially troublesome over the more muscular portions of the limbs.—Itching of the wings of the nose and of the eyes, followed by redness and very small pimples (after one month).

Sleep and Dreams.—Frequent yawning with shivering (after fifteen days).—Drowsiness in daytime (after four weeks).—Light sleep, frequently interrupted (unusual).—Habitual sleeplessness, with starting when on the point of falling asleep.—Dreams which interrupt sleep (in the beginning).

Fever.—Shivering all over the body (at the beginning).—[130.] Internal heat, with flushes of heat in the chest (after the season).—Sensation of external cold, with transient shivering followed by heat and by pricking on the skin.—Easy sweat (from the beginning).—The least exertion brings on a profuse sweat (at the last).

Conditions.—Aggravation.—(*Morning*), Eyelids feel swollen, etc.; bleeding at the nose; more frequent erections.—(*Towards evening*), Paleness, etc.—(*Evening*), Head feels too full; chilliness; when lying down, gurgling in stomach.—(*Night*), Teeth feel too long, etc.—(*After a meal*), Burning heat at stomach; tumultuous action of heart; pains in kidneys.

ACIDUM BORACICUM.

Boric acid; formula $7(B_2O_3)54(H_2O)$.
Preparation, Solution of the crystals in alcohol.
Authority. A. H. Z. 33, 15, S. J., took repeated doses of the third dil. (from Inaug. Dis. on Borax and the Borates).

Head.—Head unusually confused on waking in the morning.—A gastric headache.

Mouth and Throat.—Much cold saliva in the mouth.—Hawking.

Stomach and Abdomen.—Great nausea and heaviness in the stomach, which disappears after walking in the open air.—Retching and vomiting of tough mucus, with watery fluid which is very strongly alkaline.—Vomiting of tough fluid substances strongly alkaline (after sixteen minutes).—Heaviness and restlessness in the stomach till dinner.—Rumbling in the abdomen in the afternoon, and two scanty pasty stools.

Stool and Urinary Organs.—[10.] A pasty stool.—A moderately transient pain in the region of the ureters.—Frequent and urgent desire to urinate.—Urine nearly double the normal in amount.

Generalities and Skin.—General discomfort, which disappears after a walk of two hours.—Some time after beginning the proving of the alkaline Borates, an eruption was noticed on the right thigh, consisting of vesicles, which continually extended and became covered with crusts; in the middle, a circumscribed spot as large as a ten-cent piece, surrounded by new vesicles, which were very moist when broken (Impetigo figurata, *Willan*).—After two months, this eruption extended to the right lower leg; it then passed over to the left lower leg and disappeared, eight months after first breaking out, and two months from the time of taking any medicine.

Conditions.—Aggravation.—(*Morning*), On waking, head confused. —(*Afternoon*), Rumbling in the abdomen, etc.

Amelioration.—(*After walking in open air*), Nausea, etc., disappears. —(*After a walk*), General discomfort disappears.

BORAX.

Natrum biboracicum $(2BO_2Na.B_2O_3 10H_2O)$. Sodium biborate.
Preparation, Triturations.
Authority. 1, Hahnemann, H. Ch. Kn., 2, 281; 2, Schreter, ibid.; 3, Fischer, Z. f. V. Œst., 1857, p. 217, provings with tinct. of Borax (Borax

5 grs., Alcohol 100 drops), on pellets; 4, Dr. J., Inaug. dis., Berlin, 1845, experiments with powdered Borax.

Mind.—Voluptuous mood (after five weeks),².—Very cheerful, lively, affectionate, with desire and liking for all work, in the forenoon (sixth day),².—The child cries at intervals very violently, ceases after a few minutes, and is again contented and playful,².—Very earnest (after one day),².—Low-spirited and peevish (second day),².—* *Very anxious on riding rapidly down a hill, contrary to his custom; he feels as though it would take away his breath* (first five weeks),².—* *The child becomes anxious when dancing; if one rocks it in the arms* **it has an anxious expression of the face during the downward motion** (the first three weeks),².—Anxiety with rumbling in the bowels (after ten hours),².—* *Great anxiety, with great sleepiness; the anxiety increased until 11 o'clock in the evening*, when the person became dizzy and sleepy, and fell asleep,¹.—**[10.]** Anxiety, with weakness and trembling in the feet, and palpitation (when mesmerizing), (after three days),².—**Fright*; both he and she start up at a distant shock,².—* *Fright; he starts in all his limbs on hearing an anxious cry* (after four weeks),².—* *The baby is frightened at hawking and sneezing,².*—Dread and fear of contagion,¹. —Irritable during important business (after eight days),².—The child is fretful, whines and cries, contrary to its custom (first day),².—Very fretful in the afternoon at 4 o'clock, and peevish, although he was in good humor previously; he rebukes people for trifles, for several days (eighth day),².— * *Before the easy stool in the afternoon, fretful, ill-humored, indolent, and discontented; after it, lively, contented with himself and the world, and looking cheerfully into the future* (after twenty days),².—Violent; he scolds and swears at trifles (first day),².—**[20.]** Violent, fretful, ill-humored (first day),².—He does not become offended, and is indifferent to things which usually vex him very much (curative action), (fifteenth day),².—Pleasure and activity in his business (curative action), (after five weeks),².—At times his thoughts vanish (fourth day),².—* *He idles through the afternoon, does not really get at his work; changes from one business to another, from one room to another; does not keep at one business,².*—Disinclined to work; he does only what he is obliged to as if by force (the first five weeks),².—He is obliged to reflect a long time, until he knows everything that he has done through the day; for a long time he is not certain whether he had been at a place yesterday or to-day (sixth day),².

Head.—On walking, head confused,⁴.—The whole head confused, with stitching in left ear, evening (first day),³.—Vertigo, in the morning in bed (fifth day),².—Vertigo in the evening when walking, as if some one pushed him from the right side towards the left (fifth day),².—**[30.]** Attacks of vertigo, with loss of presence of mind (third day),².—Giddy and full feeling in the forehead in the morning, so that he immediately lost his good humor (fourth day),².—Light, clear head (sixth day),².—Heaviness in the head (first day),².—Headache, with confusion of the whole head, and sticking in the left ear (first day),².—Fulness of the head on ascending a mountain or steps (fifth day),².—Fulness in the head and pressure about the eyes, as if they were held fast, so that he can scarcely move them,².—Fulness in the head and pressure in the small of the back when sitting, together with a sleepy sensation in the eyes (seventeenth day),².—Fulness in the head in the morning, with lack of clear ideas and presence of mind, so that he is unable to perform any mental work, and has no desire for it; after walking in the open air he is better, but still feels great weakness in the feet and joints (second day),².—*Aching in the whole head, with nausea, inclination* to vomit, and trembling in the whole body, in the morning at 10 o'clock (in two female provers at the same time), (second day),[2 3].—**[40.]** Dull pressive headache in the morning, especially in the forehead (first day),[2].—During menstruation, throbbing in the head and roaring in the ears,[2].—Headache in the forehead, with sticking in the left ear, and a hollow lower back tooth on the left side, in the evening (fourteenth day),[2] ([3]).—Drawing pain in the forehead extending towards the eyes (fourth day),[2].—Pressive drawing headache in the forehead above the eyes and towards the root of the nose, at times extending into the nape of the neck; on stooping a severe pressure in the frontal bone; when writing and reading the pain becomes much more violent, with pressure in the region of the spleen (sixth day),[2].—Dull pressure in the forehead (sixth day),[2].—Pressive headache above the eyes; soon disappears when walking in the open air (fourth day),[2].—Sticking headache over the eyes and in the temples, alternating with heat and coldness, so that at one time the hands were very hot, at another quite blue, with sticking in the swollen glands in the neck, which afterwards became softer and smaller (fourteenth day),[2].—Twitching pain in the forehead, with nausea and tearing in both eyeballs, in the afternoon (first day),[2] ([3]).—Throbbing in the forehead,[2].—**[50.]** Sticking from the right temple to the left half of the forehead,[2].—Pressive sticking in the right temple (eleventh day),[2].—Rhythmical pressive dull sticking in the right temple (fortieth day),[2].—Throbbing in both temples (fourth day),[2].—Throbbing headache in both temples, especially in the right (sixteenth day),[2].—Headache in the vertex and forehead, in the evening (second day),[2] ([3]).—Boring in a small spot in the vertex (twentieth day),[2].—Tearing in the vertex in the forenoon, with a great roaring in the ears (eighth day),[2].—Stitches, transient, in the left side of the head in the vertex, afterwards transient stitches in the genitals, and in the following night lascivious disgusting dreams, in a married woman (first day),[2].—Stitches deep in the right side of the head, with discharge of pus from the right ear; stitches so violent that he involuntarily drew back his head, together with tickling in the left ear, such as precedes a discharge, followed by very acute hearing (thirty-second day),[2].—**[60.]** Tearing in the left half of the head, starting in a hollow tooth (fourth day),[2].—Throbbing headache in the occiput, as if it would suppurate there, with shivering over the whole body, lasting the whole night and following day (second day),[2] ([3]).—Pulsating rush of blood into the occiput (sixteenth day),[2].—Sensitiveness of the external head to cold and change of weather,[1]. —*As in Plica Polonica, the child's hairs become entangled at the tips and stick together, so that they cannot be separated; if these bunches are cut off they form again* (for ten weeks),[2].

Eyes.—The infant becomes very red around the eyes when crying (fourth day),[2].—Sensation in eyes as if something had fallen into them, which disappears on rubbing, first in the right eye, then in the left, four times during half the day, and returning next day at noon (seventh day),[2 3]. —Burning in the eyes and momentary contraction of them as soon as he removes the glasses (after six days),[2].—Pressive burning in the right eye, in the afternoon (third day),[2].—Pressure above the eyes from time to time (tenth day),[2].—**[70.]** Pressure in the right eye very painful, as if it would be pressed into the orbit, in the morning (after five weeks),[2].—Sensation in the right eyelid, while sitting, as if something pressed out from within, from between the skin coming from the temples; immediately followed by pressure around the eyes (fourth day),[2].—Cutting in the left eye lengthwi coming and going suddenly (thirty-seventh day),[2].—In the left eye, t' stitches in succession, evening (third day),[2] ([3]).—Itching in the eyes, with a sensation at times as if sand were in them (fourth day),[2].—*The lashes turn inward toward the eye and inflame it, especially in the outer canthus, where the margins of the lid are very sore* (sixth week),[2].—Inflammation of the margins of the lid in an infant; he rubs the eyes and at night they are agglutinated (first day),[2].—*Inflammation of the left eye in the inner canthus, with nightly agglutinations* (first days),[2].—*Inflammation of the right eye in the external canthus, with irregularity of the lashes; agglutination of the eye at night* (thirty-fifth day),[2].—At night the eyes are agglutinated with hard, dry mucus, which irritates the eyes like sand (fifth week),[2].—[80.] In the morning the eyes are agglutinated and lachrymate (fifth day),[2].—In the evening it is difficult to close the lids, and in the morning difficult to open them (fifth week),[2].—Pressive pain in the upper lid on opening the eye,[2].—Soreness in the external canthi (after five weeks),[2].—Lachrymation of the eyes (eighth day),[2].—Itching in the internal canthus, so that she must frequently rub it (first days),[2].—Tearing in both eyeballs, with a twitching in the forehead, and nausea in the afternoon,[2] ([3]).—Stitches in the eyeball, with contraction in the right upper lid (eighth day),[2].—Obscuration of the left eye in the evening; she was obliged to make great exertion, but still saw nothing (ninth day),[2] ([3]).—Sensitiveness of the eyes to the candlelight in the evening (third day),[2].—[90.] *Flickering before the eyes in the morning when writing, so that he does not see distinctly; there seem to be bright moving waves, now from the right to the left side, now from above downward, several mornings in succession* (after twenty-four days),[2].

Ears.—Inflamed hot swelling of both ears, with a discharge of pus from them (twenty-seventh day),[2].—Purulent discharge from both ears preceded by itching in the occiput (nineteenth day),[2].—A purulent discharge from the ears, with sticking headache (after thirty-two days),[2].—A previous discharge from the ears ceases (curative action),[2].—Suddenly a sensation as if the ear were enveloped or stopped,[1].—Pain in the ear; a sensitive pressure behind the right ear (after six days),[2].—Stitches in the ears (after six weeks),[2].—Stitches in the ears in the morning when washing in cold water (after three days),[2].—Stitches in the left ear, on waking unusually early (fourth day),[2] ([3]).—[100.] Stitches in the left ear, in two provers (after fourteen days),[2].—Stitching in left ear (in a man), (fourteenth day),[3].—Stitching in left ear, with headache in the forehead, and stitching in left, lower, hollow, molar tooth (in a female), evening (fourteenth day),[3].—Sore pain in the ear on boring in with the finger (thirty-second day),[2].—Itching in the left ear, and sore pain after removing the ear-wax, in the evening, when walking; at the same time a kind of sticking in the left side of the neck (nineteenth day),[2].—Difficult hearing in the left ear, in a child five years old (ninth day),[2].—Crackling in the left ear, as if thick wax were in it which stopped the ear, which then opened again, in the evening (tenth day),[2] ([3]).—Dull drumming in the left ear, as if over a subterranean vault (fourteenth day),[2] ([3]).—Ringing and piping in the right ear, which afterwards changed to a roaring (twentieth day),[2].—Roaring and ringing in right ear (eighth day),[2] ([3]).—[110.] Roaring in the ears, and much difficult hearing (eighteenth and nineteenth days),[2].—Rushing in the left ear as from a storm (third and fourth days),[2].

Nose.—The infant rubs his nose vigorously with the hands, and then the eyes (fifteenth day),[2].—(*Red and shining swelling of the nose, with throbbing and tensive sensation*),[1].—*In the upper and forepart of the left nostril, towards the tip of the nose, a small boil, with sore pain and swelling of* *the tip of the nose* (tenth day),[3].—* *Ulceration in the left nostril, in the forepart, in the tip, with sore pain and swelling of the tip of the nose* (tenth day),[2].— * *Many dry crusts in the nose, which constantly form again after being removed* (after sixteen days),[2].—Sneezing, with great painfulness; he tries to stop it, since it causes severe sticking in the right side of the chest; for three weeks (after six days),[2].—Sneezing and fluent coryza (first days),[2].—Fluent coryza with much crawling in the nose (after sixteen days),[1].—[120.] Discharge of much greenish thick mucus from the nose,[2].—Bleeding from the nose (after twenty-five days),[2].—Bleeding of the nose in the morning, and in the evening pulsating headache (after six days),[2].—Some blood is usually discharged on blowing the nose, preceded by itching in the nose (eighteenth day),[2].—Itching and crawling in the nose; he is obliged to put his finger into it (after twelve days),[2].

Face.—* *Erysipelas in the face* (after thirty-four days),[2].—* *The face of the infant looks pale, suffering, earthy* (first day),[2].—Swelling of the face with pimply eruptions on the nose and lips (first days),[2].—Swelling, heat and redness of the face, with tearing pain in the malar bone, and severe pain in the swelling when laughing (thirty-first and thirty-second days),[2].— A feeling in the right side of the face, by the mouth, as if cobwebs had formed there,[2].—[130.] Dull tearing in the left cheek, starting from a hollow tooth, with pressure in the forehead and in both eyeballs (after four days),[2].—Red inflamed swelling as large as a pea on the lower lip, with burning soreness when touched (forty-first day),[2].—Twitching of the muscles near the right corner of the mouth several times,[2].—Burning in the upper lip below the left nostril, in the morning in bed (seventh day),[2] ([3]).—Burning pain in the lower lip, soon passing away, in the evening (third day),[2] ([3]).— 4 A.M., sensation in the lower lip like the crawling of insects (fourth day),[3]. —Crawling on the lips as from beetles (second day),[2].

Mouth.—Teeth and Gums. A piece broke out of a hollow tooth of itself (after six days),[2].—The teeth seem too long (first day),[2].—Toothache in an upper hollow tooth, with burning of the cheek, which pains as if tense when touched (after seven days),[2].—[140.] Constrictive griping in a hollow tooth (after four days),[2].—*Toothache in a hollow tooth, dull griping, in wet rainy weather,* in five provers,[2].—Aching in the hollow teeth in bad weather (after forty days),[1].—Dull, pressive boring in the hollow teeth in the evening, in cool air (first day),[2].—Pressive-digging toothache, after every supper and breakfast; is relieved by tobacco smoking; for several days (after forty days),[2].—Drawing pain in the teeth,[1].—Fine intermitting stickings in all the teeth, mostly in a hollow back tooth in the left lower jaw (second day),[2][3].—Sticking toothache in a left lower hollow back tooth, with sticking in the left ear and headache in the forehead, in the evening (after fourteen days),[2][3].—Tearing from the hollow teeth into half of the head, if they are touched with the tongue, or if cold water is taken into the mouth,[2].—Tearing and griping in an upper hollow tooth, which seems to be larger than natural, so that she cannot bite or clench the teeth; with inflammation and swelling of the gum as if a gum-boil would form; in the evening the pain extends into the lower teeth, and then disappears on going to sleep (fourth day),[2].—[150.] Crawling and tickling in the lower incisors, followed by accumulations of saliva in the mouth (after seven days),[2].— Swelling of the gum for three days, with pressure in the hollow teeth in bad weather (after forty days),[2].—* *Inflamed large swelling on the outer side of t'.e gum, which pains severely (gum-boil), with dull pain in a hollow tooth; swelling of the cheek and whole left side of the face, as far as below the eye,* *where there is an elevated œdematous swelling* (smelling of Chamomilla relieves the pain), (after thirty-six days),[2].—The gums of the upper teeth bleed without pain (after six days),[2].—**Tongue.** *An aphtha on the tongue* (after thirty-three days),[2].—*Red blisters on the tongue, as if the skin were eroded; they pain on every motion of the tongue, or if anything salt or sour touches them* (after five weeks),[2].—Dryness of the tongue in the afternoon (third day),[2].—Falling asleep of the tongue, so that respiration is impeded,[3]. —Cramp in the tongue, as if stiff and gone to sleep, so that breathing is impeded thereby,[2] ([3]).—**Mouth.** *Aphthæ in the mouth* (after four weeks),[2].—[160.] *An aphtha in the inner side of the cheek, which bleeds when eating* (after thirty days),[2].—*The infant's palate was wrinkled* **and it cried frequently when nursing** (after four weeks),[2].—*The mucous membrane of the forepart of the palate is shrivelled as if burnt, and pains, especially when chewing,* for several days (after six days),[2].—Slimy mouth (first day),[2].—*The mouth of the infant was very hot,*[2].—Pain in the corners of the mouth, as if they would ulcerate (after twenty days),[2].— Copious cold saliva,[4].—**Taste.** *The taste is flat and insipid* (after five days),[2].—*She had no tast when she ate anything, for several weeks* (after eight days),[2].—The soup has no taste at dinner; it causes sweat (eighth day),[2].—[170.]* *Bitter taste; if she eats anything or swallows saliva everything tastes bitter* (second day),[2] ([3]).

Throat.—Much mucus accumulates in the throat, which he must expectorate,[2].—Tough mucus in the throat, which is difficult to loosen (after eighteen days),[2].—Much tough mucus in the throat, which he must hawk up with much exertion, so that he vomits (after six days),[2].- *Tough whitish mucus in the fauces, which is loosened only after great exertion* (for several days), (after five days),[2].—A piece of mucus streaked with blood is hawked up (after nine days),[2].—Hawking of mucus in the morning; the mucus is easily raised in lumps,[2].—Green loose mucus is hawked from the throat (after twelve days),[2].—Dryness in the throat (after five days),[2].— Roughness in the throat, as if a grater were in it,[2].—[180.] Throat rough in the morning,[1].—Burning in the throat; this causes him to swallow saliva, which is painful (ninth day),[2].—Rawness in the pit of the throat, with drawing stitches in it when coughing and sneezing, and with relief after hawking up mucus (eleventh day),[2].—Scraping in the throat, causing a dry cough (after first day),[2].—Tickling in the throat, provoking a dry cough (after four weeks),[2].

Stomach.—Appetite. Great appetite in the evening,[1].—Increased appetite for breakfast (fourth day),[2].—Appetite much less than usual (after five days),[2].—Less hunger and appetite than usual (first five weeks),[2].— Diminished hunger and appetite, frequently however hunger without real appetite (after five days),[2].—[190.] He eats very little,[2].—He has less appetite, especially for supper (after eight days),[2].—She has very little appetite in the evening for several weeks (after eight days),[2].—Loss of appetite, nausea, drawings in the head from the vertex to the temples, and drawings from the abdomen toward the groin, every evening for several days (fifth week),[2].—No appetite for dinner (after twelve days),[2].—No more desire for tobacco (second day),[2].—Thirst in the morning; he must drink a great deal (fourteenth day),[2].—Longing for sour drinks (fourteenth and fifteenth days),[2].—**Hiccough and Nausea.** The infant hiccoughs very often,[2].—Severe hiccough, which makes the throat raw,[1].—[200.] Hiccough after eating (eighth day),[2].—Nausea,[4].—Nausea during eating (after nineteen days),[2].—Nausea with periodic inclination to vomit (fifth day),[2].—Nausea in the morning, with inclination to vomit; disappears after dinner (sixth day),[2].—Nausea immediately after waking, with great inclination to vomit, which however does not follow until he drinks water, when he vomits a large quantity of mucus and some bitter substance with great exertion (seventeenth day),[2].—Nausea followed by vomiting of mucus, with heat and rapid feverish pulse (after twenty-three days),[2].—Nausea even to vomiting when riding (first day),[2].—Nausea and little appetite (fourth day),[2].—Nausea in the stomach, with pain in the sternum, from 3 o'clock in the afternoon till evening, several days in succession (after five days),[2] ([3]).—[210.] Nausea and sick feeling even to fainting, in the morning (sixth day),[2].—Frequent nausea and faintness in the afternoon (after twelve days),[2].—Nausea at the thought of eating, at noon, with coldness, drawing headache and pain in the abdomen, followed by three attacks of diarrhœa (after twenty days),[2].—*Vomiting.* Vomiting tough fluid substance,[4].—Vomiting of sour mucus, after breakfast (of cocoa), (second day),[2]. —Heaviness in stomach, diminished by walking in open air,[4].—*Epigastrium.* Pain in the stomach, as from bad digestion, on external pressure on the pit of the stomach (second day),[2].—*Pain in the region of the stomach after lifting something heavy; the pain goes into the small of the back, where it becomes sticking, so that she cannot turn without pain the whole night; in the morning better* (two days before the menses),(thirteenth day),[2]([3]). —*After eating, which he relishes, great distension, discomfort, sick feeling and ill humor;* in the evening, on going into the open air, somewhat relieved (after forty-one days),[2].—After eating apples, with mutton, fulness in the stomach, with peevishness and ill-humor; fulness in the head, as if the blood forcibly pressed into it (nineteenth day),[2].—[220.] Constrictive pain in the region of the stomach (after six days),[2].—Constrictive pain in the region of the stomach every day from four in the morning till twelve at noon, a kind of winding-up sensation, which extends to the spine, where it causes a sticking, for several days in succession,[2] ([3]).—Pressure in the stomach (first day),[3]. —Pressure in the stomach after every meal (first days),[2].—After eating pears, especially in the morning or forenoon, pressure in the pit of the stomach, with discomfort,[2].—Pressure in the pit of the stomach, which disappears on walking,[2].—Pressive-sticking in the stomach, with oppression of the chest, which compels him to take a deep breath, which, however, he cannot do on account of sharp pinching pain in the right side of the chest,[2].

Abdomen.—Hypochondria. A sensitive pressure in the region of the spleen (first day),[2].—In the left hypochondrium, a feeling as of violent pressure, as with the hands, when riding in a carriage without springs,[2]. —Pressure, and sometimes a burning, with a sensation in the left hypochondrium on deep breathing, as if something rose up into the chest from the region of the spleen, which sank down again on expiration (after six days),[2].—[230.] A pressure in the left hypochondrium, from the lowest ribs to the hip-bone, which is increased by external pressure, after a midday sleep till evening (second day),[2].—Pressive pain in the left hypochondrium, as if a stone lay there, when dancing; on continuing to dance it disappears (after fifteen days),[2].—On the second day after menstruation pressure, as from a stone in the right hypochondriac region, extending to the shoulder-blade, from which place the pain extends spasmodically into the stomach and small of the back, followed by vomiting,[2] ([3]).—Cutting in the right hypochondrium soon after breakfast, extending downward across through the bowels, followed by diarrhœa; evacuation sudden (third day),[2].—Cutting in the left hypochondrium on walking rapidly, as if a hard, sharp, movable piece were there, with a sensation in the abdomen as if only hard pieces were in it much mixed up (after six days),[2].—The drawing-sticking pain in the right side of the chest extends down into the right flank, where it becomes exceedingly painful on hiccoughing, sneezing, coughing, and yawning (three weeks),[2].—*Abdomen.* Rumbling in abdomen,[4].—Much rumbling in the abdomen at night, relieved by passing flatus upward and downward,[2].—After dinner, rumbling in the abdomen and diarrhœa (third day),[2].—Much flatulence,[2].—[240.] Much discharge of flatus,[3].—Formation of flatulence and frequent passage of it,[2].—Abdomen distended after supper (fifth day),[2].—*Flatulent distension after every meal* (after five days),[2].—Weakness in the abdomen (fourth day),[2].—*Pain in the abdomen several times through the day, as if diarrhœa would result,*[2].—Immediately after eating, pain in the abdomen, as if diarrhœa would come on ; disappears after a midday nap (second day),[2].—*Pinching in the abdomen,* at different times,[2].—*Pinching in the abdomen, with diarrhœa* (after twenty days),[2].—Pinching constrictive pain in the abdomen above the navel, so that she is obliged to bend double, then it ceases ; daily in the morning for five minutes (after eight days),[2].—[250.] Griping pains in the abdomen, with shivering and gooseflesh (after six days),[2].—During menstruation, spasmodic dragging and shooting pain in the groin,[1].—Stitching in the abdomen, in the region of the uterus, in the evening, in bed (second day),[3].—*At the time of the menses, pain in the groin like stitching and pressing;* at the next period they were absent, on account of which she received, six weeks afterwards, two pellets of *Borax* 1st, whereupon the menses appeared on the following day, with griping in the abdomen,[3].

Rectum and Anus.—Contraction in the rectum, with itching (after forty days),[2].—Stitches in the rectum in the evening (after two days),[2] ([3]). —A swollen vein in the anus as large as a pencil, and painless (second and third days),[2].—Brown mucus in the anus after the stool (after nine days),[2]. —Boring-sticking pain in the anus and small of the back (after fifteen days),[2].—Itching in the anus in the evening (seventh day),[2] ([3]).—[260.] Itching in the anus, as from hæmorrhoidal mucus (sixteenth day),[2].

Stool.—After smoking, a feeling as though diarrhœa would come on (sixth day),[2].—Frequent desire for stool, with rumbling in the abdomen and diarrhœa-like discharges (first days),[2].—Frequent desire for stool, with pinching in the bowels, and easy, pasty evacuations,[2].—Desire for stool in the morning ; at first hard, then diarrhœa-like discharge, with burning in the anus (first day),[2] ([3]).—Very soft stool in the morning ; in the evening the usual evacuation (after seven days),[2].—*Frequent very easy stool every day* (first days),[2].—Two scanty, pasty stools,[4].—Diarrhœa-like stool in the afternoon, with much wind, following a hard stool in the morning (fifth day),[2]. —Diarrhœa, two or three times, without pain (after one hour),[2] ([3]).—[270.] The child has three stools a day, the last like yellow water,[2].—Stool every hour, soft, slimy, without other symptoms (third day),[2].—Diarrhœa during the first three days (in a subject constantly troubled with constipation),[3].— Diarrhœa after breakfast, four times in succession (fourth day),[2].—*Diarrhœa six times, from the morning till 2 P.M., without pain* (fifth day),[2] ([3]).— Diarrhœa, with rumbling in the abdomen (first days),[2].—Diarrhœa sudden toward noon, with rumbling and grumbling in the abdomen (fourth day),[2]. —Diarrhœa, without pain, twice a day, followed by discharge of mucus and blood (sixteenth day),[2].—Diarrhœa immediately after eating, with weakness in the joints and legs, which is relieved after walking (first day),[2]. —The primary action of Borax is diarrhœa, followed by no stool for several days, afterwards a hard stool daily,[2].—[280.] Soft stool (first three days),[2].—Hard stool, with straining (sixteenth day),[2].—Pale mucus passes four times, with the stool once involuntarily (fourteenth day),[2].—*Soft, light-yellow, mucous stool, three times a day, with weakness and exhaustion (first days),[2].—* Green stool in the infant preceded by crying (sixth day),[2].—Tenacious, glutinous, yellowish mucus with the stool (eighteenth and nineteenth days),[2].—Reddish liquid mucus with the stool, as if it was colored with blood (twenty-first day),[2].—Passage of blood and mucus from the anus (ninth day),[2].—Passage of round worms,[1].—[290.] Constipation, with fæces like sheep-dung for ten days (after several days),[2][3].

Urinary Organs.—Pressure and sticking in the region of the kidneys, increased on turning (after three days),[2].—Dark-blue spots at the orifice of the urethra, as if the skin was off, with biting pain on urinating (after twenty-four days),[2].—The orifice of the urethra seems agglutinated with gum,[2].—Burning tension in the urethra after urinating,[2].—Smarting pain along the urethra, especially when touched (after twenty-six days),[2].—*Smarting in the urethra after urinating (fifteenth, twentieth, and thirtieth days),[2].—*The orifice of the urethra pains as if sore after urinating,[2].—During involuntary emission, cutting pain in the urethra; the semen was so thin that he thought he urinated,[2].—*Severe urgent desire to urinate, so that he can scarcely hold the urine (first days),[2].—[300.] Severe urging to urinate at night, several times (twenty-fifth day),[2].—*At night he must rise several times to urinate (after thirty-four days),[2].—After an emission, urging to urinate, and on urinating cutting in the urethra,[2].—*Desire to urinate, without being able to pass a drop, with cutting in the genitals and distension in both hips, for two hours (first day),[2] ([3]).—Frequent urinating (first days),[2].—*The infant urinates nearly every ten or twelve minutes, and **frequently cries and screams before the urine passes,** for a long time (after six days),[2].—**Hot urine in the infant** (after four days),[2].—*Pungent smell of the urine (first days),[2].—Pungent peculiar smell of the urine (first two weeks),[2].

Sexual Organs.—Male. Tensive erection in the morning on waking (fourth day),[2].—[310.] Frequent excitement of the genitals without desire for coition (first day),[1].—Stitches in the genitals, soon disappearing (first day),[3].—Sticking sore pain, especially when touched on the penis at the margin of the place where a chancre formerly existed (after twenty-four days),[2].—While resting his hands in a kind way upon a sick female he had sensual sensations without desire for coition (third day),[2].—Indifference to coition (first five weeks),[2].—He is obliged to wait a long time during coition for the discharge of semen (after five weeks),[1].—Emission with dream of coition, whereby the semen came very rapidly, which woke him,[2].—On coition, the semen passes very soon, and there is a continual irritation in the genitals (after five weeks),[1].—*Female.* Easy conception during the use of Borax observed in five women,[2].—A woman who had been sterile fourteen years on account of a chronic acrid leucorrhœa, in addition to other remedies at last took Borax; she became pregnant and the leucorrhœa improved,[3][2].—[320.] Sticking in the region of the uterus (second day),[2].—Sensation of distension and sticking in the clitoris at night (sixth day),[2].—Leucorrhœa white, like mucus, without other symptoms, fourteen days after menstruation (after fifteen weeks),[2].—*Leucorrhœa thick as paste and white, for five days (after four days),[2].—**Leucorrhœa like the white of an egg, with sensation as if warm water were flowing down,** several days (after twelve days),[2].—Menstruation appeared one day too soon, without any trouble (after four days),[2].—Menses three days too soon, without any pain (after seven weeks),[2].—Menstruation four days too early, without any trouble; only the evening and the morning preceding its appearance heaviness on the chest, with difficult breathing and much roaring in the ears (after twenty-six days),². —*Menses four days too soon and very profuse, with gripings in the abdomen, nausea and pain in the stomach, extending into the small of the back, which lasted till midnight, when a profuse sweat broke out and she fell asleep (eighth day),². —The menses omitted the second month after taking the drug, but after she had taken a dose of Borax in the sixth week appeared the next day, with pinchings in the abdomen,². — [330.] The menses, which had omitted six weeks, appeared immediately after taking Borax, lasted one day and again disappeared; it was so copious, however, that it seemed more like a hemorrhage,². —Suppression of the menses for fifty-four days, without any trouble, then they appear, without pains at first, somewhat pale; in the afternoon, however, redder and more profuse; they cease on the third day in the night and return again on the fourth (they should have appeared three weeks after taking the drug),². — Menses two days very scanty, the third day very profuse, with pale-red blood, until the sixth day, with weakness, so that she could scarcely stand,².

Respiratory Apparatus.—Tearing in the larynx, in the evening (third day),². —Dry hacking in the child,². —*Hacking and violent cough, with slight expectoration, **of a mouldy taste and of the same smell**, from the chest, with every paroxysm of cough; in the evening (third day),². —Night cough,¹. —Cough, with scraping in the throat and pressure in the chest (first day),². —*Dry cachectic cough, as in old people, especially in the morning on rising and in the evening when lying down, with sticking in the right side of the chest and right flank; washing the chest with cold water afforded the most relief, but after drinking wine the pains were aggravated; for twelve days (after three weeks),². —Cough, with expectoration of mucus, mostly in the morning, with pain in the region of the liver, which still continues until noon (fourth day),². —[340.] Streaks of blood in the mucus, when coughing up a white mucus which is difficult to loosen (eighteenth day),². —Respiration difficult (after eighteen days),². —Respiration difficult; he is obliged to breathe deeply, which he cannot do on account of stitches in the chest (the first days),². —*Every three or five minutes he is obliged to take a quick, deep breath, which is every time followed by a stitch in the right side of the chest, with a subdued painful sigh and slow expiration (after seven days),². — *Arrest of the breath when lying in bed; he is obliged to jump up and catch for breath every time he has a stitch in the right side of the chest (after seven days),². —Shortness of breath after ascending steps, so that he cannot speak a word, and when he speaks he has every time **a stitch in the right side of the chest**; so also in running or on any exertion of the body which heats him (after eight days),².

Chest and Heart.—The milk is increased (fourth day),². —Much milk flows from the breast, so that the bed becomes wet (after thirty-two days),¹. —The milk which flows from the breast becomes cheesy and curdled (the first days),². —Anxiety in the chest in the evening, in bed (first day),³. — [350] Oppression of the chest in the evening, in bed (first day),². —Heaviness on the chest, so that for a time she cannot breathe (after six weeks),². —Weakness in the chest, with dryness in the throat (ninth day),². —At every attempt to breathe the chest becomes contracted (fourteenth, fifteenth, and seventeenth days),². —Tightness of the chest, with constrictive oppression of the breath on ascending steps; he is then obliged to take a deep breath, which is accompanied every time by a sensitive drawing stitch in the right side of the chest (sixth day),². —Pressive tightness, extending from the pit of the stomach into the chest when sitting stooped; it impedes respiration and causes a sticking in the lung (seventh day),[2].—Drawing pain in a small spot in the intercostal muscles, which changes on bending toward the left side into a pain as from a severe blow,[2].—Pressure in the chest,[2] ([3]).—During a deep inspiration a sensation as if something with a burning pressure arose from the left hypochondrium into the chest and sank down again on expiration,[2].—Pressing on the chest, with scraping in the throat and cough (first day),[3].—[360.] Pain in the pectoralis major muscle, as from a hard bed, with soreness on touch, at night (third day),[2] ([3]).—Tearing from the larynx into the chest, provoking cough (after five weeks),[2].—*With every cough and deep inspiration sticking in the chest (after seven days),[2].—Stitches in the chest as from incarcerated flatus (first days),[2].—Stitches, as with fine needles, from the back of the chest, in the evening (after eight days),[2].—*Stitches in the chest when yawning, coughing, and breathing deeply (seventh day),[2].—When lying quietly stretched out upon the back the chest feels somewhat better,[2].—Pains in the chest are mostly relieved by walking slowly about the room; he then feels most comfortable,[2].—*Contractive pains in the left breast when the child nurses the right (first days),[2].—*Gripings and sometimes stitches in the left mamma, and when the child has nursed she is obliged to compress the breast with her hand, because it aches on account of being empty,[2].—[370.] Drawing pain in the right intercostal muscles if he bend forward and to the right (after six days),[2].—*With every paroxysm of cough sticking in the right side of the chest in the region of the nipple; in the evening (third day),[2] ([3]).—Stitches immediately in the right side of the chest if he raises the arm (seventh day),[2].—Stitches in the left ribs, with soreness internally in the chest,[2].—With every inspiration stitching in the left side of the chest as with a knife (second day),[2].—*Stitches between the ribs of the right side, so that he cannot lie upon that side on account of the pain, with sensitive drawing and obstruction of breathing, so that he has to catch for breath; if he lies upon the painful side the pains immediately awaken him from sleep (first four weeks),[2].—Stitching in the region of the left ribs, with aching in the chest; cough with expectoration of mucus several times during the day, especially in the morning; with a pain in the region of the liver, which also continues without the cough till noon (fourth day),[3].—If he holds the painful side with the hand, on account of the pain in the chest, it is somewhat relieved,[2].—*When coughing he is obliged to press the right side of the chest and flank with the hand, whereby the pains are tolerable (the first three weeks),[2].—Sticking pressure on the sternum after dinner, increased by deep inspiration (fortieth day),[4].—[380.] A feeling as if the heart were on the right side and were being squeezed (seventh day),[2].

Neck and Back.—Rheumatic drawing pain in the neck, which extends to the left shoulder and then into the shoulder-blade, in the evening when walking in the open air (forty-first day),[2].—Pain in the back, when sitting and stooping, as from pressure (third day),[2].—Pain in the back when walking (first day),[2].—Pain in the back, with much mucous discharge with the stool (nineteenth day),[2].—Burning in the back while sitting (fifth day),[2].—Dull backache when stooping (sixth day),[2].—Dull pressure in the back (seventh day),[2].—Pressive pain in the back on both shoulders,[2].—Stitches in the right lumbar region, increased by stooping, in the morning, while walking, relieved when sitting (first day),[2].

Upper Extremities.—[390.] Drawing and tearing pain in the shoulder and between the shoulders, so that he cannot stoop, for eight days (after five weeks),[2].—Momentary stitches as with needles in the right shoulder,[2].—Pressure on both shoulders,[3].—Burning pain in the upper arm a hand's breadth around the whole arm (second day),[2].—Sticking in the palm, with a feeling in the whole hand, extending above the wrist, as if the arm had gone to sleep, in the evening (second day),[2] ([3]).—Tearing and breaking sensation in the forepart of the right hand, as if rheumatic (after fifteen days),[2].—Burning heat and redness of the fingers, even from slight cold, as if they had been frozen (after twenty-four days),[2].—Throbbing pain in the tip of the thumb day and night, frequently waking him from sleep at night (second and third days),[2].

Lower Extremities.—Burning pain on the left thigh a hand's breadth around the whole limb (eighth day),[2].—A burning in the right thigh near the pudenda, which is increased by cough or laying the hand upon it (third day),[2].—[400.] Transient tearing in the bone of the right thigh, extending from the middle downward and up again, from morning till noon, and again in the evening (seventh day),[2] ([3]).—Erysipelatous inflammation and swelling of the left leg and foot after violent dancing, with tearing tension and burning in it, and increased burning pain when touched; on pressure with the finger the redness disappears for a moment (seventeenth day),[2].—Numb sensation with heat in the left lower leg,[1].—In the foot where the erysipelas was a tension on the back, so that standing became difficult; she was not prevented from walking (twenty-second day),[2]. —A feeling of heaviness in the feet on ascending steps, in the evening (first day),[2] ([3]).—Formication and trembling of the feet, with nausea and tendency to faintness; disappears when walking in the open air (fourteenth day),[2].—Pain in the heel, as if sore from walking,[2].—*Stitching in the sole of the foot* (in two persons at the same time), (second day),[2] ([3]).—Inflammation and itching on the balls of the little toes as from freezing (fifteenth day),[2].—Sensitive burning pain in the great toes, especially in the balls, particularly when walking (after forty-one days),[2].—[410.] Pain in the joints of the toes of the left foot on stepping, as if something pressed them (twentieth day),[2].—Frequent stitches in the corns, particularly in rainy weather (first days),[2].—Boring stitches in the corns, relieved by pressing upon them (first five weeks),[2].

Generalities.—*The infant becomes pale, nearly earthy-colored; the previously firm flesh becomes soft and flabby; he cries a great deal, refuses the breast, and frequently screams out anxiously in his sleep (first three weeks),[2].—While meditating at his work, trembling in the whole body especially in the hands, with nausea and weakness of the knees (eighth day),[2].—Restlessness in the body, which does not permit him to sit or lie long in one place (first day),[2].—After an animated conversation restlessness in the body, nausea and stupefaction and vertigo (third day),[2].—During a meal restlessness in the whole body, with nausea, so that he could only eat with effort; stretching backward afforded relief (after twenty days),[2].— She feels very weak and powerless (after five weeks),[1].—Weakness, especially in the abdomen and limbs (fourth day),[2].—[420.] Loss of power in the joints (fifth day),[2].—Prostrated, weak and tired, with heaviness in the feet (first days),[2].—Weak, indolent, fretful, thirsty after the midday sleep, with heat when walking in the open air, and worse on the head and face, with confusion of the head, pressure in the forehead and eyes, which pain on touch as if sore; together with inclination to breathe deeply, and when doing so, sticking in the intercostal muscles, with hard, quick pulse,[2].

Skin.—* *Unhealthiness of the skin;* slight injuries suppurate and ulcerate,[2].—Two hard wartlike indurations on the inner surface of the hand, after it had been beaten somewhat strongly with a stick (after thirty days),[2].

—Whitish pimples, as large as flaxseed, with red areola, on the chest and throat, as far as the nape of the neck (sixth week),[2].—Inflamed pimples on the back of the little toe, which pain like corns (fifteenth day),[2].—Papulous eruption in the face (after four days),[2].—Red papulous eruption on the cheeks and around the chin, in the infant (after five weeks),[2].—A corroding blister forms upon the nates (fifteenth day),[2].—[430.] Large herpetic spots upon the mouth, and the upper lip very scurfy, follow burning heat,[1].—Herpetic eruption on the nates of the child (after four weeks),[2].—Pustule with red areola on the middle finger of the right hand, with swelling and stiffness of the finger, which continues to suppurate and pain after the opening of the pustule (after thirty days),[2].—Old wounds and ulcers are inclined to suppurate,[2].—Long-continued suppuration of a place under the thumb nail, where she had stuck a needle, with painfulness to touch,[2].—A suppurating spot in the heel, which had been rubbed by the shoe,[2].—An ulcer in the left axilla,[1].—Violent itching and crawling on the os coccygis, so that he cannot help scratching, followed by a discharge of mucus from the anus (after thirty-two days),[2].—A feeling as if a cobweb were lying upon the skin of the hands,[2].—Itching here and there on the backs of the hands, with irritation to scratch, as if bitten by fleas,[2].—[440.] *Severe itching on the backs of the finger joints, so that he is obliged to scratch them violently,[2].—Itching on the malleoli (second, ninth, and tenth days),[2].

Sleep and Dreams.—Very sleepy and tired in the evening.[1].—Sleepiness at midday, and deep sleep for two hours (eighth day),[2].—Sleep early in the evening, and long sleep in the morning, for four weeks (after eight days),[2] —*The child at the breast sleeps more than usual, but wakes frequently* (first days),[2].—Much sleep in the twilight, but when he went to bed sleep disappeared, although during the day he had taken much exercise, and had slept but little the night previous (after seven days),[2].—Falls asleep late and wakes early (after six days),[2].—He wakes before midnight, and cannot sleep till 2 o'clock,[2].—He wakes at 1 o'clock in the night, and cannot sleep again till 4, on account of much thinking (ninth day),[2].—[450.] *She wakes uncommonly early, at 3 o'clock; she cannot fall asleep again for two hours. on account of heat in the whole body, especially in the head, with sweat on the thighs* (eleventh and twelfth days),[2] ([3]).—He wakes at 4 o'clock in the morning, and is quite wide awake, so that he goes to work with cheerfulness (after five weeks),[2].—Very wide awake in the evening,[1].—Restless sleep; she could not sleep, but tossed about the bed (twenty-first day),[2].—Restless night; he could not sleep well on account of rush of blood to the head, restlessness of the body, rumbling in the abdomen and diarrhœa (first days)[2].—*A child five years old tosses about, cries the whole night till 4 in the morning, frequently out of its sleep, and in the morning is in a whining mood; the infant frequently cries out of its sleep, and anxiously grasps its mother, as if it had been frightened by a dream* (first two weeks),[2] ([3]).—Restless sleep, with thirst and coldness (first day),[2].—He can sleep only on the left side; as soon as he turns upon the right side he is awakened by drawing-sticking pains in the right intercostal muscles (seventh day),[2].—A feeling as though he had not slept enough in the morning [1].—Voluptuous dreams (thirtieth day),[2].—[460.] At night, lascivious disgusting dreams (in a married woman), (first day),[3].—She dreams of coition, but without pleasurable sensation (fourth day),[2].—Vexatious dreams,[2].—A dream of sore throat and other diseases,[1].

Fever.—Shivering over the whole body at night and the following day, with throbbing pain in the occiput, as from suppuration (second day),[2] ([3]).--Chilliness over the whole body, especially in the back, without thirst, with flat taste, rawness of the larynx, stitches in the chest when breathing, weakness, prostration, stretching of the limbs, contracted quick pulse, together with heat, heaviness, and stupefaction, and in the head, burning of the eyes, with sensitiveness to light (twenty-third day),[2].—A chill at night, from 2 to 4, with trembling, vomiting of the food, tearing in the thighs and pain in their bones, as though they would be broken, followed after sleep by heat and thirst; afterwards, at half-past eight in the morning, bitter vomiting, followed by sweat, with diminished thirst (second day),[2].—Coldness, with headache and subsequent heat, without thirst; on walking in the open air, the headache ceases, and she feels quite well (fourteenth day),[2].—Coldness every second day, in the afternoon, with thirst and sleep, followed, on waking, by heat, with pressive pain in the inguinal ring, without subsequent sweat (thirty-eighth day),[1].—With the erysipelatous inflammation of the lower leg, first coldness, shivering, and thirst, with vomiting of food and bile, followed by heaviness in the head and throbbing in the temples, with restless sleep at night, only slumbering, and afterwards (on the sixth day) nose-bleed,[2].—[470.] Coldness in the afternoon, from 2 to 6 (after thirst in the forenoon); then until going to sleep, heat, with pressive pain in the left hypochondrium (fifth week),[2].—Coldness immediately after eating, with more thirst than appetite for dinner, and tensive drawing backward around the hypochondria, and heat suddenly rising into the head on taking a deep breath; then heat in the evening, at 6, during which he must lie down until 10, then sweat, and after the sweat thirst, for four days (fifteenth day),[2].—At one time coldness, at another heat, frequently with sweat in the face, during which coldness runs up the back, with stretching of the limbs, with weariness and sleepiness, so that he is obliged to lie down in the afternoon, without, however, being able to sleep; when walking, he drags the feet, and is fretful and taciturn,[2].—Heat if she puts the hands under the bed-covers; as soon as she puts them out she becomes cold again (fifth day),[2].—Heat in the evening, in bed, and sweat, but immediately on rising he becomes chilly (seventeenth day),[2].—Burning heat and redness of the toes, with some coldness, as after freezing (after twenty-four days),[2].—Flushes of heat frequently in the morning, with nausea and inclination to vomit (second day),[2].—*The infant has a hot head,* hot mouth, and hot palms (fourth, fifth, sixth, and seventh days),[2].—Heat in the head in the evening, when writing, with thirst and sensation as if sweat would break out (seventh day),[2].—Burning heat and redness of the left cheek (after four days),[2].—[480.] Perspiration at night,[1].—Sweat during the morning sleep; when dressing he feels cold, and is seized with a dry cough, with rawness in the chest, as after taking cold (fifteenth day),[2].

Conditions.—Aggravation.—(*Morning*), In bed, vertigo; giddy, etc., feeling in head; *at* 10 *o'clock, aching in whole head, etc.;* headache; pressure in right eye; when writing, flickering before eyes; when washing in cold water, stitches in ears; on waking unusually early, stitches in left ear; nose-bleed; in bed, burning in upper lip; hawking of mucus; throat rough; thirst; *nausea,* etc.; after eating peas, pressure in pit of stomach, etc.; pinching, etc., in abdomen; desire for stool; till 2 p.m., diarrhœa; on waking, erection; on rising, dry cough, etc.; cough, etc.; stitch in region of left ribs; on stooping, while walking, stitch in lumbar region; flushes of heat; during sleep, sweat.—(*Forenoon*), Cheerfulness, etc.; tearing in the vertex; from 4 o'clock till noon, pain in region of stomach; after eating peas, pressure in pit of stomach, etc.; tearing in thigh-bone.—(*Toward noon*), Diarrhœa, etc.—(*Noon*), Nausea, etc.; sleepiness.—(*Afternoon*), At 4 o'clock, fretful; before stool, fretful, etc.; pain in forehead; boring in eye; tearing in eyeballs; dryness of tongue; from 3 o'clock till evening, nausea, etc.; frequent nausea, etc.; diarrhœa-like stool; every second day, coldness, etc.; from 2 to 6 o'clock, coldness.—(*Evening*), Head confused; when walking, vertigo; headache in forehead, etc.; headache in vertex, etc.; stitches in left eye; obscuration of left eye; stitching in left ear; when walking, itching in left ear, etc.; pulsating headache; burning pain in lip; in cool air, boring in teeth; sticking toothache, etc.; great appetite; very little appetite; loss of appetite, etc.; in bed, stitching in abdomen; stitches in rectum; itching in anus; tearing in larynx; hacking, etc.; on lying down, dry cough, etc.; in bed, anxiety in chest; in bed, oppression of chest; stitches from back of chest; with every fit of cough, sticking in side of chest; when walking in open air, pain in neck; sticking in palm, etc.; tearing in thigh-bone; on ascending a height, heavy feeling in feet; in bed, heat, etc.; when writing, heat in head, etc.—(*Night*), Rumbling in abdomen; *urging to urinate;* sense of distension, etc., in clitoris; pain in pectoralis major; shivering; from 2 to 4 o'clock, chill, etc.; perspiration.—(*On ascending a height*), Fulness of the head; shortness of breath; tightness of chest, etc.—(*On bending forward and to the right*), Pain in intercostal muscles.—(*After breakfast*), Toothache; vomiting; cutting in right hypochondrium; diarrhœa.—(*At every attempt to breathe*), Chest becomes constricted.—(*On deep breathing*), Sensation in left hypochondrium; *stitches in chest;* pressure on sternum.—(*After animated conversation*), Restlessness, etc.—(*Coughing*), Stitches in pit of throat; *stitches in chest;* pain in right side of chest; *sticking in chest;* burning in right thigh.—(*Dancing*), Anxiety; pain in left hypochondrium; inflammation in leg.—(*After dinner*), Rumbling in abdomen, etc.—(*Eating*), Nausea; hiccough; distension, etc.; apples with mutton, fulness in stomach, etc.; pain in abdomen, etc.; diarrhœa; coldness, etc.—(*During involuntary emission*), Pain in urethra.—(*After an emission*), Urging to urinate.—(*In any exertion of body which heats*), Shortness of breath.—(*Hiccoughing*), Pain in right side of chest.—(*With every inspiration*), Stitching in chest.—(*During deep inspiration*), Sensation as of something rising into chest; *sticking in chest.*—(*Laying on of the hand*), Burning in right thigh.—(*After lifting*), Pain in stomach.—(*When lying in bed*), Arrest of breathing.—(*During a meal*), Restlessness, etc.—(*After every meal*), Pressure in stomach; *flatulent distension.*—(*While meditating*), Trembling of whole body.—(*During menstruation*), Throbbing in the head, etc.; *pain in groin,* etc.—(*On opening eyes*), Pain in upper lid.—(*On raising arm*), Immediately, stitches on right side of chest.—(*Reading*), Pain in forehead.—(*When riding*), Nausea.—(*When riding in carriage without springs*), Feeling as of pressure with hands.—(*When sitting*), Fulness in head, etc.; sensation in right eye; burning in back.—(*Sitting stooped*), Tightness from pit of stomach into chest; pain in back.—(*Sneezing*), Stitches in throat; pain in side of chest.—(*After smoking*), Feeling as though diarrhœa would come on.—(*On stepping*), Pain in joints of toes.—(*Stooping*), Pressure in frontal bone; dull backache.—(*After supper*), Toothache; abdomen distended.—(*Touch*), Pain in urethra; pain in penis.—(*On turning*), Pressure, etc., in kidney region.—(*Urination*), Tension in urethra; smarting in urethra; cutting in urethra.—(*On waking*), Head confused; immediately, nausea, etc.—(*When walking*), Pain in back; pain in great toes.—(*On walking rapidly*), Cutting in left hypochondrium.—(*In wet weather*), Toothache in hollow tooth; stitches in the corns.—(*In bad weather*), Aching in hollow teeth; pressure in hollow teeth.—(*Drinking wine*), Pains in chest.—(*Writing*), Pain in forehead.—(*Yawning*), Pain in right side of chest.

Amelioration.—(*Morning*), Pain in stomach.—(*Afternoon*), After stool, lively, etc.—(*Evening*), On going into open air, distension, etc.— (*Walking in open air*), Headache; fulness in head; heaviness in stomach; formication, etc., of the feet.—(*On bending double*), Pain in abdomen ceases.—(*After dinner*), Nausea disappears.—(*On continuing to dance*), Pain in left hypochondrium disappears.—(*Hawking up mucus*), Rawness in throat.—(*Holding painful side with hand*), Pain in chest.—*When lying quietly stretched out upon the back*), Chest feels better.—(*After midday nap*), Pain in abdomen, etc.; weakness, etc.—(*Pressure*), Stitches in groins.— (*Rubbing*), Sensation in eyes.—(*Sitting*), Stitches in lumbar region.—(*To-bacco smoking*), Toothache.—(*Walking*), Pressure in pit of stomach; weakness in joints, etc.—(*Walking slowly about room*), Pains in chest; feels most comfortable.—(*Washing chest with cold water*), Sticking in chest, etc

BOTHROPS LANCEOLATUS.

B. lanceolatus, Wagler-Dumeril; *synonyms*, Coluber glaucus, Linn. Vipera cærulescens, Laurent; Coluber megara, Shaw; Cophias lanceolatus, Merrem; Craspedocephalus lanceolatus, Gray (Trigonocephale jaune, Cuvier; Vipera jaune; *Fer-de-lance*).

An Ophidian of the family Crotalidæ, found in the Island of Martinique.

Authority. Dr. Ch. Ozanam, L'Art. Med., 19, 116 (A collection of cases (15) and general observations on the effect of the bite, quoted from Dr. Rufz, " Enquête sur le serpent de la Martinique.")

Mind.—Consecutive and long-lasting hypochondria.—Ideas confused. —Coma, becoming deeper until death ensues.

Head.—Vertigo.—Frequent dizziness.—Hemicrania.

Eyes.—*Amaurosis* (sometimes immediately after the bite).—Persistent amaurosis.—Amaurosis, without perceptible dilatation of the pupil.— Hemeralopic amaurosis; can scarcely see her way, especially after sunrise. —[10.] Pupil a little dilated.

Face.—Altered countenance.—Hippocratic countenance.—Injection, more or less dark and bluish, of the entire cutaneous surface of the face; a hue like that of cholera in the algid stage, or that in the last stage of yellow fever.

Mouth.—Trismus (after eighteen days).—*Inability to articulate, without any affection of the tongue* (after seven to fifteen hours).

Stomach.—Gastric mucous membrane dotted red.—*Thirst.*—Nausea and vomiting.—*Vomiting.*—[20.] Vomiting, followed by a nervous trembling.—Painful sensation extending to the epigastrium.—Intolerable epigastric malaise.

Abdomen.—Small intestines of a livid redness exteriorly.—Small intestines dotted red.—Mucous membrane of the small intestines, especially the jejunum, inflamed in different parts.—Small intestines of a deep blue color, confined entirely to the muscular layer.—Severe pains in the abdomen, which extend to the epigastrium and become intolerable (after a few hours).—The entire abdomen is sensitive to pressure.

Stool and Urine.—Colliquative diarrhœa.—[30.] Hæmaturia.

Respiratory Apparatus and Chest.—Trachea and bronchi

blue.—All the symptoms of *pulmonary congestion*, oppressed breathing, and bloody expectoration, more or less profuse (after three to six days).—Præcordial pains.

Heart and Pulse.—Soft, flabby heart.—Black spots on the pericardium and under the endocardium.—Pulse and respiration become slow. —Frequent and compressed pulse.

Extremities in General.—Speedy swelling of the bitten limb.—The swelling, at first pale and confined to the parts around the bite, becomes livid and involves the entire limb, both below and above the bite.—[40.] The swelling of the part bitten gradually extends to a great distance from its original seat; the limb becomes triple its ordinary size, and is soft and flabby, appearing as if distended with gas.—Enormous bloody infiltration, like that which results from a violent bruise (of the bitten limb).—The extremities become cold.—Almost entire inability to move the right arm or right leg.—Paralysis of one arm, or of one leg, only.—Severe pain in the bitten limb.

Upper Extremities.—Arm swollen from hand to shoulder.—Very considerable tumefaction of the whole limb, from the fingers to the shoulder and adjacent portion of the chest, soft, like emphysema, very sensitive, with blue spots.—After being bitten in the little finger of *one* hand paralysis began in the finger-tips of the *other* hand, and extended over the whole of that side.—Cellular tissue, and also the muscles of the forearm (where the bite was inflicted) engorged with black blood.—[50.] The bones of the forearm and hand are laid bare.—Consecutive necrosis.—Numbness in the right arm (after a bite on the right hand).—Anchylosis and deformity of the hand, which became united into one immovable bone, with the wrist and fingers packed together.

Lower Extremities.—Legs infiltrated with bloody serum.—Very extensive suppuration of the leg.—Destruction of the skin of the whole leg. —Left thigh enormously swollen, and of a bluish color, with here and there blotches of a deeper hue,[6].—Softening of the cellular tissue in the hollow of the ham, and at the posterior portion of the thigh, including one half of the limb.—Gangrene of the skin over the whole anterior portion of the right leg from the foot to the knee.—[60.] Gangrene of the muscles of the leg.—Inferior extremity of the tibia laid bare (after fifteen days).—Tibio-tarsal articulation laid open.—Paralysis of the leg.—Gangrenous ulcer on the great toe.—Intolerable pain in the *right* great toe (the patient having been bitten on the left thumb).

Generalities.—Œdematous swellings, like elephantiasis.—Infiltration of bloody serum, equally diffused throughout the substance of the cellular tissue, but better marked in the vicinity of the bites.—Very extensive suppuration.—Suppuration and sero-sanguinolent infiltration of all the tissues.—[70.] Within two or three days suppuration sets in, the skin comes off, and, if the proper incisions are not made, the part becomes gangrened; portions of cellular tissue are detached, with a reddish sanious discharge; the tendons and bones are laid bare; the joints are exposed; sphacelus invades the parts, especially the fingers; the whole limb is dissected alive; colliquation succeeds, and if the patient does not succumb to the consequences of purulent absorption, or of gangrene, amputation becomes necessary.—Remarkable fluidity, dissolved condition, of the blood. The blood is black, or rusty-looking; very fluid.—Hemorrhages of various kinds, and especially from wounds.—Very fluid black blood flows in jets at the least movement.—Capillary hemorrhage after amputation; blood discharged continuously, not by jets; very fluid and very pale.—Muscles laid bare.—The blackened muscular tissue is dissected off bit by bit.—Caries of the bones.—Emaciation.—[80.] Tetanus (after amputation).—Nervous trembling.—Opisthotonos (after fourteen days).—Convulsions and death (after two days).—Paralysis (generally incurable).—Hemiplegia of the right side (after five and seven hours).—Inexpressible lassitude.—*Weakness.* —Repeated fainting fits.—*Frequent syncope.*—[90.] Indefinable malaise; general uneasiness.—Intolerable pains in the swelling.

Skin.—Bluish skin (of the leg).—Yellow skin, as in yellow fever.— Skin as if affected by a most extensive and severe bruise.—Bloody subcutaneous and intermuscular infiltration.—Blackish, serous infiltration in the intermuscular tissue.—Many phlyctenæ are formed under the epidermis (of the bitten limb).—Phlyctenæ in the hollow of the ham.—Obstinate ulcers.—[100.] Abscess, more or less considerable.—Fistulous openings.— Wounds heal with difficulty.

Sleep and Dreams.—Drowsiness.—Very remarkable sleep or coma, which may end in death.

Fever.—Chilliness.—*Slight shivering, followed by very profuse cold sweat.* —Sometimes very great external heat.—General heat.—High fever.—[110.] Body covered with a cold and viscid sweat.—Profuse cold sweats at the beginning and end of the disease.

BOUNAFA.

(*See* FERULA GLAUCA.)

BRANCA URSINA.

(*See* HERACLEUM SPHONDYLIUM.)

BOVISTA.

Lycoperdon Bovista, Pers.   *Nat. order,* Fungi;   *Common names,* Warted Puff ball, Kugelschwamm.   *Preparation,* Triturations.

Authorities.   1, Hb, Hartlaub and Trinks, Arzneimittellehre, 3; 2, Ng., ibid.; 3, S., ibid.; 4, Petroz, Journ. d. l. soc. gal., 4, 82, symptoms observed by M. Gerard from inhaling the fumes of the burning fungus; 5, Ibid., symptoms observed by a young woman from olfaction of the tincture.

Mind.—Emotional. Talkative,[3].—Very open-hearted; she spoke of her own failings, contrary to her custom,[3].—Averse to everything after dinner,[2].—Very much exhilarated; life seems very pleasant to her, in the morning, but, towards evening, out of humor and peevish,[3].—Very courageous and vigorous; he would like to fight with everybody,[3].—Melancholy the whole day,[3].—Dull and depressed; and towards evening she became very weary,[3].—Very much depressed (after three hours); then alternating moods and (after seven hours) great sadness, amounting to melancholy,[1].— Anguish; she felt as if enveloped in a black vapor,[5].—[10.] *Great sensitiveness;* became easily offended at everything,[3].—Very apprehensive, and at the same time fretful; she was disinclined to do any work,[2].—Very irritable; everything affected her,[3].—Peevish mood, for an hour in the morning after rising (fifth day),[2].—Ill-humored, fretful, and apprehensive, with confusion of the head,[2].—Ill-humor, confusion of the head, gloominess, also peevishness and irritability, for fourteen days,[1].—Peevish, fretful, and ill-humored during a violent headache in the afternoon,[2].—Fretful, ill-humored, and indifferent to life,[3].—At one time life seemed very exciting to him, at another very hateful,[3].—In company she was lively; alone, sad, depressed, and not interested in anything,[3].—[20.] Extremely indifferent to all external objects (ninth day),[1].—*Intellectual.* Confused thoughts,[5].—Stupid feeling,[2].—Very absent-minded, so that it was impossible for her, even on great exertion, to pay attention to what one was saying or doing (after thirteen days),[1].—She is very absent-minded, makes mistakes in writing, leaves out whole syllables, and writes several words entirely wrong (after five days),[1].—Lost in thought; he often looked vacantly for several minutes,[3]. —Weak memory,[3].—He recollected only with difficulty the transactions of a few hours previous,[3].—Feeling of stupefaction at times,[3].

Head.—Confusion and Vertigo. The head is somewhat confused and heavy,[3].—[30.] The head was very much confused and dizzy after coition; he was unable to sleep for a long time,[3].—Head very much confused and empty, with drawing about the whole head, especially in the morning,[1].—Head very much confused; he could not think correctly, with heaviness and pressure in the forehead,[3].—The head was very much confused and painful on stooping, mostly in the left temple,[2].—Vertigo for several minutes,[3].—Vertigo; the whole room seemed to turn about with him,[3]. —Frequent transient vertigo,[3].—Frequent vertigo, wherewith all his senses left him,[1].—Vertigo, even to falling forward, towards evening,[3].—Vertigo, which drew him backward,[3].—[40.] Vertigo, on rising, as if everything turned around in a circle with her, and she could not trust herself to stand upright,[3].—A kind of vertigo, with stupefaction, in the morning on rising from his chair, so that he nearly fell down (second day),[1].—*Sudden attacks of vertigo and feeling of stupidity in the head, on rising; she loses consciousness for a moment, preceding and following a headache, in the morning,*[2].— Vertigo and feeling of heaviness in the head, while standing, followed by sudden jerking of the head backward,[2].—Dizziness, in the morning,[1].— Dizzy and stupid, and a feeling of whirling in the head, after rising from stooping (first day),[2].—*Sensations.* Heaviness of the head,[5].—Heaviness of the head (after a few moments),[4].—Stupefying headache, especially in the forehead,[3].—In the evening, the head is stupid and heavy, and feels as if bruised (second day),[2].—[50.] Headache, on waking, as after too much sleep,[3].—Headache, with heaviness of the head, which makes her ill-humored and unable to think continuously; the pain is increased on lying, and is most severe on waking from the midday nap, and is combined with a kind of pulsating beating in the head; its chief seat is in the forehead over the nose, which is at the same time stopped (after fifteen days),[1].—She did not dare to raise the head at night, from dread of unendurable pains, which were somewhat relieved toward morning (after twelve days),[2].— Headache as if suppurating; a raging in the whole brain, coming on in the cold air and continuing in the room at 8 A.M.,[2].—The whole head seems larger than usual, with the headache,[2].—On waking, at 3 o'clock in the morning, very violent headache, with which he feels every pulsation, and which threatens to burst the head asunder; it gradually disappears on the outbreak of sweat, especially on the head (seventeenth day),[1].—A contractive sensation and a feeling of dulness in the head, disappearing after breakfast (first day),[2].—The brain feels as if screwed together, with a heavy sensation, in the morning, disappearing in the open air (eighth day),[2].—Dull headache, frequently returning,[2].—Dull headache, with weariness,[3].—[60.] After walking in the open air, violent pressive headache, with a feeling of heaviness, mostly in the occiput, in the morning; this pain disappeared at night, but immediately returned when she went into the open air in the morning, and disappeared again in the room (fifth and sixth days),[2].—Violent pressive headache on coming into the room from the open air, on both sides, with some throbbing, in the evening,[2].—Dull pressive headache, in the morning,[3].—Head feels as if compressed by a tight bandage, but without pain (after a few moments),[4].—Tearing in the whole head, with heaviness and bruised sensation continuing almost constantly,[1].—All the pains are felt deep in the brain,[2].—*Forehead.* Painful boring outward in the left side of the forehead, at 8 P.M.,[2].—Pressure in the forehead,[3].—Heavy pressure on the forepart of the head, especially the temples,[5].—Dull headache, like a pressure, above the right eye, extending toward the temporal region,[1].—[70.] Pressive pain and a feeling of heaviness in a small spot on the left side of the forehead, deep internally and pressing upon the eye, for four minutes; the pain returns soon with redoubled severity, whereby it seems as if there were a cloud before the left eye, which disappeared by frequent wiping; in the morning on moving about,[2].—Stitches in the middle of the forehead, rather externally, in the evening (first day),[2].—First stitches, then, pressure, in the forehead,[3].—Stitches and tearing in the right frontal eminence, which extend toward the right ear,[2].—Sharp stitches in the right side of the forehead, twice in succession,[2].—Sharp stitches in the right frontal eminence, in frequent succession,[2].—Extremely painful fine stitches, deep in the forehead, in the evening (fourth day),[2].—A painful twitching in the brain, in a small spot above the right frontal eminence, which frequently remits and returns, with peevish mood, at 2 P.M.,[2].—Tearing pain in the forehead, extending to the left side of the occiput, and then back again to the forehead, and becomes seated in the left temple, where it remains several days (tenth day),[1].—Fine tearing in the middle of the forehead, rather externally, in the morning (first day),[2].—[80.] Violent unendurable tearing in the forehead, with heaviness in the head, on stooping, and burning in the right eye (fourth day),[2].—Pressive-tearing in the forehead, especially above the orbits, which extends into the root of the nose (sixth and seventh days),[1].—*Temples.* Heaviness in the temples,[3]. —Compressive headache starting from both temples,[3].—Intolerable painful pressure and throbbing in the right temple, with great fretfulness; the pain extends down to the neck, and there disappears, in the morning,[2].—Sticking and jerking in the left temple,[3].—Several fine stitches in the left temporal bone,[2].—Fine tearing in the left temple, extending towards the ear (after three-quarters of an hour),[2].—A raging or digging-tearing in the left temple, deep in the brain, in the afternoon,[2].—Violent tearing in the right temple and in the right half of the forehead, frequently intermitting (tenth day),[2]. —*Vertex.* [90.] Stupefying headache of the whole vertex, with heat in the eyes,[3].—Constant slight drawings in the whole top of the head,[1].—Pressure upon the vertex,[1].—Violent sharp stitches on the vertex; they extend over the whole head; in the afternoon,[2].—Frequent, fine, extremely painful stitches on the left side of the vertex; this place is also very painful to touch; in the evening,[2].—Violent tearing on the vertex, which is painful on touch, as if bruised, together with fine tearing on the margin of the right concha; in the morning,[2].—Bruised pain on the left side of the vertex, when touched and when not,[2].—*Parietals.* Painful pressive heaviness in the right side of the head,[2].—Beating and roaring in the right side of the head at 7 A.M., when coming into the room from the cold air,[2].—Pressure in both sides of the head,[1].—[100.] Pain as though the brain would be pressed together from both sides, in the afternoon (fourth day),[2].—Compressive pain in both sides of the head on coming into the room after walking in the cold air (eighth day),[2].—Dull pressure in the left side of the head,[3].—Sharp stitches on the right side near the vertex,[2].—Some fine stitches in the right side of the head at 7 A.M.,[2].—Sensitive dull stitches in the upper part of the right side of the head,[2].—Sudden dull stitches, like boring, deep in the right side of the head, so that she was obliged to cry out,[2].—Violent tearing in the right side of the head,[2].—Severe bruised pain in the whole right side of the head, which even affected the eye, at 10 A.M.,[2].—Painful throbbing, as in an ulcer, in the right side of the head,[2].—[110.] Headache, almost like a throbbing, on a small spot on the left side of the head, in the afternoon, at 1 o'clock,[2].—*Occiput.* Confusion and heaviness in the occiput, with inclination of the lids to fall down, and feeling as if the eyes would be drawn backwards, especially in a bright light, in the evening, together with anxiety and uneasiness of the body,[1].—Dull headache in the occiput, with tension in the temples,[3].—Pressive pain in the occiput, which extends over the vertex to the forehead, in the forenoon,[2].—Severe pressure on both sides of the occiput, from which place the pain extends to the forehead; a feeling in the occiput as if everything would protrude; in the afternoon till evening (fifth day),[2].—Pain in the occiput, as if a wedge would be pressed in,[3].—Violent sticking and tearing in the left side of the occiput, continuing a long time,[2].—Dull, boring-pressive stitches in the occiput, extending to the forehead over the left eye; in a warm room in the afternoon,[2].—Violent fine stitches in the left side of the occiput, in the morning, at 7 o'clock,[2].—Tearing in the occiput, and at the same time in the lower jaw,[2].—*External Head.* [120.] The hair falls out,[3].—Small sore spots on the scalp, with itching,[1].—Small reddish blisters, with severe itching, on the scalp,[3].—Great sensitiveness of the scalp generally to touch; she could not even endure the comb,[2].—Itching on the head as if the whole head was full of lice, especially in the morning,[3].—*Itching over the whole scalp, extending to the neck, especially if he became warm, so that he was obliged to scratch the forehead, which was not relieved by scratching,*[1].

Eye.—Objective. Redness of the eyes,[4].—Inflammation of the left eye,[3].—The eyes are closed involuntarily, though without drowsiness (after a few moments)[4].—Lost in thought; she looked a long time at one point,[2].—*Subjective.* [130.] Weak eyes, without lustre, or snap,[3].—A feeling as if something was in the right eye, with lachrymation in it (first day),[1].—Burning in the eyes, and such great heat in the cheeks that she thought they would burst,[3].—Heat in the right eye, and a painful contractive feeling in it, for an hour,[1].—Pressure in the eyes, as if something were in them; with which the left eye is red (after eight days),[1].—Stitches over the left eye, as with a pointed instrument,[3].—Excessively painful tearing, deep in the right eye, which extends above it to the forehead,[2].—Smarting in the eyes, so that he had to keep them shut,[4].—*Orbit, etc.* Tension in the left eyebrow,[2].—Extremely painful pressure and twisting deep in the right orbit; the bone is very sensitive to pressure, during menstruation,[2].—[140.] Pressive sticking in the right orbit,[3].—A sudden turning when sitting, or a sensation of a sudden current of air above the left eye, above the root of the nose,[2].—A feeling of painful contraction, with stitches over the left eye, as if the left frontal eminence would be screwed together; the pain began

at the root of the nose, and extended outward behind the left frontal eminence, with lachrymation of the left eye; afterwards the place above the
eye was sensitive to pressure; after the pain ceased heat arose over the
whole body, with a feeling as if sweat would break out during dinner (fifth
day),[2].—Sticking in a small spot above the left eye, with redness of the
cheek, without external heat, after dinner,[2].—*Lids.* Could not open the
eyes well in the morning (sixth day),[1].—The left eye was agglutinated in
the morning,[3].—The eyes were always agglutinated in the morning,[2].—
Irritation of the eyelids (second day),[4].—The canthi are red (after thirty-
two days).—*Lachrymal Apparatus.* Lachrymation, in the morning,[1].—*Vision.* [150.] It seems as though there were a veil before the
eyes, in the morning, on rising (after four days),[1].—Illusion of vision; she
feared that a person sitting near her would stick the shears into her eyes,
although she sat two steps away and was cutting paper; all her visual
perceptions were distorted; it seemed as though the shears were close before
her eyes,[3].

Ear.—Objective. Twitching in the left external ear, for ten minutes,[2].—(A copious purulent offensive discharge from the ear, which had
lasted four years, disappeared),[1].—*Subjective.* Heat and burning from
the right ear, extending down to the angle of the lower jaw,[2].—Drawing in
the ears (after three days),[1].—Stitches in the ears,[3].—Stitches in the right
ear,[1].—Tearing in front of the right ear, which suddenly disappears, after
dinner,[2].—Extremely painful tearing in the left ear, in the afternoon,[2].—
[160.] Tearing deep in the right ear, and a tensive sensation on the border
of the concha,[2].—A feeling of picking in the left ear, as though something
were lying in it,[2].—Severe itching in the ears, with some difficulty of hearing,[1].—*Hearing.* He did not hear distinctly, understood many things
wrongly, and also made mistakes in speaking,[3].—(In the ears, especially in
the right, frequent noises, like rain),[3].—Roaring in the left ear, with diminished hearing for a short time,[2].

Nose.—Objective. The septum of the nose where it unites with th[
upper lip is red and sore,[3].—*Scabby nostrils,[1].—A scab in the nostril i
frequently renewed; after removal, the sore place burns,[2].—Coryza, for a
few moments only,[4].—[170.] Stopped coryza,[1].—Stopped coryza, in the
morning, after rising, with frequent sneezing; with which she could draw
air only through the right nostril,[2].—She is frequently obliged to blow the
nose, whereby only thin water is discharged,[3].—Frequent need to blow the
nose, though but little nasal mucus is discharged,[2].—The nose is very much
stopped; troubles her in speaking,[3].—Great stoppage of the nose; she could
only get air through with great difficulty; with pressure in the temples,[3].—
At night, the nose is stopped; she cannot draw air through it (eighteenth
day),[1].—The left nostril is stopped, and a few drops of water run out of it
(seventeenth day),[2].—Fluent coryza,[3].—Fluent coryza; thin mucus is discharged from the nose,[2].—[180.] Fluent coryza, with confusion of the head,[3].
—The previously profuse, tough, yellow nasal mucus, a quantity of which was
discharged, became white and more profuse (after sixteen days),[1].—Frequent sneezing,[2].—Sneezing, in the morning, after waking,[2].—*A few drops
of blood from the nose every time on sneezing* (fifth day),[2].—*Bleeding of the
nose in the morning,[3].—Subjective.* Constant feeling of coryza in the
nose, and swelling of it (fifteenth day),[1].—Burning in both nostrils, as i
they were sore,[2].—A contraction over the nose, with a feeling of heaviness
and pressure as though the skin were too short,[3].

*Face.—*The face is very pale, in the morning, after rising,* for severa days (after fourteen days),[1].—[190.] Great changes of color in the face, which is at one time red, at another pale,[3].—Tension and heat rise into the face,[3].—*Locally.* Boring and digging in both malar bones,[3].—Cracked lips,[2].—On the inner border of the left side of the lower lip burning, as in a cut,[2].—Fine stitches, as with needles, or as from splinters, in the lower lip,[3].—Violent tearing in the left side of the lower jaw, and in one of the teeth,[2].—A feeling of throbbing on the left side below the lower jaw; she believes that a gland must be swollen,[2].

Mouth.—Teeth. The teeth are frequently coated with mucus,[1].—The teeth, gums and lips are filled with clotted blood, in the morning, on waking,[1].—[200.] Slight gnashing of the teeth, now and then, in the evening, as in a chill (after fifteen days),[1].—A hollow tooth seems longer than the others,[2].—Toothache, as if the exposed nerves were rubbed,[1].—In the evening, in bed, toothache, which was only relieved by warmth (after fourteen days),[1].—The toothache ceased on going into the open air,[1].—Painful boring in the teeth, in the evening,[2].—Digging-boring pain in a hollow tooth, with a tearing pain in the right side of the head, and stitches in the ears, very much increased by cold,[3].—Digging pain in a hollow tooth, morning and evening,[3].—Tearing-digging in the hollow teeth, extending thence into the temples, in the evening in bed,[2].—Drawing toothache, as if the roots would be torn out, in the evening,[2].—[210.] Dull drawing pain in the hollow teeth (after twelve hours),[1].—Painful drawing a few times in a hollow tooth of the right lower jaw, in the evening,[2].—Very painful drawing toothache awoke her before midnight, and lasted an hour, three nights in succession,[2]. —*Violent drawing pain in the hollow back teeth of the left lower jaw, for two evenings in succession, in bed,* which lasted till morning, during menstruation,[2].—Dull toothache, which she had not had for several years, followed by long-continued, elevated, pale swelling of the upper lip and sweat, all night, till morning, which was especially profuse on the head (after three weeks),[1].—Stitches in the sound teeth, especially at night, so that he could not sleep on account of it; the gum bled easily; the pain was relieved if he sucked the blood out of the teeth with the tongue,[1].—The stitches in the teeth extend into the eyes,[1].—Pain in the upper front teeth; they pain on touch, and do not bear chewing; with the upper lip beginning to swell, the toothache was somewhat relieved; the swelling increases so that the lip hung far over the lower one and was even with the nose; after the swelling of the lip had somewhat subsided, the left cheek began to swell; all the swollen parts were painful to touch (after fifteen days),[1].—Jerking toothache (fifth day),[1].—*Gums.* Swollen, painful gum,[3].—[220.] The gum retracts so that the teeth seem longer,[3].—An inflamed spot on the gum over a decayed root, which is painful by itself, and still more when touched, like an ulcer, with throbbing, with a feeling as if the root were too long,[2].—An ulcer on the gum, from which blood exudes on pressure,[2].—Clear blood oozes from the mouth (gum) even without sucking the gum,[1].—*As often as he sucks the gum blood comes into the mouth, with which the whole gum becomes painful,*[1].—*Tongue.* Yellow-coated tongue in the morning (after seven days),[1].—A red spot, painful to pressure, near the left ligament of the tongue, where it is united to the tongue, for several days (after thirty-five days),[2].—A small depressed ulcer on the left margin of the tongue, sore and painful to touch,[3].—In the morning, after waking, burning in the tip and a numbness on the posterior portion of the tongue, and over the whole mouth, for four mornings in succession (after thirteen days),[2].—* *Cutting pain in the tongue,* repeated several days,[1].—*General Mouth.* [230.] Offensive smell from the mouth (sixth day),[1].—(Internally in the left cheek a swelling; this disappeared and a burning blister developed on the cheek externally, filled with yellow fluid, which became flattened and dried up the next day),[3].—Great dryness in the mouth, as if she had sand in it, with thirst,[3].—Towards evening, the mouth became very dry; in the evening he was always full and satiated, and had no appetite,[3].—Numbness of the whole mouth and tongue, in the morning, after walking; it disappears after eating,[2].—The whole mouth seemed numb and burnt, in the morning, on waking, with a bitter slimy taste and soreness of the throat,[2].—Burning and heat in the mouth, without thirst,[1].—Painful tension in the mouth, in the right cheek,[2].—Sticking pain in the palate, which extends to the chin, for several minutes (first day),[1].—*Saliva.* Much collection of saliva in the mouth,[1].—*Taste.* [240.] Bad taste with much mucus in the mouth,[1].—Bitter taste,[3].—Taste of blood in the mouth,[3].—*Speech.* Stammering,[3].—He stammered at times, when reading; was not able to pronounce several words,[3].

Throat.—Sensations. Dryness in the throat, on waking, sticking on swallowing, and numbness in the mouth, disappearing after rising and eating,[2].—Great dryness in the throat, in the morning, on waking, so that the tongue seemed almost like wood,[3].—Frequent pain in the throat,[1].—*Burning in the throat,*[3].—Sore throat in the evening; painful when swallowing the saliva, as if something were sticking in the throat; he was unable to swallow food easily,[3].—[250.] Scraping in the throat, with irritation to cough (first day),[1].—Every morning, scraping in the throat, with mucus,[1].—The sleep was frequently interrupted by scraping in the throat; she was obliged to hawk up mucus,[3].—Scraping and burning in the throat, as if he had eaten something too hot,[3].—Scraping and burning in the throat, causing a dry cough,[3].—Rawness of the throat, in the morning, after rising, and in the evening, for several days,[2].—Tickling in the throat, which obliges her to cough frequently, in the afternoon, at five (third day),[2].—Slight irritation of the pharynx,[4].—Swelling of the cervical glands,[1].—Swollen cervical glands, with tension and drawing pains, for six days,[3].

Stomach.—Appetite. [260.] Constant excessive hunger; he was unable to eat enough, and was soon hungry again,[1].—(Hunger in the afternoon, contrary to custom),[3].—Hunger towards evening,[3].—She relished the food, although afterwards she had a pressure in the stomach as if she had overloaded it,[3].—Appetite without real hunger,[3].—No appetite; she was obliged to force herself to eat,[3].—No appetite for cooked food, only for bread (eleventh and twelfth days),[2].—A child loses its appetite; the whole body becomes hot, with puffy, scarlet face; it lies and vomits mucus and food; followed by excessive sweat through the night, mostly on the head, with nose-bleed twice during sleep (after twenty-seven days),[1].—*Thirst.* Great longing for water and wine,[3].—Thirst the whole day (after twenty-one days),[2].—[270.] Thirst, the whole afternoon and evening, contrary to his usual habit (fourth day),[2].—Thirst, especially in the evening,[3].—Thirst, during the chill,[2].—Thirst for cold water,[3].—Thirst for milk, in the morning (after four days),[2].—Much thirst, towards evening, as if she had eaten much salt food,[3].—Unquenchable thirst (after three hours),[1].—*Loss of thirst,*[1].—He had an unnatural thirst; previously he almost never needed to drink,[1].—*Eructations and Hiccough.* Empty eructations, several mornings, fasting,[2].—[280.] *Frequent empty eructations,* even before breakfast,[2].—Eructations, tasting of the breakfast, the whole forenoon,[3].—Eructations of gas,[3].—Inclination to hiccough; it only, however, amounts to half a hiccough, in the forenoon,[2].—Severe, long-lasting hiccough at 1 P.M.,[2]. — Frequent hiccough, an hour after dinner,[2]. — *Nausea.* Qualmishness in the stomach, as if one had not eaten for a long time,[3].— *Great qualmishness in the stomach, with inclination to vomit, in the morning; though only water was vomited; with nausea; this ceased after breakfast,[3].—Nausea,[1][5].—Nausea in the stomach, as if she would vomit, in the forenoon,[2].—[**290.**] Nausea and palpitation, worse on motion; with chilliness,[3].—Nausea and coldness, in the forenoon,[3].—Nausea, with chilliness in the morning, with sticking-tearing toothache, especially on the left side; the pains were relieved by cold water,[3].—Excessive nausea and shuddering, in the morning, so that she could not get warm; followed by vertigo, which relieved the headache,[3].—*Stomach.* Distension and fine twinges in the epigastric region; relieved by passage of offensive flatus at 8 A.M. (seventeenth day),[2].—Gurgling in the stomach, in the morning, relieved after eating (eleventh day),[2].—Gurgling on the left side, near the pit of the stomach, in the evening,[2].—A feeling in the stomach, as if one had fasted, even after eating (twentieth day),[2].—Every morning on rising, it seems as though the stomach was foul, with a nauseous taste in the mouth; after some time this disappears and he has an appetite; for fourteen days in succession,[3].—A cold feeling in the stomach, as if a lump of ice lay in it,[2].—[**300.**] Burning, externally, in the pit of the stomach, together with frequent fine stitches in it, after dinner,[2].

Abdomen.—Hypochondria. Frequent sharp stitches in the right hypochondrium, near the back,[2].—Stitches, with a peculiar indescribable pain, in the right hypochondrium (twelfth day),[2].—Some stitches in the left hypochondrium, and, at the same time, in the left elbow,[2].—Burning stitches in the left hypochondrium, on sitting bent, which disappear on becoming erect,[2].—*Umbilical.* Very transient burning internally about the navel, at 11 A.M.,[2].—Sticking colic about the navel,[3].—Stitches about the navel (after one hour),[3].—Frightful colic in the umbilical region after eating, as if knives were cutting the abdomen, for several minutes (third day),[1].—Twinges about the navel, with griping, in the morning on waking, as if he should go to stool,[3].—*General Abdomen.* Distended abdomen, with pain in it (eighth day),[1].—[**310.**] Distension of the abdomen, with rumbling in it, which disappeared after passing flatus in the morning (fifth day),[2].—Great distension of the abdomen, which constantly increases till midnight, and at last disappears after the passage of flatus (eleventh day),[2]. —Severe rumbling and noises in the abdomen, as if diarrhœa would ensue, though a diarrhœa-like stool occurred only after several hours,[3].—Much rumbling in the bowels, as from a purge, always relieved by passage of flatus,[2].—Very severe rumbling and gurgling in the abdomen, with constipation,[3].—Frequent passage of flatus,[3].—Very frequent passage of loud flatus, followed by distension of the abdomen and colic, at 5 A.M.,[2].—Much passage of flatus, after lying down in bed,[3].—Offensive flatus, especially in the morning and evening (first day),[1].—Offensive flatus, and rumbling in the abdomen, in the evening,[2].—[**320.**] Very violent pain in the abdomen, as if everything were dried up, in the evening in bed (eighth day),[1].—Cold feelings creep about the abdomen,[2].—Pain almost like burning, in both sides of the abdomen, after dinner,[2].—Tension and sticking in the upper part of the abdomen,[3].—Spasmodic pain in the abdomen, especially on inspiration and on drawing in the abdomen (after fourteen days),[1].—Colic, night and morning, with diarrhœa,[3].—(Colic, and some chilliness, always after dinner),[1].—Frightful colic, so that he was obliged to bend quite double, and could not stand erect, with high-colored urine and much thirst (after twenty-four hours),[1].—Sensations of colic in the intestines, in the afternoon, with an inclination to an evacuation,[1].—Colic-pain in the abdomen, with trembling and gnashing of the teeth, on account of coldness, especially after the stool; the pain is very violent, especially in the morning on waking, with distension of the left side of the abdomen and urging to stool; on turning about, or pressing on the abdomen, the side was relieved; it was more severe during rest; stool followed after one hour, was first hard, then fluid, with immediate relief of the pain,[3].—[330.] Twisting pain in the abdomen,[3].—Cutting pain in the forepart of the abdomen, in the morning; was relieved after eating,[1].—Cutting in the abdomen, which extends towards the stomach, and frequently intermitting in the evening; the pains are renewed the next morning and last till noon; only passage of flatus relieves them,[2].—Stitches in the abdomen, as with needles,[3].—Stitches in the abdomen on stooping,[3].—Stitches in the abdomen, with a feeling of discomfort,[3].—Violent twinges in the right side of the upper abdomen, after dinner,[2].—The abdomen is sensitive, internally and externally, so that she could not bear it touched and was obliged to walk bent (eleventh day),[2].—Pains, as from suppuration and tearing, in the abdomen, with diarrhœa and great exhaustion, on the last day of menstruation,[3].—Violent motions in the abdomen, relieved by passage of flatus; with urging to stool, in the evening (fifth day),[2].—[340.] Trembling and cutting in the abdomen, as if diarrhœa would ensue, for a quarter of an hour; relieved after the passage of flatus at 10 A.M.,[2].—*Hypogastrium and Iliac Regions.* Pain in the lower abdomen, extending from the left side to the right, as if the bowels were suppurating,[3].—Violent pain as from constriction in the right groin, relieved by stretching out the body,[2].—Pinching as with two fingers in the right groin,[2].—Frequent sharp stitches in the right groin (fifth day),[2].

Rectum and Anus.—Very violent pressing pain deep in the rectum, extending forward, after the diarrhœa,[2].—Severe itching in the rectum, as from small worms, on riding,[3].—Burning in the anus, continuing a long time, after a watery stool,[2].—Transient stitches through the perineum towards the rectum and genitals,[1].—Urging to stool without effect, with passage of flatus, at 6 A.M.,[2].—Urging to stool, when only a little thin stool of a yellowish color passed, followed by burning in the anus (fifth day),[2].—[350.] Painful urging to stool, followed by three attacks of diarrhœa, and afterwards tenesmus and burning in the anus, with prostration of the whole body (twenty-first day),[2].—After an ordinary stool, a feeling as though diarrhœa would still come on,[2].

Stool.—Diarrhœa. Diarrhœa six times during the day, with cutting pains in the abdomen (eleventh day),[2].—Diarrhœa, with pain, in the morning, with which the abdomen felt as if suppurating,[3].—Diarrhœa, with colic, in the evening,[3].—Diarrhœa, with tearing in the abdomen, and tenesmus in the rectum, at night,[3].—*Diarrhœa, frequently before and during menstruation* (nineteenth day),[2].—Quite watery diarrhœa, four times in succession, with tenesmus and burning in the anus (sixth day),[2].—Frequent fœcal diarrhœa in the morning (fourth, fifth days),[2].—[360.] Profuse diarrhœa, morning and evening,[3].—A stool three or four times a day; he was obliged to make great exertion when the stool, at first hard, then soft, passed,[2].—A soft stool followed soon after the customary evacuation,[3].—An ordinary stool, although he had had the usual stool in the morning, before taking it,[2].—Two liquid stools a day until the thirty-first day, mostly in the forenoon,² —Stool, soft in the morning, hard in the evening (second day),²—Stool normal in the morning, liquid in the afternoon (eleventh day),²—Irregular stool; it occurs at an unusual time of the day and is too hard,¹—Stool more copious than usual,³—Stool soft (sixth day), hard (seventh day),²—[370.] Stool softer and more regular than usual,²³—It seems to make a hard stool soft, as a secondary action,¹—*Constipation.* Constipation for three days,³—No stool the second day,²—No stool on the third day of the menstruation,²—Stool only every second or third day and rather hard,³—The evacuation follows with difficulty and great exertion,³.

Urinary Organs.—Pain in the region of the kidneys,³—*Urethra.* The orifice of the urethra is inflamed and agglutinated,³—Pain in the urethra on urinating, as if the urine passed over a sore place (fourteenth day),¹—[380.] Burning in the urethra when not urinating,³—Burning in the urethra on urinating,³—Burning in the urethra after every urination (second day)²—Stitches in the urethra,³—Itching in the urethra when not urinating,³—Frequent urging to urinate, but only a little urine passed,³—Frequent urging to urinate; she was obliged to rise at night to urinate, and considerable passed,³—Very frequent urging to urinate, with a profuse discharge of urine,³—After urinating, soon again frequent urging thereto; she, however, passed only a few drops,²—*Micturition.* (Frequent urinating with sudden urging),¹—[390.] Increased passage of urine in the afternoon,¹—She passed urine four times in the afternoon and much each time (after four days),²—Urine frequently intermitting on urination,²—*Urine.* Urine clear-yellow, with a slowly forming cloud,²—The urine was yellowish-green, afterwards turbid,²—Urine turbid, like gruel, with violet sediment, for several days in succession,².

Sexual Organs.—*Male.* Burning in the genital organs,³—A red, hard, painful nodule in the skin of the penis, which suppurates (fourteenth day),¹—Emissions two nights in succession, which was once associated with a voluptuous dream (in one who had never had the like before),¹—*Female.* A voluptuous sensation in the genital organs,³—[400.] Soreness on the mons veneris during menstruation,²—Some leucorrhœa for eight days,³—Leucorrhœa after menstruation,²—*Profuse leucorrhœa, of a yellowish-green color, so acrid that it almost corrodes the pudenda and thighs,³—* Very thick, mucous, tenacious leucorrhœa when walking,²—*Discharge of thick leucorrhœa, like the white of an egg, when walking,²—(*Menstruation four days too soon and more profuse than usual,* followed by some leucorrhœa),³—Menstruation eight days too early,³—Menstruation nine days too early and rather profuse (two days after taking it),²—Menstruation nine days too early and more profuse than usual,²—[410.] Menstruation two days too late, coming on in the evening, on lying down; *after midnight painful urging towards the genitals, with great heaviness in the small of the back, which was somewhat relieved the next day with discharge of blood,²—* Menstruation five days too late,²—Menstruation was less than usual and did not continue so long,²—Menstruation did not last as long as usual, and flowed mostly at night,²—*The menses flow most profusely in the morning, but scanty during the day and night,²—The menstrual blood was very watery, with weariness of the thighs,². * Traces of menstruation between the menses* (ninth, tenth, thirteenth, eighteenth days),².

Respiratory Organs.—*Larynx.* Great scraping in the larynx as if sore, extending down into the chest, with much tough mucus in the chest, which threatens to suffocate her; this mucus is raised with difficulty and tastes salty,[3].—Tickling in the larynx provoking cough,[3].—(Frequent irritation to cough from tickling in the larynx; the mucus which she expectorates is very tough and only loosened with great effort),[3].—*Voice.* [420.] Hoarseness every morning,[1].—Catarrhal voice, with roughness in the throat, the whole morning (sixth day),[2].—*Cough.* Cough, excited by tickling in the trachea, in the evening and morning after rising for several days in succession,[2].—Cough caused by tickling in the chest, which she could not suppress in the morning on entering into the room from the cold air (seventeenth day),[2].—Spasmodic cough; difficulty of breathing; deep anxious respiration; in feeble tones she called for help; when the window was raised the fresh air revived her and was very agreeable,[5].—Dry cough in the evening and morning for an hour,[2].—Dry cough in the morning after rising for half an hour (twentieth day),[2].—*Respiration.* Deep, noisy breathing,[5].—Anxious breathing,[5].—Oppressed breathing.[3].—[430.] Shortness of the breath on every exertion of the hands,[3].

Chest.—Feeling of heaviness on the chest, as if something lay upon it, and she could only breathe deeply,[3].—Cutting-burning in the middle of the chest, more externally, twice in succession,[2].—Oppression and heat in the chest, which rises into the head,[3].—Oppression in the middle of the chest, with fine stitches, on breathing,[2].—Oppression of the chest; he was frequently obliged to sigh in order to get a full breath, with which he could not bear anything on the chest, and his large waistband seemed too small,[3]. —A severe pressure extends from the pit of the stomach up into the chest after eating; better when walking, worse when sitting; sometimes with a drawing-tearing pain in the left side of the head,[3].—Stitches in the chest, extending from before backward, increased by deep breathing, during dinner,[3].—Stitches first in the middle of the chest, then in the right hypochondrium, and afterwards in the left (tenth day),[2].—*Front.* Burning on the sternum and visible pulsation, especially in the pit of the stomach,[3].— [440.] Feeling of constriction below the sternum,[3].—Pressure beneath the sternum and in the stomach,[3].—Spasmodic pressure beneath the sternum, as if the stomach were overloaded, six days in succession,[3].—Painful stitches in the middle of the sternum,[2].—Painful dull stitches, or boring, in the sternum, in the evening (third day),[2].—Stitches, frequently in succession, in the forepart of the lower portion of the chest, when standing stooped and without influencing the respiration; after dinner,[2].—*Sides.* A visible pulsation above the right mamma, near the clavicle,[3].—Stitches in the left side of the chest,[3].—Stitches in the right side of the chest, and at the same time in the right great toe,[2].—Stitches, as with an awl, in the upper part of the left mamma, extending through to the back,[3].—[450.] A burning stitch on the outer portion of the left ribs,[2].—A slow, dull stitch in the lowest ribs of the right side in the morning,[2].—Fine stitches in the forepart of the left lowest ribs, which extend up into the chest,[2].—Sharp stitches in the right side of the chest, with constant stretching, in the forenoon,[2].—Sharp stitches in the right side of the chest beneath the axilla, so violent that she cried out, in the morning, third day,[2].—Very sensitive, sharp stitches in the lower portion of the left side of the chest,[2].—Severe sharp stitches below the right ribs, alternating with stitches in the right groin,[2].

Heart.—Fulness and anxiety in the præcordial region (after one hour),[1]. —Pressure in the præcordial region, with tension in the temples, with pressure on the sternum,[3].—Sharp pain in the præcordia (after a few moments),[4]. —[460.] *Palpitation,[3].—Palpitation, with vertigo and headache,[3].—Palpitation in the heart, with congestion to the head, heat and thirst, with itching in the right eye,[3].—Palpitation, with trembling of the whole body and uneasiness,[3].

Neck and Back.—*Neck*. Stiffness in the neck, in the morning, on rising (fourth day),[1].—Painful tension on the right side of the neck, on moving the head, with twitches in the left ear,[2].—Tension and pain on pressure, as from a blow in the neck,[3].—Stitches in the nape of the neck, during rest and motion, in the evening,[2].—Sharp stitches on the left side of the neck, extending into the left ear,[2].—Tearing in the tendons of the left side of the neck,[2].—*Back*. [470.] Sticking and tearing pain on the inner border of the right shoulder-blade, with a feeling as though a piece of it would be torn off, on sitting bent, disappearing on becoming erect,[2].—Several violent stitches, as with a knife, between the shoulders, in the afternoon,[2].—(An old pain in the back, with stiffness after stooping, disappeared), (after seventeen days),° [1].—Sticking pains in the lumbar region, increased on turning the body,[3].

Extremities in General.—*Great weariness in the hands and feet the whole day*,[3].—Suddenly, great weariness in the hands and feet, in the afternoon,[2].

Superior Extremities.—Weariness in the arms, especially in the shoulder-joints,[3].—Loss of power in the left arm,[3].—The left arm felt lame and sprained, so that it was with difficulty that he could raise it above the head; the pain increased during the day so much that at last he could scarcely make any movement with the arm; after sweat in the morning, the pain was very decidedly diminished (fifteenth day),[1].—The right arm was painful and sore to the touch, with pressure in the shoulders,[3].—**Shoulder.** [480.] A previously morbid onion-like smell in the axillæ was very much increased (after three days),[1].—She could not move the right arm freely; she had no power in the shoulder-joint,[3].—Difficult to raise the right arm; she seemed to have no power in the shoulder,[3].—Sensation in the right shoulder-joint as if it was exhausted by great exertion; she had no strength at all in the arm, and if she took hold of anything it pained,[3].—Great tension in the shoulder-joint,[3].—Tension in the shoulder-joints, as if they were too short, on bending the arms backward,[3].—Violent dull stitches and tearings on the inner border of the left shoulder-blade, deep in the bone,[2].—Violent tearing in the right shoulder-joint (after twelve days),[2].—Painful piercing-tearing in the right shoulder-joint, in the afternoon (fifth day),[2].—**Arm.** Violent pain on the inner side of the left upper arm, as if it would break, in the forenoon,[2].—[490.] Violent tearing in the outer side of the left upper arm, especially in the bone, in the afternoon,[2].—Bruised pain in the right upper arm, in the bone, relieved by firmly pressing upon it, in the morning,[2].—**Elbow.** Very sensitive boring-sticking pain beneath the elbows, on the margin of the radius; it extends to the fingers, which become lame on account of it, for two minutes,[3].—Stitches in the right elbow, afterwards in the left also, in the evening,[2].—Tearing in the left elbow, in the morning (after three days),[2].—Severe tearing in the tip of the right elbow,[2].—Painful tearing in the right elbow, in the morning,[2].—**Forearm.** Paralytic and itching sensation in the radial arteries of the forearm (first day),[1].—Sticking and tearing on the inner side of the left forearm,[2].—On the inner side of the forearm, near the thumb, a very sensitive pain, as if the tendons were torn; the same sensation in the other arm, but on the outer side, in the direction of the index finger,[3].—**Wrist.** [500.] A feeling of numbness in the left wrist,[1].—Spasmodic drawing in the tendons of the left wrist,[1].—Sprained and ulcerated pain in the left wrist, in the middle of the upper surface, on a small spot only perceptible to touch or on bending the hand upward and downward,[1]. —Stitches in the right wrist three days in succession; if. she took' hold of anything, especially if she brought the thumb and index finger together, the stitches became more severe; after this ceased in the right hand, it appeared in the left, though only for a short time,[3].—Very sensitive sharp stitches in the right wrist,[2].—Tearing a hand's breadth above the wrist, and extending into it, in the morning,[2].—Tearing and throbbing in the right wrist, in the evening (seventh day),[2].—Pain, as if suppurating, in a small spot on the back of the right wrist, on bending the hand and pressing upon it,[2].—*Hand.* Trembling in the hands, with palpitation and anxiety,[3].—*Loss of power in the hands,[3].—[510.] *She had no power in the hands, especially in the right, *and almost allowed the slightest objects to fall, from weakness*,[3].—The hand is stiff; cannot easily close it; with feeling of weakness in the fingers,[3].—The left hand is heavy; she cannot move it easily,[3].—The right hand feels as heavy as a hundred-weight, together with a severe pain, as if bruised, in the place where the pulse is felt; it does not tolerate any touch,[3].—*Fingers.* (One finger after another suppurates like a panaritium; as soon as one heals, another becomes sore), (after ten weeks),[3].—Stitches in the joints of the right index finger, while working,[3]. —Violent tearing in the left thumb,[2].

Inferior Extremities.—*Hip.* An intermitting pain in the right hip, on stooping, as if the sacrum were broken,[2].—Biting, as from fleas, on the hips and on the abdomen,[3].—*Thigh.* Slight burning on the thigh, above the knee,[2].—[520.] A piercing stitch in the middle of the left thigh, on sitting down,[2].—Sore feeling in the bend of the thigh, during menstruation,[2].—Sore feeling in the bend of the right thigh; in walking, it feels as though something woollen rubbed against it,[2].—*Knee.* A feeling of weariness in the hollows of the knees,[3].—Stiffness and pain in the left knee, if he tries to stretch it out, after it has been bent for some time,[1].—Sticking pain in the left knee, especially on rising from sitting,[1].—Violent stitches in the left knee-joint, nearly the whole forenoon, on rest and motion; she thought that she could not endure it (second day),[2].—Violent sharp stitches on the inner side of the right knee, as if in the bone,[2].—Sensation above the knee-cap, as if it had been bruised,[3].—*Leg.* The right leg is very much asleep; the same in any position, for a quarter of an hour, in the afternoon (first day),[1].—[530.] The whole left leg is so sleepy, with crawling, as from ants upon it, that she cannot stand upon it,[2].—Very weary pain in the right lower leg, during menstruation,[2].—Raging or beating pain in the right fibula, with tearing extending up to the knee, in the afternoon (sixth day),[2].—Cramp in the left leg,[1].—Cramp in the calves towards morning, in bed; it was so violent that the pain continued till evening, as if the leg were too short (after fourteen days),[1].—Transient stitches in the left leg, and in the chest,[1].—Sharp stitches in the middle of the left tibia (second day),[2].—*Ankle.* Sharp stitches in the right external malleolus, together with painfulness of the inner malleolus (third day),[2].—*Foot.* Heaviness of the feet,[3].—Drawing and tearing in the right foot,[3].—[540.] Tearing dragging-drawing pain in a foot which had been sprained in childhood, as if the joint had been broken, with swelling of the foot, so that she could not put on the shoe,[3].—Pain in the forepart of the left sole, when walking, for several days (twenty-ninth day),[2].—Burning in the left sole,[3].—*Toes.* Stitches in both great toes, extending into the ankles, in the evening,[3].—Pain in the corns,[3].—Extremely violent pain in a corn, for a long time (after eighteen days),[1].—Stitches in the corns,[3].

General Symptoms.—Objective. Frequent stretching, without sleepiness,[2].—* *Very awkward; everything falls from his hands*,[3].—**Debility.** Feels very weary,[1].—[**550.**] Very weary the whole day,[3].—Very weary and exhausted, after a walk (sixth and seventh days),[1].—Great weariness, obliging her to sleep after dinner (fifteenth day),[1].—Excessive weariness, in the evening, after eating (first day),[1].—Excessive weariness, during and after dinner (fourth day),[1].—Such loss of strength that she could neither rise nor hold her head up,[5].—A sudden attack like faintness, at noon, when sitting down, as if objects turned bottom upwards (third day),[1].—When trying to walk, she fell down in a swoon; her limbs and body became stiff,[5]. —Although everything was done to restore her, she again fell down and remained motionless; she was in despair,[5].—**Restlessness.** She found no rest,[3].—[**560.**] Uneasiness, anxiety, unpleasant warmth, and heaviness in the abdomen, and alternating sensations of coldness through the whole body,[1].—**Sensations.** (He feels as if intoxicated by wine),[3].—General anxiety and weakness of body, eructations, nausea, distension in the abdomen, passage of flatus, frequent yawning, and stretching of the limbs, with irresistible desire to sleep (after two hours),[1].—Bruised feeling in the whole body, especially in the joints of the arm and the abdominal muscles, on motion and touch (fourteenth day),[1].

Skin.—*The skin of the fingers becomes unusuall dented by the instruments with which she was working (shears or knives),[3].—*Eruptions, Dry.* Goose-flesh over the whole body, with severe itching,[1].— *The corners of the mouth are broken out*,[3].—Very severely itching small spots, like a tetter, on the right side below the chin; the itching was not relieved by scratching,[3].—A painful eruption on the temple,[3].—Itching eruption on the throat,[3].—[**570.**] A small reddish swelling, hard to touch, like a boil, on the right leg,[3].—Pimples over the whole body, with very severe itching,[3].—Itching and small pimples on the head (after three weeks),[1].—Large, scattered pimples, papulous, on the forehead, without itching (seventh day),[2].—Several tensive pimples on the upper and lower lip (after twenty days),[2].—Several pimples on the left side, near the mouth, without itching,[2].—An itching pimple, which itches still worse after scratching, on the forepart of the neck,[2].—An eruption of hard, red pimples, as large as peas, which itch very much, and burn, and then disappear after some days, on the chest, on the left hand, and on the left foot; after scratching the itching is worse,[3].—*The hands are covered with small, dry, reddish pimples, which gradually disappear after a few days,[1].—Several pimples, which do not itch, on the back of the hand, and between the middle and ring fingers,[2].—[**580.**] An itching pimple above the knee,[3].—A pimple on the tibia, with a sensation as if burnt,[3].—*Eruption on both feet of small, red, rash-like pimples, with an itching-burning pain, with which the feet are covered, as far as half way up the calves; lasting two days, scratching does not affect them,[3].—*Moist.* A number of small vesicles containing water, about the left corner of the mouth (after twenty days),[2].—White blisters on the right hand, with red areola, and great itching; they disappear after half an hour,[3].—Small, red, sore, painful blisters on the backs of both feet, and at the roots of the toes,[3].—*Pustular.* (A panaritium appeared from a small prick of a needle),[3].—An itching, maturating eruption on the forehead,[3].—Maturating eruption in the left corner of the mouth, on the chin, and on the forehead,[3].—A previously existing wart developed a red point, suppurated and disappeared (after twenty-one days)[1].—[**590.**] Two longish, flattened pustules, filled with matter, under the nose, upon which a scab remained for more than fourteen days (after eleven days),[2].— An ulcer in the right ear, with pain in it, on swallowing,[1].—***Sensations, General.*** Itching on the body, on the lower jaw, on the left side, extending to behind the ear ; on the left side of the neck, on the abdomen, on the right arm, on the inner margin of the right foot, on the heel, over the whole body, especially on the hands, and on the head,[2][3].—Itching over various parts of the body, with red pimples,[1].—Itching over the whole body, in the evening, followed by the appearance of tetter (tenth day),[1].—***Local.*** Creeping, as from insects, on the back, at night,[2].—Violent itching, which always returns after scratching, on the forepart of the scalp, on the inner side of the right upper arm, and on the left shoulder,[2].—Itching, which was not relieved by scratching, on the left side of the head, on the nose, on the chest, on the abdomen, on the inner side of the right upper arm, on the inner side of the left forearm, on the right hip, on the inner side of the thigh, here and there on the limbs,[2].—Itching, which was relieved by scratching, on the forehead, on the right side of the nose, on the right shoulder, on the left hip, on the inner side of the right knee, in the hollows of the knees, in the right sole,[2].—Itching in the ear, which disappeared on boring in with the finger,[2].—[**600.**] Itching in the ears and eyes,[3].—Constant itching on the forepart of the nose, which does not disappear after scratching,[2].—Itching in the upper part of the right nostril, with ineffectual attempts to sneeze,[2].—Itching, which becomes worse after scratching, near the nose, beneath the lower jaw, below the right hip,[2].—Severe itching on the chest; after scratching, small itching pimples appeared,[2].—Itching on the left side of the chest, which caused a fine eruption ; disappeared the next day (fifth day),[2].—*Severe itching on the coccyx, so that he was obliged to scratch it till sore, whereupon a crust appeared,* which remained some days (after one day),[1].—Violent itching on the arms, always at evening, and after washing, biting and burning in them (after three weeks),[1].—Itching and biting in the arms, repeated daily, especially in the evening, and also in the morning after washing,[1].—Extraordinary itching in the right arm, for several days (ninth day),[1].—[**610.**] Burning-itching on both forearms, in the region of the pulse, not relieved by scratching, in the evening (seventh day),[2].—Violent itching on the right forearm ; the place remains red and burning a long time after scratching,[2].—Severe itching on the inner side of the right forearm, not relieved by scratching, but a number of small itching pimples appeared,[2].—Severe itching on the inner side of the left forearm ; she was obliged to scratch it till it bled,[2].—Violent itching on the right knee, which disappeared only after scratching a long time,[2].

Sleep and Dreams.—Sleepiness. Much yawning, in the evening,[3].—Frequent yawning, with sleepiness, in the afternoon at five,[2].—*Great sleepiness early in the evening,*[3].—Very sound, quiet sleep at night, and when he arose later than usual in the morning, great weariness, especially in the limbs,[1].—Sleep after eating, quite contrary to his habit,[3].—[**620.**] Sleepiness during dinner (third day),[2].—Great sleepiness, after dinner (fifth day),[1]. —***Sleeplessness.*** Little sleep,[3].— Uneasy sleep, with much tossing about the bed,[3].—Very restless night, she awoke every hour,[2].—When he awoke at night from a very sound sleep, he did not seem to know where he was,[3].— ***Dreams.*** Sleep full of dreams,[3].—Dreams of past and future events,[3].— Many dreams of subjects of previous conversation, in a sound sleep,[3].— Tiresome dreams,[2].—[**630.**] Anxious dreams of serpents which had bitten her; that she would die; that she had a bleeding wound, etc.; whereupon she awoke and continued anxious a long time after waking (after fifth day),[2].—Vexatious dreams, and waking every moment through the night,[1]. —Frightful dreams, that she was in a cellar and the walls were falling in; that she was obliged to remain and could not get out,[2].—Dreams of danger of drowning, and that some one had fallen into the water,[2].—A dream of ghosts, whereupon she awoke frightened,[2].—Unremembered dreams (after four days),[1].

Fever.—Chilliness. He was chilly the whole day, with cold hands,[1].—She was constantly chilly on the uncovered parts, on the neck and chest, and was obliged to bind cloths about them, even at night (third and fourth days),[2].—Although she sat by a warm stove she was chilly the whole day (second day)[2].—Chilliness at 5 A.M., in bed, three mornings in succession,[2].—[**640.**] Chilliness every morning from six to nine, cold to touch externally, with griping in the abdomen, without subsequent heat, and without thirst,[1].—*Chilliness the whole evening*, she could not get warm (fourth day),[2].—Chilliness in the evening, lasting the whole night (eleventh day),[2].—A shaking chill lasting a few moments, in the evening, on lying down in a warm room (after fifteen days),[1].—Shivering and coldness, during supper,[3].—Chilliness with thirst, with tension and stitches in the throat, so that she could not turn her head easily, also with sticking in the chest,[3].— Constant cold hands and feet,[1].—Feet very cold at night, could not be warmed,[3].—*Intermitting fever of eight days' duration; severe chill every evening from seven till ten*, commencing with chilliness in the back, the first day with thirst, without subsequent heat or sweat; every time with violent drawing pain in the abdomen (after four days),[1].—Chilliness, with glowing heat of the face,[3].—*Heat.* [**650.**] Orgasm of blood, with thirst,[3].—Increased warmth in the whole body, in the afternoon (third day),[2].—Great warmth and sweat over the body, in the evening (first day),[2].—Frequent flushes of heat,[3].—Much heat and thirst, the whole day,[3].—Heat, anxiety and restlessness, the whole day,[3].—Frequent heat and oppression of the chest, so that he was obliged to be uncovered, whereupon he felt better,[3].— *Sweat.* Sweat, especially upon the chest, every morning from five to six, for eight days in succession,[3].—Profuse sweat under the arms, when walking slowly in a cold temperature (first day),[1].

Conditions.—Aggravation.—(Morning), For an hour after rising, peevish mood; head confused, etc.; on rising from chair, kind of vertigo, etc.; dizziness; on waking, at 3 o'clock, headache; after walking in open air, pressive headache; pressive headache; on moving about, pain, etc., on left forehead; tearing in forehead; tearing on vertex, etc.; 7 o'clock, on going from room into cold air, beating, etc., in right head; 7 o'clock, stitches in left occiput; itching on head; lachrymation; on rising, seems as though veil before eyes; after rising, stopped coryza; after waking, sneezing; after rising, face pale; on waking, teeth, etc., full of blood; yellow-coated tongue; after waking, burning in tip of tongue, etc.; after waking, numbness of mouth, etc.; on waking, dryness in throat; scraping in throat; after rising, rawness of throat; thirst for milk; fasting, empty eructations; qualmishness in stomach, etc.; nausea, etc.; gurgling in stomach; on rising, stomach feels foul, etc.; on waking, twinges about navel; 5 o'clock, passage of flatus, etc.; offensive flatus; on waking, colic pain in abdomen; pain in right arm; pain in abdomen; diarrhœa, etc.; fœcal diarrhœa; profuse diarrhœa; hoarseness; after rising, cough; on entering room from cold air, cough; dry cough; after rising, dry cough; stitches in right ribs; stitches in side of chest; on rising, stiffness in neck; tearing in right elbow; tearing above the wrist; after washing, itching, etc., in arms; 5 o'clock, in bed, chilliness; 6 to 9 o'clock, chilliness; 5 to 6 o'clock, sweat.—(*Forenoon*), Pain in occiput; eructations; inclination to hiccough; nausea in stomach; nausea, etc.; 11 o'clock, burning about navel; liquid stools; stitches in side of chest, etc.; pain in left arm; stitches in knee-joint.—(*Noon*), Attack, like faintness.—(*Afternoon*), During violent headache, peevish, etc.; 2 P.M., twitching in the brain; raging in left temple; till evening, pressure on occiput; in warm room, stitches in occiput; tearing in left ear; 5 o'clock, tickling in throat; hunger; sensation of colic in intestines, etc.; increased passage of urine; stitches between shoulders; weariness in hands, etc.; pain in shoulder-blade; tearing in left arm; right leg asleep; pain in right fibula; 5 o'clock, yawning, etc.; warmth in whole body.—(*Toward evening*), Out of humor, etc.; weary; dry mouth; thirst.—(*Evening*), Vertigo; head stupid, etc.; 8 o'clock, pain in left forehead; stitches in middle of forehead; stitches in forehead; stitches in side of vertex; especially in bright light, confusion, etc., in occiput; gnashing of teeth; in bed, toothache; boring in teeth; in bed, digging in hollow teeth; drawing toothache; drawing in hollow teeth; in bed, during menstruation, *pain in hollow teeth;* sore throat; rawness in throat; thirst; gurgling on left side; offensive flatus; offensive flatus, etc.; in bed, pain in abdomen; diarrhœa, etc.; profuse diarrhœa; cough; dry cough; stitches in sternum; stitches in nape of neck; stitches in right elbow; tearing in left elbow; tearing, etc., in wrist; stitches in great toes; after eating, weariness; itching all over; itching on the arms; itching, etc., in arms; itching on forearms; yawning; early, *great sleepiness; chilliness;* shaking chill; warmth, etc., over the body.—(*Night*), Pain in head, on raising it; nose stopped; stitches in sound teeth; diarrhœa, etc.; feet cold.—(*Before midnight*), Drawing toothache.—(*Toward morning*), In bed, cramp in calves.—(*Open air*), Feeling in brain disappears.—(*Bending hand and pressing on it*), Pain on back of wrist.—(*On bending arms backward*), Tension in shoulder-joints.—(*Deep breathing*), Stitches in chest.—(*Bringing thumb and index finger together*), Stitches in wrist.—(*During chill*), Thirst.—(*After coition*), Head confused.—(*Cold*), Pain in hollow tooth.—(*After the diarrhœa*), Pain in rectum.—(*During dinner*), Feeling of contraction, etc., over left eye; stitches in chest; weariness; sleepiness.—(*After dinner*), Averse to everything; sticking above left eye; hiccough; burning in pit of stomach; colic, etc.; pain in abdomen; colic twinges in upper abdomen; when standing stooped, stitches in chest; *weariness;* sleepiness.—(*Drawing in the abdomen*), Pain in abdomen.—(*After eating*), Pressure into chest.—(*On exerting hands*), Shortness of breath.—(*Inspiration*), Pain in abdomen.—(*Lying*), Headache.—(*After lying down in bed*), Passage of flatus.—(*Before menstruation*), *Diarrhœa.—(During menstruation*), Pressure, etc., in right orbit, etc.; diarrhœa; sore feeling in bend of thigh; pain in right leg.—(*After menstruation*), Leucorrhœa.—(*Motion*), Nausea, etc.; bruised feeling all over.—(*During rest*), Colic pain in abdomen.—(*On riding*), Itching in rectum.—(*On rising*), Vertigo; attacks of vertigo, etc.—(*Rising from sitting*), Pain in left knee.—(*On rising from stooping*), Dizzy, etc.—(*In room*), After being in open air, pressive headache.—(*Scratching*), *Itching of the pimple;* itching near nose, etc.—(*Sitting*), Pressure into chest; stitch in middle of thigh.—(*On sitting bent*), Stitches in left hypochondrium; stitches, etc., on right shoulder-blade.—(*Standing*), Vertigo, etc.—(*After stool*), Colic pain in abdomen.—(*On stooping*), Head confused; heaviness in head; stitches in the abdomen.—(*During supper*),

Shivering, etc.—(*Touch*), Bruised feeling all over.—(*Turning body*), Pains in lumbar region.—(*On urinating*), Burning in urethra.—(*On waking*), Headache.—(*When walking*), Leucorrhœa; pain in sole.—(*After a walk*), Weary, etc.—(*On becoming warm*), Itching over whole scalp.—(*While working*), Stitches in finger-joint.

Amelioration.—(*Morning*), Exhilarated; after sweat, pain in left arm.—(*Evening*), Cutting in abdomen intermits.—(*Toward morning*), Pain in head.—(*Open air*), Toothache.—(*After breakfast*), Qualmishness.—(*Cold water*), Toothache.—(*After eating*), Numbness of mouth; gurgling in stomach; pain in abdomen.—(*On becoming erect*), Stitches on right shoulderblade.—(*Passage of flatus*), Distension, etc., in epigastric region; rumbling in bowels; cutting in abdomen; motions in abdomen.—(*Firm pressure*), Pain in right upper arm.—(*Pressing on abdomen*), Colic pain in abdomen. —(*After rising*), And eating, dryness in throat.—(*Sucking blood out of teeth*), Stitches in teeth.—(*Turning about*), Colic pain in abdomen.—(*Vertigo*), Headache.—(*Walking*), Pressure in chest.—(*Warmth*), Toothache.

BROMIUM.

The pure elementary substance (Bromine).

Preparation. Tincture, and dilutions with distilled water.

Authorities. (1 to 17 *from Hering's résumé, Neues Archiv*, 2, 3; when the preparation used is not noted with the symptom or referred to in this list, it is understood to be the 30th); 1, Lippe, provings on himself, a young woman, and on others; 2, C. Hering, provings on himself and others, including a girl and a married woman; 3, F. Hausemann, provings on himself with different potencies, from the 30th to the 3d, for several months; 4, Schmid, a.; 5, Schmid, b.; 6, Schmid, c.; 7, Neidhard; 8, Heimerdinger, inaug. dis. Tübingen, 1837, took 5 and afterward 8 drops of Brom. in distilled water; 9, Höring, inaug. dis. Tübingen, 1838, took daily in the morning a teaspoonful of a solution of 6 drops in $\frac{1}{2}$ an oz. of water, afterward increasing doses to 9 drops; 10, Lœwig; 11, N. N.; taken from Noak and Trinks; 12, Gosewich, provings on himself and others; 13, Fournet, from Trousseau and Pidoux, took two drops in some gum arabic water; 14, Butzke, Dissert. Berol., 1828, took daily 3 to 13 drops of a solution of $\frac{1}{2}$ dr. of Brom. in 4 ozs. of water; 15, "Ch. W" (in Hering); 16, Franz, Berlin. Jahrb. f. Pharm., 1828, effects of the vapors (he also made numerous experiments on various animals); 17, Carwig (from Hering); 18, Lembke, A. H. Z., 37, 115 et seq., provings with the 1st; 19, ibid., provings with the 3d; 20, ibid., provings with the 2d; 21, ibid., provings with the $\frac{1}{20}$th; 22, Czerwiakovski, De Brom. (from Roth); 23, Glover, Edin. Med. Journ., 58, 120 (ibid.); 24, Dublin Press, 1850 (ibid.); 25, Duffield, case of poisoning, N. Y. Med. Record, 2, 323 (from Detroit Rev. of Med. and Pharm.); 26, Berridge, N. E. Med. Gaz., 9, 403, proving of Miss A. B., with the cm. of Fincke.

Mind.—He becomes averse to his business; it seems as though he must relinquish it,[1].—Lively mood in a hypochondriac,[1].—Lively disposition,[18]. —Apathy, weakness,[18].—Taciturn,[1].—Disconcerted, with increased sensation of warmth in the head,[18].—In the evening some apprehensiveness, oppression of the heart and some headache.—No action on the pulse or heart, rather upon respiration (after he had taken the drug for sixteen days increasing to fourteen drops; having taken in all 132 drops),[9].—In the evening when alone it seems as though he was obliged to look about him, and would somewhere see an apparition (from the 3d),[3].—He is unusually out of humor for five days (from the 3d),[1].—[10.] Fretfulness,[1].—Quarrelsomeness,[1].—Consciousness is not disturbed,[24].—*Desire for mental labor*,[1].—Great activity in business,[1].—Indisposition for mental work,[18].—Disinclined to read,[18].—The previous desire to read disappears,[18].—The thoughts are difficult to fix upon any object; the condition of the patient yesterday was difficult to call to mind (after six hours),[18].—Loss of ideas,[18].—[20.] Lack of ideas,[18].—Very great forgetfulness,[2].

Head.—Confusion and Vertigo. Confusion of the head,[11].—Confusion of the head as if a hoop were about it the whole day, causing vertigo,[6].—Confusion in the head the whole day (after the fourth dose),[5].—Confusion of the head, especially in the forehead; pressure on the brows and root of the nose, frequently affecting a small place above the eyes alternately in one or the other side,[6].—Confusion of the head, with heaviness (half an hour),[18].—Incipient vertigo,[18].—Commencing vertigo (first day),[19].—Vertigo, especially at evening on lying down, with confusion of the head,[1].—[30.] Vertigo, worse in damp weather,[2].—Vertigo, especially if crossing a little running water.[1].—Vertigo as soon as he steps the foot over water; the foot is drawn involuntarily in the direction of the stream,[1].†—Vertigo, with nausea (twelve minutes after 8 drops),[8].—Vertigo, with tendency to fall backward (second day), (from the 6th),[3].—Vertigo, with a feeling as if one would fall to the ground, with flushes of heat (after one and a half hours),[18].—Vertigo, with bleeding at the nose and subsequent headache (from the fumes),[10].—A slight vertigo, with nausea, continued inclination to vomit, without, however, actual vomiting, six minutes after 5 drops,[8].—Dizziness in the head (after half an hour),[18].—Dizziness in the head (second day),[18].

General Sensations.—[40.] Headache as a consequent symptom,[10].—Violent headache throughout the whole head for two hours, 3 to 4 P.M. (third day), (from first),[2].—Dizzy headache in the morning on waking, with itching over the whole body, especially on the chest and between the shoulders,[6].—Toward evening in rather damp weather pains in the bones of the head, mostly in the forehead and occiput (second day),[19].—A sensation deep in the brain soon after dinner (that was eaten with little appetite), as if apoplexy were imminent; a sensation as if he would lose his senses and have vertigo, equally severe when walking or sitting, lasting a quarter of an hour,[18].—Slight headache, with here and there vertigo,[9].—Headache, especially in the forehead, alternating with pain in the small of the back,[6].—Headache and severe stitches in the lung if he attempts to breathe deeply; he is obliged to cough frequently; the pulse is full and hard, in the beginning somewhat slow, afterwards from 80 to 85 (several hours after twenty to thirty drops),[9].—Bursting pain in the head, more on the left side (from fifth),[3].—Pressive pain over the whole head immediately,[12].—[50.] Dull pressive headache,[11].—*Forehead.* He must keep the forehead wrinkled,[18].—Confusion in the forehead,[6].—Heaviness in the forehead,[18].—Pain at times in the frontal bones,[18].—Pain in the frontal bone in the evening, with stitches in the larynx,[18].—Headache in the forehead for several days,[6].—Pain in the forehead after dinner (second day),[1].—Stupefied headache in the forehead worse during rest, disappearing during riding,[1].—Pain and pressure in the forehead (soon),[18].—[60.] Pain in the forehead, with pres-

† In a strong young man who was not otherwise nervous, C. Hg.

sure; sense of heaviness and increased warmth,[18].—The pain over the left eye extends into the forehead, with a burning sensation and an oppressive benumbing pain,[4].—Boring in the left side of the frontal bone.[18].—Severe boring in the left side of the frontal bone,[21].—Pressure in the left frontal bone, then in the right,[21].—Pressure in the frontal bone with confusion in the forehead,[21].—Long-continued pressure in the frontal bones, in the room, not in the open air (half an hour),[20].—Pressure in the forehead,[18].—Pressure in the right frontal eminence,[18].—Pressure in the forehead above the eyes,[18].—[70.] Pressure in the forehead, with heaviness in the head, with disinclination to think,[18].—Pressive pain in the forehead,[18].—Pressive pain in the forehead (second day),[19].—Pressive pain in the forehead several times, soon disappearing,[19].—Dull pressive pain in the forehead,[18].—A hot pressive headache in the forehead extending inward; throbbing and extending to the maxillary bone, at 9 A.M.,[6].—Pressive headache, as if digging over the eyes,[5].—Pressive pain in the forehead, deep in the eyes, with sensitiveness of the eyes when reading (fourth day),[19].—Dull pressive headache in the forehead in the morning, from which the eyes become affected (thirteenth day) after repeated doses,[3].—Pain in the forehead, as if everything would press outward, in the forenoon,[5].—[80.] Slight pressive pain in the forehead, especially on coughing,[18].—Tearing in the frontal bones,[18].—

Temples, etc. Rather severe pressure in the bone in the left temple (after three hours),[18].—Painful pressure in the left temple, together with a constant dizzy feeling in the head,[2].—Pressure on the vertex,[21].—Left-sided headache,[1].—Pain on the left side of the head (from 5th),[3].—Pain in the left side of the head, which extends to the left eye (from the 3d),[3] —Headache from the left ear to the left temple, aggravated by stooping,[1].—Slight drawing in the left side of the head (from the 8th),[3].—[90.] Pressure in the right anterior lobe of the brain and in the right side of the nasal bone (first day),[3].—Tearing in the right side of the cranial bones,[19].—Stitching pain through the right side of the head (from the 3d),[3].—*Headache after drinking milk,* like a severe throbbing, and a hard pulse in the left side; relieved if he lies upon the right side with his arms over his head,[12].—Trickling-crawling in the left half of the head and on the left cheek (afternoon of second day),[3].—Headache; heaviness in the occiput, *in the heat of the sun; goes away in the shade* (from the 1st),[7].—Heat in the occiput,[18].—Crawling beneath the skin of the occiput.[18].

Eyes.—Eye in General. Clonic spasms in the muscles of the eyes, in the face, and in the limbs,[11].†—Severe inflammation of the eyes,[11]. —[100.] The right eye becomes inflamed and dim, with lachrymation,[3].—Pain over the right eye with photophobia (after two and a half hours),[18].—Slight pain, frequently in and above the right eye, with some inflammation of the conjunctiva (first day), (from 1st),[2].—Distressing burning in the eyes, with spasmodic closing of the orbicularis and increased lachrymation; confusion of the head, with severe pressure upon the chest, and cough (from inhaling the vapor),[8].—Paroxysmal pressive pain in the eyes and root of the nose, as if extending from the interior of the brain toward the vertex,[6].—Sticking in the eyes and in the chest,[11].—*Stitches through the left eye,*[3].—*External Parts.* Dull, pressing, stupefied pain (a dead pain) over the left eye,[4].—Sticking sensation about the orbits,[11].—Trickling

---

† Compare twitchings in the face and hands with violent burning and scraping in the throat, etc. All the convulsions noticed in animals are only fatal symptoms and without any value. (C. Hg.)

in the left arcus superciliaris (afternoon of second),³.—[110.] The eyes will
close, as if sleepy,¹⁸.—The lids are very heavy; he can only open and keep
them open with great difficulty, with coldness of the lids (from the 3d),³.—
Stitches in the lids of the left eye when reading (second day),¹⁸.—
(*Throbbing stitches in the left upper lid, extending to the brow, the forehead, and left temple; increased by external pressure, motion, and stooping;
relieved by rest; a pain which unfits him for every work),¹.†—Biting in
the margins of the lids (one hour),²¹.—Cutting in the right inner canthus,
then in the outer,²¹.—Severe cutting in the right inner canthus; the next
day the same symptom in the left inner canthus,¹⁸.—Stitches in the canthi,¹⁸.
—Stitches in the right inner canthus,²¹.—Itching above the right external
canthus, relieved by scratching (from 8th),³.—[120.] Distended tortuous
vessels in the conjunctiva bulbi of both eyes, with stitches in the lids,¹⁸.—
Ocular conjunctiva dull and wrinkled,²⁴.—Biting in the conjunctiva palp.,¹⁸.
—Increased lachrymation (from the vapor),⁹.—*Lachrymation of. the right
eye* (from 5th),³ etc.—***Pupils and Vision.*** Pupils normal,²⁴.—A kind
of vanishing of sight when sitting and reading in the evening, as if a wind
before the eyes took away the power of sight (from the vapor),².—Daylight
is somewhat sensitive to the eyes,¹⁸.—Sensitiveness of the eyes to bright
light,¹.—Some photophobia,¹⁸—[130.] Photophobia, with pressure on moving
the eyes,¹⁸.—A gray point before the right eye moving up and down with
the movement of the eye, on looking into the distance and also near to
(one hour),¹⁸.—Lightnings before the eyes,¹.—Illusions of vision; it seemed
as though all kinds of things jumped up on the ground before her,¹.—Illusions of fantasy; it seems to him as though strange persons were looking
over his shoulder (from the 30th),¹.‡

Ears.—Pain in the right ear, appears and disappears at the same time
as a tickling on the right cheek (in the afternoon of second day),³.—Towards evening a burning sensation in the left ear, as if a coal or hot water
were in it,⁴.—Dull pain deep in the right ear,²¹.—Pressive earache, as if
internal around the ear, first in the left, then in the right, in the evening
before going to sleep,¹².—Pressure as with a plug in the upper part of the
left ear, followed by sticking in the tip of the tongue (morning of third
day),¹⁸.—[140.] Sharp stitches behind the left ear (one hour),²¹.—Stitches
deep in the right ear,¹⁸.—Stitches deep in the right ear, with heat in the
whole ear and great sensitiveness of the head to cold air (second day),¹⁹.—
Stitches in the right ear (one hour),¹⁸.—Stitches deep in the left ear,²¹.—
Throbbing in the ears,¹.—Tickling in the right lavator auris, behind the
right ear, on the lobule of the left ear, relieved by scratching (from the 8th),³.
—Tickling on the margin of the right ear (from the 7th),³.—Noise of distant rushing in the ears,¹⁸.—Continued rush in the right ear,¹⁸.—[150.]
Ringing in the right ear as if full of bells,⁵.—Constant roaring in the ears,
worse in the left (from first to third day),¹.—Roaring in the ears, and in the
morning the right ear feels closed (fourth day),¹⁹.

Nose.—Objective and Discharges. Some twitchings in the
right side of the nose (first day),³.—Severe inflammatory affection of the
mucous membrane of the nose, fauces, and respiratory organs, has been

---

† (This symptom occurred in a young watchmaker, who had suffered every two or
three weeks for several years; it generally continued three or four days. A very
marked aggravation after Bromine X, improvement in one hour and no return
after seven weeks.)° Lippe.

‡ (The provers of the last two symptoms were in different places, proved at very
different times, and did not know one another's symptoms. C. Hg.)

noticed since taking Bromine, also palpitation of the heart, frequently, at times when walking, at times on rising from chair,[1b].—Swelling and pain in the left side of the nose on pressing it, as if a boil were forming (from the 3d),[2].—Ulceration in the left nostril like crust, with tingling under it (second day),[3].—Crusts in the right nostril, second day; crusts in the nostrils, especially in the right, in the morning of third day,[3].—Much mucus in the nose, sometimes with streaks of blood, in the afternoon (second day),[18].— Much tough white mucus, mostly in the right nostril; sometimes pieces of tough yellow mucus in both nostrils (second day),[19].—[160.] Yellowish mucus from the nose, and yellowish expectoration,[18].—The nose is stopped by mucus (fifth day),[19].—Stopped nose, scanty mucus (one hour),[18].—Stoppage of the nose, together with fluent coryza, with lachrymation of the right eye,[3].—Sneezing,[18].—Sneezing (first day),[19].—Sneezing a few times,[18] [19]. —Sneezing several times (after four hours),[18].—Sneezing frequently,[18].— Violent shattering sneezing, followed immediately by stoppage of the nose (from 5th),[3].—[170.] Much sneezing, which is frequently repeated (after several days) ; nasal mucus is secreted in large quantities, especially in the posterior portion of the nares; at times the mucus is very watery, mixed with streaks of blood; at other times there is obstinate dryness in the nose,[18]. —Coryza for two days,[18].—Coryza with stoppage of the right nostril (from 8th),[3].—*Severe coryza, whereby the right nostril is stopped and sore throughout (evening of second day),[3].—Continued coryza, with discharge from the right nostril, and at the same time stoppage of it (from 3d),[3].—*Long-continued obstinate coryza, with soreness beneath the nose, and on the margin of the nose (from 5th),[3].—*Fluent coryza, in which the right nostril is more affected and more stopped, afterwards the left (from 6th),[3].—*Fluent coryza, with frequent violent sneezing; corrosive soreness under the nose and on the margins of the nose (second day), (from 6th),[3].—Several drops of blood after blowing the nose (second day),[18].—Nose-bleed after slight blowing of the nose, on the right side,[18].—[180.] On the third morning, on blowing the nose some blood from the right nostril,[18].—On blowing the nose, some blood from the left nostril,[18].—Some blood from the left side of the nose on blowing it; the blood is bright red,[18].—Nose-bleed after oppression of the chest (from fumes),[10].—Nose-bleed for twelve minutes, with relief of the chest and eye symptoms (from fumes),[8].—Awoke with nose very cold, subjectively and objectively (second and third nights),[26].—It seemed to him as if a fluent coryza would appear, with soreness in the right nostril, as if he had pulled out some hairs ; with dim eyes, and violent pain in the right ribs, and little appetite (from the fumes); the same symptoms returned afterwards, from the fumes mixed with iodine,[2].—Pain on the right side of the tip of the nose (from the 5th),[3].—Pain in the left compressor nasi on pressing upon it (from the 5th),[3].—Momentary pressure in the nasal and superior maxillary bones, and in various places in the frontal bones,[20].—[190.] Soreness in the nose, and crusts,[3].—* The whole nose is sore, and the wings of the nose swollen; a scurf forms in it, with pain and bleeding on wiping it (from 7th),[3].—Soreness and swollen feeling, first around the lamilla and then in the wings of the nose, then crusts; and also constant crustiness of the right nostril, which bleeds after removing it (from 7th),[3].—Smarting beneath the right nostril (first day),[2].—Slight crawling, at first below the left nostril, then on the right cheek (from 8th),[3].—Tickling in the nose (half an hour),[18].—Tickling in the nose, as if he would sneeze immediately,[21].—Tickling in the left side of the tip of the nose (from 7th),[3].—Tickling in the left nostril, afterwards in the right (from 8th),[3].—Itching in the nose, with continued smell of Bromine,[18].

Face.—[200.] Pale color of the face soon after eight drops,[8].—Hot unpleasant sensation in the face, especially below the nose, tickling-smarting *as from cobwebs, especially on moving the nose,* together with fluent coryza and lachrymation of the right eye (from 5th),[3].—Sensation in the cheeks, more in the right, afterwards in the left (first day), (from 30th); also in the left (from 7th),[3].—Tension in the left cheek extending to the lower jaw, at times with pressive pain extending into the left ear (second day), (from 3d),[1].—Tickling on the left cheek and left side of the head (from 7th),[2].—Tickling on the left malar bone, afternoon (second day), (from 8th),[3].—Tickling on the right cheek relieved by scratching (from 8th),[2].—Tickling crawling in the middle of the left cheek, first day, more in the left cheek (second day),[3].—Pain in the left zygoma, and stitches in the ear, then the same pain in the right side,[2].—Pain in the left zygoma in the evening, then stitching in the left ear, then pain in the right zygoma (from 7th),[3].—[210.] Pain in the upper lip as if it were bruised, and in this place, extending from the right corner of the mouth, several yellowish spots as large as the head of a pin, which seem to lie beneath the epithelium and contain a yellowish fluid; the sensitiveness of the part is not great,[18].—Burning of the upper lip, which therewith feels very smooth (from 3d),[3].—A momentary sensation as if the middle part of the upper lip and the neighboring portion of the nose were stretched,[21].—Soreness of the upper lip, with coryza and long-continued desquamation of it (from 3d),[3].—Tickling in the upper part of the right side of the upper lip; disappears on slight scratching, but returns again (from 8th),[3].—Tickling in the right corner of the mouth, afternoon (second day), (from 7th and 30th),[3].—*Slight swelling of the articulation of the left jaw, with cracking in it when chewing; *swelling and hardness of the left parotid,* which is warm to touch; rosy red swelling of the tonsils and difficult swallowing; tension and pressure in the throat, when swallowing and when not; the pain in the throat is especially increased when swallowing fluids; hawking up mucus,[1].†—Boring in the right lower jaw (third day),[18].—Very painful boring in the right lower jaw-bone,[18].—Pressure as from a dull body in the front of the left joint of the lower jaw, but deep in extending towards the lowest fossa of the left nostril, as if in the Eustachian tube; on swallowing, the motion of the superior muscles of the pharynx changes this sensation for a moment; it lasts half an hour,[21].—[220.] Some pain on the left side of the lower jaw in a hollow tooth, which seems excited by a current of air when blowing coals,[18].

Mouth.—Teeth and Gums. A hollow tooth seems too long when biting,[1].—The teeth become very blunt and remain so for some time, although he had taken two swallows of water immediately after it,[18].—Pain in the teeth of the left side,[1].—Pain in a hollow tooth of the right side, and in the left upper eye teeth (second day), (from 6th),[3].—A painful sensation in the left side of the upper jaw in a hollow tooth which was never painful before, as if toothache would develop,[18].—A peculiar sensation of commencing pain in the left side of the upper jaw; appears several times without being caused by pressing or touching the teeth,[18].—Toothache, especially in a hollow tooth of the left side of the lower jaw; the anterior half of the hollow tooth

† (In a seven-year-old girl two weeks after a normal attack of the measles; improvement began in nine hours from the dose of Bromine X, and the whole disappeared within four days.) Lippe.

pains as if sore when touched, and seems to be loose,[1].—Drawings in some hollow teeth on either side,[18].—Long-continued dull aching in a hollow tooth,[18].—[230.] Stitching pain, at first from the forehead to the lower jaw, and hence into a hollow tooth, with throbbing pain in it,[6].—Sensitiveness of a hollow tooth to cold water (one hour),[18].—Throbbing beneath a hollow tooth,[1].—External pressure relieves the toothache,[1].—The gum pains in the morning (from 5th),[2].—*Tongue and Mouth in General.* Inflammation of the tongue (in half an hour),[24].—Pimples on the posterior portion of the right side of the tongue,[2].—The tongue cannot be protruded (in four hours),[24].—Dry sensation on the tongue,[18].—Burning as from pepper under the tongue,[21].—[240.] Burning and sticking on the under surface of the tongue,[21].—Sticking on the tip of the tongue, and afterward suddenly disappearing tickling in it (from 5th),[3].—Sharp stitches in the tip of the tongue,[21].—Inflammation of the whole buccal cavity (in half an hour),[24].— Dryness in the mouth continuing half an hour,[18].—Sensation in the mouth and pharynx as after a glass of rum,[13].—Heat of the mouth ($\frac{1}{2}$ drop tinct.),[24]. —Heat in the mouth, œsophagus, and stomach, together with colic,[14].— Burning sensation in the mouth, pharynx, and stomach, with pain in the abdomen,[14].—Feeling of burning in the mouth, pharynx, and stomach ; increased secretion of mucus, inclination to vomit, severe eructations and stomachache,[14].—[250.] Burning from the mouth to the stomach, accompanied by internal heat,[11].—Sore pain ; slight smarting on the arches of the palate (second day),[2].—*Saliva and Taste.* Increased secretion of saliva every time after taking it,[9].—Increased secretion of saliva (from fumes),[9].— Increased secretion of saliva ; salivation, with increased mucus in the mouth and nose,[11].—If inhaled it increased the saliva, lachrymation, nasal mucus, caused coryza, cough, slight headache here and there, and vertigo,[9][16].— Much thin saliva,[18].—Much thin saliva (one hour),[18].—Much collection of thin saliva (one hour),[21].—Thin tasteless saliva,[18].—[260.] Tasteless saliva,[18]. —Collection of tasteless saliva (after three-quarters of an hour),[18].—Constrictive sensation in the orifice of the salivary glands, with flow of saliva,[18]. —Very disagreeable taste (immediately, from 40 drops tinct.),[23].—Very nauseous, offensive taste from six drops in half an ounce of water,[9].—Taste is very strong, peculiarly puckered, burning and offensive,[15].—Sweetish taste in the mouth (half an hour),[21].—Decided salty taste in the tip of the tongue for several minutes (one and a half hours),[21].—Sour taste,[1].—Intensely bitter taste at the tip of the tongue, without other gastric symptoms,[18].—[270.] It leaves a strong scraping taste (13 drops in water),[9].— Very acrid, scraping, offensive taste, or rather exciting nausea, if taken without water,[9].—Violent burning taste immediately after taking,[18].—Water tastes salty in the morning fasting,[1].

Throat.—In General. The throat is stiff and painful on turning the head, on the left side,[4].—In the morning, the throat is stiff, so that she cannot turn the head,[5].—A very acrid burning extending from the tongue to the stomach ; on account of which he becomes nauseated, has great inclination to vomit, the mouth becomes filled with saliva, respiration difficult and somewhat painful (from 20 to 30 drops),[9].—Sticking in the throat,[18].— Stitches in the throat, with lachrymation and flow of thin saliva,[21].— Stitches near the hyoid bone, with secretion of thin saliva ; afterwards coldness in the tip of the tongue, with flow of saliva,[18].—[280.] The throat is very sore and raw (second day), (from 6th),[3].—Scraping in the throat,[18]. —Scraping and frequent hawking of scanty mucus from the throat,[18].— Scraping and sticking in the throat, lasting two hours,[18].—*Scraping in the*

throat and a rough deep voice, continued for an hour (soon after taking),[18].—
Feeling of rawness in the throat, with severe stitches and tickling in the
larynx, lachrymation of the eyes, and a feeling as if the larynx were laced
together, in the evening (second day),[21].—*Fauces.* Chronic inflammation
of the fauces, with a dry sensation, was aggravated (from the 1st),[2].—Inflammation of the fauces and uvula, with dry cough, caused by irritation
of the elongated uvula, especially severe in the morning; yellow thick
nasal mucus, streaked with some blood, without sneezing or blowing of the
nose, both of which conditions are usually very severe, with coryza, lasting
some days, and disappearing gradually (fifth day),[18].—Fauces and uvula
are red,[18].—Fauces dark-red, the tonsils covered with much mucus, scraping-sticking sensation of rawness, some swelling of the tonsils; repeated
after several days (soon after taking),[18].—[290.] Feeling as if a small
bo´y were in the fauces, which caused hawking,[18].—Unpleasant puckered
sensation in the fauces, followed by burning and sensation as if sore,[11].—
In the fauces, at first, an unpleasant puckered sensation, followed by burning and soreness; salivation lasted a quarter of an hour, with increase of
mucus in the mouth and nostrils (soon after 5 drops),[8].—Puckering in the
fauces,[11].—Scraping in the fauces, which causes hawking,[18].—Scraping and
dryness in the fauces towards evening,[18].—*Pharynx, Œsophagus,
and Externals.* Feeling of warmth, which increases to a burning, extending through the whole pharynx into the stomach, especially distressing
in the pharynx (after 8 drops in an ounce of water),[8].—Sensation of burning and scraping in the pharynx, so violent that for some minutes there
are convulsive twitchings in the face and in the hands, with strong inclination to vomit and forcible empty retchings (after daily doses increased to
45 drops),[13].—Raw, unpleasant feeling in the pharynx (immediately),[9].—
Pressure arising from the stomach into the œsophagus,[18].—[300.] Burning
in œsophagus and stomach ($\frac{1}{2}$ drop tinct.),[23].—Swallowing is especially
painful in the whole of the right side of the fauces, which is dark-red and
without secretion of mucus,[18].—Pain in the submaxillary glands of both
sides (first day),[3].—Slight pressive pain in the left submaxillary gland
(second day),[3].—Stitches in the glands at the side of the hyoid bone,[20].

Stomach.—Appetite and Thirst. Appetite neither increased
nor diminished while taking it (for sixteen days),[9].—Good appetite and
digestion; embonpoint increases (in provers of large daily doses),[13].—
Diminished appetite,[11].—Not much appetite (fifth and sixth days),[26].—
Little appetite,[19].—[310.] Very little appetite the whole day,[18].—No appetite,[18].—Desire for acids, which aggravate the symptoms and cause diarrhœa,[1].—Aversion to the customary tobacco-smoking; it causes nausea
and vertigo,[1].—Thirst,[11].—Aversion to drinking cold water,[1].—*Eructations and Hiccough.* Eructations shortly after taking it (from
the 8th),[3].—Empty eructations,[18].—Empty tasteless eructations (first day),[19]
—[320.] Eructations of tasteless air (from 3d),[3].—Eructations taste of
bromine (soon),[18].—Empty eructations, with taste of bromine,[18].—Eructations like foul eggs (from five to seven days), (from 3d),[1].—Frequent
eructations, with vomiting, whereby much mucus is thrown up (after 5
drops),[8].—Many eructations of tasteless air and much rumbling of air in
the abdomen,[21].—Remarkably frequent empty eructations and much rumbling in the abdomen,[18].—Frequent regurgitations,[24].—Hiccough (2 drops
tinct.),[23].—*Nausea and Vomiting.* Qualmishness in the pit of the
stomach, with empty eructations,[18].—[330.] Nausea,[20].—Nausea (2 drops
tinct.),[23].—Slight nausea,[6 18].—Some nausea,[18].—At times, transient nausea,[5].

—Slight sensation of nausea in the epigastric region,[18].—Nausea toward evening, without being able to vomit; better after eating,[4].—Nausea, hiccough, increased secretion of mucus (after 2 drops),[14].—Nausea, eructations, roughness in the stomach, mouth full of saliva, slow pulse, and congestion of the chest,[14].—Great inclination to vomit, increased discharge of mucus, and profuse eructations,[14].—[340.] (Exceedingly offensive vomiting, suddenly, after allopathic doses, which were given to a patient to remove indurations in the stomach. After persistent continuance of the drug a constant retching set in, exhausting the patient even to dying; it could not be relieved by the usual methods; Lachesis, X, relieved it at once, prolonged the patient's life, and enabled him to go home and die comfortably),[2].— *Stomach.* Inflammation of the stomach; suggillations in the stomach like ulceration,[14].—Feeling of emptiness in the stomach,[1].—Emptiness in the stomach; better after eating, for which, however, he had no longings,[12].— Feeling of heaviness in the stomach,[11].—Warmth in the stomach, with confusion in the forehead (first day),[19].—Warmth and burning in the stomach, and flow of saliva,[11].—Warmth in the region of the stomach,[18].— Warmth in the stomach, immediately,[18].—Warmth in the stomach, nausea, empty eructations, increase of saliva, with pressive heaviness in the forehead, with sensitiveness of the eyes; continued for a long time,[18].— [350.] Slight attacks of pain at stomach (40 drops tinct.),[23].—Violent pain in the epigastric region, worse upon pressure, relieved by bending forward, together with a distended abdomen and flushes of heat starting from the back (first day),[19].—Severe pain in the stomach, now and then,[18].—Burning pain at stomach (in half an hour),[24].—Burning in the stomach constantly (after large doses),[9][14].—A kind of contractive cramp in the stomach at 11.30 A.M.; disappears after eating,[6].—Aching in the stomach, as if diarrhœa would ensue, followed in about an hour by a liquid stool, with some urging, although two hours before he had a normal stool, at noon (first day),[19].— Slight pressure of the stomach (after one hour),[18].—Pressure on the stomach, as from a stone, with internal heat,[6].—Constant pressure on the stomach, as of a stone (latest action),[4].—[360.] Pressure in the stomach and right hypochondrium, with sensation of fulness,[20].—Long-continued pressure in the stomach, increased by pressure with the hand,[18].—Excessive pressure in the stomach, with inclination to vomit, eructations, colic, and rumbling in the abdomen (a quarter of an hour after 10 drops),[13].—Sticking pain in the pit of the stomach, extending to the navel, increased by deep pressure, and generally seems to be deeper than the stomach (from 8 to 11 A.M.),[18]. —The pain in the stomach is increased by pressure,[18].

Abdomen.—Hypochondriac and Umbilical Regions. Sensation as of a ball in the left hypochondrium (after six hours),[1].—Pain in the left hypochondrium,[20].—Pressure upon the hypochondria is painful,[18]. —Violent cutting in both hypochondria, deep, extending to the side of the navel, especially on the left side, with a soft abdomen, increased by pressure,[21].—Transient stitches in the hypochondria from right to left,[18].— [370] Sharp stitches in the left hypochondrium,[18][20].—Sharp stitches in the right and left hypochondria,[19].—Stitches in the left hypochondrium,[21].— Sharp stitches in the left hypochondrium,[21].—Sensitiveness of the hypochondrium and epigastric region to pressure, with flow of saliva,[18].—Pulsation in the right hypochondrium in the evening,[20].—Pain in the liver,[10].— Decided pain in the region of the liver, especially on pressure and riding, with great distension and hardness of the right hypochondrium, and a feeling as if a hard body were sinking down there; lasts from ten to twelve hours (after three days),[18].—Stitches shooting from the liver toward the navel,[18].—Dull pain in the region of the spleen, extending towards the spinal column,[18].—[**380.**] The pain in the abdomen extends from the stomach to the navel, and below the short ribs (first day),[19].—Severe pain to the left of the navel, deep, increased by pressure,[21].—Pain in the region of the navel, increased by drawing in the walls of the abdomen,[18].—Cutting pain in the region of the navel, after eating, increased by pressure (after three and a half hours),[18].—Sticking pain on the left side from the navel to the inner surface of the wall of the chest, increased by pressure, morning and evening, and in the evening cuttings deep in the region of the navel, increased by pressure, lasting half an hour, with stitches extending towards the rectum, to the neck of the bladder, and along the right spermatic cord,[18].—*In General.* * *Tympanitic distension of the abdomen and passage of much wind*,[18].—The abdomen is full of wind, as is shown by percussion,[19]. —Slight twitching in the left side (from 8th),[3].—Sounds of gas in the intestines, and also in the œsophagus,[18].—Rumbling in the bowels,[11].—[**390.**] Rumbling in the abdomen,[18].—Much rumbling in the abdomen,[18].—Frequent rumblings in the abdomen,[18].—Rumbling and fermenting in the abdomen (from four to six days), (from 3d),[1].—Rumbling in the abdomen and slight pressure in the stomach,[18].—Continued rumbling, with passage of flatus and empty eructations,[18].—Flatulence,[18].—Passage of flatus (after two hours),[18].—Passage of much odorless flatus (from 8th),[2].—Pleasant sensation of warmth in the abdomen, with accelerated pulse (after 5 drops),[8]. —[**400.**] Pain in the left side for several days,[6].—*Pains in the abdomen and small of the back*, as during menstruation ; *passage of much flatus*, as was the case during menstruation,[2].—After tobacco-smoking, very violent pinching pains in the abdomen, better when pressing upon it, worse on sudden motion ; on sitting bent and pressing upon it he noticed the pain only during expiration, not during inspiration (from 3d),[3].—Slight gripings in the intestines immediately after taking, each time (after 6 to 8 drops),[9].—Severe gripings in the intestines (from 13 drops),[9].—Colic (½ drop tinct.),[23].— Colic, violent pains in the abdomen,[6].—Colic and borborygmi,[11].—Before menstruation, sticking in the abdomen, relieved by lying bent,[1].—Some right inguinal glands are much larger than usual, without pain,[21].—[**410.**] Pain in the left inguinal ring,[18].—Pain in the left inguinal canal, especially on walking, pressure, and cough,[18].—Pain in the left side of the abdomen, becomes a dragging toward the inguinal ring (from 8th),[3].—Pain in the crest of the right ilium (from 8th),[3].—Boring in the posterior portion of the left crest of the ilium,[21].—Stitches in the anterior spine of the crest of the left ilium,[21].

Rectum and Anus.—Painless hæmorrhoids (third day),[19].—Soft painless hæmorrhoid as large as a nut (second day),[18].—* *With the diarrhœa of black fæces, blind hæmorrhoids, which pain severely*, which he had had for years but were never so painful. They disappeared after nux and sulphur, but returned in fourteen days very painful, and continued for a longer time ; cold and warm washing aggravated them ; nux and sulphur did not relieve ; capsicum and the use of saliva relieved,[4].—Very frequent but ineffectual anal tenesmus (in three hours),[24].—[**420.**] Some fine stitches in the anus,[18]. —Tickling in the anus (first day),[3].—Much itching-crawling in the anus, as if something living were moving in it,[21].

Stool.—Severe urging to stool, with which much more wind than fæces is passed at 2 P.M., following the natural morning stool,[20].—Frequent desire for stool, with passage of flatus and stitches in the anus,[18].—Regular evacuation, with slight tenesmus,[8].—Diarrhœa of black fæces and painful hæmorrhoids (latest action),[4].—Violent diarrhœa relieved by black coffee,[9].—*Diarrhœa after every meal ceases, but returns after eating oysters,°[2].—Stool in the beginning more constipated than usual, then two stools in each day thinner and more copious than usual,[12].—**[430.]** Repeated pasty stools (after 144 drops taken within ninth day),[9].—Several pasty stools throughout the day, twice at night; from daily doses (eleventh day),[9].—No action on the intestines from 10 or even 20 drops, if it was omitted the following day; but pasty stools from a dose of 30 drops,[9].—Soft stool after he had had the usual one in the morning,[18].—Obliged to rise twice at night on account of thin stools if he took it after the morning hours (from 20 drops daily), (fourth and fifth days),[9].—Thin, diarrhœa-like stool an hour and a half after 13 drops; this is repeated four times till the next morning,[9].—Diarrhœa-like stool, bright-yellow, preceded by cutting and rumbling in the abdomen (fifth to seventh day), (from 3d),[1].—Mucous, somewhat diarrhœa-like stool, with much wind, the second and the following days (from 1st),[2].—Thin fluid stool,[12].—Soft stool, with disappearance of the hæmorrhoids (third day),[18].—**[440.]** Stool-like sheep-dung, with pressure in the stomach and abdomen,[6].—Stool in the forenoon hard, tough, brown, and glistening; it breaks to pieces like sheep-dung,[6].—Hard stool (second to third day),[18 19].

Urinary Organs.—Pain in the region of the bladder and in its sides, with desire to urinate (after half an hour),[18].—Some clear drops of mucus flow from the urethra (on different days),[18].—Burning in the urethra after urinating,[1].—Pressure in the prostate gland when walking (third day),[19].—Some fine stitches in the orifice of the urethra,[18].—Stitches in the urethra (fifth day),[19].—Some slight stitches in the urethra (half an hour),[18].—**[450.]** Some stitches in the urethra extending towards its orifice,[18].—Stitches in the end of the urethra (fourth day),[19].—Pulsation in the urethra behind the testicles,[19].—Frequent calls to urinate,[18].—Renewed desire to urinate, although he had urinated a short time before (after half an hour),[18].—The desire to urinate continues, with tickling sensation in the tip of the urethra,[18].—Very little desire to urinate,[18].—Dribbling of urine after urinating (from third to tenth days),[1].—After urinating some drops of urine continue to flow, which burn very much,[1].—Increased secretion of urine (2 drops tinct.),[23].—**[460.]** The secretion of urine seemed somewhat increased,[9].—Diminished urine,[1].—Urine scanty (first day),[19].—Urine scanty and dark,[18].—Urine scanty and dark (second day),[19].—Urine very scanty and dark during the whole day,[18].—Urine scanty, dark, and turbid, with a red sediment,[18].—Scanty, very dark, and very turbid urine for several days; it deposits a whitish sediment, adhering to the vessel,[18].—Urine diminished, dark at times, with a red coating on the vessel (during the whole proving),[18].—The scanty urine, which is passed after much desire, is clear and darker than usual,[18].—**[470.]** The urine becomes cloudy and decidedly ammoniacal after one hour,[18].—The urine contains large flakes of white mucus,[18].

Sexual Organs.—*Male.* Erections in the morning,[1].—Erections in the morning from 3 to 8 o'clock; for several days (from fumes),[2].—Pressure in the right spermatic cord,[21].—Pressive-pinching pain in the penis, more on the right side, in the evening (eleventh day), after repeated doses,[3].—Stitches in the glans and in the sides of the dorsum of the penis,[11].—Stitches in the glans penis,[21].—Long stitches extending through the penis to the glans,[21].—Swelling of the left testicle, with sore pain,[1].—**[480.]** Increased firmness of the testicles (from 8th),[3].—Coldness of the left testicle,[1].

—Increased sexual desire (fourth day).—Early emission during coition,[1].—Emissions the third night in a man who had none for three years,[1].—Emissions for two nights in succession,[3].—*Female.* *Loud passage of flatus from the vagina* (from fifth to eighteenth day),[1].—Sore pain in the pudenda,[1].—Before menstruation pain in the back, feeling of weakness and want of appetite,[1].—On accession and during menstruation frontal headache; a feeling on stooping as if the eyes would fall out,[1].—[490.] On the appearance of menstruation headache,[1].—Menstruation appeared too early and profuse,[1].—Menstruation appeared in twenty-one days in one who menstruated regularly,[1].—Menstruation was delayed when she took Bromine 30th on the appearance of the usual forebodings, B.,[2].—*(Menstruation, which she had every six weeks, passed without any pain ; she used to suffer every time after it had continued a few hours from the most violent sticking cramps, which continued from six to twelve hours, so that she could scarcely remain lying, followed by sore pain in the abdomen),°[2].—Clear blood, with the menses,[1].

Respiratory Apparatus.—Larynx, Trachea, and Voice.

Much hawking of scanty mucus from the larynx,[20].—*Cold sensation in the larynx, with a cold feeling when inspiring, after breakfast; better after shaving,[12].—* Constriction in the larynx,[18].—*Sticking constriction in the larynx,[18].—[500.] Pain, as if crushed, in the left side of the larynx,[18].—* Every time on swallowing saliva a stitch in the posterior portion of the larynx, with a feeling of contraction,[18].—Stitches, with pressure in the larynx,[18].—Stitches, with itching in the larynx (fourth night),[19].—Severe stitching in the larynx, with lachrymation (after five minutes),[18].—*Scraping and rawness in the larynx provoking cough,[20].—*Scraping in the larynx provoking dry cough, in the evening* (first day),[18].—* Tickling in the larynx, followed by cough,[18].—Frequent tickling in the larynx with dry cough, which is immediately followed by tickling again; during the cough pain in the left side, extending inward from the nipple,[18].— Tickling in the larynx, with irritation to cough; constrictive sensation deep in the throat, and dry cough; coppery taste on the back part of the palate; spasmodic sensation extending downward from the throat, with dry cough in the evening, and scraping in the throat (first day),[21].—[510.] Dryness in the trachea,[11].—* Contracted sensation internally in the trachea, or a feeling as if the pit of the throat were pressed against the trachea; it lasts two days (from 6th),[12].—* Tickling in the trachea on inspiring, which causes a cough,[1].—*Hoarseness,[18].—*Hoarseness is worse in the afternoon than in the forenoon (from 6th),[3].—*Hoarseness, loss of voice; he cannot speak clearly; the voice is weak and soft, with a feeling in the throat as if scraped raw (in the evening), (from 7th),[3].—*Cough.* Cough, with pain in the chest,[9].—Cough excited by scratching and tickling (from 6th),[3].—* Cough excited by deep inspiration,[1].—*Cough, with paroxysms of suffocation suddenly on swallowing (from 5 drops in half an ounce of water); respiration is very short; is obliged to catch for breath,[8].—[520.] Short cough without expectoration, with sore pain in the chest,[1].—Slight hacking cough,[2].—Hacking cough several times in the day,[2].—Violent cough, and sensation of sulphur fumes, followed by confusion of the head and dull pressive headache (from fumes),[16].—Rough cough,[11].—Racking cough, which does not allow one to speak,[11].—Dry cough,[18].—Dry cough several times,[18].—Frequent dry cough, soon after taking,[20].—Dry cough, from a continued slight tickling rawness in the throat (from 7th),[3].—[530.] Dry cough, in the morning (second day),[19].—Now and then a dry cough, with pain in the left side of the chest,[18]—Dry cough,

with sticking in the left side, extending from the left nipple into the chest,[18].
—A rough, hollow, dry cough, with great fatigue (from 3d),[3].—*Respiration. The glottis had closed with a spasm, and did not yield willingly,*[25].—
Spasmodic respiration (in four hours),[24].—Deep breathing becomes a yawning,[3].—Quick and short breathing (in half an hour),[24].—Necessity for
breathing deeply (first hour),[18].—Deep expirations now and then (after an
hour and a half),[18].—[540.] Frequent deep breathing (first day),[19].—Frequent deep expiration, when sitting (soon),[18].—*Deep forcible inspiration is
necessary from time to time,*[18].—A feeling as though he could not breathe
enough, and must voluntarily breathe more strongly (soon after taking),[18].
—*Oppression of breath immediately after taking it, with deep inspiration,
together with a sensation as if he did not get enough air into the chest, on account of which he elevates the thorax and inspires forcibly,*[18].—*Difficulty of
breathing; he cannot inspire sufficient;* when walking, even rapidly, better;
worse in the morning, better in the evening and at night (third day),[3].—
Short, difficult breathing, with prolonged inspiration and mucous râle (in
two hours),[24].—Difficult painful breathing,[11].—Frequent difficult breathing,[18].—Frequent difficult respiration (after half an hour),[18].—[550.] Respiration is very much embarrassed; he is obliged to catch for breath,[8].—
Respiratory troubles; it seems as if inspiration was prevented by an impediment in the middle of the chest (from 3d), (even after six weeks),[3].—
Impeded respiration, as from a slight pressure on the lower end of the
breast-bone (from 8th),[3].—Impeded respiration, from a slight pressure in
the pit of the stomach,[3].—Inspiration of very concentrated fumes causes
dyspnœa; for a long time the saliva, etc., is increased; it is followed by
cough and pain in the chest; after some time pain in the abdomen; after
two hours a pasty stool, which is repeated three times in the afternoon, becoming very thin; a slight hacking cough remains for several days,[9].—If
a large quantity is inspired it causes severe oppression and cough, together
with a very full pulse, which, however, is not faster than usual. The secretion of saliva markedly increased; it is followed by vertigo, frequent
bleeding of the nose, and finally a headache remains. All the conditions
disappear within four to six hours,[17].—(*An asthma, in a girl of sixteen
years, had remained for ten years after measles, so that the girl was never
able to walk rapidly nor ascend steps without being very much exhausted;
disappeared after five doses of five globules of the 30th, which she took for
proving,°[4].)— *Chest.—In General.* Swelling of the mammary glands,[1].
—Congestion to the chest,[11].—Peculiar sensation of weakness and exhaustion in the chest,[11].—[560.] The pain in the chest continues; is especially
noticed when coughing,[18].—Pain under the ribs, especially on pressure, more
in the right side,[18].—Burning in the chest, with subsequent sensation of heat,
only gradually disappearing, with ineffectual efforts to vomit,[11].—Tension.
in the chest,[1].—Slight feeling of fulness in the chest and throat, increasing
towards noon, continuing till evening, and feeling as if a soft substance
were between the lungs and the breast-bone (from 6th),[3].—A sensation of
constriction of the chest impedes respiration and is very unpleasant, with
a dry tickling cough the whole of the first day and the following days, lasting only an hour (from 1st),[2].—Paralytic drawing pain through the chest
and toward the shoulder-blade and arm (left),[3].—Feeling of anxiety in
the chest, with difficult breathing,[18].—Pressure from the chest at times,[18].—
Slight pressure upon the chest on deep inspiration,[11].—[570.] Pressure in
the upper part of the chest,[20].—Pressure in the upper part of the chest,
with difficult breathing (first day),[19].—Slight pressure in the upper part of

the chest, as if breathing was difficult,[18].—Pressure several times in the
upper part of the chest, with oppressed breathing soon after taking,[19].—
Severe oppression, cough, headache, and vertigo (from the fumes),[2].—Sticking pain here and there in the walls of the chest, uninfluenced by breathing,[20].—Stitches in the upper part of the chest, with difficult breathing and
sensation of distension (first day),[19].—*Sides and Sternum.* Pain in
the right lung (from 3d),[3].—A pain in the right side of the chest, gradually extending towards the back, lasting some hours (first day), (from 1st),[2].
—Pain in the right wall of the chest, on waking (second day),[21].—[580.]
Pain in the right side between the seventh and ninth ribs, especially on
motion,[19].—Constant pain in the right side beneath the ribs, especially on
somewhat deep pressure (after seven hours),[19].—The pain in the right side
of the chest increased very much toward evening; lifting a light weight
with the right hand increased the pain, so also walking, on account of the
increased motion of the pectoral muscles; at times the pain extends to the
dorsal muscles of the same side, and then is also increased by expiration;
this continues until he falls asleep; it awakens him at night in turning the
body; continues equally severe the next morning; only disappears after five
days; it is especially severe in the morning and evening; worse when moving the thorax; less when walking than when sitting; especially severe on
waking; rest is almost impossible,[18].—The pain on the right side under the
ribs still continues, though not so severe all the time; it is aggravated by
pressure on the sixth day; this same pain continues the following days,
sometimes so violent that even breathing becomes painful; the abdomen is
therewith distended with gas; a stooping posture and moderate pressure relieve the pain, which seems to be in the region of the gall-bladder, and
which, on deep breathing, extends to the navel; also, however deep, when
fasting, the pain is not noticed; it seems to be most severe two hours after
eating,[19].—Pain, like a pressure, in the right side of the chest,[3].—Pressive
pain in the right lung (from 8th),[3].—Pressure in the wall of the chest below
the right nipple,[21].—A sensation in several places in the right wall of the
chest, as if it were pressed from within outward; not increased by breathing, but by motion of the thorax; at 6 P.M., and several times repeated
during the evening (first day),[21].—Sticking in the right side of the chest
beneath the fourth rib, with palpitation (from 7th),[3].—*Sharp stitches in the
right side of the chest,* especially when walking rapidly,[1].—[590.] Severe
stitches between the sixth and seventh ribs of the right side, at 6 P.M. (from
the fumes),[2].—Tickling in the right side of the chest in the region of the
sixth rib (in the afternoon of second day),[3].—A tickling spot in the region
of the right eighth rib (from 8th),[3].—Transient pain in the left chest,[3].—
Very transient pain in the left lung (from 8th),[3].—Wandering pains in the
left side of the chest uninfluenced by breathing; afterwards these pains extend to the right side of the chest, where they become pressive; they then
leave the left side and continue in the right side for three days; they appear
immediately on walking, are neither increased by breathing nor by motion,
only aggravated by bending both shoulders forward, with slight flexion of
the upper part of the chest, or by turning the thorax on its axis, whence the
pain seems to be in the muscles of this region,[18].—Severe pain on the left
side under the ribs, several times; it quickly disappears; on the night of
the sixth day the same pain extends higher up, and is somewhat more violent; worse when lying bent; not increased by breathing,[19].—Pain in the
left side of the chest by the fourth rib, and tickling in the right side of the
head (from 7th),[3].—Paralytic drawing pain through the left side of the

chest towards the shoulder-blade and into the left arm (from 7th),[3].—Pressure in the left pectoral muscles,[21].—[600.] Pressure below the left clavicle,[21].—Tearing in the left clavicle,[21].—Sticking pain in the left side of the chest,[3].—Sticking pain on the left side of the chest, extending towards the arm,[6].—Transient stitches in the left side below the ribs,[19].—Pressure in the sternum,[21].

Heart and Pulse.—Palpitation of the heart,[18].—Palpitation perceptible in the region of the heart, which is noticed even without laying the hand upon it, together with forcible breathing (after three hours),[18].—Violent palpitation of the heart in the evening, so that she cannot lie upon the left side,[3].—Palpitation when walking, without cause (second day),[18].—[610.] Slight oppression around the heart and palpitation, at the same time the inspired air seems very cold, with tendency to yawn (from 3d),[3].—Pulse rather slow and hard during the two provings with large daily doses,[9].—Pulse very full, not accelerated,[10].—Pulse more frequent,[18].—Full, hard, at first slow, afterwards accelerated pulse,[11].—Pulse 64 to 70 fifteen minutes after five drops; after thirty minutes again normal,[8].—Pulse 70 after eight drops; in fifteen minutes only 62,[8].

Neck and Back.—A gland as large as a pea on each side of the neck (second day),[18].—Twitching in the left latissimus dorsi (from 8th),[3].—10 A.M., aching pain at inner border of left scapula up to neck, on moving left arm or sitting leaning to left (fifth day); it extended half way down upper arm; worse on moving arm (seventh day); nearly gone, but worse in evening (ninth day),[26],—[620.] Boring in the spinous processes of different vertebræ at various times (fifth day),[18].—Pressure in the left dorsal muscles,[21].—Wandering pressive pain in the dorsal muscles below the shoulder-blade,[18].—Tension in the right lumbar and dorsal muscles, increased by moving these parts,[21].—Sticking-tickling in the spine, more towards the right side (from 7th),[3].—Sore pain in the small of the back, unchanged on rising or on motion,[1].

Extremities in General.—Great stiffness in all the limbs at 11 A.M., better in the afternoon,[5].—Pains in the limbs, afterwards alternating with chilliness and heat,[4].—Compression in the upper arm, in the forepart of both knee-joints,[20].—Crawling in the fingers and short twitches in the muscles of the foot and the region of the knee (after a quarter of an hour); repeated from time to time; slightly perceptible the next morning; it appeared a quarter of an hour before colic and rumbling in the bowels,[13].

Upper Extremities.—[630.] Great restlessness and jactitation of the arms (in three hours),[24].—Great loss of power and weakness of the arms,[1].—Weakness in the left arm,[1].—The whole left arm feels paralyzed,[4].—Constriction in the upper extremities,[11].—Drawing in the right arm from above towards the hand, together with a paralytic sensation in the left arm,[2].†—Pain in the right shoulder (first day),[6].—Pain below the shoulder (from 5th),[3].—Painful paralytic sensation in the left shoulder, soon disappearing; afterward paralytic pain in the right shoulder-joint (from 8th),[3].—Sensation of heat in the forepart of the right shoulder-joint,[21].—[640.] When walking in the street a severe rheumatic, dull, constricting pain; it extends into the right shoulder and thence into the arm, where it disappears (second day), (from 1st),[2].—Pressure in the right shoulder-joint,[21].—

---

† In a person who had disease of the heart, he often experienced the last sensation, with palpitation and sounds in the heart which denoted changes in the valves of the left side of the heart. C. Hg.

Pressure and weariness in the left shoulder-joint,[21].—Sharp stitches in the right axilla,[18].—Burning stitches on the top of the right shoulder-joint,[21].—Bruised pain in left shoulder, afterwards in the right elbow-joint,[18].—Cracking in the left elbow-joint,[2].—Sticking in the inner condyle of the right elbow,[18].—In the afternoon a paralyzed feeling in the left arm, as after a blow, on holding the left arm bent, when walking, together with ill-humor,[12].—Sensation in the forearms, from the wrists to a little below the elbows, as if they were in a vice; afterwards a sticking pain in the fingers, which extends toward the head (seventy-five minutes after ten drops),[13].—[650.] Tearing in the arms in the evening, especially in the hands and fingers,[6].—Pressure in the left wrist,[21].—Violent pain in the right hand; once it shoots into the middle finger, with throbbing pain,[6].—The fingers of the right hand become so stiff that she is afraid she will let the dish fall which she is holding in her hand,[5].—Dead pain in all the finger-joints of the left hand; the pain extends hence to the elbow and shoulder, and pain in the upper and lower part of the arm,[4].—Hot bromine (thirty-six to forty degrees R.) placed upon the dorsal surface of a finger caused more violent burning pain than on the flexor surface; in the latter case the yellow spot soon easily disappears; in the former it remains yellow for more than fourteen days, and gradually disappears in fine scales,[9].—Pressure in the root of the left fingers,[21].—Pressure in the metacarpal bone of the right index finger,[21].—Pressure on the back of the joint between the first and second phalanges of the right fourth finger,[18].—Severe compression at the basis of the left fourth and fifth fingers,[18].—[660.] Tearing in the fingers,[11].—Tearing in the first phalanges of the right fourth and fifth fingers,[21].—Tearing through the left fourth finger and in the right third and fourth fingers,[21].—Tearing in the middle joint of the middle finger of the left hand, which obliges one to extend the fingers,[4].—Tearing asunder pain between the metacarpus and the first phalanx of the right finger,[20].—Jerklike tearings through the left thumb, at 6 P.M., in the frontal bone very frequently, through the right great toe, in the lower part of the right leg, in the right knee, with bruised pain when sitting, in the evening,[18].—Severe cutting on the back of the whole of the left fourth finger,[21].—Stitches in the fingers,[13].—Stitches on the back of the joint between the first and second phalanges of the left fourth finger continue the whole forenoon,[20].—Severe burning stitches in the tip of the left index finger,[20].—[670.] Fine stitches on the back of the right little finger, when some bright-red small spots appeared and lasted the whole day,[21].

Lower Extremities.—Weakness of the left leg,[2].—Paralytic sensation in the right leg,[3].—In the evening on going out a throbbing pain in both legs, especially in the right, with stiffness in the limb as far as the foot, and with stiffness and pain in the right great toe and in the middle toes,[5].—Stiffness in front of left thigh on walking (seventh day),[26].—Twitching in the inner side of the right knee (from 8th),[3].—Pain in the right knee and downward, with a feeling of heaviness in the right leg,[18].—Pain in the left knee and hip, worse on motion (second morning),[12].—Rheumatic pain in the left knee (from 5th),[3].—Burning pain in the left knee,[4].—[680.] Pressure in the left knee,[21].—In the right knee a dull pressive pain in the bone,[18].—Pressive pain in the bend of the right knee (from 5th),[3].—Pressure in the forepart of the left knee,[21].—Throbbing in the forepart of the right knee while sitting, lasting several minutes,[18].—A pain in the forepart of the leg, extending to the right side, like gnawing or sawing, sudden, severe, and transient,[21].—Dull pain deep in the left, then in the right leg, while sitting,[18].—Dull pressive, fatiguing pain in the bones of the left leg (second day),[18].—Pressure deep in the left leg,[21].—Pressure in the head of the right tibia,[21].—[690.] Boring in the left tibia (half an hour),[20].—Boring pain in the right tibia (after nine hours),[18].—Boring in the right tibia several times,[19].—Boring in the lower part of the right tibia,[18].—Violent boring pains at times in the left tibia,[19].—Pressure in the right tibia,[21].—Pressure with a sensation of weariness deep in the left leg, which extends through the left ankle into the foot,[21].—Pressure in the right internal malleoli,[21].—Pressure in the right ankle, especially in the inner malleoli,[21].—Pressure in the left ankle and in the bones of the right metatarsus and the bones on the back of the right foot,[21].—[700.] In the evening, when stepping, violent pain in the middle of the ball of the left foot, as if one stepped upon a hard body, with paralyzed sensation of the knee-joint and also somewhat in the hip; immediately afterwards, as this becomes better, a pressive pain in the left side of the throat near the thyroid cartilage,[12].—Tension in the tendons on the back of the right foot on bending the ankle when walking (after four hours),[20].—Drawings in the tendons on the back of the right foot,[20].—Pressure on the back of the right foot,[21].—Tearing in the tendons on the back of the right foot,[19].—Cold sensation in the left great toe,[1].—Pain in the right toes (from 8th),[3].—Almost constant pain in the fourth toe of the right foot (in the evening of second day),[3].—Pain in the tip of the right fourth toe, together with tickling on the forehead and pain in the inner side of the right knee,[3].—Cutting in the flesh near the nail of the great toe.[18].—[710.] Waking at night with crawling and coldness of the left great toe,[1].—A corn on the right little toe becomes painful and grows rapidly,[1].—Slight burning and pain in a corn on the fourth toe of the right foot, and beneath the ball of the foot (first day, repeated second day in the afternoon, and evening of eleventh day, after repeated doses),[3].

Generalities.—Embonpoint increased,[13].—If introduced into a cut it becomes unhealthy-looking, and a green decay forms about it, with an offensive odor,[11].—Cracking in the joints, in the morning after rising (second day),[3].—In the afternoon the throat, neck, arms, and legs become stiff, so that she is afraid that she would not be able to walk, with a headache extending from the occiput towards the forehead, shooting and dragging as if everything would press out in the forepart of the head,[5].—General trembling (first and second day), (from 3d),[1].—Feeling of weakness,[18].—Great weakness and loss of power,[1].—[720.] If she wakes at night, a sensation of trembling weakness as though she could not rise (sixth day),[1].—Weak and sleepy the whole afternoon and evening (second day),[18].—Great weakness after breakfast as if bruised; she is scarcely able to make the bed,[5].—Great weakness when walking, which compels her to sit down,[6].—Great exhaustion; she cannot work any more, and must lie down,[5].—The whole body is very much affected and weak, continuing a long time after all the other symptoms had disappeared,[5].—Great indisposition,[2][3].—Physical and mental indisposition during the whole proving,[18].—Sensation as of fasting; feeling of heaviness in the head, with some stiffness in the muscles of the neck,[18].—Sensation as if the flesh were loose and bruised on touch, especially on the left side of the chest,[1].—[730.] The right side suffers most,[6].—The whole left side is most affected,[4].—Many symptoms on the left side,[1].—A glass of stimulants did not relieve him,[3].

Skin.—Colors the skin yellow,[15].—It destroys the skin very rapidly, with severe burning and consequent inflammation,[15].—Several small red spots on the back of the left hand, more towards the thumb and index finger;

they sometimes itch, sometimes not, soon disappearing, and then again re-appearing; several of them change to small vesicles, which dry up within twelve to twenty-four hours, and leave a small red spot,²¹.—Papulous eruption above the right inner canthus; pains on touch; a watery discharge on pricking (from the 3d),¹³.—Pimples on the nose, and at the same time on the back part of the right side of the tongue,².—Pimples on the right ring finger, on the ulnar side of the third phalanx, without pain, only disappearing after eight weeks (first day),³.—[740.] On the anus a small pimple, painful when rubbed, which he never had before (after twenty-four hours),¹⁸.—The pimple by the anus is not a hæmorrhoid, but is seated directly in the suture just before the anus, and can be felt with the finger as a pimple seated on or beneath the skin; it pains only on strong pressure, but more on rubbing, even with soft paper,¹⁸.—*Boils on the arms* and in the face (later action),⁵.†—Severe cutting in the skin of the ball of the right great toe,¹⁸.—Stitches in the skin on the malar bone,²¹.—Stitches in the skin on the larynx,²¹.—Feeling as if something living in the skin, especially in the arms and legs,¹.—Slight prickling in the skin, with a sensation of warmth, changing to a burning, and dryness of the part after external use,¹¹.—Tickling over whole body, easily relieved by scratching,³.—Tickling on the right side of the forehead, on the left side of the occiput (from the 8th and also from the 5th),³.—[750.] Tickling on the right shoulder (from 8th),³.—Tickling on the legs,³.—Tickling on the outer side of the left thigh (in the afternoon of second day),³.—Tickling below the right knee-cap, disappears on scratching (from 8th),³.—Itching soon relieved by scratching,³.—Itching in various places in the skin that causes scratching, whereby the itching ceases, but soon reappears,¹⁸.—Itching, now here, now there, mostly in the right side of the face,³.—Itching between the fingers, soon disappearing on scratching,¹⁸.—Tickling-itching soon disappearing, always in a small spot, now in the right side, now in the left (second day),³.

Sleep and Dreams.—Yawning, early in the morning; great yawning the whole day; full inspiration causes yawning (from 3d),³.—*Continued yawning, with the respiratory troubles* (twelfth day), (after repeated doses),³.—*Continual yawning the whole day, with difficulty of breathing* (from 30th),³.—[760.] Yawning and heat in the face and nose (from 6th),³.—Very sleepy (from 3d),³.—*Very much inclined to sleep,¹⁸.—Great inclination to fall asleep,¹⁸.—Even after eight weeks, irresistible sleepiness during the day and also the whole evening; every exertion to throw it off is ineffectual,⁴.—Great sleepiness and weakness; can scarcely keep on the legs; great inclination to sit down, yet he feels better when moving about,³.—In the evening, when writing, almost irresistible sleepiness, with confusion of the head; it seems as though the scalp were too tight, or as though a band were tied around the head, with some pain in the shoulder,⁴.—When reading in the evening, he became sleepy at an unusual time, but as soon as he put out the light and tries to sleep he cannot; he lies awake for hours without cause (after the fumes),².—Very sound sleep (two nights),¹⁸.—Prolonged unrefreshing sleep in the morning,¹.—[770.] In the morning he sleeps very long, as if stupid; is unusually sluggish; he will not rise until 10 o'clock (from fumes),².—Insufficient sleep in the morning; he always falls asleep again, and when he wakes it seems almost impossible for him to rise (in

---

† (Noak and Trinks have furuncles, but in a case in which they were produced from the bromides. The thirtieth potency, however, is decisive. It is now seen that they are produced by Bromine itself. C. Hg.)

four persons), (after the 30th),[1].—Decided sopor at night, early in the evening and late in the morning; one is obliged to make great exertion to rise,[18].
—Sleep very light; he is easily awakened (two nights),[18].—He awakes bright in the morning, at 5 o'clock (curative action),[4].—Wide awake in the evening, cannot sleep,[1].—Starting in sleep,[1].—Startings and twitchings in sleep,[2].—She lies asleep with her mouth open,[1].—Dreamy night (one night),[19].
—[780.] Night full of dreams,[4].—Restless dreamy sleep,[1].—Starting from sleep the second night, on account of restless dreams, he sprang out of bed, and only came to his senses by putting his feet on the cold floor,[18].—Vivid dreams, and wide awake on waking,[12].—Vivid dreams at night; he is ascending a height,[4].—A vivid dream in the second night, as if one were climbing a steep place, etc., and moving about in the bed without waking from sleep (two nights),[18].—Vivid dreams of journeyings, climbings, quarrels, and fightings, with distinct recollection on waking,[6].—She dreams of nothing but dying, coffins, and funerals (tenth day),[1].

Fever.—Chilliness. Sensitiveness to cold air, especially when walking; immediately a cold sensation runs through the back into the legs,[18].—Sensitiveness to cold air, and chilliness on motion in the evening (second day),[18].—[790.] Sensation of coldness at times (after one and a half hours),[18].
—Very chilly, with confusion of the head; with headache extending into the left eye (from 5th),[3].—Shivering through the whole body; very chilly, with external coldness, which is somewhat relieved by the warmth of the stove (from 3d),[3].—*Violent shiverings, with yawning and stretching*, as in intermittent fever, which she had ten years before; with this the head is confused; drawing in the left tibia down to the ankle, whereby the foot becomes quite cold; *this is repeated every other day, as a chilliness with cold feet* (from 30th),[2].—Coldness in the back and limbs in a warm room, at 3 P.M. (second day),[18].—Creepings down the back (from 5th),[3].—Creeping coldness over the back,[18].—Now and then coldness over the back, with cold hands and feet (after one hour),[18].—Cold drawings down the back (from 8th),[3].—Cold shivering drawing down the back (from 8th),[3].—[800.] Chilliness in the back when sitting, several times (after five hours),[18].—*Hands cold and moist,[18].—Cold tips of the fingers,[18].—Cold, exceedingly unpleasant drawing, through the whole body, with rapid alternations of warmth, at first in the left hand and side (from 8th),[3].—*Heat.* Sensation of internal burning; it seems as if she were in a hot vapor, though without sweat, in the forenoon,[5].
—Burning sensation in the whole body, while performing moderate manual labor; a clammy sweat breaks out in the evening, twelve hours after the burning in the ear (from 80th),[4].—At 9 A.M., an internal burning; afterward it seems beneath the skin and flesh,[4].—Heat rises into the head, now and then,[19].—Increased warmth in the forehead and chest (soon),[18].—Heat of the face,[11].—[810.] Heat in the nose and on the left cheek (from the 7th),[3].—Heat in the back, which extends into the head and face,[18].—Frequent heat, extending over the body from the back,[18].—Heat of both hands (from 7th),[3].—Heat of both hands and heat of the head, with coldness in the rest of the body,[3].—The right hand is hot and full, as if distended (from 8th),[3].—Heat in the feet (from 3d),[3].—Heat in the feet, in other respects he feels quite cold,[1].—*Sweat.* Sweats easily on slight movement,[1].—Sweat in the palms,[18].—[820.] Profuse sweat in the palms (after three hours),[18].—Sweat in the palms, with increased warmth (after one and a half hours),[10].

Conditions.—Aggravation.—(Morning), On waking, dizzy, headache, etc.; pain in forehead; gum pains; fasting, water tastes salt; throat stiff; cough; *erections;* dry cough: difficulty of breathing; pain in right chest ; after rising, cracking of the joints ; 9 o'clock, internal burning.—(*Forenoon*), Pain in forehead ; 11.30 o'clock, cramp in stomach ; 11 o'clock, stiffness in limbs.—(*Afternoon*), Blood-streaked mucus from nose ; tickling on malar bone ; hoarseness ; when walking, feeling in left arm, etc.; throat, etc., become stiff.—(*Toward evening*), In rather damp weather, pains of head ; burning in left ear ; scraping, etc., in fauces ; nausea.—(*Evening*), Apprehensiveness, etc.; vertigo ; pain in frontal bones, etc.; when sitting reading, vanishing of sight ; before going to sleep, earache ; cutting in both hypochondria ; pulsation in right hypochondrium ; cutting in left side ; pain in penis ; scraping in larynx ; pain in right chest ; palpitation ; tearing in anus ; on going out, pain in legs ; when stepping, pain in ball of foot ; on motion, chilliness.—(*Evening till midnight*), *Symptoms in general.—(*Acids*), Aggravate the symptoms and cause diarrhœa.—(*Bending shoulders forward*), Pains in left side of chest.—(*Lying bent*), Pain in left side.—(*After breakfast*), Sensation in larynx, etc.—(*Coughing*), Pain in forehead ; pain in chest.—(*Crossing running water*), Vertigo.—(*Damp weather*), Vertigo.—(*Drawing in abdominal walls*), Pain in region of navel.—(*After dinner*), Apoplectic sensation ; pain in forehead.—(*After eating*), Pain in region of navel.—(*Hawking up mucus*), Pain in throat.—(*In heat of sun*), Headache.—(*On deep inspiration*), Pressure on chest.—(*Lying down*), Vertigo.—(*Before menstruation*), Sticking in abdomen.—(*After drinking milk*), Headache.—(*Motion*), *Stitches in upper lid ; pain in right side ; tension in lumbar, etc., muscles ; pain in left knee, etc.—(*On moving eyes*), Pressure.—(*Moving nose*), Sensation in face.—(*When moving thorax*), Pain in side of chest.—(*After eating oysters*), *Diarrhœa returns,°.—(*Pressure*), Stitches in left upper lids ; pressure in stomach ; pain in stomach ; cutting in hypochondria ; pain in region of liver ; pain to left of navel ; pain in left side.—(*Deep pressing*), Pain in pit of stomach ; pain in right side.—(*When reading*), Sensitiveness of eyes ; stitches in eyelid.—(*Rest*), Pain in forehead.—(*Riding*), Pain in region of liver.—(*In room*), Pressure in frontal bones.—(*When sitting*), Symptoms seem to increase ; deep inspiration ; throbbing in right knee ; pain in legs ; chilliness in back.—(*Stooping*), Headache ; *stitches in upper lid.—(*Swallowing fluids*), Pain in throat.—(*Swallowing saliva*), Stitch in larynx.—(*Tobacco-smoking*), Causes nausea, etc.; pains in abdomen.—(*Turning head to left side*), Throat stiff, etc.—(*Turning thorax on its axis*), Pains in left chest.—(*After urinating*), Burning in urethra.—(*On waking*), Pain in side of chest.—(*Walking*), Pressure in prostate gland ; palpitation ; stiffness in front of thigh ; weakness.—(*Walking rapidly*), Stitches in right chest.—(*In warm room*), Symptoms seem to increase.

Amelioration.—(*Afternoon*), Stiffness in limbs.—(*Evening*), Difficulty of breathing.—(*Night*), Difficulty of breathing.—(*Motion in open air*), Symptoms in general.—(*Alcoholic stimulants*), Cured.—(*Vapor of alcohol*), Most of the symptoms.—(*Ammonia*), Most of the symptoms.—(*Black coffee*), Diarrhœa.—(*Cough*), Pain in inguinal canal.—(*After eating*), Symptoms disappear, etc.; nausea ; emptiness in stomach ; cramp in stomach.—(*When fasting*), Pain in right side not noticed.—(*Lying bent*), Sticking in abdomen.—(*Lying on right side, with arms over head*), Headache.—(*Motion*), *Most of the symptoms.—(*External pressure*), Toothache ; pains in abdomen ; pain in inguinal canal ; pain in right side.—(*Rest*), *Stitches in left upper lid.—(*When riding*), Symptoms disappear.—(*In shade*), Headache goes away.—(*After shaving*), Cold sensation in larynx, etc.—(*Stooping*), Pain in right side.—(*Walking*), Mental and bodily conditions ; pain in inguinal canal ; difficulty of breathing ; pain in right side of chest.

BRUCEA ANTIDYSENTERICA.

See STRYCHNOS NUX VOMICA.

BRUCINUM.

An alkaloid, obtained from the bark and seeds of Strychnos Nux vomica.
Formula, $C_{23}H_{26}N_2O_4$. *Preparations*, Triturations.
Authority. Lepelletier, Gaz. des Hop., 1851 (Zeit. f. Hom. Kl., 1, 57),
effects of 0.02 to 0.90 of a gramme.
Head.—Headache.
Eyes.—Hazy vision.
Ears.—Ringing in the ears.
Stomach.—Diminished appetite.—Thirst, from dryness of the mouth.—
Nausea.—Burning in the stomach.
Urinary Organs.—Increased urinary secretion (once).
Sexual Organs.—Erections.
Upper Extremities.—Twitching of the fingers.
Generalities.—Sudden jerkings, especially of the lower extremities
(increasing in intensity with the dose), spreading generally, but not ac-
companied with trismus and tetanus, and not extending to the œsophagus
and pharynx, as is the case with strychnia.—Twitchings in the paralyzed
as well as in the healthy muscles.—General weakness.
Skin.—Formication.—Itching of the skin.
Sleep.—Deep sleep, after the attacks.—Sleeplessness.
Fever.—A fever of short duration terminates the attacks.

BRYONIA.

Bryonia alba, Linn. *Natural order*, Cucurbitaceæ. *Common name*,
White Bryony; *German*, Zaunrebe. *Preparation*, Tincture of the root,
procured before flowering.
Authorities. 1, Hahnemann, from R. A. M. L., 2, 420; 2, Fr. Hahnemann, ibid.; 3, Hornburg, ibid.; 4, Herrmann, ibid.; 5, Michler, ibid.;
6, Ruckert, ibid.; 7, Stapf; 8, Nicolai, ibid. (*Nos.* 9 *to* 40 *are from the
daybooks of the Austrian provings, Œst. Zeit.,* 3, 1); 9, Arneth, two provings with 20 to 220 drops of the tincture; 10, Arneth, two provings with a
single dose of an ounce of the 203 d. dilution; 11, Gubatta, proving with
20 to 50 drops of tincture; 12, Wm. Huber, proved (*Bryonia dioica*), beginning with the 10th dil. and gradually descending to the 3d; 13, Wm.
Huber, proved (*Bryonia dioica*), 6 to 100 drops of the tincture; 14, Wenzel
Huber, proving with the 30th and 25th decimal dil.; 15, ibid., with 15 to
100 drops of the tincture; 16, Landesmann, proving with 8 to 180 drops of
tincture; 17, ibid., with 100 drops of the 1st dil.; 18, Mayrhofer, 20 to 200
drops of tincture; 19, ibid., 120 to 1000 drops of the 1st dec. dil.; 20,
Johanna B. (girl, 21 years old), 10 to 20 drops of tincture; 21, Anna Maria
M. (a woman, 34 years old), 5 to 100 drops of tincture; 22, Reisinger, 5 to
160 drops of tincture; 23, ibid., provings with the dilutions beginning with
the 8th decimal and descending to the 1st; 24, Dr. Schwarz, 3 to 140 drops
of the tincture; 25, ibid., 20 to 300 drops of the 6th dec. dil.; 26, Dr.

Wachtl, two provings, first, with 100 drops of tincture, second, with 200 drops; 27, ibid., 1st dec. dil.; 28, ibid., 6th dil.; 29, Dr. Watzke, 25 to 80 drops of tincture; 30, ibid., 100 drops of tinct. of *Bryonia dioica;* 31, ibid., 5 to 50 drops of tinct. of *Bryonia alba;* 32, Dr. Wurmb, 20 to 300 drops of tincture; 33, Zlatarovich, 8 to 50 drops of tincture; 34, "Gary Johann," 10 drops to ½ oz. of tincture; 35, Dr. Wurstel, 6th dil. (50 to 100 drops) of *Bryonia dioica;* 36, ibid., 20 to 50 drops of tincture; 37, Aloys Loewy, 60 to 130 drops of tincture of *Bryonia dioica;* 38, ibid., one dose of 215 drops of tincture of *Bryonia alba;* 39, Otto Piper's provings (also A. H. Z., 13), 10 to 200 drops of tincture; 40, ibid., 1 to 70 drops of tincture; 41, Lembke, N. Z. f. H. Kl., 4, 75, proving with 20 to 60 drops of tincture; 42, Dr. T. Dwight Stow, H. Month., 5, 359, took 15 drops of the 1st dec. dil.; 43, Dr. E. C. Price, Am. Hom. Obs., 2, 521, proving with 30 to 50 drops of the tincture.

Mind.—Emotions, Delirium. Mental illusion; her head seemed too heavy,[2].—*Irrational talking of his business, for an hour (after half an hour),[1].—**Nightly delirium,*[1].—**In the morning at daybreak delirious* prattling about business to be attended to; this disappears when the pain commences,[1].—About 10 o'clock at night, a delirious frightful fantasy, as of soldiers cutting him down; that he was on the point of escaping; with great heat in the body, sweat (without thirst); the delirium relieved by uncovering and getting cool,[1].—*Moods.* Much crying for one and a half days,[2]. —*(*Great despondency; disinclined to think; exhaustion of the intellectual powers*),[1].—**Despondent,*[3].—A very unusual melancholy mood,[22].—[10.] * *Great depression, and very morose mood without any cause, quite contrary to his habit,*[11].—My usual lively disposition becomes changed to hypochondria, which lasts several months, without any reason,[36].—*Anxiety; he is apprehensive of the future,[4].—**Anxiety in the whole body, which compelled him to do something constantly, and wherever he went he found no rest,*[1].— Feeling of anxiety on lying down in the evening, which appeared to depend upon a constriction of the chest,[29].—**In the room he became very anxious; better in the open air,*[2].—Great anxiety, with sensation of constriction of the cavity of the chest; difficult short respiration,[11].—* *Great sense of insecurity, with mental depression, and apprehension for the future* (sixth and seventh days),[42].—**Apprehensiveness, fearfulness* (after eighteen hours),[1].—He tried several times to escape from bed,[2].—[20.] **Disposition more irritable than usual; contradiction easily provoked anger during the whole proving,*[13].—*Irritable mood (will not have his wife and children about him; wishes to be alone),[31].—**Mood at once irritable, weeping, and morose,*[1].—**Very irritable mood; inclined to fright, fear, and vexation,*[1].—**Fretful mood,*[15].—Fretful; she imagines that she cannot accomplish her work; constantly takes up the wrong piece, and always inclined to change and take another; followed by pressive headache in the forehead,[1].—Ill-humor,[22].—**Ill-humored and inclined to be angry,*[3].—Very ill-humored and inclined to be angry,[1].—**Ill-humored and quarrelsome without reason,*[33].—[30.] *Very ill-humor; troubled with needless anxiety,[33]—General ill-humor and discomfort, after a meal,[33].—**Out of humor,*[15 36]—Out of humor during and after a meal,[33].—*Morose; everything puts him out of humor,[3].—Discontent,[33].—At first despondent, at last (after five days) jovial,[5].—*Intellect.* Over-busy; she undertakes and works far too much (after twenty hours),[1].—Disinclination for work,[15 22].— Imagination very sluggish; it is impossible to make any plan for the future, even for the next day; the judgment, however, is unimpaired,[53].—[40.] On attentive reading the thoughts seemed to vanish suddenly,[36].—*So weak in mind that his ideas disappear as if he would faint, together with heat in the face, especially on standing,¹.—*Mental exhaustion,³³.—Want of memory (after four hours),¹.—She is not conscious of what she is doing, and lets everything fall from her hands (in the room),².—She was not fully conscious of what she was doing (in a room); worse when lying; lasting twenty-four hours (immediately),².—Insensibility greatly increased in the evening,³³.

Head.—Confusion. *Confusion of the head,¹³ ¹⁵ ²² ²⁶ ³³.—*Confusion of the head* (second morning),³⁷.—*Head is confused (after one hour),⁴ ¹⁵.— [50.] *Confusion of the whole head,¹³.—Slight confusion of the head,¹¹ ²³.— Head suddenly confused,¹⁹.—Transient sensation of unusual confusion of the head, though much less than from previous doses, after 210 drops (first day),⁹.—*Head more or less confused the whole day (fourth day),³².—*Confusion of the head for several days after the proving,²².—*Great confusion in the head, especially in the frontal region,²³.—Slight confusion of the head in the forehead,¹⁵.—A dull, dizzy confusion in the head,⁵.—Head confused, as if in a vice,²².—[60.] Head confused in the morning,¹⁵.—*In the morning on waking, the head is as confused and aching as if he had dissipated and been intoxicated the evening previous; does not wish to rise from bed,¹.—Confusion of the head after rising from bed,¹³.—Confusion of the head the whole forenoon (second day),¹³.—Confusion in the head until he goes to sleep,¹.—Confusion of the head without definite pain, while riding for two hours over a very rough road,¹⁵.—Confusion of the head, especially when walking; disappeared when sitting quietly,³².—Confusion of the head, relieved by empty eructations,³⁶.—Head very much confused, relieved by moving in the open air,³⁶.—Confusion and stupefaction of the head,¹³.—[70.] Head confused and heavy,¹⁵.—Head confused and heavy after a meal,³³.—More confused than dizzy in the head,¹.—Very dizzy confusion and stupefaction of the head,¹³.—Confusion in the head, with dull pain in the forehead,¹⁸.—Head very much confused, with pressure in both temples,³⁶.—Confusion of the head, with pressive pain in the temples and forehead,²³.—*Confusion in the head, with drawing in the occiput, extending into the neck before going to sleep,³³. —Confusion of the head, with pressive pain in various places, now in the temples, now in the occiput, now in the forehead,³³.—Confusion of the head, which gradually increased to a severe pressive pain, especially in the left temple; this pain reached its greatest severity at 5 P.M., and was then accompanied by nauseous vomiting, great sensitiveness of the smell, and a hissing in the left ear like the noise of boiling water; all these symptoms disappeared within half an hour after riding in a wagon,³².—*Vertigo.* [80.] Continued inclination to vertigo,¹¹.—*Vertigo,¹ ²².—Slight vertigo (after three hours),¹⁵.—*Several times momentary vertigo, as though all objects were reeling (after four hours),¹⁸.—Vertigo, as from drunkenness, the whole day (after eight days),¹.—A kind of vertigo, as if he were drunk, and as if the blood rushed furiously to the head,⁴.—Vertigo in the morning,².— Frequent attacks of vertigo during the forenoon,³⁶.—*Vertigo in the afternoon, as though the brain were turning around (eighteenth day),²⁶.—Vertigo suddenly towards midnight,³⁹.—[90.] Slight vertigo after eating,²⁶.—*Slight vertigo on raising the head from inclining it forward (after three to four hours),⁴².—*Vertigo as soon as he rises from his chair; everything turns about; after walking awhile it disappears,¹.—*Vertigo like whirling if she sits up in bed, with nausea in the middle of the chest, as if faintness would ensue,¹.—*Vertigo, as if one were being turned around, or as if everything whirled about, when standing,¹.—*So great vertigo, on standing, at 8 P.M., that he reeled backwards, and nearly fell over backwards,¹.—Vertigo and reeling of all objects while walking; the general exhaustion increased to a feeling of complete prostration,[19].—Frequent attacks of vertigo while walking in the open air, which disappeared always on sitting down,[37].—Vertigo, with feeling of heaviness; it seems as if everything were turning in a circle,[4].—Vertigo, with fulness of the head,[3].—[100.] Dizziness in the head,[27].—Dizzy and weak on waking in the morning,[15].—*Dizzy in the morning, and weak in the limbs the whole day,[1].—*In the morning on rising from bed, dizzy and whirling, as if the head were turning in a circle,[1].—On sitting (stooping) and reading, dizzy heaviness in the head, which disappears on raising up the head,[1].—Dizziness on turning the head (third day),[42].—He felt as if drunk, and would lie down,[2].—After moving when standing, she tottered to one side,[1].—On walking he reeled to both sides, as if he could not stand firmly (after forty-eight hours),[1].—*General Sensations.* Head feels light, with constant wabbling in both ears (sixth and seventh days),[42].— [110.] The head is dull; reflection is difficult,[4].—Dulness in the head, with remarkable forgetfulness,[2].—*Stupefaction of the head,[1].—*Stupefaction of the head (fourth day),[38].—Headache (after half an hour),[18].—Tormenting headache,[11].—The head is painful, especially to touch, mostly in the forepart, for twenty-four hours,[2].—Headache in the morning on waking,[1].— Headache on waking, which continued to increase, lasting all day (second day),[28].—Awoke with headache, especially over the left eye; after rising the pain extended towards the vertex and occiput, and there disappeared,[33].— [120.] *Headache commences in the morning, not on waking, but when first opening and moving the eyes,[1].—*Headache in the morning after rising, *a twitching-drawing in the malar and maxillary bones,*[1].—Violent headache in the forenoon, especially in the forehead and vertex,[33].—Headache towards evening, with all the symptoms of a commencing coryza,[21].— (Headache a quarter of an hour after every meal; it then gradually ceased, but returned after the next meal),[1].—*Heat in the head,* with continued nausea from the stomach,[13].—*Rush of blood to the head,[13].—At first the blood mounts to the head, then a pressing together of both temples follows,[1]. —He is scarcely able to turn the head on account of a feeling of fulness in it,[3].—*Heaviness in the head,[36].—[130.] *Excessive heaviness of the head* (frequently, and also after four days),[4].—*The head seems as heavy as a hundredweight,[1].—Sense of heaviness and vertigo in the head,[11].—*Great heaviness in the head, and pressure of the whole brain forward,[1].—*Violent headache, like a great weight in the head, as if he would incline it to either side, with pressure in the brain from within outward, and great desire to lie down, immediately,[1].—Oppressive headache in the afternoon,[17].—*Always on coughing, motion in the head like pressure,[1].—Pressive headache (after three hours),[15].—Pressive headache, which became so severe in half an hour that he was obliged to stop riding,[15].—*Headache, as if something pressed the skull asunder,[1].—[140.] Sensation as if the head were pressed together from both ears,[3].—Pressive headache in the morning (second day),[15].—Violent pressive headache on waking in the morning, especially seated in the upper portion of the forehead; after rising the pain extends to the supraorbital region; during the forenoon slight returns of the headache; in the afternoon quite well,[33].—*In the morning before breakfast, pain as if the head were compressed, with heaviness in it mingled with stitches; she could not raise the eyes on account of the pain, and if she stooped she could not rise up (after sixty hours),[1].—Pressive headache, more upon one side, with severe pressive sensation in the eye of the same side (in the afternoon),[6].—*A pressure in the head, as if the brain were too full and pressed outward, mostly when sitting,[1] —

(Pressure in the head on stooping),[1].—Headache pressing together, with jerks in the brain like pulsation,[1].—*Stitches in the head from the forehead to the occiput,[1].—[150.] *Stitches through the head, mostly from before backward, on stepping hard,[15].—On walking in the open air, a stitching in the head, then on the temples,[1].—When coughing, shooting through the whole head,[1].—Pain in the head, more a twitching than a throbbing, with a hot face,[1].—A throbbing headache, which affects the eyes so that she cannot see well; on motion, the throbbing in the head becomes more rapid; she thinks she hears it,[1].—*Forehead.* Whirling sensation in the right side of the forehead, and a stitch in the left side of the forehead,[1].—*Frontal headache,[18].—Dull headache in the frontal and temporal regions (soon),[9]. —Frontal headache during the whole forenoon,[18].—Slight headache in the left side of the forehead and in the occiput, with slight tension in the right side of the neck just below the mastoid process at 4 P.M.,[13].—[160.] A tension in the frontal muscles under the skin, on moving the eyes,[1].—Drawing, distending headache in the left half of the forehead and occiput, while walking about the room,[13].—Dull compression in the head, in the forehead above the eyes,[1].—In the afternoon, from a two hours' quiet nap, he felt a constrictive pain in the frontal region and heaviness in the head, which, after one hour, was relieved by washing with cold water (second day),[37].—Painful drawing in the whole forehead, with cloudiness and confusion of the head,[18].—Drawing headache in the left side of the forehead (morning of third day),[13].—Painful drawing and tension in the left half of the forehead above the eyebrow, as though a bud were slowly unfolding in the forehead, and caused a pressure upon the parts about it,[13].—Very painful drawing and tension in the left side of the forehead above the brow,[13].—Painful drawing and tension in the right frontal eminence and in the posterior portion of the right parietal bone, lasting ten or fifteen seconds, and after a quarter of an hour alternating with the same pain in the same places on the left side at 6 P.M.,[13].—Slight drawing headache in the forehead, and pressure in the occiput,[13].—[170.] Pressive frontal headache (after one hour),[15].—Pressive pain in the whole frontal region,[23].—*A pressive pain in the forehead, so that he can scarcely stoop,[3].—*Pressive frontal headache, very much increased by stooping (second day),[27].—*Headache on stooping, as if everything would fall out at the forehead,[1].†—*Pressing outward in the frontal region and left eyeball from above downward, especially on stooping, in the evening,[28].—*Headache as if everything would press out at the forehead.‡—Headache after eating, and on taking a walk a pressing outward in the forehead,[1].—Violent pressive pain in the forehead, especially toward both eyebrows after an ordinarily violent motion (afternoon of first day),[9].—*Pressive pain in the forehead and occiput, aggravated by motion,[24].— [180.] Pressive pain in the forehead, which appeared after continued reading (third day),[9].—*Pressive pain above the left eye which continued for half an hour, was followed by a dull pressive pain in the occipital protuberances, whence it spread over the whole body, and continued more or less severe the whole day; on quick motion and after eating the pain

---

† Sensation of pressing asunder accompanied that of pressing together (162. 127, 140, 148, 144) almost always, since it is felt by the brain inclosed in the unyielding skull; the organic senses cannot distinguish whether the painfulness arises from its great distension, or from the resistance of the skull, and hence either may cause the sensation.

‡ Compare 357.

became so severe that it seemed like a distinct pulsation within the head,[24].—*Digging pressure in the forepart of the brain towards the forehead, especially severe on stooping and walking rapidly; walking fatigues him very much* (after twenty-four hours),[4].—Headache, even on stooping a pressure outward in the forehead mingled with stitches,[1].—A drawing-pressive pain in the forehead over the right eye, which after two hours changed to a violent drawing pain in the diseased incisors of the same side; a quarter of an hour after this toothache had ceased the headache returned, which gradually spread over the whole forehead, and lasted all day,[21].—*Tearing in the head across the forehead, then tearing in the cervical muscles, then tearing in the right arm,*[1].—Stitches in the forehead in the forepart, with confusion of the head,[3].—Itching, needle-like stitches in the right frontal muscles,[4].—Throbbing headache in the forehead, so that he is obliged to lie down,[3].—Pain in the forehead and occiput, a kind of hollow throbbing (after two hours),[1].—*Temples.* [190.] Gurgling in both temples,[1].— Headache in the temporal and frontal regions alternating with pressive pains in the finger and wrist joints, and with griping in the abdomen,[15].— Pain in the temples, as if one pulled them by the hair,[1].—Drawing pain in the right temple (soon),[34].—Painful drawing in the left temporal region near the eye, returning several times at short intervals,[13].—*Slight drawing in both temples towards the malar bones,*[26].—**Slight drawing in the temporal bones from above downward towards the zygoma,** *especially on the left side* (after four hours); afterwards this symptom returned and extended to the left jaw,[27].—Drawing in the temporal muscles, in the muscles of the upper arm, and here and there in the body,[33].—Drawing in the temples, followed soon afterwards by copious pasty evacuations,[27].—Drawing and pressing in the left temple (after two hours),[28].†—[200.] Pressing-out pain in both temples,[1].—Pressing together in the temporal bones alternates frequently with drawing pains in the occipital protuberances,[27].—Pain in the left temporal region, as though the brain were pressed out at various places (fourth day),[32].—The head seemed as if pressed from both temples towards the forehead,[36].—Tearing-pressing in both temples (tenth day),[26].—Throbbing pressure in the head from within outward towards the temporal bones, on going to bed,[26].—*Pain in the right temple; a tensive twisting in single muscle-fibres,* lasting several seconds, very sensitive,[31].—*Drawing-tearing pain in the right temple, but mostly extending down into the upper back teeth and the muscles of the neck* (forenoon of fourth day),[26].‡—Pressive-tearing pains in the temples, which sometimes extend to the occiput, sometimes to the petrous portion of the temporal bones, and frequently change their position during the last days of the proving,[26].—Frequent sudden stitches in the head from the temporal region to the forehead,[36].—[210.] Violent stitches in both temples, which several times extended over the parietal region,[29].—*Vertex.* In the region of the crown and of the forehead dull motions in the head, which cause vertigo and cessation of ideas,[5].—Increase of pain under vertex, with soreness of scalp just over the same; painful soreness of vertex, it feels bruised (after three to four hours),[42].—A spot on the top of the head, as large as half a dollar, of burning pain, which is not sore to touch,[1].—Sensation of weight pressing on vertex (sixth and seventh

---

† Almost always the first symptom in the proving of this drug. Wl.

‡ This prover suffered from the same pain two years previously in the summer; after several days and several ineffectual remedies, it was cured within an hour by Bryonia.

days),[42].—Sensible beating in vertex, with same, and fulness within cranium, in region of cerebellum (first day),[42].—*In the morning on waking, a headache on the top of the head, a painful throbbing*,[1].—**Parietals.** Pain behind and above the ear on left side of head (thirteenth day),[43].—Throbbing-drawing pulsating pain in the parietal bone, extending to the forehead (third day),[34].—Pressing-together pain on both sides of the head,[3].—[220.] Semilateral headache; a (digging) pressure upon a small spot in the right half of the brain, like a kind of digging or tearing, extending along down the bones of the upper and lower jaws, associated with a painful submaxillary gland (after thirty hours),[1].—*On coughing, a long-continued stitch deep in the brain on the left side*,[1].—Tearing in the sides of the head (first day),[41].—Tearing in the left side of the head (after twenty-four hours),[2].—Throbbing in the right side of the head, which is perceptible externally to the hand,[1].—Piercing pain in the right parietal bone, as if torn with a sharp hook,[33].—Suddenly a drawing-throbbing pain on the right parietal eminence, which disappeared on pressure (forenoon of second day),[34].—**Occiput.** Numb sensation over the whole occiput, with a feeling as though it were enlarged,[13].—Dull pain in the occiput,[3].—*In the morning, in bed, after waking, while lying upon the back, headache in the occiput, which extends to the shoulders, like a heaviness which pressed upon a sore spot*,[1].—[230.] Painfulness of the lower portion of the left side of the occiput, aggravated by touch, at 4 P.M.,[17].—Dull pressure in the occiput,[6].—Slight pressure in both sides of the occiput,[13].—Painful pressure on the left side of the occiput, with momentary sticking pain in the left heel,[13].—*A pressive pain in the occiput, with drawing down into the neck; this pain was relieved towards noon,* but appeared in the afternoon as a pressure in the temporal bones, also frequently in the frontal and occipital regions,[27].—A tensive pressive pain in both sides of the occiput,[13].—Sharp pain in left occipital protuberance, coming and going suddenly (after half an hour to two hours),[42].—Sore feeling on one side of the occiput on touch,[3].—**External Head.** The scalp tightly drawn over the head and sensitive,[33].—Sensation as if the scalp on the posterior half of the skull were spasmodically contracted, which caused a kind of tension in the anterior half of it, for half an hour (eighth day),[26].—[240.] *Sensitiveness of the scalp towards evening*,[31].—A biting-gnawing on the scalp at night,[1].—A peculiar crawling and creeping sensation in the scalp on both sides of the ears to the distance of about an inch,[33].—Itching of the head while combing,[1].—*In the morning the hair seems very fatty,* with a cool head; the hands become fatty while combing the hair (after ten hours),[1].

Eyes.—In the forenoon sudden swelling of one eye with pain, without redness; there is a discharge of pus and the conjunctiva is dark-red and swollen,[1].—In the afternoon a sensation in the right eye as if a grain of sand were in it,[1].—Biting in the eyes as if sand (?) were in them, which causes rubbing,[1].—*Severe burning and lachrymation of the right eye*,[21].—Pressure in the eyes for sixteen days in succession,[2].—[250.] In the morning on waking a pressure in the eye, as if it were pressed with the hand, or as from a room full of smoke,[1].—Pressure in the eyes, with burning-itching sensation of the lids,[3].—**Orbit.**—Headache in a spot in the supraorbital ridge of the size of a needle (soon),[9].—A transient pain deep in the right orbit aggravated by pressure upon the eyeball,[19].—Pain as if burnt from without into the left eye (after twenty-four hours),[2].—Pain as from a burn over the left eye and on the left side of the nose, relieved by pressure,[2].—Contractive pain in the muscles of the right eyebrow,[4].—Slight drawing-pinching pain in the right eyebrow, with severe itching of the left, causing rubbing (third day),[34].—Aching in left orbit, pulsation in the same (after three to four hours),[42].—Drawing pain, beginning slowly and increasing gradually, over the left eyebrow, extending into the forehead, frequently repeated,[13].—[260.] Pressive pain above the left eye,[23].—Sensitive pressive pains all about the right eye, especially on the lower margin of the orbit, in the evening, in the open air,[33].—Slight pressing pain in the left supra-orbital region, which extended to the right side,[23].—Pressure from within outward over the right orbit into the brain, which changes to a pressure on the eyeball from above downward (after three days),[4].—Transient stitches in the eyebrows,[16].—Fine stitches above the right eyebrow,[33].—Sticking, bruising pain in the upper border of the right orbit, with a feeling of heaviness in the left (third and fourth day),[34].—*Lids.* Redness and swelling of the lids, with pressure in them for three days (after third day),[2]. —*Puffiness of the right upper lid,*[21].—The lower lid is at times red and inflamed, the upper one twitches,[1].—[270.] Swelling of the lower lid, together with pressive pain; the eyes agglutinated in the morning,[1].—Lids, especially of the right eye, swollen and somewhat reddened (second day),[32]. —In the morning the lids seem swollen and *agglutinated,*[1].—Twitching in the right upper lid,[31].—*Painless twitching drawing together in the left upper lid, with a persistent sensation of heaviness therein,*[31].—In the morning on waking he is scarcely able to open the eyes; they are agglutinated with purulent matter,[4].—Lids agglutinated in the morning, with a burning-biting in the right canthi (ninth day),[26].—The lids feel agglutinated in the morning, somewhat red and swollen, and ache as if rubbed and heated,[1].—Agglutination of the lids in the morning, and after a forcible opening he saw as through a veil, soon disappearing (third day),[37].—Slight burning in the lids of the right eye (fourth day),[58].—[280.] Pressure above the lids towards evening,[23].—Sore pain in the left inner canthus, with smarting,[1].—Sticking-itching on the margin of the right lid relieved by rubbing,[13].—Increased burning in both external canthi on touch,[33].—Itching-biting in the left external canthus,[13].—Itching in the left external canthus, together with some biting, not relieved by rubbing (after six hours),[1].—*Lachrymal Apparatus.* Frequent lachrymation,[4].—The eyes fill with tears and the lids itch, as if something were healing; is obliged to rub them,[1].—Profuse lachrymation; the white of the eye is red, lids agglutinated in the external canthus,[28].—Much lachrymation in the open air,[1].—*Ball.* [290.] Pressure on the right eyeball, more from above downward (after third day),[4].—* *Very sensitive pressive pain (coming and going) in the left eyeball, especially violent on moving the ball, with a feeling as if the eye became smaller and were retracted within the orbit,*[31].—A throbbing in the right eyeball,[2].— *Vision.* Vision as through a mist (fourth day),[38].—Dim vision of the left eye, as if it were full of water,[r].—Weakness of the eyes in the morning; if she attempts to read all the letters run together,[1].—(Presbyopia), she is able to see clearly at a distance, but not near (after twenty-four hours),[1].—Flickering before the right eye on looking out of the window after a very moderate dinner; afterwards *appearance of all the colors of the rainbow; every object seemed covered with these colors;* on closing the eye there appeared a jagged, broken, iridescent stripe, which on keeping the eye closed a long time became of a blinding white color; the left eye was not affected by this illusion; after a quarter of an hour these symptoms disappeared, but the eye remained weak for some time; after half an hour *photophobia* and confusion of the head,[33].

Ear.—Objective. Boil-like swelling before the ear, which arises after twelve hours, discharges, and becomes a yellowish scurf,[2].—Discharge of blood from the ears,[1].—*Subjective.* [300.] Sensation as if the ears were stopped and no air could enter them,[1].—Pain about the left ear,[3].—Burning in the lobules of the ear,[3].—Dull pain as if burnt, extending from without into the left ear (after six hours),[2].—A constrictive pain in the meatus auditorius, which only disappears after removing the wax with the finger, but suddenly returns again, with difficult hearing,[5].—A slight drawing pain in the right ear,[17].—Pressure in the right concha,[26].—Severe pressure on the right cartilage of the ear,[1].—Sensation in the external meatus as if the finger were pressed into it, which increases on stooping, when reading,[6].— Violent sticking in the right meatus auditorius (fifth day),[34].—[310.] Stitches in the ears (fourth day),[34].—A slight stitch when touched on the convex surface of the right ear (fifth day),[10].—If he goes into the open air or goes into the house from a walk he feels stitches, now under one ear, now under the other ear,[1].—The whole of the union of the ear with the skull is sensitive (sixth day),[10].—The border of the ear and the point of the union of the ear with the skull is so sensitive that washing is unpleasant (seventh day),[10].—The sensitiveness of the ear extends from the convex to the concave surface; the latter was decidedly red, the temperature of the ear increased. the external meatus somewhat swollen, the convex surface rather painful; during the course of the day the symptoms increased; the inner surface of the ear became hot to the touch; the swelling increased; at times severe stitches pierced deep into the ear; the heat was diminished, though only momentarily; ringing in the ear; chewing became difficult and the bony parts about the ear painful; at night it was impossible to lie upon the right side; the next day the condition of the ear was the same, only somewhat more painful; there was also a constant noise before the ear as of boiling water; the hearing itself was not impaired; pressure upon the ear, even severe, was pleasant, but warmth especially so; cracking in the ear on sneezing; the night was very restless; next day the stitches in the ear were more frequent, often when at rest, but especially on every step; hearing was somewhat diminished; cold air increased the pain in the ear; the next day, after an almost sleepless night, the swelling in the ear had decidedly increased; the hearing on the right side very much diminished, the hissing continued, the right ear felt completely stopped; the swelling and pain extended over a portion of the parotid gland into the zygoma; transient stitches extend into the head and external portion of the neck; on the two last evenings there was slight chilliness and some acceleration of the otherwise small pulse; it was interesting to notice that, while listening to harmonies of music, the high tones were heard correctly, while the lower ones seemed incorrect and even reversed; the next night was sleepless, with the exception of about two hours; it was not, however, the excessive pain that kept him awake, but he could not find a place to lay the head without the general integument over parotid being made tense, for such tension caused pain sufficient to prevent sleep; the parotid gland was especially sensitive to the touch of the steel bows of the glasses, which also caused violent burning, that lasted several seconds after removing them; this symptom, which did not disappear during the whole duration of the Bryonia ear-trouble, was at first ascribed simply to pressure, but he became convinced that the burning pain was just as violent from a light touch upon the parotid with the steel as from severe pressure; the region of the parotid gland was very much distended, and tearing pains attacked two teeth in the lower jaw (he had never suffered from toothache except when proving Colocynth); the next night was almost sleepless; the ear continued to swell, so that the convex surface continued to be more removed from the base of the ear, the margin was double its ordinary size, the external skin was very red and warmer than usual, and the hearing greatly diminished; sudden creeping shivering over the back; small, accelerated pulse; the toothache continued the whole day, with some interruption; the next night was entirely sleepless; the next day all symptoms aggravated; the following day the external ear stood out from the base of the ear; the skin, especially on the margin, thickened, dry, white, with many scales, insensible to touch, but itching exceedingly; the meatus was very much contracted, the antitragus very much thickened, hearing greatly diminished; at short intervals violent stitches pierced the auditory apparatus; cracking in the internal ear when sneezing, hawking, etc.; the region of the parotid gland greatly distended and painful even to slight pressure; burning and sensation of warmth lasted for some time after touch; the swelling extended even to the lower eyelid and the right side of the neck; toothache continues in the molar teeth of the right side of the lower jaw, it was like electric shocks and caused one to drink cold water instinctively, whereby the pain was completely relieved for a time, but returned after a few minutes with the same intensity. The next morning a severe chill attacked the back and extremities, with small, accelerated, depressed pulse; he remained in bed and took, morning and evening, six pellets of the thirtieth dilution of Rhus tox.; the symptoms lasted all day, with the same intensity; towards evening, although in friendly company, he could not rid himself of the idea that he would become delirious in the night, and spoke of all possible precautions in such a case; *indeed he could scarcely help thinking of the probably fatal issue of his sickness.* The next night he slept very little; he had headache, which extended from the region of the parotid gland into the temple; a little after midnight he had a sensation of moisture in the ear; there really was a small quantity of odorless, dark matter, like ear-wax. On the next day, the same symptoms as yesterday; took, morning and evening, a dose of Rhus; he did not leave his bed; no appetite or thirst; taste not changed; in the afternoon there was some discharge from the ear; the matter discharged was clearer than that of yesterday; the next night was still little refreshing; in addition to the toothache, which still continued, he was troubled by repeated severe stitches extending from the region of the parotid through the malar bone to the nose. The next morning, the fever had disappeared and he sat up for a few hours; the discharge from the ear was more profuse, quite clear and smelt like pus; warm injections were especially agreeable; dry warmth he could not endure, on account of the burning pain which it caused; the discharge from the ear lasted three days; on the fourth it ceased, the toothache also ceased, the hearing improved, and the nights became refreshing; the sensitiveness of the ear and also the diminished acuteness of hearing lasted a week longer; during this time portions of the integument of the ear desquamated; even after this the parotid region was sensitive to steel (from fifth to thirty-second day),[10].†—

Hearing. Difficult hearing in the left ear, as though it was stopped,[13].— Rumbling before the right ear,[1].—A chirping in the head as from locusts,[1].—Ringing in front of the left ear, as from small bells (after one hour),[2].—[**320.**] Ringing in both ears with difficult hearing for two hours,[28].—

*Roaring in the ears,[18] [27].—Roaring in the ears (half an hour),[18].—Sudden roaring in the ears,[13].—Roaring, humming in left ear, resembling the pouring of water over a dam (first day),[42].—More roaring in right than left ear (after two hours),[42].—Roaring in the ears, with accelerated pulse,[18].—A sudden very peculiar sensation in the ears, as if one heard the noise of a wind-mill at a great distance, it commences in the left ear and goes to the right; disappears in ten minutes,[33].

Nose.—Objective. *Swollen nose, with nose-bleed for several days (after five days),[2].—*Swelling of the tip of the nose, with twitching pain in it, and on touch feeling as if it would ulcerate,[1].—[330.] An ulcer within the left nostril, with biting pain,[1].—Frequent sneezing (soon after taking),[32].— Frequent forcible sneezing,[33].—Violent sneezing in the morning (after eighteen hours),[1].—Sneezing eight times in the forenoon (thirty-second day),[16].—Several attacks of sneezing at 10 P.M.,[17].—Sneezing several times in succession (afternoon of ninth day),[26].—Severe sneezing six times in succession, in the evening (as if a coryza would appear, which, however, did not), (second day),[16].—*When coughing, sneezing twice,[1].—Frequent sneezing, especially if he strokes the hand across the forehead,[1].—[340.] Violent sneezing and yawning in the morning (after forty-eight hours),[1].—Frequent sneezing; severe coryza,[23].—Closing of right and opening of left nostril, with tendency to watery discharge (after two to three hours),[42].—A sudden stopped coryza, with roaring in the left ear, and a sensation as though something were placed before it, which diminished the hearing,[13].—Copious discharge from the nose,[21].—Much mucus in the nose and bronchials,[23].— Slight, thin discharge from left nostril (fourth day),[42].—Fluid, thin, light-colored discharge from right nostril (after half an hour to two hours),[42].— Fluent coryza for eight days,[2].—Fluent coryza, with greenish discharge, preceded by repeated sneezing; this gradually diminished, lasting fourteen days (seventeenth day),[16].—[350.] Violent fluent coryza, with chilliness in the skin; stretching of the limbs, with frequent yawning,[13].—Profuse coryza, with pain in the forehead,[2].—Profuse coryza, without cough (after thirty-six hours),[1].—Very restless night on account of profuse, fluent coryza,[21].—Profuse fluent coryza, so that he speaks through the nose, together with chilliness, for eight days,[2].—Profuse fluent coryza, with much sneezing, for eight days (after forty-eight hours),[2].—Severe coryza, mostly stopped (after forty-eight hours),[1].—Severe coryza, with sticking headache; it seems to press out at the forehead, especially when stooping (after seventy hours),[1].†— The coryza was better in the open air, and discharged more in the room,[21].— A few drops of bright red blood from the left nostril (morning of third day),[16].—[360.] Discharge of red blood from the right nostril follows the vertigo,[39].—Nose-bleed (after forty-eight and seventy-two hours),[1].—Nose-bleed (after ten and sixteen days),[2].—Nose-bleed, without having stooped,[1].— *Nose-bleed, for a quarter of an hour in the morning, after rising,[1].— *Profuse nose-bleed, daily (after fourteen days),[2].—*Nose-bleed, three days in succession (tenth, eleventh, and twelfth days),[2].—Nose-bleed several times daily (for fourteen days),[2].—Nose-bleed from the right nostril (after nine days),[2].—Nose-bleed during sleep, in the morning at 3 o'clock, so that he is awakened thereby (after four days),[1].—[370.] Nose-bleed, followed by ulcerated nostrils,[1].—**Subjective.** Frequent crawling and tickling in the septum of the nose, especially on blowing it,[1].

† Compare 174, 176, H.

Face.—Objective. Paleness of the face for twenty-four hours,[2].—The color of the face was very pale the whole day,[13].—Red spots in the face and on the neck for two days,[1].—*Red, hot, soft puffiness of the face,*[2].— Great swelling of the upper half of the face, especially great swelling under the eyes and over the root of the nose, with swelling of the eyelids; was unable to open the left eye for four days (after three days),[2].—*Subjective.* Stiffness of the facial muscles, which lasted nearly two hours with varying severity, whereby it seemed as if any desired expression could be given to the face by simply pushing the muscles,[15].—Drawing in the facial muscles,[33].—(Painful throbbing in all parts of the face, which is perceptible even to external touch),[1].—*Cheeks.* [380.] Swelling of the right cheek close by the ear, with burning pain (after four days),[2].— Swelling of the left side of the face, more down along the nose, with some pain in it (with diarrhœa),[2].—A drawing pain in the left cheek (after half an hour),[16].—*Painful pressure under the right cheek-bone, relieved by external pressure* (after one hour),[4].—*Pinching pressure in the articular cavity of the right jaw, more violent on motion,*[4].—Violent tearing in the left cheek,[36].— *Twitching-tearing in the right malar bone, up to the right temple, externally sore upon touch,*[4].—Drawing-tearing pain in the left upper and lower jaws, as from a drawing toothache,[36].—*Lips.* *The upper lip and expansion of the nose swollen, red, and hot, as in beginning erysipelas;* the swelling disappeared after an hour, but the lip remained sensitive to touch,[33].—*A crack in the lower lip,*[2].—[390.] A small aphthous erosion appears on the mucous membrane of the upper lip,[13].—Twitching in both corners of the mouth, so that he could not hold his cigar,[33].—Trembling in the lower lip, followed by loss of power in it, and the lip is drawn to the left side, disappearing after ten minutes (sixth day),[26].—The lips stick together,[33].—*Great dryness of the lips, of the tongue, and of the hard palate, while the tip of the tongue was moist* (after half an hour), (from 7th dil.),[12].—Burning in the lower lip,[3].—*Lower Jaw.* A feeling in the lower jaw as if a pimple were on the bone, with a pressive pain on touch, and on turning the head (after sixty-one hours),[7].

Mouth.—Teeth. Looseness of all the teeth noticed on touch, and when biting,[1].—*The teeth seem too long,*[2].—A diseased tooth causes him to rise from bed and have it extracted; after the operation a sudden violent vertigo; this continues a long time while sitting,[37].—[400.] *Pain as if a tooth were screwed in and then pulled out,* **which is momentarily relieved by cold water,** *but becomes better on walking in the open air, together with tearing in the cheeks and pinching in the ears, at night, till 6 A.M.,*[1].—*Toothache if one takes anything warm into the mouth,*[1].—Toothache on opening the mouth; the air streams in painfully,[1].—*Toothache about 3 A.M., as if an exposed nerve in a hollow tooth were paining from cold air,* **which becomes aggravated on lying on the painless side, and then goes away if one lies on the painful cheek,**[1].—Frequent grumbling in a hollow tooth,[36].—Toothache towards evening, now tearing, now drawing; this returns every day for more than a month,[36].—Excessive toothache during rest, and especially in bed, which is relieved by chewing,[3].—Pains in the teeth and limbs, in the upper arm, wrist, thumbs, tibiæ, malleoli; on the right side they last all day, while on the left side they are transient,[34].—*On eating, a drawing-sticking toothache extends into the muscles of the neck; is especially aggravated by warmth,*[1].— Periodic drawing and tearing pains in the teeth (third day),[36].—[410.] Toothache, stitching, and twitching in the cheek, extending toward the ear, which compels one to lie down,[1].†—A hollow tooth in the left lower jaw, and the gum about it becomes sensitive to the touch of the tongue as if sore,[33].—A sore pain in the teeth, not when drinking cold drinks,[1].—Tearing in the left teeth,[36].—*Jerking toothache when smoking* (which he was accustomed to), (after one hour),[1].—Throbbing-drawing pain in the roots of the right lower incisors, and when these are relieved by pressure upon them a similar pain appears in the two upper middle incisors; afterwards the same pain in the last upper molars of the right side; the pain causes a waving sensation,[34].—In the morning after waking, a feeling as if all the back teeth were too long; they can be moved back and forth; they are so loose that she is not able to bite with them, and when she tries to bite pain as if they fell out, lasting fifteen hours (after forty-eight hours),[7].—Pain in the back teeth, only when chewing,[1].—A drawing-tensive pain in the two upper right molars, relieved by pressure with the tongue, or biting the teeth together,[34].—Drawing pain in the back teeth of the upper and lower jaw (after twenty-four hours),[4].—[420.] *Drawing, at times jerking toothache in the left upper back teeth, only during and after eating, when the teeth seem too long and wabble back and forth* (after six hours),[4].—*In the evening, in bed, jerking toothache, now in the upper, now in the lower back teeth* (for an hour); *when the pain is in the upper teeth, and they are pressed by the tip of the finger, then the pain suddenly ceases, and changes to the corresponding lower teeth* (after five days),[1].—The pains in the teeth and limbs are aggravated by lying down, and last till he falls asleep,[34].—*Gums.* Spongy gums,[1].—Dull aching in alveoli of upper jaw, right side, now jumping, and now mild (after half an hour to two hours),[42].—*The gum is painful, as if sore and raw, with painful loose teeth,[1].—*Tongue.* *Tongue coated white,[15].—*Very white-coated tongue,[1].—*Tongue thickly coated white,[24].—Tongue thinly coated yellow, with sunken raphe, or longitudinal fissure (second day),[42].—[430.] Blisters on the anterior margin of the tongue, biting and burning,[2].—A painful blister in the middle of the left margin of the tongue, disappearing after a few hours, but slightly felt for several days (twenty-first day),[16].—*Several small aphthæ on the tip of the tongue, which disappear after a few days,[33].—Tip of tongue dry; filiform papillæ are much elevated and prickle (second day),[42].—Dryness of tongue, with sensation of prominent papillæ (after half an hour to two hours),[42].—Burning pain in the middle of the tongue, followed after an hour by a hard lump as large as a pea in the same place, which lasted two days (in the evening, twentieth day),[16].—Tobacco-smoking caused burning on the tongue,[33].—Fine pricking in anterior third of tongue (after half an hour to two hours),[42].—*General Mouth.* Offensive breath,[1].—Very offensive smell from the mouth, with hawking of offensive tough mucus, sometimes in round cheesy lumps of the size of a pea (after twenty days),[34].—*Mouth and lips very dry,[33].—[440.] *Dryness in the mouth, so that the tongue sticks to the palate,[2].—*Mouth dry; drinking moistens it for a moment, but the former dryness returns in a greater degree,[33].—A dry sensation in the mouth in the morning (after forty-eight hours),[5].—Unusual dryness in the mouth in the evening; the palate, tongue, and lips, almost stick together, so that

---

† There are several symptoms of Bryonia which oblige one to lie down (compare 688, 1273, 1626), or to sit down (736), and several which are increased by walking and standing (as 848), but on the contrary, there is a secondary action, in which the symptoms are relieved by motion, and when quiet, lying, or sitting, cannot be endured, which is much more common in Bryonia.

speech is difficult,[33].—*Dryness in the mouth, without thirst,*[3].—*The inner mouth seems dry, without thirst,*[1].—Dryness of the whole mouth, excepting of the tip of the tongue (half an hour), (after 70 drops),[13].—A feeling of dryness, not on the tongue, but above, on the palate,[1].—Dry sensation in the palate at night, as though a tough mucus were on the uvula, which could not be loosened,[27].—Dry sensation in the palate after eating,[28].—[450.] A feeling of dryness only on the inner side of the upper lip and on the upper teeth,[1].—A sticking very sensitive twitching between the lower lip and gum (in the morning in bed), something like cancer of the lip,[1].—A decided disposition to aphthæ; during the proving he had several times sensitiveness in the mouth, which was not followed by aphthæ (formerly these sensations were followed by aphthæ),[10].—*Saliva.* Accumulation of saliva in the mouth,[22 23 33].—Increased flow of tasteless saliva,[13].—Much spitting of saliva,[1].—*Collection of much soapy, frothy saliva in the mouth,*[3].—Saliva runs out of the corner of the mouth involuntarily,[1].—The saliva is a few times mixed with clear blood,[36].—Profuse saliva, which causes constant spitting,[15].—[460.] Unusual flow of saliva after tobacco-smoking,[15].—*Taste.* Taste flat,[15 24].—Flat, insipid taste in the mouth,[1].—*Flat, insipid taste in the mouth, with almost no taste,*[1].—*Flat nauseous taste in the mouth (after five days),*[15].—*Taste pasty,*[22 23 33].—Taste pasty (second day),[38].—Taste very offensive, pasty, especially at the root of the tongue,[33].—Taste pasty, mealy, with good appetite, and natural taste of the food (second and third day),[34].—*Taste sweetish,*[36 39].—[470.] *Sweetish insipid taste in the mouth,*[1 23].—Sweetish nauseous taste in the mouth,[2].—Taste sweetish, insipid (several days after the proving; the appetite diminished for several days),[22].—Unpleasant salty, sweetish taste for a long time,[33].—*Bitter taste in the mouth,*[37].—*Offensive bitter taste (after drinking beer),*[15].—*Pasty bitter taste in the forenoon,*[33].—*An intensely bitter taste on the tongue,* as of the mother tincture (third day),[13].—Very bitter taste, only in circumscribed spots on the tip of the tongue,[13].—*Nauseous bitter taste in the mouth in the morning,*[1].—[480.] Bitter taste in the mouth, in the evening after lying down,[1].—*The bitter taste remains in the posterior part of the palate after dinner,*[1].—*Frequent drinking of cold water relieved the bitter taste and the inclination to vomit,*[38].—After eating, a sour, dry taste; the forepart of the mouth remains dry, without thirst; the lips are dry and cracked,[1].—Taste earthy (fourth day),[38].—In the morning, fasting, a taste in the mouth as of bad teeth or of bad meat (after twelve hours),[1].—Very unpleasant taste, with nausea, towards evening, so that vomiting was imminent,[38].—Nauseous taste soon; accumulation of bitter saliva in the mouth (after one hundred and fifty drops); a slight drawing in the right fingers and in the border of the left foot, after two hours; a dull, continued pain in the forehead, in the evening,[18].—Acrid nauseous taste in the mouth, with bitter risings from the stomach, lasting six hours (immediately after taking),[18].—*She has almost no taste for food; when not eating the mouth is bitter,*[1].—[490.] Meat does not taste good (after three hours),[15].—Tobacco does not taste good the whole day, and when attempting to smoke, profuse salivation,[15].—Offensive nauseous taste to beer, which caused nausea, inclination to vomit, and shivering over the back,[15].—*Something bitter rises into the mouth, without eructations, with nausea,*[1].—Some soup tasted bitter, and provoked an inclination to vomit; after a few spoonfuls of warm water, which tasted bitter, he vomited a yellowish-green fluid, with the remnants of food, followed by relief,[37].—*Everything tastes bitter; cannot swallow food,*[1].

Throat.—*Objective.* Posterior nares closed by swelling for several days,[39]—In the evening, the throat becomes slimy, and she becomes thirsty,[1]—Much mucus in the throat, with expectoration of transparent, tough, slippery mucus,[34]—Accumulation of foul-smelling mucus in the throat, as after eating crabs or fish,[27]—[500.] The hawking of the offensive mucus and the cheesy lumps continued for several days; especially, a large number were raised easily in the morning,[34]—Accumulation of mucus in the posterior nares caused frequent hawking (fourth day),[34]—Much tough mucus in the throat and posterior nares, causing hawking,[34]—*Subjective.* With a tolerably clean tongue, a bad taste in the throat, with offensive breath; it smells of decaying meat, just as it tastes; while eating, she does not notice it,[1]—Late in the evening there is an offensive, rancid, putrid taste in the throat,[1]—In the evening, a dry sensation in the posterior and upper parts of the throat (after forty-eight hours),[1]—The whole throat seemed dry internally, although there was much mucus in it,[15]—Rheumatic stiffness in the side of the throat, extending to the neck,[3]—Tensive stiffness of the left side of the throat,[3]—Pain in the back part of the throat, perceptible on motion,[3]—[510.] *Pain in the throat; the throat is dry and raw on empty swallowing; on drinking, this sensation disappears for a short time, but soon returns; it is worse in a warm room,[1]—Some pain in the throat, with slight redness of the pharynx and difficult swallowing (evening of third day),[18]—Pain in the throat; in the right side of the throat especially a sensation in the tonsil of a pressive pain, only on empty swallowing, together with some stitches shooting into the right ear (fourth day),[32]—A sensation in the throat as if a morsel were sticking in it; soon afterwards, as if a worm were moving in it,[15]—*The back of the throat seems swollen;* feels as if he had a severe coryza, which hinders him when reading,[3]—Slight constriction of the throat (after half an hour),[30]—Drawing, with pressure, in the throat, extending to the ear,[3]—Pressure in the throat, as if he had swallowed a hard angular body,[1]—A feeling in the throat as if a foreign body were sticking in it,[13]—Stitches internally in the throat, on coughing,[1]—[520.] A stitch internally in the throat, on external pressure and on turning the head,[1]—*Itching needle-like stitches in the throat (especially if he was walking rapidly), which irritate and cause scratching; disappear after scratching* (after twenty-four hours),[3]—Scraping in the throat,[32]—Transient scraping in the throat,[16]—A feeling as of scraping in the throat, as if he had drank strong rum,[34]—Scraping raw sensation in the throat (after five hours),[13]—Rawness in the throat,[36 39]—Creeping in the throat, with a sensation as if the throat were too narrow,[36]—*Tonsils.* Slight pain in the throat, in the left tonsil, with a full sensation in the loins, in the morning, on waking,[13]—[530.] The angina tonsillaris, with which he awoke in the morning, lasted in a slight degree the whole day,[13]—*Fauces and Pharynx.* Tough mucus in the fauces, which is loosened by hacking,[3]—He hacks and hawks yellowish mucus from the fauces,[1]—Dryness of pharynx, with smarting just behind the pomum Adami (first day),[42]—Constriction in the pharynx, as if pressed with a broad band, with frequent yawning,[13]—*Œsophagus and Swallowing.* Painful sensation in the œsophagus, more in the lower portion, as if it were contracted,[1]—Pressure in the œsophagus, as from an overloaded stomach,[17]—Constant disposition to swallow, with sharp stinging pain in external parts (right side) on a line with the promontory of larynx (after half an hour to two hours),[42]—(A sensation when swallowing as if the throat were swollen internally, or were full of mucus, which cannot be raised by hawking),[1]—*A stitch in the throat when swal-

lowing,[1].—[540.] She cannot swallow what she eats and drinks; it chokes in the throat,[1].—**Throat Externally.** Strong pulsation of the carotid,[26].—Simple pain or a pinching in a submaxillary gland (after twelve hours),[1].—Sharp rheumatic pain in tendon of trapezius (left) on turning the head to the left (after two to three hours),[42].—A transient stitch, as from a needle, in the forepart of the right side of the neck, just above the sternal end of the clavicle,[13].—On the day after the last symptom (315) he noticed only a very slight sensitiveness of the parotid, which was very slightly enlarged; he took, at 1 P.M., an ounce of the 203d dilution; repeated slight stitches in the parotid during the first three hours, followed by a stitch in the inner ear and a sensation of warmth in it, with a sensation as though an abscess would open; soon afterwards, ringing in the ears and itching in the concave surface of the ears; these stitches continued far into the night, but not so severe as to prevent his falling asleep late; the next day stitches here and there, but much more frequent itching in the ears; the sensitiveness of the parotid to steel ceased. The next day very frequent stitches, especially in the region of the articulation of the lower jaw, even when not chewing; on swallowing, a sensation of swelling in the throat, with stitches and noises in the right ear; dull pain in the forehead; pasty taste; the stitches become very irregular; in the afternoon, long-continued stitches in the hitherto healthy left ear; towards evening, great sensitiveness of the right ear, frequent stitches in it, but especially in the right articulation of the lower jaw; on the next day, pain in the throat and very slight sensitiveness in the right ear,[10].

Stomach.—Appetite. * *Unnatural hunger for six days*,[2].—Excessive hunger for fourteen days,[2].—Ravenous hunger continued into the night,[1].—Ravenous hunger, without appetite,[1].—[550.] Ravenous hunger in the morning, with thirst and flushes of heat (after thirty and seventy-two hours),[5].—Hunger, with loss of appetite,[5].—He is hungry, and eats, but does not relish it,[1].—Ravenous hunger in the morning, when fasting, with loss of appetite,[3].—*He desires things immediately, but, when offered, does not wish them*,[1].—Food smells good, but when he begins to eat, the appetite disappears,[1].—He longs for many things which he cannot eat,[1].—He longs for things which are not at hand,[1].—*Desire for acids (very much), (second day),[38].—Intense craving for oysters and strong coffee (third day),[42].—[560.] *He has no appetite for milk; but if he takes it, the appetite returns, and he begins to relish it*,[1].—No appetite,[16].—Appetite lost,[3].—Loss of appetite (fourth day),[38].—Loss of appetite for ten days,[2].—Complete loss of appetite,[21].—Loss of appetite and thirst,[24].—Loss of appetite, without bad taste (after three hours),[1].—Aversion to food,[32].—Aversion to all food,[22].—[570.] Aversion to every kind of food; even a glass of beer, before eating, is repugnant, with longing for warm broth; immediately after taking it, urging to stool, with three successive painless, liquid stools, which are discharged as from a tube; the color of the stool is greenish-brown; followed by burning pain in the rectum and on the nates,[22].—Appetite less, taste bitter,[15].—Loss of appetite for his usual breakfast, which almost nauseates him,[26].—Little appetite for dinner (second day),[32].—Aversion to tobacco, with much saliva on smoking (after one hour),[15].—**Thirst.** Thirst moderate (fourth day),[38].—Increased thirst,[23].—* *Great thirst*,[3].—*Excessive thirst*,[1].—*Great thirst for twenty-two days*,[2].—[580.] *Great thirst day and night*,[2].—*Great thirst (he was obliged to drink much cold water), with internal heat, without feeling hot externally*,[3].—*Great thirst; she can and must drink a great deal at once; the drink does not distress her*,[1].—Great thirst in the morning, on rising,[1].—Great thirst after eating, for sixteen days,[2].—*Great thirst, with longing for wine,[33].—Much thirst,[33].—Much thirst during the day, without heat,[1].—Thirst, without external heat,[3].—Thirst, especially in the morning,[2].—[**590.**] Thirst about 3 A.M., before the sweat, followed by sweetish sour-smelling sweat for four hours; before this ceased, headache appeared, consisting of pressing and drawing, which, after rising, changed to a confusion in the head,[1].—Was obliged to drink several times during the night (after thirty hours),[1].—He awoke at 11 o'clock at night with unusual thirst, which he attempted to satisfy with a few glasses of water with raspberry juice; he was in a feverish excitement, pulse accelerated, hearing sensitive to every noise, even the swinging of the pendulum of a small clock affected him unpleasantly; he tried to sleep again, but lay a long time in a dreamy half-sleep,[13].—Thirst, and after drinking wine and water pain in the stomach, aggravated by deep inspiration and pressure; soon after drinking, the previous bitter pasty taste returns,[33].—Thirst increased from drinking beer,[1].—*Thirst for very clear, cold water (sixth and seventh days),[42].—Desire for coffee,[1].—Great longing for coffee (after five hours),[2 5].—*Desire for wine,[1].—Desire for wine, which, however, caused nausea,[22].—[**600.**] Aversion to beer in the evening,[15].—At first thirst (after one hour), then loss of thirst, with cold hands and feet (after four hours),[1].—**_Eructations and Hiccough._** Eructations (after three hours),[15].—Eructations,[22].—Frequent empty eructations,[15].—Frequent empty eructations, with confusion of the head,[36].—Empty eructations, tasting of the medicine,[23].—Several empty eructations and two pasty stools during the day (second day),[13].—*Tasteless eructations,[23].—Empty tasteless eructations after eating, with dizzy confusion of the head and slight drawing headache in the left half of the forehead,[13].—[**610.**] Frequent tasteless eructations,[13].—Severe eructations after eating, from morning till evening,[1].—Frequent eructations of air,[33].—Eructations of air and rumbling on the left side near the stomach (after three hours),[13].—Constant eructations of tasteless wind,[22].—Frequent eructations of gas; hiccough after the eructations, without having previously eaten,[1].—Constant eructations, at first of the taste of the tincture, afterwards of tasteless gas, without relieving the pressure in the stomach and the distension of the abdomen,[22].—Eructations tasting of food,[1].—Frequent eructations tasting of the food,[17].—(Eructations of offensive taste in the mouth, and mucus in the throat),[1].—[**620.**] Sour eructations, and a collection of sourish water in the mouth,[1].—Frequently, at times, sourish eructations after eating,[4].—*Eructations after eating, at last bitter,[1].—Bitter eructations for ten minutes,[9].—*Bitter eructations after eating,[1].—Drinks cause no eructations. but the slightest food does, though only of air, without bad taste,[1].—(Eructations almost constantly burning, which make the mouth raw, and prevent tasting of food),[1].—Eructations of the contents of the stomach, almost without effort to vomit,[1].—She raises mucus from the stomach in the morning by a kind of gulping,[1].—In the evening (at 6) gulping up of water and mucus, like waterbrash, which rises into the chest, with coldness over the whole body,[1].—[**630.**] Food rises into the mouth, with a kind of gulping,[1].—Severe hiccough,[1].—*Hiccough after eating, and on every shock caused by it, pressure in the forehead, as if the brain shook from behind forward (third day),[28].—Hiccough after vomiting,[16]—Hiccough, afterwards eructations for a quarter of an hour (after forty-eight hours),[1].—**_Nausea and Vomiting._** Nausea,[28].—Nausea (immediately),[5].—Great nausea (after one hour),[13].—Nausea upon taste. the whole day (120 drops),[24].—Nausea soon after taking,[15].—

[640.] Nausea soon after taking, which lasted the whole evening,[32].—Nausea (immediately after taking),[40].—Great nausea, lasting several hours after taking it (120 drops),[22].—Nausea became so severe, even on looking at the bottle containing the tincture, that he was obliged to desist from taking it (second day),[16].—Every morning, two hours after rising, nausea for half an hour, with collection of water in the mouth,[1].—Nausea in the morning, after anxious dreams, without being able to vomit, with frequent empty eructations,[1].—Nausea the whole forenoon,[22].—Nausea the whole forenoon at intervals of ten to fifteen minutes,[13].—Nausea in the evening, before going to sleep,[1].—Nausea in the evening, followed by a flow of much water from the mouth,[1].—**[650.]** Nausea before midnight,[34].—In order to remove the persistent bitter taste, he frequently rinsed his mouth with water, but it always caused inclination to vomit,[22].—Nausea from tobacco (after six hours),[15].—Nausea, especially on smoking (to which he is accustomed),[3].—*He was obliged to lie perfectly quiet, because the slightest motion caused nausea, even to vomiting,*[13].—When walking in the open air, he felt so qualmish and nauseated, the limbs seemed so weak, and he felt so weak in the head, that he believed he would fall; he gasped, and warmth came into the chest, which extended to the head; this disappeared in the room, but returned in the open air,[1].—Nausea and qualmishness after drinking, in the afternoon,[1].—Severe nausea starting from the stomach, several times during dinner; it made him anxious,[31].—Nausea for twenty-four hours, with much running of water from the mouth (after five minutes),[2].—Continued nausea, and immediately afterwards ravenous hunger (after a few hours),[2].—**[660.]** A feeling of qualmishness and emptiness in the stomach,[36].—Nausea, with much salivation and frequent spitting,[15].—Nausea and creeping chills (soon),[15].—Frequent nausea, causing a shivering, with involuntary shaking of the head and closure of the lids,[13].—*Nausea and inclination to vomit* (after half an hour),[30].—Nausea, with inclination to vomit,[23].—Nausea, with inclination to vomit (after one and a half hours),[16].—Nausea, with inclination to vomit (from 60 drops),[21].—Nausea, with inclination to vomit (soon after 90 drops),[22].—Great nausea, with inclination to vomit,[19].—**[670.]** Nausea and inclination to vomit after a breakfast of coffee (soon after taking),[33].—Sudden nausea from the stomach at 9 P.M., in bed, as if it would cause vomiting, frequently repeated, followed by increased flow of saliva and a sensation in the stomach as if rancid, and scraping, without the slightest cause,[13].—Immediately after midnight, he wakes with nausea; is obliged to vomit food and bile,[1].—*In the morning, on waking, nausea and vomiting,*[1].—After eating food which had tasted good, nausea and vomiting,[1].—Nausea and vomiting, without having eaten (after one hour),[1].—Nausea, even to vomiting, especially when lying upon the right side, followed by easy empty eructations, alternating with secretion of saliva in the mouth (soon after taking), (fourth day),[12].—Sudden nausea, followed by vomiting, half an hour after eating; the vomiting was paroxysmal and with great exertion; the material was much larger than had been eaten; it was accompanied by a few drops of bright-red blood from the right nostril,[16].—Inclination to vomit,[24].—Great inclination to vomit,[13].—**[680.]** Great inclination to vomit soon followed by vomiting of a very bitter taste (soon),[38].—Sudden desire to vomit; vomiting lasted continuously for five minutes; repeated after half an hour, and again a third time after a half hour; the last was very painful; the pain consisted in extremely violent retching and constriction of the stomach; the matter vomited

seemed like chocolate, water, and mucus, and tasted of the medicine,[30].†—
She vomits solid food, but not drinks,[1].—Sour vomiting, in the morning, of
the fish which he had eaten the previous evening, which he had usually
digested easily,[31].—On coughing, vomiting of food,[1].—Frequent vomiting
of yellow and green mucus,[2].—Vomiting of mucus, in the evening (after
five hours),[1].—*In the morning (about 6), vomiting of bitter, musty, and
putrid liquid, which leaves a similar taste in the mouth,[1].—(Vomiting of
blood and lying down),[1].—When coughing, he vomited, without nausea,[1].—
Stomach. [690.] Distension of the epigastric region,[26].—Distension
of the stomach and eructations of wind (immediately),[21].—Distension of
the stomach, and afterwards of the abdomen,[21].—Painful distension of the
stomach, and afterwards of the whole abdomen, lasting all day,[21].—The
distension of the stomach increased to a slight meteorismus; rumbling,
without gripings, in the intestines; passage of offensive flatus,[22].—*Stomach
full and sensitive to pressure*,[15].—A painless throbbing-twitching to the left
of the epigastrium (like twitching of tendons and muscle-fibres), in or just
beneath the wall of the abdomen,[13].—During the last days of the proving
the digestion is very weak (little appetite, eats more from habit than from
necessity, and frequently feels a distension in the epigastric region),
(twelfth day),[26].—The stomach is empty; he is hungry, without appetite,[4].—
Feeling of great emptiness in the whole stomach; great distension of the
whole abdomen,[36].—[700.] Uncomfortable sensation in the epigastric region, with distension of the abdomen,[23].—Uncomfortable feeling in the stomach, with flatulent distension of the abdomen (two hours after taking),[33].—
Burning in the stomach,[33].—Short attacks of heartburn in the afternoon,[33].—
A glass of wine taken in the evening caused heartburn (second day),[15].—
Pressive-burning pain in the stomach,[33].—Pressive-burning pain in the stomach (after one hour),[33].—Sensitive pain in the stomach; burning constriction
caused by bending forward, aggravated by deep inspiration, without intermission; it rapidly reached great severity, together with accumulation of
saliva in the mouth; during its greatest severity there was pressive pain in
both axillæ and on the right hip; the head was confused for a short time;
this was followed by pain in the intestines and desire for stool (second
day),[33].—Burning and pressure in the stomach in short repeated paroxysms,[33].—Violent burning-twisting pain in the stomach (after two hours),[33].
—[710.] Heat in the pit of the stomach, worse during every inspiration
(first day),[42].—An extraordinary warmth in the epigastric region causes
shortness of breath, with a kind of pressive pain,[1].—Sensation in the stomach as of something sharply rancid (a quarter of an hour after 100
drops),[13].—Fulness of the stomach,[15].—Sensation of fulness in the stomach,[22].—Stomach full and sensitive, with a sensation as if heartburn would
appear,[15].—Feeling of fulness as from accumulation of flatus, which pressed
forward toward the stomach, and caused severe pressive pain, soon again
pressing backward; these symptoms, continuing more or less severe the
whole day, were relieved by walking and bending backward, increased by
bending forward (third day),[27].—*A feeling as if the pit of the stomach were
swollen*,[3].—Exceedingly unpleasant sensation as of swelling below the pit of
the stomach,[3].—Tension in the stomach and bowels,[20].—[720.] Constrictive
pain in the region of the stomach, as if the stomach were rolled into a ball,
which he believed he could feel with the hand; this pain was so marked

---

† He had taken chocolate for breakfast; afterward, vomiting very difficult, of
only saffron-yellow, tough, bitter fluid.—Watzke.

that he could not straighten up, hence he went to bed, *where he obtained relief by drawing the legs up against the abdomen;* after half an hour the sensation as of a ball in the stomach disappeared and gave place to a severe pressive pain in the left side of the chest, which impeded breathing; it seemed to him as if the left lobe of the lung had become enlarged; while lying quietly in bed with a thin summer coverlet, he soon began to sweat, and then he fell asleep,[37].—Constrictive pain in the epigastric region, which extended over the whole chest, and caused a feeling of oppression; this pain increased toward evening, so that he was not able to stand upright; vigorous rubbing of the epigastric region gave relief; he lay in bed and took a cup of warm soup, covered the stomach with warm clothing, and drew the legs up to the abdomen; scarcely was this pain in the stomach relieved, when another not less troublesome symptom appeared, urging to stool, with audible rumbling in the intestines and very offensive yellowish diarrhœa; he was obliged to rise nearly every hour for stool; the stool caused severe burning in the rectum; he was only able to sleep after 3 o'clock, and even then was awakened several times by desire for stool and diarrhœa (first night),[38].—Contractive pain in the stomach several hours after eating,[1].—Contractive pain in the stomach after eating, then cutting pain in and above the pit of the stomach, eructations, rising heat, nausea, and vomiting of what he had eaten (after forty-eight hours),[1].—Pinching in the stomach (after twelve hours),[5].—Pinching pain in the stomach, soon changing to colic pains in the bowels,[21].—Griping and tension in the stomach, which extends to the abdomen,[20].—*Stomachache, associated with anxiety,[1].—Pressure in the stomach (after three hours),[15].—*Pressure in the pit of the stomach,[1].—[730.] Pressure in the stomach after eating,[3].—*Pressure in the stomach·as soon as he had eaten, and· even while eating,[1].—*Severe pressure in the stomach, as if a stone were lying there, after eating,[28].—*Pressure in the stomach after eating; a feeling as if a stone were lying in it, which makes him fretful,[1].—Pressive sensation in the stomach after eating (second day),[27].—Pressure in the stomach when walking,[3].—Violent pressure in the pit of the stomach, when walking, immediately after supper; then pressure on the bladder and perineum; it becomes insupportable; disappears while sitting (after twelve hours),[1].—*Pressure in the stomach, as from a stone* (soon); this pressure continued after breakfast, and was followed by rumbling and griping in the intestines, together with constriction of the chest and tension in the pectoral muscles,[33].—Pressure in the stomach, with continual eructations, without relief,[22].—Pressure and burning in the stomach,[33].—[740.] Pressure and fulness in the stomach,[15].—Pressure in the stomach, with feeling of fulness,[15].—Pressure and constriction in the stomach at 4 and 5 P.M., repeated every two or three minutes (soon after taking),[31].—Pressure in the stomach, and tension, with burning, in the right side of the chest, increased by moving the arm (soon),[33].—Pressive pain in the stomach (half an hour after taking),[33].—*A sensation as though a stone lay in the stomach; the epigastric region is painful to touch (after six hours),[15].—Sticking pain with every eructation,[1].—*Cutting, as with knives, in the epigastric region (after one hour),[1].—Several attacks of sharp sticking-cutting, though only transient, pains in the pit of the stomach, returning several times at short intervals with renewed severity,[13].—Violent stitches in the stomach on deep inspiration (twenty-fifth day),[16].—[750.] Fine stitches in the pit of the stomach on walking about the room, especially noticed on deep inspiration,[13].—*The epigastric region is painful to pressure,[15].—*Epigastric region sensitive; he could not endure the clothes (second day),[38].—

* *When coughing, soreness in the pit of the stomach*,[1].—A scraping sensation in the stomach (from 3d dil.),[12].—Scraping, rancid feeling in the stomach, as of beginning heartburn, with a tensive pain in the right hypochondrium,[13].—Scraping sensation in the stomach, with eructations of tasteless gas and rumbling in the upper abdomen (from 1st dil.),[12].—Scraping sensation in the stomach, with inclination to eructations of air (after half an hour), followed by nausea arising from the stomach, as if he would vomit, with dizzy confusion of the head, frequent yawning, continuing for two hours,[13].—Scraping sensation in the stomach, eructations, rumbling in the abdomen, great nausea from the stomach, with shuddering, shivering, and convulsive contraction of the abdominal muscles, especially on each side of the epigastrium (after half an hour), (from 80 drops),[13].

Abdomen.—Hypochondria. Slight pressive sensation in both hypochondria,[23].—[760.] A tensive pain in the right hypochondrium lasting ten minutes, then disappearing with rumbling in the upper abdomen (from 3d dil.),[12].—**Tensive pain below the false ribs in the right hypochondrium, especially sensitive on deep inspiration*, lasting about ten minutes (from 1st dil.), (after half an hour),[12].—Transient, sharp stitches deep in the right hypochondrium,[13].—A sharp transient stitch beneath the wall of the abdomen in the right hypochondrium, extending toward the epigastrium (from 5th dil.),[12].—Sharp, transient stitches in the right hypochondrium, soon followed by a similar one in the epigastrium,[13].—**Some transient stitches in the right hypochondrium; painful sensitiveness of this region, especially to hard pressure and deep inspiration*,[13].—Burning pain in the abdomen in the region of the liver (after eight hours),[1].—* *Tensive pain in the region of the liver*,[1].—Long-drawn stitches in the liver while sitting (ninth day),[26].—The region of the liver was sensitive,[15].—*Umbilical and Sides.* [770.] Hard swelling about the navel and beneath the hypochondria,[1].—Transient burning in the abdomen below the navel,[33].—In the afternoon, while riding in a very jolting wagon, pinching pain above the navel extending towards the spleen,[15].—Slight griping around the navel (after quarter of an hour),[15]. —Slight, frequently repeated griping in the upper part of the umbilical region (first days),[22].—Slight griping above the navel, extending from the region of the liver to the spleen, with nausea and inclination to vomit,[15].—Severe griping around the navel,[15].—Awakened three times in the night by severe griping in the umbilical region,[16].—Violent griping in the umbilical region, which started the sweat on the forehead an hour after dinner; it gradually disappeared with passage of offensive flatus (thirty-second day),[16]. —Colic-like pain around the navel before eating,[13].—[780.] Colic-like pains around the navel half an hour after dinner, lasting half an hour, relieved by passage of flatus,[17].—Very violent attack of colic, two fingers' breadth below the navel, followed by passage of flatus after eating,[13].— Boring pains around the navel,[15].—Boring pain around the navel (after two hours),[15].—Boring, but transient pains around the navel, with chilliness (after half an hour),[15].—Slight pressive pain below the navel towards noon,[33].—Pressive pain in the region of the navel and great urging to stool, which awoke him from sleep at 6 A.M. (second day),[10].—Dull pressure in the region of the navel every time on waking, but he soon sank back into a kind of half sleep, in which he was busy with frequent fancies; this continually recurred until he awoke at six in the morning, with urgent desire for stool,[9].—Pressure on the navel, as from a button, when walking in the open air,[1].—A pressive sensation in the region of the navel was relieved by walking in the open air, but lasted in a slight degree till about 5 P.M.

(second day),[10].—[**790.**] Painful twisting, with stitches around the navel,[1].
—Twisting about the navel, with slight nausea,[31].—Rather severe bruised
sensation at the ends of the left false ribs, extending to the navel, continuing thirty hours,[9].—*Painless twitching in the left side of the abdomen between the navel and the left flank, as of twitching in the muscles of the
walls of the abdomen, followed by sticking pains deep in the left side of
the back,[13].—Tearing pains in the left side of the abdomen,[26].—Sudden
colic-like pain in the right side of the abdomen somewhat below the navel,
sticking-pinching, lasting several minutes, and followed by passage of
flatus,[13].—Stitches in the left flank (fourth day),[31].—*General Abdomen.* *Distension of the abdomen,*[28 33].—*Distension of the abdomen* (soon
after taking),[33].—*Great distension in the abdomen,* towards evening,[33].—
[**800.**] Great distension of the abdomen after eating,[33].—Distension of the
abdomen and feeling of discomfort after a simple meal (eleventh day),[26].—
Distension of the abdomen after every meal,[1].—*Distension of the abdomen,
relieved by passage of offensive flatus,[23].—The abdomen is very much distended, with an unusual uneasy feeling in it, as if menstruation would
come on,[1].—Distension of the abdomen, impeding respiration,[33].—*Distended abdomen, continued motions in the abdomen, and colic, then continued
constipation; feels as if something lay in the abdomen,*[1].—Sudden dropsy of the
bowels; is unable to breathe and must sit (after eighteen hours),[1].—The
whole abdomen very tense (second day),[36].—Very troublesome tension in
the abdomen after eating, which even made respiration difficult,[36].—[**810.**]
Tension in the abdomen, which disappears after a long walk,[36].—Tympanitic tension of the abdomen, painful, followed the next day by two pasty
evacuations, which relieved the distension,[20].—The abdomen tense and distended,[31].—Tension and distension of the abdomen, especially in the afternoon after eating (third day),[36].—Extreme tension and distension of the
abdomen and epigastric region, which was only relieved towards morning
by passing a great deal of offensive flatus,[36].—Abdomen very much retracted,[11].—Frequent twitchings and convulsive movements in the abdominal muscles on the right side,[13].—Gurgling in the bowels in the afternoon at three, followed by a moderate pasty evacuation and passage of
flatus,[13].—Rumbling in the abdomen, without pain,[23].—Rumbling in the
abdomen, especially in the forenoon,[35].—[**820.**] Rumbling, with tension in
the abdomen, after eating,[36].—Rumbling in the abdomen and sensation as
if diarrhœa would ensue,[1].—Rumbling in the abdomen and passage of
offensive flatus,[13].—Rumbling in the abdomen; griping, rather severe colic
pains in the left side of the abdomen, which cease after a few minutes, followed by passage of flatus,[13].—Rumbling in the intestines followed by three
liquid stools, without relief,[37].—Rumbling and gurgling in the intestines with
gripings, followed by two liquid stools at short intervals (soon after taking),[11].
—Frequent rumbling in the abdomen, with desire for stool, which was
softer than usual,[36].—Loud rumbling of the bowels for fourteen days,[2].—
Loud rumbling in the bowels, especially in the evening, in bed, for eighteen
days,[2].—Flatulent troubles, with constant inclination to diarrhœa,[72].—[**830.**]
Passage of much flatus,[32].—All day long discharge of flatus (third day),[42].—
Passage of much loud odorless flatus,[35].—*Passage of offensive flatus,*[17 23].—
Passage of offensive flatus (second day),[32].—Constant, or rather frequent,
short emissions of offensive flatus (after three hours to four hours),[42].—Pas-
sage of flatus in the night, preceded by loud rumbling and grumbling,[1].—
Heaviness in the abdomen,[33].—Heaviness in the abdomen below the navel,[33].
—The abdomen, especially the lower abdomen, seemed heavy while sitting,

as if it hung down upon the thighs,[33].—[**840.**] (Sensation as if a lump were lying in the abdomen),[1].—Pain in the abdomen as if one would vomit (after fifth day),[1].—Pain in the abdomen as if he had taken a purge, or as of hæmorrhoids; vomiting,[1].—*Pain in the abdomen, as if diarrhœa would ensue*, for one and a half hours (after five minutes),[12].—*All day long feeling in abdomen as though a diarrhœa would come on;* the same sensation exists in anus (third day),[42].—Pain in the abdomen on urinating,[1].—At 6, 7, and 8 P.M., sense of fulness, weight, and intestinal hypertrophy (third day),[42].— Tension in the abdomen,[22].—Pinching and pressure in the abdomen, in the region of the navel, when walking and standing,[1].—*Slight pinching and moving in the intestines, followed by watery stool, with passage of flatus; the pinchings do not disappear, but are frequently repeated during the afternoon, *with a sensation of soreness in the intestines, together with a dragging downward and outward*, with two profuse watery evacuations in one hour, followed by slight burning in the anus,[24].—[**850.**] Gripings in the abdomen,[37].—Griping in the abdomen (fifth day),[34].—Slight griping in the abdomen (fourth day),[34].—Frequent griping in various places in the abdomen,[16].—Griping in the abdomen, while walking, before a meal, followed by a liquid stool, whereby the contents of the intestines poured out as from a tube; after the meal a similar stool, followed by burning in the anus,[33].— Gripings and rumblings in the abdomen, with tympanitic distension of the abdomen,[21].—Gripings and rumblings in the bowels, with ineffectual urgings to stool,[11].—*Griping and pinching in the abdomen and in the region of the navel, as after taking cold*, for several days, and (after three days) a profuse, thin evacuation followed,[1].—Dull griping and cutting in epigastric region, prior to passage of flatus; motion and standing increase the pains (after three to four hours),[42].—The griping in the abdomen returned several times (second day), but became less severe as flatus was passed, and at last there was only rumbling in the abdomen (second day),[16].—[**860.**] A slight attack of colic after eating, followed by passage of flatus and afterwards a pasty evacuation,[13].—Slight colic at time of rising, and through forenoon (second day),[42].—The night's rest was disturbed by continuous wind colic,[21].— Colic-pain during and after dinner,[13].—Flatulent colic after supper, with pressure in the cæcum,[1].—*Colic with the stool, like a constriction and griping with the hand, which causes diarrhœa*,[1].—The colic lasted two hours and disappeared with a pasty evacuation and passage of flatus,[21].†—Spasmodic pain in the abdomen after dinner,[1].—Intermitting cuttings in the abdomen in the forenoon, as if dysentery would ensue, without stool,[1].—*Sudden painful cuttings in the intestines, with a feeling as though one were digging him with the fingers, compelling him to bend double; relieved by profuse pasty evacuations*,[25].—[**870.**] Very violent cuttings in the abdomen, with gurglings and rumblings, followed by a watery stool,[24].—Severe cutting stitches in the abdomen from below upward into the stomach (after drinking a cup of warm milk in the afternoon); the pain obliges him to bend double and is relieved after a stool,[1].—Pain in both sides of the abdomen, like a pleuritic stich,[1].—Tearing and drawing in the abdomen, especially on motion, followed by stitches, especially with stool, mostly in the evening,[1].—*Sensitiveness in the abdomen,*[24].—*Abdomen very sensitive, as if sore* (first day),[17].— Sensitiveness of the abdomen; rumbling and passage of flatus,[25].—Constant movings in the abdomen, as if a stool would follow, which, however, did

---

† The patient frequently suffered from a similar wind colic of a less severe character,[21].

not,[21].—*Hypogastrium and Iliac Regions.* Slight, crampy, cutting pain, with heat in right hypogastric region, increased by every inspiration (after half an hour to two hours),[42].—Violent colic-like pain, starting from the small of the back and extending over the whole lower abdominal region (after four hours),[21].—**[880.]** Pressure and pinching in the lower abdomen,[4].—Violent cutting deep in the lower abdomen,[32].—A sudden violent stitching in the lower abdomen from left to right, soon followed by two very painful stitches across through the chest from the left to the right side, while at dinner,[18].—Drawing in both groins, which gradually changed to a burning on the right side; afterwards this sensation extends over the inner surface of the right thigh (second day),[26].—Pressive pain in the region of the left inguinal ring every morning for half an hour for several days,[39].—Pressive pain towards the inguinal ring on sitting down,[40].—Dull stitches in the right inguinal region (fourth day),[28].—Soreness in the groin, in the overhanging folds of the abdomen,[1].

Rectum and Anus. *Slight burning with the evacuation of the stool and urine,*[27].—Long-continued burning in the rectum after a hard stool,[1].—**[890.]** Dragging in the rectum, like urging to stool, without real need for it, with slight pain in the anus,[33].—Severe stitches in the rectum as often as flatus passed; it seemed to press against the rectum (twentieth day),[34].—Itching, jerking-like coarse stitches from the anus into the rectum,[1].—Four stitches, with slight tenesmus and scanty fæces,[27].—A pulse-like jerk in the rectum (second day),[16].—A hæmorrhoid protruded, which had formed the previous night, and lasted several days (third day),[15].—Burning in the hæmorrhoidal vessels in the evening,[33].—Severe aching in the hæmorrhoidal vessels, which renders sitting difficult,[33].—Severe dragging and pressure in the hæmorrhoidal vessels, with severe transient stitches through the pelvis into the urethra,[33].—Pressure in the hæmorrhoidal vessels,[33].—**[900.]** Severe pressure and burning in the hæmorrhoids,[33].—Retraction of the anus,[33].—Slight discharge of mucus from the anus,[33].—A feeling as from a plug in the anus,[33].—At 6 A.M., sensation of plug in anus (second day),[42].—Burning pain in the anus before a meal,[33].—Burning in the anus for some time after a natural stool,[33].—Pressing towards the anus,[26].—Severe itching and burning in the anus (twentieth day),[34].—Drawing-sticking stitches in the perineum, in the evening, for half an hour; they extend to the urinary bladder, and especially to the bulbus urethræ, whereby urination was momentarily prevented (eighteenth day),[26].—**[910.]** Urging to stool without result,[37].—Ineffectual desire for stool in the afternoon (second day),[27].—Urging to stool, followed by a soft evacuation,[26].—Urging to stool, and a soft stool, although he had a natural one in the morning (after two hours),[15].—* *Urging to stool, followed by copious pasty evacuations, with relief of all the symptoms, except that the confusion of the head remained,*[32].—Violent urging to stool followed a scanty passage of firm consistence,[11].—Urging to stool without result, twice in the evening; only the day after a stool followed, after great exertion,[26].—Urgent desire for stool, but in spite of much urging only wind passed, together with rumbling in the intestines,[32].—Much straining in order to finish defecation (sixth and seventh day),[42].—With passing of flatus, sensation as though a diarrhœic stool would come on. Instant and striking is the sensation, as though he must go to stool. It seems to be a sense of pressure, heat, weight, and powerlessness of the sphincter ani and rectum (after three to four hours),[42].—**[920.]** He felt well excepting the inclination to diarrhœa, which especially came on from the slightest drafts of air (third day),[9].—On the slightest tightening of the clothes, a sensation as if he must go to stool, without any pain in the abdomen; stool somewhat soft (third and fourth days),[10].—After a crumbly stool, a sensation, with severe urging, as if the fæces could not be voluntarily retained,[33].—Urgent desire for stool, at 6 A.M.; the stool was acrid, fluid, with compact portions; during the course of the day three or four similar stools (second day),[9].

Stool.—Diarrhœa. Diarrhœa (after three days),[1].—Diarrhœa (for four days in succession every three hours), so sudden that he was not able to retain it; during the following twelve days the usual stool passed just as suddenly,[2].—Diarrhœa, without the slightest griping,[22].—Diarrhœa, mostly in the morning,[2].—Diarrhœa, at 4 P.M.,[13].—(Diarrhœa at night),[1].—[**930.**] *Diarrhœa, especially at night, and burning in the anus with every passage* (after seventh day),[2].—Painless diarrhœa, after eating,[13].—Painless diarrhœa of thin slimy fluid, at 1 P.M., after eating,[13].—Easy, painless diarrhœa of a greenish-brown liquid, preceded by a pinching pain, extending from the right hypochondrium toward the stomach, lasting several seconds, after eating,[13].—*Diarrhœa smelling foul, like old cheese,[2].—*Diarrhœa, preceded by colic* (forty-four to seventy-two hours),[2].—Diarrhœa of a green, slimy fluid, followed by loud passage of flatus,[13].—Diarrhœa twice a day; makes her so weak that she must keep her bed (after three days),[2].—It purges without other symptoms (twenty-four and thirty-eight hours),[5].—Frequent stool (after forty-eight hours),[1].—[**940.**] Frequent brown stool in an infant,[1]. —Stool softer than usual, four times in the day, followed by constipation, for several days,[40].—Three thin fluid stools, in the afternoon,[27].—Three diarrhœa-like stools without pain, but with passage of very offensive flatus (after seven hours), (from 200 drops),[18].—Liquid stool, three or four times a day, followed by a burning in the anus,[22].—Diarrhœa-like stool, two or three times a day, for several days,[22].—Two profuse liquid stools (after one hour),[15].—Two stools a day; after some days constipation,[1].†—Two soft stools in the afternoon,[15].—Two mucous stools in the evening and at night (three to twenty-seven hours).[1]‡—[**950.**] **Two pasty, offensive evacuations in the afternoon, followed by burning in the anus,[23].**—Two thin fluid evacuations in the forenoon,[27].—Two liquid stools in the evening; rumbling in the bowels; sudden urging to stool the whole day (four and five days),[11]. —Bilious liquid stools,[22].—Two copious watery stools, about 6 P.M., with tenesmus, and slight burning in the anus,[24].—A dark, not liquid evacuation, at noon,[33].—Stool at 6 A.M., very watery, followed by a similar one in half an hour (two days),[10].—A very thin stool in the morning (ninth day),[12].— Evacuation in the afternoon, with slight burning in the anus,[27].—Involuntary stool, at night, during sleep,[2].—[**960.**] The irregularity in the stools lasted a long time,[11].—Diarrhœa-like stool (after twenty-eight hours),[3].— Diarrhœa-like stool after dinner, followed in an hour by a second, with little fæces but much mucus, *followed by a burning in the anus,[27].—*Diarrhœa-like stool followed by prickling and burning in the anus,[22].—*Diarrhœa-like, bilious, acrid stools, with soreness in the anus, continuing eight days,[22].*—Diarrhœa-like passage of a thin greenish mass (at 2½ P.M.),[13].—*Soft stool in the morning* (second day),[15.36].—A soft, but not otherwise diarrhœa-like stool, at 1 P.M.

---

† More frequent primary action of Bryonia is retention of stool; its secondary action, looseness of the bowels, is more rare; when the other symptoms correspond, it permanently cures constipation, which but few remedies besides Nux vomica and Opium can do —H.

‡ These symptoms were the more noticeable, since, for some two months, the stools had been irregular, and seldom, so that he scarcely had an evacuation for two days.

(second day),[10].—Soft stool, with sharp burning pain in the anus,[1].—Pasty evacuations,[25].—[970.] *Very offensive, pasty evacuation (soon after 25 drops),[33].†—A brownish, pasty evacuation, in the morning,[13].—Soft, pasty stool soon after eating,[15].—Copious pasty stools at 2 P.M.,[15].—*Stool pasty, with much flatus, followed by hard portions, and again by soft, so that he believed that he would scarcely finish the evacuation (second day),[36].—*A pasty evacuation, with burning in the anus, soon after waking; a second fluid stool after half an hour,[33].—*In the morning, a pasty, afterwards a liquid stool, of a strong odor, followed by burning and soreness in the anus (soon after 15 drops),[33].—Very offensive, profuse stool, and cutting in the forepart of the bowels,[1].—After every meal, very liquid stools,[22].—Liquid stool after a meal, followed by transient pain in the sacrum,[33].—[980.] Watery offensive stool (fourth day),[38].—Thin bloody stool (after twenty-four hours),[2].—Constipation. *Obstinate constipation,[11].—Constipation; if an evacuation takes place, it is with the greatest exertion (third day),[36].—Constipation, with painful swelling of the hæmorrhoidal vessels,[21].—Stool retained (first day),[36].—No stool (first and second days),[18].—No stool, not the slightest desire for one (third morning),[32].—No stool, the whole day, which was never before the case (second day),[15].—Stool scanty, delayed (from second to thirtieth day),[24].—[990.] *Dry, parched stool, with effort, in the morning (second day),[42].—Stool sluggish, with a twitching and sticking in the anus (second day),[28].—The evacuations are very sluggish; although the fæces are never hard, yet the expulsion of them is only effected with great exertion,[26].—Stool copious, pasty, but passed only after a long exertion (second day),[36].—A very difficult stool,[29].—Stool very difficult (second day),[36].—Fæces thick, firm, difficult to pass,[1].—The stool, which at first was regular, became, during the latter part of the proving, difficult, and was expelled with great exertion, less than the firmness of the fæces than from the inactivity of the intestines,[26].—*Stool very unsatisfactory, only after much straining, which caused a rush of blood to the head, and a feeling of confusion in the head (fourth morning),[32].—The stool, during the first days of the proving, was very unsatisfactory, or omitted altogether, while during the latter days, there were daily frequent and very copious evacuations, almost like diarrhœa,[32].—[1000.] Stool hard (second day),[16].—A hard stool (evening of second day),[36].—Very hard stool,[1].—Very hard stool, with pressing out of the rectum, which, however, returns of itself; this is followed by a diarrhœa-like stool, with fermenting in the abdomen,[2].—The evacuations became suddenly harder, and passed with more exertion; at first, hard portions, followed by softer (third and fourth days),[36].—*Hard stool, with great exertion, with confusion of the head (third and fourth days),[36].—A hard stool at 3 P.M., with inclination to eructations,[13].—Hard, difficult stool, only for two days,[18].—Hard, unsatisfactory stool (second day),[32].—A hard, unsatisfactory stool (second morning),[32].—[1010.] Two hard, unsatisfactory stools, preceded by

† From the body getting cool, while eating or soon after eating, or from taking cold water after eating soup, or after eating stewed fruit; or from sudden change of temperature while driving, from cold to warm or vice versa; sudden severe griping in abdomen, followed by copious pasty evacuations of a dark greenish-black color, and a very offensive cheesy odor, followed by great prostration; the natural course of the attack extending over twenty-four hours, with five or six stools, and ending in a dysenteric diarrhœa; arrested in fifteen minutes by Bryonia (the potency apparently a matter of indifference, the 6th, 30th, 200th, and 50th m., having been equally efficacious). An observation many times repeated on three patients, whose habit was constipated.—C. D.

colicky cuttings in the abdomen (sixth day),[11].—Hard stool, followed by drawing and heaviness in the sacrum,[33].—The usual evacuation is hard, and the tense abdomen is not relieved after it (second day),[36].—Hard, difficult stool,[36].—Scanty, hard stool in the evening,[21].—A hard stool, with drawing and pressure in the small of the back (one hour after taking),[27].—*Stools very dry, large, and hard* (sixth and seventh days),[42].—*Morning stool large, hard, and dry* (fourth day),[42].—Stools dry, large, hard, and very dark (third day),[42].

Urinary Organs.—Bladder. Repeated transient pain as of suppuration in the region of the right kidney, in the morning in bed,[13].— [1020.] After urinating a feeling in the bladder as if he had not finished, and a few drops still pass involuntarily,[1].—A sensation as though the bladder were not entirely empty, and even after urinating, there remained a feeling of heaviness in the region of the bladder, with various cramplike motions in it (second day),[9].—After he has urinated, contraction in the bladder and a feeling as if there was a little more urine to pass,[1].— *Urethra.* Bright-red spots around the orifice of the urethra, and in many places on the glans and on the inner place of the prepuce; they were very sensitive and burned severely; the secreting gland of the prepuce became swollen, and secreted a profuse, yellowish smegma; this balanitis increased from the third to the sixth day, then gradually disappeared, with fine itching and biting on the prepuce and glans,[18].—Burning in the urethra,[1].—Burning and cutting before the urine passes (third day),[2].— A pain in the forepart of the urethra when not urinating, consisting of an itching-burning and sticking,[1].—Sensation on urinating as if the urethra were too narrow,[1].—(A pressive pain in the urethra),[1].—Fine sticking pain in the urethra,[13].—[1030.] A severe stitch in the anterior portion of the urethra in the evening,[17].—A drawing-tearing in the forepart of the urethra when not urinating,[1].—Desire to urinate, and frequent urinating, when walking in the open air (after five hours),[1].—He is not able to retain the urine long, and when he is urged to urinate, and does not immediately attend to it, there is a feeling as if the urine passed involuntarily, though this does not happen,[1].—*Micturition.* Frequent urination,[36].—Frequent and profuse urination (second day),[32].—Urination more frequent than usual,[24].—The secretion of urine is decidedly increased; the desire to urinate comes very suddenly,[27].—Frequent urinating, with burning in the urethra and a sensation as if all the urine had not been evacuated,[27].— Frequent urinating at night; the urine was scanty and hot,[15].—[1040.] Obliged to rise several times at night to urinate,[1].—Great urgency to urinate; he is obliged to rise at night,[1].—He is compelled with such haste to urinate, even when the bladder is not full, that he is scarcely able to hold it for a moment (twelfth hour),[1].—A few drops of urine pass involuntarily when moving about,[1].—Urine scanty, seldom,[25].—The urine passes hot,[2].—Urine burning,[13].—"Every time on urinating it seemed like a partial crisis,".[24]—*Urine.* Urine profuse,[39].—Urine profuse, sometimes clear, sometimes high-colored,[39].—[1050.] An unusual quantity of urine, clear yellow, nearly every half hour,[34].—Urine copious, pale-colored, especially at night,[40].—Urine unusually scanty,[33].—Urine scanty and hot,[15].— Urine rather scanty and red (second day),[42].—*Urine scanty and darker than usual,*[18].—Urine hot,[24].—*Red urine,*[1].—*Urine dark, almost brown,*[19]. —*Urine brown, like beer,*[18].—[1060.] Urine brown, without sediment,[13].— The urine showed a thick brown cloud,[13].—*The urine passed through the night deposited a white sediment; its color was reddish-yellow (third day),[37].

Sexual Organs. — Male. A sticking, burning-itching on the border of the prepuce,[1].—Stitches in the right spermatic cord (fifth day),[34]. —Painful tension extending from the right testicle along the spermatic cord into the groin,[13].—Some stitches in the testicles (immediately) when sitting,[1].—Sexual desire rather increased,[13].—Increased sexual desire; after coition there followed in the night an emission and in the morning almost painful erections (second day),[34].—Emission and strong erections in the night,[34].—*Female.* [1070.] Very severe pain in the region of the right ovary, as though there were a sore spot which caused an irritation and a dragging; this pain extended down to the thighs, while at rest,[21].—Pain in the right ovary aggravated by touch,[21].—Swelling of the left labia majora, on which a black, hard pustule rises, like a little button, without pain or inflammation,[1].—(Increase of leucorrhœa),[2].—The menses appear eight days too early,[2].—The menses appear fourteen days too early,[2].—The menses appear three weeks too early,[2].—The menses follow within a few hours, sometimes eight days too early,[1].†

Respiratory Organs.—Larynx, Trachea, and Bronchi. Slight hawking of mucus from the larynx,[33].—Sensation as of apple-seeds lodged in upper larynx, or rima glottidis (after half an hour to two hours),[42].— [1080.] At 7 P.M., while sitting, sudden scraping in larynx with dry cough several times, without apparent cause (first day),[41].—Tickling in the larynx, with dry hacking cough,[33].—Tickling in the larynx, with a violent shaking cough, lasting several minutes (ninth day),[26].—*Tough mucus in the trachea, which is loosened only after frequent hacking,[4].—Irritation to cough, as though some mucus were in the trachea; after he has coughed some time a pain is felt there mingled with pressure and soreness; the pain is worse while talking or smoking (after four hours),[4].—When he goes into a warm room from the open-air a sensation as if vapor were in the trachea, which causes him to cough; he feels as though he cannot inspire enough air* (after two hours),[4].—A scraping sensation at the lower portion of the trachea, provoking a dry cough, in the morning,[13].—Scraping irritation in the trachea causing dry cough,[13]. —A scraping sensation at the bifurcation of the bronchi, which caused a dry cough,[13].—*Voice.* Voice somewhat higher than usual,[33].—[1090.] *Voice rough and hoarse* (after four hours),[4].—*Hoarseness* (second day),[28]. —Hoarseness lasting twenty-one days,[2].—A kind of hoarseness together with an inclination to sweat,[1].—Some hoarseness, and only one tone of the voice, on walking in the open air,[1].—The hoarseness which he commonly had disappeared in the course of the day, and showed itself in the evening only after long reading aloud (second day),[10].—At times, loss of voice,[39].

Cough and Expectoration.—Scraping, painful, hacking cough in the throat, as from rawness and dryness in the larynx, in the evening after lying down in bed,[1].—(Cough, especially after eating),[1].—(Nausea excites cough),[1].—[1100.] *Dry cough,[1].—Several attacks of dry cough,[16].— *A hacking dry cough from the upper part of the trachea,[1].—Dry cough, in the morning, with coryza,[40].—Continued dry cough, especially in the morning, together with collection in the mouth like water-brash,[1].—*A dry hacking cough; single, spasmodic, forcible shocks towards the upper part of the trachea, which seems to be covered with dry tough mucus; even

† This is the primary action; Bryonia may be therefore effectual for metrorrhagia.—H.

tobacco-smoking causes it,[1].—*Dry cough, with sticking pain under the sternum,*[39].—*Dry cough, as if coming from the stomach; together with a crawling and tickling in the pit of the stomach,*[1].—He awoke after a restless night with a violent dry cough and feeling of soreness in the chest; this cough returned several times during the day, but disappeared at night; it caused a thin greenish mucous expectoration (eleventh day, gradually decreasing till thirtieth day),[16].—Cough with expectoration (immediately),[2].— [1110.] *Cough, from a constant crawling upward in the throat, followed by expectoration of mucus,*[1].—Sudden cough, as if caused by irritation in the abdomen, with expectoration of yellowish-green mucus (eleventh day),[26].— In the morning, in bed, a severe cough, which lasts a quarter of an hour, and causes a profuse mucous expectoration,[1].—Cough, with expectoration of gelatinous mucus, in the morning,[33].—Slight, hacking cough, with sensation of soreness and swelling in the pharynx and air-passages in the morning; expectoration of mucus difficult to loosen,[39].—Cough, with expectoration, in. the forenoon, for four days in succession (after thirty-four hours),[2].— Frequent expectoration of thick mucus,[33].—Frequent easy expectoration of thick mucus in the morning,[33].—Expectoration of thick mucus, almost without cough, which almost causes vomiting,[33].—He expectorates clots of blood (after three hours),[1].—*Respiration.* [1120.] Respiration more rapid while walking, with a sensation as if the upper part of the chest were too narrow,[15].—Frequent sighing,[33].—Deep sighs in quick succession,[29]. —Frequent catching for breath immediately before a paroxysm of coughing, a quick spasmodic gasp, as if the child could not catch the breath, and on this account could not cough; a kind of suffocative attack, which is followed by cough; especially after midnight,[1].—Constant disposition to sigh, and sigh deeply (first day),[42].—Impeded respiration,[1].—Asthmatic breathing (after one hour),[1].—The breathing is short; he is obliged to expire quickly,[1]. —Anxiety in the morning which seemed to rise from the abdomen, as if a purge had been taken, and as if the breathing were too short,[1].—Sudden, anxious, almost impossible breathing, on account of stitches in the chest, at first below the shoulder-blades, then below the pectoral muscles, which hinder breathing, and cause her to sit upright, and followed by stitches in the vertex,[1].—[1130.] Oppressed respiration,[33].—Oppressed breathing, with heaviness in the chest in the forenoon,[36].—Slight oppression of breathing in the middle of the upper half of the sternum, with sticking pain in the anterior wall of the chest, caused by every movement of the trunk, lasting several minutes,[13].—Oppression of breathing for a long time in the forenoon, so that the whole chest could not be expanded, with accelerated breathing,[33]. —Breathing difficult; it is relieved by walking,[1].—An attack as if nausea rose up and took away the breath, and stitching,[1].—Dyspnœa, so that he could not utter a word,[11].

Chest.—A sensation as if everything were loose in the chest and fell downward into the abdomen,[3].—Heaviness in the chest, and heaviness in the body, which disappears on eating,[1].—Painfulness of the chest,[29].—[1140.] Pain over the whole chest, with oppression, which passes off with passage of flatus, in the evening at 9 P.M.,[1].—*Internal heat in the chest,*[3].—Transient heat internally in the chest,[23].—Sensation of heat throughout chest, particularly on left side, at every inspiration (first day),[42].—Sense of fulness and stuffing throughout the chest (first day),[42].—Tension in the chest, when walking,[1].—Constriction in the upper part of the chest,[33].—Constriction of the chest; heaviness in the sternum,[33].—Constriction in the lower portion of the chest,[33].—* Constriction of the chest; she felt the need of breathing deeply *(as if the chest were stopped and she could get no air)*, *and if she attempted to breathe deeply there was pain in the chest, as if something were being distended which could not be completely distended,*[1].—**[1150.]** Constriction of the chest, as also a sore pain in the inner surface of the sternum, became more violent, and at last compelled him to get out of the wagon and rest, after riding over a rough road; the pectoral muscles also felt bruised, and every movement of the arms was painful,[15].—On going to sleep, a sensation as if the chest were too narrow; the thorax was somewhat sensitive,[31].—Pain in the chest just above the pit of the stomach, pinching, worse when sitting upon a chair and bending forward, or in bed lying upon the side,[1].—Slight drawing pain externally in the chest,[33].—Pressure over the whole chest (after twenty-four hours),[1].—Pressure on the chest, as if it was pressed by mucus, and on inspiration some stitches in the sternum, which seemed to be relieved by eating,[1].—Oppression of the chest,[1].—Great oppression of the chest,[39].—Frequent slight oppression of the chest (fourth day),[38].—Oppression in the chest, in the forenoon, while sitting and talking,[33].—**[1160.]** Oppression of the chest in the morning; he feels as if there were a coating of mucus in the chest, which could not be easily loosened,[1].—Frequent oppression of the chest, while walking, in the forenoon,[33].—Pressive pain in various parts of the chest (after one hour),[33].—Pressive pain in the lower portion of the chest, extending backward,[33].—At noon, on walking, pressing pain about the whole thorax, repeated several times in a few minutes (third day),[41].—A sticking-pressing in the chest from within outward,[1].—Transient stitches through the chest,[18].—Stitches in the chest, in the evening at 6, with oppression,[1].—An attack of stitches in the side and portion of the chest, which lasts twelve hours.[1].—*On inspiring, a stitch in the upper part of the chest through the shoulders,*[1].—**[1170.]** Severe stitches shoot through the chest several times,[18].—The tearing pains, which in the beginning of the proving were only in the head and extremities, have disappeared, and are now seated in the chest and abdomen,[26].—*Chest very sensitive, with stitches in the left side of it on inspiration, the whole forenoon* (twentieth day),[16].—The pectoral muscles do not seem free, especially on deep inspiration,[33].—The pectoral muscles pain when writing, with a sensation as if the thorax were too tight,[15].—Slight drawing in the pectoral muscles (second day),[33].—Drawing and tension in the pectoral muscles,[33].—The pectoral muscles and diaphragm are so sensitive that inspiration is difficult,[33].—The pectoral muscles are sensitive on moving the hands and on pressure,[15].—The pectoral muscles are painful to touch, as if bruised (after six hours),[15].—**[1180.]** On inspiring, pain in the angles of the ribs towards the back, with tensive pain, which is increased to a dull stitch on slightly deeper inspiration, especially below the shoulders, and mostly when stooping,[1].—(A tension across the short ribs),[1].—Stitches in the last ribs, on coughing,[1].—

Front. Great swelling of the anterior outer part of the chest,[3].—*Sensation of heaviness beneath the sternum, which extends toward the right shoulder, impeding respiration; deep inspiration was only accomplished with exertion; together with oppression in the right side of the chest, with very fine, extremely severe stitches in the right axillary glands,*[25].—Burning pain, extending backward from the inner surface of the sternum,[15].—A griping in the chest near the sternum,[1].—Pressure on the upper part of the sternum, as with the hand; she believes it cannot disappear without pain, even in the open air,[1].—Pressive pain in the centre of the breast-bone, also when inspiring, with ice-cold feet,[1].—Pinching pressure behind the sternum, more violent when breathing out or in (after five days),[4].—**[1190.]** Sticking and pressure beneath the breast-bone, increased by motion and deep inspiration (fourth day),[28].—On the slightest inspiration, a stitch, as in an ulcer, which lasts as long as the inspiration, in a small spot below the sternum, which pains like an ulcer, even on touch, but still more on raising the right arm, in the morning (after twenty-four hours),[1].—*Stitches in the sternum on coughing; he was obliged to hold the chest with the hand; *even pressing upon it caused a sticking*,[1].—Sore pain down the whole length of the sternum,[15].—Sore pain beneath the sternum,[15].—Sore sensation on the inner surface of the sternum the whole day,[15].—Soreness of the upper part of the inner surface of the sternum, especially on breathing,[15].—Soreness in all the muscles of the anterior surface of the chest; they are also sensitive to touch,[33].—Pain in the ensiform cartilage on touch, as if injected with blood, in the evening,[1].—Burning pain along the anterior insertion of the diaphragm (after half an hour),[33].—*Sides.* [1200.] A painful sensation in a spot as large as a half dollar, on the right side of the chest below the axilla, increased by touch,[13].—Burning pain in the right side of the chest (after eight hours),[1].—A short burning pain in the ribs of the right side, in a place of the size of a two-cent piece, at 9 A.M.,[13].—A tensive sensation on both sides of the chest externally, which is especially noticed on deep inspiration (after five hours),[15].—Drawing pain in the right pectoral muscles,[33].—A dull pain in the left side of the thorax and the region of the lower angle of the shoulder-blade; *it extends from behind forward :* it lasts several seconds, and causes a necessity for deep breathing (thirteenth day),[26].—Pressure in the right wall of the thorax, uninfluenced by respiration (first day),[41].—Severe pressure on the right border of the sternum, especially in the open air (sixth and seventh days),[34].—Slight pressure in the region of the false ribs, and fine stitches in the region of the navel, impeding respiration,[25].—Pressive sensation at the bend of the lower ribs of the right side, over a surface as large as a palm,[33].—[1210.] Pain in the chest, so that he had to go to bed; the pains were violent, pressive, tearing, seated between the sixth and seventh ribs on the right side near the sternum, were not aggravated by deep breathing; they continued the next day, and it seemed as if they approached pleuritic stitches; at the same time a pressive throbbing pain appeared in the right clavicle,[24].—11 P.M., while sitting, pressing pain in the left intercostal muscles (first day),[41].—Oppression of the right side of the chest prevented deep inspiration,[25].—*Pain of a sharp kind in left infra-mammary region ; worse during inspiration* (after two to three hours),[42].—Sticking pains under the lowest ribs of the left side; these lasted an hour, but gave place to sticking pains in the right loin, but as these disappeared the others also returned, and lasted till 9 P.M., gradually becoming weaker,[18].—Slight sticking pain to the right side of the sternum; the stitches extend deeper downward toward the navel; also, in the same place, constriction; on sneezing the pain becomes so severe that he is obliged to bend double,[33].—*Sharp sticking pain below the right nipple, extending outward in the thorax, only on expiration*,[4].—Sticking and throbbing in the lower portion of the right side of the chest, like a pulse,[1].—Transient stitches in both sides of the chest,[16].—Several stitches in the ribs of the right side,[27].—[1220.] Frequent stitches in the left side of the chest (second day),[38].—A momentary stitch in the left clavicle, which is followed by simple pain (behind this there is a simple aching),[1].—*Short but violent stitches in the right side of the chest, so that he was obliged to hold the breath, and could not cry out* (sixteenth day),[16].—On turning in bed, a stitch in the side of the chest on which he does not lie,[1].—Stitches in the sides in the

ribs, jerklike, on deep breathing, which disappear in the open air,[1].—
*Stitches in the right side of the chest between the third and fourth ribs, while
sitting,*[33].—Dull stitches in the region of the fifth and sixth ribs on the right
side of the sternum,[25].—Sensitive stitching in the left side in the middle of
the thorax, lasting several minutes,[18].—Fine, wandering, very sensitive
stitches in the right side of the chest, in the pit of the stomach, and in the
region of the navel, as if these places were touched here and there with a
fine-pointed instrument with several points at the same time; some of these
stitches pierced with lightning-like rapidity the right half of the chest, and
seemed more like fine cuttings (second day),[17].—A fine, transient, rather
severe stitch in the left side of the chest below the nipple, and fine needle
stitches in the pit of the stomach, the latter only noticed on very deep inspiration, or on inclining the trunk towards the right side,[13].—[1230.] Transient severe stitches at the insertion of the deltoid muscle, and in the left
side of the chest, mostly superficial in the left intercostal muscles,[24].—Drawing stitches on the right side between the tenth and eleventh ribs (in the
evening, fourth day),[34].—*Tearing stitches in the left side of the chest, which
extend from behind forward, are relieved during rest, are aggravated during
motion and on deep inspiration,*[26].—Slight pleuritic pain in right breast,
about two inches to the right of and in an intercostal space, two ribs above
the nipple of that side; worse during inspiration; better during expiration
(after two to three hours),[42].—A sore pain on the left side of the chest between the seventh and ninth ribs, in a spot of the size of a palm, rather
externally, increased by touch,[33].—Respiration normal, but the ribs painful, as if torn from their union,[24].—*A painful spot on the second rib of
the right side, extending to the sternum, as after a blow or bruise,*[33].—
Throbbing pain between the tenth and eleventh ribs in the right side, in a
spot of the size of a penny, immediately disappearing on pressure (after
one hour),[34].—Several slight electric-like shocks in a hardened nipple, for
two and a half hours, after which all trace of hardness disappeared (after
five hours),[7].

Heart and Pulse.—Aching in the præcordial region,[33].—[1240.]
Pressive pain in the præcordial region,[33].—Stitches in the præcordial region,
lasting only a few seconds,[13].—Cramp in the region of the heart (fourth
day),[34].—Slight cramp in the region of the heart, with accelerated pulse,[34].
—At 6 A.M., decided oppression in the region of the heart, without change
in its beat,[11].—*The heart beats violently and rapidly,*[11].—Palpitation
several days in succession (after twelve hours),[2].—*Pulse full, hard, and
rapid,*[13].—Pulse full, large, and quick, but not very frequent, at 9 A.M., two
hours after breakfast (second day),[47].—Pulse increased scarcely ten beats
in a minute,[24].—[1250.] Pulse 80 (after one hour),[43].—Afternoon, pulse 80
(sixth day),[43].—Pulse at three different times, since 4 P.M., has been 84
(third day),[43].—Pulse 85 (after half an hour),[43].—Pulse decreased from 94
to 87 (after thirty-five minutes); rose from 87 to 92 (after forty-eight
minutes); sunk to 87 (after one hour); to 82 (after one and two-third hours);
to 74, considerably weaker and more compressible (after three and five-sixths
hours); 75, fuller and stronger (after five and five-sixth hours),[43].

Neck and Back.—Neck. Pains in the neck, on moving it,[34].—
Pain in the nape of the neck, as after taking cold,[1].—*A pain in the nape of
the neck near the occiput, like a pain and weakness together, as if the head
were weak,*[1].—Painful stiffness of all the cervical muscles on motion, with
rawness in the throat when swallowing,[1].—* On the right side of the nape of
the neck, towards the shoulder, painful stiffness of the muscles on moving the

head,[1].—**[1260.]** Tension in the nape of the neck, on moving the head,[3].— *Drawing and stiffness in the muscles of the right side of the neck*,[33].—Pressure on the left side of the nape of the neck,[13].—Tearing pains in the muscles of the left side of the neck down to the shoulder,[33].—Sore pain on motion in the left side of the neck, and throat, and the muscles of the face, and mastication renders turning the head or chewing difficult and almost impossible (after twenty-four hours),[3].—**Back.** Feeling of stiffness every time on rising; disappeared after walking,[36].—Burning in the back,[5].—Tension in the back and sacral region in the forenoon,[33].—Constrictive pain across over the whole back, as if he were bound tightly with bands, almost like a cramp (from four to eight in the afternoon), (after forty-eight hours),[1].—*A drawing down the back* when sitting, disappearing on motion,[1].—**[1270.]** Frequent stitches in the afternoon on the left side of the back, especially violent in the left side of the chest and in the nipple, aggravated on moving the trunk or on bending the left arm backward,[13].—*Shooting stitches in the back through the chest*, in the forenoon,[33].—Stitches in the back in a very small spot between the tenth and eleventh ribs (third day),[34].—He can neither bend nor stoop on account of the pain in the back and lumbar vertebræ, a tearing, more when standing than when sitting, but not when lying,[1].—Painful sticking twitches on both sides near the spine, when sitting, especially in the morning and evening,[1].—**Dorsal.** Uncomfortable sensation between the shoulder-blades, more internally towards the posterior mediastinum, which causes frequent motion of the shoulders and trunk,[33]. —Rheumatic pain in back, between inferior angles of scapulæ (after three to four hours),[42].—Burning below and between the shoulder-blades,[5].—A spasmodic pain between the shoulder-blades almost like shivering,[1].—Tension between the shoulders,[33].—**[1280.]** A very violent drawing pressive-tensive pain in the first dorsal vertebra (where the prover had suffered fourteen years before from a wrenching of the spine) with impeded and difficult respiration ; *the pain extended through the thorax to the lower portion of the sternum*,[21].—Drawing between the shoulders,[33].—Slight drawing between the shoulders, more on the right side,[33].—Drawing and sticking between the shoulders on moving the trunk (third day),[34].—Pressure between the shoulders and opposite in the forepart of the chest, when sitting; disappears when walking,[1].—A scraping-sticking sensation in a place between the shoulder-blades, as large as a quarter of a dollar, as though a thorn were thrust into the flesh, only noticed on motion,[13].—Very violent, sudden (lightning-like) stitches in the region of the lower angle of the right shoulder-blade in the evening, and especially in bed, returning at short intervals,[24].—*Dull stitches between the shoulder-blades, extending from behind forward*, in the afternoon while lying,[27].—Violent twitching and tearing pain in the region of the last dorsal vertebra and sacrum (third day),[27].—Dull aching, and sharp, alternating pains, beneath right scapula, at its lower or inferior angle (after two to three hours),[42].—**Lumbar.** **[1290.]** Loss of sensation in the lumbar and sacral regions, in the forenoon, while walking, so that the muscles performed their functions automatically,[33]. —Pain in the right lumbar region, as after long stooping,[34].—Throbbing, tensive pain deep in the right lumbar region, just above the ilium, recurring twice at short intervals, though lasting only two or three minutes,[13].— Drawing and pressing in the lumbar region, and in the temporal bones, especially after eating,[27].—Pressure in the lumbar region,[33].—When lying upon the abdomen, a sensation in the left lumbar region of a bladder filled with air, the size of a man's fist, lying beneath the walls of the abdomen and pressing toward the surface, without pain or hardness ;† this sensation was least noticed when lying upon the back ; slight diarrhœa in the evening and morning (1st dil.),[12].—Tensive-pressive pain in the right lumbar region,[13].— Dull pressive pain in the right lumbar region (from 3d dil.),[12].—Painful pressure and fulness in the lumbar region,[13].—Drawing, sticking pain deep in the upper part of the right lumbar region,[13].—[1300.] Bruised pain in the lumbar region,[33].—Stitches in the lumbar vertebræ,[3].—Violent stitches from the third to the fourth lumbar vertebra, extending on both sides of the chest, especially on breathing (twentieth day),[34].—Dull aching in lumbar muscles (third day),[42].—Pressure and drawing in the lumbar muscles; the lumbar vertebræ by themselves seem to pain in the fore-noon,[33].—The lumbar muscles were sensitive to touch; the band of the drawers could scarcely be endured (third day),[27].—Paralyzed feeling in the small of the back,[33].—*Pain in the small of the back, which makes walking very difficult,[2].—*Pressive-drawing pain in the small of the back and loins, which made turning very difficult; it awoke him from sleep (eighth night),[12].—Sticking pain in the small of the back, and in the back, at night for six hours (after seventy hours),[2].—[1310.] Bruised pain in the small of the back and thigh,[1].—Bruised pain in the small of the back when sitting, worse when lying, less when moving,[1].—*The small of the back pains as if bruised when lying upon it,[1].—A jerklike pain in the small of the back, like a cramp, when sitting and lying,[1].—Pain in the loins, with dull pressive pain in the occiput and chilliness in the skin, awoke him at 1 A.M. (first night),[12].—Drawing pains in the loins, after a meal,[33].—Drawing pain in the loins and small of the back after eating,[33].—Bruised sensation in the loins (second day),[33].—The feeling of weariness on the right side of the sacrum, which rendered walking difficult, was very troublesome,[24].—Heaviness in the sacrum and dragging in the hæmorrhoidal vessels,[33].—[1320.] Dull, rheumatic pain, drawing lameness, in muscles of right sacro-iliac region, and in right deltoid muscle, at its centre (after two to three hours),[42]. —He was unable to lie stretched out without violent pain in the sacral region; sitting up, lifting, or turning the body increased the pain; he found himself relieved when at rest with the body bent forward; he arose out of bed with great difficulty; putting on the clothes was very difficult on account of the violent pain in the sacral region; walking in the street caused great exhaustion; going upstairs was especially troublesome; walking caused such intolerable pain that he was obliged to be taken home in a carriage; he went to bed; the pain extended from the lumbar and sacral regions in part along the spine, in part down towards the legs; on attempting to raise or stretch out the legs or to raise the body upright, the greatest pains; every slight touch of the spine, especially in the lumbar region, increased the pain; urination much increased; urine yellowish-red; fever moderate; pulse full and hard (third day),[38].—Slight tensive pain in the sacral and lumbar region, on walking,[33].—Drawing pain in the sacral and lumbar regions, with moderate fever (afternoon, second day),[38].—A sharp violent stitch on the right side of the lowest portion of the back (from 5th dil.),[12].—A persistent drawing-tearing pain, at the point of union of the ilium with the sacrum (in the evening of fourth day),[26].—Sticking-drawing in the coccyx while walking,[26].

---

† Apparently caused by a partial spasmodic constriction of a portion of the intestines distended by gas. This sensation was frequently observed during the proving and for a long time afterward, but never before.

Extremities in General.—Stretching of the limbs, in the afternoon,[6].—*Heaviness in the limbs, which seem like lead* (third day),[37].—A feeling of weariness in the limbs, with shivering in the face,[34].—[1330.] Weariness and bruised feeling in the limbs,[24].—*Weariness and heaviness in all the limbs; the feet can scarcely carry her on account of heaviness, when walking,[1].—* Weariness and stiffness of the limbs, especially of the lower,[22].— * Weakness in the limbs, which obliges him to sit,[4].—Sensation of prostration in the limbs; audible rumbling in the abdomen (fourth day),[38].—Pains in the limbs (after two hours),[18].—The well-known Bryonia pain in all the limbs and joints grew worse constantly till toward noon, especially they attacked the right side,[19].—While riding such severe pains in all the limbs that he was inclined to drink some beer (must), which relieved the pains (second day),[18].—Violent drawing through all the limbs; it is unendurable to keep the affected part still; he moves it up and down,[1].—Drawing and scraping in the long bones frequently,[18].—[1340.] Scraping pains in the long bones, especially noticed on riding,[18].—Tearing-scraping pain in all the limbs and joints, reaching a great intensity,[19].—*All the limbs seem bruised and paralyzed* (in the evening), as if he had lain upon a hard bed (after four hours),[1].—Bruised pain in the arms and legs, even when lying, worse when sitting than when walking; when lying he is obliged to move the limbs constantly on account of pain; it seems as though he would feel better by lying in some other position than that in which he is,[1].—*Swelling of the elbow-joint, and somewhat above and below it, as far as the middle of the upper and forearm, and of the soles of the feet,* for three hours,[3].—(The hands and feet felt dead at night, senseless, sleepy, ice-cold, and could not be warmed),[1].—A feeling in the upper arm and thigh as after a transient but violent exertion (afternoon of fourth day),[26].—Rheumatic pains in the tops of both shoulders and in the left knee,[39].—Pains in the thumbs and in the right great toe, the former pinching, and the latter violent sticking pains (fifth day),[34].—[1350.] Drawing, alternating in both knees, in the hips, and especially in the left shoulder, lasting only a short time,[36].—Drawing in the sheaths of the muscles of the upper and lower extremities,[27].—Drawing pain in the thumbs and great toes (immediately),[34].—Slight drawing pain in the right upper arm and in the right leg,[33].—A sensitive drawing pain, frequently returning, in the lower third of the ulna of the right forearm, which alternated with a painful drawing in the left knee,[13].— Slight drawing and tension in the upper arms and thighs,[18].—Wandering drawing pain alternating in both hips and in the right shoulder,[36].—Drawing and tearing in the joints of the forearm and metatarsus,[27].—Pressive pains with some transient stitches, now in the fingers, now in the wrist, which extend to the axilla and shift to the knee, and then alternate back and forth, so that walking becomes difficult,[15].—Drawing-sticking in right great toe and right thumb (third day),[34].—Several transient stitches in the left knee, in the first joint of the right thumb, when walking about,[18].—[1360.] Short piercing stitches, as with fine needles suddenly thrust into the bones, now in the left upper arm, now in the right leg,[33].—Tearing pain·in both elbows and both middle toes of the right foot (fifth day),[26].—Jerklike tearing in the first joint of the right thumb and the lowest joint of the right great toe (fourth day),[32].—Drawing-tearing pains frequently return, now in the upper, now in the lower extremities, now in the ligaments, now in the tendinous sheaths of the muscles, but they never last long; these pains at first seemed to appear on motion, but they also appeared during rest (fifteenth to thirtieth day),[26].—A drawing-tearing scraping pain in the little finger of the left hand and in the left great toe (after two hours),[21].—

While sitting, bruised pain in the knees, legs, arms, in single joints of the fingers and legs (first day),[41].

Superior Extremities.—Towards evening, while writing, the arm frequently goes to sleep, and long afterwards it remains heavy,[23].—A drawing through the bones of the arm, as from a thread, extending to the tips of the fingers,[1].—(Violent sticking and crawling in the left arm),[1].—A nervous tearing down the inner portion of the arm,[1].—*Shoulder.* [1370.] Unpleasant sensation in the shoulder-joints, which obliges movement of the shoulders,[33].—The wandering pains gradually became seated in the left shoulder-joint, where they lasted for an hour, but were not aggravated by touch,[18].—Paralytic feeling in the left shoulder, whereby the motion of the arm becomes difficult,[33].—Pain in the region of the acromion, as if sprained, on raising the arm (after three hours),[1].—A sticking-tensive pain in the ligaments of the left shoulder-joint, slightly perceptible during rest, but on active motion paining as if wrenched, at 11 A.M. (from 7th dil.),[12].—*A painful tension and pressure in the right shoulder, when at rest,*[13].—Drawing pain in the right shoulder,[33].—Slight drawing pain in the middle of the right upper arm; after half an hour, the same sensation in the left arm and left side of the chest,[33].—Drawing and tearing in the right shoulder, extending into the upper arm, less on motion, aggravated during rest (after four hours),[33].—[1380.] A pressive tensive-drawing pain in both shoulder-joints, together with momentary sticking and tearing, and, on raising up the arm, lameness, tension, and heaviness on the shoulder, and also at the insertion of the deltoid muscle in the upper arm,[18].—*Painful pressure on the tip of the right shoulder, worse upon touch; on deep breathing it becomes a dull sticking, which extends downward and outward to the shoulder-joint* (after ten hours),[4].—Pressure and feeling of fulness and heaviness in the shoulders,[18].—Violent stitches in the axilla, towards noon,[27].—Dull stitch across the shoulder to the arm,[3].—Tearing in the right shoulder, with increasing discomfort; this increased for half an hour, so that he must move the arm involuntarily back and forth; in the afternoon, in the open air, the arm was nearly painless; after going into the house the pains were renewed; especially troublesome was the sensation bordering on paralysis; could hold nothing firmly with the hand, and on attempting it, as in writing, the pains in the shoulder increased and became violent, even continuing after the hand was rested; on rubbing the hands together, the right one seemed thicker than the left,[33].—Violent tearing pains in the right shoulder and upper arm, so that the arm could scarcely be moved, at 6 A.M.; after rising the pain became greatly relieved, and disappeared after half an hour; at 11 A.M., while walking in the open air, the pain in the arm remained, though not so severe, and alternated with some pain in the right hip; at noon, in the arm, the pain was only in the shoulder-joint, but so violent that the arm could scarcely be moved; after half an hour it disappeared, and was followed by creeping and crawling along the ulnar nerve, with sensation of coldness in all the limbs,[33].—Frequent tearing in the right shoulder, in the knees and chest,[36].—*Arm.* Swelling of the right upper arm as far as the elbow,[1].—Feeling of heaviness in the right upper arm, with slight drawing,[23].—[1390.] Rheumatic pain in the right upper arm,[22].— The upper arm seemed too thick, in the evening; the sensation in it was diminished, with itching on the skin (second day),[26].—Slight drawing pain in the right arm,[33].—Slight drawing on the inner side of the right upper arm,[17].—Drawing pain in the right upper arm below the insertion of the deltoid, lasting two days,[16].—Drawing paralytic pain in the right upper arm; a feeling as of lead, which lasted one and a half hours,[23].—A pressure in both humeri, which prevents falling asleep in the evening,[1].—Very sensitive pains in the right arm, in the forenoon, for several hours; at noon these pains had nearly disappeared, but they returned in the afternoon at short intervals,[33].—(A stitching and jerking in the deltoid muscle),[1].—A kind of stitch in the upper arm, on raising it,[6].—[1400.] Very fine shooting, extremely painful stitches, deep in the deltoid muscle of the left arm, extending toward the surface,[24].—Tensive drawing-tearing pains in both upper arms, and along the ulna of the right arm,[21].—*Elbow.* *Swelling of the right elbow-joint, with stitches,*[3].—Slight drawing in left elbow (after three hours),[41].—Drawing and tearing in the right elbow, and along the forearm to the wrist,[26].—*A feeling in the right elbow as if the arm were broken, with a troublesome paralytic pain; it changed afterwards to a drawing pain; it extended to the shoulder-joint, and lasted all day;* a similar pain also in the right thigh (twentieth day),[34].—Stitches in the tips of the elbows, with drawing in the tendons down to the hands; the sticking is aggravated on bending the elbows,[1].—*Forearm.* Sensitive drawing and scraping in both forearms, while riding,[18].—At times, pressure, tearing, and gnawing in the forearm,[21].—In the morning, pressing and drawing in right forearm; later, in the left hand and fingers of right hand (second day),[41].—[1410.] *Tearing pain on the inner surface of the forearm, in a line from the elbow to the wrist* (after five days),[4].—Pressive-tearing pain in both forearms, which disappeared in a few hours from the left forearm, but became very violent in the right; before going to sleep, he bathed the affected arm in cold water; the next morning the pain had disappeared,[24].—*Wrist.* Pains in the wrist and thumbs (third day),[34].—*Pain in the wrists, as if wrenched or sprained, on every motion* (after twenty-four hours),[1].—*Fine stitches in the wrists if the hands became warm, and during rest; they do not disappear on motion,*[1].—*Hands.* An inflammation of the back of the hand, about midnight, with burning pain,[1].—Trembling of the hands, and distended vessels on them,[3].—He is unable to grasp tightly with the hands,[3].—Stiffness of the right hand and fingers,[13].—Painful stiffness in the left hand and forearm, as if in the ligaments and aponeuroses,[13].—[1420.] Painful stiffness of the right hand, especially on motion, and painful pressure over a hand's breadth in the region of the right nipple, especially violent during expiration (from 3d dil.),[12].—Numb and pithy sensation in the palms,[1].—Long-continued holding of the pen, and strong pressure upon any object, is painful,[15].—Sticking pain in the joints of the hands, with heaviness in them,[3].—Jerking-tearing in the metacarpal bones of the right hand, while writing (second day),[28].—*Fingers.* *A rather hot, pale swelling in the last joint of the little finger, with sticking in it, on moving the finger or on pressing it,*[1].—The third finger of the right hand had become very much swollen, and pained somewhat on pressure, still more on motion; the joint between the first and second phalanges was especially affected, similarly, but not so violently; the fifth finger of the same hand was affected the next day (fourth day),[9].—(The fingers of both hands go to sleep, as far as the wrists),[1].—Painful stiffness of the right finger-joints, especially on bending them (from 4th dil.),[12].—[1430.] Painful stiffness in the middle joint of the right middle finger, increased by bending, relieved by rubbing,[13].—Paralytic feeling in the fingers,[1].—Suddenly, after writing slowly, he noticed that the third finger of the right hand refused to work; he gave it rest, but after a time, when attempting to write again, this lame feeling had become worse (third day),[9].—*On writing, or taking hold of anything, a sensation as if the finger-joints*

were swollen and puffed; they are painful on much exertion and on touch,[15].—
Pain in the joint of the first phalanx of the right index-finger, lasting
several seconds, during rest,[13].—Pain in the root of the little finger, as if
pus were in it,[1].—Drawing in the ball of the left, afterwards of the right
thumb (fourth day),[34].—Sticking in the joint of the left little finger,[27].—
(Pain in the balls of the thumbs, like sticking and cramp),[1].—*Sticking pain
in the fingers, when writing,*[3].—[1440.] Transient tearings in the joints of
the left fingers (after two hours),[15].—Jerking-like tearing in the joints between the metacarpus and the fingers, or in the lowest joints of the fingers,
of both hands, lasting a few minutes, on motion,[6].—The phalanges are somewhat sensitive to severe pressure, with a sensation in them as if the articular
surfaces were swollen, which impeded their motion (second day),[15].

Inferior Extremities.—Great lameness and desire to keep quiet
(third day),[42].—Heaviness of the lower extremities,[33].—*The legs are so weak
that they will scarcely hold him, on commencing to walk, and even when standing,*[3].—A remarkable sensation of heaviness in the lower extremities while
walking,[26].—Drawing pain in the long bones of the leg,[1].—Drawing and
tearing in the whole of the right leg; the weariness disappears after walking
for an hour,[33].—On sitting, pressing pain in the whole left leg, especially in
the lower leg and ankle, compelling motion of the foot; lasts about two
hours; afterwards decreases on walking, and ceases (third day),[41].—*Hip.*
Slight pain in the left hip,[13].—Painful tension in the left hip,[13].—[1450.]
Slight drawing pain in the left hip,[33].—Slight drawing in the hips and
knees,[36].—Drawing pain in the hips and nates,[33].—Dull sticking pain in
the hips,[3].—*A few large stitches, like knife stitches, in the hips,*[1].—Pain in the
hip-joints, like a jerk or shock, when lying or sitting, better when walking,[1].
—Feeling in the hip-joint which makes rising from a seat difficult, but
which disappears on walking,[36].—Paralytic drawing pain in the left hip-
joint, which was relieved by pressure with the hand on walking, returning
every time on walking; every step caused decided cracking in the joints,
lasting five days (twentieth day),[34].—Pressive pain in the left hip-joint,
aggravated by motion, after half an hour; this pain extends after a little
while to the right hip, then it suddenly leaves the left hip and attacks the
inguinal region of the same side, especially the tendinous fibres which form
the inguinal ring; even after an hour there is slight sensitiveness of both
hips,[33].—Pains in right trochanter and gluteal region, of an aching, cramplike, and bruised kind, worse at every motion (third day),[42].—[1460.] Pain
in the trochanter, a sticking which makes him start on every false step;
during rest throbbing in it; the spot is very sore to touch,[1].—*Thigh.*
Tottering of the thighs, especially when going up and down the stairs (after
second day),[2].—Great weariness of the thighs, noticed even when sitting
(after eight hours),[6].—*Great weariness in the thighs, he can scarcely go up
the steps; less when going down the steps,*[6].—Stiffness in the thighs, like a
cramp, in the morning, in bed,[1].—*Great painfulness of the right thigh; the
pain comes from the head of the femur, extends along the anterior surface of
the thigh to the knee,* is most severe about the middle, and disappears in the
night; aggravated by motion, although it does not entirely disappear
during rest; on motion, the pain is drawing tearing; during rest there is a
paralytic sensation,[33].—Violent burning on the inner side of the thigh,
towards evening,[39].—A painful tension and drawing on the anterior surface
of the right thigh just below Poupart's ligament, relieved for several minutes
when at rest, and soon returning,[13].—Tensive pain on the anterior surface
of the right thigh, just below Poupart's ligament,[13].—While walking, the

tendinous expansion of both thighs seems tense, so that walking is difficult,[33].
—[1470.] Drawings in the thighs, as if menstruation would appear,[1].—
Drawing on the anterior portion of the left thigh, on the posterior portion
of the right thigh (fourth day),[34].—Drawing in the left thigh, extending
towards the hip,[36].—Clawing pains across the left thigh (fifth day),[34].—A
stitch in the upper anterior portion of the thigh,[1].—Some short, fine stitches
in the thighs, in the forenoon, now here, now there,[33].—Tearing pain in the
right thigh, on motion,[2].—Bruised pain in the middle of the thigh, and,
when sitting, a throbbing like a hammer in the same place,[1].—*Knee.*
Redness of the knee-caps,[39].—Excoriation of the hollow of the knee, for
more than a week,[40].—[1480.] *The knees totter and knock together when walking,*[3].—Weariness, especially in the knee-joints,[3].—Weariness, especially in
the knee-joint (immediately),[5].—Weariness and lameness in both knees,
aggravated by walking, relieved when at rest (second day),[26].—A weak and
paralyzed feeling in the right knee-joint, so that he almost had to drag the
foot, when walking in the forenoon (twenty-fifth day),[16].—Very weak feeling in the knees, especially on going up stairs, in the evening,[18].—The
weakness in the knees increases, and extends downwards into the middle
of the leg,[18].—Loss of power in the knees, especially on going upstairs,[18].—
Tensive, painful stiffness of the knees,[1].—*A feeling in the right knee-cap,
as if he had been kneeling a long time,*[33].—[1490.] Violent continued pain
in the knee,[39].—Pain on the right knee, on the inner condyle of the femur,[33].
—*Pain in the right knee, so that in the evening he could scarcely walk, and
was obliged to keep the leg very quiet; the inner side of the knee was very painful to touch; the next morning, while in bed, there was no pain, but after being
up awhile the pain returned,*[33].—Pains seated in the left knee, aggravated
by walking,[39].—Pains in the left knee-joint, only noticed on walking,[13].—
*Tensive sensation in the bend of the knee, which afterwards changed to a
drawing and wrenching along the crest of the fibula, lasting several minutes,*[27].
—Cramp in the knee and in the sole, when sitting, and at night when
lying,[1].—The knee-caps ache, as if they had been beaten loose,[1].—Pain on
going down stairs, as if the knee-caps would break,[1].—In the evening, digging and itching in the legs, about the knees and on the thighs; after
scratching or rubbing, small red elevated pimples appear, which cause a
burning pain; when the pimples arise, the itching ceases,[1].—[1500.] Tearing-drawing in the left knee-joint, and in the middle toes of the left foot,
in both elbow-joints, and on the flexor surface of both thighs; all these
pains are relieved during rest (sixth day),[26].—Drawing and sticking in the
left knee and calf (third day),[34].—Pressive pain in the knee, usually more
severe in the morning; begins soon after taking the drug and lasts through
the whole proving,[40].—At 9 A.M., on walking, pressing pain in the right
knee and lower leg (third day),[41].—Violent tearing-sticking in the right
knee-joint after a warm covering; when this ceased, some stitches appeared
in the left axilla,[27].—Sensitive sticking in the right knee, and in the right
external malleolus (second day),[19].—*When walking bent, sticking pain from
the hip into the knee,*[1].—A few stitches in the knee-joint (twenty-fifth day),[43].—
Fine transient stitches in the knee-joints, only on motion,[6].—*Stitches in the
knees when walking,*[2].—[1510.] Stitches in the right knee on ascending steps,
obliging him to stand still (second day),[15].—Transient stitches in the hollows
of both knees, in the afternoon, when walking,[18].—Transient stitches in the
right knee-joint, on motion (after five hours),[18].—Violent tearing stitches in
the left knee-joint, disappearing after rising (morning of fifth day),[26].—Jerklike, very painful stitches on the inner side of the left knee, repeated two

or three times, lasting several seconds,[23].—Tearing in the left knee, which extended along the tibia to the ankle, and then disappeared,[28].—(A tearing and) burning in the right knee,[1].—Reappearance of the tearing pain in the knee after eating, especially if one leg is riding over the other,[28].—Stitch-like tearing from the feet into the hollow of the knees, better during rest than during motion,[3].—*Leg.* Swelling of both legs (after forty hours),[2].— [1520.] Sudden swelling of the lower leg,[1].—Swelling, without redness, of the lower portion of the lower legs, excepting on the soles of the feet, which are not swollen,[3].—A twitching in the lower leg at night; during the day a twitching like an electric shock,[1].—Unsteadiness of the legs, and tottering when walking down the steps (after twenty hours),[1].—Heaviness in the right leg (second and third days),[33].—Heaviness and tension in the right leg,[33].—Heaviness and tension in the right leg, in the afternoon,[38].—Pain in the legs, as after walking the previous day,[33].—Severe drawing pain in the lower leg, especially in the calf, lasting for an hour, and followed by sweat in that place (after four days),[1].—Drawing and tearing in both legs, especially around the right knee, which is also painful to touch, and in the left leg,[33].—[1530.] In the evening, violent bruised sensation in the legs (first day),[41].—While sitting, bruised pain in left leg, for a moment (after two hours),[41].—Pain in the tibia and in the knee-cap, only when walking (fifth day),[34].—Burning on the anterior surface of the right tibia,[33].— Drawing-tensive pain in the tibia, extending to the right foot; it disappeared on walking,[20].—Sticking-drawing along the outer border of the tibia (third day),[34].—Tearing in the tibiæ, with swelling in the feet, and heaviness in the arms,[1].—Tearing-twitching pain in the upper part of the tibia,[1]. —Pinching tension in the left calf,[13].—Cramps in the calves, while lying,[21]. —[1540.] At night, cramp in the calves (a contractive tension), which disappears on motion,[1].—Cramp in the left calf, in the morning (after twelve hours),[1].—A dull, pressive-drawing pain in the left calf, which would not allow him to sit, and was relieved by walking (third day),[18].—*Pinching-tearing in the right calf*, very painful, but not lasting a long time, while sitting, after a meal (second day),[28].—*Bruised pain on the outer side of the left calf, on moving and turning the foot, as also on touch; during rest, a numb sensation in this place for several days* (after twelve hours),[3].—*Ankles.* Immobility of the right ankle on walking,[36].—Pain in the left ankle while sitting,[33].—Pain in the ankle and right great toe (second day),[34].—*Tension in the ankles on motion*,[1].—He dreamed that violent pain prevented walking, and on waking, found that he had a real sticking and scraping in the outer malleolus of the foot; it lasted a quarter of an hour; when it ceased, pains spread over the whole body, alternately attacking the limbs and joints, were continued a long time, lasting two hours; the sleep after midnight was restless and interrupted by fatiguing dreams, only towards morning quiet sleep, and on rising he felt slight remnants of the wandering pains,[18].—*Feet.* [1550.] *Hot swelling of the feet* (after eight hours),[1].— Top of foot still swollen a little; joint of great toe still weak and tender, and hurts a little when walking (twenty-first day),[43].—*The feet are tense and swollen in the evening*,[1].—Heaviness in the feet, in the forenoon,[33].—On rising, after eating, the feet felt as heavy as a hundredweight,[1].—Weariness of the feet, as if she had walked a long distance,[1].—The feet are weak when going upstairs,[1].—Stiffness in the feet, on rising after long sitting,[36]. —Pain deep in the right foot between the bones, so severe that he was often obliged to stop when walking; the painful place itched severely; the skin was rough; the metatarsal bones seemed swollen (after one and a half months),[34].—Burning heat in both feet as far as the malleoli, as though they were put into hot water, with painful stitches in the heels and in the corns; stiffness in the lower extremities and the nape of the neck,[13].—[1560.] Cramp in the feet at night, when lying in bed, on the back of the feet and on the heels (after six hours),[1].—Drawing pain in both feet,[36].—Drawing along the whole length of the left foot, after rising,[36].—Frequent drawing pains in the feet, with stiffness in the joints, continued several weeks,[36].— *Pain in the feet, as if sprained,[1].—Pressive pain in the metatarsal bones, several times in the afternoon,[33].—*Stitches in the feet,[3].—Sticking in the balls of both feet, with sensation of great heat, towards evening; is obliged to take off the shoes,[1].—A very sensitive tearing pain on the ridge of the right foot, which lasted ten minutes, and two hours after appeared in the left upper arm,[19].—Sudden violent tearing in the right metatarsal bones, in the forenoon, when walking, so that he is obliged to stand still, whereby the pain is relieved; it is renewed, however, on motion, and lasts five or six minutes (twelfth day),[26].—[1570.] At 2 P.M., pain quite severe; it now feels more like a bruise; the pain during the last hour has extended higher up the tendon, which is very tender to the touch, from an inch above the joint of the big toe to the bend of the ankle; (I took *Cauloph.* again this morning), (fifteenth day),[43].—*Hot swelling of the instep, with bruised pain on stretching out the foot; the foot seems tense on stepping on it, and on touch it pains, as if suppurating, like an abscess,[1].—* *Tensive pain on the back of the feet, even when sitting,[1].—Dull drawing-pressive pain on the back of the left foot; walking was very difficult, with pain at the same time in the sole of the foot (twentieth day),[34].—Tearing on the back of the right foot (first night),[2].—The last place affected was high up on the instep; the skin was swollen, and the parts beneath tender; at last, when the soreness did disappear, it seemed to go suddenly (after eight weeks),[43].—Cramp in the right heel (fifth day),[34].—Slight stitches on the inner side of the right heel,[13].—Needle-stitches in both heels, in the morning, in bed, which disappear after rising,[1].—Fine burning stitches in the left heel, at the insertion of the tendo Achillis,[27].—[1580.] Frequent tearing on the inner side of the right heel,[13].—Shooting into the heel as from a hook, two nights, immediately after lying down; sudden dull stitches in succession, for quarter of an hour,[1].—For a short time, a sore, tender sensation at the bottom of the heel when pressing upon it (twenty-fifth day),[43].—A feeling of heaviness in the soles, and a numb sensation as if they were swollen,[1].—Pinching pain in the sole of the right foot, while sitting,[33].—Cramp in the plantar muscles, sometimes at night,[39].—Pressure on the inner margin of the left sole (after one hour),[4].—Such violent sticking in both soles, that she could not step; with tension in the ankles; she could not even lie on account of tension and sticking,[2].—Knife-like stitches in the left sole,[1].—Pain, as if numb, and like a tension in the hollow of the foot, when stepping,[1].—[1590.] In the hollows of the feet, stitches on stepping,[1].—*Toes.* Painfulness of the left second toe, in the afternoon, when walking,[33].—Burning pain in the second left toe,[33].—Sticking pain in the balls of the right toes, worse when sitting, less when walking,[1].—Severe sticking, as with needles, on the lower surface of the right third and fourth toes, in the afternoon, lasting several seconds,[13]. —Several stitches extend into the toes,[3].—Fine stitches beneath the nail of the left little toe (sixth day),[28].—The left little toe pains as if sore, without anything to be seen upon it,[33].—The pain extends into the tarso-metatarsal joints of all the toes except the small one (seventeenth day),[43].—(Cloudy this morning), pain much worse, pains constantly, but worse when walking;

joints feel sprained, or like a bruise from something heavy falling across the toes; 8.30 P.M., a great deal better, does not pain when at rest now; pain twice to-day in left knee (eighteenth day),[43].—[1600.] Pain in toes rather worse; it extends up the metatarsal bone again (twenty-fifth day),[43]. —Pain in the balls of the left toes, as if bruised,[1].—The left toes become continually more sensitive; they frequently itch,[36].—*Sudden pain in the balls of the great toes;* it seemed as if he could not stretch out the toes, lasting half an hour,[36].—Violent drawing in the right great toe, extending over the back of the foot, and upward to the middle of the tibia; a similar pain at the same time in the left forearm,[34].—Sticking and pressure in the balls of the great toes, also pain in them as if frozen,[1].—Stitches through the tip of the left great toe (fifth day),[34].—Sore feeling near the middle of the tarsal bone of great toe, left foot, before getting up in the morning; on walking down to my office (about six squares) after breakfast, the foot became so painful in that region that I could scarcely walk; the further I walked the worse it became: I felt as if the ligaments had been sprained; I forgot that I had taken *Bryonia,* and supposed I was getting the rheumatism; I took a few globules of *Cauloph. 3d;* it soon got better, the pain passed off with a comfortable sensation of burning, very much like an injured part does "when it stops hurting." On walking out about 11 A.M., the pain returned again, but was not so intense as in the morning, when it was so severe as to make me walk lame. This time it also affected the right foot slightly in the same place for a short time; took *Cauloph.* again, when it again got better, but came back slightly at night (fourteenth day),[43].—Foot a great deal better to-day, it only pains now when walking; the pain has moved down into the large joint of the great toe; it feels when I stand or step on that foot as if the joint had been sprained; sometimes it has felt when treading with that foot, as if the joints were *giving way or spreading apart* (sixteenth day),[43].—A very slight degree of pain in joint of big toe this morning, still aggravated by walking. For several days the skin over the tarsal bone of the big toe has been swollen and inflamed; it has nearly disappeared this morning. The soreness appears to be in the sheath of the tendon, but principally in the *periosteum* and *ligaments;* there does not appear to be that *swelling of the joints, stiffness,* and *dread of motion* that usually characterizes rheumatism; but *motion always increases the pain* (nineteenth day),[43].—[1610.] Large joint of great toe continues to hurt me when walking; yesterday the corresponding joint of the next toe pained also; sometimes it is perfectly easy when at rest, sometimes it is not; the sensation is still that of having been sprained (twenty-fourth day),[43].—The joint is better, but there is a great deal of soreness all along the top of the metatarsal bone of great toe; there is also swelling, redness, and great engorgement of the veins, so much so that I am afraid of a permanent varicose condition of them. Took Hamamelis, 3d dil., 2 drops, and used tincture externally (twenty-sixth day),[43].—The hitherto painless corn grows and pains, mostly when stepping, though also during rest,[1].—Drawing pain in a corn on the left little toe,[34].—Burning-sticking pain in a hitherto painless corn, only on very slight touch; the pain immediately ceases on severe pressure,[1].—The corns pain as if sore, on slight touch, even in bed,[1].

General Symptoms.—Objective. On walking, he was obliged to bend considerably forward (second day),[38].—When the pain disappears, the part trembles and the face becomes cold,[1].—* *When walking, especially after rising from sitting, and when beginning to walk, unsteadiness of all parts of the body, as if all the muscles had lost their power; on continuing to walk it became* *better* (after forty-eight hours),[1].—***Restlessness.*** Restlessness,[33].—[1620.] Nervous excitement in the middle of the day,[33].—At night she tosses the hands and feet about until 10 o'clock, as in anxiety; she lies, as in consequence, with cold sweat on the forehead, and sighs; followed by weakness,[1].—***Fatigue.*** Feel lazy and indisposed to work (sixth and seventh days),[42].— Indolence and general discomfort (after one hour),[33].—* *Very tired and prostrated*,[23].—He became fatigued very soon on walking in the open air; especially troublesome was ascending steps; he was obliged to rest frequently (second day),[37].—On walking in the open air she was not tired, but when she walked in the room she became so tired that she was obliged to sit or lie down,[1]. —* *Weariness*,[1].—* *Great weariness in the morning*,[31].—* *Great weariness in the afternoon*,[28].—[1630.] * *Great weariness and sweat over the whole body after a slight exertion* (after three hours),[15].—Weariness in the afternoon, followed by two liquid stools without tenesmus,[11].—Weariness when sitting, less when walking,[1].—Great weariness, when waking from sleep,[1].—* *Weariness, prostration, in the whole body*,[13].—* *Uncommonly wearied and prostrated* (after four hours),[18].—After a heated walk and rapid cooling, the same weariness, chilliness, bruised sensation, and wandering pains in the whole body that are felt after taking cold,[34].—* *General weakness*,[3]. —Weak, indolent, weary, and sleepy,[2].—*She is weak; the arms and feet ache; if she does any work the arms sink down; if she goes upstairs she can scarcely get along*,[1].—[1640.] * *Great weakness and exhaustion*,[21].—Weakness very great,[19].—*The feeling of weakness becomes very great, especially great fatigue after a long walk*,[18].—She feels weakest when walking in the open air,[1].—Great weakness when walking (eleventh day),[26].—Unusual weakness and prostration towards evening,[18].—Unusually weak and heavy in the morning, after rising (second day),[16].—The symptoms disappeared after a short rest while quiet in bed, except the weakness and the very depressed mood, which continued the whole day,[11].—*Loss of strength on the slightest exertion*,[1].—**On rising, great exhaustion and weakness, which increased during the forenoon while walking, so that he had to drag himself about;** *on going upstairs there was excessive weakness in the knees and legs* (second day),[18].—[1650.] * *General prostration* (forenoon of second day),[38].—General prostration (after half an hour),[18].—The general prostration was relieved after a short rest,[18].—* *Great prostration and uneasiness*,[11].—Great prostration and weariness, with slight feeling of anxiety,[18].—**On rising from bed, he was attacked by faintness,** *with cold sweat and rumbling in the abdomen*,[1].—***Sensibility, Acute.*** Painful sensitiveness here and there in the body, in the left knee, in the left hip, in the loins, though only noticed when walking,[13].—Sensitiveness of the skin,[13].—***Sensations.*** Always after taking the medicine, I would feel light, vigorous, and active, or I might say supple,[43].—General discomfort, weariness, so that even the clothes feel oppressive (soon after taking),[33].—[1660.] General sick feeling,[24].— Soon after waking from the midday sleep, he felt sicker, all the symptoms were increased, and he was out of humor,[1].—* *Every spot in the body is painful when taken hold of, as if bruised, or as if suppurating, especially in the pit of the stomach, and especially in the morning*,[1].—Pain all over the body, as if the flesh were too loose (for sixteen days),[2].—The pain affected every portion of the body, even to the feet, *especially on the right side*,[34].—Transient pain in several parts of the body, in the metacarpus, metatarsus, the ribs, and clavicles,[33].—Pain in the joints, especially worse after walking,[18].— Painless drawing back and forth in the affected parts,[1].—Slight drawing pains here and there in the body,[34].—Drawing pains at 10 P.M., while at rest in bed, wandering through all the limbs and joints of the body, most violent and continued in the middle of the left side, where it caused stitches, impeding respiration,[18].—[1670.] *Drawing rheumatic pains in various parts of the body, especially in the insertion of the left ligamentum patellæ, on the anterior portion of the right leg, and in the nape of the neck, at different times during the day (fourth day),[34].—*Transient drawing and tension in almost all the limbs and joints; the pains were most sensitive in the left wrist; they were only transient, and soon moderated in the knees, ankles, and neck, but remained longest in the left shoulder-joint; they appeared equally during rest and motion; during the latter a sensation of chilliness was felt,[18].—Same pains as before described, not only in the joints, but also in the forearms, upper arms, thighs, and legs, along the course of the long bones, in the phalanges of the fingers and toes, and in the neck; the drawing-scraping pain in the long bones was combined with transient fine stitches,[18].—Pressive-drawing pain in the periosteum of all the bones, causing apprehension, as in the onset of ague, in the forenoon (after twenty-four hours),[1].—A pressing in the whole body, especially on the chest,[1].—Stitches over the whole body, as with needles,[1].—Stitches in the affected part,[1].—Stitches, which cause her to start, in the affected parts,[1].—Some stitches here and there, especially in the right eye and left arm,[16].—Two stitches in various parts of the body, at different times (third and following days),[16].—*Stitches in the joints, on motion and on touch,[1].—[1680.] In the affected parts, stitches if one press upon them,[1].—In the evening, dull stitches from before backwards, and also a similar sensation in the abdomen, a hand's breadth above the navel,[27].—Jerking stitches here and there, on the vertex, on the wrists and elbows, especially frequent and violent in several places on the forehead, with sensitiveness of the teeth,[31].—Frequent tearings in various parts of the body, especially in the toes and in the right shoulder, with a feeling as if motion was difficult,[36].—In the morning, unable to lie in bed; every part on which she lay was sore,[1].—In the morning, feels bruised and lame, particularly in right hip (fourth day),[42].—(Painful throbbing in the vessels of the whole body),[1].—Pains arise during rest, disappear after motion; others, however, during motion, and disappearing during rest,[34].

Skin.—*Yellow skin of the whole body, even of the face (after twelve days),[2].—Small red spots in the skin of the arms and feet, which pain like burning nettles; on pressure they momentarily disappear,[1].—[1690.] *A red, round, hot spot on the cheek on the malar bone,[1].—Round red spots, as large as peas and larger, in the skin of the arm, without sensation; they do not disappear by pressing upon them,[1].—Cracking of the skin and formation of thin crusts,[39].—**Eruption, Dry.** *Eruption over the whole body, especially on the back as far as the neck, which itched so violently that he was obliged to scratch it,[1].—Eruption on the lower lip outside the border, with itching-biting pain as from salt,[1].—Eruption below the left corner of the mouth, with smarting pain,[1].—A biting-itching eruption around the throat, especially after sweating,[1].—Eruption on the abdomen, and on the back as far as the neck, and on the forearms, in the forepart of the night and in the morning, causing a burning and biting pain,[2].—Dry eruption on and in the hollow of the knee, which itches at evening; seems red; scratching causes a biting pain,[2].—*A red, elevated, rashlike eruption over the whole body, in a mother and her infant; in the infant it appeared after two days, in the mother after three days,[2].—[1700.] Rash on the arms, on the front of the chest, and above the knees; it becomes red in the evening, itches, and burns before she lies in bed, but when in bed, after she becomes warm, the rash and itching disappear,[1].—Red nettlerash on the throat,[2].—The glans is covered with a red pimply rash, which itches,[1].—Red rash on the upper portion of the forearm,[2].—Eruption of small red pimples,[39].—A pimple as large as a pea in the left lower lid, painful to touch for sixteen days (after twenty-four hours),[2].—(A pimple on the chin, with sticking pain on touch),[1].—A small pimple in the right corner of the mouth, or rather on the lower lip, which bleeds profusely from time to time, for six days,[2].—Pimples appear on the abdomen and on the hips, which burn and itch, and when she scratches smarting results,[1].—Several inflamed pimples on the back and face, especially on the forehead; they do not pain, but itch on strong pressure, and leave a sore sensation for some time,[33].—[1710.] Pimples between the right thumb and index finger; every touch causes a fine stinging pain,[1].—Pimples, which are somewhat painful, on the thigh (fourth day),[10].—The aphthæ on the inner surface of the lip bled somewhat,[13].—A small tetter on the right cheek (after fourth day),[2].—*Moist.* A vesicle on the vermilion border of the lower lip, with burning pain,[1].—Vesicular eruption, with burning in the middle of the upper lip; it was nearly round and of the size of a penny, and looked like a hydroa,[18].—An eruption began upon the sacral region, extended over the back, chest, and forearm, consisting of more or less diffused groups of rashlike pimples, as large as the head of a pin, pointed with white semi-transparent vesicles; these gradually dried, the spots desquamated, and left a red color for a long time; there was no pain, only sometimes, on especially active motion, a slight itching, easily relieved (the last weeks of the proving),[31].—(Moist, exuding eruption on the legs),[1].—*Pustular.* (Itchlike eruption only on the joints, on the inner surface of the wrists, in the bends of the elbows, and externally on the condyles of the elbows, especially externally on the knee, as also on the hollow of the knee),[1].—A soft boil in the inner canthus of the left eye; matter flows from it from time to time, for ten days (after six days),[2].—[1720.] Hard boil behind the ear, which frequently changes its size (after twenty-four hours),[2].—Small suppurating spot on the lower lip, with burning pain on touch,[2].—A pustule under the knee, which pains and sticks when touched,[1].—(White pustules on the sole of the foot, with a pain like a bad ulcer; the foot was red, and he could not walk on account of pain),[1].—*Ulcers.* (The discharge from an ulcer colors the linen blackish),[1].—Chilliness in an ulcer, with pain as if it had been affected by too great cold,[1].—Tearing pain in an ulcer,[1].—(Ulcerated cartilage of the ears),[1].—*Sensations.* During a slight mental excitement (in laughing), a sudden sticking (itching) burning over the whole body, as if he had been stung with nettles, or had a nettlerash, though nothing could be seen upon the skin; this burning appeared even when merely thinking of it, or if he became heated,[1].—A sore painful spot begins to burn violently,[1].—[1730.] A burning pain in the skin on the right side of the first dorsal vertebra, in a place as large as a quarter of a dollar, as if this part had been touched by nettles, for half an hour (eleventh day),[26].—Burning pain in the skin on the outer margin of the left knee-cap, lasting several seconds, and frequently returning,[17].—A tension of the skin of the face on moving the facial muscles,[1].—Paroxysmal drawing in the skin under the lower jaw on the right side, and the inner side of the left leg, and groin, and knee,[34].—In the morning, after rising, a biting pain in the region of the scab of an ulcer, which increases on standing, is relieved on sitting, and disappears on moderate motion,[1].—Itching-biting in the left inner canthus, as from sand, at

3 P.M. (first day),[13].—A throbbing in the vicinity of the crust of an ulcer, which resembles a sticking (after dinner),[1].—(Crawling in the hands, as if asleep),[1].—A crawling-creeping, as from a mouse, from the axilla to the hip,[1].—Itching on the scalp and about the anus,[33].—[1740.] Itching on the border of the left upper lid, mingled with burning and tearing,[1].—Itching at the union of the first and second phalanges of the fingers of the left hand without any apparent cause (fourth day),[9].—Itching in the hips and thighs (after forty-eight hours),[2].—An itching, as if something was healing, in the hollow of the knee, with sweat in this place, at night,[1].—Burning-itching and continued stitches in various parts, in the evening after lying down in bed (after two hours),[1].—Sticking-itching here and there over the body,[13].—A sticking-itching below the right upper lid, as from a stiff hair, relieved by rubbing,[13].—Immediately before going to sleep, during the day or in the evening, tearing-itching in various places on the soft parts of the body, or digging burning-itching stitches,[1].—Tickling-itching (during the day) on the arms, hands, and feet, with rashlike pimples,[1].

Sleep and Dreams.—Sleepiness. *Very much inclined to yawn; frequent yawning the whole day,*[1].—[1750.] Yawning,[13].—Yawning almost all day,[40].—*Frequent yawning,*[3 15 39].—Frequent yawning towards noon (second day),[36].—Frequent yawning, sneezing,[15].—Sudden yawning before dinner, with much thirst,[6].—Continual inclination to sleep for three days,[2].—Sleepiness,[33].—Sleepiness, immediately after eating,[3].—Sleepiness on waking was almost irresistible (second morning),[34].—[1760.] Great sleepiness, even in the daytime, for several days in succession,[2].—Great sleepiness during the day, with great inclination to a midday sleep; on waking, all the limbs were asleep,[1].—*Great sleepiness and constant yawning, though he had slept well the previous night,*[22].—Great sleepiness in the afternoon,[22].—*Much sleepiness during the day when alone,*[1].—*So sleepy that he wishes to sleep the whole day,* for thirteen days in succession,[2].—She slept the whole day, with excessively dry heat, without eating or drinking, with twitching in the face; she let the stool pass six times involuntarily, which was brown and very offensive,[1]. —Very sound sleep during the night (perhaps owing to sitting up late for two or more nights), (second day),[42].—He slept soundly the whole night, and continued sleepy through the whole day; the next night he slept uneasily, and the day after was lively,[1].—Difficult to wake from sleep in the morning,[34].—[1770.] In the morning he cannot rise from bed, and wishes to lie a long time (without being weak),[1].—Three hours' sleep after eating (contrary to custom), and very vivid dreams; after waking dull stitches and pressure in the chest near the sternum, in the region of the fifth rib,[27].—In former years, when young, a sensation of invigoration, not only after awaking, but even during sleep; a certain feeling of comfort; this sensation had disappeared during my residence in Vienna (for three years), but it returned again very marked for six nights, from massive doses of Bryonia,[9].—*Sleeplessness.* *Sleeplessness on account of uneasiness in the blood and anxiety* (was obliged to rise from bed); the thoughts crowded upon one another without heat, sweat, or thirst,[1].—(Tired, and yet cannot sleep; when he tries to sleep he loses his breath),[1].—*Loss of sleep at night, on account of uneasiness in the blood;* tossed about the bed,[1].—*Loss of sleep, before midnight,*[1].—Restless sleep, full of thoughts,[5].—*Loss of sleep before midnight,* with frequent urinating (second day),[34].—Restless sleep, with confused dreams; tossed from side to side,[3].—[1780.] *Night restless; he could scarcely sleep for half an hour, and* during his slumbering was **continually busy with what he had read the evening previous** (first night),[9].—Night very restless,[22][31].—The night was very restless; anxious dreams; about three o'clock she cried out in her sleep,[1].—*Night very restless, disturbed by frightful dreams; frequent waking and falling asleep* (second and third day),[36].—Very restless sleep at night, with much sweat,[31].—The night's rest disturbed; she only slept towards morning,[21].—*Uneasy sleep and frequent waking, in consequence of troublesome dreams* (third night),[32].—At night uneasiness in the blood; he slept late and not soundly,[1].—He was unable to sleep several nights on account of heat; the bed covers seemed too hot, and on uncovering he felt too cool; still without thirst and almost without sweat,[1].—*He could not sleep well; a warmth and anxiety in the blood prevented it until 12 o'clock,*[1].—[1790.] The child was unable to sleep in the evening; could not get quiet; it rose again from bed,[1].—*He could not sleep before midnight on account of a frequent shivering sensation, which crept over one arm or foot, followed by some sweat,*[1].—He was unable to sleep before 2 o'clock; he was obliged to turn back and forth in the bed like a child that had been deprived of its rest; in the morning after waking he was still very sleepy,[1].—He slept only before midnight, then not again; remained quite wide awake; felt great weariness when lying, which increased in the legs on rising, but soon afterwards disappeared,[1].—She only slept at four in the morning, and then dreamed of dead persons,[1].—She tosses about the bed until 1 o'clock; she cannot sleep on account of anxious heat, yet has no perceptible external heat,[1].—Waking early in the night,[1].—She woke every hour all night and remembered her dreams, and when she fell asleep again she dreamed again just as vivid, and remembered it just as well after waking,[1].—In the evening, in bed, she awoke after a short sleep with a twisting sensation in the pit of the stomach, which caused nausea, threatened to suffocate her, so that she was obliged to sit up in bed,[1].—He woke suddenly before 3 A.M., and broke out into a slight perspiration, which lasted till morning, wherewith he lay most comfortably on the back, and only slumbered a little, with dryness of the forepart of the mouth and lips, without thirst (after eight hours),[1].—[1800.] *He started from an anxious dream and screamed out,*[1].—Sleep did not refresh him; in the morning on waking he was still very tired; the weariness disappeared on rising and dressing,[1].—Startings in sleep, which wake her,[1].—*In the evening, before falling asleep, she starts up in fright,*[1].—Startings on falling asleep every evening in bed,[1].—He talked irrationally when waking from sleep,[1].—Moaning in the sleep, about 3 A.M.,[1].—(He makes motions with his mouth in his sleep as if he were chewing),[1].—Towards evening while asleep she drew her mouth back and forth, opened the eyes, distorted them, and talked irrationally, as if she were wide awake; she spoke distinctly, but hastily, as if she fancied that many other persons were about her; looked freely about, talked with absent children, and desired to go home,[1].—The sleep was very remarkable; he seemed conscious that he was sleeping; consciousness was apparently emancipated from the realm of sleep, which overpowered the other senses (analogous to somnambulism?); this condition caused him the more anguish, since consciousness became weaker, and at last was entirely lost as in faintness; from this anguish arose an internal cramp, which caused a return to complete consciousness, which had the effect of making him wide awake; after waking, the arm upon which he was lying was senseless and stiff, which, however, soon disappeared (second night),[1].—[1810.] Somnambulistic condition,[8].—She rose at night from her bed in her dream, and went to the door as if she would go out,[1].—Awakened in the night by shouts and laughter of students living with me; I found myself out of my bed, in the opposite corner of the room, lying upon the bed covers spread upon the floor, without knowing how I got there; it must have happened in deep sleep, from which I was only aroused sufficiently to get back to bed without being able to give connected answers to questions put to me. In the morning I ascertained that for several nights while asleep I had disturbed others by cries and groans without being able myself to remember more than heavy dreams. My sleep for about three weeks had been unusually sound; though I had always enjoyed sound sleep, yet I was usually awakened by every slight noise in my room, while lately I had not been conscious of persons entering my room, and could be aroused from sleep only by shaking. I only knew that during this time I tossed about restlessly in my sleep, because I had been conscious of knocking against the wall several times in a not very gentle manner (thirty-third night),[16].—**Dreams.** During sleep much dreaming,[13].—Sleep disturbed by dreams for several days,[22].—Frequently awakened from sleep by dreams,[37].—Pleasant dreams during the night (second day),[42].—Very vivid dreams, so that he remembered everything after waking (sixth and seventh nights),[10].—Very vivid remembered dreams after midnight,[31].—Night disturbed by vivid dreams; awakened frequently, and every time had a feeling of chilliness in the toes,[32].—[1820.] *In his dreams he was busy about his household affairs,[1].—The night was disturbed by restless dreams (first night),[18].—Frequently awakened by restless dreams, or by involuntary motion of the legs, which caused immediately great pain (second night),[38].—Many confused and indistinct dreams, in which he was very active,[13].—Night disturbed by confused and anxious dreams,[36].—Anxious dreams,[1].—* *Very vivid dreams the whole night of anxiety and care about his business,[1].—Frequently awakened by unpleasant dreams and obliged to urinate (second and third night),[37].—Dreams of dispute and vexation,[1].—He dreamed while awake that he tried to toss some one out of the window,[1].—[1830.] Numerous indistinct dreams of battles in which the prover took part, during the night (from 3d dil.),[42].—On waking he could not free himself from his dream; he still continued to dream waking,[1].

Fever.—Chilliness. Continued chilliness (after two hours),[15].—Chilliness, the whole of the first day, all over,[1].—Chilliness toward evening,[18].—Chilliness in the evening before lying down,[1].—*Chilliness in bed in the evening after lying down,[1].—Chilliness in the open air and dread of it,[1].—Chilliness on waking,[1].—Chilliness while walking up a steep mountain, followed by unusual sweating and weariness,[14].—[1840.] Paroxysms of fever; lying down, chilliness, yawning, nausea; then sweat without thirst, from 10 P.M. till 10 A.M.,[1].—Chilly in the open air,[2].—*After the midday nap he was chilly; the head confused,[1].—After a walk in the open air, she gets chilly in the room; she was not chilly in the open air,[1].—Chills over the whole skin,[1].—Creeping chill (after two and a half hours),[15].—Chills towards evening,[1].—Frequent chills while walking on a hot day,[15].—Violent chill, with such great prostration that she could not leave the bed for three hours; this unusual weakness lasted three days,[21].—Violent shaking chill, through the whole body, as in an ague, which compelled her to lie down, with sticking pain in the left side above the hips, as if an abscess would break there, though without thirst and without subsequent heat (after forty-eight hours),[7].—[1850.] Cold sensation and discomfort through the whole body,[38].—Shivering,[1].—Shivering over the whole body, especially over the back,[15].—Violent shivering was suddenly caused by a draft of air from turning in bed; he wrapt himself closely in the bed; the dorsal, pectoral, and abdominal muscles twitched convulsively; the extremities trembled;

the chill seemed especially to concentrate itself in the interior of the chest; it lasted ten minutes, gradually diminishing, but immediately reappeared on moving the body or putting a limb out of bed (first night),[13].—A peculiar shivering sensation while washing (after tenth night),[9].—Excessive shivering, and nausea; aversion to tobacco-smoking,[15].—Slight chilliness, followed by heat,[23].—Chilly sensation, with sudden general heat (after half an hour),[1]. —Chilliness, with great heat, in the afternoon while walking,[15].—In the afternoon shivering, then heat, together with chill; the chill was on the chest and arms (but the arms and hands were warmer than usual); the heat was in the head, with throbbing pulse-like pain in the temples, much aggravated in the evening; the shivering, heat, and chill were without thirst,[1].— *Partial.* [1860.] Chilliness in the face,[22].—Chilliness on the arms,[1].— Creeping chilliness in back, from above downward (after half an hour to two hours),[42].—Creeping chills in the lower extremities in the evening, in bed, especially on the thighs; even the skin felt cool,[27].—Creeping chills in the left thigh in the evening,[28].—Creeping chills over the left leg (second day),[28].—He felt coldness down the whole right side,[1].—A cold sensation over the back, which extends forward, together with severe pressure in the pit of the stomach, soon after eating; afterwards this cold sensation extends over the shoulders and forearms,[27].—Cold sensation along the whole spine, with drawing pressure in the back and lumbar muscles, and a necessity to suddenly straighten up, lasting the whole day, and only relieved by motion,[27].—Shivering, which started in the neck and extended down the spinal column, but lasted only a short time,[15].—[1870.] Frequent, violent shivering in the back,[13].—Shivering through the back and coldness over the whole body,[13].—The shivering in the back became very violent and intense; with it the eyelids involuntarily closed (after 50 drops),[13].—*Heat.* Sensation of heat through the whole body,[15].—*Immediately after lying down in bed in the evening, sensation of heat, with external heat over him, without thirst, through the whole night; he turned from one side to the other; did not dare to uncover any part, because it immediately caused violent pain in the abdomen, a painful griping-sticking or a sticking-griping, as if flatus moved spasmodically here and there, with loss of sleep from a multitude of crowding thoughts; in the morning this condition disappeared, without his noticing any flatulence,[1].—Flushes of heat,[3].—Heat, without thirst,[1].—Heat of the body, without thirst,[1].—In the morning, repeated dry heat all over,[1].—*Dry heat at night,[1].—[1880.] Sudden dry heat, on every motion, and every noise,[1].— Dry heat spread over the whole body; especially the hands, feet, and face burned; the circulation was very much excited, over one hundred pulsations to the minute; confusion of the head, pressing-out pain in the occiput and neck, roaring in the left ear, violent coryza, the left nostril stopped, and from the right a discharge of a thin watery substance; slight angina tonsillaris; loss of thirst and appetite; transient stitches below the left nipple, as if in the pleura costalis; pressive pain in the loins; continued erection of the penis without desire; single fine stitches in the left testicle; burning pain in the region of the lower third of the right ulna; during this heat-stage he slept quietly, and awoke about midnight quite bright and active, with copious sweat over the whole body, after which all symptoms disappeared (first night), (after 70 drops),[15].†—Only internal heat, with un-

---

† I hesitated to ascribe this catarrhal fever to the action of Bryonia, because sometimes after taking cold I was subject to a catarrhal angina, especially in cold, wet weather; in this case I had, however, taken no cold, the weather was fine and

quenchable thirst,[1].—Internal dry, burning heat, without previous coldness, extending over the whole body, with dryness of the tongue, lips, and palate; loss of thirst, prostration, and extraordinary weakness in the whole body, especially in the extremities, the pulse full, accelerated, the skin as dry as parchment and rough,[3].—*Partial.* *Internally great warmth; the blood seems to burn in the veins,[1].—*Heat in the interior of the body* (especially in the abdomen),[3].—*Heat in the head in the morning; it seems warm before the head,[1].—*Heat in the head in the forenoon; feels as though it would come out at the forehead,[1].—Heat in the head at 3 p.m., with pressure in the frontal eminence,[15].—*Heat in the head and face,[3].—[1890.] Flushes of heat over the face,[3].—Heat in the face, toward evening,[1].—Heat of the face, and, after light work, profuse sweat of the face,[15].—*A feeling of heat in the face, with redness and thirst** (after three hours),[4].—Extraordinary warmth in the region of the pit of the stomach caused excessive thirst, but not dryness in the throat,[1].—Heat in the abdomen (and over the whole inside of the body),[3].—Heat in the chest and face,[3].—Along the spine, where there was yesterday a cold sensation, appeared to-day increased warmth; the skin was hot to the touch and somewhat sensitive and even transpiring on slightest motion (second day),[27].—Sensation of heat in the palms and in the forearms; she was obliged to put them out of bed in the morning; after some hours a cold sensation in them,[1].—Heat only in the lower limbs, and frequent attacks; it seems as if she stepped into hot water,[1].—[1900.] Heat of the knee, perceptible externally,[39].—*In the evening, hot and red cheeks, with chill all over, with goose-flesh and thirst,[1].—Heat in the evening, in the external ear, followed by shivering and shaking in the thighs (after four hours),[1].—Paroxysm of fever; in the forenoon heat (with thirst); after a few hours (in the afternoon) chilliness without thirst, with redness of the face and some headache,[1].—*Sweat.* Profuse sweat six nights in succession,[2].—Profuse sweat while walking, which runs in streams from the face,[33].—Profuse sweat after moderate exercise in the open air; it continued afterwards while at rest, and after changing the linen the sweat flowed in streams from the face and the whole body; together with so great acceleration of respiration that he could only speak in broken and jerk-like words,[33].—Profuse sweat of the whole body, also of the head, while lying in bed,[2].—*Profuse night-sweat after 3 a.m.,* for twenty nights in succession,[2].—He is obliged to go to bed early (by 9 a.m.); after a time a copious sweat breaks out, after which the previous symptoms disappear in the same order in which they appeared, only vertigo continued somewhat longer, lasting half an hour,[11].—[1910.] *Sweat in the morning,[1].—Sweat towards morning, especially in the feet,[1].—Some sweat towards morning after waking,[1].—General sweat on waking,[13].—He sweats while eating,[2].—*He sweats on the slightest exertion,[2].—*Sweat breaks out easily on the slightest exertion, also at night,[1].—He sweats all over when walking in the cold air,[1].—An anxious sweat prevents sleep,[2].—Slight perspiration in bed from evening till morning, with which he only slept from 12 till 3,[1].—[1920.] Transpiration suppressed,[24].—Very profuse warm sweat over the whole body, even dropping from the hair,[2].—Sweat which seems like oil when washing, day and night,[2].—*Sweat sour** (sometimes towards midnight),[39].—

warm, and I had been busy in the house, so I was forced to ascribe this fever to Bryonia, especially as the accompanying symptoms were for the most part the same as those observed from repeated provings of Bryonia. I should also note that this was the third time during this short proving that I was feverish, and each time had nightly aggravations.

*Sour-smelling, profuse sweat, during a good night's sleep,[1].—Sweat in the axillæ,[1].—Warm sweat in the palms,[1].

Conditions.—Aggravation.—(*Morning*), At daybreak, delirious; head confused; on waking, head confused, etc.; vertigo; on waking, *dizzy, etc.; on waking, headache;* when first opening eyes, headache; after rising, headache; pressive headache; on waking, pressive headache; before breakfast, pain as if head compressed; on waking, headache on top; in bed, after waking, while lying on back, headache in occiput; hair seems fatty; on waking, pressure in eye; agglutination of lids; weakness of eyes; sneezing; sneezing, etc.; after rising, nose-bleed; during sleep, at 3 o'clock, nose-bleed; dry sensation in mouth; in bed, twitching between lower lip and gum; nauseous taste in mouth; fasting, taste in mouth; on waking, pain in tonsil, etc.; *ravenous hunger;* on rising, great thirst; about 3 o'clock, before sweat, thirst, etc.; raises mucus from stomach; two hours after rising, nausea, etc.; after anxious dreams, nausea, etc.; on waking, nausea, etc.; sour vomiting; about 6 o'clock, vomiting; every time on waking, pressure in region of navel; pain in left inguinal ring; 6 o'clock, desire for stool; diarrhœa; *soft stool;* brownish evacuation; pasty evacuations; in bed, pain in region of right kidney; scraping sensation in trachea; in bed, severe cough; cough, etc.; hacking cough; expectoration of mucus; *dry cough, etc.;* anxiety in chest; oppression of chest; twitching near spine; 6 o'clock, pains in right shoulder, etc.; pressing, etc., in forearm; stiffness in thighs; pain in knee; 9 o'clock, on waking, pain in right knee, etc.; cramp in calf; stitches in heels; weariness; after rising, weak, etc.; on rising, exhaustion, etc.; whole body painful; every part laid on, sore; feels bruised, etc.; dry heat all over; heat in head.—(*Forenoon*), Attacks of vertigo; violent headache; headache; swelling of one eye, etc.; pasty taste; nausea; rumbling in abdomen; slight colic; cutting in abdomen; cough, with expectoration; *oppressed breathing, etc.;* while sitting and talking, oppression in chest; while walking, oppression of chest; tension in back, etc.; stitches in back; while walking, pains beneath scapula; while walking, loss of sensation in lumbar, etc., regions; lumbar vertebræ pain; pains in all limbs, etc.; stitches in the thighs; when walking, weak, etc., feeling in right knee; when walking, tearing in metatarsal bones; pain in periosteum; heat in head; heat, etc.—(*Toward noon*), Pain below navel; stitches in the axilla.—(*Noon*), On walking, pain about thorax.—(*Afternoon*), Vertigo; oppressive headache; pain in frontal region; sensation in right eye; after drinking, nausea, etc.; attacks of heartburn; while riding in a jolting wagon, pain above navel; after eating, tension, etc., of abdomen; at 3 o'clock, gurgling in bowels, etc.; after drinking warm milk, stitches in abdomen; ineffectual desire for stool; 4 P.M., diarrhœa; while lying, stitches between the shoulder-blades; stretching of the limbs, stitches in hollows of knees; heaviness, etc., in right leg; pain in metatarsal bones; when walking, painfulness of toe; sticking in toes; weariness; great sleepiness; while walking, chilliness, etc.; shivering; 3 o'clock, heat in head.—(*Toward evening*), Headache, etc.; *sensitiveness of the scalp;* pressure above lids; toothache; unpleasant taste; pain in epigastric region; distension of abdomen; unusual weakness, etc.; *chilliness;* heat in face.—(*Evening*), On lying down, feeling of anxiety; insensibility; on stooping, pressing outward in frontal region, etc.; on going to bed, pressure in head; in open air, pains about right eye; 10 o'clock, attacks of sneezing; in bed, toothache; dryness in mouth; after lying down, bitter taste in mouth; throat becomes slimy, etc.; late, offensive taste in throat; at 6 o'clock, gulping up of water, etc.; before going to sleep, nausea; nausea; at 9 o'clock, in bed, sudden nausea, etc.; vomiting of mucus; in bed, rumbling in bowels : at 6, 7, and 8 o'clock, sense of fulness, etc., in bowels ; tearing, etc., in abdomen ; burning in hæmorrhoidal vessels ; stitches in perineum ; stitch in urethra ; after lying down in bed, cough ; at 9 o'clock, pain over chest, etc.; at 6 o'clock, stitches in chest ; pain in ensiform cartilage ; twitches near the spine ; in bed, stitches in right shoulder-blade ; on going upstairs, weak feeling in the knees ; pain in right knee ; digging, etc., about the knees, etc.; bruised sensation in legs ; dull stitches ; after lying down in bed, itching, etc., in various parts ; before lying down, chilliness ; *in bed, after lying down, chilliness ;* pain in temples during fever ; in bed, chills in lower extremities ; chills in left thigh ; immediately after lying down in bed, sensation of heat, etc.; heat and red cheeks ; heat in external ear.— (*Night*), At 10 o'clock, delirious fantasy ; gnawing on scalp ; pain in tooth, etc.; dry sensation on palate ; thirst ; at 11 o'clock, wakes with thirst ; griping in umbilical region ; passage of flatus ; diarrhœa ; diarrhœa, etc.; *frequent urinating ;* urine copious ; sticking pain in back ; when lying, cramp in knee, etc.; cramp in calves ; when lying in bed, cramp in feet ; immediately after lying down, shooting into heel ; itching, etc., in hollow of knee ; dry heat ; sweat.—(*Toward midnight*), Sudden vertigo.—(*Before midnight*), Nausea.—(*After midnight*), Wakes with nausea ; gasping for breath, etc.; vivid dreams.—(*Open air*), Aversion to ; lachrymation ; stitches in ears ; pressure on border of sternum ; *chilliness*.—(*Slightest draughts of air*), Inclination to diarrhœa.—(*On walking in open air*), Attacks of vertigo ; stitches in the head ; qualmish, etc.; pressure on navel ; desire to urinate, etc.; hoarseness, etc.; soon fatigued ; feels weakest.— (*Ascending stairs*), Loss of power in knees ; stitches in right knee ; feet weak ; weakness in knees, etc.—(*While ascending a steep mountain*), Chilliness.—(*After drinking beer*), Offensive taste ; thirst.—(*Bending forward*), Fulness in stomach, etc.—(*Bending body to right*), Stitches in pit of stomach.—(*Bending elbows*), Stitches in tips of elbows.—(*Bending fingers*), Stiffness in finger-joints.—(*Blowing nose*), Crawling, etc., in septum of nose. —(*Breathing*), Pressure behind sternum ; soreness of upper sternum ; stitches between lumbar vertebræ.—(*When chewing*), Pain in back teeth.— (*After breakfasting on coffee*), Nausea, etc.—(*Cold air*), Pain in ear.—(*On coughing*), *Motion in head ;* shooting through head ; stitches in throat ; vomiting of blood ; vomiting without nausea ; soreness in pit of stomach ; stitches in last ribs ; stitch in sternum.—(*Descending stairs*), Pain in knee-caps ; vertigo.—(*During dinner*), Severe nausea ; colic-pain ; stitching in lower abdomen.—(*After dinner*), Griping in umbilical region ; colic-like pains ; colic-pains ; spasmodic pain in abdomen.—(*After drinking*), Bitter taste returns.—(*While eating*), Pressure in stomach.—(*After eating*), Slight vertigo ; pressing outward in forehead ; pain above left eye ; toothache ; dry sensation in palate ; sour, etc., taste ; thirst ; *eructations*, etc.; severe eructations ; sourish eructations ; bitter eructations ; hiccough ; constant nausea ; *pain in stomach, etc.; pressure in stomach ;* attack of colic ; distension of abdomen ; tension in abdomen ; rumbling, etc., in abdomen ; attack of colic ; *painless diarrhœa ;* soft stool ; cough ; heaviness in chest, etc. ; drawing, etc., in lumbar region ; when one leg is riding over the other, pain in knee reappears ; immediately, sleepiness.—(*During and after eating*), Toothache.—(*After extraction of tooth*), Vertigo.—(*On expiration*), Pain below right nipple ; pressure in region of right nipple.—(*On passing flatus*), Stitches in rectum.—(*Slightest food*), Causes eructations.—(*Attempting to hold anything firmly with the hand*), Pains in shoulder.—(*After going into house*), Tearing in right shoulder renewed.—(*On going into house from a walk*), Stitches under the ears.—(*Inspiration*), Heat in pit of stomach ; pain in hypogastric region ; sensation of heat throughout chest ; stitches in sternum ; stitch in upper chest ; stitches in left chest ; pain in angles of ribs ; stitch below sternum ; pain in infra-mammary region ; pain in right breast.—(*Deep inspiration*), *Pain in stomach ;* stitches in stomach ; stitches in pit of stomach ; pain in right hypochondrium ; pectoral muscles do not seem free ; sticking, etc., beneath breast-bone ; sensation in sides of chest ; stitches in ribs.—(*Lifting*), Pain in sacral region.—(*Lying*), Pains in teeth ; pain in small of back ; jerklike pain in small of back ; pain in hip-joints ; cramps in calves.—(*Lying on side*), Pain in chest.—(*Lying on right side*), Nausea. —(*Lying on painless side*), Toothache.—(*During a meal*), Out of humor.— (*After meals*), Out of humor ; head confused, etc. ; headache ; distension of abdomen ; liquid stools ; pain in loins.—(*During slight mental excitement*), Burning over whole body.—(*Motion*), The symptoms ; pain in general ; throbbing in head ; pain in forehead ; pressive pain in forehead, etc. ; *pressure in articular cavity of jaw ;* nausea ; griping, etc., in epigastric intestines, etc. ; tearing, etc., in abdomen ; sticking, etc., beneath breast-bone ; stitches in left chest ; sticking between shoulder-blades ; *pains in wrists ;* stiffness in right hand ; pains in finger ; twitching of fingers ; tearing in finger-joints ; pain in left hip ; pains in right trochanter, etc. ; painfulness of right thigh ; pain in right thigh ; stitches in knee-joints ; stitches in right knee-joint ; tension in ankles ; stitches in the joints ; chilliness reappears ; sudden dry heat.—(*Quick motion*), Pain above left eye, etc.—(*Moving the part*), *Pain in left eyeball ;* pain in left shoulder-joint.—(*On moving head*), Tension in nape of neck.—(*On moving eyes*), Tension in frontal muscles.— (*Moving trunk*), Stitches in back ; drawing, etc., between shoulders.—(*Moving arm*), Pressure in stomach, etc.—(*On moving and turning foot*), Pain in outer side of left calf.—(*Noise*), Sudden dry heat.—(*On opening mouth*), Toothache.—(*Pressure*), Stitch in throat ; pain in stomach.—(*Putting limb out of bed*), Chilliness reappears.—(*Attempting to raise body upright*), Pain in sacral region.—(*On raising head from forward inclination*), Slight vertigo.—(*On raising arm*), Pain in region of acromion.—(*Attempting to raise or stretch out the legs*), Pain in sacral region.—(*After continued reading*), Pain in forehead.—(*During rest*), Especially in bed, toothache ; drawing, etc., in right shoulder ; pain in finger-joint ; numb sensation in calf.— (*While riding*), Pains in all the limbs ; pains in the long bones ; drawing, etc., in forearms.—(*Rinsing mouth with water*), Inclination to vomit.—(*On rising*), Stiff feeling in back ; after eating, feet feel heavy ; after long sitting, stiffness in feet.—(*After rising*), Drawing along left foot.—(*Rising from bed*), Confusion of head.—(*On rising from chair*), Vertigo.—(*In room*), Anxiety ; unconscious of what she is doing ; coryza ; after walking in open air, gets chilly.—(*Sitting*), Pressure in head ; stitches in right chest ; *drawing down back ;* twitches near spine ; pressure between shoulders, etc. ; pain in small of back ; pain in the arms, etc. ; pain in hip-joints ; cramp in knee, etc. ; pains in knees, etc. ; bruised pain in knees, etc. ; after a meal, tearing in right calf ; pain in left ankle ; pain in sole of right foot ; pain in balls of right toes ; weariness.—(*On sitting down*), Pain in inguinal ring.— (*On sitting up in bed*), Vertigo, like whirling, etc. ; pain in sacral region. —(*After midday sleep*), All symptoms ; *chilly, etc.*—(*When smoking*), Toothache.—(*Sneezing*), Pain to right of sternum.—(*Going up and down stairs*), Tottering of thighs.—(*Standing*), Weakness of mind ; *vertigo ;* after moving, tottered to one side ; pinching, etc., in abdomen ; griping, etc., in epigastric intestines ; tearing in back ; pain in region of scab of ulcer.—(*Stepping*), Stitches in ear ; stitches in hollows of feet ; corn pains.—(*On stepping hard*), Stitches through head.—(*Stooping*), Pressure in the head ; frontal headache ; *headache, as if everything would fall out of forehead ;* pressure in forepart of brain ; when writing, sensation in external meatus ; sticking headache.—(*On sitting stooping*), Dizzy heaviness in head ; pain in chest. —(*Walking stooped*), Pain from hip to knee.—(*On stroking hand across forehead*), Sneezing.—(*After supper*), Flatulent colic, etc.—(*When swallowing*), Stitch in throat.—(*After sweating*), Eruption around throat.—(*Talking*), *Pain in trachea.*—(*On the slightest tightening of the clothes*), Sensation as if he must go to stool.—(*Tobacco*), Burning on tongue ; flow of saliva ; *nausea ; pain in trachea.*—(*Touch*), Pain in right ovary ; sensation on right chest ; pain in sacral region ; *pressure on right shoulder ;* pain on outer side of calf ; pain in corn ; stitches in the joints.—(*Turning body*), Pain in sacral region.—(*On turning head*), Dizziness ; stitch in throat.—(*On turning head to left*), Pain in tendon of trapezius.—(*On urinating*), Pain in abdomen ; sensation as if the urethra were too narrow.—(*After vomiting*), Hiccough.—(*On waking*), Great weariness ; talked irrationally ; chilliness. —(*Walking*), Confusion of head ; vertigo, etc. ; reeled to both sides ; pressing outward in forehead ; pinching, etc., ir abdomen ; griping in abdomen ; respiration more rapid, etc. ; tension in chest ; *pain in sacral region ;* drawing in coccyx ; stitches in left knee, etc. ; heaviness in lower extremities ; pain in left hip-joint ; weariness, etc., in knees ; pains in left knee ; pains in knee-joint ; *stitches in knees ;* immobility of right knee ; pains in toes ; pain in great toe ; especially after rising from seat, and when beginning to walk, unsteadiness of the body ; *fatigue ;* weakness ; exhaustion, etc. ; painful sensitiveness in body ; pain in the joints ; frequent chills ; profuse sweat.—(*Walking rapidly*), *Pressure in forepart of brain ; stitches in throat.*—(*While walking about room*), Headache in left forehead, etc. ; stitches in pit of stomach ; back very tired.—(*Warmth*), Toothache.—(*In warm room*), Pain in throat.—(*On going into warm room from open air*), *Sensation as of vapor in the trachea.*—(*On taking anything warm into the mouth*), Toothache.—(*On taking warm broth*), Urging to stool, etc.—(*While washing*), Shivering ; sweat like oil.—(*After drinking wine and water*), Pain in stomach.—(*When writing*), Pectoral muscles pain ; tearing in bones of right hand ; *pain in fingers.*

Amelioration.—(*Afternoon*), In open air, tearing in right shoulder. —(*Open air*), Anxiety ; coryza ; stitches in ribs.—(*Walking in open air*), Pain in tooth ; pressure in region of navel.—(*Bending backward*), Fulness in stomach, etc.—(*Chewing*), Toothache.—(*Drinking cold water*), Bitter taste, etc.—(*Uncovering and getting cool*), Delirium.—(*Descending steps*), Weariness in thighs.—(*Drawing legs up against abdomen*), Pain in region of stomach.—(*Eating*), Bad taste in throat ; stitches in sternum.—(*Empty eructations*), Confusion of head.—(*Profuse evacuations*), Cutting in intestines ; all symptoms.—(*After three watery evacuations*), All symptoms, except weakness.—(*Expiration*), Pain in right breast.—(*Passage of flatus*), Relief ; colic-like pains ; distension of abdomen.—(*When lying*), Feels better.—(*Lying on painful cheek*), Toothache goes away.—(*On taking milk*), Appetite returns.—(*Motion*), *Drawing down back ;* pain in small of back ; drawing, etc., in righ shoulder ; cramp in calves ; cold sensation along spine.—(*Motion in open air*), Seemed to afford relief.—(*Moving affected part*), Drawing through all the limbs.—(*Pressure*), Pain over left eye, etc. ; *pressure under cheek-bone ;* pain in right side ; pain in left hip-joint.—(*On* *severe pressure*), Pain in corn immediately ceases.—(*On raising head*), Dizzy heaviness disappears.—(*Rest*), Stitches in left chest; tension, etc., on anterior surface of thigh; weariness, etc., in knees; drawing in knee-joint, etc.; tearing from feet into hollows of knees; symptoms disappear, except weakness; general prostration.—(*Rest with body bent forward*), Pain in sacral region.—(*After riding in a wagon*), Confusion of head, etc., disappears. —(*Rising from bed*), Pains in right shoulder; stitches in knee-joint; stitches in heels.—(*Rubbing the part*), Pain in epigastric region; stiffness in finger. —(*Sitting*), Confusion of head; pressure in pit of stomach; pain in region of scab of ulcer.—(*On sitting down*), Attacks of vertigo disappear.—(*Walking*), Vertigo; fulness in stomach, etc.; pressure in stomach; immediately after supper, pressure in stomach, etc.; difficult breathing; stiff feeling in back; pressure between shoulders; pain in hip-joints; feeling in hip-joint; pain in tibia; pain in left calf; pain in balls of right toes; weariness.— (*Continuing to walk*), Unsteadiness of the body.—(*After a long walk*), Tension in abdomen.—(*After becoming warm in bed*), Rash, etc., disappears.— (*Washing with cold water*), Pain in frontal region, etc.

BUFO.

Rana Bufo, L. *Nat. order*, Bufonidæ, of the Batrachian family of vertebrate animals. *Common names*, Toads; (German) Die Kröte; (French) Le Crapaud commun. *Preparation*, Trituration of the poison from the cutaneous glands, obtained by irritating the animal.

Authorities. 1, Desterne, Journ. d. l. Soc. Gal., 2d series, 4, 289 (symptoms without reference to cause or time); 2, Aëtius, "De nox. animal. morsu," effects of bite, from Desterne's compilation; 3, Sennert, "La Med. du Prophete," effects of eating toads (ibid.); 4, Ambroise Paré, "De la Morsure du Crapaud," xxxi, 773, effects of taking the poison in wine (ibid.); 5, J. L. Hannemann, effects of venom applied to the sound skin (ibid.); 6, Standigelius, "De la crainte," etc., effects of venom spirted into the eye; of bathing in water taken from a pool frequented by toads (ibid.); 7, Schelammer, effects of momentarily introducing a toad into the mouth, without touching (ibid.); 8, Paullinus, "Ephemerides," effects of toads taken into the stomach, by eating the spawn on herbs, also effects of the venom injected into the eye, also effects of the bite, also effects of an infusion of roasted toads powdered (ibid.); 9, Brandelius, effects of a toad jumping into the mouth and entering the stomach during sleep (ibid.); 10, Schrœckius, effects of swallowing the ovules of a toad in muddy water (ibid.); 11, Gavini, Correspondence Scientif., effects of venom injected into the eye; 12, Houat, Nouvelles Données de Mat. Med., I, p. 41; 13, Archive (Homœop.), 14, 2, 102, effects of repeated doses of the 30th potency of the venom; 14, Struvius (from Desterne), effects of a live toad in the stomach; 15, Hencke, A. H. Z., Mon. Bl., 1, p. 18, effects of 30 drops (of the tincture?).

Mind.—Emotions. Constant feeling of intoxication,[12].—After eating he is always as if intoxicated,[12].—Paroxysms of fury, which cease as soon as he sees any one,[12].—Propensity to bite,[11].—The child runs like mad,[11].—Inclination to get drunk, and he takes pleasure in being intoxicated,[12].—Desires solitude, and yet is afraid of being left alone and dying forsaken,[12].—Aversion to strangers,[12].—Dislike to conversation,[12].—[10.] Howling, constant crying,[11].—Sadness, full of restlessness and apprehension,[12].—He is anxious about the state of his health; is afraid he will die or that some other misfortune will happen to him,[12].—Excessive anguish,[12].— Very easily frightened; a bird or insect flying by causes a start,[12].—Fear of animals,[12].—Fear of catching diseases,[12].—Very sensitive disposition,[12].— Choleric disposition,[1].—Nervousness; excessive irritability,[1].—[20.] Irritable, impatient humor,[1].—He is irritated and weeps about the merest trifle,[12].—He is irritable, anxious about his state of health, with great dread of death,[12].—Impatience and ill-humor,[12].—Ill-humor when going to sleep at night, and on waking in the morning,[12].—Defiance, duplicity, spitefulness,[12].—Anger, with desire to strike and destroy,[12].—Alternate complaining and crying in the case of a child,[11].—Varying mood; taciturn, hypochondriac,[12].—Apathy sort of stupidity, with regular pulse,[11].—*Intellect.* [30.] Enfeebled intellect,[12].—Little disposed to work,[1].—Great difficulty in collecting his ideas,[12].—He mistakes words; often he only half pronounces a word and gets angry when not understood,[12].—After an attack, imbecility, palpitation of the heart, trembling of all the limbs, spasmodic movements of the intestines, colic and pains, which extend into the groins,[12]. --Idiocy, mania, furious insanity,[12].—Absence of mind; want of memory,[12]. —After the dizziness, stupefaction, sometimes lasting for a minute, and obliging him to seek support,[1].—Coma, which lasts two days,[11].—Stupor and inability to speak, which last two years,[11].

Head.—Vertigo and General Sensations. [40.] Vertigo,[3,4].— Vertigo with tottering, so that he requires support.[12].—Dizziness; the head is as if carried along by the motion of waltzing,[1].—Dizziness, especially in the morning, with weakness, as after losing blood,[1].—The dizziness appears only in the morning, three or four times, especially after a meal,[1].—Constant shaking of the head and arms,[11].—Numbness of the head, with sensation of intoxication and great somnolence,[12].—Heavy, stupefying headache, with sensation as if the scalp and ears were burned by an acid,[12].— Heaviness and weight of the head, so that he has to support it,[12].—Heaviness of the head,[6].—[50.] Pains in the head, extending to the maxillary sinuses,[12].—Neuralgic pains running through the whole head, and affecting the eyes and nape of the neck,[12].—Headache with vertigo, trembling of the whole body, dimness of sight, eructation, nausea, and vomiting,[12]. —*Great heat in the interior of the head, with sensation as if the brain were boiling,[12].—Sanguineous congestion, with deepseated pains in the brain,[12].—Sensation as if the cranial bones were separated,[12].—Pressive and contractive pains in the interior of the head,[12].—Pressive and throbbing pains in the head, with frontal heaviness,[12].—Sensation of a great weight on the head, with lancinating pains in the sinciput and eyes,[12].—Stitches and prickings in the brain,[12].—[60.] Sensation of shaking, as if a heavy ball was in the head,[12].—Hammering pains from the eyebrows to the cerebellum,[12].—Hammering sensation in different parts of the head, with commotion of the whole brain,[12].—Throbbing and lancinating pains, as if there were an abscess in the head,[12].—Sensation of shivering and of vibration in the head, accompanied by fluent coryza,[12].—Sensation as if the head were full of water,[12].—The pains in the head increase for three or four minutes, and then diminish during the same time,[1].—Headache on waking, at 3 A.M., for two days in succession,[1].—Headache in the afternoon, after breakfast, continuing into the night and preventing sleep,[1].—Headache in the afternoon and at night, preventing sleep,[1].—[70.] Headache in the evening towards 5 o'clock, for an hour and a half, obliging him to lie down,[1].—Aggravation of the head symptoms by movement,[1].—Excessive headache after drinking spirits,[12].—The beating of the heart increases the headache and seems to correspond with it,[1].—Headache during work, when sitting,[1].—Headache better at night and by lying down,[1].—The epistaxis relieves the headache,[1].—*Forehead, Temples, and Vertex.* Weight in the forehead and eyelids; disturbed vision; sparks before the eyes, pain at the heart; cold sweat on the head and in the hair; coldness of the body, especially the feet, and such piercing colic as almost to cause fainting; at the same time burning thirst, vomiting after drinking; vomiting of food, then of bitter and acrid matter; the least movement aggravates the headache and brings on the nausea and vomiting,[1].—Headache in the forehead and vertex, with soreness of those parts when touched, during eight days; the soreness is worse in the evening towards 4 or 5 o'clock,[1].—After a hard and curled stool, accompanied with protrusion of hæmorrhoids, headache in the forehead, heaviness in the eyelids, and nausea,[1].—[80.] Lancinations from the interior of the head to the forehead and eyes,[12].—Clawing-digging pain in the left temple when walking, lasting one hour (after three-quarters of an hour),[13].—Alternate movements of traction and relaxation in the temples,[12].—Stitches in the temples, with constriction of the throat,[12].—Headache on waking, towards 3 A.M.; the pain affects the left temple and vertex; those parts are sore to touch,[1].—Pressure in the temples, as if the head were compressed by bands of iron,[12].—Sensation as if a hot vapor rose to the top of his head,[12].—*Parietals, Occiput, and External.* Hemicrania of the right side, ceasing when the nose bleeds,[1].—Semilateral headaches, with nausea, depression, and inclination to lie down, especially in the evening,[12].—Headache, sometimes on the right side, sometimes on the left,[12].—[90.] Lancinations in the cerebellum, making the head fall backwards; loss of consciousness and falling down; tonic and clonic spasms; turgescence and distortion of the face; convulsive agitation of the mouth and eyes; bloody salivation; involuntary emission of urine; repeated shocks through the whole body; the lower extremities are in more violent motion than the upper; face bathed in perspiration,[12].—Falling off of the hair,[3].—Complete baldness,[12].—The hair changes color and decays,[12].—A great deal of dandruff and scales on the scalp and all over the body,[12].—Copious sweat of the hairy scalp; all the head is soaked with it,[1].—Frequent and oily sweats on the head, especially in the evening,[12].—Sour and disagreeable smell of the hair,[12].—Great sensitiveness of the scalp,[12].—Burning-itching and shuddering in the scalp,[12].

Eyes.—[100.] Frightful and squinting look,[4].—The eye is somewhat bloodshot from the penetration of the venom,[11].—Inflammation of the eyes and lids,[12].—Sensation as from cold water on the eyes,[12].—Spasmodic pains in the eye,[11].—Drawing in the eyes, with dimness of vision,[12].—Pressive and crampy pains in the eyes, with dazzling and vertigo,[12].—Lancinating and drawing pains in the eyes,[12].—Lancinating and beating pains in the eye, which had been poisoned by the venom,[8].—Sensation as if the eyes were full of sand,[12].—[110.] Directly after the poison has been cast into the eye itching, redness, swelling, dimness of vision; very painful lancinating pains; stinging; these last two symptoms last a long time,[6].—A whitish-looking crust over the brows,[13].—Ulceration of the lids,[12].—Large scabs on the eyelids,[12].—Swollen and burning eyelids,[12].—The eyes open more widely,[6].—Inability to keep the eyelids open,[11].—Continual winking,[12].—Convulsive beating of the eyelids,[12].—The eyelashes fall out,[11].—[120.] Burning pains at the corners of the eyes, with ulceration and suppuration of these parts,[12].—Considerable lachrymation,[12].—Ulcers on the cornea,[12].—Pupil with red and white reflections,[12].—Pupil dilated and apparently vacillating,[12].—The sight, previously at times weak and disturbed, becomes excellent, and this condition lasts ten months,[1].—Myopia,[12].—Presbyopia,[12].—Dimness of vision,[38].—Loss of sight,[4].—[130.] Photophobia,[12].—He cannot look at bright objects,[12].—All objects appear crooked,[12].—Appearance of a veil before the eyes at exactly 3 or 4 o'clock P.M., with smarting in the eyes and lachrymation,[1].—Muscæ volitantes,[12].

Ears.—Ears swollen and scabby,[12].—Inflammatory swelling of the ears and parotids,[12].—Warty excrescences on the ears,[12].—Desquamation, ulceration, suppuration, and bleeding of the concha of the ears,[12].—Ulcers and abscesses in the ears,[12].—[140.] Herpetic eruption behind the ears, with intolerable itching,[12].—Purulent discharge from the ears,[12].—Sensation of burning heat in the ears,[12].—Distensive pains in the ears, as if an animal was trying to force its way out,[12].—Feeling as if the auditory canal were stopped up by concretions,[12].—Crampy pains in the interior of the ears,[12]. —Stitches and digging in the ears, as from a foreign body in them,[12].— Pulsative pains in the right ear, with a sensation as if there was hot vapor in it,[12].—Pressing on the submaxillary glands relieves the internal pains of the ears,[12].—Very sensitive hearing,[12].—[150.] The least noise annoys him; even music is unbearable,[12].—Attacks of deafness,[12].—Hardness of hearing; he hears, and especially understands words, with great difficulty,[12].—Crackling, roaring, and tingling in the ears,[12].—The symptoms of the ears often coincide with those of the eyes and of the head,[12].—The contact of water aggravates all the ear symptoms,[12].

Nose.—Nose swollen, red, and covered with pustules,[12].—After coryza, crusts in the nose,[1].—Liability to cold in the head,[12].—Stoppage of the nose, with sensation as if it were clogged up,[12].—[160.] A great deal of sneezing in the evening, on going to bed,[1].—Frequent sneezing in the evening; obstruction, with heaviness in the head and eyelids,[1].—He blows clear water from the nose,[1].—Fluent coryza, with frequent sneezing,[12].—Coryza, with great dryness of the nose,[12].—Coryza in the morning, with sneezing three or four times in succession,[1].—The secretion from the coryza has a bad smell,[1].—The coryza ceases after a sweat, in the morning, in bed,[1].— Considerable mucous secretion, which is dry or soft, and extremely fetid,[1]. —The secretion of mucus, of an exceedingly offensive smell, continues for twelve days,[1].—[170.] Discharge of yellowish, greenish, and grayish mucus, of a putrid odor, especially in the evening and after being in the open air,[12]. —Blowing of blood from the nose,[1].—Epistaxis,[1].—Epistaxis, principally morning and evening,[12].—He bleeds from the nose nearly to fainting,[12].— Heat and great itching in the nostrils; constant desire to bore in the nose,[12]. —Burning in the nostrils,[1].—Burning, lancinating pains in the nose, extending to the forehead,[12].—The cold air, when breathed, seems to corrode the nostrils,[12].—Ulcerated nostrils, as if burnt,[12].—[180.] Throbbing and gnawing pains in the nasal bones,[12].—Strong odors are annoying, especially that of tobacco,[12].—Loss of smell,[12].

Face.—Altered expression,[11].—Thin, bony face, with large eyes, red, or sunken, and with circles round them,[12].—Face pale, yellow, or gray,[12].— Face in places white and pale, or red and gray,[12].—Face every now and then flushed with heat,[1].—After an attack of dizziness the face becomes flushed, the heart feels compressed, the chest seems squeezed in a vice,[1].— Red face, as after a vapor-bath,[12].—[190.] Inflammation and puffiness of the face; the eyes appear lost in their orbits,[12].—Inflammation, swelling, and caries of the facial bones,[12].—Lancinating pains in the face, with bruised sensation in the bones,[12].—Throbbing and heat of the face, as from being too near the fire,[12].—Water and dampness are very disagreeable to the face, and cause pricking,[12].—Very painful cramps felt from the head to the cheeks, and *vice versa*,[12].—Swollen, thick, hanging lips,[12].—Lips contracted, dry, chapped, bleeding, very painful,[12].

Mouth.—Teeth and Gums. The teeth decay and break easily,[12]. —The teeth fall out,[3].—[200.] The teeth feel long and loose,[12].—The teeth seem to sink into the gums when eating,[12].—Toothache, especially in the evening and at night,[12].—Boring pains in the teeth,[1].—Pulling pains in the teeth, with contraction of the jaw and compression of the teeth,[12].—Lancinating, boring, and digging pains in the teeth, excited by cold air, change of temperature, and movement,[12].—Swollen gums, bleeding very easily,[12]. —Hard swelling of the gum, with pain as if forcing out the back teeth, which seemed too long, with increased secretion of saliva at night; the symptoms prevented sleep; laying the arm hard on the cheek prevented the pain for a short time (after fifty-three days),[15].—Inflammation, abscess, and ulcers of the gums,[12].—Pains as if the gums were burned,[1].—[210.] Tongue covered with a loose, pasty, yellowish coat,[15].—Black tongue,[4].— Tongue cracked, and often of a bluish color,[12].—Tongue thick, hard, and full of small burning pimples,[12].—Large pimples like abscesses under the tongue, with great difficulty in eating,[12].—Tongue difficult to move,[13].— Easy biting of the tongue, which bleeds readily,[12].—Desire to drink and moisten the tongue, although it is covered with saliva,[12].—*Mouth in General and Saliva.* Cracks and exfoliation of the walls of the cheeks,[12].—Erysipelatous inflammation of the entire mouth,[12].—[220.] The mouth smells offensively,[23].—Very bad-smelling breath, especially in the morning,[12].—Pain in the palate and in the right margin of the tongue, with complete aversion to tobacco,[15].—Mouth burning, as if from an acid,[12].— Scraping dry sensation on the palate and back of the mouth, painful on empty swallowing, lasting three weeks (after three days),[15].—Cold liquids aggravate all the symptoms of the mouth,[12].—Very copious salivation,[12].— Abundant, frothy saliva,[1].—Mouth full of thick mucus,[12].—*Taste and Speech.* Insipid and disagreeable taste of the food, especially in the morning,[12].—[230.] In the morning, nauseous, sweetish taste, for a quarter of an hour, with clammy mouth, continuing while he remains in bed,[1].— Bitter taste (not of food),[15].—Peculiar, biting, bitter taste, as from radishes, in the back of the mouth (immediately, lasting several hours),[15].—Salty and bloody taste in the mouth,[12].—Constant taste of blood in the mouth,[12]. —Bitter, sour, bloody, nauseous, coppery, insipid, salty, strong, or oily taste in the mouth,[12].—Desire for milk, dainties, even brandy, to remove the bad taste in the mouth,[12].—Tobacco does not taste as good as usual ; nausea and vomiting after long smoking ; smoking in the forenoon caused overpowering desire to sleep, lasting six weeks (after three days),[15].—Stammering,[4].— Difficult, impeded, and unintelligible speech,[12].—[240.] Hears what is said without being able to answer or move,[1].

Throat.—Inflammation and swelling of the throat and tonsils,[12].— Convulsive movements and constriction of the throat, with sensation as if there was a stone there,[12].—Something seems to come down from the head into the throat,[1].—Mucus descends from the nasal fossæ into the throat,[1].— Accumulation of much viscid mucus in the throat, with constant taste of blood,[12].—Constant inclination to hawk,[12].—Dryness of the throat in the morning,[1].—Raw feeling and lancinating pains in the throat,[12].—The air, in passing through the throat, seems impregnated with a corrosive acid,[12].

—[250.] Throbbing pains, as from an abscess, in the tonsils,[12].—Inflammation and dryness of the pharynx and œsophagus,[8].—Difficult and painful deglutition; he can hardly swallow his saliva,[12].—Painful swelling of the submaxillary glands of the right side,[15].

Stomach.—*Appetite and Thirst.*—Excellent appetite,[1].—Violent hunger, even after eating, especially in the evening,[12].—In the morning after breakfast, often feels hungry, as if he had eaten nothing,[12].—Would like to be in the country and eat pot-herbs,[12].—Desire for pastry and dainties,[1].—Desire for confectionery and acid fruits,[12].—[260.] Fastidious in eating,[12].—Dislike to salted or hot food,[12].—Loss of appetite, with thirst,[12]. —Aversion to food and drinks,[11].—Loathing of food,[1].—Irregular appetite, which ceases after the first mouthful,[1].—Slight thirst during a meal, while the cough continues,[1].—Urgent thirst for cold sugared water,[1].—***Eructations, Hiccough, Nausea, and Vomiting.*** Incessant eructations, evening and morning,[12].—Eructations tasting sour, bitter, or nauseous,[12].—[270.] Eructations tasting like spoiled eggs for three or four hours, after eating fresh bread and pastry,[1].—Sugar-water and milk cause eructations and nausea,[12].—Fetid risings,[8].—Risings during the day, with some acidity,[1].—Regurgitation and heartburn after every meal,[12].—Hiccough,[2 8]. —Frequent hiccough,[12].—Phlegm, followed, especially in the morning, by bitter, bilious vomiting,[12].—Abundant phlegm, which rises, especially in the afternoon, and seems to afford relief,[12].—Nausea for five minutes, half an hour, or an hour after a meal, three or four times, on different days,[1].— [280.] Nausea, with weight and pressure in the epigastric region,[12].—Nausea, with feeling of intoxication, especially morning and evening,[12].—Horrible loathing,[6].—Incessant inclination to vomit,[6].—Violent vomiting,[4].— Yellow, green, or blood-streaked vomiting,[12].—Brownish vomiting, and sometimes of bright blood,[12].—Vomiting almost immediately after eating,[12]. —Vomiting after a meal, especially in the afternoon,[12].—Vomiting, with urging to stool,[12].—[290.] After drinking, vomiting of what has been eaten, followed by two other bitter and acid vomitings, during the headache,[1].— Vomiting of food, bile, and mucus, with bloody taste in the mouth, and tensive and crampy pains in the stomach and abdomen,[12].—**Stomach in General.** Difficult digestion, especially of the morning meal,[12].—Feeling of weakness and faintness in the stomach,[12].—Sensation of emptiness in the stomach; also of heat and cold alternately,[12].—Burning in the stomach, especially after eating,[12].—Burning, crampy, and pinching pains in the stomach,[12].—Heat and drawing in the stomach, extending to the back, with scraping in the epigastric region,[12].—Fulness, heaviness, and distension of the stomach,[12].—Cramps in the stomach,[14].—[300.] Cramps in the stomach arresting digestion,[12].—Cramps in the stomach from the least movement,[12]. —Pretty severe and prolonged cramp in the stomach, for a quarter of an hour after breakfast,[1].—Stomachache, with burning and lancinating pains extending to the liver and heart,[12].—Drawing in the stomach, as if from hunger, but without appetite, with very strong beating of the heart, shortly followed by headache,[1].—Lancinations, contraction, and shocks in the stomach,[12].—Great sensitiveness of the epigastric region,[12].—Scraping and excoriating pains in the stomach, with a feeling as if stones were being forced through the cardia,[12].—Formication and gnawing sensation in the stomach,[12].—Wine aggravates the stomachache, and causes vomiting,[12].

Abdomen.—[310.] Burning and contraction in the hepatic region,[12].— Cramps in the liver, which force him to writhe and to cry out,[12].—Digging and gnawing sensation, with neuralgic pains at the liver and stomach, especially at night,[12].—Throbbing pains, with sensation of swelling and tearing at the liver,[12].—Beating and lancinating pains in the liver, as from an abscess, and accompanied with bilious vomiting,[12].—Every movement of the body aggravates the pains in the liver,[12].—Inflammation and swelling of the spleen, with pressive and lancinating pains, ineffectual urging to stool, constipation, and disposition to be frightened,[12].—Inflammation of the bowels, with distensive pains, inflated abdomen, colic, and diarrhœa,[12]. —Enlarged and hard abdomen,[12].—Inflation of the abdomen, with heat and lancinations, especially on the left side,[12].—[320.] Encysted tumors of the mesentery,[12].—Flatulence,[1].—Fetid flatulence,[1].—Flatulence and eructations for ten days, especially after a meal,[1].—Copious emission of flatulence in the morning, preceded by borborygmi, with empty feeling in the stomach,[1]. —Sensations as if cold balls were running all through the intestinal canal,[12].—Burning in the bowels, as from an eruption,[12].—Tensive pains, with extreme weariness at the abdomen, extending into the hypochondria,[12]. —Daily pain in the abdomen, on the fortieth day after taking the medicine, after the ulcers on the finger and tibia had healed, especially in the morning and after drinking milk, and also from smoking tobacco; it was not very violent, but a very troublesome, digging-cutting pain (so that he thought of being poisoned),[15].—Cramps in the bowels, which seem twisted and knotted up,[12].—[330.] Colic in the daytime, four or five hours after a meal, with borborygmi, at various intervals and lasting several hours,[1].—Violent colic, with convulsive movements of the limbs and jaws,[12].—Lancinating colic, so violent as nearly to cause fainting, with burning thirst, cold sweat in the hair, followed by four stools, increasingly liquid,[1].—Colic, with tearing sensation in the bowels, borborygmi and flatulence, which often rises from the bowels into the stomach,[12].—Pressive pains in the abdomen,[1].—Great heaviness of the abdomen, with sensation as if the bowels were pressed and crushed,[12].—Great sensitiveness of the abdomen; the least pressure causes severe stitches,[12].—Accumulation of serum, like ascites, in the hypogastric region,[12].—Dull colic in the lower abdomen,[1].—Inflammation and swelling of the inguinal glands,[12].—[340.] Swelling of the inguinal glands,[12].— Enormous scrofulous buboes on the groins,[12].

Rectum and Anus.—Prolapsus recti, even between stools,[12].— Erysipelatous swelling of the anus,[12].—Blind hæmorrhoids, with great pain,[12].—Hæmorrhoids, with discharge of blood, and sometimes of purulent matter,[12].—Frequent protrusion of very painful hæmorrhoidal knobs,[12].— Reappearance of hæmorrhoids, with loss of clear red blood and a feeling of comfort, in the case of a female disposed to piles,[1].—In consequence of straining at stool there escapes from the hæmorrhoidal tumor a jet of blood, the quantity of which may perhaps be estimated at 150 grammes; after this trifling hæmorrhage sense of fatigue,[1].—Itching and burning at the anus,[12].

Stool.—[350.] Stool every two days,[1].—Frequent urging to stool for three or four days, but resulting in only one very scanty evacuation daily. To this state succeeds, for three or four days, four daily stools, accompanied with colic and flatulence,[1].—Five stools in one day,[1].—Several daily stools,[12]. —Two stools in the day, which are yellowish, soft, but consistent,[1].—Stools at night, towards two or three o'clock, A.M.,[1].—Diarrhœa, often accompanied with inclination to vomit,[12].—Watery diarrhœa, with copious urination and canine hunger,[12].—Dysentery,[8].—Diarrhœic stools, with tenesmus and heaviness,[12].—[360.] Diarrhœic stools, sometimes involuntary, with burning in the abdomen, and especially in the rectum,[12].—Whitish stools, as in icterus,[9].—Yellowish, liquid stools,[1].—Yellow diarrhœic stools mixed with dark substances,[12].—Brown stools, of a very bad smell,[12].—Bloody diarrhœic stools, sometimes followed by very liquid whitish stools,[12].—Hard, difficult stools,[12].—Stool sometimes hard, sometimes soft, sometimes both together,[15]. —Thin stools,[11].—Semi-liquid stools after a meal, for three days; one or two daily, morning and evening, without colic; followed three or four days after by an obstinate hæmorrhoidal tumor, the size of a filbert, and situated outside the margin of the anus; the appearance of this tumor is preceded by smarting, three or four days before,[1].—[370.] Lumbrici in the child's stools,[11].—Ascarides and lumbrici,[12].—Constipation; frequent ineffectual urging to stool,[12].—Suppression of stools; the whole body is cold, while the head is burning hot,[1].

Urinary Organs.—Sensation as if the neck of the bladder were obstructed by polypi,[12].—The bladder feels swollen, with constant desire to urinate,[12].—Soft concretions in the kidneys and bladder,[12].—Nephritic colic,[12].—After every urination, painful stitches in the kidneys and bladder; weakness and depression,[12].—Pulsative and lancinating pains in the kidneys, often with hæmaturia,[12].—[380.] Ulcers in the urethra,[12].—Profuse discharge of yellow and gray mucus from the urethra, with painful weariness and weakness in all the lower portion of the body,[12].—Cutting pains, as from a knife, all along the urethra, with inclination to apply the hand there,[12].—Great smarting in the urethra, especially after urinating,[12].—Too frequent urination,[12].—Urine frequent and copious, of a normal color,[11].—Clear urine with liquid stools,[1].—Whitish urine, with chalky sediment,[12]. —Red urine,[1].—Urine brown, smelling strong, like fish-brine,[15].—[390.] Urine full of glairy mucus,[12].—Scanty urine, of a yellow-ochre color, with yellowish sediment, coincident with some pains in the loins; after the pains in the loins, the urine is clearer and very abundant; micturition four times in a night,[1].—Urine scanty, thick, yellowish, depositing a sediment, and diffusing a strong ammoniacal smell, during constipation,[1].—Turbid and grayish urine,[12].—Suppression of urine,[14].

Sexual Organs.—Male. He applies the hands to the genital parts,[11].—The least motion aggravates the pains in the genitals,[12].—Penis swollen, red, and burning,[12].—Hardly any erection,[12].—Obstinate impotence,[12].—[400.] Impotence all night, in the case of a man thirty-two years old,[1].—Burning pains in the prepuce,[12].—Pimples of a tuberculous appearance at the scrotum,[12].—Inflammation of the testicles, with sensation as if a tumor were forming there,[12].—Atrophy or hypertrophy of the testicles,[12]. —Pains in the testicles, as if they were pulled and twisted, and sometimes as if they would return into the abdomen,[12].—Increased venereal appetite,[12].—He seeks solitude that he may abandon himself to onanism,[12].— Complete absence of venereal desire,[12].—Aversion to coition,[12].—[410.] Speedy ejaculation without pleasure, sometimes with spasms and painful weakness of the extremities,[12].—The ejaculation is tardy, or altogether wanting,[12].—Frequent nocturnal emissions followed by debility,[12].—Involuntary discharge of semen,[2 3].—**Female.** Hard tumor and polypi of the uterus,[12].—Ulcers and fissures at the os uteri,[12].—Inflammatory swelling of the womb,[12].—Metrorrhagia,[12].—Liability to abortion,[12].—Difficult, painful and tedious parturition,[12].—[420.] Sensation as if something rose from the uterus to the stomach, with nervous agitation and spasms,[12].—Distensive and burning, or crampy, digging, or gnawing pains in the womb,[12].—Griping and contraction of the uterus, like labor-pains,[12].—Severe stitches, like stabs, in the uterus,[12].—The uterine pains are aggravated in the morning, by walking, and by too long sitting,[12].—Hydatids of the ovaries,[12].—Swelling and great sensitiveness of the ovarian region,[12].—Sensation of burning heat, and of stitches, in the ovaries,[12].—Violent cramps in the ovarian region, extending into the groins,[12].—Itching of the vulva, causing frequent pollutions,[12].—[430.] Leucorrhœa, without smell, with no itching, and clear as water,[1].—Purulent and very offensive leucorrhœa,[12].—Leucorrhœa, especially in the evening, with colic, burning in the hypogastrium, torticollis, and general cramps.[12].—Before and after the menses, yellow, thick, or whitish leucorrhœa; leucorrhœa like cream, or the washings of meat,[12].—Discharge of blood between the menses,[12].—Before menstruation, headache, nausea, colic, itching, and burning in the uterus and vagina,[12].—Menses too early and too profuse,[12].—The menses are only three days too early, in the case of a woman who generally has them eight, ten, and even twelve days too early,[1].—The menses are six days too early,[1].—The menses, which usually anticipate the regular period by four days, are now eight days too soon,[1].—[440.] Menses accompanied with headache, during two days, but the pain shifts about a good deal,[1].—During menstruation, contractions in the hypochondria, pains in the liver, palpitation, chilliness all over, especially in the legs, strong venereal desire, stitches in the splenic region, painful weariness, weakness, and general malaise,[12].—After the menses, heaviness and bad temper,[12].—Menses of clotted, or very fluid and pale blood,[12].

Respiratory Apparatus. — Membranous productions in the larynx,[12].—Ulcers and tubercles in the larynx,[12].—A great quantity of mucus obstructs the larynx and bronchi,[12].—Burning sensation, and bleeding fissures in the larynx, with severe, jerking, and suffocative cough,[12].—Sensation of contraction in the windpipe, and of heaviness in the chest,[12].—Sense of compression of the larynx, with great difficulty in breathing,[12].—[450.] After having cold feet, prickings in the larynx exciting a cough all day, and especially in the evening; the cough continues all night,[1].—Throbbing, lancinating, and excoriative pains in the larynx,[12].—Obstinate hoarseness,[12].—Severe cough, excited by a constant tickling in the larynx,[12].—Cough caused by a pricking in the larynx, only at night, and for several nights running, towards 1, or 3, or 4 o'clock, A.M.,[1].—Cough excited by a stinging in the larynx, following coryza,[1].—Thick cough, especially on waking, in the morning and in the evening, with cold sensation, followed by great heat, and congestion to the chest,[12].—Cough after meals or from any emotion,[12].—Motion increases the frequency of the cough, although it is equally troublesome during rest,[1].—Violent cough, provoking vomiting,[12].—[460.] Hoarse cough, with tearing sensation in the chest,[12].—Deep, hollow cough, with lancinating and bruised pains, especially in the left side of the chest,[12].—Dry, hacking cough, seemingly ameliorated by more frequent alvine evacuations,[1].—Dry cough, with burning in the larynx and chest,[12].—Cough, with expectoration of mucus and blood, or of blood only,[12].—The cough occurs in the daytime, before a meal and in the room; it ceases during the night,[1].—Clear, viscid expectoration, often without cough,[12].—Copious expectoration, frothy, whitish, yellow, grayish, or greenish, and purulent,[12].—Whistling respiration,[12].—Whistling, difficult, rattling respiration,[12].—[470.] The lungs seem always in want of air,[12].—Attacks of paralysis of the lungs, and of suffocation,[12].—Gradually increasing difficulty in breathing,[2].—*Difficult and noisy breathing,[12].—Suffocation at night, towards 3 A.M., with restlessness in all the limbs, trembling of the hands, legs, and head; it seems as if everything, even in the head, were unsteady,[1].

—The patient cannot catch breath, and pants like a dog after too much running,[4].—Dyspnœa, with inability to remain lying down; he is obliged to sit bent forward in order to breathe,[12].

Chest.—Inflammation and swelling of the breasts,[12].—Engorgement of the breasts,[12].—Small knotty indurations and tumors, like scirrhus, on the breasts,[12].—[**480.**] Large abscess forming sinuses in the breasts,[12].—Milk vitiated, and often mixed with blood,[12].—Sensation as if the breasts were drawn towards the abdomen,[12].—Boring, lancinating, digging, crampy, pinching, and gnawing pains, in the mammary and axillary glands,[12].—Granulations and tubercles in the lungs,[12].—Inflammation and swelling of the lungs, especially on the left side, with severe, tiresome cough,[12].—Weakness of the chest, with feeling as if it would collapse,[12].—Feeling of rumbling and of numbness, beginning at the cardiac region and extending through the chest,[12].—Oppression of the chest,[3 8].—Oppression in the afternoon, two days running; the chest and heart feel tightly compressed,[1].—[**490.**] Oppression and loss of breath when going upstairs,[1].—Oppression of the chest, with palpitation, especially when walking rather fast, or in going upstairs,[12].—Burning heat in the chest, as if there were a furnace in it,[12].—Pressive pain in the chest, in a small spot, now here, now there, when walking (after five hours),[15].—Cutting pains in the whole chest, accompanied by tickling and pricking,[12].—Painful stitches in the chest, which check respiration,[12].—Violent, sharp, short stitches, which impede respiration, as if piercing the deep pectoral muscles and the mammary gland, mostly on the right breast, several times a day at different times, lasting ten days (after twelve days),[15].—Violent itching, which seems to come from the lungs, and often shifting about in the chest,[12].—Feeling as if there were two swellings at the upper part of the sternum, appearing to grow larger when in bed, impeding the respiration, and causing pain in swallowing anything, even saliva,[1].—Smarting in the upper third of the sternum,[1].

Heart and Pulse.—[**500.**] The heart-beats are sometimes quick, sometimes slow, intermittent, or irregular,[12].—Palpitation of the heart, at intervals,[6].—Palpitation of the heart, sounding in the ears like drum-beats,[12].—Palpitation of the heart after a meal, with interval during which the person feels as if going to be ill,[1].—Four days after getting chilled, pain at the heart every two hours of the day; straining to vomit; cough with expectoration, tinged with clear red blood; about 8 o'clock the next morning, the cough, the red expectoration, and the pain at the heart return; towards the fifth day, the sensation of having two swellings ceases, but the cough and hoarseness remain,[1].—Feeling as if the heart was very large, and plunged in a vessel of water,[12].—Lancinating and pulling in the region of the heart, as if it were being distended,[12].—Pains as if pins were thrust into the apex of the heart,[12].—Sensation of scraping and weight in the heart,[12].—Trembling feeling at the heart,[12].—[**510.**] Shocks and digging at the cardiac region, with great oppression, especially in the evening, after meals, and from movement,[12].—He has to press upon the cardiac region, to allay the pains,[12].—Hard, frequent, irregular pulse, much quicker and more agitated evenings than mornings,[12].

Neck and Back.—On waking, stiff neck, arthritic pains, and aggravation of all the pains,[12].—The pains in the head affect the nape of the neck, which feels as if compressed,[1].—Boring pains, with painful weariness in the loins; he has to lie on the back for relief,[12].—Pains in the loins so violent that they prevent breathing; they very nearly cause fainting; a red-hot iron seems to pierce the loins; the violence of the pains renders the least movement impossible; this symptom appears in the morning, two days running; the first time it lasts five or six minutes, and two or three minutes the second day; the following day, dull pains in the loins, as from a strain in the back, preventing him from straightening himself, or stooping down; during the pains in the loins, the urine is scanty, of the color of yellow-ochre, thick, with a yellowish sediment; the pains in the loins last five or six days,[1].—Pains in the loins, lasting six or seven days, followed by a very violent trembling of both legs at once, in the morning, and giving way of the legs, from weakness, for two days together,[1].—Distensive pains, with sensation of swelling and discomfort in the loins,[12].

Extremities in General.—Trembling of the limbs,[12].—[520.] In the case of a child the legs are drawn up so as to touch the buttocks,[5].—Limbs easy to move,[13].—Numbness and deadness of the limbs on waking in the morning,[12].—Pinching-digging pains, drawing about as if in the periosteum, not continuing long, and always affecting the middle of the long bones (after five days), lasting twelve days,[15].—Contractions and very painful cramps, from the extremities of the limbs to the trunk,[12].—Contractions in right arm and leg,[12].—Cramps and startings in the limbs,[12].—Lancinating, digging, and tensive pains with great weariness in the limbs,[12].

Upper Extremities.—Inflammatory tumors on the arms,[12].—The upper extremities go to sleep when lightly lying upon them; after a few days also the lower extremities, lasting fourteen days,[15].—[530.] Heaviness of the arms, with great difficulty in moving them,[12].—Painful weariness of the arms, with violent pain in trying to move them,[12].—Paralytic weakness of the arms and hands,[12].—Burning, lancinating pains in the bones of the arms,[12].—After the poison has touched the right hand sharp burning and swelling of the arm, which is colored yellow on a black ground,[8].—Bruised pains in the arms, legs, and loins, especially during movement,[12].—Bruised and crushing pains in the arms, especially the joints,[12].—Digging, pinching, pressive pain in the right arm, which is seated in the deltoid muscle, on the slightest attempt to raise the arm, though by no other motion of the arm, and not when taking hold of it or during rest, lasting fourteen days (after fifth day),[15].—Digging, throbbing, periodic pain on the inner surface of the right ulna, lasting five days (after second day),[15].—Drawing pains in the arms, especially in the evening, at night, and on waking in the morning,[12].—[540.] The lightest covering on the arm annoys and feels uncomfortable,[12].—Pulsative and lancinating pains, with erysipelatous swelling of the arms and hands,[12].—Digging pains in the elbow-joint,[12].—Swelling of the wrist and of the finger-joints, with burning pains and strong pulsation in these parts,[12].—Hands and fingers often numb and stiff, with disposition to become crooked,[12].—Panaritium, attacking even the bones of the fingers,[12].—An insignificant bruise of the right little finger, which he got fourteen days after taking the medicine, became on the third day very painful and suppurated; a few days afterwards the finger became again inflamed, caused tearing-drawing pain along the whole arm and redness of the finger along the lymphatics extending to the axilla, in which small granular swellings appeared and were painful, especially to motion and touch; in thirty-six hours the inflamed lymphatics become swollen as if they had been injected; the lymphatic glands in the axilla become hard and painful and swollen as large as beans; the arm was heavy and painful, and had to be carried in a sling; a few olfactions of Hepar sulph. 1st, relieved the lymphatic swelling in one night, and the corrosive pain in the ulcer in the little finger and the ulcer under the nail of the thumb within ~~twenty-four hours~~,[15].—Superficial, slightly developed, hot, bluish-red swelling, painful to touch, on the lower border of the left thumb-nail; afterwards it suppurates, with throbbing-digging pain; the suppuration involves half of the nail; the pain afterwards becomes gnawing; the skin scales off several times; the throbbing-digging pain of this ulcer extends into the joint of the index finger and metacarpal bones of the left hand (after second day), lasting several weeks,[15].

Lower Extremities.—Feeling as if a peg were driven into the joints of the hips, knees, and feet, and prevented them from moving,[12].—Staggering gait, more like jumping than walking,[12].—[550.] Great weakness of the legs, so that on rising up they give way under the weight of the body,[12].—Lancinating pains, with painful weariness in the hips and legs, especially when walking or changing position,[12].—Aching weariness of the thighs when walking,[15].—Cord-like swelling, as in *phlegmasia alba dolens*, from the groins to the popliteal region,[12].—Tophus on the knees and feet,[12].—Swelling of the knees, with pulsative and distensive pains,[12].—Burning and dryness in the knee-pan,[12].—Pains of dislocation in the knees and feet,[12].—Lancinations in the knees, especially when walking,[12].—Bruised pain in the knees; he has to squat down,[12].—[560.] Inflammation, swelling, and great brittleness of the leg-bones,[12].—Gouty swelling of the legs,[12].—Swelling of the legs, especially in the evening and after walking,[12].—Deep-red swellings, like bruises, on the legs,[12].—Varicose swellings in the legs,[12].—Trembling of the legs,[1].—Uneasiness and irritation in the legs; he has to move them constantly; he knows not what to do with them, nor what position to take for relief,[12].—Heaviness of the legs, with sensation of pulling in the joints,[12].—The legs easily get numb,[12].—Feeling of stiffness in the right leg that begins above the right knee, where it is most marked (ten minutes),[15].—[570.] Weakness of the legs, even to falling, for more than eight hours,[1].—Violent cramps in the legs, which draw up with a start, towards 4 or 5 A.M.,[1].—Cramps in the legs and toes, especially on stretching them out in bed at night,[12].—Aching in the middle of the right tibia as from a blow, when standing, lasting all day (after one hour),[15].—The weakness is accompanied with a crampy pain in the calf, which is worse when moving and ceases when at rest,[1].—Arthritic swelling of the feet,[12].—The feet are apt to turn in walking, and the ankles to be sprained,[12].—The feet, which were constantly cold, become burning hot,[1].—Burning, lancinating, and pulsative pains in the feet, with constant sensation as if the shoes were too tight,[12].—Digging pain in the ungual phalanges of the three last toes and on the inner malleolus, with corrosive itching on the inner border of the right foot (after second day),[15].

Generalities.—[580.] Inflammations and sanguineous congestions, especially of the chest, throat, and head,[12].—Swelling of the whole body,[2].—Obesity,[12].—Progressive emaciation, even to consumption and death,[9].—Constant emaciation, with good appetite,[12].—Emaciated body, with bloated abdomen,[12].—Swelling and induration of the glands,[12].—Swelling, ulceration, and curvature of the bones,[12].—Malignant tumors of an erysipelatous character,[12].—Arthritic nodes,[12].—[590.] Nervous attacks, with laughing and weeping together,[12].—Pandiculations,[11].—Jactitation of tendons,[11].—*Convulsions,[8].—Epileptic convulsions in the evening, at night, and sometimes in the morning, as well as at the period of the new moon,[12].—Attacks of tetanus,[12].—Great sensitiveness to cold air and to wind,[12].—He has every moment to change his position,[12].—Fits of muscular exaltation, in which he has to move the arms about forcibly,[12].—Restlessness all over, with great physical and moral agitation,[12].—[600.] He cannot keep still, is constantly restless, although movement aggravates the pains,[12].—Desire to move about and take gymnastic exercise in the evening,[12].—Uneasiness and weakness, especially mornings, with inability to move about,[12].—Languor, laziness, no desire for any occupation; if he does anything it is only mechanically,[12].—On waking great lassitude and drowsiness, as if he had not slept,[12].—With the headache general feeling of fatigue, nausea, and cold feet,[1].—Great fatigue and profuse sweat after the least exertion,[12].—General weakness, often accompanied by palpitation and vertigo,[12].—Great weakness, with sensation as if the bones would give way under their own weight,[12].—In the midst of a meal, sense of general debility, kind of total prostration, with inability to speak or move, dimness of sight, and distress at the region of the heart; this attack lasts five minutes, and passes off without leaving any traces,[1].—[610.] Gradual failure of strength,[6].—Sinks back in an arm-chair motionless, but without loss of consciousness,[1].—Faint feeling every now and then; the head feels the reaction from it; it passes off like an effect of intoxication,[1]. —Faint feeling, as from hunger, in the morning and during the day, before a meal,[1].—Syncope,[3].—Fainting fits, especially after meals, and in the evening,[12].—Faintness after breakfast,[1].—Pains sometimes on the right side, sometimes on the left, but rarely on both sides at once,[12].—Frequent cramps, doubly painful in the cold air, in the evening, and in the morning,[12].—On going to bed he is attacked with cramps, formication in all the limbs, and with neuralgic pains, especially of the head, which cause anguish and prevent sleep,[12].—[620.] Frequent dislocated pains,[12].—Pains of dislocation, especially in the wrists,[12].—Sensation as if bitten in various parts of the body,[12].—Pulsative pains in the joints,[12].—Disposition to lie on the left side; feels better so than when on the right side,[1].

Skin. Swelling and redness of the whole body, as in general erysipelas,[12]. —Skin bloated and tense, or loose and flabby,[12].—The whole surface becomes pale and swollen, as in dropsy,[3].—The patient becomes yellow,[4][9].— The skin takes on a deep yellow tinge,[2].—[630.] Skin of a yellow tinge, as in jaundice,[12].—Skin greenish, and always looking dirty or oily,[12].—Skin moist, or dry and stiff as parchment, and affected by every change of temperature,[12].—Every slight injury, even the prick of a pin, suppurates, with corrosive pain,[15].—Very unhealthy skin, excoriating and chapping easily,[12]. —The skin of the face tans quickly, and is easily excoriated and torn,[12].— Scabs and cracks in the face,[12].—Chaps and fissures on the hands,[12].—Excoriation between the buttocks and the thighs,[12].—*Eruptions, Dry.* Acne rosacea,[12].—[640.] Miliary eruptions and urticaria,[12].—Very smarting miliary eruption on the penis, pubis, and scrotum,[12].—Burning eruption like nettle-rash on the hands,[12].—A large quantity of scales on the face, which are constantly renewed, with intolerable itching,[12].—Furfuraceous herpes, with great itching of the legs and thighs,[12].—Eruption of little pimples on the skin, after contact with the saliva or urine of the toad,[3].— Pimples like small furuncles,[12].—Small, white pimples, lasting only for a day,[12].—Red and very painful pimples on the forehead,[12].—An erysipelatous attack, in a woman subject to the complaint for many years, was on the point of breaking out, when it was cut short immediately by a few doses of the remedy; subsequently, two pimples appeared on the right temple, on the side most frequently attacked by erysipelas; these pimples, the size of a small lentil, ended in a rounded head; the whole temporal region in the middle of which they were situated was red and swollen. This redness disappears on pressure with the finger, but returns again immediately; at the same time it is always painfully sensitive to cold, and the sensation it causes is identical with that which marks the onset of erysipelas; this eruption lasts seven days; it is accompanied at its first appearance, for two nights successively, by difficult and broken sleep; afterwards return of the pimples on the temples, with sensation when they first break out, as if the skin were pinched,[1].—[650.] Subcutaneous pimples on the cheeks,[12].—After a coryza, small herpetic pimples on the upper lip,[1].—Pimples like small-pox on the glans,[12].—Warts, mostly on the backs of the hands,[12].—*Eruptions, Moist and Pustular.* Erysipelatous eruption on different parts,[12].—Phlegmonous erysipelas of the face,[12].—Phlegmonous erysipelas, which leaves the face disfigured,[12].—Erysipelas of the legs,[12].—Herpes, furfuraceous, moist, crusty, and yellowish,[12].—Acute herpes of the face,[12].— [660.] Herpetic eruptions, burning, and sanious oozing of the vulva,[12].— A small vesicle, surrounded by an erythematous blush, appears near the left wrist; this small vesicle excites a burning itching. It discharges a little serum, and is then succeeded by a small abscess like a boil, with fever and lancinating pain of the forearm, and of the corresponding upper arm, extending to the axilla,[1].—A corrosive vesicle on the inner surface of the first phalanx of the right index finger, very painful (after seven days); it lasts ten days, when the skin in this place scales off,[15].—A small vesicle caused corrosive pain in the middle of the right tibia, with a red areola, and after a few days a whitish-gray, thick, fatty scurf formed, which from new exudations enlarged until it reached the size of a quarter of a dollar, and was surrounded with a broad red areola; at times on touch, and even without cause, corrosive pains attacked this tetter; the crust dried in about fourteen days and desquamated, leaving a reddish-brown spot with shiny scaling skin (twenty-sixth day),[15].—Large blisters in palms of hands and soles of feet, three inches in circumference, yellow; the fluid was yellow and excoriating; this was repeated in several places,[13].—Very painful blisters and corns on the feet,[12].—Phlyctenæ and pemphigus,[12].—Phlyctenoid eruption; thick and sanious scabs on the scalp,[12].—Phlyctenæ on the lips,[12]. —The whole body is covered with pustules like those of a bad case of scabies,[7].—[670.] Eruptions like the itch, lichen, and prurigo,[12].—Boils and abscesses,[12].—Eruption like small boils on the cheeks and neck,[12].—The skin-symptoms are aggravated in the evening and at night,[12].—*Sensations.* Sensation of tension and of shuddering in the skin,[12].—The skin feels as if stretched to bursting,[12].—Formication and torpor on different parts of the body,[12].—Tickling on the skin, as from insects, or drawing a feather over it,[12].—Great sensitiveness of the skin and bones of the face,[12].— Intolerable itching, which ends in smarting, all over the body, and is aggravated on going into the open air,[12].—[680.] The itching is relieved by the friction of the body-linen; it is followed by smarting, especially when it has been thus allayed,[1].—Violent itching in the afternoon, towards 4 or 5 o'clock, in the whole outer surface of the thighs and legs, for eight successive days, always at the same hour,[1].—Great itching of the cheeks,[12].—Intolerable itching at the nape of the neck,[12].—Corrosive itching on the left leg and knee-cap, which compels rubbing, lasting several days (after second day),[15].

Sleep and Dreams.—Fits of drowsiness coming on after eating, and in the open air,[12].—Drowsiness, with agitation and sleeplessness; he is constantly turning in bed,[12].—Great sleepiness, especially in the morning, after breakfast, or after being in the open air,[12].—Invincible drowsiness after a meal,[1].—Very heavy sleep, with congestion to the head,[12].—[690.] Sleep tardy, or too prolonged in the morning, with dreams, nightmare, and great fatigue on waking,[12].—Insufficient sleep; he awakes too early,[12].—Wakes too early, 3 or 4 o'clock A.M.,[1].—Wakes up every few moments,[1].—Wakes up sad, or very joyful,[12].—Sleep with talking, cries and groans; he awakes sobbing,[12].—Restless sleep, with starting awake, fright, palpitation, etc.,[12].—Sleeplessness in the evening and at night,[12].—Sense of fatigue during sleep, and of numbness in every limb, obliging him to change his position frequently,[1].—Many dreams, fantastic, and generally frightful,[12].—[700.] Dreams of travel, of projects, and of greatness,[7].

Fever.—He desires warmth; is always cold, especially in the limbs,[12]. —Obstinate coldness in bed at night,[12].—Shivering all over after stool, aggravated in the evening,[1].—Coldness, shiverings, trembling, and vertigo, especially on going into the fresh air,[12].—Coldness and shivering, with moisture of the skin, nervous excitability, and trembling,[12].—Chilly sensation in the calves, which precedes a cramplike pain in that part,[1].—Chilliness and numbness of the feet,[12].—Alternations of heat and cold rising like waves from the lower part of the body,[12].—Heat and burning all over, accompanied by passing shiverings,[12].—[710.] General sensation of heat and turgescence, followed by contraction and icy coldness of the whole system,[12]. —Fever with shivering, increase of muscular strength, and delirium, especially in the evening,[12].—Feverish heat all over, excepting the feet, which remain constantly cold, day and night, during four days,[1].—Calor mordax, with embarrassed head, burning of the neck, throat, and chest; agitated pulse, great thirst,[12].—The heat of the fire is distressing to him,[1].—Fever is developed, the extremities become burning hot,[2][3].—Quotidian evening fever, with great depression,[12].—Tertian fever, with general painful weariness, great hunger, and urgent thirst,[12].—Quartan fever, with intense heat and violent delirium,[9].—Heat which rises into the face,[1].—[720.] Great heat, contraction, and digging in the loins,[12].—Burning heat of the hands for three weeks,[1].—Sensation as if the legs and feet were held over a pan of burning charcoal,[12].—Burning hot feet,[1].—The skin is burning, red, and crimpled in different places,[12].—Aggravation of the fever in the evening, at night, and sometimes in the morning,[12].—The body is almost always moist with perspiration,[12].—Cold sweats,[4].—Sweat in the morning, in bed,[1].—In bed, on waking up in the morning, general moisture,[1].—[730.] Excessive perspiration during sleep, especially towards morning,[12].—Debilitating, sour-smelling perspiration, especially in the morning, in bed,[12].—Night-sweat, especially on the head, chest, and back,[12].—Copious sweat after the slightest exertion,[12].—Copious sweat, with weakness, and often with morbid hunger,[12].—Frequent perspiration of the hands,[12].—Sweat mostly on the hams,[1].

***Conditions.*—Aggravation.**—(*Morning*), On waking, ill-humor; dizziness, etc.; after a meal, dizziness; on waking, at 3 A.M., headache; coryza; bad-smelling breath; insipid taste of food; nauseous, etc., taste; dryness of the throat; after breakfast, feels hungry; vomiting; emission of flatulence; pain in abdomen; pains in uterus; towards 1, 3, or 4 A.M., cough; on waking, cough; on waking, stiff neck, etc.; *pains in loins;* on waking, numbness, etc., of limbs; after breakfast, sleepiness; in bed, sweat; in bed, on waking, general moisture; in bed, perspiration.—(*Afternoon*), After breakfast, headache; rising of phlegm; after a meal, vomiting; oppression; towards 4 or 5 o'clock, itching.—(*Evening*), Towards 5 o'clock, headache; towards 4 or 5 o'clock, soreness in forehead, etc.; semilateral headache, etc.; sweats on the head; on going to bed, sneezing; mucus from nose; toothache; hunger; leucorrhœa; cough; shocks, etc., at cardiac region; pulse quicker; swelling of the legs; fainting fits; skin symptoms; after stool, shivering; fever, etc.—(*Night*), When going to sleep, ill-humor; headache; toothache; digging, etc., in liver, etc.; pains in arms; skin symptoms.—(*Towards morning*), During sleep, perspiration.—(*Open air*), Mucus from nose; itching; fits of drowsiness; sleepiness.—(*When ascending stairs*), Oppression, etc.—(*On going to bed*), Cramps in legs, etc.—(*After breakfast*), Faintness.—(*Cold air*), The pains; pains in teeth; coldness, etc. —(*Cold liquids*), Mouth symptoms.—(*Dampness*), Most symptoms.—(*After eating*), As if intoxicated; almost immediately, vomiting; turning in the stomach; fits of drowsiness.—(*After exertion*), Sweat.—(*Hearty food*), Most symptoms.—(*Great heat*), Most symptoms.—(*Strong liquors*), Most symptoms.—(*Lying on back*), All the pains.—(*Before a meal*), Cough.—(*After a meal*), Regurgitation, etc.; nausea; flatulence, etc.; semi-liquid stools; cough; palpitation, etc.; fainting fits; drowsiness.—(*Meat*), Most symptoms.—(*Before menstruation*), Headache, etc.—(*During menstruation*), Contraction in hypochondria, etc.—(*After menstruation*), Heaviness, etc.— (*Drinking milk*), Pain in abdomen.—(*Movement*), Head symptoms; headache; toothache; cramps in stomach; pains of liver; cough more frequent; pain in calf.—(*Odors*), Most symptoms; (*On changing position*), Pains in hips, etc.—(*On slightest attempt to raise arm*), Pain in deltoid muscle.—(*In room*), Cough.—(*Sitting*), During work, headache; pains in uterus.—(*Smoking tobacco*), Nausea, etc.; pains in abdomen.—(*Drinking spirits*), Headache.—(*When standing*), Aching in right tibia.—(*Change of temperature*), Toothache.—(*Walking*), Pain in temple; pains in uterus; pain in chest; pains in hips, etc.; rawness of thighs; lancinations in knees; swelling of cheeks; the pains.—(*Walking fast*), Oppression, etc.—(*Contact of water*), Ear symptoms.—(*Windy weather*), Heat.—(*Wine*), Stomachache.—(*Working in water*), Most symptoms.

Amelioration.—(*Morning*), In bed, after a sweat, coryza ceases.— (*Night*), Headache; cough ceases; on stretching out in bed, cramps in legs; in bed, coldness.—(*Keeping bent over on one side*), The pains.—(*Epistaxis*), Headache.—(*Friction of body-linen*), Itching.—(*Lying down*), Headache.—(*Lying on left side*), Feels better.—(*Lying on back*), Pains, etc., in loins.—(*Pressing on submaxillary gland*), Pains in ear.

BUFO SAHYTIENSIS.

A South American toad, to which this name has been given by Dr. Mure, in his Pathogenesie Brazilienne.

Mind.—Aversion to work, with unfitness for it, the whole afternoon (first day).—Gay, lively (thirty-ninth day).—Very gay in the evening; disposed to talk about cheerful things (thirty-eighth day).—Careless (twentieth day).—Sadness; he shuns society (thirty-ninth day).—Gloomy and silent mood (thirty-ninth day).—He is unable to act with decision; he forms projects and does not accomplish them (thirty-ninth day).—Heightened imagination (thirty-ninth day).—Weakness of mind and memory, less in the evening (thirty-ninth day).—[10.] Lazy and discouraged (twentieth day).—Not disposed to study (after three days).—He is apt to forget things he had been occupied with a moment before (seventeenth day).— Weak memory (after twenty days).

Head.—Extreme heaviness of the head, at 2 o'clock (first day).— Heaviness of the head after a walk (thirty-ninth day).—Long-lasting headache (thirty-ninth day).—Pressure on the right side of the forehead (thirty-ninth day).—Sharp stitches in the left temple (thirty-ninth day).— (Sense of weakness in the whole left side of the head), (thirty-ninth day).— [20.] Large red pimple on the occiput (thirty-sixth day).

Eyes and Ears.—The orbits feel larger and as if in contact with the orbital walls (after seventeen days).—Almost continual expansive pressure in the orbits, and sensation of external itching; he is obliged to rub his eyes with the palm of his hand (after two days).—The upper portion of the orbits seems to be in contact with the orbital walls, especially at night (after twenty days).—The eyes are red, and smart (seventeenth day).—The eyes smart, and are painful to touch (nineteenth day).—Pain in front of the lobe of the left ear (thirty-ninth day).

Stomach and Stool.—Pricking at the pit of the stomach (thirteenth day).—Easy stools (third day).

Sexual Organs, Chest, and Back.—Constant erections without desire (after four days).—[30.] Painful sensation under the false ribs (thirty-ninth day).—Pressure at the cartilages of the false ribs (fourteenth day).—Itching on the lumbar vertebræ (twentieth day).—Pain at the sacrum, worse when rising, stooping, or sitting (after two days).

Extremities.—Pricking in the tips of the right fingers and left toe (thirty-ninth day).—Pinching at the inside of the left elbow (thirteenth day).—Pain in extensor muscles of right arm (thirty-ninth day).—Acute pain in the right wrist (thirty-ninth day).—Crampy pain at the outer side of the right leg (thirteenth day).—Pain at the inner part of the right knee (third day).—[40.] Ganglion on the sole of the right foot (thirty-ninth day).—Prickling at the right big toe (twelfth day).

Generalities and Skin.—Less active than usual (after three days).—Excoriation of the left masseter muscle, discharging a little sanguinolent humor (thirty-ninth day).—A former fungus bleeds (seventeenth day).—Red pimple, which breaks and leaves a black spot in its place (thirteenth day).—Pimples on the forehead (thirty-ninth day).—Pimple on right wrist (thirty-ninth day).—A black spot on the right outer ankle, which had remained after a pimple, continues (twentieth day).—Formication of the lower jaw (twentieth day).—[50.] Formication in the lumbar region (thirty-ninth day).—Violent itching (thirty-ninth day).—Itching almost all over (after three days).—Itching on the face (after two days).—He is obliged to rub his face in the morning (twentieth day).—Violent itching at the lips (second day).—Itching at the pubis (second day).—Itching about the anus (twentieth day).

Sleep and Dreams.—Drowsiness (thirty-ninth day).—Sleeps for an hour in the middle of the day, contrary to habit (thirty-ninth day).— [60.] No sleep (eleventh day).—Dreams every night, but on waking, does not recollect what they were about (thirty-ninth day).—Poetic and philosophical dreams (thirty-ninth day).

Conditions.—Aggravation.—(*Morning*), Obliged to rub face.—(*Rising*), Pain at sacrum.—(*Sitting*), Pain at sacrum.—(*Stooping*), Pain at sacrum.—(*After a walk*), Heaviness of head.

Amelioration.—(*Evening*), Weakness of mind, etc.

BUXUS.

Buxus sempervirens, L. *Nat. order*, Euphorbiaceæ. *Preparation*, Tincture of the young leaves and twigs.

Authority. Br. Journ. of Hom., 11, 158, effects of an infusion taken every six hours for eight days, for the purpose of producing an abortion, which it failed to do.

Strong forcing pains, like those of labor, in the lower part of the abdomen, which varied greatly in intensity, and lasted from twenty or thirty seconds to a minute or longer.—Pretty frequent desire to urinate, but no increase in amount of urine emitted.—Slight increase in frequency of pulse.—Slight degree of nausea on one or two occasions.

CACAO.

Theobroma cacao, Linn. *Nat. order*, Sterculiaceæ. *Tribe*, Buettnerieæ.

Common name, Cocoa (chocolate in part). *Preparation*, Trituration of the seeds (crude).

Authority. Marvaud, Aliments d'epargne.

In order to ascertain the effect of the active principles (aromatic essences and theobromin) contained in Cacao upon the nervous system and its dependencies, it was necessary to separate those principles, as far as possible, from the fatty substances (Butter of Cacao) of which the beans are so largely composed.

With this view, we prepared a decoction of powdered Cacao in boiling water, and conducted our experiments with this liquid.

By placing ourselves under the influence of a decoction highly charged with aromatic principles, and made from powdered Cacao well roasted, we ascertained that this beverage produces an excitement of the nervous system similar to that caused by a strong infusion of black coffee; since these effects are insignificant if a decoction of the raw bean is employed, it is natural to attribute them to the aromatic essences which are developed in the Cacao by the process of roasting.

A still wider difference is observed when we compare the effects on the circulation respectively produced by a decoction of powdered Cacao roasted, and one of the same substance in a crude state. In the former case, the sphygmographic tracing indicates an excited state of the circulation, as shown by an accelerated pulse, *with increased fulness and diminished arterial tension.*

When, on the other hand, an infusion of the raw bean is made use of, the action of the theobromin predominates, and *an entirely different character of pulse* is the result, as may be placed beyond doubt by examining the following traces, obtained from a single individual.

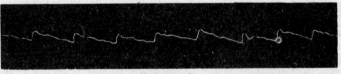

Normal pulse.

In explaining the nutritive value of Cacao, we must take into account the presence in this substance of a special alkaloid, theobromin, whose physiological effects are identical with those of caffein and theiu (as we

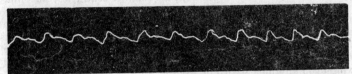

Pulse five minutes after a decoction of the roasted bean. (Action of the aromatic essences.)

have proved by numerous experiments), and which, retarding the organic waste in the same way as the active principles of coffee and tea, place

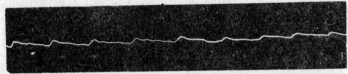

Pulse fifteen minutes after a decoction of the crude bean. (Action of Theobromin.)

Cacao high up among " les aliments d'épargne ou antidéperditeurs " (the conservative substances, or those which check tissue-waste).

CACTUS.

Cereus grandiflorus, Haw. (Cactus grandiflorus, Linn.)

Nat. order, Cactaceæ. *Common name*, Night-blooming cereus. *Preparation*, Tincture of the flowers and young twigs.

Authority. 1, Rubini (translated by Dr. Ad. Lippe); 2, Hencke, A. H. Z., 86, 173, proving with the 1st dil.; 3, ibid., proving with the 3d; 4, ibid., proving with the 6th; 5, ibid., proving with the tincture; 6, Lembke, N. Z. f. H. Kl. 12, 2, proving with the tincture; 7, Dr. John H. Fitch, The Medical Eclectic, 1, 190, proving with 7 to 20 drops of tincture; 8, ibid., proving with one dose of 195 drops of tincture; 9, Dr. Burt, West. Hom. Obs., 3, 239, proved 100 to 600 drops of the 3d dec. dil., under the name of "Cactus serpentarius."

Mind.—Slight delirium at night; on waking up, it ceases for a time, but begins again as soon as he goes to sleep (seventh day),[1].—Talking nonsense while asleep at night; on awaking, he talks unconnectedly (tenth day),[1].—*Love of solitude;* he avoids those around him who wish to comfort him (ninth day),[1].—Felt decided impulses to swallow large and unwholesome portions of medicine (first day),[8].—Continued taciturnity; he will not answer repeated interrogations (third day),[1].—Decided repugnance to take any more medicine (first day),[7].—Was affected with impulses to do something facetious, which were repelled (first day),[7].—Impulses to do something bordering on the grotesque (first day),[7].—Depression and languor during the whole day,[1].—[10.] *Sadness, taciturnity, and irresistible inclination to weep* (first six days),[1].—*Hypochondriasis and invincible sadness* (first six days),[1].—Profound *hypochondria;* he is unwilling to speak a word (fourth day),[1].—Unusual *melancholy,* for which he himself can give no reasons (first four days),[1].—Anxiety returning in the evening (first fifteen days),[1].—Extraordinary irritability; the smallest contrariety puts him into a passion (fifteenth day),[1].—Feeling of semi-remorse at having done something wrong (first day),[8].—Feeling of having done violence to myself (first day),[8].—*Fear of death extreme and continuous; he believes his disease to be incurable (seventh day),[1].—Disposition to do deliberately whatever was undertaken (first day),[7].—[20.] Felt a considerable degree of difficulty in fixing upon anything settled or fixed in what he was pursuing; when conclusions were arrived at, however, they were to the mind quite satisfactory (first day),[7].

Head.—Vertigo, from sanguineous congestions to the head (after ten days),[1].—On retiring to his room, felt some unsteadiness of gait, almost amounting to staggering, a reeling sensation,[7].—At night, sensation as if the brain was attached to the skull, grown fast (first day),[7].—Feeling of emptiness in the head (second day),[1].—Violent pain in the head, insufferable, from congestion to the head (fourth day),[1].—Excessive pain in the head, which causes such anxiety that he cannot stay in bed (first day),[1].—Pain in the head, with great prostration and weariness,[1].—Dull frontal headache (after four hours), (600 drops),[9].—Pressing pain in the forehead, day and night, for two consecutive days,[1].—[30.] In the evening, a constant pressing pain in the left side of the forehead, lasting until he went to sleep, and felt at night on waking twice (first day),[6].—Pressing pain in the forehead, increased by bright light, and on hearing loud voices or noises,[1].—Pressure in the forehead during the whole day, at intervals; worse in the room than in the open air (first day),[6].—Jerking-tearing in the forehead, and throughout the limbs (first day),[6].—Sensation of heavy weight in the right temple and on the right eyebrow, diminished by pressure,[1].—Strong pulsations in the temples, as if the skull would burst,[1].—Continued and tormenting pulsation in the temples and ears, which is exceedingly annoying, and causes hypochondriasis (first eight days),[1].—Pulsating pain in the temples, becoming intolerable at night (second day),[1].—Tensive pain in the vertex, which returns periodically every two days (in the first twenty days),[1].—**Pressing pain in the head, as if a great weight lay on the vertex,**[1].—[40.] *Sensation of weight on the vertex, with dull pain, increased by the sound of talking and by any noise,*[1].—**Heavy pain, like a weight, on the vertex,** *which diminishes by pressure,*[1].—Very severe pain in the right side of the head, which increases to a great degree when raising the head from the pillow, for many days in succession (after three days),[1].—Very severe pain in the right side of the head, which is increased by the sound of talking and by a bright light (first five days),[1].—A troublesome pressure on the right parietal bone (3d dil.), (second day),[3].—Pressure in the left parietal bone (first day),[5].—Pressive pain in the left parietal bone, in the morning, after rising (second day),[5].—Pressive pain in the left parietal bone, in the forenoon, more internally (6th dil.), (first day),[4].—*Pulsating pain, with sensation of weight in the right side of the head, continuing day and night, so severe as to make him cry out with a loud voice* (after four days),[1].—On retiring, felt some heaviness and pain, not severe, however, affecting the posterior region of the brain, increased by lying on the back with the head touching the pillow. Instantly relieved by lying on the side, so that the occipital portion of the skull did not come into contact with anything hard or otherwise (first day),[7].—[50.] Complained most bitterly of its producing constant dull pain in the cerebellum; if the remedy was omitted, the pain would cease, but would return as soon as its use was resumed,[9].—Pain and drawing in the occiput, increased by the motion of the head,[1].—Painful drawing in the aponeurotic covering of the occiput, ameliorated by bending the head backward,[1].—Felt at times pressure in the occiput, not severe, and relieved by quick exercise or mental activity (first day),[7].

Eyes.—Weakness of sight recurring periodically; objects appear to be obscured,[1].—Weakness of sight for many days in succession; objects appear as if clouded (first four days),[1].—Dimness of sight; at a few paces' distance he does not recognize his friends,[1].—At a short distance he does not recognize any one, not even a friend,[1].—Momentary loss of sight (first day),[1].—Loss of sight; there appear circles of *red light* before the eyes, which dim the sight (sixth day),[1].

Ears.—[60.] Pulsations in the ears, continuing day and night (first six days),[1].—Hearing diminished by the buzzing in the ears; it is necessary to speak in a loud voice to be understood (first day),[1].—Noise in the ear, like the running of a river, continuing all night (first day),[1].

Nose.—Dry and very unpleasant coryza; he must breathe, during the night, with his mouth open,[1].—Fluent and very acrid coryza, which makes the nostrils sore,[1].—*Profuse epistaxis*, which ceases in a short time,[1].

Face.—*Paleness of the face* and emaciation (first six days),[1].—Face flushed (after four hours), (600 drops),[9].—Face bloated (acceso) and red, with pulsating pain in the head (twelfth day),[1].

Mouth.—Fetid breath in the morning (third day),[1].—[70.] Scraping in the palate for an hour after taking (first day),[5].—Sensation of having swallowed something unpleasant (after quarter of an hour),[7].—For some minutes a soapy taste in the mouth (after one hour),[7].—Slimy, weedy taste, not so distinctly soapy as the night before (second day),[7].

Throat.—Felt an accumulation of mucus in the throat, which was expectorated (immediately),[7].—Constriction of the throat, which excites the frequent swallowing of saliva (eighth day),[1].—Scraping on the soft palate (6th dil.), (first day),[4].—Constriction of the œsophagus which prevents swallowing; he must drink a great quantity of water to force anything down into the stomach (sixth day),[1].

Stomach.—Appetite good, better than usual,[8].—At breakfast, appetite better than usual (second day),[7].—[80.] Great appetite, but weak and slow digestion (twentieth day),[1].—*Complete loss of appetite; he cannot take the least morsel of food (third day),[1].—Want of appetite and loss of the taste of food, which disappears after a few hours (second day),[1].—Want of appetite and nausea for many days; it is only by an effort that he can swallow a few mouthfuls (first fourteen days),[1].—Great thirst, which causes him to drink much water (first day),[1].—Nausea in the morning and all day long (seventh day),[1].—*Copious vomiting of blood*,[1].—*Severe gastroenteritis,* cured in five days,[1].—Bad digestion; all food causes weight in the stomach, and so much suffering that he prefers to remain fasting,[1].—Very slow digestion; even after eight or ten hours the taste of the food rises up in the throat,[1].—[90.] Acrid acid in the stomach, which rises in the throat and mouth, and makes everything he attempts to eat *taste acid* (fourth day),[1].—A feeling of emptiness in the stomach, with good appetite and natural stool (fifth, sixth days),[5].—Sensation of something disagreeable at the stomach (second day),[7].—Sensation of violent burning in the stomach (first five days),[1].—Sensation of great *constriction* in the scrobiculus, which extends to the hypochondria, constricts them, and impedes respiration (fourth day),[1].—Sensation of heaviness in the stomach,[1].—Sensation of great weight in the stomach, which continues many days (during the first eight days),[1].—*Sensation of weight in the stomach,* which soon goes off, but reappears every time the medicine is taken (first fifteen days),[1].—Oppression and weight in the stomach (fourth day),[1].—*Strong pulsation in the scrobiculus (first eight days),[1].—[100.] *Continuous and annoying pulsation in the stomach,[1].—Very troublesome pulsation of the cœliac artery, after dinner, which lasts three hours, and corresponds with the pulsation of the right temporal artery,[1].

Abdomen.—Wandering pains in the umbilical region, which cease and recur periodically (fifth day),[1].—Sharp, cutting pains in the umbilicus (after half an hour), continuing about one hour after stool,[9].—Severe cutting pains in the lower umbilical and hypogastric regions, lasting about an hour (after thirty-five minutes),[9].—The abdominal parietes, when touched with the hand, impart a burning sensation, and are much hotter than the other parts of the body (third day),[1].—Borborygmus in the bowels, before the alvine evacuations,[1].—Slight pain in bowels (after four hours), (600 drops),[9].—Very violent pains in the bowels, almost causing him to faint, which continue, more or less, during the day (seventh day),[1].—Soreness, with distension of the abdomen (third day),[7].—[110.] Distressing sensation in the bowels, as if a serpent was turning round, here and there, in the bowels (fourth day),[1].—Sensation of painful constriction in the groins, extending around the pelvis,[1].

Rectum and Anus.—Swollen varices outside the anus, which cause much pain,[1].—Stool, followed by blood from piles (first day),[7].—*Copious hemorrhage from the anus,* which soon ceases,[1].—A peculiar sensation in the anus, as if the rectum was swollen; it caused a scraping during the stool and a prickling sensation (second and third days),[2].—*Sensation of great weight in the anus, and a strong desire to evacuate a great quantity; however, nothing passes (fifteenth day),[1].—Pricking in the anus, as from sharp pins, which ceases on slight friction,[1].—Great itching in the anus, which causes him to rub the part very often,[1].

Stool.—Morning, diarrhœa of very loose fæces, preceded by very great pain, eight motions from 6 to 12 A.M.; no motion in the afternoon (seventh day),[1].—[120.] Bilious diarrhœa, with pain in the abdomen; eight evacuations in one day (third day),[1].—Bilious diarrhœa, with four or five evacuations in one day, always preceded by pain (during the first eight days),[1].—Mucous diarrhœa, preceded by drawing pains; three motions in the day (twelfth day),[1].—Watery diarrhœa, very abundant each time; passages during the morning hours always preceded by pains and borborygmus (ninth day),[1].—Soft stool, followed by quite severe pains in the hypogastrium (after four hours), (600 drops),[9].—Mushy stool (after three hours),[9].—Dry, hard stool (second day),[9].—Evacuation of hard, black fæces, immediately on taking the remedy, in a man who had been constipated for some days.; on the following day bilious evacuations (first day),[1].—Had with difficulty a hard stool; afterwards a discharge of fluid blood from the anus, which continued to drop a moment or two (second day),[7].—Constipation during all the first six days,[1].—[130.] Constipation, as if from hæmorrhoidal congestion,[1].—During the early part of the proving felt a tendency to constipation, with hard stools and bleeding piles; the bleeding after stools; after the second or third day this passed into a more loose condition of the bowels, mushy stools, and felt no more of the piles,[7].

Urinary Organs.—Constriction of the neck of the bladder, which at first prevents the passage of the urine; but when he strains much he urinates as usual (tenth day),[1].—Redness at the orifice of the urethra,[8].—*Insupportable irritation in the urethra, as if he should pass water constantly,[1].—Heat in the urethra, which, increasing gradually, becomes insupportable (fifth day),[1].—Great desire to pass water, and though he tries a long time, he is unable to pass any at all (first day),[1].—*Frequent desire to urinate, with an abundant flow of urine, each time, during the night (first six days),[1].—Desire to urinate; after he had endeavored to do so for a long time he at last succeeds in passing water abundantly (first day).—*Urine very much increased; he must pass water very frequently, and each time discharges it in great quantity,[1].—Involuntary escape of urine in bed, at night, whilst asleep, at 5 A.M. (first night),[1].—[140.] Urine passed by drops, with much burning (fourth day),[1].—Urine more copious than usual (first four days),[1],—*Very profuse urine of a straw color (first day),[1]. —Urine more scanty than usual (fifth and sixth days),[5].—Passed about half a pint of urine, having the odor of freshly drawn green tea (immediately),[8]. —*Urine reddish, turbid, very abundant,[1].—Urine, on cooling, deposits a red sand,[1].

Sexual Organs.—Male. Tendency to congestion to the urinogenital system, early in the proving,[8].—Toward evening priapisms (first day),[8].—Just before retiring slight priapismal symptoms (first day),[7].— [150.] In one or two instances strong sexual desire, with priapisms,[8].—About 12 M. copious seminal emission, after strong sexual desire (third day),[8].— **Female.** Pain in the uterus and its ligaments, periodically returning every evening, and increasing gradually until 11 P.M., when it is much worse; it then ceases until the following evening for many successive days (after fourteen days),[1].—Painful sensation of constriction in the uterine region, which gradually extends upwards, and in a quarter of an hour reaches the stomach, and causes the sensation as of a great blow in the veins, that makes the patient cry out, after which it rapidly goes off (on the first day after taking one globule of the 100th potency),[1].—Pulsating pain in the uterus and ovarian regions, like an internal tumor suppurating; the pain extends to the thighs, and becomes insupportable; then it ceases completely, and occurs on the next day at the same time, and so on, for many successive days (after fifteen days),[1].—*Menstruation eight days too soon (it happened usually some days too late), (third day),[1].— Menstruation scanty, and ceasing when she remains lying down,[1].—Menstruation of black, pitchy blood, rather abundant,[1].—Menstruation with most horrible pains, causing her to cry aloud and weep (fifth day),[1].—Very painful menstruation, accompanied by great prostration of strength; she is obliged to remain in bed for three days (eighth day),[1].—[160.] Menstruation, which was usually preceded by very strong pains, comes this time without any pain, and very copiously,[1].

Respiratory Apparatus. — *(Bronchitis speedily cured),[1].— *(Chronic bronchitis, **with rattling of mucus**, which, becoming acute in consequence of a cold, causes great anxiety and suffocation; it is rapidly relieved, and the acute state ceases very soon),[1].—*(Chronic bronchitis, of many years' standing, with rattling of mucus, continuous day and night; oppression of breathing on going upstairs, and inability to lie horizontally in bed, which is rapidly cured),[1].—Obstinate, stertorous cough, worse at night,[1].—*Spasmodic cough, with copious mucous expectoration,[1].—Dry cough, from itching in the larynx (first night),[1].—Cough, with thick expectoration, like boiled starch, and very yellow,[1].—*Catarrhal cough, with much viscid expectoration,[1].—*Hæmoptysis, which soon ceases,[1].—[170.] Congestive asthma, which soon passes away,[1].—Short inspiration (after first day),[6].—Short breathing when walking, also when going upstairs, with palpitation of the heart (fourth day),[5].—*Oppression of breathing, as from a great weight on the chest (third day),[1].—Slight oppression of breathing when walking (third day),[2].—Prolonged oppression of the respiration, with great anxiety (first eight days),[1].—Chronic oppression of the breathing, which increases in the open air, and soon goes off again,[1].—Difficult breathing (first day),[5].— *Difficulty of breathing; continued oppression and uneasiness, as if the chest were constricted with an iron band, and could not dilate itself for normal respiration (first eight days),[1].—Periodical attacks of suffocation, with fainting, cold perspiration on the face, and loss of pulse (first eight days),[1].— [180.] *Inspiring fresh air is very reviving (second day),[6].

Chest.—*Sanguineous congestion in the chest, which prevents him from lying down in bed (third day),[1].—(*Pneumorrhagia, renewed every four, six, seven, or eight hours, accompanied each time with convulsive cough, and expectoration of two or three pounds of blood; is at once relieved, and ceases entirely in four days),[1].—For a moment, at night, pain in the nerves, running from the left axilla to the pectoral region adjoining (first day),[7].— *Sensation of constriction of the chest, as if bound (fourth day),[1].—Constriction in the upper part of the chest, which hinders respiration (first fifteen days),[1].—*Painful sensation of constriction in the lower part of the chest, as if a cord was tightly bound around the false ribs, with obstruction of the breathing (sixth day),[1].—Feeling of constriction in the chest, which prevents free speech; and when forced to speak, the voice is low (weak), and hoarse (tenth day),[1].—Oppression of the chest, with loss of breath (first four days),[1].—Oppression in the left subclavian region, as if a great weight prevented the free dilatation of the thorax (fourth day),[1].—Pressive pain in the upper part of the side of the chest (first day),[5].—Sensation in the chest as if some one were pressing and holding it tightly; under the delusion that this was the case, the patient cried out, "Leave me alone!" (third day),[1].—[190.] A pressive pain in the chest, that impedes respiration and causes deep breathing; is worse in walking and on going upstairs; is very troublesome on account of palpitation of the heart,[2].—*Sensation of great constriction in the middle of the sternum, as if the parts were compressed by iron pincers, which compression produces oppression of the respiration, aggravated by motion (first ten days),[1].—Sharp, wandering pains in the thoracic cavity, very annoying, especially in the scapular region (first fifteen days),[1].—Pain in the left breast, which is increased by touching, and relieved by gently raising it (first twelve days),[1].—Painful drawings in the muscles of the left side of the chest, which extend to the shoulder-joint, and impede respiration and the free use of the arm,[1].—Pressive pain in the left side of the upper part of the chest, between the second and third ribs, when sitting quietly, impeding respiration, and causing deep breathing, lasting several minutes (second day), (from 3d dil.),[3].—Several violent stitches in the right upper thorax,[6].

Heart and Pulse.—*Increased action of the heart, and on walking, pulsation in the chest with anxiety; lasts the whole forenoon (first day),[5].— *Rapid, short, irregular beats of the heart, on rapid motion,[6].—Several violent, irregular beats of the heart, on slow walking, rising from a chair, turning suddenly (fourth day),[6].—[200.] *Several violent, irregular beats of the heart, with sensation of pressure and heaviness in the region of the heart (after one hour),[6].—Many violent beats of the heart on walking the room slowly;

with tightness of chest and deep breathing (second day),[6].—The beating of the heart and the pulsation of the chest were worse when lying on the back, more perceptible and audible than when lying on the side, together with anxiety and restlessness at night,[5].—Violent palpitation and pulsation in the upper part of the chest, at night in bed (first day),[5].—Fast walking does not cause palpitation of the heart; on the other hand, it is brought on by a rapid motion, such as suddenly stooping, or rising from a chair, as well as by any excitement (first day),[6].—The palpitation occurs very frequently during the day, and always at the commencement of any motion whatever, such as stooping, rising, turning around; but walking for some time does not bring it on; it is accompanied by an anxious sensation in the chest, rising into the throat (second day),[6].—*Palpitation of the heart, continuous day and night, worse when walking, and at night, when lying on the left side* (first six days),[1].—Palpitation of the heart, on standing and sitting; anxious sensation in the heart (after first day),[6].—Palpitation, and feeling of oppression at the heart, on sitting, and lying in the evening, in bed, especially when lying on the back,[6].—* The palpitation of the heart consists of small, irregular beats, with necessity for deep inspiration; slight excitement or deep thought is sufficient to produce this condition,*[6].—[210.] Nervous palpitation of the heart, augmented gradually on the occurrence of the catamenia,[1].—*Dull, heavy pains in the region of the heart*, increased by (external) pressure (second day),[1].—*Sensation of constriction in the heart, as if an iron band prevented its normal movement* (first ten days),[1]. —For a moment, just before going to his room to retire, a slight drawing sensation in the region of the heart,[7].—* Very acute pain, and such painful stitches in the heart as to cause him to weep and to cry out loudly, with obstruction of the respiration* (first eight days),[1].—*Pricking pain in the heart*, impeding respiration and the motion of the body (fourth day),[1].—Sensation of very annoying movement, from before backward, in the cardiac region,. as if a reptile were moving about in the interior; worse by day than by night (first ten days),[1].—On waking at night, and changing position, the heart symptoms were felt, as in the daytime,[6].—The heart symptoms are repeated very often to-day; when commencing to walk, they are often so violent that he must stand still, and inspire deeply several times; this also occurs on ascending steps quite slowly, and even on descending; so that the condition becomes somewhat annoying (third day),[6].—Later in the day,. the heart-symptoms again appeared, several times very violently, so that he had to stand still and inspire deeply, on which the heart's action became quiet and he could go on; this symptom was often noticed, also, on rising from a chair, etc.; and toward evening, even a sudden movement while sitting, was sufficient to cause several violent, irregular beats of the heart (fifth day),[6].—[220.] The pulse was hard and sudden, without being frequent (first day),[5].—Pulse completely lost, for many days, in a man affected with chronic hypertrophy of the heart; immediately after taking the remedy, the pulsation returns, *with an irregular rhythm, and intermitting, as before,*[1].

Back and Extremities in General.—Pain in the lower part of the muscles of the back on the right side, extending into the gluteals, in the morning before rising, continuing the whole day (third day),[5].—Toward evening, single violent pains in the limbs appear, but soon cease (second day),[6].—Drawing in the fingers, toes, knees, and ankles (fifth day),[6].

Upper Extremities.—After retiring, and before going to sleep, a drawing pain, for ten or fifteen minutes, in the left axilla and neighboring portion of the chest anteriorly, affecting the nerves,[7].—Sensation of great constriction in the shoulders, so that he could not move (fifth day),[1].—Tearing in the left shoulder-joint (6th dil.), (first day),[4].—Transient tearing pains in the joints, now in the shoulder, now in the elbows, now in the fingers, for the most part on the right side (fourth day),[5].—Painful weariness and heaviness of the arms (fifth and sixth days),[1].—[230.] Formication and weight in the arms, which cannot be raised freely; worse in the left arm,[1].—Pain in the muscles of the right upper arm, of the thorax, of the calves, of the soles of the feet, now and then during the day (second day),[5]. —Numbness of the left arm, and troublesome pricking in the little finger (first night),[5].—Tearing through the left arm (first day),[6].—A drawing-tearing in the right arm, early in the morning, on waking, and lasting through the forenoon; after rising, it extends into the right side (6th dil.), (second day),[4].—Œdema of the hands, worse in the left,[1].

Lower Extremities.—Great weariness and heaviness of the legs, and unusual sleepiness in the morning, on rising, after a quiet sleep, lasting about two hours (second day),[2].—Violent pain in the right knee, extending from the knee-cap to the outer side of the leg; the slightest motion of the leg increased the pain; it awoke him at night; lasted an hour (first night),[5]. —Pains in the knees and forehead, with necessity to inspire deeply, and single, irregular beats of the heart (after one hour).—Œdema of the legs up to the knees; the skin is shining, and pressure with the fingers leaves an impression for a long time),[1].—[240.] Œdema of the feet up to the inferior third of the legs, which soon goes off),[1].—Cramplike pain in the sole of the right foot, several times during the day, when walking (3d dil.), (third and fourth day),[3].

Generalities.—In the evening, the muscles did not accurately obey the will, whether owing to defective vision or other causes. Had noticeable ill-luck in performing accurately what he undertook in anything requiring precision, either on account of perfect sight or execution. Played a game of croquet very badly (second day),[7].—He cannot remain still when sitting; he throws his legs about here and there involuntarily,[1].—For several days, marked restlessness, and haste in his actions; he seemed to be too late everywhere, never to be in time, and always behindhand in his business; at the same time, agitation at the heart, with feeling of oppression,[6].— General weakness, so that he does not venture to speak,[1].—Great weakness for many successive days; he does not venture to walk at all,[1].—*Such great weakness, that he does not venture to do anything, not even to walk through the room,[1].—*General weakness,* with sadness and bad humor,[1].— Great corporeal depression; he does not trust himself to stand on his feet,[1]. [250.]—*Great prostration of strength,* so that he must remain in bed, not feeling able to use his legs,[1].—General discomfort (fifth day),[5].—General malaise, and such weakness as to be unable to rise from his seat,[1].

Skin.—Dry scaly herpes at the outside of the right elbow, without itching, of one and a half inches in breadth (thirtieth day),[1].—A similar dry, scaly, herpetic eruption on the outside of the left elbow (after forty-eight days),[1].—Dry scaly herpes, two inches broad, on the left internal malleolus, without itching (after twenty-four days),[1].—A similar dry, scaly herpes on the right internal malleolus (after thirty-eight days),[1].—Every evening very troublesome itching, like the stings of insects, on the chest and abdomen, compelling one to rub; relieved in bed on going to sleep; it was not noticed during the day (third to sixth day). The same itching appeared even during the day and disappeared at evening (two provings), (first day),[2].—Itching on the abdomen and on the calves in the evening on undressing (3d dil.), (second day),[3].—Very violent itching, causing him to scratch the lower part of the tibia (after twenty-one days),[1].—[**260.**] Violent itching on the ankles (twentieth day),[1].

Sleep and Dreams.—Slept well every night during the whole time of the proving,[8].—Sleepiness as after severe illness (fifth day),[5].—Felt rather drowsy, laid down early, and slept well all night with his clothes on (first day),[8].—At about daylight, undressed himself, and went to sleep again (second day),[8].—Awoke, feeling refreshed; in fact, better than usual (second day),[7].—Awoke, feeling splendidly (second day),[7].—Restless sleep at night (fifth day),[5].—The forepart of the night sleepless on account of rush of ideas, afterwards restless sleep (second night),[5].—Interrupted sleep at night; the next morning he feels fatigued, as if he had not slept at all (twentieth day),[1].—[**270.**] He cannot sleep in the first hours of the evening, and when then he falls asleep he awakens suddenly (first eight days),[1].—Sleeplessness in the evening and at night, from arterial pulsations in the scrobiculus and right ear (second night),[1].—Sleeplessness at night, without apparent cause (first night),[1].—Protracted sleeplessness during forty-eight hours, with pulsations in both ears (third day),[1].—Sleep disturbed by voluptuous dreams and painful erections (first night),[5].—Had an erotic dream, with emission of semen (second day),[8].

Fever.—Slight shivering, which passes off quickly towards 2 P.M. (first day),[1].—* *General chilliness,* so severe as to make the teeth chatter, which lasts three hours, and does not go off, although he lies down, and covers himself over with many blankets (first day),[1].—Great chilliness towards ten in the evening (first day),[1].—Great coldness at night, which lasts half an hour (first day),[1].—[**280.**] * *Coldness in the back and icy-cold hands,* which remained so for half an hour, although he took warm soup, and his face and hands became hot (after two and a half hours),[6].—Burning heat, which causes shortness of breath and madness, so that he cannot remain quiet in bed; this heat succeeds the chill of three hours' duration, and continues during twenty hours (first day),[1].—Scorching heat in the course of the night, with much pain in the head, great dyspnœa, and inability to remain lying (first day),[1].—Great heat in the head, and heat of the face, as if he had been before a strong fire, which causes madness and horrible anxiety (first day),[1].—Insupportable heat in the abdomen, as though something burned him internally (after two days),[1].—Copious perspiration, which follows the hot stage (first day),[1].—Slight fever and pain in the head, which develops itself after a very short chill; it lasts but a short time, and terminates with slight perspiration, at 4 P.M. (first day),[1].—* *Quotidian intermittent fever, which recurs every day at the same hour for many successive days.* At 1 P.M., a slight chill, then burning heat, dyspnœa, and very great pulsating pains in the uterine region, terminating in very slight perspiration. From 11 P.M. till 12 A.M., the next day, complete apyrexia (after thirteen days),[1].

Conditions.—Aggravation.—(*Morning*), After rising, pain in parietal bone; fetid breath; diarrhœa; early, on waking, tearing in right arm.—(*Toward evening*), Priapism; pains in limbs.—(*Evening*), Anxiety; pain in left forehead; itching on chest, etc.; on undressing, itching on abdomen, etc.; toward 10 o'clock, chilliness.—(*Night*), Delirium; sensation in brain; pain in temples; cough in bed, palpitation, etc.; when lying on left side, palpitation of heart; heat, etc.—(*Open air*), Oppression of breath.—(*Ascending stairs*), Short breathing; pain in chest.—(*After dinner*), Pulsation of cœliac artery.—(*Bright light*), Pain in forehead; pain in right side of head.—(*Lying on back*), *Palpitation of heart*, etc.—(*Lying on back, with head touching pillow*), Pain in occiput.—(*On occurrence of menstruation*), Palpitation of heart.—(*Motion*), *Constriction in sternum;* palpitation of heart.—(*Rapid motion*), Palpitation of heart.—(*Moving head*), Pain, etc.; in occiput.—(*Noise*), Pain in forehead; weight on vertex.—(*Periodical*), Pain in vertex; pains in umbilical region; *pains in uterus*, etc.; *attacks of suffocation;* fever.—(*Pressure*), Pains in region of heart.—(*Raising head from pillow*), Pain in side of head.—(*Rising from chair*), Beating of the heart.—(*In room*), Pressure in forehead.—(*Sound of talking*), Weight in vertex; pain in right side of head.—(*Touch*), Pain in left breast.—(*Turning suddenly*), Beating of the heart.—(*Walking*), Short breathing; oppression of breath; pain in chest; *beating of the heart;* palpitation of the heart; pain in right sole.—***Amelioration***.—(*Inspiring fresh air*), Is very reviving.—(*In bed*), On going to sleep, itching on chest, etc.—(*Bending head backward*), Drawing in occipital aponeurosis.—(*Quick exercise*), Pressure in occiput.—(*Deep inspiration*), Weight over the heart;° heart-symptoms.—(*Lying on side, so that occiput did not touch anything*), Pain in occiput.—(*Mental activity*), Pressure in occiput.—(*Pressure*), Sensation in temple, etc.; pain on vertex.—(*Gently raising the part*), Pain in breast.

CADMIUM SULFURATUM.

Sulphide of Cadmium (CdS).   *Preparation*, Triturations.

Authorities.   1, Petroz, pathogenesis, Jour. d. l. Soc. Gal. 5, 15 ; 2 Burdach, took half a grain at once, Hufeland's Jour., vol. 64, 1827 (Frank's Mag., 2, 771).

Mind.—Horror of solitude,[1].—Horror of work,[1].—Anxiety,[1].—Anxiety before going to stool,[1].—Apprehension at the approach of anybody,[1].—Excessive irritability,[1].

Head.—Inflammation of the brain,[1].—Apoplexy,[1].—Lancinations in the head,[1].—[10.] Hammering in the head,[1].—Tingling, digging, and drawing in the head,[1].—Pulsation in the temples,[1].—Pain in the vertex,[1].

Eye.—Scrofulous inflammation of the eyes,[1].—Cicatrix on the cornea,[1].—Hollow eyes,[1].—Blue circle around the eyes,[1].—Lancinations in the eyes from within outward,[1].—Rending pains in the eyes,[1].—[20.] Tension in the eyebrows,[1].—Pressure above the eyes,[1].—Burning lachrymation,[1].—Dilatation of one pupil, and contraction of the other,[1].—Inability to read small type,[1].—Hemeralopia,[1].

Ear.—Pressure behind the ears,[1].—Lancinations in the ears,[1].—Lacerating pain in the ears,[1].—Abnormal hearing, alternating with abnormal vision,[1].—[30.] Sounds echo in the head,[1].—Clucking in the ears,[1].

Nose.—Caries of the nose,[1].—Ulceration of the nostrils,[1].—Obstruction of the nose by swelling,[1].—Epistaxis,[1].—Numbness of the nose,[1].—Tightness at the root of the nose,[1].—Tension in the nose,[1].—Lacerating pain in the nose,[1].—[40.] Ulcerative smell,[1].—Cancerous smell,[1].

Face.—Gloomy countenance,[1].—Vexed look,[1].—Grayish complexion,[1].—Crawling sensation in the face,[1].—Yellow spots on the cheeks and nose,[1].—Swelling of the lips,[1].—Spasmodic motion of the upper lip,[1].—Trembling of the jaw,[1].

Mouth.—[50.] Salivation,[2].—Food tastes salt,[1].—Pitchy taste,[1].—The symptoms of the mouth are aggravated during deglutition,[1].

Throat.—Constriction of the œsophagus,[1].

Stomach.—Thirst. Thirst,[1].—In bed, at night, thirsty and hot,[1].—***Eructations.*** Rancid eructations, especially at noon,[1].—***Nausea and Vomiting.*** Nausea,[1].—Nausea at the chest, in the mouth, in the abdomen, generally accompanied with red face and trismus,[1].—[**60.**] Gagging and retching up of tough mucus, every few minutes,[2].—Vomiting,[1].—Vomiting food, bile, and mucus,[2].—Vomiting of acid matter, of black or yellowish matter, accompanied with cold sweat on the face, and griping,[1].—***Stomach.*** Violent pains in stomach and navel, and urging to stool,[2].—Burning pain in the stomach,[1].—Cutting pain in the stomach,[1].—Gastric symptoms aggravated during pregnancy; in drunkards; after cramps in the stomach; after drinking beer; in the forenoon,[1].—The symptoms of the stomach and hypochondria are aggravated by walking, or carrying burdens,[1].

Abdomen.—Lancinations in the left hypochondria,[1].—[**70.**] Inertia in the abdomen,[1].—Stretching pain in the abdomen,[1].—Compressed feeling in the abdomen,[1].—Pressure in the sides of the abdomen,[1].—Lancinations in the abdomen,[1].—Bruised pain in the abdomen,[1].—Pulsation in the abdomen,[1].—Griping in the lower bowels,[1].

Urinary Organs.—Griping in the region of the kidneys,[1].

Respiratory Organs.—Cough, with loss of consciousness, agitation, red face, pain in the stomach, or vomiting of bile,[1].—[**80.**] Interrupted breathing during sleep,[1].—On waking, want of air,[1].

Chest.—Swelling of the external chest,[1].—Inflamed nipples,[1].—Rheumatic pain in the external chest,[1].—Drawing in the external chest,[1].—Feeling as if the lungs adhered to the chest,[1].—Weakness of the chest,[1].—Feeling of dilatation in the chest,[1].—Contraction in the chest,[1].—[**90.**] Painful blows in the chest,[1].—Tingling in the chest,[1].—The chest symptoms are aggravated by a squatting posture,[1].

Heart.—Beating near the heart,[1].

Neck.—Pain in muscles of neck, as from the efforts to vomit,[2].

Superior Extremities.—Suppuration of the axillary glands,[1].—Stretching of the arms,[1].—Swelling of the arm-bones,[1].—Sensation of swelling of the arms,[1].—Tension in the forearm,[1].—[**100.**] Gnawing in the hands,[1].—Tearing pain in the metacarpal joints,[1].—Jerking of the fingers,[1].

Inferior Extremities.—Rheumatism of the lower limbs,[1].—Boring in the lower limbs,[1].—Digging in the lower limbs,[1].—Lancination in the joints of the lower limbs, and in the toes,[1].—Numbness of the thighs,[1].—Trembling in the knee,[1].—Cramps in the knee,[1].—[**110.**] Pressure in the knee,[1].—Tearing pain in the legs,[1].—Cramp of the calf,[1].—Pain as if sprained,[1].—While asleep, the feet are agitated by shocks,[1].—Heaviness of the feet,[1].—Chilblains,[1].

General Symptoms.—He lies with the head low, and the hands under it,[1].—Jactitations; startings of the limbs,[1].—Restlessness,[1].—[**120.**] Weakness after vomiting,[2].—Weakness of affected parts, with horripilation,[1].—Cutting pains in the joints,[1].

Skin.—Blueness of the skin,[1].—Red spots on the extremities,[1].—Brown spots on the chest,[1].—Brown spots on the elbow,[1].—Yellow eruption,[1].—Chronic eruption of the forehead, on the nose, and around the mouth,[1].—Aphthæ on the lips,[1].—[**130.**] Scaly, tearing, damp, suppurating herpes,[1].—Herpes on the temples,[1].—Erysipelatous inflammation of the nose,[1].—Erysipelas of the mammæ,[1].—Boils on the nose,[1].—Boils on the buttocks,[1].—In bed, at night, itching,[1].—Itching when touched, and during cold,[1].—Itching ameliorated by scratching, which excites a voluptuous feeling,[1].

Sleep and Dreams.—Sleepiness in the forenoon,[1].—[**140.**] Drowsiness when sitting,[1].—Somnolence, with broken dreams,[1].—He sleeps with his eyes open,[1].—Moaning and smiling during sleep,[1].—Nightmare,[1].

Fever.—Horripilation, after drinking,[1].—Horripilation, with hot hands,[1].—Coldness, even when near the fire,[1].—Icy coldness,[1].—Coldness after sleeping, and after walking,[1].—[**150.**] Coldness, with heat in the hands,[1].—Fever, before midnight,[1].—Sweat in the axillæ,[1].—Sweat in the palms,[1].

Conditions.—Aggravation.—(*Morning*), Symptoms in general.—(*Forenoon*), Symptoms in general; gastric symptoms; sleepiness.—(*Noon*), Eructations.—(*Night*), In bed, itching.—(*Before midnight*), Fever.—(*Open air*), Symptoms in general.—(*After exposure to a draft of air*), Symptoms in general.—(*Ascending stairs*), Symptoms in general.—(*Carrying burdens*), Symptoms of stomach and hypochondria.—(*Cool air*), Symptoms in general.—(*After cramps in stomach*), Gastric symptoms.—(*During deglutition*), Symptoms in general.—(*After drinking*), Horripilation.—(*After intoxication*), Symptoms in general.—(*Looking steadily*), Symptoms in general.—(*Lying down*), Symptoms in general.—(*Fit of passion*), Symptoms in general.—(*During pregnancy*), Gastric symptoms.—(*After reflection*), Symptoms in general.—(*After running*), Symptoms in general.—(*Sitting*), Symptoms in general; drowsiness.—(*After sleep*), Symptoms in general; coldness.—(*Squatting posture*), Chest symptoms.—(*In sunshine*), Symptoms in general.—(*Vexation*), Symptoms in general.—(*On waking up*), Symptoms in general.—(*Walking*), Symptoms in general; symptoms of stomach and hypochondria; coldness.

Amelioration.—(*While eating*), Symptoms in general.

CAINCA.

Chiococca racemosa (L.) Jacq. *Nat. order*, Rubiaceæ. *Preparation*, Tincture of the root.

Authorities. 1, Dr. Koch, took the infusion, A. Z. f. Hom., 2 (day-books, translated in N. Am. J. of Hom., 2, 50); 2, Wimer, ibid., took an infusion; 3, Ibid., a young man took 150 and 200 drops of the tincture; 4, Ibid., a young man took 100 to 700 drops of the tincture; 5, Ibid., the same prover took, at another time, 20 to 150 drops of the tincture; 6, Dr. Lippe took the 2d dilution.

Mind.—Feeling of anxiety, with increased warmth of the lower abdomen (soon after),[3].

Head.—**Vertigo.** Vertigo,[2].—Symptoms of giddiness and sickness (after four hours),[4].—On going upstairs, he became giddy,[5].—Giddiness, with vomiturition,[5].—**Sensations (in general).** Heaviness of the head,[2].—Very violent headache,[2].—Severe headache, particularly in the occiput, forbidding reading and every intellectual exertion,[6].—**Sensations (local).** Pressure in the sinciput,[4].—[**10.**] Darting pains in right half of sinciput,[4].—Forepart of the head uneasy,[4].—Heaviness, pressure, and uneasiness of front of head,[4].—Piercing pain in right temple (after four hours),[4].—Feeling of weight and pressure in occiput,[4].

Eye.—As his eyes gave him so much pain, as the sight was considerably impaired, and both upper eyelids began to be again œdematous, he found himself forced to give up taking the medicine, and to employ anti-dotes,[5].—Burning in the eyes,[6].—Increased sensibility of the eyes,[2].—*Lids.* Right lower eyelid œdematous, afterwards a minute pustular point was dis-cerned, which again disappeared,[4].—Œdema of left upper eyelid, lasting five days; it then became red and wrinkled, and there was considerable itchiness in it at intervals,[5].—*Ball.* [20.] Pressure in eyeballs,[5].—Pressure in the eyeballs from above downwards and from below upwards, with sensa-tion as if the eyeballs were pressed upwards, and the light fell only from above, with troubled vision for five minutes, returning after half an hour,[5]. —*Vision.* Photophobia (seventh to tenth days),[6].—On waking from afternoon sleep, he could not, for a quarter of an hour, see clearly in the open air, from a mist before the eyes (after eight hours),[4].—Before 12 o'clock, as it were clouds before the right eye (second day),[4].

Ear.—Intolerable hissing in the ears,[2].—Roaring and buzzing in the ears, as if from a swarm of insects in the air,[2].

Nose.—Violent catarrh of thin mucus, excoriating the nose, especially in the daytime (twelfth to eighteenth days),[6].

Face.—Heat of the face,[2].

Mouth.—Teeth. After dinner, obliged to clean the teeth of a great quantity of paplike mucus,[5].—[30.] In evening, tearing pains in the teeth of the upper jaw,[4].—*Tongue.* Tongue coated with mucus,[2].—Tongue furred white (seventh to sixteenth days),[6].—Tongue exceedingly dry, with a white and very dark coating,[2].—*General Mouth.* Offensive smell of the breath,[4].—On awaking, offensive smell of the mouth (second day),[4].—*Sa-liva.* While it was taken, there was considerable salivation,[1].—Saliva seemed no longer to be secreted,[2].—*Taste.* Taste perverted,[2].—Taste in the whole mouth like that of the sloe, bitter, the teeth set on edge,[2].—[40.] Mucous, insipid taste,[4].—Drug tasted like apple-wine, first sweetish, then bitter and burning,[2].

Throat.—Ulcers in the throat to the Eustachian tube (eighth, ninth, and tenth days),[6].—Inflammation of the throat (seventh day), with foul-smelling salivary flow (eighth, ninth, and tenth days),[6].—Distressing dry-ness in throat (soon after),[3].—Through the day, some roughness of the throat,[4].—Obliged to hawk often from irritation of the upper part of the throat,[5].—Burning and grating pain in throat,[2].—Rawness of throat, with taste like that of pepper in it,[4].—Rawness and dryness of throat, requiring frequent clearing of it,[4].—[50.] Grating feeling of rawness in throat, which afterwards became drier, so as to make him hawk (immediately),[4].—Grat-ing sensation in throat (after first dose), which increased more and more as the doses followed quickly on one another. If the doses are large and fre-quent, this feeling becomes so distressing that it might well drive one mad, if one were to take large quantities in the form indicated all through the day,[1].—Feeling of scraping in throat, forcing him to cough,[4].—*Pharynx.* Burning in the pharynx, at first with sensation as if from pepper,[4].—Dry burning heat in pharynx,[2].—Feeling of itchiness and scraping in pharynx and œsophagus,[4].—*Œsophagus and Swallowing.* Cold feeling down the œsophagus,[4].—Burning in the œsophagus while swallowing the tincture,[4].—Dysphagia beginning at the upper and back part of the throat,[5].

Stomach.—Appetite and Thirst. In the evening, appetite good,[4].—[60.] Absence of appetite,[2].—Less appetite than usual for dinner,[5]. —No appetite for supper,[1].—Thirst,[2].—*Eructations.* Eructations,[4].— Eructations, as after small doses of tartar emetic,[2].—Much tasteless eruc-tation, dryness of the throat, trembling of the hands,[4].—*Nausea and*

Vomiting. Slight qualms (after half an hour),[5].—Some nausea,[4].—Constant vomiturition,[2].—[**70.**] Vomiturition and slight shivering, for half an hour (after each dose),[2].—Violent vomiting (from three spoonfuls); it soon abated, however (second day),[1].—*Stomach.* Much wind came off the stomach,[4].—Feeling of cold in the epigastric region,[4].

Abdomen.—Hypochondria. Stitches in and through the spleen,[4]. *—Umbilical.* Felt a degree of warmth about the umbilicus,[2].—Pain under the umbilicus, with desire to go to stool,[4].—*General Abdomen.* Fulness of the abdomen (second day),[4].—Although a stool had already been passed, the abdomen soon became full and distended,[4].—Fulness of the abdomen, with inclination to vomit, and turgescence at upper part, increased by clearing the throat,[5].—[**80.**] Inflation and uncomfortable feeling in the abdomen, with tenderness to touch, especially under the umbilicus,[4]. —After eating, perceptible pulsation of abdominal aorta during rest,[4].— Rumbling in bowels,[4].—Gurgling and rumbling in the abdomen,[4].—Towards evening, some wind passed without relief,[4].—Slight pains in abdomen,[4].—Slight pinching pains in belly,[4].—Slight colic, with borborygmus,[2]. —Cuttings in the abdomen (second day),[4].—After breakfast and dinner, cutting abdominal pains (second day),[4].—[**90.**] Cutting pains in abdomen before evacuation of the bowels,[4].—Cuttings in abdomen, with calls to make water (after four hours),[4].—Tenderness of the abdomen on touching it and bending backward (after four hours),[4].—*Hypogastrium.* Hypogastrium swollen (after one hour),[5].—Hypogastrium distended, but soft,[4].

Rectum and Anus.—Inclination to go to stool, with pressure at the anus,[4].—Frequent calls to stool, with escape of nothing but air (soon after),[3].—Burning at the anus (second day),[5].—In the evening on lying down to sleep, lively tickling in the anus, obliging him to scratch frequently,[4].

Stool.—Fecal evacuations increased, occurring two or three times a day, of semifluid consistence, yellow color, preceded by cutting pains in the belly, but moderate and of short continuance,[3].—[**100.**] Fecal diarrhœa (after four hours). In about nine hours the diarrhœa returned, followed by rumbling in bowels,[4].—Three stools between morning and midday, first hard, then softer like pap, and less highly colored (second day),[5].— Two soft dark-colored stools in the day,[4].—Immediately after rising, a copious, soft stool (second day),[4].—After dinner, a soft stool,[4].—Stool delayed till 2 P.M., then natural; some partially digested food was evacuated at the same time (second day),[4].—After increased colicky pains, fecal diarrhœal stool, mixed with many small air-bubbles (after six and eight hours),[4].— Paplike stool, followed by short colicky pains, which returned periodically throughout the day, never lasting more than half a minute (after a quarter of an hour),[4].—A somewhat hard stool (he was previously constipated),[1].— Scanty stool, followed by itching at the anus (after eight hours),[4].

Urinary Organs.—Urethra. [**110.**] Slight feeling of uneasiness, while the desire to pass urine continued (second day),[1].—Burning in the glandular portion of the urethra,[5].—Constant desire to micturate (first day),[1].—*Micturition.* In the morning, difficulty in making water, afterwards accompanied by burning in the glandular portion of the urethra; at noon with burning at the orifice of the urethra, and unremitting desire to make water (second day),[5].—Passed much urine, though he had done so twice in the afternoon,[1].—8.30 A.M., a pretty large quantity of urine was passed, though this had been done already at 7 o'clock (after a few minutes),[1].—The evacuation of urine had taken place three times to a considerable amount; and then had set in an increasing nisus to make water without any uneasiness (second day),[1].—Another discharge of urine, which was passed in tolerably large quantity, and of a lighter tint than the first (after half an hour),[1].—A good deal of colorless water passed (second day),[1].—Scanty evacuation of urine, which was of a dingy brown, exciting burning heat in the urethra, almost with strangury,[4].—[120.] Urinary secretion not increased, but frequently evacuated,[2].—Urine passed with erection of the penis, fiery, and causing a burning pain in the urethra (soon after),[3].—*Urine.* Polyuria of some months' duration disappeared (on the tenth day),[6].—Renal secretion still abundant, and clearer in color (after eight days),[1].—Urine not increased, but darker in color,[4].—Urine through the day is strongly saline; has an animal smell, not unlike sausage-soup,[5]. —The urine had the disgusting taste of the root,[1].

Sexual Organs.—In the evening, continual drawing in the testicles and spermatic cord, with flaccidity of the scrotum, and feeling as if it were enlarged, after half an hour, with pain, such as to make him go to bed unusually early. During the passing of the urine, which had a pungent smell, the pains increased (third day),[5].—Horridly excited sexual impulses, for a week after,[6].—In the night he had fearfully lascivious dreams, with erections, restlessness, and was finally awaked towards morning by an emission (second day),[6].

Respiratory Organs.—Larynx and Trachea. [130.] Inclination to cough,[4].—Accumulation of easily detached portions of mucus in the trachea (seventh to twelfth day),[6].—Violent heat in the trachea (seventh to tenth day),[6].—*Voice.* Hoarseness,[4].—Voice hoarse and hollow,[2]. —Hoarseness and roughness (seventh to tenth day),[6].—Hoarseness, vomiturition, and colic ceased after the occurrence of diarrhœa (after thirty hours),[2]. —Aphonia (eighth to ninth day),[6].—*Cough.* Tickling cough, with tough greenish-gray expectoration, waking him at 3 A.M. (twelfth to eighteenth day),[6].

Chest.—Constriction of the chest,[4].—[140.] Constriction of chest (after four hours),[4].—Constriction and pressure on chest,[4].—Peculiar shooting and beating pain over the trunk,[2].—*Sides.* Piercing pain in middle part of right side of chest,[4].—Dartings in middle third of right side of thorax,[4].— Pricking pain in lower third of right side of chest, with feeling of weight there (after five hours),[4].

Heart and Pulse.—Tension in the præcordia, which did not prevent him, however, from moving about,[5].—Pulse accelerated during the whole day, especially after the siesta,[4].—The pulse, though increased in frequency to 55, was quite uniform (second day),[1].—Pulse full, rather than accelerated,[2].—[150.] Pulse 54 (after a few minutes),[1].—Pulse became small, and sank to 50 (second day),[1].

Superior Extremities.—Pricking pain in left hand,[4].

Inferior Extremities.—Stretching of lower limbs,[4].—Heaviness of the lower limbs,[4].—*Feet and Toes.* Feeling of lassitude in soles of feet,[5].—Constant pressure in the lower third of the under part of right foot,[4].—Acute pricking under nail of great toe,[4].

General Symptoms.—Slight uneasiness (after a few minutes),[1].— Weakness,[4].—[160.] After dinner, weakness so as to make him lie down,[5].

Sleep and Dreams.— Sleepiness. Yawning,[4]. — *Yawning;* stretching of the limbs, with cramplike feeling of the lower extremities,[4].— Sleepiness in morning,[4].—Somnolence,[4].—Yielded to his desire to sleep (after eight hours),[4].—*Sleeplessness.* Sleepless during the whole night,[2]. —Sleep very restless, with lascivious dreams,[6].

Fever.—Heat. Heightened temperature of the body,[5].—Warmth all over the body,[2].—*Sweat.* [170.] Moist skin; sweating even when at rest (second and third days),[2].—He perspired more easily than usual with him,[4]. —In the evening, he sweated all over on moving in the least, and in the cold,[5].

Conditions.—Aggravation.—(In daytime), Catarrh.—(*Morning*), Difficulty in making water, etc.—(*Afternoon*), 4 to 6 o'clock, symptoms in general.—(*Toward evening*), Passage of wind.—(*Evening*), Pains in upper teeth; on lying down to sleep, tickling in anus; sweat.—(*Ascending stairs*), Giddiness.—(*After breakfast*), Abdominal pains.—(*Clearing throat*), Turgescence of upper abdomen.—(*After dinner*), Mucus on teeth; abdominal pains; drawing in testicles, etc.; weakness.—(*After siesta*), Pulse accelerated.—(*On waking*), From afternoon sleep, mist before eyes.

Amelioration. —(Evening), Appetite good. — (*After diarrhœa*), Hoarseness, etc., ceased.

CAJUPUTUM.

Oleum Cajuputi (obtained by distillation of the leaves of Melaleuca leucadendron, L.). *Natural order,* Myrtaceæ.

Authority. Dr. C. Ruden, Hahn. Month., 6, 66, proving of 6 to 10 drops of the oil.

Mind.—Feeling as if I did not want any one to speak to me (after twenty-four hours).—Do not want to be spoken to; feel better in the society of ladies; do not like to talk with the men, but can laugh and make free with the women (am naturally bashful), (after two hours).—Feel sad and down-hearted, as if I could cry (after two hours).

Head.—Frontal headache, especially in the eyes, worse on bending forward (third day).

Eye.—Pain in the right eye (after two hours).—" He looks around the eyes as if he had taken too much liquor."—Pain over the left eye (after six hours).—Sticking pain above the orbital arches, relieved by pressing the hand on the parts, worse on removing the hand (after ten minutes).—Could not see on going out of doors; rubbed his eyes to bring sight (at midnight).

Nose.—[10.] Nose is most prominent; it looks as if it were large and extending out from the face, on looking down.

Face.—Sensation of burning in the face (had same sensation last night).—Pain through the left malar bone (after six hours).

Mouth.—Tongue looks white and rough; feels as if it were scalded, and as if the skin would peel off; it looks like a calf's tongue.—Tongue moist, feels as if scalded, looks white and rough.—Much water in the mouth; want to spit a great deal (after twenty-one hours).—Taste in the mouth between sour and bitter (after twenty-one hours).—Always had salty taste, *now* have sweetish taste (after twenty-one hours).

Throat.—Burning in the throat down to the stomach.

Stomach.—Some appetite, but when I get what I had previously desired, then I do not want it (after twenty-four hours).—[20.] No appetite. —No appetite (after one hour).—No appetite (after twenty-one hours).— No appetite (second day).—No thirst (after one hour).—No thirst (second day).—Nausea.—Smoking tobacco makes me feel like vomiting (after twenty-one hours).

Abdomen.—Griping pain in the bowels on riding.

Rectum and Anus.—Itching around the anus.

Stool.—[30.] Diarrhœa, watery, yellowish, although while taking the medicine I was costive (second day).—Diarrhœa by day, *and worse by night;* bowels moved about ten times (second day).

Urinary Organs.—Passed water, the first for thirty hours (after eighteen hours).—Urine dark-red, and smells like that of cats (after eighteen hours).

Sexual Organs.—Erections, with great desire for an embrace (after four hours).

Chest.—Pain across the chest (after one hour).—Soreness across the chest, with pain in the left shoulder (after one hour).—The lungs felt loose and that I must hold them together by pressing on them, on riding (after ten hours).—Pain in the right side below the ribs.—Pain in the right lung.

Heart and Pulse.—[40.] Pulse 74.—Pulse 70.

Extremities in General.—Joints feel enlarged, with some pain (after twenty-one hours).

Superior Extremities.—Sensation in the arms, as if they were tied to the body, especially the left one (after one hour).—Left arm feels as if it were out of joint; cannot raise it without pain (after two hours).—A pain, as if the joints were enlarged, in both shoulders (after twenty-one hours).—Pressure on the inside of shoulder-joint gives sharp pain, which seems to act most on the left side (after two hours).

Lower Extremities.—Weakness and pain in both knees, so that it was with great difficulty that I could walk, on going to supper. Went to bed without supper, and was better on lying down.—Stitching pains through both knees, on rising in bed (never had such pains before), lasting quarter of an hour (at midnight).

General Symptoms.—Languid.—[50.] Tired and sleepy.—Felt as though I could not get myself together, and could not find my clothes for some time, although they were quite near; better in the open air, at 10 P.M.—Feel all over as if poisoned (after twenty-one hours).

Skin.—An eruption as thick as measles, all over the arms and body, and upper portion of the legs (third day).—Intense itching, aggravated by scratching, lasting two hours (after five hours).

Sleep and Dreams.—Wanted to sleep with his arms locked under his head, for the first time.—Sleep, with amorous dreams, without emissions.

Fever.—Feels cold, and cold sweat all over the body (after one hour).—Very (uncommonly) profuse and weakening sweat.

Conditions.—*Aggravation.*—(*Night*), *Diarrhœa.*—(*On bending forward*), Frontal headache.—(*On riding*), Pain in bowels; loose feeling in lungs, etc.—(*Scratching*), Itching.

Amelioration.—(*In open air*), Felt as though he could not get himself together, etc.—(*In society of ladies*), Feels better.—(*Lying down*), Weakness, etc.—(*Pressure*), Pain above orbital arches.

CALADIUM.

Caladium seguinum, Vert. (Arum seguinum, Linn.) *Nat. order,* **Araceæ.** *Preparation,* Tincture of the root.

Authorities. 1, Hering, Archiv f. Hom. Hielk., 11, 2, 161;† 2, Schreter, Neu. Archiv., 3, 3, 153, proving with the 30th dil.; 3, Dr. Chairou, L'Union, 1863 (Schmidt's Jahrb., 119, 289), case of poisoning by the root; 4, Berridge, Am. J. Hom. M. M., 8, 126, a man proved the 200th dil.; 5, ibid., a woman proved the 200th dil.

Mind.—Emotional. Extreme excitement,³.—Loud cries about an illness, like a child, with inconsiderate prattlings, after many days,¹.—He is very apprehensive about his health, and about everything apprehensive and anxious (after a fever, for several weeks),¹.—Apprehensiveness, before going to sleep,¹.—Fear of cutting himself while shaving (eleventh day),².—Becomes easily angry at everything,¹.—*Intellectual.* Very forgetful; he cannot remember if what he ought to have done and written during the day is really accomplished until he convinces himself of it,².

Head.—Confusion and Vertigo. Confusion and whirlings in the head,¹.—Vertigo, after some walking (second day),².—[10.] Vertigo and nausea, in the morning, with stitches in the pit of the stomach (after fourteen days),¹.—*Sensations.*—Occasional heat in the head,².—Heat ascends from below into the head and becomes an internal glowing heat (after two hours),¹.—Pressive headache after the midday sleep, or after lying on the side; disappears when sitting,¹.—Drawing-tearing, extending to the head,².—Bursting headache, especially in the forehead (sixth day),².—*Forehead.* Boring pain in the forehead,².—*Temples.* Boring and sticking in the left temple, relieved by pressure,².—On waking, stupefying pressure in the right temples (fifth day),².—Sticking in the right temple, especially in the right eye,².—*Occiput.* [20.] Drawing in the occiput (first day),².—*External.* Pimples on the hairy scalp behind the ear, sensitive when touched,².

Eye.—Burning in the eyes,¹.—Sensitive, stupefying pressure in the eyes and forehead, with heat in the face, and restlessness he can hardly control, while smoking tobacco; followed by much hawking of mucus and slimy vomiting, with urgency to stool,².—The eyes close from sleepiness before dinner, with tension in the temples (second day),².—Pressure in the eyeballs, with painful sensitiveness when touching them, soon after rubbing his abdomen with Calad. (fifth day),².

Ear.—Sensations. Pains in the ear, during a fever (after seventh day),¹.—Burning on the external upper margin of the ears, without redness or heat (fifth day),².—Throbbing in the right ear, and a sensation around it as if warm water were flowing about it in a circle (after five days),².—Tickling and itching in the right ear, evenings,².—*Hearing.* [30.] Extremely sensitive to noise, especially if he wishes to sleep (after three, four days),¹.—When going to sleep he is waked by the folding of paper; he is sensitive to it (fifth day),².—Something seems to be put before the ears which makes him deaf,¹.—Twittering in the ears,².—Roaring in the ears, frequently during the day,².

Nose.—Sudden burning in the upper part of the nose, then a long-continuing irritation to sneezing, and at last violent, as from pepper; short sneezing, followed by fluent coryza (in the evening), (first day),¹.

---

† 1 began with half a drop, and experienced most of the symptoms a few hours after taking it, or during the day; those that appeared later I have always marked with the number of the day; larger doses produced no more symptoms than the smaller, only more severe. An exceedingly healthy feeling appeared after twelve or twenty-four hours; all the symptoms seemed to disappear, but they always returned again; in many provers on the fourteenth day there were quite new symptoms.

Face.—Biting-burning stitches in the cheek,[1].

Mouth.—Teeth. After vomiting, the teeth seem too long; insipid taste on the tongue, herbaceous, with a scratchy sensation in the throat, as of something sharp (second day),[2].—Toothache, mornings and evenings,[2].—Toothache, in the evening, that wakes him from his sleep again in the morning,[2].—[40.] Boring toothache, with stitches in the ear,[2].—Drawings through the left back teeth from above downward (after a few hours),[1].—*General Mouth.*—Mucous membrane of the mouth uniformly very red; the curtains of the palate exceedingly red, not swollen; the uvula slightly swollen,[3].—The mouth is sticky and herby (after several hours),[1].—Burning in the mouth and fauces,[3].—Sensation in the mouth as if burnt with creasote,[2].—*Taste.* Milk tasted sour and was repugnant,[3].—*Throat.* Scratchy in the throat, with dry sensation, with much hawking of mucus,[2].—Tickling in the throat, with cough (after one hour), often renewed during the day,[2].—Dryness in the fauces and pharynx, not in the mouth, without thirst, and with *aversion to cold water* (after one and several hours),[1].

Stomach.—Appetite and Thirst. [50.] Sensation of hunger, soon after taking,[2].—Evenings, after the theatre, he is hungry, contrary to custom, but eats nothing; nausea in the morning while half asleep, a sensation like faintness, as if he had over eaten and must vomit; when fully awake this sensation ceased (second day),[2].—Takes his breakfast with hunger and relish, but is hardly satisfied when he becomes discouraged and uncomfortable; head exceedingly confused, and he grows sleepy (fifth day),[2].—Has great desire to smoke, and relishes it uncommonly (fourth day),[2].—He only eats because the stomach is so hollow, without hunger, but very hastily, and is immediately satisfied,[1]. —Thirst, with dry lips, wakes him at night,[1].—Longing for beer, without decided thirst; he was not able to drink water throughout the proving,[1].—Does not drink the whole day,[1].—After eating, he drank only because it seemed so dry in the stomach, which sensation could not be called thirst; it was quite different from it,[1].—*Eructations and Hiccough.* *Frequent eructations of very little wind, as if the stomach were full of dry food* (after twelve hours),[1].†—[60.] Incomplete eructations, because they are hindered by burning pressure in the abdomen,[1].—Hiccough continues for some time,[2].—*Nausea.* After, and while smoking his accustomed tobacco, nausea and inclination to vomit,[2].—While smoking a cigar, sudden inclination to vomit; he must stop smoking; at the same time urgency to stool, so that he thought he could scarcely retain it, yet is obliged to strain hard to get rid of the pappy yellow stool (second day),[2].—Nausea, with confusion of the head,[1].—*Stomach.*—Pain deep, internally, when pressing on the pit of the stomach (after several hours),[1].—A constant sensation as if a bird were fluttering in the stomach and trying to escape, causing nausea in the stomach, but without retching, from morning till afternoon (very soon),[5].—Burning in the stomach, which is not relieved by drinking (after one hour); it continues the whole evening after drinking tea and chocolate (several hours after eating),[1].—Dull internal burning in the stomach and upper part of the abdomen; at last it becomes a very severe pressure, extending upward under the breast, and then a gnawing, in the orifice of the stomach, which prevents deep breathing and eructations (after several hours),[1].—[70.] Pressure in the pit of the stomach impedes respiration and causes cough,[1].—Cuttings, as with glass, across the pit of the stomach,[1].—

† From this characteristic, Caladium cured several asthmatic attacks.—C. Hg.

Cuttings in the pit of the stomach and in the left flank; disturbed him at midnight so that he could no more sleep,[1].—Stitches, as with needles, deep in the pit of the stomach,[1].—Stitches in the pit of the stomach, which is drawn inward with every stitch; worse when sitting; it makes him weak and nauseated (Ignatia relieves),[1].—Throbbing in the pit of the stomach, after walking; it makes him very tired,[1].

Abdomen.—Hypochondria. Stitches, jerkings, and pressure in the region of the spleen,[1].—*Umbilical.* Spasmodic cutting in the abdomen, at the navel; must bend himself double,[1].—*General Abdomen.* Abdomen very hard, distended, painful to pressure,[3].—Scanty, offensive flatus,[1].—[80.] Felt, three or four times, a sensation as if a long worm were writhing in the region of transverse colon or transverse duodenum,[4].—He eats a sour plum that does not agree with him, and is followed by a drawing in the abdomen; he begins to smoke a cigar, which he is at once obliged to lay aside, as it causes nausea and inclination to vomit, although he has only taken a few whiffs; soon after, the inclination to vomit is increased, and followed by a corrosive, acid vomiting, with much mucus, and a part of some cocoa he had taken; he is hungry not long after, and eats bread and butter with relish (second day, forenoon),[2].—If the pain extends into the abdomen it leaves behind a dull pressure,[1].—Sudden twisting pain in the abdomen, in the evening (first day),[1].—The abdomen is painful to touch, especially the region of the bladder (one hour),[1].—Violent throbbing, especially on the right side, above the navel,[1].—Violent pulsating in the upper part of the abdomen,[1].

Rectum and Anus.—Sticking in the rectum,[2].—Stitches as of knives, in the rectum (first day),[2].—Stitches in the rectum, soon after stool (second day),[2].—[90.] Mornings, urgency to stool; passage of noisy flatus at first; is compelled to strain hard to eject the soft pappy stool (second day),[2].

Stool.—Diarrhœa. Frequent desire for a soft, pasty, yellow stool (first day),[2].—Seven stools, at first watery, afterward thicker (three hours),[1].—Soft stool, after one hour, followed by passage of blood; later, moving about, and burrowing in the abdomen; hæmorrhoidal symptoms, an hour after a second stool, with passage of blood after the evacuation (after two hours),[2].—Soft stool, yellow, pasty; he was scarcely dressed after the movement before he was obliged to go again (third day),[2].—Mucus passes after the stool, and later, a thin fluid flows from the anus (for three days),[2].—After stool, thin red blood passes in considerable quantities,[2].—*Constipation.* Stool omits the first day, with a feeling of diarrhœa, in the evening,[1].—*Very scanty pasty stool,*[1].

Urinary Organs.—Bladder. Region of the bladder painful to touch; without desire to urinate, the bladder seems as if full, followed by moderate urination,[1].—[100.] Spasmodic drawing sidewise, from the bladder towards the penis, or deep behind and near the bladder,[1].—*Urethra.* Burning in the urethra, with and without urinating (sixth day),[2].—Stitches in the urethra, evenings (after third day),[2].

Sexual Organs.—Sexual organs seem larger, as if puffed, relaxed and sweating; the skin of the scrotum seems thicker than usual (after two hours),[1].—Glans very red, covered with fine red points, very dry, which causes a desire to rub it; the prepuce is very much swollen along its margin, sore and very painful (after second day),[1].—Prepuce swollen, sore on the margin, with biting on urinating, compelling him to rub it frequently,[1].—After coition, the prepuce remains retracted, does not cover the glans, with pain and swelling,[1].—Sore corrosive pain on the prepuce,[1].—The symptoms of the prepuce soon disappear after Mercurius 2d, but they return the same as ever after coition, and continue for two months,[1].—Erection mornings, without any desire (eighth day),[2].—[110.] Erections, when half asleep, mornings, that ceased when fully awake,[2].—An erection in the morning and cohabits, but suddenly his desire ceased, and he did not know if there was an emission or not,[2].—Painful erections, without sexual desire; it alternates one morning with desire, with relaxed penis,[1].—Incomplete erection; it seems as though it were broken, with which the semen emits too soon,[1].—No erection, even after amorous caresses (first day),[2].—Impotency ; the penis remains relaxed during excitement and sexual desire (first night),[1]. —Dull burrowing in the penis,[1].—During an embrace, no emission and no orgasm; penis less hard than usual,[1].

Respiratory Organs.—Larynx. The epiglottis and adjacent parts decidedly swollen, and exceedingly painful to pressure,[3].—*Larynx and trachea seem constricted, so that it impedes deep breathing; *and the attacks of cough seem to originate above the larynx*,[1].—[120.] When asked where he suffered, he pointed to his larynx, then to his mouth, and lastly to his stomach,[3].—He desires to cough, but the heaviness in the pit of the stomach will not permit it,[1].—*Voice.* He was unable to speak a word, apparently on account of the swelling of the vocal cords, or on account of the continual cough,[3].—*Cough.* Weak, toneless cough ; at night, prevents sleep ; continues the next morning,[1].—Incessant cough of a hoarse sound,[3].— The cough was not spasmodic, was without expectoration, and aggravated if he attempted to speak a word,[3].—Cough in slight, weak, sensitive paroxysms, with expectoration of small lumps of mucus,[1].—Continued weak cough ; after the expectoration of lumps of mucus, the chest seems hollow and empty,[1].—*Respiration.* Respiration very incomplete, inspiration catching ; on inspiration, the sinking in of the pit of the stomach was very noticeable,[3].—Respiration difficult and oppressed ; he grasped his throat with his hand every moment,[3].

Chest.—[130.] On straightening up, cracking below the last ribs, as if they had been dislocated and snapped back again,[1].—Oppression of the chest, with burning in the stomach ; the oppression also continues afterwards,[1].—Dull sticking in the right side of chest, with oppression ; worse on the left, better when lying on the right side, evenings, in bed (fourth day),[2].—Pressive sticking in the left side of the chest, near the sternum,[2].— Stitches, in a small spot between the left nipple and shoulder, as with needles, very deep internally, without influencing respiration or motion,[1].— Stitches in the chest, in the evening,[1].

Heart and Pulse.—A peculiar throbbing below the heart, not palpitation, only perceptible on applying the hand,[1].—Hard, full, jerking pulse (after six hours),[1].

Back.—Stitches in the back, as if from incarcerated flatus (forenoon, sixth day),[2].—The sacral region and back feel bruised ; in the morning, on rising,[1].—[140.] Pains in the sacrum, mornings, a kind of weakness, as if he had not sufficient strength in the sacrum; stitches even on certain movements, especially when walking,[2].—Boring and burrowing in the sacrum and anus (sixth day),[2].

Superior Extremities.—Drawing-pinching pains between the bones of the forearm, and behind the tendo Achillis,[1].—Feeling in palms, like pins and needles, similar to what is felt when the ulnar nerve is struck, or, by some people, when looking down from a height ; this lasted till sleep, causing her to rub them hard, towards evening (second day),[5].—All the fingers felt very large, like sausages; she could not use them well; they felt as if they were going to be paralyzed; this lasted till middle of the next day (first day),[5].

Inferior Extremities.—Sudden violent pain in the left knee, as if it would be torn asunder; it cracks on stepping, preventing walking (second day),[1].—Cramp in the soles, at night,[1].—When standing, his knees feel weak and tremble; is obliged to sit down,[2].—Sticking in a corn (first day),[2].—Stitches in a corn of the left little toe (after five minutes),[2].- - [150.] Stitches in a corn, left foot, and in the left eye, often during the day,[2].

General Symptoms.—Restless during the forenoon, not inclined to anything, afterwards very busy and forgetful,[2].—Dread of motion; wishes to lie down the whole time, though he is strong enough when he makes an effort,[1].—Must lie down and close the eyes, when it seemed as if he were rocked (after four hours),[1].—Faintness after writing, when reflecting, lying, and on rising up,[1].—Stitches, as from insect-bites, pain very much; they itch and burn afterwards,[1].—Evenings, after eating fish pickled in vinegar, feeling unwell, discomfort, and distension of the abdomen; relieved when walking, worse when driving (seventh day),[2].—Throbbing in the abdomen, after internal heat; very much prostrated (after three hours),[1].

Skin.—Eruptions, Dry. Nettle-rash eruption on the chest; it alternates with asthma, for several weeks,[1].—Nettle-rash on the inner side of the forearm, consisting of very red pimples, which itch and burn very much, after three to four days, when it disappears, immediately; *great oppression of the chest, so that he could scarcely get the breath, as if mucus would suffocate him,* without anxiety; especially after eating, and after a midday nap,[1].—[160.] Painful pimples on the septum of the nose, in the right nostril,[2].—Pimples on the mons veneris, and on the left ear,[2].— *Moist.* Rash, with white vesicles, on the wrist, forearm, and elbow; it itches in the heat, at night, burns internally after scratching, the twelfth day. Carbo relieves it for some time,[1].—*Pustular.* White, suppurating pimples, with red areolæ, appear here and there on the body, with an itching sensation, sore to the touch (after seven days),[2].—A carbuncle had formed on the buttock, that pained him severely, when sitting. When the external application of Calad. was discontinued, the pain of the carbuncle ceased,[2].—*Sensations.* On the skin, especially in the face, frequent sensations, as if a fly were crawling there,[2].—Sudden, violent, corrosive burning frequently in small places in the skin, on the cheeks, nose, toes, and in other places; obliges touching, always on the right side (without any contact with the juice of the plant), (after one hour),[1].—Stitches in the skin of the forehead, as if with needles,[2].—Itching of the fingers, especially when lying down at night,[2].

Sleep and Dreams.—Sleepiness. Sleepy very early in the evening; cannot keep awake,[1].—Grows sleepy and fretful again at 7 in the morning, and would like to return to bed,[2].—Sleepy in the morning, after rising; his eyes close while walking in the open air, with nausea and qualmishness in the stomach, like a sensation of emptiness, with weakness and prostration in the knees,[2].—*Sleeplessness.* [170.] He is obliged to lie down during the day, but is unable to sleep; he shivers, and is dizzy,[1].—Cannot get asleep till 1 at night (second day),[2].—Sleep at night restless, with confused dreams,[1].—Restless night, with heat; is obliged to uncover, with light sleep, like slumber. Excessive erections, at 4 in the morning, without desire; deep sleep towards 6 o'clock, so that he can scarcely rouse himself, with vivid dreams of persons whom he has not seen for years,[2].—Everything troubles him in sleep,[1].—[**180.**] *He groans and moans anxiously in sleep,* so that he wakes the neighbors several times in the night, and for several nights,[1].—Violent starting in sleep,[1].—*Dreams.* During a confused sleep, everything comes to his mind which he had forgotten while awake,[1].—Very clear, vivid dreams,[1].—Restless, anxious dreams,[2].—Dreams of dead persons, and events of past years, so vivid that when he awakes, he falls asleep again directly, and continues to dream of them,[2].

Fever.—Chilliness. Chilly in the evening, without thirst; coldness extends from the abdomen to the feet; they are icy cold, as also are the fingers,[1].—Chilliness over the back and whole body, with drawing pains in the left little finger, that feels as if full and gone to sleep, besides a pulled, stretched sensation in the whole body (second day),[2].—*Heat.* Fever the ninth day; heat with thirst, in the evening, till midnight; it again wakes him, when it disappears,[1].—Fever after seven days; heat with thirst; violent pain in the ear; swollen submaxillary glands, and constipation,[1].—Internal feverish heat, exhausting sweat, as from oppressive heat (after one hour),[1].—Internal fever disappears during sleep,[1].—Heat of the hands, face, and abdomen, with cold feet before midnight; after midnight, the abdomen is cold, the feet hot, without thirst,[1].—[**190.**] Heat before midnight, chill after midnight,[1].—Heat after the midday sleep, then sweat, then chill in the open air,[1].—Fever on the twelfth and thirteenth days; in the evening, till midnight, coldness with thirst, catching in the chest, therewith he feels sleepy; it wakes him again about midnight, and then disappears, together with throbbing in the chest and coryza (Ignatia cured),[1].—*Sweat.* Perspiration toward evening, with prostration, yawning, and sleepiness (sixth day),[2].—On account of perspiration after heat, flies trouble him very much, being allured by the sweat (first day and afterwards),[1].—Excessive perspiration on the scrotum (after five days),[2].—The sweat relieved all the symptoms (first day),[1].

Conditions.—Aggravation.—(*Morning*), Vertigo, etc.; till afternoon, sensation in stomach; urgency to stool, etc.; erections; on rising, small of back, etc., feel bruised; pains in sacrum; 7 o'clock, sleepy, etc.—(*Forenoon*), Restless, etc.—(*Toward evening*), Perspiration.—(*Evening*), Tickling, etc., in ear; hungry; pain in abdomen; stitches in rectum; sticking in side of chest, etc.; stitches in chest; after eating pickled fish, feels unwell, etc.; chilly; till midnight, heat, etc.—(*Night*), Thirst, etc.; cramp in the soles; when lying down, itching of the fingers.—(*Midnight*), Cutting in pit of stomach, etc.—(*After coition*), Symptoms of the prepuce return.—(*Driving*), Feeling unwell, etc.—(*After eating*), Oppression of chest.—(*Lying*), Faintness.—(*After lying on side*), Headache.—(*When reflecting*), Faintness.—(*On rising up*), Faintness.—(*After the siesta*), Headache; oppression of chest.—(*Sitting*), Stitches in pit of stomach.—(*Sleep*), During the day, all the symptoms.—(*Before going to sleep*), Apprehensive.—(*Attempting to speak*), Cough.—(*After stool*), Sticking in the rectum; mucus passes.—(*Tobacco smoking*), Pressure in eyes, etc.; cramp in the soles; when lying down, itching of the fingers.—(*Walking*), Vertigo; throbbing in pit of stomach; stitches in the sacrum.—(*After writing*), Faintness.—(*Lying on right side*), Sticking in right side of chest.—(*Pressure*), Boring, etc., in left temple.—(*When sitting*), Headache disappears.—(*During sleep*), Internal fever disappears.—(*Sweat*), All symptoms.—(*Walking*), Feeling unwell, etc.

CALCAREA ACETICA.

Calcium acetate, $CaC_2H_3O_2$.
Preparation, Triturations.
Authorities. 1, Hahnemann (Chr. Kr., 2); 2, Fr., ibid.; 3, Htn., ibid.; 4, Lgh., ibid.; 5, Stf., ibid.; 6, Sol., ibid.; 7, Gr., ibid.

Mind.—Disinclined to talk without being morose (after six and a half hours),[3].—He is lively and desirous to be with people and to talk with those about him (after ten hours),[3].—Sadness, almost to weeping, with solicitous care for the present and future,[4].—Anxious disposition, as though something evil were impending or to be dreaded in the future, with constant inclination to work,[4].—Anxious thoughts, which came and went, before going to sleep in the evening; with which the objects seemed like different objects; he dreaded the dark, and made an effort to look at the light; all of which was relieved after the passage of flatus,[1].—Anxiety about the present and future, with deep thought, with indifference to objects about him, though not without inclination to work,[4].—Apprehensive, sad mood, as though he were awaiting some depressing news,[4].—As soon as he was quiet and thoughtful, he became fretful and sleepy, and averse to everything,[2].—Very fretful and disinclined to talk; as soon as he went into the open air he felt better, but it returned in the room with increased headache,[2].—[10.] Fretful, peevish, and very irritable, and completely indifferent to the most important objects; he performed all his work with aversion and as if compelled to do so,[4].—Anxious the first part of the day; during the last part of the day lively and contented with himself,[4].—Fretful and peevish the whole day; in the evening good-humored and talkative,[4].—Loss of will-power, although he feels strong (seventh day),[1].

Head.—Vertigo. Slight impending vertigo (after a quarter of an hour),[3].—Vertigo as if his body did not stand firmly (after six hours),[6].—Vertigo on walking in the open air (after twenty-six days),[4].—Vertigo on walking in the open air, as if he would fall to the right side (after two hours),[4].—An attack of stupefying vertigo; the head inclined forward to the left side, during rest and motion (after three-quarters of an hour),[4].—**Sensations.** Shattering in the brain, on stepping, like an echo in the head,[1].—[20.] Stupid feeling in the head, as if he had turned in a circle for a long time, 3 to 4 P.M.,[4].—Great heaviness in the head, with severe jerks in both temples, and painfulness in the whole head, which disappeared on rising up (after nine and a half hours),[3].—Drawing pain in the right side of the forehead, above the eye, and in the occiput, on exerting the mind (second day),[2].—Drawing and pressive headache in the left supraorbital region, or in the temporal bone,[2].—Pressive pain in the whole head, especially in the temples (after nine hours),[3].—Drawing, pressive, at times, also, tearing, headache, now in the forehead, now in the occiput, now in the temples, which disappears on pressing upon the parts or on exerting the mind (third day),[2].—**Forehead.** Pressive headache, in the right frontal eminence, which extended to the right eye, and compelled him to involuntarily close it (after one and a half hours),[3].—Pressive headache in the forehead, especially above the left eyebrow, on walking in the open air,[4].—Stupefying pressive pain in the right side of the forehead, especially increased on stooping (after fifty hours),[4].—Stupefying pressive pain in the whole forehead in the morning after rising from bed, as though he had not slept enough, or had been dissipating through the night (after twenty-four hours),⁴.—[30.] *Stupefying pressive pain in the forehead* with confusion of the senses and obscuration of the whole head *while reading;* he was obliged to stop while reading and did not know where he was,⁴.—Boring-sticking pain in the left side of the forehead, when sitting, which immediately disappeared on walking, standing, and on touch (after twelve hours),⁴.— Intermitting needle stitches in the left side of the forehead, during rest or motion,⁴.—Boring stitches in the middle of the forehead, extending into the brain (after three hours),⁶.—Dull pressive stitches on walking, which especially affect the left side of the forehead, but disappear after continuing to walk,⁴.—*Temples.* Cramplike pain in the right temple (after six hours),⁶.—Cramplike pain in the left temple (after eight and fourteen hours),⁴.—Pressure in the left temporal bone, as if it were pressed in, internally and at the same time externally (after seven and a half hours),³. —Pressure in the right temple, close to the eye, as if something hard pressed upon it (after five and a half hours),³.—Pressing-out pain in the left temporal region, and on the whole left side of the head, as also on the right side of the occiput,³.—[40.] *Drawing-pressive pain in the right temporal muscle,* also in the evening, at times with pressure on the upper row of teeth; on pressing upon the temple the pain changes into a pressive headache in the forehead,².—The drawing-pressive headache about the temple was always increased after eating, and even while eating, with great sensitiveness of the teeth when chewing, as though they were loose and would be bent over,².—Digging stitches in the left temple, near the eyebrow, on moving the lower jaw (after five hours),⁴.—Dull pressive stitches inward from both temples (after twenty-four hours),⁶.—Rhythmical intermitting, boring, knifelike stitches extending upward into the left temporal region, which disappear on touch and when sitting,⁴.—*Vertex.* Pressure on the vertex, extending into the eye,¹.—Fine stitches in the vertex externally (after seven hours),⁶.—Severe throbbing in the upper part of the head in the region of the vertex as from an artery, with cutting shocks extending outward,⁶.—*Parietals.* Feeling on stooping, every time, as if headache would commence in the right side of the head,³.—Violent jerklike stitches in the whole right half of the brain, which often return and leave behind a pressive, bursting sensation,³.—[50.] Pulsating stitches in the left parietal bone (immediately),⁶.—*Occiput.* A feeling in the occiput as if it would be pressed asunder,³.—Pressive pain, suddenly shooting through the occiput, which only gradually disappeared,³. — Jerklike pressing from within outward, in the left side of the occiput, which extends down into the neck (after fourteen hours),³.—Drawing-pressive headache in the left side of the occiput, with stiff feeling in the neck,².—Sore pain on the occiput, when touched, as if the place were suppurating,⁴.—*External.* Tickling-itching on the scalp, which causes scratching, with painfulness of the roots of the hairs on touch,⁴.—Crawling and itching on the scalp, not relieved by rubbing (after ten hours),⁶.—The whole scalp is painfully sensitive on moving the frontal muscles back and forth (after one and a half hours),⁶.

Eye.—Violent inflammation of the eyes; the white of the eye is entirely red, with much matter in the eyes, especially in the external canthi the whole day; the external canthi are sore and ulcerated for fourteen days (second day),¹.—[60.] Violent tearing-stitching in the right eye, as though it would become inflamed,⁶.—Severe itching of the eyes,¹.—*Orbit.* Boring-stitching on the upper margin of the orbit (after five hours),⁶.— Fine twitching in the upper margin of the orbit, extending down to the nose,[1].—*Lids.* Hardened matter in the canthi for two days (after ten hours),[4].—Agglutination of the eyes in the morning, on waking from sleep (after twenty-four hours),[4].—Stickiness of the lids on moving them, with pressure in the canthi, especially in the external one (after fifty-five hours),[4]. —Burning in the left upper lid, extending to the inner canthus (after six hours),[3].—Sticking in the outer and inner canthi,[2].—Itching-stitching in the inner canthi, which disappeared on rubbing (immediately),[6].—[70.] Itching in both corners of the eyes,[1].—Tickling-itching in the right external canthus, which compelled rubbing (after twenty-five hours),[4].—*Pupil.* Pupils at first dilated, then contracted,[4].—*Vision.* Farsightedness in one naturally nearsighted; he could distinguish all objects at a distance, the whole day,[4].

Ear.—Twitching in the cartilage of the ear (after forty-eight hours),[6].— A feeling in the right ear as if something was put before the drum, without diminished hearing (after fifteen hours),[4].—Cramplike feeling on the back of the concha (after nine hours),[3].—Stitches in the ears,[1].—*Hearing.* Sensitiveness to noise, in the evening on falling asleep,[1].—Slight whizzing in both ears, with confusion of the whole head, immediately (after half an hour),[6].

Nose.—Objective. [80.] Pimples in both nostrils, with scabs,[1].— Frequent sneezing, without coryza,[4].—Coryza, with painful sensitiveness of the nose, and internal heat in the head (after seventy-two hours),[6].—Fluent coryza, with much sneezing (after twenty-seven hours),[1].—Fluent coryza, with headache (immediately removed by camphor), (after five days),[1].— Stopped coryza, with frequent sneezing (after seventy-two hours),[4].—*Subjective.* Gnawing pain at the root of the nose (after one hour),[6].

Face.—Yellow face,[1].—*Cheeks.* A feeling of tension in the right cheek, as if it were swollen (after second day),[2].—Dull pain in the muscles of the left cheek (after two hours),[4].—[90.] Pulsating throbbing on the cheek-bones (after two hours),[6].—Pressive pain in the right upper jaw, when chewing (after three hours),[3].—Violent tearing in the right upper jaw (after nine hours),[3].—*Lips.* Much moist scurf below the right angle of the mouth,[1].—Roughness and dryness of the lips, especially of the upper, as if it would crack (after forty-nine hours),[4].

Mouth.—Teeth. Gnawing toothache in the upper back teeth, as though they would be hollow; in all positions (after six hours),[4].—Stitches in the teeth,[1].—Throbbing toothache, with sensitiveness of the teeth to touch, and swelling of the gum, which pained when touched (after seven days),[1].—*Gums.* Boring in the gum of the right side of the upper jaw, followed by swelling, with pressive-drawing in the right temporal muscles,[2]. —Fine stitches in the gum of the whole upper jaw (after two hours),[4].— [100.] Blisters on the tongue, with burning pain and heat in the mouth,[1]. —*Tongue.* Dry sensation on the tongue (after five days),[1].—A feeling of rawness and soreness in the tongue, which is coated white,[4].—Rawness and scraping on the back of the tongue, which provokes cough, but does not disappear after coughing (after twelve days),[6].—*Saliva.* Dryness in the mouth, as from chalk,[2].—Accumulation of much mucus in the mouth; he could not swallow it fast enough (after one and a half hours),[4].—*Taste.* Food, especially meat, has little taste,[2].

Throat.—Throat hoarse and rough, for three days (after twenty-four hours),[1].—Sensation of much mucus in the fauces on swallowing, with dryness in the mouth (after one and a half hours),[4].—Violent sticking on the right side of the upper part of the œsophagus, when not swallowing (after three-quarters of an hour),[3].—[110.] Swelling of the submaxillary glands, with pressive sensation in them,[2].

Stomach.—Thirst. Thirst, with dryness of the throat,[1].—Thirst in the morning,[1].—Severe thirst, with desire for cold drinks, especially for water; he was obliged to drink a great deal, for eight hours (eighth to fifty-fifth day),[4].—*Eructations and Hiccough.* Frequent empty eructations,[4].—Constant sour eructations,[3].—*Sour, offensive eructations,*[4].—Frequent hiccough,[4].—Much hiccough, for a quarter of an hour (after five hours),[6].—*Nausea.* Nausea, with eructations and accumulation of water in the mouth, with a kind of vertigo in the head (immediately),[3].—[120.] After drinking milk in the morning, nausea arose from the stomach, as from a foul stomach,[1].—Nausea, with cough and a kind of heartburn, awoke him at midnight,[1].—Dull pinching-retching just below the pit of the stomach (immediately),[3].—*Stomach.* Anxiety in the pit of the stomach (after six hours),[6].—Anxiety, as if it arose from the pit of the stomach, when sitting, with immediate burning in the abdomen, which soon disappeared when walking or standing (after twenty-six hours),[4].

Abdomen.—Hypochondria. Violent pinching in the hypochondriac region and chest, which here and there ends in small stitches (after half an hour),[3].—Tensive pinching pain in the whole hypochondrium, and in the pit of the stomach (after ten hours),[3].—Griping in the hypochondriac region below the pit of the stomach, with chilliness over the whole body,[1].—Griping-twinging sensation in the whole hypochondriac region, extending to beneath the breast-bone, where it becomes sticking, and causes eructations (after three-quarters of an hour),[3].—*Umbilical.* Griping in a small spot below the navel, which becomes a gurgling, on rubbing with the finger (after half an hour),[3].—*General Abdomen.* [130.] Audible rumbling in the right side of the abdomen, as if diarrhœa would follow,[4].—Frequent audible rumbling and crawling, extending outward in the right side of the abdomen, as from flatulence, which is passed,[2].—Loud rumbling and gurgling in the abdomen, as from emptiness,[4].—Pinching, almost cramplike pain in the walls of the abdomen, in the right groin, in a small spot, only when speaking; also painful to pressure with the finger (after eight hours),[3].—Cutting pain in the abdomen every morning, also in the evening and night; it ceased after eating, and left behind a gurgling in the abdomen,[1].—Tearing in the abdominal muscles, increased by inspiration,[6].—*Hypogastrium and Iliac Regions.* Griping deep in the lower abdomen, as if in the region of the bladder, frequently repeated, and always associated with passage of flatus,[3].—Pressure in the lower portion of the abdomen, which causes confusion of the head,[1].—Pressive tension in the left groin (after eight hours),[3].—Sore pain in both groins, as if the glands would become swollen, especially felt when walking; on touch there seems to be slight enlargement of the glands (after ten hours),[4].—[140.] Swelling of the glands of the left groin (after twenty-two days),[1].—Tearing in the inguinal glands, when sitting and walking (after nine hours),[2].—Pinching on the crest of the ilium,[6].

Rectum and Anus.—Twinging in the end of the rectum when at stool, with loud rumbling and gurgling in the abdomen,[6].—Pressure in the anus,[6].—*Severe itching in the anus,*[1].

Stool.—Diarrhœa. Diarrhœa, not exhausting, two, three, or four times a day, for several days (after second day),[1].—Frequent stools, the first is solid, afterwards pasty, then thin, with difficulty; constipation the two following days,[4].—During the day three soft stools,[4].—*Constipa-*

tion. Constipation for two days (seventh day),[1].—[150.] No stool (second day),[2].

Urinary Organs.—Urethra. Frequent desire to urinate, with scanty discharge (after twenty-six hours),[4].—Frequent urging to urinate, with profuse discharge,[4].—**Urine.** The urine becomes turbid after standing, like gruel,[6].

Sexual Organs.—Male—Penis and Testicles. Tickling-itching on the prepuce, which caused rubbing (after nine hours),[4].—Tickling-itching at the end of the glans, compelling rubbing (after ten hours),[4]. —The left testicle is drawn spasmodically up to the abdomen, and is painful to touch, with painful pressure and pain in the left groin,[1].—**Emissions.** Frequent emissions,[1].—Emissions at night,[2].—Two emissions the first night, with voluptuous dreams,[3].—[160.] Two emissions in one night, without voluptuous dreams,[4].—**Female.** Discharge of blood from the uterus of an old woman who had not menstruated for several years; in the last quarter of the moon (after seven days),[1].—Itching of the pudenda,[1].—The usual leucorrhœa was increased,[1].

Respiratory Organs.—Loud rattling in the air-passages on expiration, as from much mucus in the chest (after thirty-seven hours),[4].—Tickling irritation in the air-passages, which provokes cough,[4].—The cough became loose, and large pieces, like purulent matter, were expectorated,[7].—Difficult breathing, which was relieved by bending the shoulders backward,[1].

Chest.—Anxiety in the chest, as if it were too narrow, with short breath, especially when sitting, with pressive pain in the chest, especially on inspiration; the heart beat anxiously and trembling,[6].—Constrictive, anxious sensation the whole day, as if there was not room enough in the chest to breathe, with stoppage of the nose (after thirteen days),[1].—[170.] Very anxious constriction of the chest and difficult breathing, like a tension in the lower portion of the chest; the breathing was affected for almost an hour almost to suffocation, both on motion and when sitting (after thirty hours),[4].—Cutting pain from within outward in the lowest ribs, aggravated by inspiration,[6].—Broad stitches in the pectoral muscles on every beat of the heart,[6].—Itching stitches in the chest, worse on expiration, disappearing on rubbing (after forty-eight hours),[6].—**Sides.** Long stitches in the right side beneath the ribs (after thirteen hours),[3].—Sharp stitches in the right side of the chest from within outward, without affecting breathing (after seven hours),[6].—Sharp stitches in the left side beneath the axilla, from within outward, worse on inspiration (after two hours),[6].

Heart.—Sticking-drawing pain in the præcordial region (after nine and a half hours),[2].

Back.—Dorsal. Sharp pain on the inner side of the shoulder-blade,[6]. —Severe stitches from the thoracic cavity out through the spine, between the shoulder-blades,[6].—[180.] Dull jerks from the posterior wall of the thorax to between the shoulder-blades, synchronous with the beat of the heart, with great anxiety (after eight hours),[6].—**Lumbar.** Severe needle-like stitches in the middle of the spine, almost cause crying out, on walking in the open air, somewhat relieved when standing,[3].—Cutting, pressing-out pain in the right lumbar region, which only transiently disappears on touch,[2].—**Sacral.** Sticking in a place above the sacrum, on touch,[1].—Sharp stitching in the sacrum, and at the same time in the leg above the ankle (after two hours),[6].

Superior Extremities.—Shoulders. Pain in both shoulders,[1]. —Severe stitches in both axillæ (after four days),[6].—**Arm.** Pinching pain (with tearing) in the muscles of the upper arm (on walking in the open air),[4].—Tearing-stitching in the muscles of the left upper arm, when sitting,[4].—Fine jerkings in the left upper arm,[6].—[**190.**] Tearing-jerking in the upper arm (after seven hours),[6].—*Forearm.* Cramplike tearing in the muscles of the left forearm (after forty hours),[4].—Cramplike pain in the forearm, in front of the elbow-joint (after one hour),[6].—Cramplike pain in the outer side of the left forearm near the wrist (after one, thirteen, and twenty-nine hours),[4].—Tearing pressure in the muscles of the left forearm during rest and motion (after three hours),[4].—Fine tearing and boring stitches in the muscles of the left forearm,[4].—*Wrist.* Pain as if sprained just above the wrist, worse in rest than on motion,[4].—Sharp stitches in the external condyle at the wrist,[6].—Crawling and sticking in the wrist,[6].

Inferior Extremities.—Hip. Drawing, sprained-like pain in the hip-joint, when walking,[2].—[**200.**] Cutting in the socket of the hip-joint, when sitting (after three hours),[6].—Tearing in the hip-joint and about the anterior crest of the ilium, extending into the groin, on motion,[2].—Pinching-jerking on the posterior side of the hip-joint, worse in rest than on motion,[6].—*Thigh.* Pressive-sticking on the inner side of the left thigh, when sitting (after three hours),[3].—Cramplike stitches in the muscles of the right thigh, when standing and walking, disappearing when sitting,[4].—Sharp stitches on the outer side of the thigh above the left knee (after three hours),[6].—Tearing stitches on the inner side of the thigh above the knee, when sitting (after twelve hours),[2].—Tearing pain on the inner side of the thigh, on motion,[2].—Bruised pain in the muscles of the thighs, when walking,[1].—Soreness between the nates, when walking,[1].—*Knee.* [**210.**] An inflamed swelling below the patella,[1].—Pain in the left knee-joint, evening during rest,[1].—Pain in the knees, when turning or touching them,[1].—Drawing cramplike pain on the knee-cap (after second day),[2].—Pain as if sprained in the left knee-cap, when sitting, disappearing when walking and standing (after twelve hours),[4].—Sharp stitches in the right knee-joint (after four hours),[6].—Bruised pain just below the patella, on walking in the open air (after thirteen hours),[4].—*Leg.* Drawing in the legs, extending to the tips of the toes,[1].—Bruised pain in the leg, especially in the lower leg, when lying,[2].—Bruised pain in the leg, as if wearied; he was obliged to change frequently from one place to another,[6].—[**220.**] Tearing-jerking in the forepart of the leg below the knee, during rest,[6].—Cramplike pain close to the tibia, when sitting,[4].—Pressive pain in the left tibia near the ankle, when walking in the open air (after fifty-two hours),[4].—Intermitting pressive pain in the calf,[2].—*Ankle.* Swelling of the left external malleolus,[1]. —*Foot.* Cramplike pain in the left sole (after five hours),[3].—Cramp in the soles after walking, which became better on continuing to walk, and disappeared when sitting,[1].—Cramp in the soles and toes at night, and on drawing on the boots, during the day (eleventh day),[1].—*Toes.* Severe stitching in the left little toe, as if outside of it (after fourteen hours),[3].— Intermitting, cramplike, needle stitches in the right toes when sitting and standing, but disappearing when walking (after half an hour),[4].—[**230.**] Sharp stitches in the last joint of the great toe, during rest (after twenty-four hours),[6].

General Symptoms.—Very weary from want of sleep, during the day; he is, however, unable to sleep,[1].

Skin.—Eruptions, Dry. A pimple beneath the lobule of the ear, on account of which there is tensive pain in the joint of the jaw, on chewing,[1].—Pimples in the middle of the cheek that became moist after scratch-

ing, and were followed by greenish crusts (after forty-eight hours),[4].—
Pustular. A pustule above the left eyebrow,[4].—An ulcer on the cheek, with sticking pain,[1].—**Sensations.** Fine crawling in the face beneath the eye and on the side of the nose,[6].—Itching-crawling on the upper lid, which after rubbing immediately appears on another spot, near by (after one hour),[6].—Itching-tickling on the border of the left hand, with irritation to scratch,[4].—Itching-sticking tickling, in the right palm, provoking scratching,[4].—[240.] Itching returned in a spot where there had been a tetter, several years previous (after five days),[1].—*Itching below both calves,*[1]. —Tickling-itching on the index finger, with irritation to scratch,[4].

Sleep and Dreams.—Sleepiness. Frequent yawning, as if he had not slept enough (after fifty-six hours),[4].—Great sleepiness and fretfulness, in the evening,[2].—Great sleepiness in the morning with fretfulness and pressive headache in the whole forehead (after two days),[2].—**Sleeplessness.** Restless sleep, with talking in it, and frequent waking,[3].—He was unable to sleep nearly the whole night; tossed about, and sweated over the whole body (after ten hours),[4].—Frequent waking from sleep, as though he had slept enough,[4].—Frequent waking from sleep, as from some disturbance,[4].—[250.] He frequently awoke from sleep, on account of tossing about, and thinking; he thought he was lying turned around in bed,[4].— **Dreams.** Dreams vivid, confused, not recollected,[4].—Very vivid dreams of previous transactions, with long deep morning sleep,[6].—Dreams vivid, full of strife and anger,[4].—Frightful, shuddering dreams,[4].—Dreams of sick people, and dead people, with violent weeping in the sleep (in one who never dreamt),[5].

Fever.—Chilliness. Frequent chilliness with yellow color of the skin,[1].—Shivering over the whole body, as though he had taken cold, with frequent yawning,[4].—Shivering over the whole back (after twenty-four hours),[4].—Shivering over the whole body, with warmth or heat of the forehead and face, and cold hands (after three, forty-eight hours),[4].—**Heat.** [260.] External heat, with internal chilliness, even on lying down (after seventy-two hours),[1].—Glowing heat and redness of the face, with hot forehead, cold hands, and great thirst, for several hours,[4].—**Sweat.** Exhausting sweat, day and night, for three days,[1].—*Sweat every morning* (after seven days),[1].

Conditions.—Aggravation.—(*Morning*), After rising from bed, pain in forehead; thirst; after drinking milk, nausea; sleepiness, etc.—(*Evening*), Before going to sleep, anxious thoughts, etc.; on falling asleep, sensitiveness to noise; during rest, pain in knee-joint; sleepiness, etc.— (*Night*), Cramp in the soles, etc.—(*Walking in open air*), Vertigo; headache in forehead; stitches in spine; pain in muscles of arm; pain below patella; pain in left tibia.—(*When drawing on the boots*), Cramp in the soles, etc.—(*Eating*), Headache about temples.—(*Expiration*), Stitches in the chest.—(*Inspiration*), Pain in chest; pain in ribs.—(*When lying*), Pain in leg.—(*On exerting the mind*), Pain in side of forehead, etc.—(*On motion*), Tearing in hip-joint; pain in inner side of thigh.—(*While reading*), *Pain in the forehead.*—(*Rest*), Pain above the wrist; jerking in side of hip-joint; jerking in leg; stitches in great toe.—(*When sitting*), Pain in left forehead; anxiety; tearing in inguinal glands; anxiety in chest; stitches in muscles of upper arm; cutting in hip-joint; sticking on inner side of thigh; stitches on inner side of thigh; pain in knee-cap; pinching close to tibia; stitches in toes.—(*When speaking*), Pain in walls of abdomen.—(*When standing*), Stitches in muscles of thigh; stitches in toes.—(*On stepping*), Shattering in the brain.—(*During stool*), Pinching in rectum, etc.—(*Stooping*), Pain in right forehead; feeling in head.—(*On touch*), Sticking above the sacrum; pain in knees.—(*When turning the parts*), Pain in the knees.—(*On walking*), Stitches in head; sore pain in groins; tearing in inguinal glands; pain in hip-joint; stitches in muscles of thigh; pain in muscles of thigh.— (*After walking*), Cramp in the soles.—(*Water*), After working and washing in, the symptoms are aggravated or renewed,[1].

Amelioration.—(*Evening*), Good-humored, etc.—(*Open air*), Fretful, etc.—(*Bending shoulders backward*), Difficult breathing.—(*After eating*), Pain in abdomen ceases.—(*Passage of flatus*), Anxious thoughts, etc.—(*Inspiration*), Tearing in abdominal muscles.—(*Exerting mind*), Headache.—(*Pressure*), Headache.—(*On rising up*), Heaviness in head, etc., disappears.—(*On rubbing*), Stitches in chest.—(*When sitting*), Stitches in left temporal region disappear; stitches in muscles of thigh disappear; cramp in soles disappears.—(*Standing*), Pain in left forehead; burning in abdomen; stitches in middle of spine; pain in left knee-cap.—(*Touch*), Pain in left forehead; stitches into temporal region.—(*Walking*), Pain in left forehead; burning in abdomen; pain in left knee-cap.—(*After continuing to walk*), Stitches in head; cramp in soles.

CALCAREA CARBONICA.

Calcium carbonate ($CaCO_3$). *Preparation*, For Hahnemann's provings, trituration of the middle layer of the oyster-shell. For Dr. Koch's provings, precipitated carbonate of lime from a solution of chalk in hydrochloric acid, is triturated with an equal quantity of sugar of milk; twenty parts of this are mixed with one hundred parts of alcohol, and this is termed the tincture.†

Authorities. 1, Hahnemann, Ch. Kr., 2; 2, Franz, ibid.; 3, Gross, ibid.; 4, Hartmann, ibid.; 5, Langhammer, ibid.; 6, Rummel, ibid.; 7, Stapf, ibid.; 8, Wislicenus, ibid.; 9, Schreter, ibid.; (10, Omitted); 11, A man, aged 31, took the tincture, Hygea, 5, 318 (Dr. Koch's preisschrift); 12, A woman, aged 26, took the tincture, ibid.; 13, The same person proved the 1st, 2d, and 3d dils.; 14, A maid, aged 17, proved the tincture, ibid.; 15, The same girl proved the 1st dil.; 16, A man, aged 40, proved the tincture, ibid.; 17, The same man proved the 1st and 3d dils.; 18, Knorre, A. H. Z., 6, 33, fragmentary symptoms, dose not given; 19, Robinson (B. J. of Hom., 25, 322), a young man proved the 1000th, 200th, 30th, 12th, and 6th, in rotation, and afterward the 1st X trit.; 20, A young woman proved the 3d X trit., ibid.; 21, A young man proved the 30th, ibid.; 22, A young man proved the 30th, ibid.; 23, A woman proved the 30th, ibid.; 24, Dr. Lillie gave a boy, aged 12, Calc. potentized higher from the 2000th, Berridge, Fragment. Provings, Am. J. of Hom., M. M., 8, 125; 25, A man took the 107th (of Fincke), ibid.; 26, Dr. L. W. B., took the 107th (Fincke), ibid.

Mind.—Emotional. Illusion of fancy when going to sleep, as if she heard noises and clattering about her bed, which caused shuddering,[1].— As soon as she closes the eyes, in the evening, in bed, a swarm of fancies present themselves to her,[1].—*Great desire to be mesmerized*,[1].—Repugnance, aversion, disgust for most persons,[1].—*Disinclination for every kind of labor*,[1].

---

† Neither of these preparations consists of *pure Calcium Carbonate.*

—Dread and aversion to labor, with great irritability, and heaviness of the feet,[1].—Loneliness is very oppressive, with coldness of the face, hands, and feet,[1].—Much crying (in an infant, whose mother had taken Calcarea),[9].—Cries and complains about the long-past offences,[1].—[10.] Weeping about trifles, with a sensitive, irritable mood,[1].—Weeping when remonstrated with,[1].—*Moods.* Sad, despondent mood, with irritable inclination to weep,[1].—She became sad, and was obliged to weep, from every walk in the open air,[1].—*Despondent and melancholy,* in the highest degree, with a kind of anguish,[1].—Melancholy, not exactly a sad feeling, about the heart, without cause, with a kind of voluptuous trembling of the body,[1].—Sorrowful and peevish; she looked upon everything from the worst side, and imagined everything evil,[1].—She is very hypochondriac; she thinks that she is deadly sick, nevertheless can complain of nothing,[1].—Despairing mood, with dread of disease and suffering, with foreboding of sad events,[1].—She despaired of her life, and believed that she must die, with a most sad mood, and weeping, and frequent sudden attacks of general heat, as if hot water had been dashed over her,[1].—Anxiety in the afternoon, subsequent to nausea in the forenoon, with headache,[1].—[20.] At night, she was very anxious and raving; she started up anxiously in a dream, with trembling on waking out of it (after twenty days),[1].—Anxious at night, as if she would become insane, followed by shuddering chilliness for a few minutes, and a sensation as if the body were dashed to pieces,[1].—Anxious, restless, and busy mood; she is undertaking many things but accomplishing nothing; after this activity, she is very much exhausted,[1].—Anxious about every trifle, and lachrymose,[1].—*Great anxiety and palpitation,*[1]. —*Frightened, apprehensive mood, as if some misfortune were about to happen to him, or some one else, which he could in no way overcome* (after twenty-three days),[1].—Every near sound frightened him, especially in the morning,[1].—*Fearful and restless, as if something evil would happen* (after four days),[1].—*She feared that people would observe her confusion of mind,*[1].—*She feared she would lose her reason,*[1].—[30.] Dread and anxiety of the future, with fear of consumption,[1].—Irritable, weak, and despondent, in the morning, after a little work,[1].—Fretful, with persistent obstinacy for three days (after twenty-eight days),[1].—Frequent attacks of irritability and anxiety,[1].—Very peevish after a few hours,[1].—Peevish, without cause, especially in the morning,[1].—*Peevish without cause,* for two evenings in succession,[1].—Very peevish and irritable (after taking cold),[1].—So peevish about trifles that she was dizzy the whole evening, and went to bed early, but could not sleep (after twenty days),[1].—Peevish about trifles, and very irritable, in the morning, before the stool; he gets angry at everything,[1].—Frequently peevish, and she spits out saliva,[1].—Peevish and restless,[1].—[40.] Obstinate disposition,[1].—Obstinate, depressed mood,[1].—Insupportable and sullen mood,[1].—Everything is disagreeable, with great peevishness,[1].—The thought of former vexations provokes him to anger,[1].—Impatient and desperate,[1].—Unnaturally indifferent, unsociable, taciturn (after eight days),[1].—*Intellectual.* Thoughts vanish; his memory is short,[1].—She misplaces words and easily chooses a wrong expression,[1].—Great weakness of the imagination; during a slight effort in speaking, it seemed as if the brain were paralyzed, especially in the occiput; he could no more think nor recollect what had been said; with confusion of the head,[1].—[50.] Very forgetful (after forty-eight hours),[1].—On stooping or moving the head, it seemed as if she did not know where she was,[1].—Loss of consciousness, with anxious oppression of the stomach, from which she was suddenly awakened as by a violent fright,[1].—In the evening, two attacks of loss of consciousness, when walking; she would have fallen to the floor, if one had not caught her (after five days),[1].—Loss of consciousness, with illusion as regards place; it seems as if the room were a bower,[1].—Stupefaction, like unconsciousness of external objects, with waving tingling on the upper part of the head,[1].

Head.—Confusion. Confusion of the head (first day),[16].—The head feels confused,[1].—*A dull, continued confusion of the head,*[1].—*Sudden confusion of the head, as if it were too full,*[1].—[60.] Painful confusion of the head, so that she did not understand what she had read, did not comprehend what was spoken,[1].—Confusion in the head, in the morning, on waking,[1].—Confusion of the head, in the morning, on waking, with trembling through the whole body, and rush of blood to the head,[1].—Great confusion of the head, after the midday nap,[1].—Confused trembling condition of the head (first day),[6].—Stupefaction of the head, like vertigo, the whole afternoon (after twenty-four days),[1].—Stupefaction of the head at night, on account of which he awoke; it continued to get worse until it almost amounted to faintness, followed by trembling of the limbs and weariness, so that he was unable to fall asleep again,[1].—Insensibility and bluntness of the whole head, as in a severe coryza,[1].—*Vertigo.* A feeling of vertigo, as if he were raised up and pushed forward,[1].—Vertigo from vexation,[1].—[70.] Vertigo and painful turning of the head, as if in a circle, in the morning, when rising; especially very dizzy when walking and standing, with chilliness and needle stitches in the left side of the head,[1].—At night, excessive vertigo, with flickering before the eyes, which lasted till midday,[1].—Very transient vertigo, mostly when sitting, less when standing, and still less when walking,[1].—During menstruation, vertigo, on stooping, and rising up again,[1].—Severe vertigo when stooping, followed by nausea and headache,[1]. —Vertigo in paroxysms, after stooping, when walking and standing; she was obliged to steady herself,[1].—***Vertigo, on suddenly turning the head,** *and also when at rest,*[1].—** Vertigo, on walking in the open air, as if he would tumble,* **especially on suddenly turning the head,**[1].—** Vertigo after walking, when standing, and looking about, as if everything were turning around with her,*[1].—Vertigo, even to falling down, with weakness,[3].—[80.] Dizziness and loss of sense, after turning in a circle,[1].—Dizziness in the head, in the morning, after rising, with nausea and roaring in the ears, and feeling as if he would fall down in consequence (after twenty-two days),[1].—So great dizziness, in the forenoon, that everything seemed in a half dream,[1].—Dizzy tottering, in the evening, when walking in the open air, so that he staggered to and fro,[1].—*Sensations.* ** Warm streaming of blood from the pit of the stomach to the head, twice,*[1].—**During menstruation,* **rush of blood to the head, and heat in it,**[1].—**Rush of blood to the head,* with heat in the face (two hours after dinner),[1].—**Rush of blood to the head,* with heat of the face, seven hours after a meal,[1].—Rush of blood to the head, with discharge of blood from the anus, for several days in succession,[1].—Congestion of blood to the head and chest, preceded by painful stiffness in the spine,[1].— [90.] Great affection of the head, the day after coition,[1].—Great dulness in the head, every morning, on rising from bed,[1].—Heaviness and heat of the head, almost only in the forehead,[1].—Heaviness in the head, in the morning, on waking, for several hours (after twenty hours),[1].—Great heaviness of the head, in the morning, on waking, with heat in it; both are much aggravated on moving the head and on raising it (after twenty-seven hours),[1].—*Constant fulness,[1].—Shivering in the brain, on severe motion, with dull tearing pain (twelfth day),[1].—Painful shivering in the brain, especially in the left side of the occiput, on slightly shaking the head, and on every step,[1].—Icy coldness in and on the head (after four hours),[1].—*The head becomes cold very easily, which causes headache, as if a board lay upon the head, with pressive pain in it, and chilliness of the whole body (after six days),[1].—Heat about the head, in the evening,[1].—[100.] Headache the day before menstruation,[1].—Headache, also vertigo, every morning on waking,[1]. —In the forenoon, first, headache, which continually increased, with rapid sinking of the strength, so that he could scarcely reach the house, with great heat in the forehead and hands, with much thirst for acid drinks; then, after lying down, ice-cold hands with rapid pulse (after twenty-one days),[1].—Pain in the head, as though the skin were detached, extending downwards upon the neck,[1].—Headache, with nausea (after twelve days),[1].— *Feeling of fulness in the head, constantly,[1].—The head hurts as if tense,[1].— During every cough, the head is painfully shattered, as if it would burst out,[1].—Digging and pressure in the head, which extend to the eyes, the nose, the teeth, and the cheeks, with great sensitiveness to noise, and attacks of faintness,[1].—Painful dragging, from within outward, in the whole head, with a feeling as if the brain were pressed together (fifteenth day),[1].— [110.] Drawing headache, extending upward from the neck,[1].—Pressive headache, mostly in the forehead, increased in the open air,[1].—Sticking headache, extending outward to the eyes (the first days),[1].—Sticking pains in the brain, with a feeling of emptiness of the head, for three days (after twenty-eight days),[1].—Stitches in the head,[1].—Stitches in the brain,[17]. Transient stitches, here and there, in the head,[1].—Stitches in the head, in the evening, with stitches in the limbs,[1].—Stitches in the whole head, for half an hour, if she rises up from lying flat on the back, and also after stooping,[1].—During the cough, stitches in the head,[1].—[120.] Several stitches through the head, with great chilliness,[1].—During the cough, painful shootings in the head, like tearings,[1].—Tearing on the head and in the eyes, with redness of the whole face, every afternoon, from three or four till nine or ten,[1].—Jerks in the head, momentarily,[1].—Single jerks or shocks through the brain,[1].—Throbbing headache in the middle of the brain, every morning, and continuing the whole day,[1].—Stitch-like throbbing in the head, when walking rapidly,[1].—**Forehead.** *Heaviness in the forehead, aggravated by reading and writing,[1].—Headache in the forehead,[11].—Headache in the forehead, over the nose,[1].—[130.] Painful, full sensation in the forehead, with throbbing in the temples,[1].—Sharp tensive pain in the forehead,[1].—Pinching pain in the forehead,[6].—Stupefying, pressive aching in the forehead, as in vertigo, during rest and motion (after one and a half hours),[1]. —Boring pain in the left side of the forehead externally, after walking in the open air,[1].—Dull pain in the forehead, with confusion of the head, in the morning, on waking, with dry coated tongue (after five days),[6].—Violent dull headache, first in the forehead, then also in the occiput, for several days (after eight days),[1].—Stitching-like tearing in the forehead,[17].—Pressure in the forehead,[1].—Pressing in the forehead (after four days),[1].—[140.] Violent pressive headache in the forehead (first day),[13].—Pressive headache in the forehead, as if it were very thick there,[1].—*Painful pressure in the forehead, extending down into the nose (evening of first day),[12].—Pressive pain in the forehead (about noon, first day),[13].—Pressing out in the forehead, very severe, and causing vertigo, relieved by pressure of the cold hand, and disappearing on walking in the cold air (after nine days),[1].—

Sticking headache, in one-half of the forehead, which is better when lying,[1].
—Four stitches in the left side of the forehead, at 11 a.m. (second day),[15].—
Tearing in the left frontal eminence (first day),[16].—Throbbing pain in the
forehead,[1].—Sticking-throbbing pain on the right frontal eminence,[11].—
Temples. **[150.]** Swelling in the right temple, in the morning, which at
evening had disappeared (after fifteen days),[1].—Swelling below the left
temple (after fifteen days),[1].—At first dull, then pressive headache, in the
temples, in the morning on waking, with many empty eructations,[6].—
Pinching-drawing pain in the left temple, towards the parietal bone, with
heat of the face,[6].—Pressure in the temples, every day, for eight days,[1].—
Sticking pain in the left temple (in the nervus temporalis profundis),[11].—
Frequent stitches in the temples (after seven days),[1].—Stitches in the left
temple (second day),[11].—Stitches inward through the left temple, and again
outward through the right (after five hours),[1].—Tearing pain the whole day
in the temples, the orbital bones, and the cheeks, which become much
swollen,[1].—**[160.]** Spasmodic jerking pain in the right temple,[1].—Slight
creeping, as of formication on the left temple (first day),[11].—***Vertex.***
Tension in the upper part of the head,[1].—Drawing pain in the upper part
of the head,[1].—Pressure in the head, now in the upper part, now in the temples (after twelve days),[1].—Stupefying pressure in the upper part of the
head, as after rapidly turning in a circle (after twenty-four days),[1].—Spasmodic pain, extending from the forehead to the vertex (after taking cold),
(after six days),[1].—Almost constant drawing pain beneath the vertex,[1].—
Drawing pain beneath the vertex, and in the temples, which seems to come
up from the back,[1].—Spasmodic drawing beneath the vertex, in the upper
part of the head, with stitches in the temples, and heat in the ears (after
forty-eight hours),[1].—**[170.]** Violent, pressive pain in the vertex,[19].—Severe
pressive pain in the vertex, awakens him every morning at 5 o'clock, and
after an hour disappears,[1].—Pressure in the vertex and forehead, after
dinner,[1].—During menstruation, pressive pain on the vertex,[1].—Violent
pressing outward, almost sticking pain, in the region of the vertex, while
stooping (after fourteen days),[1].—When walking in the open air, a pressive
headache in the vertex, which continued until going to sleep,[1].—***Parie-***
tals. Swelling on the right side of the head, without pains (after fifteen
days),[1].—Heat in the left side of the head,[1].—A numb spot externally, on
the right side of the head,[1].—Headache only on the side on which he had
just been lying (a burning?),[1].—**[180.]** *Frequent one-sided headache, always*
with much empty eructation,[1].—Tension and pressure in the right side of the
head, as from a blunt instrument pressed downward through the head, by
paroxysms,[1].—Compressive pinching headache on the left side,[1].—Drawing
pain in the whole right side of the head, in the zygoma, and in the jaw
(after four days),[1].—Sudden pain in the left parietal bone, as if the bone
were hacked to pieces, with shivering over the whole body,[6].—Pressive headache on the parietal bones, apparently more in the bones (immediately after
taking), (first day),[11].—Sticking headache on the right side, extending into
the eye,[1].—*Sticking headache in the left side,* above the temple (after two
days),[1].—Stitches in the upper part of the right side of the head, extending
to the right eye (after twenty-nine days),[1].—Shooting pains in both sides of
the head, with nausea,[20]. **—*Occiput.*** **[190.]** Crackling, audible for several
minutes, in the occiput, towards midday, followed by warmth in the neck,[1].
—Heaviness and pressure in the occiput (after thirteen hours),[1].—Headache in the occiput, whenever she ties anything tightly about the head,[1].—
Drawing pain in the occiput, always towards the side to which he moved

the head; disappeared after sneezing (after twelve days),[1].—Gnawing sensation in the occiput,[1].—Tensive pressure in the occipital bone,[11].—Cutting pain in the occiput, and in the forehead, as if something sharp were pressed into them, aggravated by walking, and by pressure with the hand (after third day),[1].—Stitches in the right side of the occiput (after eleven days),[1]. —Itching on the occiput,[1].—*External.* The hair falls out on combing,[1].— [200.] Much eruption on the head,[6].—Eruption on the scalp, with swelling of the glands of the neck,[1].—The scalp at the vertex becomes scaly,[1].— Thin moist scurf on the scalp (after twelve days),[1].—Several places on the head pain when touched (after fourteen days),[1].—*Itching on the scalp,*[1].— *Itching on the head, every night, on waking,*[1].—Itching on the scalp, when walking in the open air,[1].—Burning-itching on the scalp (after thirteen days),[1].—Burning-itching, as from nettles, with severe crawling on the scalp, and the lower portion of the face, in the evening, before going to sleep,[1].

Eye.—[210.] Right eye became much inflamed; lids glued together,[21]. —Purulent mucus (gum) is constantly in the eyes; she is obliged to wipe them frequently,[1].—Twitching and throbbing in the eyes, by paroxysms (after twenty days),[1].—The eyes are affected and watery (after seven days),[1]. —A sensation as if fat were in the eyes,[1].—A feeling as if something painless were moving on the right eye,[11].—The eyes pain so that she is obliged to close them, with a feeling as if she ought to press them in (after eight days),[1].—*A painful sensation as if a small foreign body were in the eyes* (after seventeen days),[1].—Cold feeling in the eyes (immediately),[1].—Burning of the eyes (second day),[11].—[220.] Burning in the eyes, when closing the lids,[1].—Burning in the eyes, on the head, and in the throat (after seven days),[1].—Burning and itching in the eyes (after eight days),[1].—Sensation of heat in the eyes, with heaviness in the upper lids,[1].—Tension in the muscles of the eyes, on turning them, and exerting them by reading,[1].—*Severe pressure, day and night, as if a grain of sand were under the upper lid,[1].— Pressure in the eyes, in the evening,*[1].—Pressure and burning in the eyes, with lachrymation,[1].—Pain in the eyes, as if they were pressed in,[1].—Sticking pain in the right eye, as if a foreign body were between the lower lid and the ball,[11].—[230.] Sticking and biting in the eye,[1].—Severe stitch in the eye, which had a lachrymal fistula,[1].—Stitches in the left eye, as from a foreign body (second day),[11].—Stitches in the eye and in the head (during menstruation), (after eight days),[1].—Tearing in the left eye,[17].— Biting in the eyes (after seven days),[1].—Soreness of eyes,[25].—*Itching in the eyes,* in the evening, but pressure in the morning,[1].—*Orbit.* Swelling under the left eye, without pain,[1].—Severe stitches over the right eye, in the supraorbital nerve (evening of first day),[13].—*Lids.* [240.] Swelling of the lower lid, in the morning, after rising,[1].—*Swelling and redness of the lids, with nightly agglutination; during the day they are full of gum, with a hot sensation and smarting pain and lachrymation* (after eleven days),[1].—Redness of the margins of the lid,[1].—Spasmodic trembling of the lower lid,[11].—The left lower lid was spasmodically moved downward towards the internal canthus,[11].—*Twitching in the upper lids,* with a sensation as if the eye were moving of itself (after eighteen days),[1].—She was obliged to wink when reading; the eyes kept continually closing (they were red and watery),[1].— Dry matter on the margins of the lids and in the canthi,[1].—*Agglutination of the eyes,*[1].—Agglutination of the eyes, in the morning, on waking (third day),[11].—[250.] Lids agglutinated in various places, in the morning (second day),[11].—*The lids are agglutinated with gum in the morning, the eyes look watery*, and pain if she looks at the light (after twenty-four hours),[1].—During menstruation the eyes become agglutinated, with lachrymation, together with heaviness of the head and inability to fix the thoughts,[1].—Smarting pain in the lower lid,[1].—*Itching on the margins of the lids*,[1].—Inflammation and swelling of the left canthus and lower lid, with sticking and throbbing pain and itching all about (after ten days),[1].—*Burning in the inner canthus*, with stitches near it,[1].—*Stitches in the inner canthi*, with alternating stitches and throbbing in the eyes, and after the pain disappeared, frequent blowing of the nose,[1].—Itching in the canthi,[1].—*Itching in the right inner canthus*,[1].—*Lachrymal Apparatus.* [260.] Lachrymation (second day),[11].—Lachrymation of the right eye (seventh day),[11].—Profuse lachrymation of the right eye, with burning (third day),[11]—Lachrymation in the morning,[1].—Lachrymation in the evening (after five days),[1].—*Lachrymation on writing*,[1].—Biting water runs from the left eye, which is red,[1].—*Conjunctiva.* Redness of the white of the eye,[1].—Redness of the white of the eye, with pressure in the eyes (after twenty days),[1].—Some blood oozes from the white of the eye, which is very red, but painless,[1].—*Ball.* [270.] Stiffness of the left eyeball, in the morning, after rising; is unable to move it without an unpleasant sensation,[1].—*Pupil.* Dilated pupils,[1].—*Vision.* Small objects seem more distinct than large ones,[1].—*Farsightedness;* she was obliged to wear convex glasses when reading,[1].—*Farsightedness;* formerly she saw both far and near objects distinctly, now she is unable to recognize anything fine near her; cannot thread a needle (first nine days),[1].—It seemed as though a shadow passed before the eyes, with very dilated pupils, *so that one side of objects was invisible;* she saw, for example, only one eye in a person,[1].—Dimness of vision; she felt the need of closing the eyes without being sleepy (after six days),[1].—Dimness of the eyes, after getting the head cold (after six days),[1].—Sudden blindness, immediately after dinner; he was unable to see the table, even, by which he sat; together with anxious sweat and nausea, and an appearance of a bright shiny light before the eyes; after an hour's sleep it disappeared,[1].—The light blinds her,[1].—[280.] The sunlight hurts the eye and causes headache,[11].—The glare of the candlelight is sensitive to the eyes and head,[1].—Letters dance before the eyes,[1].—Appearance of flickering and sparks of fire before the eyes, in the morning, on waking,[1].—Flickering before the eyes, and weakness of them,[1].—He saw a halo around the light and the moon,[1].—In the dark, she seemed to see electric sparks before the eyes,[1].—Black spots float before the left eye (second day),[11].—At times, she saw a black spot before the left eye, which disappeared after a few minutes,[1].—A black point accompanied the letters, when reading,[1].—[290.] During physical exertion she often saw black spots before the eyes (after eleven days),[1].—Like feathers before the eyes,[1].—It seemed like a veil before the sight in both inner canthi, which disappeared with lachrymation,[1].—A darkness or blackness passes before the eyes at times,[1].—Frightful visions appear on closing the eyes,[1].

Ear.—Objective. Great swelling of the right ear,[1].—Swelling of the left ear, with itching,[1].—Swelling of the inner ear and the right side of the face, with profuse secretion of the ear-wax,[1].—*Swelling in front of the left ear, which pains like a boil when touched*,[1].—Profuse purulent discharge from both ears,[19].—[300.] A little water trickles from the ear (with which he hears well), while it is difficult to hear with the other ear (which has good wax),[1].—*Subjective.* Sensation of fanning before the left ear,[1].—Flapping in the ear, as if a piece of skin were loose in it,[1].—Burning pain around the ear,[1].—*Heat within the ears*, like hot blood (after twenty-nine days),[1].—Heat streams out of the left ear (after five days),[1].—The bones behind the left ear seem swollen, and itch; the parts pain on touch as if suppurating,[1].—Cramplike pain in the ear (after seven days),[6].—Drawing, dull pain in the ears,[1].—Pressure in the ears,[1].—[310.] *Crushing in the ears when swallowing* (first days),[1].—Pain in the ear, as if something pierced through it,[1].—Shooting in the ear, when sneezing,[1].—Sticking in the left ear,[11].—Sticking and pain in the right ear,[1].—Stitches behind the left ear (in the morning, third day),[15].—Stitches in the left ear and in the temples, which disappeared during rest with closed eyes,[1].—Tearing stitches in the right ear (after three days),[1].—Tearing behind the left ear,[17].—Tearing in the left ear,[17].—[320.] Twitching in the right ear, with a hissing noise, every minute, and so violent that the whole body twitched with it,[1].—*Pulsation in the ears* (first day),[1].—Crawling in the right ear (after seven days),[1].—Burning-itching in both ears,[1].—*Hearing.* Sensitiveness in the brain to a shrill sound,[1].—Bad hearing (first three days),[1].—*Hard of hearing for a long time,[9].—When blowing the nose very hard, something comes before the ear, so that she cannot hear well (on swallowing, it disappears),[1].—Noises in the left ear and in the head,[1].—Humming in the left ear,[1].—[330.] *Singing in the ears, followed by crackling in them,[1].—Singing at one time, at another cracking in the left ear,[1].—*Singing and roaring in the ears,[1].—Ringing before the ears,[1].—A cracking in the ear, when chewing,[1].—A grunting in the ear, when swallowing,[1].—A loud roaring in the ears, with difficult hearing, in the morning (second day),[1].

Nose.—Objective. Inflammation, redness, and swelling of the forepart of the nose,[1].—*Swelling of the nose, especially at the root, frequently appearing and disappearing* (after six days),[1].—Swelling of the right wing of the nose, with painfulness to touch,[1].—[340.] *Sore, ulcerated nostril, preceded by frequent sneezing,[1].—Pimple in the right nostril, only painful on moving the muscles of the face and nose; the wing of the nose is red and itches externally and internally,[1].—Painful pimple in the left nostril, with itching-stinging pain,[1].—A red spot on the tip of the nose,[1].—Twitching in the external muscles of the nose (after fourteen days),[1].—*A smell from the nose as of bad eggs, or of gunpowder* (after one hour),[5].—Coryza; it affects him in every limb,[1].—Severe coryza, which disappeared after two days and changed to a violent colic, lasting several days (after seventeen days),[1].—*Severe coryza, with headache* and oppression of the chest (tenth and sixteenth day),[1].—Severe coryza, with heat in the head, and cough (after thirteen days),[1].—[350.] *Violent coryza,* for eight days (after thirty-six days),[1].—Violent coryza, with pain in the lower abdomen,[9].—Fluent coryza,[22].—Fluent coryza for three days, with ulceration of the left nostril (after nine days),[1].—Fluent coryza with great weariness,[1].—Profuse fluent coryza,[1].—*Profuse fluent coryza* (almost immediately and after four days),[1].—Excessive fluent coryza, followed much ineffectual sneezing,[6].—*Stopped coryza* (first and twelfth day),[1].—Severe stopped coryza, with headache (after thirty-two days),[1].—[360.] *Stopped coryza, with sneezing* (first seven days),[1].—*Attacks of stopped coryza, with sneezing,* for several weeks,[1].—Frequent sneezing, daily,[1].—*Frequent sneezing, without coryza,[1].—Much sneezing, in the morning,[1].—Profuse discharge of mucus from the nose, while it is stopped (fourteenth day),[1].—Profuse bleeding of the nose (after ten days),[1].—Nose-bleed, in the morning (seventh day),[1].—Severe nose-bleed, as in a profuse venesection, almost to faintness,[9].—Some nose-bleed, at night (thirteenth day),[1].—[370.] Blackish blood is blown from the nose,[1].—Stopped nose (after eighteen days),[1].—*Complete stoppage of the nose, in the morning, on rising,[1].—Stoppage of the nose, with coryza,[1].—*Subjective.* The skin of the nose seems covered with oil (after twenty-five days),[1].—Dryness of the nose (after twenty-two days),[1].—Nose dry the whole day (first day),[11].—*Dry nose at night; moist during the day,[1].—Tensive pressure above the nasal bones, as if they were swollen,[11].—Sore, painful, swollen, and erysipelatous-looking nose; it is quite hard to the touch, and attended with much frontal headache,[22].—[380.] Soreness of the right nostril,[1].—A sore pain on the border of the nostrils, and especially in the septum of the nose,[1].—The almost sore nostril stings and pains on touch,[1].—Itching of the nose, internally and externally (after two days),[1].—*Smell.* The sense of smell is very sensitive (after twenty-two days),[1].—The smell is blunted,[1].—**Very offensive smell in the nose* (after twenty-five days),[1].

Face.—Objective. **The color of the face is pale,* with blue rings around the eyes (first day),[1].—**Pale, lean face, with deepseated eyes surrounded by dark rings* (fourteenth day),[1].—*Yellowness of the face,*[1].—[390.] Frequent excessive redness and heat of the face,[1].—Continued puffy redness and heat of the face,[1].—Swelling of the face, without heat, with needle-stitches here and there,[1].—Right side of face much swollen, and covered with pimples,[21].—Twitching of the muscles of the face,[1].—*Subjective.* Pain in the face, followed by swelling of the cheeks, whereupon the pain disappears (after ten days),[1].—Burning in the whole of the face,[1]. —The face feels swollen, especially under the eyes and around the nose, without visible swelling,[1].—Tearing in the bones of the face and head,[1].—Prickling in the face and neck,[1].—*Cheeks.* [400.] Painless swelling of the cheeks, in the morning, on rising (second day),[1].—With pinching, contractive pain, the right cheek is drawn spasmodically sideways (after thirty days),[1].—Stitches in the right cheek, very violent, the whole day (after five days),[1].—Tearing in the left cheek-bones,[1].—Tearing in the left cheek-bones (first day),[16].—*Lips.* **Swelling of the upper lip, in the morning,*[1].—The lips and mouth were spasmodically drawn together, so that she could not open them,[1].—Cracked lips, with a cracked, smarting tongue (after forty-eight hours),[1].—The upper lip was cracked,[1].—Eruption in the lower portion of the red lip (after thirty-two days),[1].—[410.] At first, slight drawing in the lower lip; afterward it became as if dead, white and numb, without feeling, as though it were thick and would hang down (for five minutes),[7].—Stitching-itching about the upper and lower lip,[1].—*Lower Jaw.* *Swelling of the glands under the lower jaw,[1].—On the left side of the lower jaw, great swelling with drawing pains (after twelve days),[1].—Tearing in the lower jaw (first and second days),[16].

Mouth.—Teeth. Protrusion of a swollen tooth; only when she bites upon it it pains very much,[1].—Looseness of an old stump with swollen gum, with sore, sticking pain when touched,[1].—*Offensive smell from the teeth,*[1].—**Inclination to gnash the teeth as in a chill,*[1].—The teeth feel too long,[1].—[420.] Toothache at night, more like a pressure, or rush of blood to the teeth, beginning immediately after lying down (first three nights),[1].—Pain in the teeth from heat or cold, **but mostly caused by a current of air,* day and night, with running of much saliva from the mouth, and sticking extending to the ears and eyes, which prevented her sleeping at night (after eight days),[1].—During menstruation, an attack of toothache,[1].—Boring toothache, with stitches extending to the nasal bones, day and night, with swelling of the gum and cheek,[1].—During menstruation, a boring in hollow teeth, which becomes a pulsation on stooping (after sixteen days),[1].—Dull toothache, in the evening on lying down (as soon as she lays the head down), lasting one hour, followed by sleep,[1].—Drawing in the teeth,[1].—Drawing in the first upper left teeth,[11].—Drawing pain in the front teeth, lasting several minutes, and returning by paroxysms (after seventeen days),[1].—*Immediately after menstruation, toothache*, drawing and sticking day and night, worse if she inclined the head to the right, or to the left, or backward; it prevented sleep or awoke her out of sleep (after fifty days),[1].—[**430.**] Boring-drawing pains in most of the back teeth, at night,[1].—*Gnawing toothache*, worse in the evening,[1].—Biting pain in the teeth,[1].—Drawing-cutting in all the teeth (after eleven days),[1].—Boring-sticking toothache, extending to the eye and ear, excessively increased on riding in a wagon (twenty-second day),[1].— At first, stitches in the last back teeth, two hours after eating, followed by boring, relieved by eating,[1].—Severe stitches in a tooth, extending to the right eye and right temple; only during the day; with inclination to touch the tooth with the tongue, which causes every time a severe stitchlike jerk in the tooth, so that she starts, and it shakes her (first five days),[1].—Tooth-ache in all the teeth (as from fine needle stitches), *much aggravated by the entrance of cold air;* it awoke him from sleep at night,[1].—A thrust in the teeth, as from a fist,[1].—Tearing in the teeth,[17].—[**440.**] Tearing in the teeth, as if the roots would be torn out (after twenty hours),[1].—Tearing in the teeth, extending to the head, to the temples, mostly at night,[1].—Tearing in the first left upper back tooth,[11].—Single tearings in hollow teeth, at half hour intervals, most severe on taking anything warm; also at night, tear-ing through the whole cheek,[1].—The teeth pain, as if sensitive on slight touch,[1].—Jerking toothache (twenty-fourth day),[1].—Jerking in the left teeth, and in the left side of the head,[1].—Throbbing toothache in an incisor, only when eating,[1].—Much tickling toothache in a hollow tooth,[1].—***The teeth cannot endure the air or any coldness,**[1].**—[450.]** *Toothache if cold air or cold drinks enter the mouth,**[1].—The toothache was aggravated by noise,[1].—*Swelling of the gum* of a hollow tooth,[1].—Swelling of the gum (and of the jaw); especially near a broken tooth a pimple swells, from which pain extends into the ear,[1].—Painful swelling of the gum without toothache, also with swelling of the cheek, which is painful to touch (after three days),[1].—Pustules on the gum above one of the back teeth, like a dental fistula (after taking cold?), (after twenty-four days),[1].—An ulcer on the gum (after fourteen days),[1].—*Bleeding from the gum*, even at night (second and third day),[1].—At night, tearing pain in the gum, and on biting a feeling as if the teeth were loose,[1].—Soreness of the gum, with painful-ness in the roots of the teeth,[1].—[**460.**] Throbbing in the swollen gum,[1].— Severe pulsation in the gum,[1].—The gum itches,[6].—***Tongue.*** Swelling of one side of the tongue, which makes swallowing difficult,[1].—Blisters on the tongue, which hinder him in eating,[1].—* *White-coated tongue* (first days),[1]. —Thick, white-coated tongue, with a feeling as if it were raw and sore,[1].— Tongue difficult to move,[1].—Dryness of the tongue, in the morning on wak-ing (after thirteen days),[1].—The tongue pains along the side and on its lower surface, especially when chewing, swallowing, or spitting (seventh day),[6].—[**470.**] **Pain beneath the tongue, when swallowing, on the left side behind the hyoid bone,*[6].—Violent burning on the tongue, and in the whole of the mouth,[1].—**Burning pain on the tip of the tongue, as from soreness; she could take nothing warm into the mouth on account of pain* (after six hours),[1].—***General Mouth.*** The mouth is slimy in the morning; it is not relieved by rinsing (after twenty-four hours),[1].—In the mouth, swelling of the right cheek, forming a thick nodule, with drawing-tearing pain in it, every evening,[1].—Blisters in the mouth, which open and form ulcers (after twelve days), (after anger?),[1].—Blisters in the mouth, and ulcers form from them on the inner surface of the cheek (after taking cold?),[1].—Small blisters on the inner side of the cheek, where the teeth touch it,[1].—Dryness in the mouth (after one and a half hours),[5].—Great dryness of the mouth and tongue, with a raw, sticking sensation,[6].—[480.] Swelling and inflammation of the palate; the uvula is dark-red and full of blisters,[1].—Sticking in the palate,[1].—Dry sensation in the palate, which obliges him to hawk up mucus,[1].—*Saliva.* In the forenoon, the saliva frequently collects in the mouth, with nausea (fourth day),[1].—Sour taste of the saliva, which she continually spits out (second day),[1].—Much mucus in the mouth, with a dry sensation,[6].—*Accumulation of much mucus in the mouth,* though it does not cause spitting,[1].—*Taste.* Sweet taste as of sugar in the mouth, day and night (twelfth day),[1].—Flat, watery taste in the mouth; the taste of food is unnaturally sensitive,[1].—*Offensive taste in the mouth,* in the morning, as of a foul stomach,[1].—[490.] Bitter mouth (second day),[16].—Bitter taste, in the morning two hours after rising,[1].—Bitterish taste in the back part of the throat (fifth day),[1].—Impure, bitter taste in the mouth,[1].—*Sour taste in the mouth,*[1].—Sour taste in the mouth, and much tough saliva,[1].—Sour taste of all food, without a sour taste in the mouth (after taking cold?),[1].—Metallic taste, taste of lead in the mouth, in the morning (sixth day),[1].—Taste of iron in the mouth,[1].—Inky taste, in the morning on waking,[1].—[500.] Everything tastes unsalted,[1].—Salty taste in the mouth, and much thirst (after some hours),[1].—Fecal taste in the mouth and fauces,[1].—Taste blunted,[1].—*Speech.* Speech is difficult,[1].—He moves the mouth as if he would speak or scream, but cannot utter a word,[1].

Throat.—Mucus in the throat, which tastes like iron,[1].—Hawking of mucus in the morning,[1].—Relaxed throat, with roughness and hoarseness,[25].—Sensation in the throat as if something rose up and stuck (first day),[11].—[510.] The throat is dry and bitter the whole day, especially in the morning,[1].—During menstruation, severe burning in the throat, with hoarseness,[1].—After every meal, almost unendurable burning in the throat lasts several hours, with or without eructations,[1].—*Pain in the throat, as from internal swelling, extending to the ears* (after fourteen days),[1].—A feeling as if a worm were gnawing in the throat; continues till she goes to bed (at 4 P.M., first day),[14].—Sticking and pressure in the throat, on swallowing,[1].—*Stitches in the throat when swallowing;* she is not able to swallow bread,[1].—Severe stitches in the throat, extending to the ear, when swallowing, and still more when speaking,[1].—Sore throat, with difficulty of swallowing,[22].—Sore throat, as from a lump in it, when swallowing,[1].—[520.] Sore throat, with swelling of the glands under it,[1].—A feeling as if the throat and uvula were raw and sore,[1].—Rawness and soreness of the whole throat; he could scarcely swallow anything (after twenty-nine days),[1].—Rawness and burning in the throat, with a sensation as if the œsophagus, as far as the opening of the stomach, were raw and sore,[1].—Tickling in the throat, as if a very small object were lying there, which excites cough (first day),[11].—*Uvula.* Swelling and dark redness of the uvula,[1].—Pain in the throat, as if the uvula prevented swallowing, even on empty swallowing; less pain when speaking, and none at all when lying in bed,[1].—*Tonsils.* *Swelling of the tonsils, with elongation of the palate, *and a feeling as if the throat were too narrow when swallowing,* sometimes a feeling of soreness with stitches (after five days),[1].—Whitish-yellow ulcers on the right tonsil,[1].—*Pharynx.* A feeling as though a foreign body were in the pharynx, which constantly obliged him to swallow (after fifteen days),[1].—[530.] *A feeling in the pharynx, in the afternoon, as if the food remained sticking in it and could not get into the stomach, with a kind of nausea,[1].—*Spasmodic contraction of the pharynx,[1].—Pressure in the pharynx after swallowing,[1].—During menstruation, a sore throat; a sore pain in the pharynx, on swallowing, on the uvula and behind it,[1].—**Swallowing.** Inclination to choke in the œsophagus, without nausea, with accumulation of water in the mouth, like water-brash,[1].—Obstruction in the throat, on swallowing, as from a pressing substance,[1].—Swallowing is difficult, as if the tongue were swollen posteriorly,[11].—Pain in the throat on swallowing (third day),[13].—**Throat Externally.** *Hard swelling of the submaxillary glands, as large as hen's eggs, with painful tension when chewing, and sticking pain when touched (after forty-one days),[1].

Stomach.—Appetite and Thirst. *Ravenous hunger, in the morning,[1]. — [540.] *Ravenous hunger, with weak stomach,[1].—Great appetite, with great weakness, in the evening,[1].—Much appetite for wine, which she never before liked,[1].—Great desire for salt things,[1].—He relishes milk,[4].—Daintiness,[1].—*Loss of appetite; but when he began to eat he relished it (first day),[11].—Complete loss of appetite (after twenty-four hours),[1].—The appetite is slight; she feels an acidity in the stomach,[1].—She will eat nothing cooked,[1].—[550.] Does not relish his accustomed tobacco; smoking causes headache and nausea,[1].—*Great thirst,[1].—Great thirst, in the afternoon (after three hours),[1].—Much thirst and brown urine,[1].—Great thirst for beer,[1].—**Eructations and Hiccough.** Eructations of air,[11].—Eructations of wind (first day),[11].—*Eructations of food,[1].—Eructations like hiccough,[1].—Many eructations, in the morning, even on waking and fasting,[1].—[560.] Eructations at night, on waking,[1].—Severe eructations at night when lying; she was obliged to rise in order to be relieved,[1].—Many eructations after eating,[1].—*Frequent eructations tasting of the food,[1].—After every meal, eructations tasting of the food,[1].—Eructations, even after six hours, tasting of the food eaten at dinner,[1].—Eructations tasting of bile, in the afternoon,[1].—Eructations of brownish-sour fluid, with burning, extending upward from the pit of the stomach (eighth and ninth days),[1].—Eructations of bitter, acrid fluid,[11].—Sour eructations in the morning,[1].—[570.] Acid eructations late in the evening,[1].—Bitter eructations,[1].—Rancid eructations; scraping heartburn,[1].—Heartburn (after one hour),[1].—Acidity of the stomach rises up as far as the pharynx; a kind of heartburn, the whole day,[1].—After taking milk, water rises from the stomach (waterbrash),[1].—Waterbrash with colic (after twenty-four hours),[1].—*Tasteless fluid rises into the mouth (evening of first day),[12].—The milk taken in the morning regurgitates sour (after three days),[1].—Hiccough the whole day till evening (twenty-ninth day),[1].—**Nausea and Vomiting.** [580.] Faintish nausea, frequently,[1].—Nausea, the whole day, as in a previous pregnancy (third day),[12].—Nausea, as if an emetic had been taken; it continues until she goes to bed (evening, first day),[12].—Nausea, as if one would vomit, at 6½ P.M. (first day),[12].—Nausea, which lasts until the afternoon (first day),[13].—*Nausea in the morning (after two hours, and after five days),[1].—Nausea, every morning, with diminished appetite,[1].—*Nausea in the morning fasting, with qualmishness and shuddering,[1].—*Nausea in the pit of the stomach, in the morning, fasting, with blackness before the eyes so that he was obliged to sit down,[1].—Nauseated feeling, in the forenoon,[1].—[590.] Great nausea, in the pit of the stomach, in the afternoon, as from great emptiness in the stomach,[1].—Nausea, in the evening, with very restless sleep,¹.—At dinner, after he is scarcely half-satisfied, he becomes nauseated ; the food that he has eaten rises into the mouth, with nauseous taste, and suddenly eructations follow for three hours (after twenty days),¹.—During menstruation, nausea, and ineffectual urging to stool,¹.—Nausea, before a stool,¹.—Nausea, with anxiety (after eight days),¹. —*Nausea, with flow of sour water from the mouth,¹.—Nausea and qualmishness, at 11 A.M.,¹.—Nausea, with vomiting of food, weakness and faintness, and loss of consciousness,⁹.—*When he had eaten almost enough, he became nauseated, which however disappeared if he once ceased eating (ninth and twelfth days),¹.—[600.] Milk does not agree with him ; causes nausea,¹.—She feels sick, but is unable to bring up anything,²⁰.—Qualmishness in the stomach, with accumulation of saliva in the mouth (after three hours),⁵.— Severe retching in the stomach, like a cramp, for two hours, on account of which she could not remain in bed, but was obliged to rise,¹.—Vomiting in the morning, followed by nausea, the whole day, with digging pain in the abdomen,¹.—*Vomiting of sour water, at night,¹.—Black vomiting (after nine days),¹.—Stomach. *Swelling of the epigastric region, toward the left side,¹.—Pain in the stomach (first day),¹⁶.—Feeling of warmth in the stomach (first day),¹¹.—[610.] Burning in the stomach,¹.—Sharp burning pain in the stomach (third day),¹¹.—Burning in the stomach, as from acrid fluid (second day),¹¹.—*Burning extending up into the throat, after every meal, especially after the use of hard dry food,¹.—Sudden pain in the stomach, as though it would be distended,¹.—Fulness of the stomach in the afternoon,¹.—After thin fluid food, in the evening, he feels stuffed, with much spasmodic pressing,¹.—Constrictive pain in the stomach, for several days, at times with pressure after eating,¹.—Cramp in the stomach and abdomen, cutting and constricting,¹.—Severe cramp in the stomach, in the afternoon, until sweat broke out all over,¹.—[620.] Cramp in the stomach, at night, which awoke him,¹.—Cramp in the stomach, with nauseous eructations, and yawning (after three-quarters of an hour),¹.— Griping in the pit of the stomach,¹.—Gnawing-griping in the stomach, extending from the chest,¹.—Gnawing and a sensation of jerks in the stomach,¹.—*Pressure in the stomach (first day),¹¹ ¹⁶.—*Pressure in the stomach, even when fasting,¹.—*Pressure in the stomach the whole day (after seven days),¹.—*Pressure in the stomach, as if something were lying heavy and solid in it,¹.—*Pressure in the stomach, as if a lump were in it, after a moderate supper, lasting one hour,¹.—[630.] *Pressure transversely across the stomach,¹.—*Severe pressure in the pit of the stomach, when pressing upon it, and after the stool, in the forenoon,¹.—Pressure in the stomach, in the evening, before lying down, like a retching,¹.—Spasmodic pressure in the stomach, after supper, and when this passes off, a feeling in the intestines as though he would have diarrhœa, which however does not come on (seventh and eighth days),¹.—Pressure and oppression of the pit of the stomach,¹.— Pressure in the stomach, with accumulation of saliva in the mouth,¹.— Stitches transversely across the epigastric region,¹.—Stitches in the pit of the stomach, on breathing (forenoon, first day),¹⁶.—Stitches in the epigastric region, after dinner (after nine days),¹.—Stitching pain in the pit of the stomach, on pressing on it, especially severe after stool,¹.—[640.] Sore pain in the stomach,¹.—*The epigastric region is painful to touch,¹. Frequent jerks in the pit of the stomach, with the anxiety,¹.

Abdomen.—Hypochondria. Tension in the hypochondria,¹.— *Tight clothes about the hypochondria are unendurable,¹.—*A feeling as if laced below the hypochondria, with trembling and throbbing in the epigas-

tric region,[1].—Sharp griping in the left hypochondriac region,[1].—Drawing pain extending from the right hypochondrium towards the symphysis pubis,[1].—Transient stitches in the right hypochondriac region, in the forenoon, lasting one hour,[1].—Stitches in the right hypochondriac region, which extend to the back, in the evening (thirtieth day),[1].—[650.] Attacks of pressive throbbing in the left hypochondrium, lasting a quarter of an hour, frequently through the day, during rest and motion,[1].—Tensive pain in the hepatic region,[1].—Tension and pressure in the hepatic region, as if it were very much enlarged, even to bursting,[1].—Drawing pain in the posterior portion of the hepatic region, extending towards the back, like tearings,[1].— Dragging pain in the hepatic region (seventh day),[1].—*Pressure in the hepatic region, on every step, when walking,*[1].—Smarting-sticking pain in the hepatic region, in the last false ribs,[1].—*Stitches in the hepatic region, during or after stooping,*[1].—Pressive pain in the liver, especially at night, when a hardness is also more distinctly felt,[1].—Raw pain in the liver,[1].—*Umbilical.* [660.] Loud rumbling around the navel, when eating,[1].—Now a burning, now a sticking pain, below the navel, extending into the groin, which is distended, worse on the left side,[1].—Burning pain below the navel, for several hours, in the afternoon,[1].—Pinching and dragging just below the navel, after supper, increased when walking, and followed by distension,[1].—Pressive pain in the abdomen, below the navel, in the morning, after rising, like a pressing inward upon the abdomen, with constipation (after twelve days),[1].—Spasmodic twisting and griping around the navel (after four days),[1].—Stitches transversely through the abdomen, below the navel, on inspiration,[1].—*General Abdomen.* *Abdomen very much distended,*[1].—*Abdomen distended, hard,*[1].—Abdomen very much distended, hard, after dinner,[1].—[670.] On walking in the open air, visible distension of the abdomen,[1].—Distension of the abdomen and stomach, after eating and drinking a little,[1].—Distension of the abdomen, soon after dinner, not after supper, when, however, she had eaten considerable,[1]. —Great distension of the abdomen, with colic, frequently during the day,[1]. —Abdomen distended, full; constriction of the rectum, which retains the flatus,[1].—Enlargement and elevation on the right side of the abdomen (in the hepatic region?); a pressure is constantly felt there, especially when sitting, and a heaviness; she cannot lie upon this side; with incarceration of flatus,[1].—Twitching in the abdominal muscles during stool,[1].—Much fermentation in the abdomen,[1].—Gurgling in the left side of the abdomen, with uneasiness in it, without pain,[1].—*Constant rumbling in the bowels,*[1].— [680.] Much rumbling in the abdomen,[1].—Rumbling in the abdomen, both on inspiration and expiration,[1].—Rumbling in the abdomen, followed by eructations,[1].—Continued rumbling in the left side of the upper abdomen (after four days),[1].—Much accumulation of flatus in the abdomen, for several nights (after five days),[1].—Incarceration of flatus very frequent, with rumbling in the abdomen (after nineteen days),[1].—Incarcerated flatus, with much vertigo (after six days),[1].—Incarceration of flatus, with pain in the small of the back (after nineteen days),[1].—Passage of offensive flatus,[1]. —Pain in the abdomen, above the hips, when walking and breathing (after six days),[1].—[690.] Slight pain and trembling in the small intestines, with pain in the small of the back, and dragging towards the rectum, as if a stool would follow,[11].—Frequent burning in the abdomen,[1].—Fulness of the abdomen, especially after eating,[1].—Fulness in the abdomen, in the evening, so that she could scarcely move, with severe colic,[1].—Tension in the abdomen (first days),[1].—*Tension in the abdomen, with distension,* the whole afternoon, without sensation of flatus, which disappears after passing wind (twentieth day),[1].—Tension in the abdomen, when sitting, and during great exertion,[1].—Tension in the muscles of the upper abdomen, when leaning backward, with painfulness of the upper abdomen when stroked with the hand, as if the skin were sore (tenth day),[1].—Constrictive pain in the abdomen, extending to the small of the back (after forty days),[1].—Constriction of the abdomen, extending up to the chest, immediately, in the morning, lasting one hour (eighteenth day),[1].—[**700.**] Constrictive pain in the upper part of the abdomen, so that she was obliged to walk bent, especially excited by deep breathing (after a few days),[1].—Constrictive sensation in the abdomen and pit of the stomach, with appetite at times great, at times small,[1].—Pinching sensation in the bowels, with diarrhœa,[22].—Griping in the abdomen (first day),[1].—Griping in the abdomen, extending from the navel, during dinner (eighteenth day),[1].—*Frequent severe cramp in the intestinal canal, especially in the evening and at night, with coldness in the thighs* (eighth and twenty-ninth days),[1].—Much colic at night, without diarrhœa (twelfth day),[1].—Colic after supper,[1].—During menstruation, when the discharge ceased for some hours, constrictive griping colic,[1].—Frequent colic through the day, lasting several minutes, like griping, followed by nausea,[1].—[**710.**] *Frequent attacks of colic*, after the disappearance of a severe coryza that had lasted two days, with great weariness and sickly look of the face, lasting several days, and then suddenly and completely relieved by bathing in cold water (after nineteen days),[1].—*Drawing in the abdomen*, with uneasiness in it, in the morning, on waking,[1].—Pressure in the abdomen, extending downward from the pit of the stomach,[1].—During menstruation, drawing-pressive pain, with stitches, in the abdomen and other parts of the body, now here, now there, with an uneasiness amounting to faintness (after ten days),[1].—Twisting in the intestines,[1].—Cutting in the left side of the abdomen, which disappeared on the passage of a soft stool,[1].—Violent cutting in the abdomen, in the morning, on waking,[1].—Twisting-cutting pain in the abdomen,[1].—Stitches in the abdomen (after seventeenth day),[1].—Violent stitches in the abdomen (third day),[11].—[**720.**] Stitches in the left side of the abdomen, extending to the small of the back, worse in the evening, and after turning the body, or on stooping,[1].—Transient stitches in the abdomen, especially on inspiration,[1].—Stitches as with needles in the abdominal muscles below the ribs, from within outward, especially on inspiration,[1].—Stitches in the bowels, extending through the back, with impeded respiration,[1].—Tearing in the abdomen, extending towards the genitals,[17].—Jerklike tearings down the sides of the abdomen (after thirty-six days),[1].—In the middle of the abdomen, excessive soreness from nausea, without inclination to vomit, for a quarter of an hour (after twenty-seven days),[1].—Griping-crawling in the abdomen, extending towards the uterus, for several days, with passage of bloody mucus with the stool (seventeenth day),[1].—

Hypogastrium and Iliac Regions. Pain in the lower abdomen, even when walking a few steps, with a feeling of heat in the whole body (after five days),[1].—Tension and cutting in the lower abdomen (after fifteen days),[1].—[**730.**] Griping in the lower abdomen (after eight days),[1].—Griping deep in the lower abdomen, in the region of the bladder, with pain on every step, as if the internal parts were dragged down by a weight,[9].—*Pressure in the lower abdomen, on physical exertion*,[1].—Pressure in the lower abdomen, with sticking in the pit of the stomach, extending downward,[1].—Severe pressure in the lower abdomen, and a hard stool (first days),[1].—Pressive pain in the lower abdomen, with nausea, lasting eight days,[1].—Stitches in the lower abdomen,[1].—Sore pain in the lower abdomen, with painful tension, on holding one's self erect or bending the body backward (after sixteen days),[1].—Tearing in the left pelvic bones,[17].—Pulsation in the pelvis, along the course of the rectum (first day),[11].—[740.] Heaviness and drawing pain in the groin,[1].—Dragging in the groin, in the hernia, in the rectum, and the back, with stitches in the chest,[1].—Cutting pain in the groin, about the pubis (after twenty-one days),[1].—Twitching pain in the right groin, when sitting (after eighteen days),[1].—Soreness in the groin, as from being shaken (after twenty-four hours),[1].—Stitches in the inguinal region, as if a hernia would protrude,[1].—Fine pain, like needle-stitches in the upper part of the left inguinal region, as if in the peritoneum (first day),[1].—Smarting pain in the right inguinal region,[1].—*Small swollen glands in both groins,[1].—Sensation of swelling in the inguinal glands,[6].— [750.] Tension in the glands of the groin, even when sitting (after forty days),[1].

Rectum and Anus.—*The rectum, with its hæmorrhoids, protrudes during stool,*[1].—Protrusion of a large hæmorrhoid,[1].—The hæmorrhoids protrude, and pain very much on walking, less during stool,[1].—*Swollen hæmorrhoids protrude and cause pain during the stool, which is not hard,*[1].—Hæmorrhoids as large as nuts, appear with itching in the anus, and constipation ; they often last two or three days (on this account, he took Sulphur three times, which relieved, but they returned on renewing the proving),[16].—The hæmorrhoids become suddenly swollen,[1].—The hæmorrhoids swell and protrude daily, during the first days, afterwards not again,[1].—The hæmorrhoids are swollen and painful, when sitting, and discharge blood,[1].—Hemorrhage from rectum, several days,[18].—[760.] *Passage of blood from the rectum,*[6].— Pin-worms from the rectum,[6].—A pin-worm crawls out of the rectum, and causes itching,[6].—Troubles from pin-worms in the rectum,[1].—Gurgling in the rectum,[1].—*A feeling of heaviness in the lower portion of the rectum,*[1].— *Burning in the rectum,*[1].—*Burning in the rectum, in the morning, after a copious stool,*[1].—*Cramp in the rectum, the whole forenoon, a griping and sticking, with great anxiety, so that she was not able to sit, but was obliged to walk about* (after ten days),[1].—Drawing and cutting in the rectum, with a feeling of heat in it, after a natural stool,[1].—[770.] Severe pressure in the rectum (after some hours),[1].—Pressure in the rectum, as in diarrhœa,[1].— Pressure in the rectum, in the evening, when sitting (after twenty-two days),[1].—Continued pressure in the rectum, and oppression of breathing, after a stool,[1].—Twisting, almost dragging-down pain, in the rectum, soon after eating,[1].—Stitches towards the rectum (after thirteen days),[1].—A pain in the rectum as if it were torn, with a stool that is not hard,[1].—Twitching in the rectum,[1].—Tensive-twitching pain in the rectum, without a stool, in the evening,[1].—*Crawling in the rectum, as from worms,*[1].—[780.] Inflamed, burning, painful, grape-like eruption in the anus (after nineteen days),[1].— Much loss of blood from the anus, during the stool, in the evening,[1].— Hemorrhage from the anus, accompanying a severe coryza,[1].—Moisture oozes from the anus, smelling like herring brine,[1].—*Burning in the anus, also during the midday nap,*[1].—*Burning in the anus, during stool,*[1].—Burning and dry sensation in the anus,[1].—Twistings in the anus, and painful dragging in the rectum,[1].—After the stool, drawing cuttings in and about the anus,[1].—Sticking sore pain about the anus, externally,[1].—[790.] Stitches in the anus during coition,[1].—Soreness of the anus and between the thighs,[1]. —Transient smarting pain in the anus (sixteenth day),[1].—Crawling in the anus,[1].—Burning-itching in the anus, after a stool,[1].—Constant desire for stool, which can only be accomplished with great exertion, when only a very little passes (after twenty-four hours),[1].—Ineffectual urging to stool (eighth day),[6].—Urging, as in diarrhœa, though with a natural stool,[1].—Painful urging to stool, day and night,[1].

Stool.—Diarrhœa (the first eight days),[1].—[**800.**] Diarrhœa-like stool (first, third, and fifth days),[1].—*Frequent passage of stool, at first hard, then pasty, then liquid*,[1].—Stool at first thin, then crumbling, without colic,[4].—Hard, black stool (after four days),[1].—*Hard, undigested stool*, and not every day,[1].—Hard stool, with mucus, burning when passing,[1].—Unusually thick, formed stool,[1].—*Undigested stool*, rather thin (sixth day),[1].—*Undigested, hard, intermitting stool*,[1].—Stool scanty, mixed with blood (after twenty-six days),[1].—[**810.**] Diminished stool (after twenty-four hours),[1].—*Perfectly white stool*,[1].—White stool, streaked with blood, with great ill-humor and much colic, caused by breathing and touching,[1].—*Offensive stool, like bad eggs*,[1].—A pin-worm during the stool,[1].—Constipation,[6].—*Constipation* (seventh, eighteenth, and twenty-fourth days),[21].—*Constipation the first day;* she has no stool without an injection,[1].—Increased constipation, from day to day,[1].—Great constipation; he had to take castor oil,[19].—[**820.**] Extreme constipation,[19].—No stool, with constant urging; with confusion of the head,[1].

Urinary Organs.—Kidneys and Bladder. Aching in the kidneys and lumbar region, when riding,[1].—Pressive pain in the region of the kidneys,[1].—Pain in the bladder, and cutting, on urinating, through the night (eleventh day),[1].—*Urethra.* Pain in the urinary passages, after getting the feet slightly wet,[1].—*Burning in the urethra, when urinating*,[1].—Burning in the urethra, and constant desire to urinate after urinating,[1].—Burning and sore pain in the urethra, on urinating,[1].—Burning in the urethra, before and after urinating,[1].—[**830.**] Cutting in the urethra, when urinating (the first days),[1].—Stitches through the female urethra,[1].—Cutting stitches in the urethra, with ineffectual urging to urinate,[1].—Fine tickling stitches through the urethra (second day),[11].—Frequent desire to urinate, soon after urinating, with a scanty discharge,[1].—Desire to urinate, especially when walking,[1].—The child desires to urinate, without urine following immediately; at another time, he was not able to retain the urine but allowed a few drops to pass,[1].—Urging to urinate; it seems as though he could not hold the urine,[1].—*Micturition.* *Very frequent urinating (after eight hours),[1].—Frequent urinating (in an infant whose mother had taken Calcarea),[9].—[**840.**] Frequent and copious urinating, forenoon and afternoon,[6].—An unusual amount of watery urine, the whole day,[1].—Nocturnal enuresis (after three days),[1].—*Frequent urinating at night*,[1].—Urinating frequently the whole night,[1].—Urinating at night, with burning in the orifice of the urethra,[1].—Much sour-smelling urine at night,[1].—A sensation as though he could not finish urinating, as though some urine remained in the bladder,[1].—Some urine always remains in the bladder after urinating, which runs out after he thinks that he has finished,[6].—Trickling of urine after urinating,[1].—[**850.**] Involuntary passage of urine, on every motion during menstruation,[1].—*Urine.* *Very dark-colored urine without sediment*,[1].—Pungent odor to the urine,[1].—Very offensive urine (second day),[1].—Offensive, pungent odor to the urine, which is very clear and pale (twenty-fifth day),[1].—*Offensive, dark-brown urine, with a white sediment*,[1].—Much mucus passes with the urine, like leucorrhœa, but which is not noticed at other times,[1].—The urine becomes turbid after a short time, and deposits a whitish, flaky sediment; a fatty pellicle forms on the surface, and the urine smells fatty (sixth day),[11].—Profuse sediment of white mealy-like powder, in the evening (after eleventh day),[1].

Sexual Organs.—Male. The prepuce is inflamed and red, with a burning pain on urinating, and on touch (fourth day),[1].—[860.] *Inflammation of prepuce and frænum, and orifice of urethra, with a little yellow pus between frænum and glans;* gone next day (first day),[24].—Severe burning in the tip of the glans (after ten days),[1].—Cutting pain in the tip of the glans (fourth day),[1].—Severe stitches in the glans (after three days),[6].—During coition, such violent tickling on the forepart of the glans, that he was obliged to withdraw the penis,[1].—Itching in the forepart of the glans, especially after urinating (after twenty-eight days),[1].—Erections in the morning, after rising, with much inclination for coition (sixth day),[1].—Frequent erections, at night (second day),[11].—Incomplete erections at night,[11].—Unpleasant twitching in the penis, in the morning and evening, in bed,[1].—[870.] The scrotum hangs down relaxed,[1].—A sore spot on the scrotum,[1].—Severe itching on the scrotum,[1].—Pain in the spermatic cord, as if contracted,[1].—Pressive pain in the right testicle,[1].—Pressive or bruised pain in the left testicle (after twelve days),[1].—Crushing pain in the testicles,[1].—Stitches in the testicles (previously indurated), at intervals of two minutes,[1].—Cutting-smarting in the testicles, starting from the groin,[1].—*Sexual desire much increased,*[1].—[880.] Very great sexual desire (after twenty-one days),[1].—Great desire for coition, especially when walking, in the forenoon (after seventeen days),[1].—Sexual desire, in the evening (second day),[11].—*Excessive sexual desire, caused by lascivious fancies, wherewith the penis failed in erection, which was only induced by rubbing; scarcely had coition taken place when the semen was emitted; this was followed by excessive weakness and great excitability of the nerves; he was discontented and angry, and the knees seemed to give way from weakness* (fourth day),[1].—Prostatic fluid flows after the urine,[1].—Prostatic fluid is discharged after the stool, and after the urine,[1].—Emissions frequently, during the first eleven days, in a man forty-three years of age, who had had none for eighteen years,[1].—*Emissions, during the first days frequently, then continually less,*[1].—Emissions the first night, followed by an improved condition,[1].—Emissions at night, which are very slight and incomplete (first day),[11].—[890.] Two emissions in one night,[19].—Emission very late, during coition (after seven days),[1].—No ejaculation of semen, at the orgasm, during coition, but it is slowly discharged afterwards,[1].—The usual emission during an embrace, but without any thrill of enjoyment (fifth day),[1].—*Female.* Voluptuous sensation in the female genitals (in the afternoon, without cause), with orgasm, followed by great weariness (after seven days),[1].—Burning-sore pain in the genitals,[1].—Burning-biting, with soreness in the female genitals,[1].—Itching and sticking in the female genitals,[1].—Moisture, like profuse sweat, in the fold between the pudenda and thigh, with biting,[1].—Inflammation, redness, and swelling of the pudenda of a little girl, with purulent discharge without pain, when urinating,[1].—[900.] Sore pain in the pudenda, after urinating,[1].—Burning in the labiæ, two days before menstruation (after thirty-nine days),[1].—Itching on the external and internal labiæ,[1].—Leucorrhœa like mucus (fifth and sixteenth day),[1].—*Leucorrhœa like milk* (the first three days),[1].—*Milky leucorrhœa,* which is usually discharged when urinating,[1].—Discharge of bloody water from the vagina of an old woman, with pain in the back, as if the menses would reappear,[1].—Discharge of blood, nine days previous to menstruation, lasting two days (after twelve days),[1].—*Menstruation.*

Menstruation appears the first time two days too early (after fourteen days); but the next time it appears on the thirty-second day (after forty-six days),[1]. —*Menstruation three days too early (after seventeen days),[1].—[910.] *Menstruation four days too early, *lasting eight days*,[1].—The usually regular menstruation appears immediately after taking *Calcarea, about seven days too early*,[1].—The menses, which had been long suppressed, appeared at the new moon (in one thirty-two years of age), (after six days),[1].—Menstruation, long since ceased, reappears at the new moon, in one fifty-two years of age (after six days),[1].—The usually too profuse menstruation was moderated (curative action),[1].—Menstruation unusually profuse, twice in succession, and brought with it a small fœtus, with a kind of labor-pain, like an abortion, with a great desire for stool, and cutting and pressure in the lower abdomen,[1].

Respiratory Organs.—Larynx. Mucus in the larynx, which is loosened by hawking,[1].—*Whistling in the larynx, in the evening, after lying down*,[1].—The larynx is rough, especially in the morning,[1].—Rawness of the larynx, with pain on swallowing,[1].—*Voice.* [920.] *Painless hoarseness, so that she was scarcely able to speak, in the morning* (eleventh day),[1].— *Cough and Expectoration.*—Hacking, hoarse cough, which, to the sound, was not caused by mucus,[1].—Constant short, hacking cough, in single hacks,[1].—*Tickling cough, as from a feather in the throat*,[1].—*Cough caused by a sensation as if a plug stuck in the throat and moved up and down*,[1].— Spasmodic cough, in the evening,[1].—*Night cough* (after six days),[1].— Night cough, during sleep, without waking,[1].—At night, severe cough on waking, for two minutes,[1].—Constant forcible, scraping cough at night, in bed, after the first waking (about 10 o'clock), (seventh day),[1].—[930.] Constant cough at night, with hoarseness (after thirty-nine days),[1].—*Cough caused by eating*,[1].—*Cough provoked by inspiration*,[1].—*Cough always caused by playing on the piano*,[1].—Cough mostly in sleep, together with stopped, then fluent coryza,[1].—*Cough, with coryza*,[1].—Hard, dry cough,[23].— *Dry hacking cough, in the evening, especially in bed (after two days),[1].— *Dry cough, especially at night*,[1].—*Dry cough at night after midnight, so that the heart and arteries throb*,[1].—[940.] *Very violent cough, at first dry, afterward with profuse salty expectoration, with pain as if something had been torn loose from the larynx*,[1].—Cough and expectoration the whole day,[1].— *Cough with expectoration during the day, but none during the night*,[1].— *Cough in the morning, with yellowish expectoration* (after five days),[1].—In the morning, after he had choked himself, he was obliged to cough violently, which caused expectoration of blood several times, followed by stitches in the palate,[1].—Much cough, with mucous expectoration, in the evening after lying down, and at night; during the day only a little and dry cough,[1].— Cough, with much tough, tasteless, odorless expectoration, morning and evening, in bed,[1].—Cough, with much expectoration of thick mucus, at night,[1].—*During a violent cough, in the evening, he raises and expectorates something sweet*,[1].—*Expectoration of mucus, with a sweetish taste*,[1].— [950.] Mucous expectoration, in the morning, with hacking,[1].—Expectoration of mucus, at night, with scraping in the throat,[1].—*Expectoration of blood, when coughing and hawking, with a rough and sore sensation in the chest*,[1].—Expectoration of blood caused by a short hacking cough, with vertigo and unsteadiness of the thighs, when walking rapidly,[1].—*Respiration.* Hot breath, with heat in the mouth, without thirst,[1].—*Frequent need to breathe deeply*,[1].—*Was obliged to breathe deeply, which caused sticking, now in the right, now in the left side of the chest, or hypochondrium,[1].—*Excessive urging to take a deep breath*, with great distension and contraction of the abdomen, and pain in the abdomen and chest (after three days),[1].—Desire to hold the breath,[1].—Tightness of breath in the chest, with stitches in it,[1].—[960.] *Shortness of breath on going up the slightest ascent*,[6].—Short breath, worse when sitting than when moving,[1]. —Short, almost sobbing breathing, when asleep after previous weeping,[1].— Difficult respiration (after seven days),[1].—Difficult loud breathing, through the nose, when walking,[1].—Loss of breath on lying down, followed by whistling respiration,[1].—Loss of breath when walking in the wind; the oppression of the chest also continues in the room, and increases as soon as she walks a few steps,[1].

Chest.—*Mucus in the chest*, without cough (after some hours),[1].—Weakness in the chest, after some loud speaking,[1].—*Anxiety in the chest*,[1].—[970.] Tightened sensation of fulness in the chest, in the morning on rising, as if he could not sufficiently expand the lungs by breathing; disappearing after some expectoration,[1].—Tightness of the chest; breathing fails her,[1].— *Tightness of the chest, as if she were filled too full, and with blood*,[1].—Tightness of the chest immediately after rising in the morning; he was unable to walk two steps without being obliged to sit down (after twenty-four days),[1].— Tightness of the chest in the forenoon, on walking in the open air (after forty-eight hours),[1].—Oppression of the chest, after a stool,[1].—*Oppression and tension of the chest*,[1].—Pressure in the chest, especially below the right nipple,[1].—*Cutting in the chest, on inspiration*, after a few hours,[1].—*Sticking pain in the chest (first evening),[13].—[980.] Fine sticking pain around the whole chest, in the region of the fourth and fifth ribs,[11].—Stitches in the chest, extending to the throat, for several hours,[1].—Stitches in various parts of the chest, with oppression (seventh day),[11].—A stitch causes shuddering, extending from the hepatic region into the chest (after ten hours),[2].— Stitches through the chest, from the left to the right side, with a feeling of contraction; he breathed with difficulty, and on breathing the stitches were more violent (after four days),[1].—Jerking stitches in the chest, mostly on the left side,[1].—*Sore pain in the chest, especially on inspiration*,[1].—*Sore pain in the right mamma on the slightest touch*,[1].—*The whole chest is painfully sensitive to the touch and on inspiration*,[8].—Raw pain in the chest after much speaking and walking, as also on coughing,[1].—[990.] *During the cough pain in the chest as if raw*, evenings and nights,[1].—*The mammary glands pain as if they were suppurating, especially on touch*,[1].—Discharge of milk from the breast of an infant (after forty-eight hours),[1].—Oppression on the forepart of the chest, even when not breathing,[1].—Pain in the sternum, as if pressed,[1].—Stitches through the chest, across the sternum, from before backwards,[11].—*Sides.* Swelling and external heat of the right breast,[1].—Glandular swelling of the right breast, with pain on touch,[1].— Swelling and inflammation of the left mamma, with fine stitches in it (fourth day),[1].—Pain in the ribs of the right side,[17].—[1000.] Tension in the ribs of both sides, extending across to the pit of the stomach (second day),[16].—Cramp in the left intercostal muscles; she was obliged to bend suddenly towards that side in order to relieve it,[1].—Gnawing pain in the left side of the chest, as if externally on the ribs and sternum, only slightly aggravated by inspiration (after one hour),[8].—Oppression and sticking pain in the region of the fifth and sixth ribs of the right side (after three-quarters of an hour), (first day),[1].—Paroxysmal pressure in the right side of the chest after motion, lasting one hour,[1].—Stitches in the region of the fifth to seventh ribs, in the left side (first day),[11].—Stitches in the region of the seventh and eighth ribs of the left side (second day),[11].—Stitches and drawing in the left side of the chest, extending to the left submaxillary gland,[1].—Stitches in the left side of the chest, especially in the evening (after eleven days),[1].—Stitches deep in the right side of the chest. in the evening, especially on breathing,[1].—[1010.] *Stitches in the left side of the chest,* on almost every respiration, usually disappearing by rubbing (after a few hours),[1].—Stitches in the left side of the chest, on breathing and on raising the body,[1]. —Tearing under the ribs of the left side,[17].

Heart and Pulse.—Anxiety about the heart (second day),[1].—Spasmodic contraction in the region of the heart, impeding respiration, followed by severe shocks (after sixteen days),[1].—Painful pressure in the præcordial region,[1].—*Palpitation,*[1].—*Great palpitation,*[1].—*Palpitation and anxiety,* in the evening, in bed, before going to sleep,[1].—Palpitation, with restless sleep, at night,[1].—[1020.] Great palpitation of the heart after dinner,[1].—Palpitation of the heart after eating, felt without laying the hand upon the chest,[1].—Palpitation in the midday sleep while sitting, which wakes him,[1].—During a walk palpitation and pain in the chest (after nineteen days),[1].—Severe palpitation, with anxious dread that he might have organic disease of the heart,[1].—Severe palpitation, with excessive anguish and restless oppression of the chest and pain in the back; she makes a loud sound as if every breath would leave the body, with coldness of the body and cold sweat,[3].—Excessive palpitation, with irregular pulse,[1].—Stitches in the heart, which prevent breathing and leave a pressive pain there,[1].—Pulse rapid, without feverishness,[1].

Neck and Back.—Neck. *Hard swelling of the cervical glands* (after thirteen days),[1].—[1030.] *Painless swelling of the glands, of the size of a hazelnut, in the neck, on the margin of the hair* (after five days),[1].—Swelling and painfulness of the lowest cervical vertebræ,[1].—The neck feels stiff,[1].—The neck feels stiff, on stooping,[1].—Effects of taking cold; stiffness in the neck, and cervical muscles; stitches in the neck and in the head, over the eyes, with cough (soon),[1].—Pain in the neck, with stiffness,[11].—*The glands of the neck pain,*[1].—*Pain in the neck, on turning the head, as if a tumor would protrude there,*[1].—Itching sticking burning, in the neck and between the shoulder-blades, with heartburn (after five days),[1].—Sudden pain in the neck, as if burnt, on twisting and turning the head,[1].—[1040.] Tension in the neck, so that she could not turn the head,[1].—Sticking pain in the neck,[11].—Tearing in the muscles of the neck,[17].—Stiffness in the nape of the neck and throat,[1].—Stitches in the nape of the neck, and shoulder-blades, with confusion of the head,[1].—Tearing in the nape of the neck,[17].—Tearings in the nape of the neck (first day),[16].—Tearing in the nape of the neck (second day),[16].—Swelling on the left side of the neck, with painfulness on touch, or turning the head, with internal soreness of the throat,[1].—Swelling in the glands on the left side of the neck, as large as a pigeon's egg, with sticking pain in the throat on swallowing,[1].—[1050.] Stiff sensation in the side of the neck,[6].—Tearing in the sides of the neck,[17]. —*Back.* Pain in the back,[17].—Intolerable pain in the back,[1].—The spine pains on bending backward,[1].—Painful stiffness in the spine, with indolence and heaviness in the legs. in the morning on waking, and after rising (after seventeen days),[1].—Pressive pain in the middle of the back and beneath the shoulder-blades (after twenty-seven days),[1].—Pain as if wrenched in both sides of the back,[1].—Stitches in the back (first day),[1].—Bruised pain in the back and chest,[1].—[1060.] Spasmodic, jerking pain, extending from the left side of the back to the anus,[1].—Painful jerks in the right side of the back, on breathing, with chilliness, and cold creepings (after seven days),[1].—*Dorsal.* Twitching in both shoulder-blades, and on the chest,[1]. —Pressure beneath the right shoulder-blade extending upward,[1].—Stitches in the right shoulder-blade (at 9 A.M., second day),[15].—Stitches in the left shoulder-blade, in the præcordial region (second day),[1].—Itching stitches in the right shoulder-blade,[1].—Pinching constriction between the shoulder-blades (after thirty days),[1].—*Drawing pain between the shoulder-blades,*[1].— *Pressure between the shoulder-blades, which on motion impedes respiration,*[1].— [1070.] Pressive pain in the spine, between the shoulder-blades, with short breath and aggravated by breathing, with painfulness in the bones of the spine on touch,[1]. — Burning-sticking pain in the back, between the shoulders,[11].—Cutting pain between the shoulder-blades, during rest (after six days),[1].—Stitches between the shoulders,[17].—Tearings between the shoulder-blades (after three hours),[1].—Tearing between the shoulder-blades (first, second, and third days),[16].—Tearing between the shoulder-blades,[17].— Drawing pressive-tearing pain between the shoulder-blades,[11].—Single fine stitches in the upper part of the back, during inspiration,[1].—*Lumbar.* Pain in the small of the back,[17].—[1080.] Pain in the small of the back,[11 17].— Pain in the small of the back (second day),[11].—Pain in the small of the back (third day),[16].—*Pain in the small of the back* (after six and eight days),[1]. —*Pain in the small of the back, so that he could scarcely rise from sitting,*[1].— Pain in the small of the back, as from lifting,[1].—Pain in the small of the back, from lifting a heavy weight,[1].—Pain in the small of the back, in the morning, immediately after rising,[1].—Severe pain in the small of the back; she could neither sit nor lie,[1].—Drawing in the small of the back (after four hours),[1].—[1090.] Drawing pain in the small of the back, when sitting,[1].— Dragging in the small of the back, towards the rectum,[1].—Tearing in the small of the back (first, second, and third days),[16].—Tearing in the small of the back,[17].—Pains in the lumbar region, and in the iliac bones, as if menstruation would come on (third day),[12].—The spine in the region of the kidneys is painful on stretching, as after lifting,[6].—Sticking pain in the left side of the sacrum, while walking (second day),[11].—Drawing in the coccyx (third day),[16].—Sticking pain in the coccyx (first day),[11].

Extremities in General.—Single involuntary motions and twitching in the right thigh, in the left shoulder and left arm,[1].—[1100.] Prostration and weariness in all the limbs (evening of first day),[12].—**Great weakness and weariness of all the limbs,* especially in the feet; it lasts till she goes to bed (evening of first day),[12].—Painless drawings in the limbs, in the afternoon,[1].—Shooting pains throughout the limbs, both upper and lower; he began to imagine he was going to have rheumatic fever,[19].— Tearings in the limbs,[1].—Slight tearing pains in the extremities (fifth and sixth days),[16].—Painless twitching of single limbs, during the day,[1].— Violent sticking-drawing pains in all the joints (first day),[11].—Drawing pressure in the joints,[6].—Slight sticking pains in the joints (second day),[11]. —[1110.] Sticking pain in the joints, on great exertion only (eighth day),[11].— Tearing stitches in various joints (third day),[11].—**Paralytic bruised pain in the long bones, and in the joints of the limbs, also in the small of the back, on motion; even when sitting and standing the back pains as if beaten, and the muscles of the legs are sore to touch,*[1].—Tearings in the arms and legs, though always only in a small spot,[1].—The hands and feet go to sleep,[1].— Burning in the palms and soles,[1].

Superior Extremities.—Slight sticking-tearing pains in the arms (fifth day),[11].—**The arms pain as if bruised, on moving them or taking hold* of them,[1].—*The arm goes to sleep if he lies upon it, with pains,[1].—*Cramp in the whole of one or the other arm, for a quarter of an hour (after fifth day),[1].—[1120.] Twitching or sticking pain in the arm and wrist at night, which prevented sleep,[1].—Uneasiness and anxiety in the joints of the arm and wrist,[1].—Burning paralytic pain in the whole of the right arm, from the finger-joints to the shoulder (after six days),[1].—Tearing below the right arm (first and second days),[16].—Tearing in the right arm from above downward,[1].—Drawing-tearing in the right arm, from the shoulder to the hand (after three hours),[1].—Jerking pain in the right arm, in the evening (thirteenth day),[1].—*Weakness and a kind of paralysis of the left arm; it is difficult to move or raise it; it will fall down of itself,[1].—Severe wrenching pain on moving the left arm (second day),[12].—Tearing in the left arm (second day),[16].—[1130.] Tearing in the left arm,[17].—*Shoulder.* Pain in both shoulders and in the elbows, as after great fatigue,[1].—Pressure on the shoulders (after twenty-four hours),[1].—Pressive pain in the right shoulder-joint, only during rest, not when raising or moving the arm,[1].—Shooting pains under left shoulder,[20].—Stitches in the right shoulder after dinner,[11]. —Tearing in the shoulders,[17].—Tearing in the shoulders (third day),[16].— Tearing in the left shoulder and elbow-joint (after fourteen days),[1].—The shoulder-joints disturb him at night, at the commencement of sleep; he was obliged to lay the arm above the head,[1].—[1140.] The shoulder-joint pains in the evening and at night,[1].—Sticking pain in the right shoulder-joint,[11].— Sticking pain in the left shoulder-joint,[11].—*Stitches in the left shoulder-joint*, the whole day (after four days),[1].—Tearing in the left shoulder-joint (first day),[16].—*Arm.* Partially paralyzed condition of the muscles of the upper arm,[11].—The upper arm pains just below the shoulder-joint, so that he cannot raise it high up, nor put it across the back,[1].—Pain in the middle of the upper arm, as if the flesh were tightly adherent to the bone,[1].— Drawing pain in the left upper arm, when sitting (and sewing),[1].—Sticking pain in the right humerus, followed by trembling of the arm with stitches of various muscles,[11].—[1150.] Stitches in the upper arm, beneath the arms, in the back, and in the limbs,[1].—Tearing pain in the middle of the upper arm in a small point,[1].—Tearing in the right upper arm (first day),[16].— *Elbow.* Sticking pain in the right elbow-joint (second day),[11].—Tearing in the elbows,[17].—*Forearm.* Swelling of the forearm and back of the hand, with tension on motion,[1].—Drawing pain in the left forearm,[1].— Drawing pain in the forearm, extending from the bend of the elbow to the wrist, mostly during rest,[1].—Painful pressure in the muscles of the forearm when walking, which immediately disappears on touch, standing, and sitting (after a quarter of an hour),[5].—*Spasmodic tearing pain on the outer side of the forearm*, extending from the elbow to the wrist, as soon as he takes hold of anything with the hand,[1].—[1160.] Tearing in the right forearm (first day),[16].—Tearing in the left forearm (first day),[16].—Tearing in the left forearm,[17].—*Wrist.* Drawing pain in the wrists and metacarpus,[1].—Jerklike drawings in the wrist, and thence up the arm, even in the morning, in bed,[1]. —Feeling as if sprained in the right wrist,[1].—*Pain as from a sprain in the right wrist, or as if something had been wrenched or dislocated,[1].—Pain as if sprained in the right wrist, with sticking and tearing in it, on motion,[6].— Stitches like tearing in the right wrist,[17].—Stitches in the left wrist (second day),[11].—[1170.] Violent stitches in the left wrist (third day),[11].—Tearing in the wrists,[17].—Tearing in the right wrist (second and third days),[16].— Tearing in the left wrist (second and third days),[16].—Tearing in the left wrist,[17].—Sticking-tearing pain in the wrists (sixth day),[11].—Jerking shocks in the wrists,[1].—***Hand.*** Distended veins on the hands, with burning sensation on the back of the hands,[1].—*Trembling in the hands,* lasting several hours, in the afternoon (second day),[1].—The hand was painful in the morning, and completely relaxed,[1].—[1180.] *Cramp in the hands,* at night, lasting till morning on rising,[1].—Cramp in the left hand,[1].—Drawing pain in the hands,[1].—Sticking in the palms, in the morning, in bed, for two minutes,[1].—Violent sticking pain in the metacarpal bones of the left hand (first day),[11].—Piercing stitches in the left metacarpal bones,[11].—Tearing in right hand (first day),[16].—Tearing in the left hand (first and second days),[16]. —Tearing in the left hand,[17].—Tearing in the left metacarpus (third day),[16]. —[1190.] Tearing pain in the palms,[1].—***Fingers.*** *The finger-joints became much swollen,*[19].—Spasmodic contraction of the fingers,[1].—Involuntary twitching of the left thumb,[1].—*The fingers become dead,*[1].—*The third middle fingers become dead; they are white, cold, and senseless, preceded by slight drawing in them* (after three hours),[7].—Severe pain in the knuckles, as if cauterized,[1].—*Pain in the finger-joints, as if they were swollen, on waking from sleep in the evening, without visible swelling,*[1].—On stretching out the fingers, they seem tense and bent inward, as if stuck together,[1].— Cramp in the fingers, without their being drawn inward,[1].—[1200.] Cramplike pain in the last joint of the index finger,[5].—Cramplike pain between the third and fourth fingers of the right hand,[4].—Drawing in the second joint of the left index finger (second day),[16].—Sticking pain in the left finger-joints (seventh day),[11].—Sticking pain in the first joint of the left index finger,[11].—Piercing-sticking pain in the first phalanx of the right index finger (second day),[1].—Piercing-sticking pain in the last phalanx of the right middle finger (first day),[11].—Tearing in the finger-joints (after twenty-eight days),[1].—Tearing in the first joint of the left thumb (first day),[16].—Tearing in the second joint of the left thumb,[16] [17].—[1210.] Tearing in the left thumb (third day),[16].—Tearing in the first joint of the left thumb,[17].—Tearing in the first joint of the left thumb (fourth day),[16].— Tearing in the left index finger,[17].—Tearing in the first joint of the left index finger (first day),[16].—Tearing in the second joint of the left index finger (first day),[16].—Tearing in the right middle finger,[17].—Tearing in the right and left ring fingers,[17].—Tearing in the first joint of the left ring finger (first day),[16].—Tearing in the second joint of the left ring finger,[17].— [1220.] Tearing in the second joint of left ring finger (third day),[16].— Tearing in the first joint of the right little finger (second day),[16].—Tearing in the first joint of the left little finger (first and second day),[16].— Tearing in the second joint of the left little finger,[17].—Transient tearing in the tips of the fingers,[1].—Jerking pain in the fingers,[1].—Several hang-nails,[1]. —Commencing suppuration around the nail of the right index finger (after six days),[1].—Suppuration around the nail of the middle finger,[1].

Inferior Extremities.—Muscular twitches in the legs and around the pelvis,[1].—[1230.] Severe twitches and spasmodic drawings of the extremities, at night, awake him from sleep (first day),[11].—*Unusual weariness in the lower extremities,* at noon, especially in the ankles (fourth day),[11].— *Painful weariness of the legs, especially of the thighs, as after a long walk* (seventeenth and nineteenth days),[1].—The legs are weary and bruised, especially the joints (after twenty days),[1].—*Weakness and trembling in the legs, especially above and below the knees, after coition,*[1].—Tearing in both legs, from the hip to the ankle (after fourteen days),[1].—Bruised pain in the joints of the legs,[1].—***Hip.*** Numb sensation on the right hip and thigh, with a feeling as though those parts were brittle, as if short and small,[1].—

Tension in the hip-joint, with drawing pain in the hip-bones, during a walk, in the evening,[1].—Wrenching pain in the left hip-joint (third day),[11].— [1240.] Stitches above the right hip,[1].—Stitches in the hip-joint, extending up from the knee-cap, when stepping on beginning to walk,[1].—Stitches in the hip-joint, on stooping,[1].—Dull stitches in the left hip-joint, aggravated by motion,[11].—Tearing in the hip-joints,[17].—Suppurating pain in both hip-joints, when walking in the room,[1].—*Thigh.* *Weariness and a feeling of stiffness in the anterior muscles of the thigh, in the morning, on beginning to walk,[1].—Weakness in the thighs and groin, when walking,[1].—Pain in the nates, as if suppurating, on touch, less when sitting than when walking (after forty-eight hours),[1].—Drawing pain in the muscles of the legs, on the back of the thighs, and in the calves, in the evening (after thirty-six hours),[1].—[1250.] Drawing spasmodic pain on the right nates, extending towards the anus,[1].—Cutting pain in the upper part of the left thigh, as from over-distension of the muscles, especially on motion,[1].—Stitches in the thigh, in the knee, and in the heel, only at night,[1].—Painful twitching in the right thigh, in a small spot,[1].—Painful muscular twitches in both nates, when sitting and standing,[1].—Tearing in the thighs,[17].—Tearing in both thighs (second day),[16].—Tearing in the right thigh,[17].—Tearing in right thigh (first day),[16].—Tearing in the left thigh,[17].—[1260.] Tearing in the left thigh (second, third, and fourth days),[16].—Bruised pain in the muscles of the right thigh, after walking,[1].—*Knee.* *Swelling of the knees,*[1].—Numb sensation in the knees during the afternoon nap, which disappeared on waking,[1].—A feeling in the knee as though she could not stretch out the leg enough (after sixteen days),[1].—Weariness in the knees, at night,[1].—Great weariness in the knees and ankles, after a warm bath (third day),[11].—Pain, as from weariness, in the knees (seventh day),[11].— Pain in the knee-cap, on rising from sitting (fourth day),[6].—Tension below the knee, on kneeling,[1].—[1270.] Tension in the right knee-joint,[17].—Pain, as if sprained, in the right knee (after fourteen days),[1].—Pressive pain in the knees,[1].—Dull pressive pain in the knee-cap,[1].—Sticking pain in the knee, at noon, when riding (third day),[11].—Sticking and throbbing pain in the left knee, in the morning, more when sitting than when walking; he was obliged to limp,[1].—Transient stitches in both knees (first day),[11].—Stitches in the left knee, lasting half an hour (after five days),[1].—Dull drawing-sticking pain in the patella (seventh day),[11].—Tearing in the knees,[17].— [1280.] Transient tearings in the knees,[1].—Tearing and tension on the inside of the knee, on rising from sitting,[1].—Tearing in the right knee (first day),[16].—Tearing in the left knee (second day),[16].—Stitchlike tearing in the left knee,[17].—Tearing pain about the knee, just above the hollow of the knee,[1].—Tearing in the right knee-joint,[17].—Tearing in the right knee-joint (first and second days),[16].—Tearing and tension in the right knee-joint,[17]. —Bruised pain in the knee (tenth day),[1].—*Leg.* [1290.] Erysipelatous inflammation and swelling of the lower leg, with chilliness of the body,[1].— Jerking of the lower leg,[1].—A stitching jerk in the right leg, so that he was suddenly jerked upward (after thirty days),[1].—*The legs go to sleep, in the evening, when sitting,*[1].—Numb sensation in the left leg (after seven days),[1].—Heaviness in the legs (after eight days),[1].—Uneasiness in the legs, with much eructations,[1].—Tension in the leg, from the foot to the knee, as though the bone had gone to sleep, with a pressive cramp in the stomach,[1]. —Cramp in the right leg for an hour, with drawing inward and pain of the foot (after four days),[1].—Tearing in the left leg,[17].—[1300.] A stitching-crawling on the lower leg,[1].—Cramp in the muscles, near the tibia, at night,[1].—Drawing and crushed pain in the tibiæ,[1].—Pain, as from a sprain, in the anterior tibial muscles, when walking (after twenty-one days),[1].— Dull pressive pain in the muscles near the tibiæ, when walking,[1].—Cuttings over the tibia,[1].—Tearing in the right tibia (first day),[16].—Tearing in the left tibia (second day),[16].—Sticking-tearing pain in the tibiæ and calves (sixth day),[11].—*The lower leg is painful in the calf, on walking and stepping*, or on touch and on bending the foot,[1].—[1310.] Tension in both calves (first day),[11].—Tension in the right calf,[17].—Tension in the calf,[1].—*Violent cramp in the calves, at night,*[1].—*Cramp in the calves and hollows of the knees, on stretching out the legs* (when drawing on the boot), which is relieved on bending the knee, but returns on stretching it out again,[1].—Cramp in the calf and foot, if he moves very much, with sticking pain,[1].—Tearing-drawing in the calf,[1].—Stitches and weakness in the calf,[1].—Tearing in the calves,[17].—Tearing in the right calf (first day),[16].—[1320.] Tearing in the left calf (first and fourth days),[16].—Tearing in the tendo Achillis,[17].—Tearing in the left tendo Achillis,[17].—***Ankle.*** Great weariness in the ankles (first day),[11].—Weariness in the ankles, especially on standing (first day),[11].— Pain in the left ankle, as if it were tightly bound around,[1].—Pain in the ankle, as if it were broken, when walking, especially in the afternoon,[1].— Pain in the right malleolus, when stepping, as if the foot would be put out of joint,[1].—Tension in both inner malleoli,[1].—Tearing in the ankles,[17].— ***Foot.*** [1330.] Swelling of the feet, lasting eleven days,[1].—*Sweat of the feet, toward evening,*[1].—*So great weariness of the feet that it seems as though they could not bear the body, and the knees would bend* (second day),[11].— Such great weariness in the feet, at 7 P.M., that she believed that the feet would break to pieces; lasted till she went to bed (first evening),[14].—Burning in the feet, in the evening,[1].—Drawing pain in the feet at night, which awakes her,[1].—Pain, as from a sprain, in the left foot (after thirteen days),[1].—Tearing in the feet,[17].—Tearing in the right foot,[17].—Tearing in the left foot (third day),[16].—[1340.] Tearing in the anterior part of the left foot (first and fourth days),[16].—Very violent tearing in the anterior part of the left foot,[17].—Tearing in the right metatarsal joints (second day),[16].— Inflammatory swelling on the back of the left foot, with burning pain, and severe itching all about,[1].—Suddenly, a very hot feeling on the back of the left foot, and on the leg, as if hot air were blown upon them,[1].—Rheumatic pain in the sole of the left foot,[11].—*Burning in the soles,*[1].—Burning in the soles of the feet, at night,[1].—*Cramp in the left sole,*[1].—Severe cutting on the outer side of the right sole, in the evening and through the whole night (after ten hours),[1].—[1350.] Severe tearing in the soles,[1].—Tearing in the sole of the right foot (first day),[16].—Painful sensitiveness of the soles, even in the room, as if softened by hot water, with great painfulness when walking,[1].—Pain in the soles, as from suppuration,[1].—Blisters appear on the left heel, when walking, which become a kind of large boils, with sticking and itching pain (after eight hours),[1].—Visible twitching in the left great toe, in the evening, in bed,[1].—*Cramp in the toes,*[1].—The toes pain, as from a tight boot,[6].—Stitches in the great toe,[1].—Tearing in the toes,[1].— [1360.] Transient tearings in the toes,[1].—Tearing in the great toe,[6].—Tearing in the left great toe (first day),[16].—Violent pain on the tip of the right great toe (after twenty-one days),[1].—Severe burning in the tip of the great toe (after twenty-one days),[1].—Burning pressure beneath the nails of the great toes,[1].—Sore burning pain in the corns,[1].

General Symptoms.—Objective. Inclination to stretch, in the morning,[1].—*Twitching of the muscles,*[1].—*Trembling in the body,*[11].—[1370.]

Trembling of the body (second day),[11].—Trembling in the body, on waking, with spasmodic twitches of various muscles in the thigh and arm (second day),[11].—Trembling in the morning,[1].—Continual trembling of the whole body, which became worse when she went into the open air,[1].—Anxious trembling, with weariness,[1].—She started so much from the slight prick of a needle in the finger, that she became nauseated; the tongue, lips, and hands became very white and cold, with coldness of the forehead and face, with obscuration of sight, uneasiness, flushes of heat, and trembling; she was obliged to lie down (mesmerizing relieved her at once), (after eighteen days),[1].—*Epileptic attacks;* while standing at his work he fell suddenly to the ground sideways, without consciousness, and on returning to consciousness found himself lying with outstretched arms; this was followed by heat and some sweat (after nine days),[1].—*Congestions of blood,*[1].—*He becomes tired very soon, from bodily exertion,*[1].—*After walking, he becomes fatigued,* even to feverishness, and is attacked with chilliness and thirst,[1].—[1380.] *Easily strained; pain in the small of the back; he could not lift anything heavy,*[1].—*Such great weariness that the person is not able to walk* (second day),[12].—Unusual weariness, which was better when walking,[1].—Very weary and sleepy the whole day (after eleven days),[1].—Weakness (first day),[13].—Great general weakness in the evening, lasting half an hour,[1].—Weakness and weariness, after dinner (after nine days),[1].—*Very weak from speaking;* she was obliged to cease,[1].—A feeling of weakness, after a stool,[1].—*Very weak and sick, for several days after coition,*[1].—[1390.] Weakness during the day, so great that she scarcely knew how she could bear the oppressive anxious condition; breathing the fresh open air, only, refreshed and strengthened her (after twelve days),[1].—Weakness, with yawning (after four days),[1].—*Great loss of strength,*[1].—**Great loss of power on walking,** *especially in the limbs, with exhausting sweat,*[1].—Exhaustion and weariness in the limbs, especially in the knees,[1].—*Great exhaustion on waking in the morning from a deep sleep, so that the confused and sleepy condition continues even after rising from the bed,*[1].—**She was unable to go upstairs,** and became very much exhausted from it (after fourteen days),[1].—She lay for ten days in the greatest exhaustion, so that she could neither move about nor do any work; with most violent attacks of convulsive laughter,[1].—Attack of faintness in the evening, with blackness before the eyes when sitting,[1].—Attacks of faintness, with coldness and indistinct vision (after three days),[1].—[1400.] Attack of faintness, with great drops of sweat on the face,[1].—Much uneasiness, so that he was obliged to move the hands and feet,[1].—Great uneasiness in the evening, especially in the limbs; he was unable to lie still,[1].—Bodily restlessness does not permit her to lie long in one place,[1].—Restless motion of the whole body, on account of suppressed eructations,[1].—Extremely restless in the evening, after nausea in the afternoon, whereby she was very absent-minded,[1].—Restless disposition, with gloominess and anxiety,[1].—Restlessness, and orgasm of blood,[1].—He found it necessary to walk a great deal,[1].—The skin of the whole body is very sensitive to touch, mostly in the feet,[1].—***Sensations.*** [1410.] *Takes cold very easily,*[1].—Rushing of blood in all the veins, in the morning, on waking from a restless sleep; the veins are swollen, with a bruised sensation in the whole body,[1].—Uncomfortable feeling in the evening, such as one feels before an attack of ague,[1].—Very much indisposed; the hands and feet were frequently cold; paleness of the face and frequent palpitation; all of which was relieved by motion,[1].—Attack of general depression, with confusion of the head, vertigo, pain in the small of the back, and chilliness of the whole body, for six hours (after twenty-two days),[1].—Sick feeling in the whole body; she was obliged to spit a great deal, and dreaded the open air (after twenty-two days),[1].—A very sick feeling, the day before menstruation; a trifle caused the greatest fright,[1].—After a walk, sick, hoarse, with oppression of the chest,[1].—The parts on which he has lain during the afternoon nap go to sleep,[1].—*Great heaviness of the body,[1].—[1420.] A feeling of painful tension over the whole body,[1].—During a walk, a drawing sensation in the whole body, extending into the head, which obliged her to sit down (after thirty days),[1].—In various places of the joints and muscles, more or less severe sticking pains (second day),[11].—Severe pulsation of the vessels, especially in the chest, after dinner; pulse rapid (second day),[11].—The pain was very intense, but disappeared quickly,[1].—The chronic troubles were worse and better every other day,[1].

Skin.—Skin inflames or suppurates easily from injuries,[1].—*Eruptions. Dry.* Eruption of red elevated spots of the size of a pea and larger, mostly on the cheeks and elbows, with great heat, much thirst, and little appetite; they disappeared the third day and left a dark spot, as if congested with blood; in an infant whose mother had taken Calcarea,[9].—*Nettle-rash*, which always disappears in the cold air,[1].—*Many very small warts appear here and there*,[1].—[1430.] White spots on the face, with itching,[1].—Eruption of white spots and some scattered red patches, on wrists, backs of hands, thighs, legs, and ankles, with violent irritation,[19].—Eruption on the nose,[1].—On left ala nasi (externally) a red, swollen spot, tender on touch, and on moving muscles of nose,[26].—Large dark-red itching spots on the lower legs, with some swelling in them,[1].—Scurfy spots on the lower leg, with burning during the day (after twenty-four hours),[1].—Rashlike eruption in the face, about the eyes and on the nose,[1].—Violent irritation about the chest, back, neck, and shoulders, and in the calves of the legs; a reddish rash was partly developed all over the back and chest,[19].—*Red stripes on the tibia, consisting of nettle-rash elevations, with severe itching and burning after rubbing* (after seven days),[1].—Fine rash on the skin and neck, with itching,[1].—[1440.] *Eruption on the feet, itching, violent biting, causing scratching, bleeding when scratched, and changing to a nettle-rashlike eruption,[16].—Itching pimples on the forehead, with itching in the whole of the face,[1].—Eruption of small painless pimples over the whole face (after five days),[1].—Many pimples in the whole of the face, with severe itching,[1].—Itching pimples on both cheeks, on the malar bones, for several weeks,[1].—Pimples beneath the right corner of the mouth,[1].—Pimples on the upper lip,[1].—*Scurfy pimples on the border of the red portion of the lower lip,[1].—Stinging-burning pimple on the border of the labia (after eight days),[1].—Pimples on the lower part of the chest, with smarting on rubbing,[1].—[1450.] *Papulous eruption on the forehead*,[1].—Papulous eruption around the mouth and in the corners of the mouth,[1].—Papulous eruption in the middle of the chin,[1].—Papulous eruption on the small of the back and on the nates,[1].—Papulous eruption on the thighs (after eleven days),[1].—A wart in the bend of the elbow inflames, pains like a boil, then dries up and disappears,[1].—*Moist.* Itching vesicular eruption over the whole body, especially over the hips,[1].—*Eruption behind the right ear, which becomes moist,[1].—Erysipelas on the cheeks (which are thick),[1].—A tetter speedily reappears,[1].—[1460.] An old tetter beneath the axillæ, in the bend of the left elbow, and in the hollow of the knee, reappears (after twenty days),[1].—Vesicular eruption grouped on the back of the hand, with severe itching; it obliges scratching involuntarily; the vesicles are clear, without areola, filled with clear fluid; a dark point forms at the tip; they gradually dry and the skin desquamates; if the vesicles are scratched, they become enlarged and seem like nettle-rash; cold relieves the itching (the prover had suffered for two years, during great heat in the summer, from an insignificant vesicular eruption on the back of the hand), (seventh day),[11].—*Pustules and Ulcers.*—Boil on the margin of the hair on the forehead (first day),[1].—A boil on the back of the left hand, with sticking pain on touch,[1].—*A painful boil on the last phalanx of the fourth finger* (twice from different doses),[9]. —A pustule on the back,[1].—*Unhealthy ulcerating skin; even small wounds suppurate* and do not heal again,[11].—Wartlike growths (behind the ears) become inflamed and ulcerate,[1].—The corner of the mouth ulcerated, for fourteen days,[1].—The right corner of the mouth is ulcerated and pains as if sore,[1].—[1470.] A smarting, oblong, transverse ulcer on the lower surface of the penis, which burns severely, with profuse hæmorrhoidal sweat on the scrotum and peritoneum (second day),[11].—An old ulcer on the thigh becomes painful, with throbbing, with drawing about it, and begins to be offensive like bad eggs (after seven days),[1].—Several ulcers on the lower legs (after seven days),[1].—*Sensations.* The damp open air does not agree with her; the skin is immediately affected by it,[1].—Burning in the skin, with itching over half the back, on the nates and posterior surface of the thighs (after ten days),[1].—Stitching in the skin, as from needles,[1].—Itching on the skin,[1].—Itching over the whole body (after twenty-three days),[1].—Violent itching over whole body,[18].—Itching of the dry, hot skin, as if it had been sprinkled with salt and ashes,[1]. [1480.] Severe itching of the sweating parts, especially between the shoulder-blades,[1].—Itching in the concha,[1].—Itching behind the ear, with dizziness in the head, after scratching,[1].—Itching about the mouth, on the nose and on the nates,[1].—Itching externally on the chest (after ten days),[1].—Itching and itching pimples on the back,[1].—*Itching on the thighs* (after twelve days),[1].—Itching on the right thigh (first day),[16].—Itching on the malleolus of the diseased foot,[1].—*Much itching on the lower leg and foot*,[1].—[1490.] Itching about the ankle and below the calves (after thirteen days),[1].—*Severe itching in the whole face;* she was obliged to scratch it constantly (first seven days),[1].—Severe itching on the back, on the pit of the stomach, the neck, chin, the left eye, the scalp, the mons veneris, and the scrotum, in the evening, in bed,[1].—Severe itching in the lower part of the thighs, at night,[1].—Burning-itching on the left arm, from morning till evening,[1].—Burning-itching on the fingers of the left hand (after thirteen days),[1].—Burning-itching on the nates,[1].—Burning-itching on the left thigh, from morning till evening,[1].—A burning-itching on the right tibia,[6].—Violent burning-itching on the malleoli of the right foot, from morning till evening (after fifteen days),[1].—[1500.] Fine sticking-itching on the thighs,[1].—Sticking-itching in a small spot on the left thigh (after twenty days),[1].—Tickling-itching on the margin of the right lower jaw, with desire to scratch,[5].

Sleep and Dreams.—Sleepiness. Frequent yawning,[1].—Continued yawning, with sleepiness (after four days),[1].—Long-continued, almost endless yawning, followed by shattering throbbing in the head, abdomen, and chest, with great heat of the face,[1].—*During the day, sleepiness and weariness;* he fell asleep several times in the forenoon (ninth day),[1].—Sleepy and weary through the day, with chilliness and headache,[1].—Sleepiness in the morning,[1].—In the morning, when he should rise, he was still sleepy and weary; could hardly get awake,[1].—[1510.] *Sleepy very early in the evening (after three hours),[1].—* *Weary sleepiness in all the limbs in the evening, with chilliness;* he was unable to escape sleep; he did not, however, sleep soundly, but continually awoke (for sixteen hours); in the morning much sweat and dryness in the throat, without thirst (after four days),[1]. —Sleepiness, with nodding, after dinner,[1].—* *Great inclination to sleep after supper,*[1].—Very long sleep at noon,[1].—He seemed to fall suddenly four times into a sweet sleep, with nausea, in the evening, from 7 to 9, with blackness before the eyes, which still continued while lying down, without vomiting,[1].—Overpowering sleep, after eating, followed by chill and tickling cough,[1].—* *Difficult to arouse himself, in the morning, on waking,*[1].—

Sleeplessness. * *When she went to bed late she could not get to sleep; she felt as though she could not get rested,*[1].—* *Frequently very late falling asleep in the evening,*[1].—[1520.] Cannot get to sleep at night, and when asleep soon wakes again,[1].—*Difficult to get asleep on account of many involuntary thoughts,*[1].—Was unable to sleep before midnight, on account of mental activity,[1].—Was unable to get to sleep at night before 2 or 3 o'clock,[1]. —She was unable to sleep before 12 o'clock, but tossed restlessly about,[1].— He was unable to get to sleep for a long time in the evening, and could not free himself from lascivious or vexatious thoughts; they followed him even in the morning after waking,[1].—Night restless, full of dreams,[11].— Restless sleep, with sweat,[1].—Restless sleep towards morning (after fifteen days),[1].—Restless, half asleep at night, with dry heat and confusion in the head and constant waking, as in fever,[1].—[1530.] He tossed about the bed the whole night,[1].—At night, soon after falling asleep, he rose out of bed and worked with the hands, with open eyes, without consciousness,[1].—The child rises up in bed after midnight and calls "father;" begins to cry and tries to spring up; the more one talks to him the worse become his cries and resistance; he rolls upon the floor and will not be touched,[1].—Frequent waking from sleep,[1].—Anxious waking at night; frequent anxious dreams (after thirty-six hours),[1].—Anxious waking after midnight and difficult breathing (twelfth day),[1].—Uneasy waking, in the evening, in bed, full of frightful fantasies (sixth night),[1].—He could not sleep long in the evening, because he was too hot, although only lightly covered in a cold room (after eleven days),[1].—Sleep only from 1 to 2 or 3 o'clock, then she could sleep no more, and was wide awake,[1].—Unrefreshed, after waking in the morning,[1].—[1540.] In sleep she laid the arms above the head,[1].—Starting up in the evening, soon after falling asleep, till she was wide awake,[1].— Jerking of the upper part of the body on going to sleep in the evening, with jerking extending into the head, followed by roaring and hissing in the ears,[1].—In sleep he often chews and then swallows,[1].—Snoring the whole night in a stupid-like sleep, from which he could not be wakened, with constant tossing about; profuse sweat in the face before falling asleep,[1]. —Screaming at night, with restless sleep,[1].—Crying out and starting from anxious dreams,[1].—Talking during a dreamy sleep (after ten days),[1].— Confused talking in the sleep, with restlessness from dreams and heat,[1].—

Dreams. Sleep at night full of dreams,[1].—[1550.] Half waking dreams in the evening, soon after falling asleep, with great anxiety,[1].—Vivid dreams all night,[1].—Amorous dreams at night (first day),[11].—A voluptuous dream the night before menstruation,[1].—Confused, anxious dreams,[1].—*Several anxious dreams in each night,* for seven nights in succession,[1].—An anxious dream, toward morning, of fire and death,[1].—Anxious dream that he would be bitten by a dog, which awoke him, after which he fell asleep again, and was again awakened by the same anxious dream, and several times every night,[1].—*Anxious and frightful dreams, from which he was unable to free himself on waking,*[1].—Frightful dream, as though he would fall or be thrown down,[1].—[1560.] *Frightful dreams the whole night,* and at last a sensual dream with an (extremely seldom) emission (after ten days),[1].—At night frightful things present themselves to her, and she is unable to keep them off,[1].—Dreams of dead people and smell of corpses,[1].

Fever.—Chilliness. Great sensitiveness to the cold air; the feet seem dead, in the evening,[1].—Goose-flesh in the thighs and legs, on the slightest contact of cold air, so great that it was painful,[1].—Shivering, at first over the face, with which the hairs stood on end, then over the whole body, with chilliness,[6].—Very chilly in the evening,[1].—She became chilly if she got out of bed,[1].—Frequent external chilliness, on the ears,[1].—*Great internal chilliness;* she was obliged to wrap up the cold hands, but the feet were warm,[1].—[1570.] Continued severe chilliness, the whole day (second day),[15].—Constant chilliness and coldness, with pale sickly look,[18].—Great constant chilliness, with much thirst,[1].—*Chill in the evening,* for several hours (after ten hours, thirteenth day),[1].—Chill for a quarter of an hour, two evenings, without subsequent heat or sweat,[1].—Chill, in the evening, in bed,[1].—Chill in the evening, in bed, so that he was unable to get warm, though covered with a feather bed, as though he had no warmth in his body (after thirty days),[1].—Shaking chill at night,[1].—The evening before menstruation, after supper, a severe chill, followed by colic, lasting the whole night,[1].—Internal chill, with restlessness and trembling anguish,[1].—[1580.] Coldness and numb sensation on the side of the back on which he had lain, during the midday sleep,[1].—He felt very feverish, and was obliged to stay at home for three days; his teeth chattered, and though he sat over the fire, he was quite cold,[19].—Cold feet, after eating,[1].—*Paroxysm of fever, in the forenoon; chill and heat alternating,*[1].—Paroxysm of fever; now chilliness, now heat; she was obliged to lie down,[1].—Paroxysm of fever, in the evening; chill externally, with internal heat and great thirst; even in bed he was chilly, and sweating at the same time; he could not get warm; at last profuse sweat (after ten hours),[1].—*Heat.* Orgasm of blood, in the morning, on waking, after a restless sleep, for several mornings (first day),[1].—*Much orgasm of blood, at night, with many dreams,*[1].—*At night, orgasm of blood, with restless sleep, especially during menstruation,*[1].—In the evening, in bed, he became immediately warm, and sweat the whole night,[1].—[1590.] Frequent transient heat,[1].—Transient heat, two or three times a day, general, though most in the face and hands; it attacked her while sitting, as from anxiety, with sweating of the face and hands, for ten minutes,[1].—Almost constant heat, which at first caused weariness and anxiety, lasting until sweat broke out,[1].—*Severe heat in the head, and great orgasm of blood,*[1].—Very much heated, in the morning, after rising,[1].—Heat for several evenings, from 6 to 7 o'clock,[1].—Dry heat, towards morning (after six days),[1].—Dry heat, at night (after twelve hours),[1].—Fever, from morning till noon or afternoon; first, tearing in the joints and heaviness in the head, then weariness, which scarcely allowed her to rise from bed; with heaviness of the limbs, stretching, heat, and sensation as if she would sweat, with trembling and uneasiness in all the limbs,[1].—Paroxysm of fever, every forenoon, at 11 o'clock, without thirst, and without previous chill, lasting one hour; she felt hot, and was hot to touch, with red face; followed by anxiety and slight sweat, especially on the hands and feet, and in the face; for four days in succession (previous to menstruation),[1].—[1600.] A feeling of heat in the interior of the body,[1].—*Internal heat at night, especially in the hands and feet, with dry tongue, in the morning*, without thirst, with external heat in the head (sixth and seventh days),[1].—Heat in the chest and head, with chilliness of the rest of the body, the whole day (after twenty-four days),[1].—Fever-heat, with burning first, then alternating with chill,[1]. —Unaccountably feverish; first hot, then cold,[20].—*Sweat.* Profuse sweat during the day, in the cold air,[1].—*Sweat breaks out frequently through the day,*[1].—Almost constant sweat,[1].—**Sweat during the day, on the slightest exertion,**[1].—Sweat in the morning (the next morning),[1].—[1610.] Sweat in the morning, for three mornings in succession,[1].—**Profuse sweat in the morning,** *for several mornings in succession,*[1].—*Night-sweat*, especially before midnight, with cold limbs,[1].—*Much sweat through the day, when walking,* and also at night,[1].—A kind of anxious sweat, with some nausea,[1].—Sweat of the whole face, at supper,[1].—Night-sweat, on the back,[1].—Night-sweat, only on the limbs, which feel clammy (after a few days),[1].—*Sweat of the palms*, on the slightest exertion,[1].—Sweat on the knees,[1].—[1620.] *Sweat of the feet,*[1].

Conditions.—**Aggravation.**—(*Morning*), Near sounds frighten him; irritable, etc.; peevish; before stool, peevish, etc.; on waking, confusion of the head; when rising, vertigo, etc.; after rising, dizziness; on rising from bed, dulness in head; on waking, headache; throbbing headache; on waking, pain in forehead, etc.; swelling in temple; on waking, headache in temples; at 5 o'clock, pain in vertex; pressure in eyes; after rising, swelling of lower lid; lachrymation; after rising, stiffness of the eyeball; on waking, appearances before eyes; roaring in ears, etc.; sneezing; nose-bleed; on rising, stoppage of nose; on rising, swelling of cheeks; swelling of upper lip; dryness of tongue; mouth slimy; after rising, bitter taste; metallic taste, etc., in mouth; on waking, inky taste; hawking of mucus; throat dry, etc.; hunger; eructations; sour eructations; *nausea; nausea, etc.;* vomiting, etc.; after rising, pain in the abdomen; immediately, constriction of abdomen; *drawing in abdomen, etc.;* on waking, cutting in abdomen; after copious stool, burning in rectum; after rising, eructations; twitching of the penis; *larynx rough;* hoarseness; *cough;* in bed, cough; mucous expectoration; on rising, sense of fulness in chest; tightness of chest; stiffness in spine, etc.; on waking, and after rising, *sleepiness;* immediately after rising, pain in small of back; hands pain, etc.; in bed, sticking in the palms; on beginning to walk, weariness, etc., in muscles of thigh; more when sitting; pain in knee; *inclination to stretch;* on waking, *trembling of body;* trembling of body, etc.; great exhaustion; on waking, rushing of blood; *on waking, difficulty in rousing;* orgasm of blood; after rising, much heated; sweat; *profuse sweat.*—(*Forenoon*), Nausea; dizziness; headache, etc.; at 11 o'clock, stitches in forehead; saliva collects in mouth; nauseated feeling; when pressing on the part, and after the stool, pressure in pit of the stomach; stitches in right hypochondriac region; cramp in the rectum; frequent, etc., urinating; when walking, desire for coition; on walking in open air, tightness of chest; *paroxysm of fever.*—(*Toward noon*), Crackling in occiput.—(*Noon*), Very long sleep.—(*Afternoon*), Anxiety; stupefaction of the head; from 3 or 4 o'clock till 9 or 10, tearing on the head, etc.; feeling in the pharynx; thirst; eructations; nausea; cramp in stomach; burning below navel; *tension of abdomen, etc.;* frequent, etc., urinating; drawing in limbs; *trembling in hands;* when walking, pain in ankle.—(*Evening*), Peevish; when walking, loss of consciousness; when walking in open air, tottering; heat about head; stitches in the head; burning-itching, etc., on scalp; *pressure in eyes; itching in eyes;* lachrymation; on lying down, toothache; toothache; swelling of right cheek, etc.; great appetite, etc.; acid eructations; nausea, etc.; feels stuffed, after eating; pressure in stomach; stitches in hypochondriac region; fulness in abdomen; *cramp in intestinal canal;* stitches in side of abdomen; when sitting, pressure in rectum; pain in rectum; during stool, blood from anus; in bed, twitching in penis; after lying down, mucus in larynx; spasmodic cough; especially in bed, dry cough; after lying down, much cough; in bed, cough; during cough, sweet expectoration; during cough, pain in chest; stitches in left chest; especially on breathing, stitches in right chest; before going to sleep, palpitation, etc.; pain in right arm; shoulder-joint pains; on waking from sleep, pain in finger-joints; during walking, tension in hip-joint; pain in muscles of legs; when sitting, legs go to sleep; burning in feet; in bed, twitching in great toe; great general weakness; attack of faintness, etc.; uneasiness; restless, uncomfortable feeling; in bed, itching on back, etc.; in bed, uneasy waking, etc.; soon after falling asleep, starting up; *chilly; in bed, chilly;* in bed, becomes warm, etc.; heat.—(*Night*), Anxious, etc.; stupefaction of the head, etc.; vertigo; on waking, itching of scalp; nose-bleed; pains in back teeth; tearing in teeth; tearing through cheek; pain in gum; on waking, *eructations;* vomiting of sour water; cramp in stomach; pain in liver; *cramp in intestinal canal;* colic; pain in bladder, etc.; *frequent urinating; cough;* on waking, cough; much cough; cough; expectoration of mucus, etc.; during cough, pain in chest; palpitation, etc.; pain in arm, etc.; at commencement of sleep, shoulder-joints disturb; shoulder-joints pain; *cramp in hands;* twitches, etc., of the extremities; stitches in the thigh, etc.; weariness in knees; cramp near tibia; cramp in calves; burning in soles; cutting on right sole; itching in the thigh; shaking chill; orgasm of blood, etc.; dry heat, etc.; *internal heat,* etc.; *sweat.*—(*After midnight*), Dry cough. —(*Toward morning*), Anxious dream; dry heat.—(*Every other day*), Chronic troubles.—(*Air*), Teeth cannot endure it.—(*Open air*), Headache; trembling of the body.—(*On ascending a height*), **Shortness of breath.**—(*On bending backward*), Spine pains.—(*On getting out of bed*), Became chilly.—(*On breathing*), Stitches in pit of stomach; pain in abdomen; stitches in left chest.—(*Deep breathing*), Pain in upper abdomen.—(*Chewing*), Pain in tongue; tension in submaxillary glands.—(*When closing eyelids*), Burning in eyes.—(*During coition*), Stitches in anus; tickling in glans penis.— (*After coition*), Weak, etc.—(*Coldness*), Teeth cannot endure it.—(*Cold air*), Toothache.—(*After getting head cold*), Dimness of eyes.—(*Coughing*), Stitches in head; shootings in head; raw pain in chest.—(*At dinner*), Nausea; griping in abdomen.—(*After dinner*), Pressure in vertex, etc.; immediately, blindness; stitches in epigastric region; *abdomen distended;* distension of abdomen; palpitation; weakness, etc.; pulsation of the vessels; sleepiness.—(*Eating*), Throbbing toothache; eructations; rumbling around navel; fulness in abdomen; pain in rectum; cough; palpitation of heart; sleep; cold feet.—(*After eating and drinking*), Distension of abdomen.—(*On exertion*), Pressure in lower abdomen; sweat of the palms.— (*During great exertion*), Tension in abdomen; pain in the joints.—(*Inspiration*), Stitches through abdomen; stitches in abdomen; stitches in abdominal muscles; cough; cutting in chest; *pain in chest;* stitches in back. —(*On kneeling*), Tension below knee.—(*When leaning backward*), Tension in muscles of upper abdomen, etc. —(*After every meal*), Burning in throat; eructations; especially after hard, dry food, burning.—(*Before menstruation*),

Voluptuous dream.—(*During menstruation*), *Rush of blood to head*, etc.; pain on vertex; eyes become agglutinated, etc.; attack of toothache; boring in hollow teeth; burning in throat, etc.; sore throat; nausea, etc.; when the discharge ceased for some hours, colic; pain in abdomen.—(*After menstruation*), Immediately, toothache.—(*Milk*), Water rises from stomach; nausea. —(*Motion*), Pressure in right side of chest; pain in long bones, etc.; pain in arms; pain in wrist; stitches in hip-joint; pain in left thigh.—(*Moving head*), Does not know where she is; heaviness of the head, etc.—(*Noise*), Toothache.—(*Pressure*), Pain in occiput; especially after stool, pain in pit of stomach.—(*Raising head*), Heaviness of head, etc.—(*Raising body*), Stitches in left chest.—(*Reading*), Heaviness in forehead.—(*On respiration*), *Stitches in left chest;* jerks in back; pain in spine.—(*During rest*), Pain between shoulder-blades; pain in shoulder-joint; pain in forearm.—(*When riding*), Aching in kidneys, etc.—(*Riding in a wagon*), Toothache.—(*On rising from sitting*), Pain in knee-cap; tearing, etc., in inside of knee.— (*Rising up from lying on back*), Stitches in head.—(*Shaking head*), Shivering in the brain.—(*Sitting*), Enlargement, etc., of abdomen; tension in abdomen; pain in groin; pain in hæmorrhoids; short breath; and sewing, pain in left upper arm.—(*When going to sleep*), Illusions of fancy.—(*During the midday sleep*), Moisture from the anus; while sitting, palpitation.— (*After midday sleep*), Confusion of head; sensation in knees.—(*Sneezing*), Pain in occiput; shooting in ears.—(*Speaking*), Stitches in throat; pain in chest.—(*Spitting*), Pain in tongue.—(*Standing*), *Vertigo;* weariness in ankles.—(*Stepping*), Shivering in the brain; pressure in hepatic region; stitches in hip-joint; *lower leg painful.*—(*Before stool*), Nausea.—(*During stool*), Twitching in abdominal muscles; burning in anus.—(*After stool*), Oppression of breathing; itching in anus; oppression of chest; feeling of weakness.—(*Stooping*), Did not know where she was; during menstruation, *vertigo;* stitches in head; pain in region of vertex; stitches in hepatic region; neck feels stiff; stitches in hip-joint.—(*On stretching*), Spine painful. —(*On stretching out leg*), Cramp in calves.—(*At supper*), Sweat of face.— (*After supper*), Pressure in stomach; colic; *inclination to sleep.*—(*Swallowing*), Pain in tongue; pain beneath tongue; pressure in pharynx.—(*Touch*), Pain in submaxillary glands; pain in mammary glands; pain in nates.— lower leg painful.—(*After turning in a circle*), Dizziness.—(*On suddenly turning head*), Vertigo.—(*On twisting and turning head*), Pain in neck.— (*On urinating*), *Pain in urethra.*—(*After urinating*), Itching in glans.— (*From vexation*), Vertigo.—(*On beginning to walk*), Stitches in hip-joint.— (*When walking*), Vertigo; pain in occiput; after supper, pinching, etc., below navel; pain in abdomen; pain in hæmorrhoids; desire to urinate; difficult breathing; palpitation, etc.; pain in sacrum; pressure in muscles of forearm; weariness in thighs, etc.; pain in tibial muscles; *lower leg painful;* drawing sensation in body; *sweat.*—(*When walking fast*), Throbbing in head.—(*Walking in open air*), Sadness, etc.; vertigo; pain in forehead; headache in vertex; itching on scalp; visible distension of abdomen.— (*When walking in the wind*), Loss of breath.—(*When walking in room*), Pain in hip-joints.—(*After walking*), Vertigo; pain in chest; pain in muscles of thigh; sick, etc.—(*After warm bath*), Weariness in knees, etc.— (*Writing*), *Heaviness in forehead; lachrymation.*

Amelioration.—(*Fresh air*), Weakness.—(*Bending toward left side*), Cramp in intercostal muscles.—(*Bending knee*), Cramp in calves.—(*Cold air*), Nettle-rash.—(*On walking in cold air*), Pressing out in forehead disappears.—(*Bathing in cold water*), Attacks of colic.—(*Pressure of cold hand*),

Pressing out in forehead.—(*Eating*), Stitches in back teeth.—(*After expectoration*), Sensation of fulness of chest disappears.—(*Lying*), Headache in forehead.—(*Motion*), Indisposition.—(*Rest with closed eyes*), Stitches in left ear, etc.—(*Rubbing*), Stitches in left chest.—(*Sitting*), Pressure in muscles of forearm; pain in nates.—(*Standing*), Pressure in muscles of forearm.—(*Touch*), Pressure in muscles of forearm.—(*Walking*), Weariness.

CALCAREA CAUSTICA.

Aqua Calcis (in part). *Preparation*, To one part by weight of quicklime (CaO), add five parts of distilled water (to be securely corked in a *warm* bottle); when quite cool, add five parts of alcohol, shake frequently for several days, after which, decant the clear liquid.

Authorities. 1, Dr. A. W. Koch, prize essay, Hygea, 5, 270, a man thirty-one years old, took 3 to 6 drops of the tincture; 2, Ibid., took the 1st and 2d dilutions; 3, A married woman, twenty-six years old, ibid., took 2 to 6 drops of the tincture; 4, Ibid., took the 1st and 2d dilutions; 5, A maid, seventeen years old, proved the tincture, ibid.; 6, Ibid., proved the 1st and 2d dils.; 7, A man, forty years old, proved the tincture, ibid.; 8, Ibid., proved the 1st and 3d dils.; 9, Wife of last, forty years old, proved the tincture; 10, A maid, seventeen years old, proved the tincture; 11, Ibid., proved the 1st dil.; 12, A man, twenty-five years old, proved the tincture; 13, Ibid., proved the 1st and 2d dils.; 14, A maid, sixteen years old, proved the tincture; 15, A maid, twenty-five years old, proved the tincture; 16, A woman, thirty-two years old, proved the tincture; 17, A maid, twenty years old, proved the tincture; 18, Dr. Keil, Zeit. f. H. Kl., 3, 149, a woman took a spoonful of Aqua Calcis, night and morning, for several days (as a tonic!); 19, Liedbeck, A. H. Z., 42, 26, proving of Aq. Calcis.

Mind.—Thought very difficult (second day),[7].

Head.—*Confusion.* Confusion of the head (first day),[2 7 14].—Confusion of the head (second day),[13].—Confusion of the whole head (first day),[9]. —Head very much confused (after two hours),[12].—Head very much confused, especially on the left side (first day),[2].—Confusion in the head (in the evening, first day),[7].—Head much confused (in the evening, when drinking beer), (first day),[1].—In the evening, after drinking his usual beer, the head became so confused that he could scarcely hold it up (second day),[1].—[10.] Head much confused, evenings, in bed, especially on the left side (after drinking beer), (first day),[1].—Head confused, the whole afternoon, as after intoxication (second day),[2].—Confused head, in the forenoon, especially on the left side, with periodic stitches; the headache is pressive, so that mental labor is very difficult (third day),[1].—Head very much confused; dull pressive pain in the forehead, extending to the occiput, so that he could scarcely attend to his business (second day),[1].—Confusion in the head, with pressure in the forehead, and transient stitches in the temples (second day),[2].—Feeling in the head as if she were foolish (fourth day),[15].—Headache, so that (as she expresses it), she cannot think any more (third day),[14].—*Vertigo.* Vertigo (first day),[12 15 16].—Vertigo, as if the room were turning in a circle; she thinks she will fall from the chair (first day),[5].—Vertigo (in the evening, first day),[13].—*Sensations.* [20.] Severe pain in the head (first day),[17].—Heat in the head (first day),[10].—Stitches in the head, from before backward (second day),[8].—General pressive headache (first day),[12].—Violent pain in the head, on stooping, as if the brain followed the force of gravitation (third day),[4].—Tearing in the head (third day),[8].—Tearing from the occiput to the forehead (fifth day),[12].—*Forehead*. Very confused head, in the forehead (first day),[16].—Pain in the forehead and above the eyes (first day),[7].—Frontal headache (first day),[9].—[30.] Frontal headache, especially above the eyes (first day),[10].—Transient pressive pain in the forehead,[3].—Sticking pain in the left frontal eminence (after two hours),[2].—A violent sticking pain from the right eye to the frontal eminence, so that the eye waters, at dinner (third day),[2].—Stitches in the whole of the frontal sinus, and in both temples (second day),[6].—Dull stitches in the left side of the forehead and temple (second day),[2].—Tearing in the forehead, above the eyebrows (first day),[5].—Tearing pain in the left frontal eminence (after two hours),[5].—Tearing in the frontal sinus (first day),[14].— Throbbing pain in the frontal sinus, so that one is constantly obliged to contract the skin of the forehead, which affords relief (second day),[6].—[40.] Severe throbbing pain in the forehead, at 9 P.M. (second day),[6].—*Temples*. Sticking pain in the left temple, at $6\frac{1}{2}$ P.M. (first day),[6].—Tearing-sticking pain in the left temple (first day),[2].—Tearing in the right temple (first day),[1].—Tearing pain in the left temple, extending to the left frontal eminence (after one hour),[1].—*Vertex*. Dull pressive headache, in the middle of the upper part of the skull (first day),[7].—*Occiput*. Pain in the occiput (first day),[9].—Dull rheumatic pain in the occiput (evening, at 5), (first day),[1].—Pressive pain in the occiput (first day),[12].—*External*. A feeling as if the hairs were pulled up (first day),[5].—[50.] Transient sensation, as if the hairs on the forepart of the head were pulled up (evening, first day),[3].

Eye.—A pain in the right eye, as if a foreign body were under the upper lid; stitches extend thence to the forehead, and the conjunctiva of the lids is red (sixth day),[2].—Feeling in the left eye, on rising in the morning, as if a thorn were in it, so that she must rub it; she was unable to open it (second day),[6].—Burning in the eyes, in the evening, by candlelight (second day),[3].—While reading in the evening, at 10, burning of the eyes (second day),[1].—Tearing in the eyes (in the afternoon, first day),[13].— *Orbit*. Paroxysmal boring pain on the upper orbital border of the right eye (first day),[3].—Stitches along the course of the supraorbital and supratrochlear nerves (immediately after taking),[2].—Transient tearing pain from the supraorbital border of the left orbit to the inner canthus, and down to the wing of the nose, at 6 P.M. (first day),[3].—*Lids*. Violent pains in the upper lids, so that every motion is painful (first day),[3].—[60.] Severe pressure and heaviness in the lids (first day),[9].—Tearing pain in the inner canthus of the right eye, extending down to the upper lid, with a feeling as if the eyeballs would become swollen (first day),[9].—*Lachrymal Apparatus*. Lachrymation of the right eye (fifth day),[2].—Lachrymation in the open air (third day),[2].—*Conjunctiva*. Redness of the conjunctiva of the lids (first day),[3].—*Ball*. Pain in the eye, as if the ball would be pressed out (first day),[12].—Stitches in the eyeball (first day),[12].—Tearing stitches through the eyeballs (first day),[12].—*Vision*. Photophobia (first day),[3].

Ears.—Tearing in the right mastoid process (first day),[8].—Dull pain in both ears (second day),[2].—[70.] Bursting pains within the left ear (at 9 P.M., first day),[1].—Severe tension and pressure in the internal portions of the ear (first day),[12].—Pinching-sticking pain in the left ear, extending to the opening of the Eustachian tube, in the throat, at 5 P.M. (second day),[2].

—Violent sticking-drawing pains within the left meatus anditorius, extending outward (immediately),[1].—Violent sticking, pressing-out pain in the internal portion of the left ear; this continues, more or less severe, some time,[1].—Sticking pains through the left and right ears (evening, second day),[1].—Dull sticking in the left ear, as from a foreign body (first day),[2].—Tearing through the inner portion of both ears (first day),[7].—*Hearing.* Ringing and roaring in the ears (third day),[13].

Nose.—Coryza, especially of the left nostril (second day),[2].—[80.] The nose has been dry for two days; it discharges a thick tough mucus (third day),[1].—Stitches from the left wing of the nose, at the angle extending to the internal canthus (first day),[4].

Face.—Tearing in the right cheek-bone (first day),[8].—The inner surface of the lips very red, with injected vessels,[18].—Stiffness in the joints of the jaws (first day),[10].—Very violent pain in the right articulation of the jaw, which was somewhat swollen, fourth day; the next day the joint was immovable, and the cheek swollen; the third day, violent pain on moving the jaw; the pain was relieved in the evening, and the night was quiet; the right cheek was still greatly swollen; disappeared after two days,[3].—Rheumatic nervous pain in the right articulation of the jaw, on pressure (this might be attributed to the fact that the person had worn a neckcloth through the whole winter, and had left it off the last three days),[4].—Tearing in the left half of the lower jaw (second day),[6].

Mouth.—Teeth. Severe toothache, every night, at 2 o'clock, as it the tooth was fuzzy and too large, together with tensive pain in the left ear, as if something was sticking in it (fourth to sixth day),[2].—Dull tearing toothache in a hollow tooth (first day),[2].—[90.] Transient tearing pain in the left lower incisors (first day),[1].—The back teeth feel fuzzy (first day),[9].—Severe pain in the hollow back teeth; they seem too large (third day),[1].—The back teeth seem too large, and are somewhat painful (first day),[10].—Drawing pain in an upper hollow back tooth of the left side, and a feeling as if it were too large (first day),[2].—Dull tearing-sticking pain in two hollow back teeth, which seemed enlarged (first day),[1].—*Tongue.* Tongue greenish-yellow, and thickly coated (fifth day),[12].—*General Mouth.* Offensive mouth (fourth day),[1].—Mouth offensive, especially the posterior portion, on the arches of the palate, with mucus (fourth day),[2].—Dryness of the mouth,[16].—[100.] The palate feels as if mucus was upon it but none is expectorated (first day),[1].—*Taste.* Mouth bitter (fifth day),[12].

Throat.—Mucus in the throat, which is difficult to raise, almost causing vomiting; for two days (second day),[9].—Hawking of granular glutinous material (like cooked rice), which collects in the larynx and trachea (for fourteen days),[4].—Pain in the throat, on rising; swallowing is difficult (second day),[5].—Burning in the fauces and œsophagus, caused by water,[18].—A feeling in the pharynx as if a bone were sticking in it (first day),[1].—Was scarcely able to swallow (first day),[17].

Stomach.—Appetite. Severe hunger three hours after eating (first day),[1].—Loss of appetite (third day),[12].—[110.] Loss of appetite for beer (second day),[2].—*Eructations.* Many eructations (first day),[1].—Eructations tasting of the food, and also sour and bitter (first day),[1].—*Nausea.* Nausea (second and fifth days),[12].—Nausea, with eructations of frothy fluid, after eating some bread (after one hour),[4].—Nausea, which is followed, after half an hour, by vomiting of sour fluid, half an hour after dinner (first day),[6].—*Stomach.* Burning in the stomach,[18].—Tensive feeling in the stomach (first day),[1].—Spasmodic contraction of the stomach (second day),[12].—[120.] Oppression above the epigastric region, and in the hypochondria (first day),[7].

Abdomen.—Hypochondria. Sticking pain in both hypochondria, especially severe in the left (first day),[1].—Pain on the left side of the region of the spleen, as if a ball were turning on its axis (second day),[4].—
General Abdomen. Rumbling in the abdomen (first day),[5].—Rumbling in the abdomen (fifth day),[12].—Constrictive pain in the abdomen, extending towards the uterus (first day),[5].—Griping in the abdomen (first day),[14 15 17].—Griping in the abdomen (first day),[17].—Griping in the abdomen (fifth day),[12].—Griping in the abdomen, with flatulence, at noon (second day),[2].—[130.] Violent stitches in the intestines, like fine knife-stitches (he often had this symptom when not proving), (second day),[1]. — Violent stitches in the small intestines when bending forward (second day),[2].—Tearing in the abdomen (after half an hour),[12].—Slight tearing pain in the abdomen (after one hour),[12].

Rectum and Anus. The usual hæmorrhoids seemed to be smaller (second day),[1]. — Hæmorrhoids trouble (first day),[13]. — Sticking-tearing motions in the rectum, extending towards the anus (first day),[12].—Crawling in the rectum and anus (second day),[13].

Stool.—Diarrhœa. Stool twice and painless (second day),[2].—Three thin stools before breakfast, and one again after breakfast (second day),[5].—[140.] Stool always very painful, as if a nail were scratching in the anus (since the beginning of the proving, until the last two days, when it was no longer painful, and the hæmorrhoids were very small),[2].—Thin, pasty stool, with much mucus, immediately after breakfast (second day),[1].—Passed many pieces of a tapeworm (first day),[15].—*Constipation.* No stool (first day),[1 2].

Sexual Organs.—Male. Emissions in the night (first day),[1].—
Female. Menstruation eight days too early,[4].

Respiratory Organs.—Larynx. Stitches in the larynx (first day),[14].—Dull stitches in the left half of the larynx (third day),[2].—*Voice.* Hoarseness (first day),[14].—Hoarseness with pain in the throat (first day),[17]. —[150.] Hoarseness; a feeling of rawness in the tráchea; cough (first day),[15].—*Cough and Expectoration.* Cough, with stitches in the chest (first day),[17].—Cough, with expectoration of mucus and blood (third day),[13].—Cough, with some expectoration of blood, hoarseness, and pain in the throat (first day),[16].—Expectoration of mucus streaked with blood (fourth day),[13].

Chest.—Pressure on the chest, which disappeared after half an hour; it felt as if all the blood had stagnated in the abdomen, as after nightmare (third day),[1].—Pressive pain in the chest (third day),[13].—Sticking pain in the region of the sixth and seventh ribs, increased by inspiration, without cough; it changes to a tearing, its seat being in the intercostal muscles and pleura costalis (first day),[1].—Stitches in the chest (first day),[16].—Stitches in the chest, on inspiration, with some cough at noon (second day),[14].—[160.] Biting in the nipple, without eruption (first day),[4].—*Sternum.* Oppression across the sternum (second day),[13].—Pressive sticking pain beneath the sternum, above the præcordial region and the hypochondrium (fourth day),[1].—Stitches across over the breast-bone (second day),[2].—
Sides. Sticking pain, in the left side of the region from the fifth to the seventh rib, after dinner (first day),[2].—Stitches in the right side, in the lowest ribs (first day),[8].—Stitches below the right short ribs (third day),[6].—Stitches in the left side of the chest (second day),[2 14].—Stitches in the left

side of the chest (second day),[14].—Stitches in the left side of the chest, between the sixth and seventh ribs (first day),[1].

Neck and Back.—Neck. [170.] Stiffness of the neck (first day),[10].—Stiffness of all the muscles of the neck (second day),[1].—Neck stiff from noon till evening (first day),[9].—Stiffness in the back of the neck (first day),[7].—Tension in the muscles of the neck, on both sides (first day),[12].—Aching and stiffness in the neck, half an hour after rising (third day),[6].—Tension and stiffness in the nape of the neck and occiput (second day),[1].—Tearing in the neck (third day),[8].—Tearing in the muscles of the neck (first day),[18].—Sticking-tearing pain in the muscles of the neck; continues the whole day (third day),[7].—[180.] Tearing in the nape of the neck, with stiffness (first day),[7].—*Back.* Tearing in the back (first day),[7].—*Dorsal.* Violent pains in the shoulder-blades, extending into the small of the back, when sitting (second day),[4].—Peculiar pain like rheumatism in both shoulder-blades (first day),[3].—Rheumatism in the right shoulder-blade, at 10½ P.M. (third day),[2].—Sensation in both shoulder-blades as if they were fuzzy, and had gone to sleep, at 8 P.M. (second day),[3].—Sticking in the shoulder-blades (third day),[6].—Tearing in both shoulder-blades, between the shoulders, then through the neck and occiput as far as the forehead (first day),[5].—Tearing between the shoulders (first day),[8].—Tearing between the shoulders (second day),[8].—[190.] Tearing between the shoulders (third day),[8].—Rheumatic pain between the shoulder-blades, with stitches, on breathing, and oppression, extending forward to the sternum (first day),[9].—Tearing between the shoulder-blades (first day),[7].—*Lumbar.* Stitches in both lumbar regions (first day),[5].—Pains in the small of the back (first day),[1389].—Pain in the small of the back (fifth day),[12].—Pain in the small of the back, on waking, relieved on moving about (third day),[1].—Slight rheumatic pains in the small of the back, neck, and upper arm (second day),[1].—Drawing in the small of the back (first day),[13].—Drawing pains in the small of the back (first day),[9].—[200.] Pressive-drawing pain in the small of the back (in the morning, second day),[1].—Violent sticking pain in the small of the back (first day),[5].—Sticking in the small of the back, at 6½ P.M.,[6].—Tearing pain in the small of the back (first day),[78].—*Sacral.* Tearing in the coccyx (first day),[7].—Tearing in the coccyx (third day),[8].

Extremities in General.—Trembling in the limbs (first day),[12].—Trembling in the extremities (first day),[1].—Trembling in the extremities, and weariness, worse in bed (possibly the result of the day's exertion), (first day),[1].—[210.] Trembling of the limbs, she could not continue her work ; the symptom disappeared after eating a piece of bread (first day),[3].—Great trembling in the arms and feet (second day),[6].—Great weariness of the limbs (after one and a half hours),[3].—Rheumatic pain, alternating in all the joints (third day),[2].—Slight rheumatic pains in the left arm and in the feet (first day),[1].—Wandering pains in the extremities (third day),[12].—Pains in the hands and feet, after a foot-bath (third day),[3].—Drawing-tearing pain in a joint, when exerting it, or in an unaccustomed position (seventh day),[2].—Tearing in the right upper arm and right thigh (first day),[7].

Superior Extremities.—Tearing in the left arm (third day),[8].—[220.] Tearing under the left arm (first day),[8].—Tearing in the right arm (third day),[7].—*Shoulder.* Slight rheumatic pain in the right shoulder (third day),[2].—Rheumatic pain in the left shoulder (first day),[1].—Tearing in the right shoulder (first day),[578].—Sticking-tearing pain in the right

shoulder,[2].—Slight rheumatic pain in the right shoulder-joint (second day),[1].
—Rheumatic pain in the left shoulder-joint, at 10 P.M. (second day),[2].—
Aching in the left shoulder-joint on hanging down the arm (second day),[6].
—Tearing-drawing pain in the left shoulder-joint, which extends over the
whole upper arm and becomes so violent that it is difficult to raise the arm;
it is chiefly seated in the deltoid muscle, in the fascia, and in the shoulder-
joint, lasting three hours (immediately after taking),[1].—[230.] Tearing in
the right shoulder-joint (first day),[9].—Slight tearing in the right shoulder-
joint (twenty-first day),[7].—Tearing in the left shoulder-joint (first day),[7].—
Tearing in the right axilla (first day),[8].—Tearing in the left axilla (first
day),[7].—*Arm.* Rheumatic pain in the biceps, deltoid, and elbow-joint of
the right arm (first day),[2].—Stitches in the left upper arm (first day),[7].—
Tearing in the left upper-arm (first day),[7].—Transient dull tearing pain in
the left upper arm, from the shoulder to the elbow, after dinner (first day),[4].
—*Elbow.* Stitches in the right elbow (first day),[2].—[240.] Stitches in
the tip of the right elbow (second day),[6].—Tearing in the elbows (first
day),[8].—Very marked tearing in the left elbow-joint (first day),[7].—*Forearm.* Tearing in the right forearm (second day),[8].—Tearing in the left
forearm (third day),[8].—Drawing-tearing pain in the left forearm, as if in
the bones, or in the intercostal ligament (first day),[2].—*Wrist.* Stitches in
the left wrist and metacarpal joints (second day),[2].—Tearing in the right
wrist (first day),[8].—Tearing in the left wrist (first day),[8].—Tearing in the
left wrist (third day),[8].—*Hand.* [250.] Paralyzed condition of the right
hand, so that he is unable to raise it; the hand will follow the force of
gravitation, at 5 P.M. (first day),[5].—Tearing in the left hand (first day),[8].—
Tearing in the left hand (third day),[8].—Tearing in the left metacarpus
(second day),[7].—*Fingers.* Sticking-tearing pain in the right thumb, at
10 P.M., when in bed (first day),[2].—Tearing in the first joint of the right
thumb (second day),[8].—Tearing in the second joint of the right thumb
(second day),[8].—Tearing in the left thumb (first day),[7][8].—Tearing in the
first joint of the left thumb (first day),[8].—Tearing in the first joint of the
right index finger (first day),[7].—[260.] Tearing in the second joint of the
left index finger (first day),[8].—Drawing-tearing pain in the first joint of
the left index finger, which changes to a dislocating pain, after dinner (first
day),[2].—Tearing in the left middle finger (first day),[7].—Tearing in the first
joint of the right little finger (first day),[7][8].—Tearing in the first joint of the
left little finger (first day),[7][8].

Inferior Extremities.—Severe tension in the lower extremities
(third day),[12].—*Hip.* Transient stitches in the right hip, without moving
(second day),[1].—Wrenching pain in the right hip-joint (second day),[8].—
Stitches from the right hip-joint down to the middle of the thigh (third
day),[2].—Severe stitches in the right hip-joint, on walking, 5 P.M. (first
day),[5].—[270.] Tearing in the right hip-joint (first day),[11].—Sticking pain
in the left hip-joint, when walking, and in the open air (first day),[2].—
Tearing in the left hip-joint (first day),[8].—*Thigh.* Tearing in both thighs
(second day),[8].—Tearing in the right thigh (first day),[8].—Tearing in the
right thigh (second day),[7].—Tearing in the right thigh (fourth day),[8].—
Tearing in the left thigh (second day),[8].—*Knee.* Tearing in both knees,
extending down through the feet (first day),[5].—Stitches in the right knee
(second day),[6].—[280.] Tearing in the right knee (third day),[8].—Tearing
in the hollow of the right knee (first day),[7].—Tearing in the left knee
(second day),[8].—Tearing in the left knee, at 6 P.M. (first day),[6].—Tearing
and sticking in the left knee (first day),[2].—Tension in the right knee-joint

(first day),[7].—Violent sticking pain in the right knee-joint, on stepping, continuing in bed on moving it, at 10 P.M. (fourth day),[4].—Tearing in the right knee-joint (first day),[7][8].—Tearing in the right knee-joint (third day),[8].—Tearing in the left knee-joint (first day),[8].—*Leg.* [290.] Tearing in the left leg (third day),[8].—Tearing in the lower part of the right tibia (first day),[6].—Tearing in the right side of the tibia of the right leg, down to the toes, at 5 P.M. (second day),[5].—Tension in the calves (second day),[8].—Tearing in the right calf (first day),[8].—Tearing in the left calf (second day),[8].—Tearing in the left tendo Achillis (third day),[8].—*Ankle.* Tearing in the left ankle (first and second days),[8].—*Foot.* Tearing over part of the right foot (first day),[8].—Stitches in the sole and in the forepart of the right foot (first day),[7].—[300.] Tearing in the left heel (first day),[8].—*Toes.* Aching in the first phalanx of the right great toe, on moving the joint (second day),[6].—Sticking pain in a corn on the left third toe (third and fourth days),[1].

General Symptoms.—Weariness (first day),[15].—Great weariness (first day),[12][16].—Great weariness (third day),[12].—Extreme weariness, so that he must lie down, and was only free from the troubles in the throat and cough after eight days,[17].—In the morning, on rising, weary and peevish (second day),[2].—Great prostration and trembling of the body (first day),[1].—On waking, felt as if he had been intoxicated (second day),[2].—[310.] In the morning he felt unwell, as if he had been intoxicated the day before (he had drunk wine the evening previous), (second day),[1].

Skin.—Very fine rashlike eruption on the forehead, without biting (second day),[4].—Six brownish-red, isolated, or partly confluent spots like flea-bites, of the size of a penny, in the lower part of the tibia; the skin somewhat swollen; lasting fourteen days (second day),[2].—Biting vesicles, filled with lymph, in various parts of the body (first day),[8].—Biting-itching eruption, with a red areola filled with purulent lymph (fifth day),[2].—Severe itching and sticking in the skin, especially in the neck and back; small vesicles appear filled with lymph, and surrounded by a red areola (sixth day); the next day the eruption extends to the chest, throat, and behind the ears and occiput,[3].

Sleep and Dreams.—*Sleepiness.* Yawning (first day),[1].—Much yawning (first day),[1].—Great sleepiness in the evening (first day),[7].—Night quiet, until morning, when a severe tension of the skin wakes him (first day),[12].—*Sleeplessness.* [320.] Night restless, with many dreams (second day),[9].—Night restless, with many dreams (third day),[2].—Night very restless (second night),[1].—Night restless with confused head (first day),[9].—Night very restless, tossing hither and thither, loss of sleep, head much confused (first day),[1].—Night restless, sleepless; continued toothache in a left upper hollow back tooth, also with earache (second day),[2].—Night restless, sleepless, with many dreams, which could not be remembered the next morning (second day),[2].—Restless sleep at night, with dreams (first day),[7].—Restless sleep, with anxious dreams (first day),[7].—Sleep restless, full of unpleasant dreams (first day),[2].—[330.] Night quite sleepless, full of dreams, much tossing about in bed (third day),[2].—Nightmare and restless dreams (third night),[1].

Fever.—Chilliness. Shivering down the back (first day),[9].—Severe chill (first day),[17].—Violent chill, in the evening, on going to bed (first day),[4].—Very violent chill at 7 P.M., lasting half an hour (first day),[3].—Severe shaking chill, with chattering of the teeth, at 7½ P.M. (first day),[6].—Chilliness for several weeks, in summer,[19].—A severe chilliness, on rising,[3].

—Great chilliness of the whole body in the evening, on going to sleep (first day),[3].—[340.] Continued chilliness, followed by heat at noon (fifth day),[12].—Severe shaking chill at 7 P.M., lasting an hour, followed by severe heat in the head, lasting half an hour (first day),[5].—*Heat.* Severe burning of the skin, before going to sleep (in the evening, first day),[13].

Conditions.—Aggravation.—(*Morning*), On rising, feeling in eye; pain in small of back; on rising, weary, etc.—(*Forenoon*), Confused head.—(*Noon*), Griping in abdomen; stitches in chest, etc.; till evening, neck stiff.—(*Afternoon*), 5 o'clock, pain in ear.—(*Evening*), Confusion of head; when drinking beer, head confused; in bed, after drinking beer, head confused; vertigo; pain in occiput; sensations as if hairs were pulled up; by candlelight, burning in eyes; while reading, at 10 o'clock, burning of eyes; on going to bed, chilly; on going to sleep, chilliness; before going to sleep, burning of the skin.—(*Night*), 2 o'clock, toothache.—(*In open air*), Pain in hip-joint.—(*In bed*), Trembling in the extremities, etc.—(*When bending forward*), Stitches in the intestines.—(*After eating bread*), Nausea.—(*At dinner*), Pain from right eye.—(*After dinner*), Nausea; pain in rib-region.—(*On hanging down arm*), Aching in shoulder-joint.—(*Inspiration*), Pain in rib-region; stitches in chest.—(*Pressure*), Pain in jaws.—(*On rising*), Pain in throat.—(*After rising*), Aching, etc., in neck; chilly.—(*When sitting*), Pains in shoulder-blades.—(*On stepping*), Pain in knee-joints.—(*On stooping*), Pain in head.—(*On waking*), Pain in small of back.—(*On walking*), Stitches in hip-joint; pain in hip-joint.

Amelioration.—(*Evening*), Pain in articulation of jaws.—(*After eating bread*), Trembling of limbs disappears.—(*On moving about*), Pain in small of back.

CALCAREA CHLORATA.†

Calcium chloride, CaCl. *Preparation,* Solution of the freshly prepared substance, at first in water, afterward in alcohol.

Authority. Cattell, B. J. of Hom., vol. 11, 168.

Glandular swellings; faintness, anxiety, and weakness; trembling and giddiness; [glandular indurations and swellings soften and disappear]; scrofula. The respiration quick, snoring; increased secretion of mucus, perspiration, and urine; nausea and vomiting; diarrhœa; præcordium tender; pulse accelerated. Failure and trembling of the limbs; giddiness; pulse small and contracted; cold sweats, convulsions, paralysis, and insensibility.

(Vogt, Pharmak.; Beddoes, Daneau's Annals, 1; Med. Gaz., 35, 64.)

CALCAREA IODATA.

Calcium iodatum; Iodide of lime, CaI. *Preparation,* Triturations.

Authorities. 1, Dr. W. Jas. Blakely, Hah. Month., 3, 267, proving with half a grain of the crude; 2, ibid., proving with the 1st trit.; 3, ibid., proving with the 2d trit.; 4, M. J. L., 30 years old, proving with the 2d trit.; 5, ibid., proving with the 1st trit.

Mind.—Indifferent to anything which may happen (after three-quarters of an hour),[4].

---

† Chlorata must not be confounded with Chlorica.

Head.—Lightheaded (after three-quarters of an hour),[4].—Slight giddy headache (after eight and three-quarters hours),[4].—Sensation as though my head wasn't, yet was (after three-quarters of an hour),[4].[†]—Slight pain in the head, with heaviness over the eyes and nose (after four hours and five minutes),[5].—Fulness of the head (after three and a half hours),[5].—Attack of the same dull headache as he experienced after the first dose (immediately),[2].—On waking in the morning, he had still the same dull aching as he had the previous night (after ten hours),[2].—***Forehead.*** Very severe headache over the forehead and in the temples, while riding against a cold wind (after one and a half hours),[2].—[10.] Fulness in the forehead, aggravated by stooping,[2].—Severe aching in the forehead, afterwards most severe in the left temple,[2].—Severe dull aching over the forehead and sides of the face, worse in the right temple,[2].—Severe dull headache in the forehead (after five minutes),[1].—Constant dull pain in the forehead, ever since first taking the drug (third day),[1].—Severe dull pain in the forehead and over the right side of the face, with dull pain in the first upper molar tooth on the same side, on waking in the morning (after ten hours),[3].—Dull heavy pain in the forehead (after ten minutes),[2].—***Temples.*** Severe headache in both temples, while making the 2d cent. trit.,[2].—Constant dull pain in the temples, ever since first taking the drug (third day),[1].—Severe dull headache in both temples, especially in the right (after five minutes),[1].—[20.] Dull pain in both temples, especially in the left, and over the root of the nose (after half an hour),[3].—Sharp piercing pain in the right temple (after ten minutes),[2].

Eye.—Pain over the eyes (after eight and three-quarters hours),[4].

Ear.—Numbness and ringing in the ears (after one hour),[4].

Mouth.—Dry furred feeling on lips and tongue (after one and a quarter hours),[4].—Mouth and gums burn like fire (after five minutes),[1].—Bitter taste in the mouth, but not disagreeable, like myrrh (after one hour and forty minutes),[5].—Bitter taste, partially relieved by tobacco (after two hours),[5].—Taste at first sweetish, afterwards slightly astringent and metallic,[2].—Astringent taste, like alum (after five minutes),[1].

Stomach.—[30.] Inclined to belch wind (after one hour),[4].—Slight hiccough (after one hour),[4].—Slight nausea (after one and a quarter hours),[4].

Abdomen.—Rumbling in the bowels, with discharge of wind (after one hour and five minutes),[4].—Constant evacuation of large quantities of wind downward,[2].—Evacuation of large quantities of wind, after rising (after ten hours),[3].—Slight pain in the abdomen,[3].

Heart and Pulse.—Pulse regular and soft, 80,[1].

Neck.—Stiffness of the back of the neck (after eight and three-quarters hours),[4].—Stiffness of the neck continues (after forty minutes),[5].

Superior Extremities.—[40.] Dull, heavy lameness in the posterior surface of the right arm,[2].—Severe laming pain in the external portion of the right arm, with numbness of the hands and fingers,[2].

Inferior Extremities.—Tired feeling in the lower limbs, especially in the calves of the legs,[1].—Pain across the anterior surface of the upper third of both thighs, as if he had been beaten,[3].

General Symptoms.—Easy, indolent feeling (after three-quarters of an hour),[4].—Weariness of the whole body,[1].

Skin.—Itching in various parts of the body, disappearing and reappearing in other parts, only relieved after much scratching (after one

---

† As I did not see the prover again, I cannot explain this "sensation."—W. J. B.

hour),². —Persistent itching on the right elbow, followed by the same on the left knee,².

Conditions.—**Aggravation.**—(*Morning*), On waking, pain in forehead, etc.; after rising, evacuation of wind.—(*While riding against a cold wind*), Headache over forehead, etc.—(*Stooping*), Fulness in the forehead.
Amelioration.—(*Tobacco*), Bitter taste.

CALCAREA PHOSPHORICA.

A mixture of the basic and other phosphates of lime, prepared by dropping dilute phosphoric acid into lime-water, as long as a white precipitate is formed; this precipitate is collected and triturated. (Hering, in Correspondenzblatt, 1837).

Authorities. 1, Hering, collection of provings with the crude, 1st and 2d triturations, Correspondenzblatt, Allentown, Pa., Feb. 8th, 1837; 2, Bute, ibid.; 3, Green, ibid.; 4, Humphrey, ibid.; 5, Additional symptoms from Hering's résumé, N. Am. J. of Hom., New Series, vol. 2, p. 232; 6, Schréter, N. Archiv., 3. 3. p. 153, proving with the 300th potency.

Mind.—Emotional. Easily excited (from the 2d),¹.—Likes to be alone,⁵.—She wishes to be at home, and when at home to go out; goes from place to place,⁵.—A child of fifteen months, with a big head and open fontanels, took from a trituration of a drachm, C. ph., with half an ounce of milk-sugar, half a teaspoonful, in the evening. Soon violent screaming, grasping with hands in great agony, towards his mother; cold sweat, most in face; whole body cold; lasted nearly two hours; next day, as well as usual; 6 P.M., another spell, lasting only fifteen minutes. Mother did not give another dose. Sooner than expected the fontanel closed. (1852, N. N.),⁵.—With the drowsiness, gloomy mood, inability to think, headache, singing in ears, sweat in face, prostration of limbs,⁵.—After vexation, depressed, as if lame; cannot work, hardly walk; gets a looseness of bowels,⁵.—Anxiousness, with other complaints,⁵.—Anxiety of children; in pit of stomach; with bellyache; with chest complaints; with palpitation,⁵.—Feels as if she had been frightened,⁵.—[10.] Great ill-humor and dread of labor; will absolutely do nothing that he should (from the 2d),¹.—Very much out of humor, disinclined to speak, prefers not to be asked questions, and to be left alone, after disagreeable news (nineteenth day),⁶.—*Peevish and fretful children,*⁵.—Grows very violent, if his opinion is differed from, or if contradicted, so that he is vexed not to have been able to control himself (seventh day),⁶.—Violent, irritable, and snappish; it affects him most to hear that some one has done wrong; indignation rises in him, and he would like to avoid the conversation (seventh day),⁶.—A communication in which some one is justly reproached concerning his conduct, affects him very disagreeably; he grows violent, and holds up his faults to himself (fifth day),⁶.—Unpleasant news makes him beside himself; sweat breaks out; inclined to indignation and anger,⁵.—Unpleasant news makes him beside himself; he can seriously think of nothing, cannot collect his thoughts, and gets into a general sweat about it (ninth day),⁶.—Stupid indifference.; cretinism,⁵.—*Intellectual.* He has a clearer oversight, and more distinct views of many things (eighth day),⁶.—[20.] Indisposition to work, also to mental work,⁵.—Obtuse intellect; difficulty in performing intellectual operations; cannot clearly distinguish,⁵.—Writes wrong words, or the same words twice,⁵.—Forgetfulness; forgets what he did a short time ago,⁵.—A lack of definiteness of memory (Jones),[5].—Complete loss of memory, so that he does not know at all what he has just done, or what he should do (from the 2d),[1].

Head.—Vertigo. Some vertigo and nausea towards noon (first day),[4]. —With his dinner, vertigo and loss of memory (Neidhard),[5].—Vertigo, when getting up or rising from sitting,[5].—Stooping causes vertigo, rush of blood to the head, dull pain in head,[5].—[**30.**] Vertigo, staggers when walking in the open air, with drawing in the nape of the neck in windy weather (sixteenth day),[6].—While walking, vertigo; running from the nose; bones of pelvis, hip-joint, thigh, knees, and ankle-joint ache,[5].—*During* catamenia, vertigo and throbbing in the forehead, blood rushes to the head; throbbing headache, increasing after; over os pubis, pressure; want of appetite; bellyache and diarrhœa; backache, shooting; lower limbs weary; over-fatigued; going upstairs, feels stiff all over,[5].—Vertigo, with other ailments; a dull headache, nausea; complaints of eyes, neck; limbs ache; with costiveness of old people; with leucorrhœa before catamenia; in motion, walking in the open air; worse in windy weather,[5].—Vertigo, with confusion of the head (twenty-first day),[6].—Old people stagger when getting up from sitting,[5].—Staggering, dizzy when walking, with drawing in the nape of neck, and confusion of the head (nineteenth day),[6].—**General Head.** Acute hydrocephaloid, with cholera infantum (Rauc),[5].—Heat in head; burning on top, running down to the toes,[5].—Headache, like a confusion all over on the inner sides of the skull (from the 2d),[1].—[**40.**] Headache, in the morning, on waking, a heavy painful confusion, as if close to the bone, from within and without, worse on the vertex; aggravated by bodily exertion; it seems to disappear on mental exertion, and return on bodily exertion; relieved by washing with cold water (from the 2d),[1].—Headache like a fulness, a painful pressure of the brain against the skull, most severe on the top of the head; it returns regularly almost every ten seconds; at last it becomes continuous, but is still more severe every ten seconds; aggravated on motion, especially on stooping, even on changing the position while sitting; especially worse on sitting up after lying down, also on rising after sitting, when it is accompanied by vertigo; better while lying still, and after stooping (from the 2d),[1].—Fulness; pressure and dulness of head; worse from pressure of the hat,[5].—*After* catamenia increases, throbbing headache; want of appetite; backache and aching in the lower limbs; whites,[5].—Headache, with hot head and face, together with ill-humor and indolence (from the 2d),[1].—Some headache, with flatulence in the abdomen (after the 2d dose),[4].—Headache, with gastric symptoms, with uterine complaints, or following other sensations,[5].—Headache, in the morning, with sore throat (from the 2d),[1].—Headache not aggravated by drinking wine, but afterwards severe on going into the open air; relieved by scratching the head, but only while scratching (from the 2d),[1].—All great exertions increase the headache or bring it back,[5].—[**50.**] Every step is felt in head, in sacrum,[5].—Headache better at first, from going out (from the 2d),[1].— After the meals, more after dinner, headache or drowsiness, weariness, itching, etc.,[5].—**Forehead.** Headache over forehead, with a tearing pain in the hands and arms, most in wrists and right middle finger,[5].—Headache worse from changes of weather, extending from the forehead to nose, from temples to jaws, with some rheumatic feeling from collar-bone to wrists,[5].— **Vertex.** Headache on top of head, behind ears, with a drawing in muscles of the neck to the nape of the neck and back of head,[5].—*Crawling sensations run over top of head,* **as if ice were laying on upper part of occiput; the head is hot, with smarting of the roots of the hair,**[5].—**Parietals.** Headache in the afternoon, with dread of labor; some pressure on both sides towards the back; just the same in the open air, relieved for awhile after supper, though continuing somewhat during the evening (crude),[1].—Stitching pain in left side of head; sleepiness during day,[5].—Throbbing headache through both sides, most after quick motion,[5].—*Occiput.* [60.] Aching, drawing pains around the lateral protuberances of the occiput,[5].—*External Head.* Affections of the skull,[5].—Sore pain; drawing, rending, tearing in the bones of the skull, most along the sutures of the skull, particularly between the frontal and parietal bones, or around the temporal bones,[5].—Scalp sore, hurts; creeping, numbness, cold crawl; coldness on occiput, head,[5].—Tight feeling; tension in scalp of forehead,[5].—Itching on the scalp, provoking scratching, for several evenings (crude),[1].

Eye.—Eyes red; capillary vessels visible in streaks from corners to cornea,[5].—As if something came into his eyes; renewed if others talk about it,[5].—Sensation in the eye, as if something were in it; *he always feels it anew, if even after several days it is only mentioned* (from the 2d),[1].—(For several days there is a frequent sensation as if something were in the left eye; it seems to move about in the eye, but is mostly felt towards the inner canthus and also in the upper part of the ball; nothing can be seen, and it often disappears after a short time; it is very troublesome and annoying; in the morning there is matter in the inner canthus; afterwards, there is some swelling and redness in the upper part of the inner canthus), (from the 2d),[1]. —[70.] Sticking-pressive pain in the left eye, extending to the upper orbital border, in the mornings, on waking (nineteenth day),[6].—The left eye pains, as if from a blow (fifth day),[6].—A pain, as if struck in the left eye; he must press it gently and hold it until it ceases (thirteenth day),[6].— Itching sensation in the eyes (crude),[1].—Itching of the eyes, as if there were sand or hair in them (fifth day),[6].—Itching in the left eye; he must rub it, in the evening (third day),[6].—In the air, eyes worse; coryza, hoarseness, cough,[5].—Using eyes by gaslight hurts them,[5].—Writing, and especially reckoning, by candlelight, affects the eyes very much (tenth day),[6]. —*Orbit.* Pressure above the eyes and towards them,[5].—*Lids.* [80.] Hot feeling in lids; sweat of the brows on lids,[5].—Violent painful biting sensation in the left eyelid, towards the external canthus, compels violent rubbing, which causes pain, but does not relieve; in the afternoon (from the second),[1].—*Lachrymal Apparatus.* Lachrymation and confusion of the head, with yawning (seventh day),[6].—Eyes water, most with gaping,[5]. —*Ball.* Squinting; distortion of eyeballs, as if it were from pressure; eyeballs seem distended; they protrude somewhat,[5].—Eyeballs hurt, aching as if beaten,[5].—*Vision.* *Cannot read; light hurts, particularly candlelight,*[5].—More nearsighted than usual, as if dim before the eyes, as from small, round, grayish spots (fifth day),[6].—Letters change in little black points, or small round gray spots, or as if a little bird was flying from right to left,[5].—Veil over eyes; eyes misty,[5].—[90.] Glimmering, glittering, fiery circles; dreams of fire,[5].

Ear.—Objective. Inner and outer ear swollen; red, sore, itching,[5].— Excoriating discharge from ears,[5].—*Subjective.* Burning pain in a small spot over the right ear, highly sensitive to the slightest touch,[5].—A severe, violent, burning pain in a small spot above the right ear (when scratching the head on account of itching); it is exceedingly sensitive to the slightest touch; after a time it suddenly disappears (crude),[1].—Aching, pressing, tearing, rending, in and around the ears, most behind or below,[5].—All the bones behind and around the ears ache and hurt, shooting outwards,[5].—

Pressive pain in the cartilage of the left ear, as if it were being squeezed together with the fingers (eleventh day),[6].—Cold feeling in the ears, coldness followed by throbbing, by heat, with hard hearing; outer ears cold; cold and aching, or hot and aching,[5].—Heat of inner and outer ear,[5].— **[100.]** Earaches, tearing, shutting, jerking pain, in alternations, or with other rheumatic complaints,[5].—Soreness in ears and around,[5].—*Hearing.* Difficult hearing, with all other ear symptoms,[5].—Singing and other noises, most in right ear,[5].

Nose.—*Objective.* Point of nose icy cold,[5].—A small, very painful ulcer forms on the right side of the septum of the nose; he cannot well blow his nose, on account of a sore pain in it; opens the second day, but does not heal till the fifth day (twenty-third day),[6].—Dry yellow mucus in the nose, which must be removed with the fingers (fourth day),[6].—Frequent sneezing (seventh day),[6].—Very frequent sneezing during the whole time (eleventh day),[6].—Frequent violent sneezing, with running from the nose, with nasal mucus and flow of saliva (from the 2d),[1].—**[110.]** Sudden sneezing, and soreness on the margins of wings of nose; fluent coryza during the afternoon,[5].—Interrupted sneezing, afterwards sneezing with coryza (fifth day),[6].—In the evening, three or four times, sudden sneezing, followed by sensation of soreness in the nostrils, with relief of the headache (crude),[1].—Coryza, fluent, in a cold room; stopped in warm air and out of doors,[5].—Fluent coryza, in a cool room; after driving out, stopped catarrh in the hot air, outside (fifth day),[6].—Very profuse, fluent coryza; three handkerchiefs a day; discharge thick, yellow, sometimes watery, with sore nostrils (twenty-first day),[6].—In the open air, on warm days, nose stopped; coming in a cool room, the nose runs,[5].—Chronic catarrh in scrofulous children,° [5].—Streaks of blood; *nose bleeding, afternoon,*[5].—Thin bright-red streaks of blood on the mucus from the nose, while sneezing (from the 2d),[1].—*Subjective.* **[120.]** Sometimes a sensation as if something had got into the nose (like a crumb, while eating), which could not be got out (from the 2d),[1].—Biting-stinging in anterior angle of left nostril; later, right nostril, sneezing and lachrymation (Jones),[5].—Tickling in the nose and sneezing,[5].—Itching and a kind of soreness within the right angle of the nose near the tip (crude),[1].

Face.—Face pale, sallow, yellowish, earthen,[5].—*Pain in face, particularly in upper jawbone, from right to left; extends from other parts to face, or from face to other parts,*[5].—Pain in the processus zygomaticus,[5].—*Swollen upper lip; painful, hard, burning,*[5].

Mouth.—*Teeth.* (Slow, backwards in teething, also in closing of fontanels),[5].—(Slow dentition, with cold tremors and emaciation), (G.),[5].— **[130.]** Teeth cannot bear chewing,[6].—(Carious teeth, cannot bear the fresh air),[5].—Pains in eye-teeth and stomach-teeth,[5].—Toothache, with other complaints,[5].—In an upper hollow root on the right side, sensation as if something had got into it that she strives to remove. The loose root is sensitively painful when touched, yet he has a desire to touch it; every minute renews the pain (twenty-first day),[6].—Raging toothache in an upper root, left, extending into the upper jaw (fifth day),[6].—Sensitiveness in an upper hollow root, right, with desire to suck it with the tongue, which increases the pain,[6].—Sensation as if something were sticking into the lower incisors; it feels like a small painful swelling of the gum (crude),[1].—Dull drawing stitches in a hollow upper back tooth, left side, afternoon (third day),[6].— Shooting in molar teeth; all the hollow teeth cannot bear the air,[5].—**[140.]** Jerking toothache in a hollow back tooth, right, after a bit of pear had got into it (fourth day),[6].—*Tongue.* Tongue white, furred on the root; most in the morning,[5].—Mornings, a whitish coated tongue, with furrows on it, as if split; insipid sweetish taste after the ice cream of the day before (seventh day),[6].—When swallowing, pain in tongue, fauces, pharynx, chest, and pit of stomach,[5].—Tip of the tongue feels as if sore or burnt (fourth day),[6].—*Tip of tongue sore, burning, little blisters,[5].—**General Mouth.** Dryness of mouth and tongue, into choanæ, with salivation, with or without thirst,[5].—Contraction in the right half of the mouth, as if from something hard; teeth also feel contracted, and as if a draught of wind came from their roots (eighteenth day),[6].—A sore spot inside of right cheek, in two provers, distant in time and space, and from different preparations (Jones and B.),[5].—**Saliva.** Saliva copious and acid (crude),[1].—[150.] Saliva running with fluent coryza,[5].—**Taste.** Flabby, sweetish taste,[5].— Bitter taste; particularly wheat bread tastes bitter (Cate),[5].—*Bitter taste in the morning, with headache,[3].—Bitter taste at the setting in of the catamenia,[5].—Foul taste and smell,[5].—All day, especially mornings, offensive taste and coated tongue (ninth day),[6].—Disgusting taste when getting awake; worse when hawking,[5].—Insipid, disgusting taste when waking; tongue thickly coated white (fifth day),[6].

Throat.—Hawking and inclination to vomit after breakfast (eighth day),[6].—[160.] Hawking up phlegm in the evening, at night, and in the morning, with gagging,[3].—When they talk, they constantly hem and hawk,[5].—Much mucus; is often compelled to hawk in his sleep, to raise the mucus (evenings, twentieth day),[6].—Much mucus, with excessive hawking and sore pain in the throat, late in the evening (twenty-third day),[6].—Dryness in the throat, at night,[5].—Throat dry, sore, scrapy (twentieth day),[6]. —A sensation in the throat as after much weeping or after running, a kind of contraction (from the 2d),[1].—Pains and burning from other parts towards the throat,[5].—Burning in pit of throat,[5].—Pain on the sides of throat; aching on pressure up to the ear, or from ear to shoulder, worse when turning the neck, also when swallowing,[5].—[170.] Sore aching in throat; worse when swallowing,[5].—Drawing in the inner throat, in the left eye, and in the left row of teeth (nineteenth day),[6].—Sore throat and running of the nose,[5].— Sore throat in the morning, on waking, worse in the right side, low down in the fauces, more towards the back; worse when swallowing; it disappears after rising and at breakfast; warm drink causes no pain (from the 2d),[1]. —In the evening, sore throat, with tickling cough, increasing after going to bed,[5].—Throat pains as if sore; rough when swallowing, as if sore and painful; worse evenings (nineteenth day),[6].—Sensation of soreness in the throat, and swelling of the left tonsil, with sensitiveness to the touch; relieved in the evening by moistening it with fruit (eighteenth day),[6].—Throat rough and scrapy, as if he would have a sore throat; sensation of dryness in a warm room (fifth day),[6].—Roughness in the throat (twenty-first day),[6]. —Tickling-crawling in the throat that excites a dry cough (sixth day),[6].— **Tonsils.** [180.] Pain in the right tonsil (after mustard), (from the 2d),[1]. —Sore pain in the left tonsil, when yawning,[6].—**Fauces.** Fauces and uvula red and swollen; warm drink does not hurt,[5].—Sensation of weakness or emptiness in fauces and throat,[5].—**Swallowing.** Difficult empty swallowing, with scratching in the throat; food is easy to swallow (seventh day),[6].—Saliva hurts to swallow, not food,[5].—**Throat Externally.** Aching, sore pain in the region of parotid gland,[5].

Stomach.—Appetite and Thirst. Appetite better than for a long time previously (crude),[1].—*Unusual hunger at 4 P.M.,[5].—Infants want to be put to the breast all the time,[5].—[190.] Has much desire and appetite for coffee and wine (fourteenth and fifteenth days),[6].—Great desire for tobacco-smoking; headache relieved (crude),[1].—Diminished appetite at noon, with headache in the afternoon; more appetite in the evening, when the headache became better (from the crude),[1].—No appetite from noon to noon, but if thinking about it, she wants to eat,[5].—Complete want of appetite, before or with catamenia,[5].—Feels no real desire for his accustomed smoking, nor does he relish it properly during the first two weeks (fourteenth day),[6].—Much thirst, with a dry mouth and tongue, after part of the day,[5].—*Eructations.* After breakfast, belching, hawking, gagging, nausea,[5].—Belching, all forenoon, with qualmishness,[5].—Sour belching and gulping up,[5].—[200.] *After belching, a burning in epigastrium,*[5].—Heartburn, one or two hours after dinner (Cate),[5].—Heartburn up into the throat; sore in right groin, and a kicking-quivering over the os pubis,[5].—*Nausea and Vomiting.* Nausea after drinking coffee, and an incipient heartburn and exceedingly unpleasant sensation, together with confusion of the head, headache, and great ill-humor (from the 2d),[1].—Nausea, rising from the pit of the stomach, when moving; better at rest; followed by headache and lassitude,[5].—Nausea lasting two hours, with vertigo and headache, worse when stooping; dull confusion of the head, with confusion of the thoughts,[4].—Nausea from smoking or after drinking coffee,[5].—Nausea when smoking as usual, inclination to vomit; tobacco itself does not taste right for several days (fifth day),[6].—He gags several times as if to vomit, mornings, with hawking of mucus (seventh day),[6].—Vomiturition from hawking phlegm,[5].—[210.] *Children vomit often and easy,[5].—Vomiting of food after eating, as if sharp, corroding, and sore in the throat, with a sensation as if the teeth were dull and too long, after ice-cream (evenings, eighth day),[6].—Vomiting, with trembling of hands,[5].—*Stomach.* Flabbiness of stomach,[5].—*An empty, sinking sensation at the epigastrium,* 7 P.M.,[5].—Indescribable uneasiness in region of stomach,[5].—*Burning* in epigastrium; in region of navel; *in whole abdomen,* rising up into the chest, into the throat,[5].—*Burning at the stomach and rising of water into the mouth* (waterbrash),[5].—*Stomach feels expanded,*[5].—Violent cramp in the stomach, a kind of pressure as if he had eaten something hard to excess that presses his stomach, with a sensation of qualmishness and nausea before dinner (twelfth day),[6].—[220.] One hour after dinner, dull pain in stomach, .with soreness when pressing upon it; one or two hours after dinner, heartburn and other gastric symptoms,[5].—Pressure in stomach; lessening when she rests,[5].—Sharp cutting or cramplike pain in stomach, with headache,[5].

Abdomen. — Hypochondria. Throbbing in right hypochondrium; lessened after belching or passing wind,[5].—Sticking in the region of the liver during a long inspiration as if from flatus (twelfth day),[6].—Stitches or shooting in region of liver, when taking a deep breath,[5].—Sharp pain in region of spleen,[5].—*Umbilical.* Emptiness or sinking around navel or in whole belly,[5].—Complaint like in the first period of pregnancy; a drawing aching in region of navel, extending to the sacral region; worse in the forenoon,[5].—Cutting pain in the abdomen around the navel, a kind of wind colic, and eructations of some herb that he had eaten at dinner; after drinking cold water, the pains are violently renewed, evening (fifth day),[6].—[230.] Two hours after eating ice cream in the evening, colic-like pains about the navel (sixth day),[6].—*Aching soreness and pain around navel;* lessens after fetid wind passes off,[5].—*General Abdomen.* Much flatulence and rumbling in the abdomen, with some pain, after two doses of the 1st; the same, also much more severe, after a third dose, together with confusion of the head, which soon increased to a dull pain, which was always more sensitive on stooping; this continued more or less severe the whole day, until a thin evacuation followed, preceded by sensitive pain; quite well the next day,[3].—Meteorismus, and pain in the abdomen, followed by stool and immediate relief of the symptoms (from the 2d),[3].— *Wind passes off, with a stench,[5].—Difficult passage of flatus, followed by slight relief (from the 2d),[1].—Motion in abdomen as if something alive,[5].— Abdominal pains, with headache, earache, hot face, pain in groins, looseness of bowels, weary legs, crawls; or in alternation with headache, burning throat, uterine pains, lassitude,[5].—Severe pain in the abdomen, with flatulence, with unusually frequent stools, at first natural, afterwards soft (third and fourth days),[4].—External wall of the abdomen asleep, numb, quivering, aching, etc.,[5].—[240.] Pinching, shooting stitches, running, kicking; moving in left side of belly,[5].—*On every attempt to eat, bellyache, (G. Bute),[5].—Bellyache less after passing wind, after stool, or after leucorrhœa,[5].—A pressure in abdomen, with difficulty of preventing escape of urine,[5].—After drinking cold water, cutting in abdomen,[5].—Cutting pains in the abdomen two hours after eating honey, relieved by passage of flatus (seventh day),[6].—Griping in the abdomen and sensation of discomfort after eating fruit (fourteenth day),[6].—Before appearance of menses, griping and rumbling in bowels and leucorrhœa,[5].—Eating ice-cream in the evening gives him the colic, and he has to vomit the next morning,[5].— *Cutting, pinching, sharp colic, followed by looseness,[5].—[250.] Severe pain in region of transverse colon, 3 P.M.,[5].—*Hypogastrium and Iliac Region.* Over os pubis a drawing pain from right to left; passing of some blood, followed by earache from left to right (female),[5].—Warm feeling in the groins; burning aching pain,[5].—Aching soreness, cutting, drawing in left groin, later in right,[5].—Throbbing, stinging, ticking, soreaching, pressing, drawing upwards in symphysis, downwards in thighs,[5].— Sacro-iliac symphysis in walking, as if separated,[5].

Rectum and Anus.—Sore aching in anus when getting up in the morning,[5].—After supper pressure in rectum, with a stool; the first hard, the last thin,[5].—Stitches in the rectum, evenings (eighth day),[6].—Single stitches in rectum towards the anus, or shooting in anus,[5].—[260.] Itching in the rectum (eleventh day),[6].—Itching, sticking, and cutting in the rectum (fourth day),[6].—Itching, tickling, prickling in the rectum, with a desire to draw it in very much, without having had a stool all day, evening, in bed (fifteenth day),[6].—On the fourteenth day, a hæmorrhoidal aggravation as on the eighth day,[6].—Protruding piles, aching and itching, sore; oozing out of a yellow fluid,[5].—Warmth, burning, pulsating in anus; bearing down towards anus,[5].—*Sore feeling in anus, worse outside, with stitching, burning, throbbing,[5].—Itching in anus; most in the evening,[5].—Shooting through perinæum into the penis (Jones),[5].—Heaviness and urging to stool, with costiveness, or after looseness,[5].

Stool. — Diarrhœa. [270.] Diarrhœa, after cider (crude),[1].— *Diarrhœa, in which there were many small white points, or flakes, like pus, scarcely perceptible (third day), (crude),[1].—*Very offensive diarrhœa (from the 4th),[2].—She was taken with diarrhœa and pain in the ball of the thumb (from the 4th),[2].—Diarrhœa after vexation,[5].—*During first dentition diarrhœa, with much wind,[5]. — *Juicy fruit or cider causes diarrhœa,[5].—Watery looseness day and night, with an urging after the stool, every fifteen minutes,[5].—Stool, etc., morning and evening.[5].—Two stools, mornings and evenings, the last with much blackish blood, mucus, and some bloody fibrinous, membranous pieces (twenty-seventh day),[6].—

[280.] Two stools in the morning with but little blood and much less mucus than usual (tenth day),⁶.—Three stools with excessive protrusion of hæmorrhoids that are sensitively sore and throbbing. After the third evacuation tenesmus and urgency as if more were to pass.; no stool the two following days (fourteenth day),⁶.—*Mornings, copious, soft stool; renewed urgency directly on wiping, after which a little more was evacuated. Dull drawing in the nape of the neck, in the afternoons (fourth day),⁶.— Pappy stool mornings after awaking, with dark, at first clotted, afterwards liquid blood ; a half hour after diarrhœa with tenesmus. Three hours later urgency to stool again, when nothing was passed but some mucus tinged with blood, with much greater protrusion of hæmorrhoids than during the previous six days, with scraping, cutting, and itching pain in them; they do not recede for some time (distinct aggravation, eighth day),⁶.—Must go to stool directly after rising ; on previous day two hours later, with much less discharge of blood than before (sixth day),⁶.—Unusual but scanty stool in the evening, *with very much flatulence* (crude),¹.—Evenings after driving a whole day, a second stool, with somewhat more blood than usual (thirteenth day),⁶.—No blood with the light properly formed stool, only so from colored mucus (seventh day),⁶.—Stool soft, mixed with blackish blood, more than formerly (after an hour),⁶.—After omitting stool for two days, an evacuation, with more blood than for some time past (seventeenth day),⁶. —[290.] Bleeding after stool, or with a soft stool followed by slime ; protrusion of piles after short buzzing in ears ; very weak feeling in male sexual parts,⁵.—After the copious morning stool with blood, renewed urgency when wiping himself, upon which he passed a few soft small pieces without blood (second day),⁶. — Diaper reddish-yellow (Boecker),⁵. — *Constipation. No stool* (ninth to twenty-first day),⁶.—No stool, and scraping sore pain in the anus, especially when walking in the evening (twelfth day),⁶.

Urinary Organs.—Kidneys and Bladder. Pain in the region of the kidneys, when lifting, digging, blowing the nose, frequently so violent as to cause crying out (from the 4th),².—*In region of kidneys, violent pain when lifting and when blowing the nose.* Pain in back, jerking, rending, cutting, shooting,⁵.—Violent pain in bladder, and all neighboring parts,⁵.—Sore aching in bladder, worse after micturition,⁵.—A painful sensation in the neck of the bladder, like that when having the stream suddenly stopped,⁵.—[300.] While urinating, drawing in bladder upwards (female) ; burning in urethra, hardness (male),⁵.—Frequent pressure in the bladder ; he is often compelled to pass a little clear, pale urine (fourteenth day),⁶.—Pressing pain, most on right side of bladder,⁵.—Before urinating, cutting in bladder, pressing down, cutting in urethra,⁵.—Shooting in the mouth of the bladder,⁵.—*Urethra.* Orifice of the urethra somewhat inflamed and agglutinated. A quantity of urine spirts out after urinating (fourth day),⁶.—When urinating, the urethra expands very much, swells and grows hard, with burning, towards evening (third day),⁶.—Cutting pains in urethra,⁵.—Cutting pain in the urethra, when not urinating (fourteenth day),⁶.—*After urinating,* cutting and burning in urethra (male) ; pressing and cutting in bladder, deep into the left (female) ; relaxation and weakness of the organs (male),⁵.—[310.] Sticking in the urethra when not urinating,⁶.—Frequent urging to make water (Cate),⁵.—Frequent urgency to urinate ; always some dropping of urine afterwards (sixth day),⁶.—*Micturition.* Passage of urine more copious than usual (third and fourth days),⁴.—Frequent, copious passage of urine, with weakness and weariness,⁴.

—Frequent urinating, evenings while in bed (fifteenth day),[6].—*Large quantities of urine, with sensation of weakness* (Gf.),[5].—Urinating at 2 o'clock in the night; he believed it was morning; clean taste in the mouth, followed by slumbering till morning, when he awoke with an insipid, disgusting taste in his mouth,[6].—When urinating, fine streams spirt sideways in every direction, from the vigorous stream; together with slight cutting in the urethra (fourth day),[6].—*Urine.* Dark urine, warmer than usual, and of penetrating odor,[5].—[320.] Urine dark-colored, hot, smelling like strong tea (from the 4th),[2].—Very dark urine in the afternoon, something very unusual (from the 2d),[1].—More urine, with flocculent sediment,[5].

Sexual Organs.—Male. Penis swollen hard, evenings, and the urethra much distended when urinating (fifteenth day),[6].—Erection, while riding in a carriage, without desire,[5].—Erection, painful, with burning in urethra, and a tension in the penis, in the evening,[5].—Excessive erections, when driving for any length of time, but without desire (thirteenth day),[6]. —The genito-urinary organs seem generally affected after the passage of a stool and urine (crude),[1].—Cutting-drawing pains in the glans, extending towards the tip, only while sitting; not very severe, but an exceedingly unpleasant sensation (from the 2d),[1].—Shooting in the root of penis and bladder (Brugger),[5].—[330.] Towards morning, special desire for coitus; together with very unusual orgasm; after rising, general well feeling, and appetite, which he did not usually have in the morning, and though there was some headache left over from the previous day, still there was more desire for work (crude),[1].—Sexual desire first increased; with others, decreased (male),[5].—At 1 o'clock, in the night, excessive emission, with a voluptuous dream (eighth day),[6].—*Female.* *Weakness and distress in the region of the uterus, and the uterine displacement; aggravated by the passage of stool and urine,*[5].—*Aching in uterus,* in the morning (female),[5].—A pressing in uterus; more sexual desire; ache in neck of bladder; prostration,[5].—Cutting pain in uterus through to the sacrum (female),[5].—Swelling of external parts and vagina, when awaking,[5].—Clitoris erect after urination, with desire,[5].—Whites, cream-like, pass from her in the afternoon, unconsciously,[5].—[340.] Whites two weeks after catamenia, or from one term to another,[5].—Voluptuous feeling, as if all the female parts were filling up with blood; she feels the pulse in all the parts, with increased sexual desire,[5].—*Over mons veneris a pressure upwards,* a throbbing or other sensations (female),[5].—Pressive-drawing and sore feeling, as if catamenia should appear; aching pressure in uterus and vagina, in the loins; flushes of heat; fatigued from going upstairs; pain from right groin into the left hip,[5].—Pains from navel and other parts drawing to the vagina,[5].—Pain in vagina, with flushes and faintness,[5].—Burning in vagina, with pain on both sides of bladder and uterus; burning like fire up into the chest,[5].—After nose-bleeding, aching in vagina,[5].—Labia sore, aching; warm feeling between externals; stitching pain in inner labia,[5].—*Before catamenia,* great sexual desire, followed by a copious flow; headache three to seven days before; griping and rumbling in bowels; stitching pains in left side of head; whites, and sleepiness during the day,[5].—[350.] Nymphomania; all organs in erection, with insatiable desire, particularly before catamenia,[5].— Catamenia too early (five to eight days), with girls, and bright blood; two weeks too late, with a widow, blood too dark; seventeen weeks too late, first bright red, then dark, last lochia-like and fetid. Blood dark, especially with rheumatic patients,[5].—Menses every two weeks, black and clotted; menorrhagia,[5].—Less catamenia, more whites, like *white of eggs,* day and night; worse in the *morning*, after rising; of a sweetish odor; increased whites, and with a stool of a bad odor,[5].

Respiratory Organs.—Larynx. He has to hawk or to hem if he wants to talk clear,[5].—Burning in larynx, after the same feeling on back part of tongue,[5].—**Voice.** Hoarseness and cough, day and night,[5].—Evenings, husky and hoarse, with inclination to vomit; is obliged to hawk in order to speak distinctly (twelfth day),[6].—Husky voice; mucus in the throat prevents him from speaking distinctly; is obliged to hawk whenever he wants to speak, in the evening (eleventh day),[6].—**Cough.** Cough in the sunny half of the day, 6 A.M. to 6 P.M.,[5].—[**360.**] Tickling cough and lachrymation of the left eye (fifth day),[6].—Dry cough, with hoarseness and soreness, and dryness in the throat,[5].—**Respiration.** Involuntary sighing,[5]. —*Involuntary sighing at times* (Cate, C. Hg., Liggen),[5].—(He was frequently obliged to take a deep sighing breath), (crude),[1].—Desire to take a deep breath, to sigh; with it a pain in the chest; shooting in liver,[5].— *Breathing more frequent, short and difficult,*[5]—Short breath and cough,[5].— Lifting child up from cradle, suffocative fits (down, Borax),[5].—Suffocating attacks of a male child of six months, after nursing; more often after crying, and after being taken out of the cradle; breathing ceases; head turns backwards; face blue; fighting with hands and feet; after attacks, greatly relaxed; some days none, some days several attacks,[5].

Chest.—[370.] Pain on a small spot, from coughing; with short breath,[5]. —Burning sensation in chest, from below up into the throat; sometimes downwards,[5].—Constriction of breast; difficult breathing in the evening, better when lying in bed, worse again when rising in the morning, with great pain in the chest when breathing,[5].—* *Contraction of the chest and difficult breathing, evening till 10 P.M.; better on lying down, worse when getting up,*[5].—Dull aching in chest, and sore to the touch,[5].—Pressing ache in the chest; most below and upwards,[5].—Over the clavicle sore, cutting; pain in throat, soreness, glands hurt,[5].—**Front.** Creaking on the left side of the sternum, like a cracking in the joints (from the 2d),[1].—Sharp pain, like an instrument passed through end of breast-bone, during the day,[5].—Tearing, pressing, and shooting in breast-bone,[5].—[**380.**] Sore pain on the sternum,[5].— **Sides.** Pains where the cartilages and ribs meet,[5].—Hardness, soreness, pressure in right side,[5].—Pressure and soreness in left side,[5].—Stitch in left side, while breathing,[5].—Shooting pain in the left chest, going through the shoulder,[5].—With inhalation, shooting in left breast and right temple; with breathing, inhaling, and exhaling, a shooting in chest; most with a deep breath,[5].—Beating on a small spot on left side of chest,[5].—Collar-bone sore; first left and then right,[5].—Sharp pain in region of sixth rib; first on right side, later on left fourth and fifth rib, coming and going; takes the breath away; most with a deep breath, during the day,[5].—[**390.**] A tumor like a walnut in left mamma,[5].—In left mamma, a hardness, like a walnut, sore to pressure; with a man of eighteen years,[5].—Milk watery, thin, neutral,[5].— Milk acid, *not* alkaline; acts on blue litmus,[5].—Milk changeable, from the alkali to the neutral, or to the acid,[5].—External feeling of warmth in mammæ, towards the left arm,[5].—Child refuses the breast; the milk has a saltish taste; trying it, the taste remains long in the mouth, 3ᶜ Jenichen. Next day, milk sweet (Pehrson, Guernsey),[5].—Pressing, tearing, rending, drawing contraction; pinching, shooting, burning in mammæ,[5].—*Mammæ sore to the touch,*[5].—Nipples aching, sore,[5].

Heart and Pulse.—[400.] Sharp pain in region of heart, with inhaling, interferes with breathing,[5].—Sharp cutting, shooting, in region of heart; interrupts breathing,[5].—Feels beating of pulse, not frequent but quick; while sitting, he feels it in the nape of neck and left chest,[5].

Neck and Back.—Neck. Muscles of neck hurt up to occiput; first right, then left,[5].—*A slight draught of air is followed by rheumatic pain in neck, stiffness and dulness of head,*[5].—* Cramplike pain in the neck; first on one side, then the other (Cate, r to l?),*[5].—Stiffness in the nape of the neck (ninth day),[6].—On exposure to a slight draught, violent rheumatic drawing pains in the nape of the neck, with a kind of stiffness and dulness of the whole head (thirteenth day),[6].—*Back.* *Backache and uterine pains,*[5].—Back and lower limbs ache less after motion,[5].—[410.] Drawing in back and limbs, with gaping, stretching, bending backwards; worse evening and morning, getting awake, on moving about,[5].—With inhalation, a sudden jerking pain in back,[5].—*Dorsal.* Pains and aches in and near, between, and *mostly below the shoulder-blades,* throbbing, pulsating, jerking,[5].—Tensive pain below the right shoulder-blade, extending forward (from the 2d),[1].—*Lumbar.* The small of the back, knees, thumbs, are especially affected,[4].—Sore aching in left loin,[5].—*Sacral.* In sacrum numbness and lameness,[5].—Sharp sacral pains, lameness,[5].—Severe pain above the sacrum, and in the hips, soon after taking it (from the 4th),[2].—* In the union of sacrum and hip-bone, sacro-iliac union, a soreness, as if separated,*[5].—[420.] Pain and aches, soreness, pressive, tearing, and shooting in os coccygis,[5].

Extremities in General.—Trembling of arms and hands, with other complaints, particularly uterine,[5].—Weariness in all the limbs during pregnancy,[5].—*Pains flying about in all parts of rump and limbs, after getting wet in rain,*[5].—*Aching in all the limbs, with weariness,*[5].—Mornings after waking, the extremities have gone to sleep, especially the hands and feet (after disagreeable news the day previous), (twentieth day),[6].

Superior Extremities.—Trembling in arms and hands (two girls), (also Cate and *),[5].—Paralysis of the whole left arm, lasting an hour (from the 4th),[2].—Dull pain in arms; first left, then right, from shoulder to fingers; from clavicle down to the wrist,[5].—Pain and numbness of the left arm, in the afternoon (after taking the drug in the morning), (from the 2d),[5].—[430.] All the bones of the arm ache, particularly in the thumb,[5].—Soreness, burning, itching under the arms,[5].—*Shoulder.* Pain and aches in shoulder and shoulder-blades,[5].—Rheumatic pains in shoulders, chest, and other parts, after getting wet in the rain (Jones),[5].—Sore aching, bruised pains in shoulder, or down the arm,[5].—*Arm.* A very sensitive pain from the left elbow-joint to the shoulder (from the 4th),[2].—Rheumatic pain in upper arm near shoulder-joint; cannot lift the arm,[5].—Sensation like a hot stitch in the right upper arm above the bend of the elbow (twenty-second day),[6].—*Elbow.* Burning in the right elbow, as if from the bite of ants (thirteenth day),[6].—Through elbows, shooting, usually first left, then right,[5].—[440.] In elbow, as if the joint had been struck,[5].—*Forearm.* Cramplike pain in forearm; sore, bruised feeling; tearing,[5].—Pain, as if broken, in the right forearm bones (fourth day),[6].—Breaking pain in the right forearm, then in the left (fifth day),[6].—*Wrist.* Sudden pressive pain in both wrists, worse in the left, lasting a long time (after eleven hours), (from the 4th),[2].—Pain in right wrist, with lameness, as if beat; cramplike and other pains when moving or using it,[5].—*Hand.* Hands tremble; she is sick; heart beats; fear of bad news; after this, trembling and weak,[5].—Trembling of hands, with headache; pain in chest, bellyache,[5].—Hands asleep,[5].—The right hand feels as if pounded, and gone to sleep in bed (fifth day),[6].—[450.] Paralysis of the left hand and arm,[2].—Burning-sticking in the left metacarpal bones, towards evening (ninth day),[6].—Pressive pain in the left hand and in the left metacarpal bones (twenty-second day),[6].—*Fingers.* The thumbs moved spasmodically,[5].—Paralysis of all the finger-joints (from the 4th),[2].—Pain in single fingers,[5].—Pain in the fingers of the right hand when writing, in the evening (third day), (from the 4th),[2].—(Pain in the first joint of the little finger, which it had already had for a long time), (from the 2d),[1].—Breaking pain in the third phalanx of the right third finger (twenty-third day),[6]. —In right thumb, all the joints as if luxated or sprained,[5].—[460.] Sticking pain, as if with a hot needle, in the tip of the left thumb (fourteenth day),[6].—Raging, twitching pain in the first joint of the left little finger (seventh day),[6].—Points of thumb and finger sore,[5].—The right little finger pains goutlike, as if bruised and swelled, worse when touched or moved ; afternoons during the finest warm weather; it was only a little windy (fourth day),[6].—* *Ulcerative pain in the roots of the finger-nails of the right hand, especially in the middle finger* (from the 4th),[2].—Pains as if ulcerated around the nails,[5].

Inferior Extremities.—The child does not stand any more,[5].— Stepping motion of lower limbs,[5].—*Lower limbs, abdomen, and sacrum asleep ; cannot get up from the seat,[5].—*Lower limbs fall asleep, with a restless, anxious feeling ; has to move them to jump out of the carriage; also at night,[5].— [470.] *Legs tired, weak, restless, crawling, tingling,[5].—Lame feeling of lower limbs, tired, heavy,[5].—In damp, rainy, cold weather, dull pain in lower limbs,[5].—*Hip.* Caries, hip-joint, heel, with stinking pus,[5].—In the hip-bone, tearing, shooting, drawing,[5].—Shooting or stitches from the hip-bone up or down; worst from the ischium down, jerking, drawing, with a warm feeling,[5].—*Thigh.* Going to sleep of the gluteal muscles, with restlessness in the lower limbs; he is constantly obliged to move them and change his position ; at the same time a feeling of anxiety, he wants to jump out of the carriage ; if he turns upon the right side, half lying, the nervus ischiadicus pains as if pressed, and he is obliged to sit up erect (during a longer drive at night), (twenty-third day),[6].—On rising after sitting a short time, the right buttock feels as if gone to sleep, and this sensation extended through the entire leg down into the toes (fourth day),[6].—Buttocks and backside asleep, with an uneasiness,[5].—Sore aching in buttocks ; warmth, heat, burning, itching, oozing pimples; after scratching, scurfs continue to itch,[5].—[480.] Day after a snowstorm, buttocks as if beaten, with lameness,[5].—In the nates lameness, as if beaten ; after a storm all kinds of pain, with soreness ; most from right to left, but alternating most on right side,[5]. —Aching and soreness of thighs,[5].—Sharp pain in the tendons on the inside of thighs, more when walking,[5].—While nursing her fifth child during sixth month (taking four drops of 4th in water), labor pains down in the thighs, with an involuntary stool, and passing some blood. A strong, healthy woman, never before having catamenia during nursing (Bute),[5].— *Knee.* Pains above the knee,[5].—Knees painful when walking, as if scraped, when touched by the pants; later he found red pimples on the knees that caused the pain (eighth day),[6].—Pains in the knees worse when walking ; first left, then right (observed in fifty-four symptoms),[5].—Boring in the right knee, worse from stretching ; most at night,[5].—Knees pain as if sprained ; sore when walking,[5].—[490.] Sharp pain in the knees,[4].—Sharp pain in both knees when walking, in the afternoon (second day), (from the 4th),[2].—Shooting through the left thigh to the knee ; stirring above, down to ankle-bones; toes too thick,[5].—Violent pain below the hollow of the knee, worse when taking boots off,[5].—Pain beneath the hollow of the knee every time it is strongly bent, as for example, on drawing on the boots, exceedingly painful; it makes the use of the whole limbs uncertain, as for example, when walking or jumping,[1].—Tendons in the hollow of the knee as if too short,[5].—Tensive drawing in the left popliteal space when raising or stretching out the foot, as if the tendons were too short, relieved by continued walking (fourth day),[6].—*Leg.* Feels blood run from the knee down to the feet,[5].—Tearing in left lower leg from the knee down to the feet; dry, crusty tetters cover the leg,[5].—Rending pains in the bones of the left leg, as if broken, alternating sympathetically with the right hand (fourth day),[6].—[500.] Contraction around the left calf, as if he were tied there (seventh day),[6].—Cramp pain in calves, drawing, rending, shooting, warm feeling,[5].—*Cramp in calves, on a small spot inside, when walking,[5].*—Pain in the calves, rending, tearing, drawing, shooting,[5].—Pain in the right calf, so violent that he could scarcely raise the leg, in the morning (third day), (from the 4th),[2].—Drawing pains in shin-bones,[5].—A pain in the head of left tibia caused by a kick returns; the spot became so sore that he could not bear it touched; it disturbed the sleep, coming on every night; gradually an exostosis formed and remained (Freitag),[5].—*Ankle.* Ankle-joint as if dislocated,[5].—Rending, tearing, shooting in ankle-joint,[5].—*Foot.* Weakness in the feet after coition (twenty-first day),[6].—[510.] Left foot went to sleep while driving, and crawling in the sole of it like formication (fifth day),[6].—Cramplike pain in the feet, most in the ankle-joint,[5].—In the right metatarsal bones, stitches, as if with needles, when stepping down (tenth day),[6].—Tearing pain in the left metatarsal bone (fifth day),[6].—*Toes.* Twitching of the big toes; the little toe drawn inward,[5].—Old (gouty) pain in the left great toe, with inclination to crack the joints, which, however, he did not do (crude),[1].

General Symptoms.—Objective. Phosphatic diathesis (G.),[5].—Rachitis; fontanels wide open; diarrhœa; emaciation,[5].—Rheumatism returning with cold weather, leaving her with the warm season,[5].—Distended veins (from the 4th.),[2].—[520.] After fractures, when they do not ossify, or the callus does not form, smaller doses of the stuff are required to form a callus, are followed by the formation of one, containing one hundred times more of the C. ph.,[5].—Disposition to stretch,[5].—Constant stretching,[5].—Convulsive starts when the child lies on his back, which cease when lying on its side,[5].—Extensors more affected than flexors, in all the limbs,[5].—Stiff in bed in the morning; can hardly turn,[5].—The greatest weariness; tired from going upstairs; does not want to rise from sitting,[5].—*Weariness when going upstairs; wants to sit down; hates to get up,[5].*—Weakness, with other symptoms,[5].—Great weakness and weariness, soon after taking; sharp pains in the stomach and in the knees, with headache, which lasted a whole day; on the next morning pain in the right great toe, worse when walking, lasting the whole day; after a few days he repeated the dose, which caused the pain in the stomach and the headache, with diarrhœa; the pain in the stomach continued the next day, was very severe at times, with a watery diarrhœa and burning stools; the diarrhœa continued the third day, with violent pain in the stomach on every attempt to eat anything; much better the fourth day; quite well the fifth day (from the 4th.),[2].—[530.] Soon after taking it she felt weak and prostrated, with flushes of heat in the head, nervous weakness; three hours afterwards she was attacked by severe pain in the right knee, on account of which she could scarcely walk; she felt as though she had received a blow on the inner side of the knee, which caused at the same time a violent pain and sensation of soreness, which lasted two days; the second dose taken some days afterwards had the same effect, aggravated by bending the knee; her twelve-year old daughter had the same symptoms from the same dose, only more severe; she had together with weakness, severe headache, pain and sensation of soreness of the thigh, which after a time extended into the left knee and there lasted twenty-four hours; after the disappearance of the pain the knee still remained sensitive to touch, as if beaten; her ten-year old son was also affected by a violent pain in the left knee, extending to the sole of the foot; her infant, who had just began to stand, would not stand any longer, and it was plainly to be seen that he had been affected by the paralyzing power of the drug through his mother's milk (from the 4th),².—Restlessness, spasmodic motion of limbs; worse when lying on back, better lying on side,⁵.—Sensitive to slight touch,⁵.—*Subjective.* She feels in general very uncomfortable (from the 4th),².—After taking cold, liable to rheumatic pains in all her joints,⁵.— Feeling of lameness of the flexors; sudden aching of the extensors of all the limbs,⁵.—Painless gnawing, with quivering, jerking, and heat; full of fear,⁵.—Trembling feeling, then toothache, and uterine pains,⁵.—Ailments from grief, disappointed love,⁵.—Pains in various parts of the body, frequently shooting along the muscles into the joints,⁴.—[540.] Pain in bones, particularly shin-bones,⁵.—Bones affected along the sutures (see head), or where bones unite, symphysis; also in the pelvis (see falling of womb),⁵.—Most pain in joints, afterwards in the bones,⁵.—Pain in all the joints; most left side; later and less the right,⁵.—Sharp pain in the tendons,⁵. —The tendons are sore when stretching and bending,⁵.—*Sensations mostly on small spots,*⁵.—Sore pain, first right, then left,⁵.—Places hurt by a shock become sore to the touch; on a place burnt twenty-three years ago a tetter forms, an exostosis; old scars exulcerate,⁵.—The symptoms remaining the longest with the provers appear in the morning hours,⁵.—[550.] The sunny half to the dark half like 5 3,⁵.—The last half of the day stands to the first half like 5 7,⁵.—In bed, pains in bones or joints,⁵.—Every cold causes pains in joints, and *where bones unite and form a symphysis or suture* (C. Hg.),⁵.—She is very much worse after taking a light cold,⁵.—* *On every little cold she is much worse; rheumatic pains and displaced uterus,*⁵.—During moderate motions of single limbs most of the painful symptoms appear, and get easier after lying down,⁵.—Pains after great exertions are worse when lying down,⁵.—Pressure worse, head, chest, belly, limbs,⁵.—The symptoms occur after the second dose and gradually diminish until the fourth day, when they disappear,⁴.—[560.] *Right to left,* sutures of frontal and lateral bones; *earache,* stopped up; cold feeling; jugular bones ache, upper jaw pains; toothache; bellyache; aching in groins, above the os pubis, mammæ, neck, chest, back, armpits, arms, elbows, forearms, hands, fingers, buttocks, thighs, above knees, shin-bones, calves, heels, big toes, toes,⁵.—Right upper, left lower; pain in bones (Schreter),⁵.

Skin.—General. After a cold foot-bath becomes red, with prickling like nettles,⁵.—After a cold river-bath, red as a lobster over the whole body, with biting and prickling, as of nettles (fourteenth day),⁶.—Skin dark-brown, yellow, with grown people; in a child of ten days,⁵.—*Eruptions. Dry.* Pimples on the forehead (eighth day),⁶.—Pimples on the ears,⁵.— Pimple on the scrotum, sore to the touch (fourth day),⁶.—Pimples in region of joints,⁵.—Pimples inside of forearm,⁵.—[570.] Pimples on back of hand, on wrist,[5].—An itching pimple on the back of the left hand; the itching ceases after scratching, evenings (third day),[6].—A pimple on the right ankle, sore to the touch (twelfth day),[6].—Tetters on lower legs, peeling off scaling,[5].—*Pustular.* Scrofulous ulcers; lax and lazy,[5].—A suppurating pimple behind the left ear, sore to the touch (twentieth day),[6].—Suppurating pimple on the nape of the neck, sensitively painful to the touch (tenth day),[6].—On the back of the left metacarpal joint a suppurating pimple, sore to the touch (eighth day),[6].—Furuncle between the right eyebrow and upper lid; eye inflamed; lids falling or closed, most in the morning,[5].—Small furuncle near anus to the right, with much pain; cannot sit; has to stand or lie on left side; discharges blood or pus, and remains a painless fistula (two provers),[5].—[580.] Large ulcers above or around the ears and in the region of parotid gland,[5].—*Sensations.* Itching and burning as from nettles,[5].—Itching and burning over the whole skin (from the 4th),[2].—Itching, biting; most on places years before affected,[5]. —Sticking-drawing of the skin on the right side of the thorax, especially when raising the arms (tenth day),[6].—Very unpleasant formication over the whole abdomen, for an hour and a half (five hours after taking 8 drops of the 4th),[2].—Itching on point of nose,[5].—Itching between the third and little finger of the left hand (seventh day),[6].—On the buttocks stinging on little spots; itching, burning, sore spots, oozing scurfs,[5].—[590.] Burning-itching of outer ear in a warm room,[5].

Sleep and Dreams.—Sleepiness. * Gaping, with irresistible drowsiness all forenoon,[5].—* Cannot get awake in the early morning (J. C. Morgan),[5]. —Gaping, with tears in eyes,[5].—Sleepiness all forenoon, before and at dinner,[5].—Great sleepiness; he can hardly pull open his eyes, during morning service (after three hours),[6].—Before dinner, very sleepy, with yawning (fifth day),[6].—Drowsy all day (Jones),[5].—Sleepy before dinner; falls asleep while eating; and after dinner, while sitting, falls in a deep sleep,[5].— All evening asleep,[5].—[600.] Sound sleep in the evening; early waking from sleep (crude),[1].—*Sleeplessness.* No sleep till 2 or 3 o'clock (from the 2d),[1].—Cannot go to sleep, must turn and toss; his body itches; frequently lies on his stomach, and does not go to sleep till after 2 in the morning (fifteenth day),[6].—Wakeful a long time, evenings,[6].—Mornings awoke earlier than usual (eighth day),[8].—Early waking, feeling well,[5].—Early waking, mornings, with erections, without desire, after which he fell into a sleep, in which he heard everything that passed about him, without being able to rouse himself. He dreamed of journeys beset with obstacles,[6].—Starting in sleep,[5].—In sleep, starting as from fright,[5].—Very restless sleep; tosses about a great deal (nineteenth day),[6].—[610.] Sleep disturbed, most before midnight,[5].—*Dreams.* Many dreams, quite unusual, with thoughts about many events (crude),[1].—Dreams very vivid, most from late events or last readings,[5].—Vivid dreams every night, that seem like actual events. Mostly of journeys in regions where he has been (eleventh day),[6].—Dreams of occurrences of the day before (sixth day),[6].—Dreams of objects about which he had read the evening before (eighth day),[6].—Dreams at night of meeting old friends, and of journeys (seventh day),[6].—Dreams of travelling (Schreter, Behlert, Cate),[5].—Sleep, with many dreams of dangers, though without fear (from the 2d),[1].—Dreams of fire, though without many flames (from the 2d),[1].

Fever.—Chilliness. [620.] Shivering, with a hot face, with bellyache,[5].—*Frequent creeping shiverings*, with motion of the scrotum not like that after urinating (crude),[1].—Ears cold ; point of nose cold,[5].—Frequent crawls all over ; crawls on the head,[5].—Chill in the morning after dressing, with cough and coryza,[5].—Chill, with uterine pains,[5].—Outdoors, a shaking chill,[5].—When going in the cold she feels chilly,[5].—Especially chilly when going into the cold air (from the 2d),[1].—Cool feeling toward eyes ; behind eyes,[5].—[630.] Cold in lower part ; face hot,[5].—*Heat.* Gets hot, with other complaints,[5].—The warm room is oppressive (from the 2d),[1].—Heat runs from the head down to the toes,[5].—Dry heat in the evening ; hot breath, beating of heart ; mouth and tongue dry, without thirst ; gaping, stretching, etc.,[5].—Heat in face, in the evening,[5].—Heat in face, with the chill, or with other complaints,[5].—*Sweat.* Copious night-sweats ; *on single parts*, towards aud in the morning,[5].—*Sweat on parts, wakens in the night,*[5].—Cold sweat on the face ; body cold,[5].—[640.] Dry skin, moist on hands,[5].—Palms of hands sweating,[5].

Conditions.—Aggravation.—(*Sunny half of day*), 6 A.M. to 6 P.M., cough.—(*Morning*), Pain in head ; pain in heart ; pain in back ; bad taste ; on waking, headache ; after waking, pain in left eye ; tongue white, etc.; bitter taste ; offensive taste, etc.; when waking, insipid, etc., taste, etc.; on waking, sore throat ; gagging, etc.; when getting up, aching in anus ; after waking, pappy stool ; *aching in uterus ;* when rising, difficult breathing ; contraction of chest ; getting awake, drawing in back, etc.; after waking, extremities have gone to sleep ; pain in calf ; in bed, stiffness ; inflammation of eye.—(*Forenoon*), Belching, etc.; pain in region of navel ; drawing in nape of neck.—(*Noon*), Diminished appetite.—(*Afternoon*), Headache ; nose-bleed ; 4 P.M., hunger ; pains in little finger ; when walking, pain in knees.—(*Towards evening*), When urinating, urethra expands etc.,—(*Evening*), Most complaints ; after going to bed, sore throat, etc.; pains in throat ; stitches in rectum ; in bed, itching, etc., in rectum ; stitching in anus ; especially when walking, pain in anus ; while in bed, frequent urinating ; painful erection, etc.; *voice husky,* etc.; difficult breathing ; drawing in back, etc.; when writing, pain in right fingers ; dry heat ; heat in face.—(*Night*), Dryness in throat ; boring in knee ; towards and in morning, sweat on single parts.—(*Towards morning*), Desire for coitus.—(*Fresh air*), Pain in carious teeth ; (*Open air*), Headache ; eyes worse ; nose stopped.—(*On exposure to slight draught of air*), Pains in nape of neck, etc.—(*When walking in open air*), Vertigo, etc.—(*After belching*), Burning in epigastrium.—(*Bending knee*), Pain beneath hollow of knee.—(*After nose-bleed*), Aching in vagina.—(*When blowing nose*), Pain in kidneys.—(*After breakfast*), Hawking, etc.—(*Deep breathing*), Shooting in chest ; pain in region of sixth rib ; stitches in region of liver.—(*Writing by candlelight*), Especially reckoning, affects eyes very much.—(*After cider*), Diarrhœa.—(*After coffee*), Nausea, etc.—(*After coition*), Weakness in feet.—(*Cold air*), Chilliness.—(*After cold bath*), Becomes red, etc.—(*After drinking cold water*), Pain in abdomen renewed ; cutting in belly.—(*After taking cold*), Liable to rheumatic pains ; pains in joints, etc.; much worse.—(*In cool room*), Nose runs.—(*In damp, cold weather*), Pain in lower limbs.—(*After dinner*), Heartburn ; pain in stomach, etc.—(*After every attempt to eat*), Bellyache.—(*Great exertion*), Headache.—(*After eating fruit*), Griping in abdomen, etc.—(*Eating juicy fruit*), Diarrhœa.—(*When getting up*), Vertigo.—(*When hawking*), Disgusting taste.—(*After honey*), Cutting in abdomen.—(*After ice cream*), Vomiting, etc.—(*On inspiration*), Shooting in breast, etc.; pain in region of heart.—(*When lifting*), Pain in region of kidneys.—(*Lifting up child from cradle*), Suffocative fits.—(*Lying*), Some complain more ; pains after great exertion.—(*Lying on back*), Aggra-

vates; convulsive starts.—(*After meals*), More after dinner, headache, etc.—
(*Before menses*), Griping, etc., in bowels, etc.; sexual desires, etc.; nymphomania.—(*At setting in of menses*), Bitter taste.—(*During menses*), Vertigo,
etc.—(*Between menstrual periods*), Whites.—(*Motion*), Headache; nausea;
drawing in back, etc.; pain in wrist, etc.—(*During pregnancy*), Weariness
in all limbs.—(*Pressure*), Pains in head, etc.—(*While riding in a carriage*),
Erections.—(*Riding on horseback*), Complaints in eyes, back, and thighs.—
(*When rising from sitting*), Vertigo; old people stagger; headache; buttocks feel as if gone to sleep; drawing in popliteal space.—(*On sitting*),
Some complain more; pains in glans penis.—(*Sitting up after lying down*),
Headache.—(*When stepping down*), Stitches in metatarsal bones.—(*Stooping*), Vertigo, etc.; headache.—(*After storm*), Pains in buttocks.—(*Stretching*) Boring in knee; tendons sore.—(*After supper*), Pressure in rectum,
etc.—(*When swallowing*), Pain in tongue, etc.—(*If others talk about it*), Sensation in eye renewed.—(*Taking boots off*), Pain below hollow of knee.—
(*Thinking about it*), Complaints in general.—(*Tobacco smoking*), Nausea.—
(*While urinating*), Drawing in bladder; burning in urethra.—(*After urinating*), Aching in bladder; cutting, etc., in urethra; pressing, etc., in
bladder; relaxation, etc., of the organs; erection of clitoris.—(*After vexation*), Depressed, etc.; diarrhœa.—(*While walking*), Vertigo, etc.; pains on
inside of thigh; pains in knees; knees sore; cramp in calves.—(*In warm
room*), Sensation of dryness in throat; burning-itching of outer ear.—
(*Change of weather*), Particularly when the snow melts, with east winds,
symptoms in general; headache.—(*After getting wet in rain*), Pain in
shoulders, etc.—(*In windy weather*), Drawing in nape of neck; vertigo.—
(*Yawning*), Pain in tonsil.

Amelioration.—(*After leucorrhœa*), Bellyache.—(*After lying down*),
Better; headache; pain in stomach; pain in belly; oppressed breathing;
contraction of chest, etc.—(*Lying still*), Headache.—(*Lying on belly*),
During restless night, better.—(*Lying on side*), Easier.—(*After motion*),
Aching in back, etc.—(*After quick motion*), Throbbing headache.—(*After
passing wind*), Bellyache.—(*While scratching head*), Headache.—(*After
stool*), Bellyache.—(*After stooping*), Headache.—(*After supper*), Headache.
—(*Tobacco smoking*), Headache.—(*Walking*), Some complain less.—(*Continued walking*), Pain in popliteal space.

CALCAREA SULPHURICA.

Calcium sulphate, CaSO$_4$.
Preparation, Triturations.
Authority. Dr. Clarence Conant, Trans. Am. Inst. of Hom., 1873. 1,
proving with the 30th; 2, proving with the 200th.

Mind.—Emotional. Good spirits, but inclined to solitude (twenty-
first day),[2].—Special good nature, late in afternoon (first day),[1].— Excessive
gayety of spirits, in the afternoon (twenty-seventh day),[1].—Good spirits;
best about 6 P.M. (ninth and thirteenth day),[2].—Hilarious good humor
always after taking drug, with eructations and sour taste (second day),[1].—
Great depression of spirits (forty-eighth day),[1].—Excessive, bitter melancholy, with distressing apprehensions of evil to loved ones (forty-ninth day),[1].
—Inclined to brooding, gloomy melancholy; easily aroused to take part in
conversation, etc., but never cheerful (fourteenth day),[2].—General low-
spiritedness, especially in the afternoon and evening (twentieth day),[1].—

[10.] Excessive grieved melancholy, in afternoon and evening (forty-seventh day),[2].—Rather gloomy and moody in evening, and very weary (fiftieth day),[2].—Excessive melancholy all day, but easily diverted (twelfth day),[2].—Very low-spirited in early evening, then more cheerful, then "blue" again (fifty-sixth day),[2].—Very irritable late in afternoon, less so in evening (twenty-fourth day),[2].—Quarrelsome (fourth day),[2].—*Intellectual.* Good spirits, but a dazed state of mind in evening (twentieth day),[2].—Suddenly, after lunch, lose all memory and power of thought, can scarcely remember what I was going to do; old issues, which have been long decided, are presented to mind, and I can't recall my decision (forty-seventh day),[2].

Head.—Spasmodic throbbing headache, mostly in right frontal region, in morning (twenty-third day),[2].—Headache and inflammation of eyes (thirty-fourth day),[1].—*Forehead.* [20.] Frontal headache (sixth day),[2].—Frontal headache, in morning and evening (thirty-second day),[2].—Frontal headache in the afternoon, worse on right side (third day),[2].—Worse after afternoon nap, having frontal headache and some influenza (fourth day),[2].—Slight frontal headache (twenty-fifth and twenty-sixth days, etc.),[1].—Slight frontal headache, passing to temporal region in evening (thirty-first day),[1].—Slight frontal headache, with some fever but no sweat (thirtieth day),[1].—Severe frontal headache (ninth day),[2].—Severe frontal headache, worse in the forenoon (thirty-fifth day),[1].—Severe frontal headache in evening (twenty-fifth day),[2].—[30.] Severe frontal headache after dinner (thirteenth day),[2].—Severe frontal headache, worse after dinner and in evening (fifty-fifth day),[2].—*Vertex.* Darting pain in vertex in the afternoon, after dinner (forty-third day),[1].—Neuralgic pains in left side of head and forehead, an hour after tea; soon passed (tenth day),[1].—*External Head.* Hard, tender swellings on scalp, in edge of hair (thirty-second day),[1].—Pimples appear on scalp (seventh day),[1].—Pimples on scalp disappear and leave a yellow scab (eleventh day),[1].

Eye.—Inflammation of eyes, most about 6, and less at 10 P.M. (second day),[1].—Inflammation of eyes at night (seventeenth and eighteenth day),[1].—Slight inflammation of the eyes (thirty-second and thirty-fourth day),[1].—[40.] Slight inflammation of the eyes, in the forenoon (fifth day),[1].—Considerable inflammation of the eyes (thirty fifth day),[2].—Severe inflammation of the eyes, worse in the corners of the eyes and in evening (forty-eighth day),[1].—Eyes smart in afternoon and in evening (thirty-eighth day),[2].—Eyelids smart, especially in inner corners, and in morning (forty-sixth day),[2].—Conjunctivæ of eyes yellow (eighteenth day),[2].—Pressing pain in left eyeball (second day),[1].—Cutting pain in left eyeball, with some soreness; in the evening (third day),[1].—*Vision.* Sees only half an object late in evening (forty-ninth day),[2].

Ear.—Takes dark-brown wax from right ear in morning (ninth and fourteenth day),[2].—[50.] Wipes blood from concha of left ear, in morning after usual bath (twenty-fourth and twenty-eighth day),[1].—Earache in the left ear in the morning, relieved by taking a lump of dark-brown wax from ear (forty-fourth day),[1].

Nose.—Pinched appearance about the nose in the morning (second day),[2].—Tendency to influenza and sneezing, disappearing in the open air (first day),[1].—Slight influenza, usually in the morning,[1].—Slight influenza in the evening (third day),[2].—Very little expectoration but considerable influenza, disappearing in open air, and worse in the right nostril (twenty-eighth day),[2].—Considerable coryza, especially in evening (forty-ninth and fiftieth day),[2].—Watery coryza from anterior nares; posterior nares closed tight (twenty-third day),[2].—Watery coryza in open air, slightly excoriating (forty-second day),[2].—[60.] Excoriating coryza in open air, soon disappearing in the house and after washing face in cold water (forty-sixth and forty-seventh day),[2].—Dry coryza, left nostril, in the forenoon; right nostril discharges white watery mucus in small quantities; at night this reversed, left nostril discharges, and right nostril is dry (twenty-eighth day),[1].—Always blow yellowish or greenish mucus from nose in morning after bath (forty-sixth day),[2].—Blow streaked mucus from nose in morning after bath (fifty-sixth and fifty-seventh days),[2].—Very little blood-streaked mucus from left nostril after bath (thirty-ninth and fortieth day),[2].—Right nostril stopped (mostly posteriorly), day and evening (twenty-second day),[2].—Right and left nostrils alternately open and stopped with transparent w tery sticky mucus (twenty-ninth, thirtieth, thirty-first, and thirty-second days),[1].—Edges of nostrils slightly sore, as if excoriated (fifty-seventh day),[2].

Face.—Faceache all night on right side (forty-seventh day),[2].—Vague pains in right side of face and right upper back decayed molar, which is somewhat tender (thirty-fifth day),[2].—[70.] Neuralgic pains in right upper jaw, proceeding from a decayed molar tooth; inside of gum swollen and sore; great aggravation by gently stroking the gum (eleventh day),[1].—Darting, neuralgic pains in right side of face (sixteenth day),[2].—Tooth seems to cause neuralgic faceache in both jaws of right side, mostly in evening (forty-ninth day),[2].

Mouth.—Teeth and Gums. Toothache just after dark (fifty-fifth day),[2].—Tooth aches at night in sleep (fifty-third day),[2].—Toothache immediately aggravated by cold water, but at last relieved by it (fifty-second day),[2].—Right upper back teeth decayed. Molar very sensitive to cold air, water, etc., and tender (seventeenth and twenty-fourth day),[2].—Gums bleed easily while brushing them (fifty-fifth day),[2].—*Tongue.* Tongue yellow-coated at base (twenty-second day),[1].—Tongue seamed with a deep red line in its centre, antero-posteriorly (twenty-seventh day),[1].—[80.] Slightly puckered sensation at base of tongue (third day),[1].—*General Mouth.* Soreness of left side of roof of mouth at dinner, as if burned; better at tea (sixth day),[2].—*Taste.* Slightly soapy taste in mouth (second day),[1].—Sour, bitter taste (third day),[1].—Sour, acid taste always after taking drug (third day),[1].

Throat.—Throat red and sore internally (twenty-second day),[1].—Throat longitudinally inflamed in strips, like ulceration (twenty-seventh day),[1].—Profuse expectoration of yellowish mucus from throat and right posterior nares (twenty-seventh day); scanty (twenty-eighth day),[1].—Expectoration from posterior nares (fifteenth, sixteenth, seventeenth, and eighteenth days),[2].—Pharynx very red and sore (twentieth day),[2].

Stomach.—Appetite and Thirst. [90.] Ravenous appetite (twenty-ninth, thirtieth, and thirty-first days),[1].—Ravenous appetite (second day),[2].—Excessive appetite and thirst, and soreness of mouth externally (second day),[1].—Hunger decreases; marked desire for green, acid fruits and vegetables (fifth day),[1].—Hunger less, but marked desire for fruit as before (sixth day),[1].—No appetite for meat (twenty-third day),[1].—Marked thirst in the forenoon (twentieth day),[1].—Great desire for tea and claret, the latter unusual at night (first day),[1].—*Eructations.* Bitter eructations in the morning after bath (fiftieth day),[1].—Sour, bitter eructations at night (twelfth day),[1].—*Nausea.* [100.] Slight nausea (second and third days),[1].—Slight nausea in the evening after taking the drug (second day),[2].—Increased nausea and slight colic about noon (second day),[1]. —Increased nausea, as from tobacco, and painful consciousness of œsophagus from mouth to stomach (second day),[1].—*Stomach.* Indigestion during breakfast relieved by hot cocoa (thirty-third day),[1].—Indigestion after breakfast (seventeenth and thirty-first days),[1].—Indigestion twenty minutes after breakfast (tenth day),[1].—Indigestion in morning after breakfast, followed by pressure on bowels, as if to diarrhœic stool (thirty-fifth day),[2].—Indigestion after breakfast and forty minutes ride in city cars, followed by diarrhœic stool, with great tenesmus and pain in abdomen, leaving a hot feeling of anus and bowels (twenty-first day),[2].—Indigestion after dinner and breakfast (thirty-fourth day),[1].—[110.] Indigestion an hour after tea (tenth day),[1].—Slight indigestion after dinner, at 2.30 P.M. (sixteenth day),[1].—Severe indigestion after breakfast (thirty-second and thirty-eighth days),[1].—Severe indigestion after breakfast (ninth and twelfth days),[2].—Severe indigestion soon after breakfast (fourteenth day),[1].—Sensation of weight in stomach and chest in the morning, relieved by dinner (forty-seventh day),[1].—Pain and soreness at stomach (third day),[1].—Dull vague pains and external soreness in stomach at night, about 10 P.M. (twenty-ninth day),[1].—Wandering pains in stomach and abdomen (second day),[1].—Vague cramps in the stomach in the afternoon (second day),[2].— [120.] Colic in epigastrium in afternoon (twenty-fourth day),[2].—Severe colic in stomach in evening, relieved (*pro tem.*) by drinking cold water, with a sensation of constriction in stomach, followed by stool, with some colic; after stool much flatulence and eructations (forty-ninth day),[2].— Colic in stomach after breakfast (second day),[1].—Stomach externally sore (thirty-second day),[1].

Abdomen.—Hypochondria. Pain in the left hypochondrium in afternoon, followed by dull pain or cramp in stomach (eighth day),[2].— Cramps in hypochondria from about 10 A.M., all day, disappearing late in the evening (second day),[2].—Cramps in hypochondria late in evening (thirteenth and fourteenth days),[2].—Cramps or colic in hypochondria, at night after retiring (fourth day),[2].—Cramps in hypochondria, with great restlessness after retiring at night (fourth and fifth days),[2].—*General Abdomen.* Considerable putrid-smelling flatus (fourth day),[2].—[130.] A single burst of putrid flatus in the afternoon, an hour after dinner (nineteenth day),[1].—Flatulence in afternoon (twelfth day),[1].—Flatulence two and a half hours after tea (tenth day),[1].—Flatulence and eructations after bath (forty-seventh day),[1].—Severe attack of incarcerated flatus after dinner, distending abdomen, and causing colic; somewhat relieved by walking and singing; distension and consequent discomfort continued during afternoon and evening (thirty-eighth day),[1].—Cramps in abdomen and flatulence at night (twenty-first day),[2].—Colic in the morning on rising (sixth day),[2].— Colic in abdomen on rising (forty-seventh and forty-eighth days),[1].—Colic in abdomen in morning after bath (ninth day),[2].—Colic in abdomen and aching weakness in back while riding; soon passed; same later also in afternoon (seventh day),[2].—[140.] Colic after ice water; soon passed; *very* unusual (tenth day),[1].—Sharp colic in abdomen on rising (twenty-fifth day),[1].—Darting colic in abdomen, late at night before retiring (nineteenth and twentieth days),[1].—Pressure on bowels, as if to stool (second day),[1].— Pressure on bowels, as if to stool, and constriction of the anus after breakfast (seventh day),[2].—*Hypogastrium.* Voluptuous burning-aching sensation in the exterior pubic arch, late in afternoon (eighth day),[2].—Pain . in right side of pelvis, followed by weariness, nausea, and pain in the stomach (fifth day),[1].—Colic in lower part of abdomen, in morning, after bath (seventh day),[2].

Rectum and Anus.—Sensation of constriction at anus (twenty-second day),[2].

Stool.—Diarrhœa. Stool in the morning, with excoriating sensation in the anus (forty-fourth day),[1].—[150.] Stool in morning, leaving slight soreness in the anus (fifty-first day),[2].—Stool in afternoon, with great tenesmus (seventeenth day),[2].—Stool in the afternoon, in one short thick piece, with great tenesmus (forty-sixth day),[1].—Stool in afternoon, preceded by pain in left side of chest and abdomen (sixth day),[2].—Stool in the afternoon, with slight colic in abdomen (forty-first and forty-second days),[1].—Stool in afternoon before dinner, leaving a sensation as of more egesta to be evacuated ; a second stool in evening before tea, leaving soreness of anus (sixtieth day),[2].—Stool in afternoon, preceded by single brief spasm of sharp cutting colic in abdomen, with excoriating, burning, and stinging sensation at anus during stool, and soreness of same after stool (twenty-seventh day),[2].—Stool at 3.50 P.M., with cutting pain in abdomen (second day),[1].—Stool in evening ; sphincter feels lame ; strained soreness (fifty-seventh day),[2].—Stool in evening, preceded by a single spasm of cutting colic in the stomach, with tenesmus (twenty-eighth day),[2].—[160.] Stool in evening, with excoriating sensation in anus, and shooting colic in left inguinal region (eighteenth day),[2].—Stool at night, followed by soreness and dull pain at the pit of the stomach (twentieth day),[1].—Stool at night, large, hard pieces ; tenesmus at close of stool ; convulsive shuddering during passage, which leaves smarting-burning in the anus (seventeenth day),[1].—Loose, pappy, light-brown, painless stool in morning (thirty-fourth day),[2].—Loose, lumpy, blackish-brown stool in the forenoon, leaving sore feeling in stomach and abdomen (thirty-second day),[1].—Rather loose stool in the afternoon (forty-eighth and forty-ninth days),[1].—Rather loose dark stool in the afternoon (second day),[2].—Loose stool in evening, with sharp cutting colic in lower part of abdomen ; two spasms of this colic (forty-fourth day),[2].—Loose stool at night (thirty-ninth day),[1].—Profuse light-colored stool in the morning on rising, with tenesmus and excoriating sensation in anus, preceded by cutting colic in the epigastrium (twenty-fourth day),[2].—[170.] Profuse stool in the forenoon ; large pieces, and the latter part loose and blackish ; looseness of bowels during stool, and of stomach all day (thirtieth day),[1].—Stool at 11.40, scanty, of light color, with pain at stomach, followed by soreness of anus (third day),[1].—Scanty, hard, dark stool in evening (a single large piece), (twelfth day),[2].—Second stool at 10 P.M., scanty, loose, black, and undigested, preceded by pricking colic in the abdomen (sixth day),[1].—Small, slowly passed stool, with slight tenesmus (thirty-second day),[2].—Small stool (a single piece), with darting colic in lower part of the abdomen, leaving constricted sensation and great soreness in anus (forty-second day),[2].—Small stool in morning, with excoriating sensation (tenth day),[2].—Small, dark stool in the forenoon (fifth day),[2].—Small, dark stool in afternoon (eighth day),[2].—Small stool in afternoon, with marked tenesmus (seventh day),[2].—[180.] Small, hard stool in the afternoon, with cutting pain in the abdomen during stool (thirty-fourth day),[1].—Two stools, both small and undigested ; one in the forenoon and one about 1.50 P.M. (twenty-eighth day),[1].—Small, easy stool in evening (thirtieth and thirty-first days),[2].—Very small, hard, but painless stool at night (forty-first day),[2].—Stool at 10.30 P.M., small, with smarting anus and darting pains in rectum, and sensation as if something was retained in it (first day),[1].—Hard stool, passed with great urging in the rectum, and excoriating sensation at the anus, preceded by sharp pains in the rectum (fortieth day),[2].—Hard, small, dark stool in the forenoon, with tenesmus (fourth day),[2].—Stool in forenoon hard, dark-brown, with burning in, during, and after stool (thirty-sixth day),[1].—Hard, dark stool in the forenoon, leaving smarting in ano, and sensation in rectum of more egesta to be expelled (thirty-eighth day),[1].—Hard stool at night; large pieces, leaving sensation in the rectum of more egesta to be expelled, and slight burning in the anus (nineteenth day),[1].—[190.] Stool at night, hard, of great bulk and large pieces, passed with great pain, leaving smarting of the anus (fourteenth day),[1].—All stools dry and hard (forty-second day),[2].—Pappy, excoriating stool late in evening (thirty-seventh day),[2].—Stool half normal (except being light color), and second half loose and nearly black, in the forenoon (sixth day),[1].—Stool very light color, followed by vague darting pains in region of external pubic arch, at 11 A.M. (twenty-fourth day),[1].—Dark, profuse, painless stool in evening, with tenesmus (fourteenth day),[2].—Stool at night, very light-colored (twenty-second day),[1].—*Constipation.* No stool (fifth, seventh, eleventh, etc., etc., days),[1].—No stool (first, third, eleventh, fifteenth, etc., etc., days),[2].

Urinary Organs.—Urine lighter in color and *not* offensive in smell (second day),[1].—Urine very pale, and micturition slightly painful (eighth day),[1].—[200.] Retained or suppressed urine, from 6 P.M. yesterday till 2 P.M.; no pain or unpleasant sensation; urine when voided (about a teacupful), of a very pale color,[2].

Sexual Organs.—Uneasy feeling of genital organs (second day),[1].—Bruised pain in testes late in afternoon, as if they had been crushed or injured (fifth day),[2].—Drawing sensation in spermatic cord and left testicle in the morning; the same again from 5 to 6 P.M., with almost irresistible amorous fancies and desires, both pure and impure (forty-fifth day),[1].

Respiratory Organs.—*Larynx.* Sensation of dust in larynx, about 11.30 A.M., with soreness increasing all day and evening (twenty-first day),[1].—*Voice.* Hoarseness (twenty-third and twenty-fourth days, etc.),[1].—Hoarseness increased (twenty-sixth day),[1].—Slightly hoarse in evening (eighth day),[2].—Marked hoarseness towards night and in evening (thirty-first day),[1].—Hoarseness, less in open air and in evening (twenty-third day),[2].—[210.] Hoarseness, with sore tight cough in evening (twenty-first day),[1].—*Cough and Expectoration.* Cough once or twice on rising (thirtieth and thirty-first days),[1].—Two or three coughs in the morning before bath, on rising (thirty-fifth day),[1].—Cough in the morning after bath (thirty-second day),[1].—Cough three or four times after bath, in the afternoon (thirty-third day),[1].—Cough, leaving strained sensation in lungs and slightly rasped feeling in throat; seems to arise from itching of throat (twenty-third day),[1].—Light, rare cough (twenty-first day),[2].—Tight, short, rasping cough, leaving a strained sensation in head and chest (twenty-fourth day); same, but less frequent (twenty-fifth and twenty-sixth days),[1].—Sharp, short, dry cough (twenty-second day),[1].—Expectoration in the morning on rising (thirty-sixth day),[1].—[220.] Expectoration in the morning after bath (fifth day),[2].—Expectoration most in evening, when left nostril is stopped (fourteenth day),[2].—Expectoration and influenza only in the house; relieved in cold or open air (thirtieth day),[2].—Expectoration in open air, influenza in house (thirty-first day),[2].—Expectoration of mucus; discharge from left nostril is yellow, as it is *at times* also from the throat (twenty-sixth day),[1].—Expectoration and influenza *not* markedly better in open air (twenty-ninth day),[2].—Expectoration and influenza only notice-able in the forenoon for about two hours after rising, and a little in evening (thirty-seventh day),[1].—Some lumpy white expectoration in evening with the coryza (fiftieth day),[2].—Some expectoration and coryza; posterior nares not so tightly closed; coryza yellowish or greenish (twenty-fourth day),[2].— Very scanty expectoration, mostly in morning after bath (eighth day),[2].— [230.] Scanty expectoration, mostly in evening (forty-ninth day),[1].—Scanty expectoration from posterior nares in the morning, with a few tight coughs (third day),[2].—Scanty expectoration of mucus, transparent early in the day, yellowish from about 12 to 3 P.M.; transparent again towards night, from throat and nares; thin transparent mucous discharge from left nostril, and slight lachrymation of left eye (twenty-fifth day),[1].—Scanty expec-toration of white mucus from the throat (forty-eighth day),[1].—Slight ex-pectoration of transparent stringy mucus, in the forenoon (nineteenth day),[1].—A *little* greenish-yellow expectoration (thirty-eighth day),[2].—Fre-quent expectoration of small quantities of transparent mucus (twenty-first day),[1].—Profuse slimy expectoration (thirty-second day),[1].—Profuse ex-pectoration of transparent, tasteless, slightly viscid mucus all day; less after nightfall (sixth day),[1].—Profuse expectoration of transparent sticky mucus from throat and posterior nares (twenty-ninth day), scanty (thirtieth and thirty-first days),[1].—[240.] Profuse expectoration of yellowish, slightly viscid mucus from throat and posterior nares (twenty-fourth day),[1].—Pro-fuse yellowish expectoration from posterior nares, and influenza in house (thirty-second and thirty-seventh days),[2].—Profuse expectoration and eruc-tations in morning (ninth day),[2].—Mucus detached from throat and pos-terior nares with great difficulty (thirty-third day),[1].—*Respiration.* Strong desire to be in the open air, and feels better there (sixth day),[1].— Desire for night air, but weariness while in it, in the evening (fifth day),[1].

Chest.—Oppression and rawness of chest (twenty-third day),[2].—Pain in apex of left lung (second day),[1].—Dull, throbbing pain in apex of left lung (first day),[1].—Chest lame and raw behind sternum, with nausea in forenoon, reaching a climax about 1.30 P.M. in a small, close, crowded room, witnessing an operation, then deadly nausea and vertigo; could hardly get into the street, where in about fifteen minutes felt much better (twentieth day),[2].—[250.] Severe, dull, superficial pain or weight in the left side of the chest at the lower end of the gladiolus (fortieth day),[2].

Neck and Back.—Painful rigidity of right side of neck in the after-noon; the same in back of neck later (third day),[2].—Rheumatic pain in left side of neck (forty-seventh day),[1].—Vague rheumatic pains in right scapular region in afternoon (thirty-fourth day),[2].—Backache (in dorsal region), in afternoon, and in evening after retiring, causing great discom-fort and restlessness (twelfth day),[2].—Weakness of back, stiffness of hands, and puffiness of the fingers, in the forenoon; joint of second finger, left hand (between second and third row of phalanges), swollen, and very sen-sitive to lateral pressure (fifth day),[2].—Weakness of middle of back (second day),[1].—Small of back weak; only noticed when lying on back, but great disposition to lie down and stretch out (second day),[2].

Extremities in General.—Some rigidity in legs, shoulders, arms, and hands, and in feet in evening, especially in right foot (twelfth day),[2].

Superior Extremities.—Growing painful rigidity of arms, shoul-ders, and back, from forenoon till late in afternoon, not noticeable in even-ing (fifth day),[2].—*Shoulder.* [260.] Shoulders stiff in morning (tenth day),[2].—Shoulders, back (over scapulæ), and forearms very stiff; can't move them without great discomfort, almost pain, worse in morning, better walking (forty-second day),[1].—Painful rigidity of muscles of shoulder and back; noticed when putting on or off a coat (thirty-seventh day),[1].—Shoulders and arms rigid and painful to touch; it is painful to put off or on a coat; worse in the morning and evening, better in open air and walking; darting pain from elbow to wrist, diagonally across the arm (forty-first day),[1].—Neuralgic pains in shoulder, extending to wrist and back of hand (third day),[1].—Sharp darting pain in left shoulder about 6.45 P.M. (first day),[2].—*Wrist.*—Sharp pain in ulna at wrist several times during evening (first day),[2].—*Hand.* Backs of hands inflamed, as if sunburned (sixth day),[1].—Numbness of hands, with sticky sensation (first day),[1].—Hands somewhat rigid in afternoon, especially right hand (twenty-first day),[2].—[270.] Rigidity in both hands, disappearing in afternoon (thirty-ninth day),[1].—Distressing uneasiness (*barely pains*) in hands (twenty-second day),[2].—Pain in hands late in evening (eleventh day),[2].—Painful cramps in right hand, and stiffness and numbness of little finger in afternoon (twenty-third day),[2].—Darting pains in hands when holding anything (fifteenth day),[2].—Vague shooting pains in hands; worse towards night (seventeenth and eighteenth days),[2].—*Fingers.* Fingers puffy and stiff in the morning (forty-seventh day),[1].—Right little finger numb and stiff for awhile in the morning (thirty-third day),[2].—Fingers very stiff and rigid; dreamed of trying to catch and hold an eel, and was unable, because of stiffness of fingers (thirty-ninth day),[1].—Middle finger of left hand stiff and puffy in afternoon; some pain in metacarpal bone and phalanx of the same finger (fifty-second day),[2].—[280.] Painful rigidity of thumb of left hand, and puffiness of fingers in the afternoon; mainly fingers of right hand (third day),[2].—Pain in right thumb and wrist late in the afternoon (forty-seventh day),[1].—Sharp pain (a half hour or so) in right thumb, extending to wrist (forty-sixth day),[1].—Exquisite soreness of left forefinger under nail (twelfth day),[1].—Bruised right thumb under nail; applied Arnica tincture; pain and lameness from thumb to elbow (nineteenth day),[1].

Inferior Extremities.—Thigh. Painful rigidity of thighs in morning; worse in afternoon, and worst early in evening (fourteenth day),[2].—*Knee.* Weariness of knees, after walking, usually felt in calves of legs (second day),[1].—When at bath, in morning, lameness of inner side of left knee (forty-seventh to fifty-first day),[2].—Inner posterior part of left knee very lame, when stooping or walking fast (fifty-seventh day),[2].—*Leg.* Legs somewhat stiff (fifteenth day),[2].—[290.] Legs stiff, and fingers puffy and stiff, in morning (nineteenth day),[2].—*Foot.* Feet slightly swollen and tender (thirty-first day),[1].—Vague pains in left foot, as if rheumatism would set in (twenty-eighth day),[2].—Feet very tender (thirty-fifth day),[2].—Ball of left foot, opposite fourth toe, suddenly becomes tender while walking, and continues so all day (twenty-seventh day),[2].—*Toes.* Pain in fourth toe, right foot, as if asleep, while lying down, with sweat (first day),[1].

General Symptoms.—Objective. Lazy (eighth day),[2].—General languor; feel absolutely indefinitely unwell all over (forty-fifth day),[2].—General lassitude (twenty-second day),[2].—General lassitude from about 2 P.M. (first day),[2].—[300.] General lassitude till towards evening, when livelier (second day),[2].—Extreme lassitude, feeling as if going to be sick, with slight fever, no perspiration, in the evening (sixth day),[1].—Very weary and stupid all day; could easily fall asleep, although not in want of rest (thirtieth day),[1].—Weakness in left side (second day),[1].—

Restless and weary (forty-eighth day),[2].—Great restlessness and sadness, in evening (eleventh day),[2].—Very restless and unhappy; melancholy easily diverted, but instantly relapses; worse in evening, better about noon (sixteenth day),[2].—Great restlessness in afternoon and evening, with sadness, dislike to talk; petulant; desire to weep and to be miserable, alone, and unhappy; moderately cheerful in morning; change not sudden, but between 2 and 3 P.M. (seventh day),[2].—*Sensations.* Excessive weariness and sleepiness between 10 and 12 A.M. (fifteenth day),[1].—Poorly in the morning, and lively in the evening (third day),[2].—[310.] Stiff and weary all over, especially in the posterior part of the left knee (fifty-fifth day),[2].—General painful rigidity, especially in legs, in morning; hands and shoulders involved in afternoon, especially the right hand (eleventh day),[2].

Skin.—Eruptions, Dry. Pimple appears on top of right ear (twelfth day),[1].—Hard swollen pimple on left cheek (ninth day),[2].—Many little matterless pimples under beard and hair, which discharge blood when scratched (thirty-seventh day),[1].—Pimple on right arm is inflamed, hard, and sensitive, deep into flesh; has a small black depressed head, which may be forced to the surface by gentle pressure; feels like a vaccine pustule (to prover), and appears as if about to exude matter when gently pressed (third day),[2].—Itching eruption on back between scapulæ, on breast about sternum, and somewhat on face (second day),[1].—*Moist.* Three small, yellow, blister-like sores, which burn and smart when touched, on right side of lower lip (twenty-first day),[1].—*Pustular.* Pimples under beard discharge an oily transparent matter (thirty-eighth day),[1].—Pimples and lip-sore have dry yellow scab, and itch (forty-fourth day),[1].—[320.] A small boil, just over left eye, and a second small boil on forehead, far above left eye, nearly in hair (forty-first day),[2].—Sore on lip tender, and gives rise to a binding-drawing sensation on lip, extending obliquely downward towards the right 'corner of the chin (twenty-sixth day),[1].—Sore on inside left corner of mouth, and one inside upper lip, just to right of centre; better towards night (thirty-first day),[1].—Sore on lips better, but ulcer-like (twenty-third day),[1].—Sore on lip tender, and discharges bloody matter (twenty-fourth day),[1].—*Sensations.* Pimples itch (forty-eighth day),[1].—Itching of back, between the scapulæ (second day),[1].—Burning-itching in top of wing of left ear (third day),[1].

Sleep and Dreams.—Sleepiness in afternoon, and nap from 6.30 to 7.40 P.M. (first day),[1].—Nap about 4 P.M., with sweat (first day),[2].—[330.] Took nap, and awoke perfectly miserable; feel weak and languid; no pluck, but suffer an intolerable lassitude (seventh day),[2].—Wakefulness in evening (first day),[1].

Fever.—Chilliness. Very cold in the morning, before breakfast (thirty-ninth day),[1].—Suffered from cold while taking usual bath (twenty-fifth day),[1].—*Heat.* Throbbing of heat, as if about to burst into a sweat (first day),[1].—Pulsations or throbbings of heat, as if about to burst into a sweat, in the afternoon and evening (first day),[2].—Flushes or pulsations of heat during dinner; no sweat (fifth day),[2].—Great heat and sweat during afternoon and evening (ninth day),[2].—Slight fever, with cold sweat (fifth day),[1].—Slow fever and slight inflammation of the eyes (thirty-third day),[1].—[340.] Heat in forehead and eyes (no sweat), with painful consciousness of testes; soon passed (seventh day),[2].—Sensation of great heat in face and eyes, but parts are really cool; relieved in open air, for which I have great desire (twenty-second day),[2].—*Sweat.* Perspiration throughout the evening (first day),[1].—Increased sweat of hands (sixteenth day),[2].

Conditions.—Aggravation.—(*Morning*), Headache; frontal head-ache; eyes smart; after bath, mucus blown from nose; after bath, eructa-tions; sense of weight in stomach, etc.; after bath, colic, etc.; stiffness in shoulders; fingers puffy; at bath, lameness in knee; *cold.*—(*Forenoon*), Frontal headache; thirst.—(*Noon*), Nausea, etc.—(*Afternoon*), Melancholy; irritability; after lunch, loss of memory, etc.; frontal headache; heat, etc.—(*Evening*), Melancholy; dazed state of mind; frontal headache; late, sees only half au object; coryza; faceache; colic in stomach; hoarseness; rigidity of thigh; restless, etc.; heat, etc.; perspiration.—(*Night*), Inflammation of eyes; faceache.—(*Towards night*), Pains in hands.—(*Open air*), Coryza.—(*After breakfast*), Colic in stomach.—(*After dinner*), Incarcerated flatus.—(*After ice-water*), Colic.—(*Lying on back*), Weakness in small of back.—(*Noise*), Affects him very much.—(*Stooping*), Knee lame.—(*Stroking gum*), Pains in jaw.—(*After walking*), Weariness of knees.—(*Walking fast*), Knee lame.—(*After working and washing in water*), **Aggravation and renewal of the symptoms.**

Amelioration.—(*About noon*), Restless, etc.—(*Toward evening*), Lassitude.—(*Evening*), Irritability; in air, feels better.—(*Night*), Symp-toms in general.—(*Open air*), Symptoms in general; tendency to influenza, etc.; hoarseness; expectoration, etc.—(*After breakfast*), Better generally.—(*Hot cocoa*), Indigestion.—(*Cold air*), Expectoration, etc.—(*Drinking cold water*), Colic in stomach.—(*Washing face in cold water*), Coryza.—(*Dinner*), Sense of weight in stomach, etc.—(*After dinner*), Better generally.—(*Eat-ing*), Symptoms in general.—(*Singing*), Incarcerated flatus.—(*After tea*), Better generally.—(*Walking*), Incarcerated flatus; stiffness in shoulders.

CALENDULA.

Calendula officinalis, Linn. *Nat. order*, Compositæ. *Common name*, Marigold; German, Todtenblume. *Preparation*, Tincture of the leaves and flowers.

Authorities. 1, Franz, Archive für Hom. Heilk., 17, 3, 169; 2, Dr. Price, Am. Hom. Observer, 6, 327, effects of a tablespoonful of the tinc-ture.

Mind.—Disposition, during the chill, anxious, morose, and solicitous,[1].—Great irritability; he is easily frightened; hearing is very acute (after he had smelled of camphor),[1].—Fretful, sleepy, dreamy,[1].

Head.—Confusion of the head, as after a night's debauch; in the morning, heaviness of the head, as after a long illness (third day),[1].—Dull sensation, especially in the upper part of the occiput,[1].—Headache in the forehead, after eating, with sensation of heat in it,[1].—Dull, pressive sensa-tion in the occiput,[1].

Eye.—Lids very much swollen (after one hour),[2].—Dryness and biting in the margin of the lids, as from smoke,[1].—[10.] The white of the eye is inflamed, with pressive headache, now in the forehead, now in the temples, when lying down, not when sitting and standing,[1].—Pupils dilated (after one hour),[2].

Ear.—Sticking pain in the ears during the fever-heat; the adjacent parts are very red,[1].

Face.—Sensation of swelling extending from the lips to the eyes and forehead, accompanied by a burning-stinging sensation (after one hour),[2].—Sensation as if the lips were swollen; from the lips it spread to the sides of the nose; increased rapidly in intensity (immediately),[2].—Drawing-tensive pain in the glands before the left ramus of the lower jaw, on moving the head,[1].

Mouth.—Speech scarcely recognizable (after one hour),[2].

Throat.—Bitter taste of mucus in the throat, before eating; food, however, tastes natural,[1].—Pain in front beneath the chin, on motion and pressure; and at the union of the clavicle with the sternum (eighteenth day),[2].—Rheumatic drawing pain in the right side of the throat, which is increased on bending the neck to the right side, and on raising the right arm; it extends to the shoulder, in the morning (second day),[1].—[20.] The submaxillary glands are swollen and painful to the touch, as if suppurating; the axillary glands are also painful to touch (fourth day),[1].—The submaxillary glands pain on touch, as if swollen, and at times cause a tensive pain, which, especially on swallowing, becomes a pressure in the throat (afternoon, second day),[1].

Stomach.—Diminished appetite for dinner, though he relishes the food when he eats,[1].—Hiccough, after smoking,[1].—Attacks of nausea, at times, in the forenoon,[1].

Abdomen.—A boring-digging pain, deep in the region of the navel, when walking,[1].—Dull, coarse stitches in the middle of the right side of the abdomen, on moving; they disappear during rest,[1].

Stool.—A stool in the morning, preceded by griping and anxiety in the abdomen, and accompanied by a chill,[1].

Urinary Organs.—Tearings, at times in the urethra, during a chill,[1].—Frequent micturition; urine white as water, is very hot and burning,[1].

Respiratory Organs.—[30.] Very deep inspiration, with heat in the chest and face,[1].—Great efforts were made to inflate the lower lobes of the lungs, which were only successful when sitting up (after one hour),[2].

Chest.—Pressive-drawing pain in the left side of the chest, and on the breast-bone, with stitches in the right side of the chest (second day),[1].—Pressure and oppression in the left side of the chest, in the evening, when lying in bed,[1].—Drawing pressure in the left side of the chest, when standing, during inspiration,[1].

Heart and Pulse.—Pulse irregular and diminishing rapidly (after one hour),[2].

Neck and Back.—Pressive-drawing pain between the shoulder-blades,[1].—Pressive pain beneath the right lower tip of the shoulder-blade, with a sensation as if everything were suppurating and bruised (afternoon, second day),[1].

Extremities in General.—Drawing-pressive tension in the wrists and ankles, during rest,[1].

Inferior Extremities.—Tired, weary feeling in the lower extremities (after one hour),[2].—[40.] Pains in the knees, while sitting, in the outer side, as if bruised,[1].—Burning-tearing pain in the upper part of the calf, while sitting,[1].—Drawing-pinching pain on the inner border of the sole, while sitting,[1].

General Symptoms.—Very restless at night, he gets rest in no position; he continually wakes; is obliged to urinate frequently, and drinks very much,[1].—A wound becomes raw and inflamed anew,[1].—A wound is painful, in the morning, as if bruised, with smarting and throbbing in it, as if it would suppurate,[1].—The rheumatic, drawing pains appear only during motion, and are very slight,[1].

Skin.—Eruption of small vesicles, in the left corner of the lower lip,[1].

Fever.—Chilliness. Chilly the whole morning, and very sensitive to the air (second day),[1].—He feels shivery, and has a kind of goose-flesh, while the skin seems warm to touch,[1].—[50.] Shivering in the back, with pressure in the last true ribs of the left side, with movements in the epigastric region and abdomen as if he would faint,[1].—Hands and feet cold (after one hour),[2].—Chilliness in the hands and feet, the whole forenoon, without thirst, together with drawing, pressive, rheumatic pains through the whole body; the ribs ache as if squeezed together and bruised, sometimes after eating (in the morning, second day),[1].—*Heat.* Great heat, the whole forenoon, with much sweat; he feels qualmish in the chest, and the axillæ are very hot,[1].—Heat in the afternoon, with creeping chills and great thirst; drinking, however, causes every time shivering and a shaking chill,[1].—Great heat, in the evening, in bed,[1].—Great heat, in the evening, in bed; he begins to sweat; especially the feet burn very much and sweat,[1].—The heat abates after 5 P.M., without shivering, even in the open air, the head feels freer, the breathing easier, and the voice stronger and deeper,[1].—The heat continues unabated after 5 P.M.; only that cold drinks cause shivering,[1].—Flushes in the forehead, in the evening (after eight hours),[1].—[60.] Sensation of heat in the face after eating, of the hands and feet, and an hour afterwards, thirst (second day),[1].—Towards evening, a feeling of heat in the otherwise cold hands and whole body, with creeping chills, without thirst, and almost dread of drinking, while sitting (after nine and a half hours),[1].

Conditions.—Aggravation.—(*Morning*), Heaviness of head; wound painful; chilly.—(*Forenoon*), Attacks of nausea; chilliness in hands, etc.; heat, etc.—(*Afternoon*), Heat.—(*Toward evening*), While sitting, feeling of heat, etc.—(*Evening*), When lying in bed, pressure in left chest; in bed, heat; flushes in forehead.—(*Night*), Restless, etc.—(*Bending neck to right side*), Pain on side of throat.—(*During chill*), Nearly all symptoms appear; anxious, etc.; tearings in urethra.—(*After eating*), Headache in forehead, etc.—(*When lying down*), White of eye inflamed, etc.—(*On moving*), Stitches in abdomen; rheumatic pains.—(*Moving head*), Pain in glands before jaw.—(*During rest*), Tension in wrists, etc.—(*While sitting*), Pains in knees; pain in calf; pain on border of sole.—(*After smoking*), Hiccough. —(*When standing*), During inspiration, pressure in left side of chest.— (*When walking*), Pain in region of navel.

*Amelioration.—*Feels best when walking about, or when lying perfectly still.

CALTHA.

Caltha palustris, Linn. *Nat. order*, Ranunculaceæ. *Common names*, Marsh Marigold, Cowslip (American). *Preparation*, Tincture of the whole plant when in flower.

Authority. Spiritus, Rust's Magazine, 1825, as quoted by Roth, Mat. Med., 1, 326.

*Mind.—*Anxiety and restlessness.

*Head.—*Vertigo (second day).—Vertigo and roaring in ears (after half an hour).—Headache; dull drawing, from occiput over to forehead, with vertigo (after half an hour).

*Eye.—*Eyes dim.—Lachrymation.—Pupils contracted.

*Face.—*Face pale, yellowish.—Prodigious swelling of the face.—[10.] Face swollen, especially around eyes.—Swelling of face, white, soft, and puffy; extended some over whole body (second day).—The swelling of the face does not subside until the eighth day.

Mouth.—The tongue is covered with a very thick, dirty-white coating. —Peculiar disagreeable impressiom on back of tongue (third day).

Stomach.—Very great thirst (second day).—Nausea (after half an hour).—Vomiting, very painful (after half an hour).—Griping pains in epigastric and umbilical regions (after half an hour).

Abdomen.—Abdomen distended.

Stool.—[20.] Diarrhœa (after half an hour).—Copious alvine evacuations, with emissions of a good deal of flatulence (second day).

Urinary Organs.—Painful burning in urethra.—Burning pain when urinating.—Dysuria (after half an hour).—Urine scanty and very red.

Heart and Pulse.—Small, quick, and contracted pulse (second day).—Pulse small, hard, rapid, sometimes intermitting.

Extremities in General.—Heaviness and numbness of the limbs (seventh day).—Pain of stiffness and tension in the joints.

Inferior Extremities.—[30.] Tottering gait.

General Symptoms.—Trembling in whole body.—Very great restlessness; the children roll on the ground in their agony.

Skin.—Red spots on feet and legs.—The inner surface of the thighs is covered with dry pustules (papulæ?), which cause itching and a painful tension, when walking. This pain extends into the whole thigh. The pustules remain three weeks, then desquamate and disappear.—Large bullæ of pemphigus, in different parts of the body, especially on the limbs, back, and face, surrounded by a red ring, and itching a great deal. These bullæ vary in size; but the largest are not bigger than an almond, and are filled with a serous liquid. On the third day, these bullæ are transformed into crusts, and on the seventh day of the disease, and fourth of the eruption, they begin to fall off (third day).

CAMPHORA.

Cinnamomum Camphor, Fr. Nees; Laurus Camphora, Linn. *Natural order*, Lauraceæ. *Preparation*, Tincture of the gum.

Authorities. 1, Hahnemann, R. A. M. L., vol. 4; 2, Franz., ibid.; 3, Hartmann, ibid.; 4, Hermann, ibid.; 5, Stapf, ibid.; 6, Wislicenus, ibid.; 7, Alexander, Exp. Essays, p. 227, proving with large doses, *quoted by Hahnemann;* 8, Collin, Obs. circa morbos, III, 148, proving with large doses, ibid.; 9, Cullen, Mat. Med., from grs. xl, in a female maniac; 10, De Meza, Compend. Med. Pract., p. 3 [not obtainable], ibid.; 11, Geoffroy, Mat. Med., IV, 30, general statement from authors, ibid.; 12, Griffin, Dis. de Camph. viribus, proving with large doses, ibid.; 13, Heberden, Med. Transact., I, 471, effect of large doses in patients, ibid.; 14, Hergt, Hufeland's Journ., XXVII, 1, 151, from 3 grs. twice a day, ibid.; 15, Hoffmann, Opera Omnia (Geneva, 1740), VI, 60, general statement from observation, ibid.; 16, Hufeland's Journ., I, 428, from large doses in a rheumatic patient, ibid.; 17, Koolhaas, Med. Not. Zeit., 1799 [not obtainable], ibid.; 18, Loss, Obs. Med., p. 314, from continual smelling, in a man of 40, ibid.; 19, Murray, App. Med., IV, 584, general statement from authors, ibid.; 20, Ortel, Med. Pract. Beob., I, 1 [not obtainable], ibid.; 21, Ponteau, Melange de Chir., p. 184, in a woman three weeks after labor, ibid.; 22, Quarin, Meth. Med. Febr., p. 51, occasional effects of large doses on fever patients, ibid.; 23, Sommer, Hufeland's Journ., VII, 87, from gr. 8–12 in lead-colic, ibid.; 24, Sponitzer, Hufeland's Journ., V, 3, 16 [observation not found], ibid.; 25, Unzer, Med. Handbuch, II, 25 [not obtainable], ibid.; 26, Whytt, works, p. 646, from gr. xxx, ibid.; 27, Tode, Acta H., IV, 4, 188, from gr. v in commencing fever, ibid.; 28 to 33, Provings of Jörg and his class with the tinct. and crude drug (when not mixed with magnesia), Jörg's Materialien; 34, Delander, experiment with twelve grains, Frank's Mag., 3, 463; 35, Schreter, N. Archiv. f. Hom., 3, 1, 183, symptoms from the X taken in water; 36, Lembke, provings with the tincture, N. Z. f. H., Kl., 10, 161, and 169; 37, ibid., proving with the 200th; 38, B. F. Joslin, M.D., proving with the 200th, U. S. Med. and S. J., 3, 146; 39, Dr. Norton, proving with the tincture, 10 to 40 drops, repeated 6 times in 5 days, B. J. of Hom., 17, 465; 40, Dr. B. Fincke, Hom. Month., 2, 12, provings with the 22^m; 41, ibid., with the 1st. trit. (one grain); 42, Dr. Berridge inhaled crude camphor, N. Eng. Med. Gaz., 9, 401; 43, Dr. Hiller, symptoms from a man who took about a scruple daily for more than a month, on account of excessive sexual desire, A. H. Z., 33, 381; 44, Klingbon, A. H. Z., 33, 381, a man took an ounce in some brandy; 45, Siemerling, Frank's Magazine, 1, 30, a rheumatic man took two drs.; 46, Frank's Mag., 4, 12, a man with cancer of the lip took four ounces, containing 160 grs., which had been ordered for rubbing his rheumatic shoulder; 47, Eickhorn, Lond. Med. Gaz., 11, 722, effects of 120 grs. at a dose; 48, Kohler, Schmidt's Jahrb., 159, 240, a woman took 200 grs. for a "bilious colic and diarrhœa;" 49, Toothaker, Hom. Times, 5, 284, effects of about half a wineglass of a saturated solution; 50, Trousseau and Pidoux, Trait. Mat. Med., effects of 5 to 18 decigrammes; 51, Wildberg, Jahrb., 1837, effects of 35 grains, quoted by Cattell, B. J. of Hom., 11, 527; 52, Wendt, of Breslau, effects of a large dose, quoted by Cattell, B. J. of Hom., 11; 53, Mesarguel (Arabian), effects of six drs. at one dose, from Leadam, B. J. of Hom., 8, 391; 54, Pharm. Journ., 26, 557, effects of a small quantity of camphorated oil on a boy 20 months old; 55, Dr. Beck, Practitioner, 2, 61 (from St. Louis Med. and S. Journ.), poisoning of a child 3 years old, by the gum; 56, Braithwaite, Med. Times and Gaz., 1, 658, poisoning by 30 grs.; 57, Reynolds, L. and Ed. M. J. of M. S., 1846, poisoning of a man from eating bits of gum (in all about 1 to 2 drs. in a few minutes); 58, Journ. de Chim. Med., 1860, a woman took 12 grs. in brandy to produce abortion; 59, Schaaf, Ed. M. J. of M. S., 1850, poisoning of three children, each taking half a teaspoonful of the gum; 60, Klingelhöffer, Lond. Med. Rec., 1, 654 (Berlin Kl. W.), effects of 30 grs.; 61, Hahn. Month., 9, 301, effects of two tablespoonfuls of the tinct.; 62, Lancet, 1874, p. 105, effects of from 25 drops to a teaspoonful of a concentrated solution; 63, Emerich, Hom. Archiv., 2, 36, effects of wearing it in flannel bands; 64, Beebe, Med. Invest., 9, 17, poisoning from a large piece of the gum; 65, Aran, N. Z. f. H. Kl., 1, 98, effects of a clyster of camph.; 66, Hom. Vierteljahrsch., 8, 107, effects of a clyster taken for priapism; 67, Christison, cited by Harley, Practitioner, 2, 213, effects of 40 grs.; 68, Orfila, cited by Harley, l. c., effects of 40 grs. in olive oil; 69, Harley, l. c., from Journ. de Chim. Med., 1860, effects of 180 grs.; 70, Harley, l. c., effects of two tablespoonfuls of camphorated oil (Ol. oliv., ʒj; camph., ʒss.), on an adult female; 71, effects of a few pieces of crude camphor, taken for the cure of seminal emissions, Hom. Vierteljahrschrift, 1, 231.

Mind.—Emotional. *Agitation,[52].—Great excitement,[51].—Excitement, as of intoxication (after three hours),[45].—Great excitement, almost amounting to frenzy (after two hours),[57].—Rage, with foaming at the mouth,[7].†—Often felt as if he ought to kill people, when in the street; never felt a disposition to kill any of his own family, but thought he ought to kill somebody,[49].—Delirium,[16].—Slight delirium, attended with somnolency and a small, languishing pulse,[63].—A little delirium,[59].—[10.] Active delirium,[66].—Most furious delirium, being with difficulty restrained in bed by two men (after one hour),[58].—Delirium, with pain in stomach,[51].—Delirious, but when spoken to gave rational answers (after three hours),[70].—Gestures and conversation very strange and wild,[57].—Talked wildly, constantly repeating the same sentence (after one hour),[56].—He talks irrationally, and proposes absurd things,[25].—He beats himself on the chest, and falls into a faint,[9].—Strips himself, and tries to jump out of window,[51].—Stripped naked, he danced wildly about, and attempted to jump out of window,[57].—[20.] He is averse to all external objects, they excite in him a repelling fretfulness,[1].—Aversion to all kinds of work,[26].—Calm opiate effect on mind and brain (after two hours),[29].—Voluptuous ideas (after eight days),[35].—Lively mood (after half an hour),[29].—Greatly exhilarated (soon after),[57].—Disposition to cry frequently, he knew not what for, but would frequently find himself crying when at work or when walking about,[49].—The child creeps into a corner, howls and cries; everything that is said to him is taken as if one were ordering him, and he were considered naughty and would be punished,[1].—Uttered a strange scream, a sort of howl, leaped from bed, apparently in great agony, and bent on something desperate (after half an hour),[49]. —Depressed, sad, out of humor,[35].—[30.] Depressed, irritable, despondent,[35]. —During the first day the disposition was indolent and depressed during the coldness and chill; but after twenty-four hours his disposition became continually better, even during the pains,[3].—*Indescribable wretchedness,[49]. —*Anxiety,[1 52 63]. — *Great anxiety,[66]. — *Very great anxiety,[15]. — **Great anxiety and extreme restlessness,** *tossing about in bed; attempted to stand, but he lay down again,[49].*—Excessively fearful, especially in the dark,[49].— *Dread of being alone in the dark,[49].*—Indescribable dread of being drawn upwards,[49].—[40.] Afraid of the mirrors in the room, lest he should see himself in them; so excessive was this fear at times in the night that he would have got up and broken the mirrors, only that he was still more afraid to get up alone in the dark; was never afraid of anything before, either by night or day,[49].—Was found much excited, screaming loudly, "I shall not faint! I shan't faint, for if I do, I will have fits and never come out of them!"[61].—Children irritable,[62].—Very irritable and fretful, every word irritates and excites him; during the first days,[35].—Fretful, anxious, at night, with frightful visions,[43].—Desire to dispute; self-willed,[1].—In a few moments after taking I awoke with an indescribable feeling of uneasiness and most deadly nausea produced by the taste and smell of the Camphor. I could not lie; the thought continually occurred, as in delirium, "I am dead! No, I am not dead! but indeed I must be dead!" and thus I flew round about myself like a top, with no other feeling than for the strong smell of the Camphor. The external world existed for me no longer. My thoughts were gone; one single fearful one remained; I imagined myself transferred to another world; for me all else was extinguished. I sat up in bed, but all about me had indeed disappeared. I was alone in the great

---

† During unconsciousness. See S. 61.

universe, the last of all things. My ideas of the world, God and religion, now seemed to me to have existed only in my imagination; the earth, upon which yesterday I lived and moved, had run its appointed course, and I was the final and solitary fragment of the whole creation. There was no other feeling in my soul than that of my hopeless, endless damnation. I sank back upon the bed, *believing that I was the spirit of evil in a world forsaken of God.* Faith and hope were gone. There was here no longer any God, or rather the Infinite himself, like all his works, had ceased to be. My misery was boundless; time itself was no more; in short, I suffered such fearful anguish as no fancy can comprehend. What soul could paint to itself my everlasting dwelling as the Evil One, alone in a vast universe, without faith or hope, and my heart forever broken by unimagined tortures? I rose suddenly from the bed, rushed to the window, and threw it up. It was a night in September; all nature lay quiet, illuminated by the moon, with the clear stars looking down. The sight increased my despair; poor nature extinguished; the sky transparent and lifeless; the earth was still in the dim, dead light. I could not bear it. The sense of touch was gone, and my eyes protruded from their sockets. For a moment I resolved to throw myself from the window and sweep through the domain of my infernal kingdom, but a weak glimmer of reason held me back. I tried to weep, but my eyes were dry; my hands could no longer grasp anything, and I felt no moisture in my eyes. I tried to pray, but the words sounded hollow from my chest, like reverberations from a cracked vessel. A fearful terror seized me, and I knew not whither to fly. I cried out aloud, "And so I am indeed dead; that hell I used to think about is no fiction, but a reality which I am doomed to experience forever. And yet I confessed this very morning, and no heavy sin rests upon my conscience." And then came doubts about my doctrinal views, for I had never been of strong faith. Thus hopelessly devoted to everlasting damnation I recollected some syrup, a sort of stomachic elixir, which was in my closet, and felt for it in the dark; but, oh, horror! my hand no longer perceived resistance, my whole body was insensible and dry as marble, and I was conscious of no internal warmth. In my ever-growing terror I sought to recall sensation, even if it were pain, and tore the skin of my face and hands, but it was useless; I felt no more.

I ran to the mantle-piece and struck a light. I saw it, came to myself, and the thought came over me that after all it might be only a dream,—a horrible vision of the night. I left the light burning, again lay down, and took a book, that I might drive away the fearful images; but scarce was I in bed before they returned, and with them a renewed desire to throw myself from the window. I started up, ran out, and fell prostrate, with a loud shriek for help, not far from the door of a neighbor. Persons came out, and seeing my desperate condition, were about to bring me a cordial, but I could not bear to be alone. Fearing some new misfortune, I seized my neighbor and held him fast, that he might not leave me. They gave me a few swallows of Moldavia water, which were followed by nausea and efforts to vomit. Next day they told me they could not stay in my room for the smell of camphor; on this account they brought me down stairs into the street, that I might breathe the fresh air, while they were making some tea for me. The sight of the sky, the pale moonlight, renewed my torturing fancies. I pressed close to my neighbor, and implored him to talk to me, that I might be freed from them, but terrified at my terror, he could find no topic for conversation. We went upstairs again, and tea was given me to drink. It tasted cold, though the woman next day assured me it was fairly boiling. Violent vomiting then came on, without any relief to my mania; they read to me, but I could not follow the train of ideas; my own thoughts absorbed me. After the vomiting I began to feel a little cold; I became more quiet, was put to bed and fell asleep. Next morning I visited again the scene of my night visions, and attempted to drive away my morbid impressions by force of will. I went to my business in town, but the attacks returned. Again I felt my sense of touch disappear; my eyes started out of their sockets, convulsive movements attacked my head, and I could not get warm. A physician prescribed some quieting mixture. In the evening I attended the theatre; but scarce could the excitement of the crowd, the music, and the play beguile my thoughts.

What I have related took place, not in a half-waking state, but clear and distinct, with full conviction of their reality, and so vividly that I perfectly recollect the smallest incident. I suffered all, not only in a higher degree than I can express, but also in an inconceivably longer duration. As I lay stretched on my couch, as the evil demon, and suffered all the anguish of a condemned and God-forsaken soul, the time seemed an eternity, and the most painful thought was that I was forever deprived of the Divine protection, and of every consolation and every hope. Nothing remained to me but the conviction of my everlasting damnation.

Since that time I have been subject to these attacks of terror at night, when I am alone. I feel a tendency to self-contemplation; outer things vanish, and I behold myself in spirit freed from matter. *I am constrained to this agonizing self-contemplation, in spite of every effort of the will, and every opposition which my thoughts can make.* In consequence my nervous irritability is greatly increased, and I sleep but little and very restlessly, which is quite the reverse of my former habit. The pollutions have much diminished in frequency, but I often wake terrified by nightmare; I shriek and call for help, because it seems that a murderer stands at my bedside. I dare not drink either tea or coffee, lest the phantasms of that fatal night return; I cannot then sleep at all. My temper is irritable and peevish, with an inclination to despair and suicide. I am afraid to go to sleep; and when I think it near it suddenly flies from me, my eyes open wide, and I fall into self-contemplation and mystical and dismal trains of thought. The source of my annoyance is not the presentation of images, but of feelings simply, without any mixture of the visible; it is my personal self, my unembodied spirit. By day I am quite quiet; night and solitude are my terrors. I still have faith and reason enough left to see in all this nothing but the phenomena of a morbid state,[11].—An indifference whether the world uses one well or ill (after two hours),[39].—*Intellectual. Thought.* Unusually clear-headed (soon after),[57].—Never felt better; ideas never more lively or clearer; it appeared as if the intellectual powers were increased; champagne never brought on a more pleasing intoxication (after half an hour),[47].—[**50.**] Intellectual dulness,[39].—The intellectual powers became much disturbed,[34].—A tumult of crude ideas floated through his mind,[67].—The ideas were confused, delirium,[10].—*Memory.* Want of memory,[63].—Complete loss of memory, after an attack of catalepsy, with loss of consciousness, followed by vomiting (after three hours),[6].—*Cognition.* Stupefaction of the senses, like fainting,[25].—Unconsciousness,[65].—Unconscious for several hours,[62].—Falls down, without consciousness, with howling cries,[44].—[**60.**] Loss of consciousness,[1].—Loss of consciousness,[7] [25].†—

---

† Original corrected by **Dr. Hughes.**

Loss of consciousness, during which he was attacked with violent convulsive fits, and maniacal frenzy,[67].—Sometimes complete loss of consciousness, at others recovered senses,[59].—Insensibility,[9].—The senses vanish,[7].—The senses disappear (after a few minutes),[1].—Coma,[7 58 62].—Coma (after half an hour),[48].—Stupid coma and delirium,[5].†

Head.—Confusion and Vertigo. [70.] Confusion of the head,[28].—Confusion of the head, with perfectly clear consciousness,[5].—Confusion of the head, changing to vertigo (after one hour),[31].—Confusion of the head, which soon changed to a vertigo,[30].—Slight confusion of the head (after two hours),[39].—Slight confusion of the head, especially in the anterior portion,[33].—Head confused, burning hot,[46].—*Vertigo,*[7 8 25] etc.—Vertigo; was obliged to steady himself, it seemed as if he could not stand still,[4].—Vertigo, so severe that he was obliged to sit down, to avoid falling (fourteenth hour after 16 drops),[28].—[80.] Vertigo, so severe that the knees knock together, and he nearly falls (soon after 20 drops),[28].—Vertigo, returning at various times,[12].—Short attacks of vertigo, after repeated inclinations to vomit,[16].—Frequent short attacks of vertigo,[16].—Vertigo, when sitting,[36].—Vertigo, with tendency to fall forward, when walking,[37].—*Vertigo and heaviness of the head, especially on stooping,*[31].—Vertigo, with sparks before the eyes,[46].—Said she had no pain, but her head turned round (after three hours),[70].—Seized with giddiness, for the relief of which she went out of her room, but the giddiness increased and compelled her to return,[60].—[90.] Giddy, confused, and forgetful (after one hour),[67].—Giddiness and dimness of sight (after twenty minutes),[51].—*He staggered as if drunk,*[4].—He staggers from side to side, when walking, and is obliged to steady himself, in order to stand still,[6].—*General Head.* The head is thrown back,[65].—The head was spasmodically drawn sideways towards the shoulder (after a few minutes),[1].‡—[Inflammation of the brain (fatal)],[22].—*Rush of blood to the head* (after six hours),[1].—*Great rush of blood to the head,[26].§—*Congestion of the head,[34].—[100.] Lightness in head,[51].—Head felt rather light,[47].—Head heavy,[52].—*Heaviness in the head,*[11].—Heaviness of the head, especially the vertex,[36].—*Heaviness of the head, with vertigo; the head sank backward* (after ten minutes),[4].—*Dizzy heaviness of the head* (after twelve hours),[4].—Stupefying feeling in the head, like the effects of laudanum (after two hours),[39].—Headache,[16 58 69].—Headache, beginning in the frontal region and extending to the occiput,[28].—[110.] Headache, in the morning, after rising, for several days in succession,[2].—Headache, with burning pain in stomach, eructations, great thirst, and a sense of formication in the extremi-

---

† Quoted from author's only to question it.

‡ The effects of a large dose given to a child, on account of which the senses vanished; all parts of the body became deadly cold, etc.—H.

§ The vertigo at first, and loss of consciousness, together with general coldness of the body, seem to be the primary action of a large dose of camphor, and point to a diminished afflux of blood from the heart to the distant portions of the body: while the rush of blood to the head, heat in the head, etc., are the reaction of vitality, just as much as the previous opposite condition is the supposed primary action. So slight inflammation, which appears suddenly, may be removed by the palliative, cooling effects of the primary action of camphor taken internally; but long-continued inflammations cannot be so removed. The continued or even frequently repeated use of camphor is not seldom followed by obstinate inflammation of the eyes, which is persistent, as one of the secondary or reactionary conditions of the organism. Although I cannot deny that an external application of camphor acts homœopathically in acute cases of inflammation of the eyes, yet I myself do not approve of it, since judging by experience, I never treat such cases by external applications.—H.

ties,[60].—Headache, with drawings in the right side,[35].—Sudden headache (soon after),[57].—Severe headache,[25].—Very severe headache,[46].—Intense headache, which confined him in bed for several days,[62].—Intense headache and giddiness,[52].—Violent headache,[36].—Heat in the head, and tearing headache, soon passing off and disappearing on pressure (after eleven hours),[2].—**[120.]** *Headache, as from constriction of the brain,*[1].—*Transient headache, as if the brain were compressed from all sides,* only felt during half consciousness, when he was not paying attention to his body; if he became conscious of his pain and thought of it, it immediately disappeared (after four and a half hours),[2].—*A contractive pain at the base of the brain, especially in the occiput,* and above the root of the nose, which continues without cessation, whereby the head is leaned to one or the other side; a pain which is very much increased by stooping low, lying down, or by external pressure; with coldness of the hands and feet, hot forehead, and coma vigil,[1].—Towards evening, felt aching in middle of head, from the forehead backwards, which lasted through the evening and next day,[49].—Drawing sensation all around head, as if the nerves of the head were all drawn up; drawings for some minutes, then remissions, then drawings again,[49].—Dull headache extending from the forehead to the temples, after three hours; this pain returns after a larger dose the next day, increases gradually all day, reaches its greatest severity at evening; it is frequently accompanied by transient stitches in both temples and in the orbits; very much relieved in the afternoon, during a walk in the open air,[28].—Pressive sensation in the head,[5].—Pressive headache from within outward, immediately,[6].—Fine tearing in the head, especially in the forehead (after seven hours),[3].—Pressive tearing headache,[1].—**[130.]** Headache, as if bruised, or as if the brain were sore,[1].—Headache; cutting jerks shoot from the forehead and temples to the middle of the brain, returning after short intervals, immediately after lying down (after half an hour),[6].—Throbbing in head,[51].—Throbbing headache,[1].—***Forehead.*** Heaviness and heat in the forehead, worse when walking,[36].—Troublesome heaviness in the forehead,[33].—Heat in the forehead,[36].—Heat in the forehead, especially in the vertex,[36].—Slight headache in the forehead, which gradually became more violent, and accompanied by stitches, apparently starting in the temporal bones, and returning every five minutes,[28].—*Dull headache above the frontal bone, with nausea,*[1].— **[140.]** Pressure in the forehead,[36].—Pressure in the middle of the forehead (after three and a half hours),[4].—Pressure and heaviness in the upper forehead,[36].—Pressure on the right side of the forehead,[36].—Pressure in the left side of the forehead,[36].—Tearing pressure and pressing from within outward in the left side of the forehead (after seven and a half hours),[4].—A pressive though not painful sensation in the forehead, changing after half an hour to a confusion of the head,[29].—In the evening, pressive headache over the left eye (after nine hours),[2].—Pressive headache, alternating in the forehead and at the sides (second day),[33].—Tearing-sticking headache in the forehead, and pressure on the upper part of the frontal bone (after four hours),[2]. —**[150.]** Throbbing-stinging headache in the forehead, which continues through the night, with general dry heat, without thirst,[1].—Fine tearing pain in the left side of the forehead and left side of the occiput (after half an hour),[4].—Throbbing headache, in forehead,[63].—Throbbing headache in forehead, over root of nose, with heat (after one and a half hours),[40].— ***Temples.*** Throbbing of the temporal arteries, and distended jugular veins,[34].—Boring headache in the temples, especially during the morning nap; returns daily, during the whole proving; after waking, it ceases, and is followed by pain in the teeth,[35].—Boring headache in the right temple, ending with a stitch, which extends with great severity into the eye and tooth, lasting three seconds and returning after three seconds, in the morning, on waking (second day),[35].—Tearing pressure in the right temple (after one hour),[4].—Throbbing pressure in the temples,[5].—Fine tearing in the right temple and forehead (after one and three-quarter hours),[4].— *Vertex.* [160.] Dull pressure in the region of the vertex,[36].—Severe pressure on the right side of the vertex,[36].— *Parietals.* Pressure by jerks, in the head, over the left ear,[36].—Single violent stitches in the right half of the brain (after four hours),[1].— *Occiput.* Uneasy feeling at back of head (second day),[60].—Pressure in the occiput,[5 36].—Cutting pressure from the left side of the occiput towards the forehead (after half an hour),[4].—*Throbbing in the cerebellum,[45].— *External Head.* Scalp intensely hot,[55].

Eye.—Objective. *Eyes staring,[66].—[170.] He looks at one staring, and wondering without consciousness (after two hours),[6].—[Staring inflamed eyes],[22]. — *Staring, distorted eyes,[1]. — *Eyes hollow* (after three days),[58].—Blue circles around eyes,[63].—Eyes brilliant,[52].—Eyes glittering,[46].—Distorted eyes,[20].—Eyes inflamed,[63].—Inflammation of the eyes (after ten hours),[1].— *Subjective.* [180.] A feeling of tension in the eyes (after three-quarters of an hour),[4].—Soreness or tense, stiff feeling in eyes and eyelids all day,[39].— *Orbit, etc.,* Pressure above right eye,[37].— Pressure on the muscles of the right eyebrow (after three-quarters of an hour),[4].— *Lids.* The eyelids are covered with many red spots (after twenty-four hours),[6].—Twitching of lids,[63].—Eyelids, in constant agitation, and half closed, showed the eyeballs turned upwards and outwards,[59].— Visible jerking and twitching of the upper lid (after thirty-six hours),[2].— Transient burning in the eyelids,[33].—Burning in edges of lids,[36].—[190.] Biting and sticking in the lids (after five hours),[2].—Biting at the edges of the lids,[36].—Smarting in the lids,[36].—Biting-itching in the lids,[5].—Frequent twitching in the external canthus (after twenty-eight hours),[2].—Biting in the external canthus (after half an hour),[1].— *Lachrymal Apparatus.* Lachrymation in the open air,[5].— *Conjunctiva.* Conjunctivæ injected,[51]. —Conjunctiva injected (after two hours),[57].—Very red spots on the white of right eye, without pain (after twenty-four hours),[6].— *Ball.* [200.] The eyeballs were turned outward,[1].—Pressing-out pain in the right eyeball on moving it (after two hours),[2].—Sensation in the left eyeball as from pressure and pushing upon it from behind (after two and a half hours),[2].— *Pupil.* Pupils inclined to dilate rapidly,[36].—Pupils dilated,[51 66].—Pupils dilated (after one hour),[56].—Pupils dilated (after three hours),[70].—Dilated pupils (after five hours),[1].—Pupil not much dilated; scarcely sensible to light (after two hours),[57].—Contracted pupils,[1 36].—[210.] *Excessively contracted pupils* (after thirty-five minutes),[4].—Pupils contracted, then dilated,[63]. —Pupils normal, insensible,[44].— *Vision.* Clearer vision,[36].—Dimness of vision,[51].—Obscuration of sight,[25 26].—Frequent obscuration and many illusions of vision,[46].—Sight indistinct, with ocular hallucinations,[52].—Photophobia and sensitiveness of vision,[63].—Eyes sensitive to the light,[36].—[220.] He could not endure the light (after half an hour),[1].—Objects quivered before his eyes,[67].—On reading script in the forenoon, the letters ran together so that he could only read with great difficulty; after ceasing to read a bright circle appeared before the eyes,[35].—Objects seem glittering,[63].— Flickering before the eyes,[45].—Flickering before the eyes (third day),[35].— Sensation of increased light,[36].—*Sensation as if all objects were too bright and glittering* (after five hours),[1].—Dazzling light before eyes,[51].—Sparks and fiery wheels before eyes,[63].—[230.] Darkness before eyes, as if objects were encircled in a cloud,[63].—Small black spots float before the eyes,[36].— Hallucinations of vision,[66].—Wonderful forms float before the eyes,[25].— On closing the eyes, while slumbering, fanciful objects appear before him, which sometimes seem too thick, sometimes too thin; this alternates with the pulse (after two hours),[1].

Ear.—The lobules of the ears are red and hot,[5].—*A dark red ulcer, as large as a pea, in the left external meatus auditorius; on touch he feels a sticking pressure* (after twelve hours); *it suppurates* (after thirty-six hours),[4].— Burning in the ears,[36].—Sticking in the ear from a draught of air or wind,[35]. —Stitches in ears,[63].—[240.] Stitches deep in the left ear,[36].—A kind of tearing in the left ear (after one hour),[1].—Tearing behind and above the ears,[36].—Ringing in the ears,[34 51 63].—[Ringing in the ears],[7].†—Singing in the left ear,[36].—Roaring in the ears,[45].

Nose.—Objective. Obstruction of nose in right side, then secretion of thin mucus (immediately),[41].—Nose stopped, or running, or bleeding,[63]. —Sneezing (twice),[36].—[250.] *Coryza* (after ten hours),[1].—Stopped coryza,[1].—In the morning, on rising (and evenings on going to sleep?), discharge of thin mucus from the nose, without sneezing, and without real coryza (after eighteen hours),[1].—Bleeding from the nose (after four hours),[31].—Moderate nose-bleed (at 7 A.M., second day),[30].—*Subjective.* The air of the room, breathed through the nose, seems cooler, when walking,[36].—Sudden, momentary boring in the right side of the nose,[36].—Drawing in the left side of the nose,[36].—Violent stitching, or crawling, from the root of the nose almost to the tip,[36].—In the anterior corner of the nostril, a stinging pain, as if the place were ulcerated and sore (after two hours),[1]. —[260.] Itching in nose,[63].—Itching in left nostril,[36].

Face.—Objective. *Paleness of the face,*[1 51 63].—The countenance, naturally red, was pale (after six hours),[60].—*Face pale and livid* (after three days),[58].—*Countenance pale and haggard* (after two hours),[57].—*Face pale and anxious* (after three hours),[70].—*Countenance pale, distorted, sunken,*[66].—Very pale face, with at first closed, afterwards open, staring eyes, with the eyeballs turned outward (after two hours),[6].—Excessive paleness of face, with a fixed and stupid look,[59].—[270.] *Face and hands deathly pale,*[61].—*Bluish color of the face,*[65].—Flushing of face,[69].—Face flushed and expression wild (after one hour),[56].—*Redness of the face,*[36 52 58]. —[Very red face],[22].—Face red, puffy,[44].—Face scarlet-red and puffy,[46].— Black in face,[62].—In morning, disturbed countenance, with blue rings around eyes (second day),[40].—[280.] Lineaments relaxed, expressionless,[63]. —Slight twitchings of the face,[59].—The face, alternately pale and livid, was the seat of incessant spasmodic movements,[59].—Spasmodic distortion of the facial muscles, with froth from the mouth,[20].‡—Face hot to the touch,[36]. —Burning in the face,[36].—*Cheeks.* Redness of the cheeks and lobules of the ears,[1].—Stitching in left cheek,[36].—Boring in right zygoma,[36].—Drawing in the left zygoma,[37].—*Chin.* [290.] Stitching in the chin,[36].—Closure of the jaws (trismus),[1].—Tensive pain in masticators,[63].—Drawing in the angle of the right lower jaw,[36].

Mouth.—Teeth and Gums. A little froth about the teeth, which were firmly clenched,[59].—Painful looseness of the teeth (after ten hours),[1]. —Transient toothache, now in one, now in another tooth,[35].—*The teeth seem*

---

† Just before losing consciousness.
‡ From several grains of Camphor injected into the median veins.

too long, with cutting toothache, which seems to originate from the swelling of a submaxillary gland,[1].—Drawing in hollow lower back teeth,[36].—When walking, drawing in decayed upper incisors,[36].—[300.] Continual toothache for several weeks; gnawing and boring in nearly all the back teeth, though especially in the hollow teeth, aggravated by coffee or alcoholic drinks, and also if even a soft piece of bread touches the affected teeth; relieved by drinking cold water; if, however, cold water is held in the mouth, it aggravates the pain, as also does cold air; together with longing for beer, which affords him relief, as also tobacco-smoking,[35].—On going into the cold, or windy air, with the toothache, a stitch shoots from the tooth into the eye,[35].—Toothache; transient, cutting shootings through the gum to the roots of the incisor and canine teeth (after a quarter of an hour), (from smelling),[6].—During coition the toothache ceases, immediately after which he sleeps quietly for the first time,[35].—Gums loosened, of a livid color,[43].— *Tongue.* Tongue thick, spongy, fissured, covered with much tough yellowish mucus,[43].—Tongue dry, or covered with aphthæ,[63].—Sensation of dryness on the back part of the tongue, like a scraping, with much saliva,[5]. —*Tongue cold,* flabby, trembling,[66].—Very decided burning on the edge of the tongue and hard palate,[36].—[310.] Tongue felt swollen and numb,[61]. —Biting sensation in the end of the tongue, as from pepper,[36].—*General Mouth.* The breath had the odor of camphor (after six hours),[60].—Offensive odor from the mouth in the morning, which he himself noticed (after twenty hours),[1].—The mouth dry; is compelled to drink frequently,[28].— Dryness of the mouth excessive the whole day (after 16 drops),[1].—Dryness in the mouth, with thirst,[33].—The mouth very dry, with increased thirst,[29]. —Continued dryness of the mouth, with increased thirst,[28].—A cold sensation rises into the mouth and to the palate (after four to six hours),[2].— [320.] The sense of coolness changed to that of sharpness and burning (after half an hour),[50].—Unpleasant warmth in the mouth,[7].—Sensation of heat in the mouth and stomach,[19].—Sensation in mouth, as after eating peppermint lozenges, and the same in stomach (immediately),[50].—Whole mouth interiorly, with tongue, gums, and palate, feels as if swollen,[41].—Severe burning on the palate, extending down into the pharynx, that obliges her to drink, but is not relieved by any amount of drinking (immediately after smelling),[6].—Single coarse stitches in the palate (after four hours),[1].—A dry scraping sensation on the palate,[5].—*Saliva.* Flow of saliva (after a few minutes),[34].—Continual collection of saliva in the mouth (after half an hour),[4].—[330.] *Collection of saliva in the mouth, which is at times slimy and tenacious* (after one and a half hours),[4].—Profuse secretion of watery saliva,[5].—Frothing at the mouth,[65].—Froth issued from the mouth (after a few minutes),[1].—Foaming at mouth,[62].—*Taste.* Taste bad,[63].—*Increased taste of all food; broth tastes very strong* (after two hours),[1].—The taste itself is natural, but everything that he tastes, and even the customary tobacco, tastes bitter (after thirteen hours),[2].—The food tastes bitter, meat still more so than bread (the eructations during and after eating tasting of camphor), (after four hours),[2].—Tobacco has an offensive, bitter taste (after two hours and three-quarters),[2].—*Speech.* [340.] When roused, he had scarcely any power to articulate (after twenty minutes),[61].—Great difficulty of speech and thought,[61].—*Speech feeble, broken, hoarse,*[43].

Throat.—Heat in throat,[59].—Burning heat in throat, mouth, and stomach,[58].—Painful drawing and stiff sensation in the side of the throat and neck, when walking in the open air (after five hours),[2].—Sore throat (at night) when swallowing, and even more when not swallowing, as if the throat were sore and torn up, with a sensation as if she had eaten rancid substances,[1].—Scraping in throat,[63].—Slight scraping in the throat,[36].— *Burning in the pharynx and stomach*,[45].—[350.] Repeated short stitches at back and toward left side of pharynx,[42].—Slight warmth in the œsophagus and stomach, extending over the whole body (soon),[29].—Drinking difficult,[44].

Stomach.—Appetite and Thirst. Total loss of appetite (after six hours),[60].—Aversion to the accustomed tobacco-smoking without its tasting badly; he soon becomes averse to it, even to vomiting,[1].—*Thirst*,[59]. —*Great thirst (after six hours),[60].—Continued thirst, with frequent drinking,[28].—Longing for drinks, without thirst,[1].—Loss of thirst (first twenty-four hours),[6].—[360.] Loss of thirst (first thirty-six hours),[4].—**Eructations.** Frequent eructations,[36].—Frequent eructations tasting of camphor,[36].—Occasional eructations having a strong odor of camphor,[60].—*Empty eructations frequently after eating, and almost continuous* (after three hours, and later),[4].—Eructations and gulping of the contents of the stomach,[1].— **Nausea and Vomiting.** Nausea,[7 12 37].—Nausea (after one and a half hours),[40].—Nausea, with accumulation of saliva,[5].—Nausea and inclination to vomit, which disappeared every time after an eructation (after a quarter of an hour),[2].—[370.] Nausea and vomiting, especially mornings,[63]. —Retching,[44].—Constant retching,[59].—Vomiting,[59 64], etc.—Profuse morning vomiting of sour mucus disappeared during the whole proving of Camphor,[35].—Vomiting of yellow, watery liquid, smelling of camphor,[66].—Vomited black-streaked fluid smelling strongly of camphor,[62].—Bilious vomiting colored with blood,[12].—She drank some coffee, which excited vomiting,[60].— **Stomach.** Digestion is impeded,[9].†—[380.] Impaired digestion,[53].—Feeling like hunger in stomach (after twenty minutes),[50].—Severe gastric pains,[62]. —Pain in the stomach,[1].—Pain in the epigastric region,[16].—Pain, at first moderate, but afterwards very intense, in the epigastrium, radiating all over the belly and into the limbs, accompanied by uterine tenesmus,[69].— Gradually increasing pain in epigastrium, loins, and bowels, with strangury and vomiting (after ten hours),[58].—Sense of coolness in stomach (after one hour),[50].—*Coldness only in stomach*,[61].—Sensation of heat in stomach,[69].— [390.] Violent sensation of heat in stomach,[52].—Burning in the stomach,[12 25 26], etc.—Violent burning in the stomach,[46].—Sensation in the pit of the stomach as if it were distended and bruised, with fulness of the abdomen (after twenty-five hours),[2].—A sensation in the region of the pit of the stomach as if the abdomen were distended at this point, and the diaphragm thereby pressed upward; this sensation was accompanied by oppression of breathing,[32].—*Pressive pain in the pit of the stomach, or in the anterior part of the liver*,[1].—An oppressive sensation, with a feeling of warmth in the pit of the stomach,[32].—Stitches in the stomach (after five minutes), (from 28 drops),[29].

Abdomen.—Hypochondria. *Constrictive pain below the short ribs, extending to the lumbar vertebræ*,[1].—Pressive pain in the hypochondria (after one hour),[1].—[400.] Stitch in hepatic region, from before backwards, worse in running (second day),[49].—**Umbilical.** Sensation of hardness and heaviness in the abdomen, above the navel,[5].—Pressure and burning above the navel,[43].—Slight cuttings in the region of the navel, followed by passage of flatus, inclination to stool, and urging to urinate,[33].—**General Abdomen.** Abdomen retracted,[55].—Transient ascites,[14].—Movements in the intestines, and in the afternoon, frequent passage of offensive flatus; and, during the next night, from 1 to 2 o'clock, violent pressive pain, located in the cœliac ganglia, so severe that he feared that inflammation would

---

† Not found.

ensue, which caused great anxiety and sweating,[33].—Flatulence,[63].—Flatulent troubles in the abdomen,[1].—Slight discharge of flatulence,[36].—[410.] Copious emission of flatulence,[37].—Much discharge of flatulence, when walking,[36].—At first, passage of much flatus, and after several hours, in the morning, pressure in the abdomen as of distension from flatulence,[1].—Pain in abdomen, as if she would get diarrhœa, which, however, did not come (second day),[40].—* Cold sensation in the upper and lower portion of the abdomen (after fourteen hours),[4].—Burning in the abdomen, which is distended,[43]. — Violent burning heat in the upper and lower abdomen (after four hours),[4]. —Pinching pain in the lower portion of the abdomen, especially in the umbilical region (after seven and a half hours),[4].—Cramplike pain in abdomen, with diarrhœa following several times (after one and a half hours),[40].— Pressure and tension extending downward from the diaphragm; after half an hour, it changed to a pain in the region of the cœliac ganglia, which remained for several hours,[33].—[420.] Pressive pain, which seems to be in the region of the cœliac ganglia, so severe in the evening that he broke out into an anxious sweat; it seemed as if a very acute inflammation would attack the organs of the abdomen; this irritability extended up to the lungs, and caused cough, with a painful sensation on the inner surface of the spinal column, extending upward from the diaphragm,[33].—Cutting colic, at night (after five hours),[1].—Drawing bruised pain, more internally than externally, especially on inspiration, in the whole right side of the abdomen, extending into the region of the liver and into the chest (after three and a half hours),[2].—A scraping acrid sensation, now on each side, now on the left of the abdomen, sometimes more in the posterior, sometimes in the anterior portion of the abdomen; it approached a burning, and after a few hours changed to a grumbling pain in the region of the cœliac ganglia,[35].—

Hypogastrium and Iliac Regions. Pain in lower abdomen,[65].— Burning heat in lower abdomen (after one and a quarter hours),[4].—Burning-sticking in a surface as large as the hand, below the anterior crest of the ilium, extending to the groin,[2].—Drawing in the left side of the lower abdomen, with a tensive bruised sensation (after twelve hours),[2].—Sticking-drawing heaviness, which is distinctly felt on pressure in the right side of the lower abdomen,[2].—Hard pressure in the left side of the lower abdomen (after one hour),[4].—[430.] Itching-crawling in the right groin, which disappears on rubbing (after quarter of an hour),[6].

Rectum and Anus. The rectum seems contracted, swollen, and painful, on passing flatus,[1].—Pressive sensation along the rectum, with urging to urinate, not only in the bladder, but beginning in the kidneys, and extending along the ureters to the bladder, with a dragging sensation along the spermatic cords to the testicles, and a general feeling of turgescence in this part of the body,[33].—Smarting in the rectum,[5].—Urging to stool (after four hours),[4].—Urging to stool; the stool is of the usual hardness, but only a little passes, followed by very violent urging again, and a scanty discharge again (after one hour),[4].

Stool.—Diarrhœa. Two stools the first day, preceded by some griping in the abdomen; the second day, no stool; the third, a rather hard and difficult stool,[2].—Stool dark-brown, thin and scanty,[33].—Stool hard and retarded,[36].—Stools sour,[63].—[440.] Stool increased during the first days, afterwards passed only with much exertion and great pressure, and also much flatus passed with as much difficulty as the hardest stool; this usually preceded the evacuation,[35].—*Constipation.* Constipation,[1].—Constipa-

tion, for five to eight days,[43].—Extremely costive at stool the day after,[7].†
—Stool sluggish and incomplete,[33].—The fæces were passed with difficulty,
not without exertion of the abdominal muscles, as if the peristaltic motion
of the intestines was diminished, and at the same time the rectum was contracted (after twenty-four hours),[1].

Urinary Organs.—Bladder. Diminished power of the bladder;
the urine passes very slowly, without any mechanical hindrance (after
twenty hours),[1].—**Urethra.** Once, for a few minutes, a hot burning in
the urethra, like the effects of Cantharides,[39].—Sticking-burning on urinating,[35].—Frequent desire to make water,[59].—[450.] Frequent desire to make
water, with some pain in course of spermatic vessels (after two hours),[57].—
Micturition. *Micturition* frequent and *difficult;* urine clear,[51]. —Almost
involuntary urination, and pain as if the passage of urine in the urethra
has a contraction from before backward,[1].—Involuntary urination, after
severe urging to urinate,[1].—Urine passed in large quantity, probably in
consequence of much water having been drunk,[65].—Urine increased, of a
dark-brown color,[33].—Urine profuse, colorless, frequent, almost every five
minutes,[43].—*Diminished urination*,[36].—Scanty urine, without difficulty,
during the first hours, but after several hours (in the afternoon), a biting
pain when urinating, which lasts several days, in the posterior portion of
the urethra; this is followed by pressure in the bladder, like a renewed
desire to urinate,[2].—No urine passed during the first ten hours,[6].—[460.]
Retention of urine for twenty-four hours, the bladder being full,[58].—Retention of the urine, with urging to urinate; tenesmus of the neck of the
bladder,[1].—Retention of urine (the first twelve hours), with constant pressure in the bladder and desire to urinate, when, however, none passes; but
after twenty-four hours frequent urination of the usual amount, though
more in the aggregate is passed; after forty-eight hours, still more frequent
and more copious urination,[4].—*Painful urination*,[1].—*Burning urine*,[1].—
Strangury,[66].—Strangury, almost immediately,[13].—The urine passes in a
thin stream,[1].—The urine passes in a very thin stream, as in stricture of
the urethra (after two and a half hours),[4].—Urine dribbles,[1].—[470.] He
is unconscious of the urinary symptoms afterwards,[51].—**Urine.** Urine
quite clear, but having, as well as the perspiration, a very strong odor of
camphor (after two hours),[57].—Yellowish-green, turbid urine, of a musty
odor (after ten hours),[6].—Red urine,[1].—Red urine (very rarely),[15].—Urine
brown,[33].—He passes turbid urine, which, on standing, becomes very turbid
and thick, of a whitish-green color, without depositing a sediment,[4].—Urine
contains sugar, is pale, odorless, contains mucus, without sediment,[43].—
Urine with white or red sediment,[63].

Sexual Organs.—Male. Weakness in the genitals, and want of
sexual desire (first two days),[6].—[480.] Pressure in the left side of the
mons veneris; at the root of the penis, in the groin, when standing (after
ten hours),[2].—Pressing-out sensation in the mons veneris, in the groins, at
the root of the penis, as if a hernia would protrude (after twelve hours),[2].—
Sticking-itching on the inner surface of the prepuce,[4].—Incomplete erection,
with weak venereal desire, which soon again vanished (after one hour),[50].—
Erections completely impossible for a year and a half (taken on account of
satyriasis); scrotum relaxed, not even contracted by cold,[43].—Impotence,[53] [63],
etc.—During the first two days laxity of the scrotum, want of erections,
want of sexual desire, but after forty-eight hours far more violent erections

than usual,[4].†—A contractive sensation in the testicles,[5].—Increased sexual desire,[19].—Sexual desire seemed to be increased during the first days (curative action),[35].—[490.] In the night, experienced unusual sexual ardor, with continued delusions respecting the object of embrace,[39].—Inclined to nightly emissions,[1].—Emissions for several nights (after sixty hours),[2].—Nocturnal pollution, without dreams,[36].—*Female.* Os uteri enlarged and hot,[58].—Severe labor-like pains as in parturition,[13].‡—Abortion,[58].—Slight discharge of blood from vagina,[58].—Sexual orgasm,[17].—Menstruation too profuse,[63].—[500.] Courses had ceased entirely,[61].—Increased sexual desire during the first days, in a woman,[35].

Respiratory Organs.—Larynx, Trachea, and Bronchi.
Mucus in the air-passages; it makes the voice husky and is not removed by hacking, or clearing the throat,[1].—Pain in the air-passages, and bronchial tubes, mostly in coughing, and even when hacking and clearing the throat,[1].—Complains of a contractive sensation in the larynx, as from sulphur-fumes,[20].—*Cough.* Short cough, from scraping in the throat,[36].—Hacking, dry cough,[63].—Dry, hacking cough, especially in the forenoon, which lasts more than fourteen days,[35].—*Respiration.* Respiration hurried,[51].—Breathing hurried, and at times greatly labored (after two hours),[57].—[510.] Deep and slow respiration,[1].—(Short inspiration and expiration, during sleep),[1].—Respiration short and snoring,[59].—Respiration impeded,[44].—Breathing labored (after three days),[58].—Heavy, slow, difficult respiration (after one and a quarter hours),[4].—Oppressed, anxious, sighing respiration,[20].—Choking sensation,[65].—*Suffocative dyspnœa, as if it arose from a pressure in the pit of the stomach* (after one hour),[1].—It threatens to suffocate him and constrict the larynx,[23].—[520.] *Almost complete arrest of breathing,*[1].—*The breathing seems to have almost entirely ceased,*[9].

Chest.—Contraction of chest,[63]. — Oppression of chest,[63]. — Painful sensation in the chest, like stitches,[5].—Stitches in chest, especially left side, often extend to spine,[63].—Stitches in the chest, and hacking cough, as if caused by a cutting cold sensation deep in the air-passages (after two hours),[2].—The stitches in and about the chest become worse every day,[2].—Fine stitches in the nipples (after two hours),[1].—Fine tearing pain near the right nipple, extending down into the pelvis (after four and a half hours),[4].—*Front.* [530.] Pressure in the upper part of the sternum, as from a load,[2].—Pressure on the breast-bone when standing (after twenty-seven hours),[2].—Soft pressure internally in the chest, under the sternum, with difficult breathing, and a cold sensation, which rises from the chest into the mouth (after twenty-nine hours),[2].—*Sides. Stitches in the left side of the chest, when walking* (after half an hour),[2].—Internal trembling of the left side of the chest, and of the left arm, when lying upon the left side; it ceases on turning to the right side (second day),[35].

Heart and Pulse.—*Præcordial anxiety,*[43] [45].—*Great anxiety in the præcordial region,*[46].—*When very loudly spoken to, he complained of indefinable distress in the præcordial region; sensation of severe coldness and*

---

† The want of sexual desire, erections, and emissions are, as we see from these observations, only the primary action of camphor, hence it acts only as a palliative, if one prescribes for excessive sexual desire, erections, and frequent emissions, which have already lasted a long time; there then follows an increase of the disease on account of the reactionary effect of the organism.—H.

‡ From gr. xl, in enema.

irresistible sleepiness,[66].—Spasmodic stitches in the region of the heart with oppression of the chest, when lying on the left side; on turning to the right side it ceases (second day),[35].—***Heart's Action.*** Heart's impulse hard, but regular,[44].—[**540.**] Palpitation,[63].—*Palpitation of the heart,[1].—*He felt and heard the throbbing of the heart against the ribs, after eating (after four and three-quarter hours),[2].—*Heart beating very slowly, and intermitting,[61].—***Pulse.*** Pulse accelerated,[29 36].—Pulse accelerated,[19].†— Pulse accelerated from 70 to 79 (after a few minutes),[34].—The pulse becomes accelerated by ten to fifteen beats and tense (from the continued use of large doses),[16].‡ — Pulse accelerated twenty beats (100),[33]. — Pulse accelerated by twenty-three beats (after three hours),[7].§—[**550.**] Pulse very much accelerated, but undulating, and without strength,[66].—Excessive frequency of pulse,[66].—Pulse frequent, *full* and hard, or *soft*,[52].—Pulse frequent and scarcely perceptible (after twenty minutes),[57].—Very rapid pulse,[22].—After the administration of gradually increased doses of camphor the pulse became very rapid, for several days (nearly ten), without increase of the temperature,[16].—Pulse gradually becomes rapid,[12].—Pulse ten to fifteen beats more rapid than usual (after one hour),[29].—Pulse almost 90, but difficult to count (after one hour),[56].—Pulse between 90 and 100, small and irregular (after six hours),[60].—[**560.**] Pulse 108, and feeble (after four and a half hours),[70].—Pulse 120, and feeble (after three hours),[70].—Pulse 180, small,[51].—Pulse 180, and small (after two hours),[57]. —Pulse slow, small, hard, almost suppressed; with fever and sweat, full,[63].— Pulse slower by three beats,[7 12].—Pulse slower by ten beats,[7 9 16].—The pulse sank ten beats below the normal (after one and a half hours),[35].—Pulse fell from 72 to 60 (after half an hour),[50].—Pulse 60 (after twenty minutes),[50].—[**570.**] Pulse fell to 56 (after two hours),[50].—Pulse irritable in the evening,[28].—Pulse hard and full,[44].—Full rapid pulse,[1].—Pulse fuller and larger,[36].—Pulse full, irritable,[16].—Pulse was small, in accordance with its frequency,[47].—Pulse small and weak,[15].||—Pulse small, weak, and quite frequent,[47 68].—Small hard pulse, becoming slower and slower,[1].—[**580.**] Pulse small, slow; sixty beats to the minute (after twelve hours),[4].—Pulse extremely small (76 to 80),[65].—Pulse weak and thready (after three days),[58].—**Pulse very weak, scarcely perceptible*,[9].—Pulse imperceptible at wrist,[61].—Pulse could not be counted (after half an hour); the next day extremely weak,[48].

Neck and Back.—Neck. Stiffness in nape of neck,[36].—Tensive pain in the muscles of the nape of the neck and lower portion of the neck; worse on every motion and on turning the neck (after fifteen hours),[4].— Drawing on left side of nape of neck, toward the shoulder,[36].—Stitches in the neck, near the right shoulder, on motion (after one and a half hours),[2]. —[**590.**] Tearing pain in the nape of the neck, on bending the head forward (after two hours),[1].—Several painless drawings in the cervical vertebræ, on motion,[5].—Creeping sensation in the left side of the neck, above the clavicle,[36].—Swelling of cervical glands,[63].—***Back.*** Violent pain in the back, all day,[36].—Pain in course of spine,[51].—Painful tearing along the medulla spinalis,[45].—***Dorsal.*** Tearing pressure on the anterior margin of the shoulder-blade, which renders motion of the arm difficult (after

† From gr. xl.
‡ The large doses are 40 to 60 grs.
§ After recovering from loss of consciousness.
|| Not found.

thirty-two hours),[2].—*Drawing, painful stitches through the shoulder-blades, and between them, extending into the chest on moving the arm, for two days* (after twenty-four hours),[2].—**Lumbar.** Pressure in the small of the back,[43].—[**600.**] Tired feeling in the small of the back, when walking,[36].—**Sacral.** Sensation of sticking coldness in the sacral region, which passed with lightning-like velocity along the side of the vertebræ to the nape of the neck, and over the whole body, alternating with a feeling of transient heat,[66].

Extremities in General.—Stretching of limbs,[63].—Trembling limbs,[63].—Convulsive agitation in the limbs, after the tetanic stiffness,[54].—Violent cramps in extremities (after three days),[60].—Limbs as heavy as lead,[43].—*The limbs are difficult to move*,[1].—General painful sensitiveness in limbs,[63].

Superior Extremities.—Arms more convulsed than lower limbs,[59].—[**610.**] Pressure and drawing on the inner side of both arms, during rest of the parts, ceasing while moving them,[36].—Heaviness in the left arm,[36].—Sensation of fatigue in the left arm,[36].—The pain immediately begins again during rest of the arms; also in the right arm, when *that* is at rest,[36].—Tired feeling in the left arm, commencing at the left shoulder, extending into the wrist; relieved by motion of the arm,[36].—Tearing on the inside of the left arm, passing at times into the thumb and index finger,[37].—**Shoulder.** Pressure on the top of the shoulder (after two hours),[2].—Violent pressure on top of right shoulder,[36].—Drawing pain in the left shoulder,[35].—Bruised pain in both shoulders,[36].—**Arm.** [**620.**] Tearing pressure in the middle of the posterior portion of the right upper arm,[4].—Jerking, fine tearing from the middle of the inner surface of the left upper arm to the middle of the forearm (after three-quarters of an hour),[4].—Drawing in the muscles of the left upper arm, when walking,[36].—Tearing in the muscles on the inner side of the left upper arm,[37].—**Elbow.** *Painful pressure in the right elbow-joint, more violent on leaning upon it, when it extends into the hand* (after one and a half hours),[4].—Bruised pain in right elbow, wrist, and fingers,[36].—**Forearm.** Tired feeling from the left elbow into the hand,[36].—Pressure in right forearm,[36].—Tearing pressure on the inner surface of the left forearm,[4].—Stitches in the forearm (after one and three-quarters hours),[2].—[**630.**] Bruised pain in the lower part of the left forearm,[36].—Painful pressure on the inner surface of the left forearm (after one and three-quarters hours),[4].—Tearing pressure in the left radius, somewhat above the wrist (after seven hours),[4].—**Wrist.** Violent, continued, pressive pain in the flexors of the left wrist,[36].—**Hand.** Trembling in the hands, especially noticed when writing,[30].—Constant movement of the hands (after six hours),[60].—**Fingers.** Pain in the last joint of the thumb, as if sprained, on moving it (after twenty hours),[1].—Drawing in the left fingers, especially in the joints,[37].—Drawing in the ball of the left thumb,[36].—Drawing-stitching in the second joint of the left index finger,[36].—[**640.**] Tearing in the third left finger,[37].

Inferior Extremities. Tottering, weariness, and heaviness of the lower limbs (after one hour),[4].—The gait was tottering,[34].—The legs are difficult to move and weary,[1].—Could walk with difficulty (after six hours),[60].—Tired feeling in the legs, especially in the knees, when sitting,[36].—Pressure and drawing on the inner side of both legs, extending to the ankles, during rest of the parts, ceasing while moving them,[36].—**Hip.** *Cracking and creaking in the hip, knee, and ankle-joints*,[1].—Pressure in right hip-joint,[36].—**Thigh.** Pain in the posterior portion of the thigh, above the hollow of the knee, as after a long walk,[2].—[650.] When walking, painful sensation of stiffness in the outer side of the right thigh,[39].—Internal coldness through the right thigh, as if cold air blew on it,[36].—Drawing in the gluteus maximus, in the upper part, at its attachment to the crest of the ilium, as if it would make the leg lame,[2].—Drawing bruised pain in the thighs, after walking (after five hours),[2].—*Drawing bruised pain in the right thigh, and on the inner side, near and below the patella; he fears that the leg will bend forward suddenly* (after four and a half hours),[2].—Pressure deep in the whole right thigh,[36].—Tearing in the thighs (after twenty-eight hours),[2].—**Knee.** The knees feel as though they would suddenly bend forward, and as if beaten (after twenty-six hours),[2].—Heaviness and pressure in both knees, when sitting,[36].—Pain in right knee, as if fatigued,[36].—[660.] Sensation of coldness in right knee, extending into the foot, when sitting,[36].—Severe heat in right knee,[36].—Pressive-drawing below the patella, on the inner side of the knee (after thirty hours),[2].—Pressure in the right knee,[36].—Pressing in the left knee,[36].—Tearing in the knees, below the patella, mostly when walking (after six hours),[2].—Stitches in the right patella, while sitting (after half an hour),[2].—**Leg.** Heaviness in the legs,[36].—The leg goes to sleep, when sitting and bending the knee, with cold sensation (after twenty-one hours),[1].—Sensation of numbness in the right leg,[36].—[670.] Pressure in left leg,[36].—Pressure above in right leg,[36].—Pressure below ,in left leg,[36].—Heaviness in the lower leg, as from a weight hanging from the knee-joint, and dragging downward,[4].—Pressure in the middle of the inner surface of the left lower leg,[4].—Pressure in the left lower leg, above the malleolus and posteriorly,[4].—Stitching in the calves,[36].—Drawing in left calf,[36].—Pressure in the centre of the left calf, when walking and sitting,[36].—Fine stitching in the left calf,[36].—[680.] Stitching, when walking, on both sides of the tendo Achillis,[36].—**Ankle.** Pain in the ankle, as from a sprain or strain, in the morning, on rising and walking (after eighteen hours),[1].—Pressive-drawing pain below the right ankle-bone, when standing, between the malleolus and the tendo Achillis; on moving the foot, it becomes a tearing (after four and a half hours),[2].—Pressure in the ankles,[36].—When walking, the pressure is worse in the ankles; when sitting, in the knees,[36].—**Foot.** Trembling of the feet,[1].—Tremulous tottering and unsteadiness of the feet,[1].—Great weariness of the feet, when walking; the leg feels bruised and as if tense,[5].—Numbness in right foot,[36].—Violent drawing in right foot,[36].—[690.] Tearing in the forepart of the left foot, in the tips of the toes, and under the nails, when walking (after ten hours),[2].—*Drawing-pinching pain on the backs of the feet, especially on moving them,*[2].—*Tearing-pinching pain on the back of the foot, extending along the outer side of the calf to the thigh* (after thirteen hours),[2].—Drawing on the back of the foot,[36].—Tearing pressure on the back of the right foot,[4].—Burning and stitching in the sole of the right foot,[36].—Pressure on the sole of the left foot,[36].—Stitching in the ball of the left foot,[36].—**Toes.** Numbness of right toes,[36].—Pressure in right toes,[36].—[700.] Sore pain in the knuckles of the toes, and in the corns (after twenty-six hours),[2].—Prickling in the tips of the left toes, then of the right,[36].

General Symptoms.—Objective. Appears drunk,[51].—Extreme emaciation,[43].—Flesh and strength decreased,[43].—It predisposes to inflammations,[11].—Distension of the arteries,[36].—Relaxation and heaviness of the whole body (after twenty-five minutes),[4].—After the violent symptoms had diminished, in about twenty minutes, he lay quiet for the next three hours, muttering incoherently to himself, and following with his eyes the motions of persons about the room,[56].—General excitement of the muscular power (soon after taking),[34].—[**710.**] *He is hasty in his actions and speech,[1].—* *Often easily startled when awake, and then feels throbbings or palpitations,[49].—* Trembling,[7 25].—Trembling, which prevented writing,[33].—Trembling, mostly of the heart,[20].—Subsultus tendinum and insensibility,[51].—Spasms,[8].—Spasm which was like an epileptic spasm (after one-quarter of an hour),[48].—*Convulsions,[65].—* Convulsions,[7 22].†—[**720.**] Convulsions in children,[63].—True convulsions, with loss of consciousness, more or less prolonged,[59].—Strong convulsions,[55].—Violently convulsed,[62].—Violent convulsions,[27].—Violent convulsions, with disordered expression of countenance; livid aspect,[59].—Most violent general convulsions, especially of the hands and feet, so that five men could scarcely hold him,[44].—Clonic convulsive movements, at intervals of a few seconds, sometimes a minute,[59].—*Convulsive circular motion (rotation of the arms),[1].—Several times the body curled itself up into a ball, and was projected out again with great activity,[59].—[**730.**] Perfectly stiff, and in an early stage of opisthotonos,[54].—Cataleptic rigidity, with loss of consciousness, for a quarter of an hour, followed by relaxed sinking down of the whole body, so that he could scarcely be held upright for a quarter of an hour; followed by vomiting, after which consciousness returned (after two and a half hours),[6].—Falls from his chair in a kind of epileptic fit, which lasts about ten minutes (after twenty minutes),[51].—He rubs his forehead, head, chest, and other parts; does not know who he is; he leans against something, his senses leave him, he slides, and falls to the ground, stretched out stiff; the shoulders bent backward, the arms at first somewhat bent, the hands bent outward and somewhat clenched, the fingers spread apart; afterwards all parts are stretched out stiff, with the head bent to one side, the lower jaw open, stiff, the lips drawn inward, the teeth clenched, the eyes closed, incessant twitching of the facial muscles, cold all over, without breathing, for a quarter of an hour (after two hours),[6].—Languid and listless (after twenty minutes),[67].—Lassitude,[36].—Unusual lassitude and depression of spirits,[15].‡—Weariness,[36].—Complaints of weakness,[44].—Felt weak (after four and a half hours),[70].—[**740.**] Great weakness,[66].—Remarkable weakness,[65].—*Excessive weakness,[10].—Peculiar sensation of weakness (morning),[37].—Great prostration and weakness, almost faintness,[61].—Attacks of prostration, with faintness and total relaxation of all the limbs,[66].—*Great exhaustion,[51].—General exhaustion and suppression of urine for three months (after twenty minutes),[51].—Slight faintness (after half an hour),[50].—Attacked with a dreadful feeling of faintness, shivering, and numbness (soon after),[61].—[**750.**] Fell down insensible (after two and a half hours),[54].—Paralytic relaxation of the muscles,[1].—For several days partially paralyzed,[62].—Restlessness,[63].—Very restless at night; jumps and tosses about,[49].—She tosses anxiously about the bed, with constant weeping,[16].—Insensible to touch,[44].—**Subjective.** General comfortable feeling (after one hour),[50].—General discomfort,[63].—*Discomfort of the whole body* (after three hours),[4].—[**760.**] Uncomfortable sensation through whole body,[63].— Inexpressible discomfort of the whole body (after half an hour),[4].—Deathlike sensation,[65].—Intoxication,[8 10 12] etc.—Symptoms of intoxication,[69].—Drunkenness,[63].—Feeling as if drunk, with staggering (soon after),[2].—Symptoms like delirium tremens, such as optical delusions, fright, screams, hideous sights, and he buried head in pillow,[64].—At night, felt as if he could fly, or rather as if he must be and was being drawn up

† In Alexander's case during loss of consciousness.　　‡ Corrected.

into the air, in spite of himself,[49].—Feeling of dryness in and over the body, especially on the head and in the bronchial tubes (after two hours),[1].— [770.] Pain in the periosteum of all the bones,[1].—Nervous drawings, with something like a shivering,[49].—Rheumatic sticking pain in all the muscles, especially between the shoulders,[1].—Tearing stitches here and there in joints,[63].—Most of the pains of camphor during the first days only exist under a condition of partial attention (so tearing in various parts of the body only occur when falling asleep) and disappear, especially the headache, as soon as he becomes conscious that he has the pain and pays attention to it; on the contrary, on the succeeding days he is only able to bring on the pains by thinking of them, or he notices them much more when paying strict attention to himself, and feels best when he is not thinking of himself,[2].

Skin.—Skin appeared in general to be pale and moist, and heat of surface diminished,[59].—Skin shrivelled, relaxed, often cold,[63].—Skin became leathery, dry, burning, without a trace of sweat,[43].—Erysipelatous inflammation,[1].†—Erysipelas (from the external use),[24].—Vesicles on neck and chest,[63].—[780.] Very dry skin, even in bed, with good appetite,[16].—Acute drawing in the skin, above and below the left clavicle,[36].—Stitches in the skin of the right forefinger, on the side of the last joint,[36].—Itching here and there over the body, in the evening, after lying down in bed (after six hours),[1].—Severe itching (from the external use),[24].—Itching in the palms of the hands (after five hours),[2].—Continually increasing itching on the backs of the hands and knuckles, with sticking pain, relieved by scratching (after four and a half hours),[2].—Itching on the knuckles and between them (after twenty-five hours),[2].

Sleep and Dreams.—Sleepiness. Yawning,[63].—Yawning and sleepiness,[12].—[790.] Frequent yawning,[5].—Much yawning, when walking, without sleepiness,[36].—*Sleepiness*,[1 36].—Sleepiness, towards noon, with marked confusion of the head,[29].—Weary with sleep; it seems as though he should fall asleep (after one hour),[4].—He became overpowered by sleep at 7 P.M., and slept for more than two hours; on waking he did not know that he had been awakened in the meantime and had spoken to some one, though he was usually awakened by the slightest noise; after waking the headache was relieved, but he continued to feel sleepy,[28].—Sleep deep, prolonged, refreshing,[28].—Stupid slumbering, with pinching headache, great heat of the whole body, with distended veins, very rapid breathing, and bruised pain in the back, without thirst and with natural taste,[1].—Sleep during the first night very sound and deep, could scarcely get awake in the morning; in the night following, he awoke at midnight, and was unable to fall asleep again, but in the morning he could not arouse himself on account of sleepiness,[35].—**Sleeplessness.** Sleeplessness,[36 43].—[800.] Loss of sleep,[11].— The usual evening sleep, which he had taken upon a sofa, is omitted,[35].— Restless sleep,[36].—Sleep restless, he was continually awakened by thirst,[33]. —Distressed sleep, with fearful dreams, visions, spectres, etc.,[49].—Starts in his sleep,[49].—Snoring during sleep, on inspiration and expiration,[1].—He murmured and sighed during sleep,[1].—Talking in the sleep, the whole night, in a low tone,[1].—Crying out and starting up in sleep,[63].—**Dreams.** [810.] Sleep full of dreams,[63].—Dreams about projected occupations,[2].— Anxious dreams (fourth day),[38].—Dreams during the first day very confused; afterwards active dreams, and later, anxious dreams, of dying, etc.;

---

† From the external application of camphor.

he also dreamed about circumstances which had been the subject of conversation the day previous, especially in the morning,[35].

Fever.—Chilliness. *The body generally quite cold,[1].*—Coldness of the body, with paleness,[9].—*Coldness of the skin,[65].*—Skin cold and insensible (after three days),[58].—Cold skin, covered with clammy, inodorous perspiration,[66].—Shivering,[63].—[**820.**] Shivering and chilliness, in the evening when lying down,[35].—Shivering, chilliness, and creeping goose-flesh over the whole body, for an hour (immediately),[2].—Slight shivering, with paleness of the face,[12].—Sensitive to cool air,[63].—In the evening, great sensitiveness to cold over the whole body, and headache, as from constriction of the brain, with pressure over the root of the nose (after twelve hours),[2].—*He is excessively sensitive to the cold air,[1].*—Great aversion to the cold air ; it affects him very unpleasantly ; he is obliged to wrap himself up warmly, and even then is chilled through and through,[35].—He is unable to endure slight cold, from which either a chill results, or cutting pain in the abdomen, with a diarrhœa-like passage of blackish-brown or black fæces, like coffee-grounds,[1].—Frequent cooling, especially in the pit of the stomach,[15].—Chilliness (after ten hours),[1].—[**830.**] Chilliness over the whole body (after a quarter of an hour),[4].—Chilliness over whole body (after one and a half hours),[40].—Chilliness over the whole body (after two and a half hours), followed (after one and a half hours) by increased warmth of the whole body,[4].—Chilliness and shivering, with goose-flesh ; *the skin of the whole body is painfully sensitive, and sore to the slightest touch,*[1].—Great chilliness,[63].—Excessive chill,[43].—*Shaking chill and chattering of the teeth,*[20].—Coldness and drawing through the whole body, with cold arms, hands, and feet (after four and three-quarters hours),[2].—Coldness for an hour, with deathly paleness of the face,[21].†—When walking, the internal coldness increases,[36].—[**840.**] Continually complaining of freezing,[61].—(Paroxysm of fever ; severe chill, with gnashing of the teeth, and much thirst ; he sleeps immediately after the chill, with frequent wakings, almost without the slightest subsequent heat),[1].—Agreeable coolness through the whole upper region of body, especially in stomach and œsophagus,[50].—Cold sensation internally, first on the right side, then on the left, as if a cold liquid were flowing from the head downward,[36].—Forehead, cheeks, and hands cold (after six hours),[60].—Chilliness on the cheeks and in the back,[5].—Chilliness in back,[36].—Frequent chilliness in the back,[5].—Internal chilliness within the scapulæ,[36].—Chilliness over the back, mingled with warmth, as if sweat would break out,[5].—[**850.**] When walking, alternate chilliness and heat in the small of the back,[36].—Internal coldness in the region of the loins and small of back, worse on walking even a few steps,[36].—Extremities cold,[44][55].—Extremities cold (after twenty minutes),[51].—Hands and feet cold (after three hours),[70].—The hands become cold when walking,[36].—Cold hands and fingers,[36].—Sensation of internal coldness, extending from the knee into the foot, when sitting,[36].—*Heat.* Increased temperature,[33].—Increased heat of the skin,[36].—[**860.**] Burning heat of skin,[52].—Pleasant warmth through the whole body (after three hours),[2].—*Increased warmth of the body, with redness of the face* (after three-quarters of an hour),[4].—Began to feel warmer and warmer till he experienced a burning heat, and at the same time heart throbbed more and more frequently till it was impossible to count the pulse (after half an hour),[47].—Heat all over body (after one and a half hours),[40].—*Heat of the*

---

† From sixty grains given for colic ; the pain disappeared, but this condition supervened. On recovering from it she was well.

whole body, which becomes excessive when walking (after five hours),[4].—On waking in the morning, peculiar sensation of heat over the whole skin, as if going to sweat,[36].—Heat, burning, and dryness of the skin,[43].—Heat, with trembling,[7 25].—[Great heat (after some time)],[15].†—[**870.**] Early symptoms soon followed by great heat and a quicker pulse,[68].—Glowing heat, with full, rapid pulse,[46].—Heat was unendurable, and aggravated his condition,[46]. —Body hot and sweating,[44].—Feeling as if he had been very much heated, together with heat and rush of blood to the head,[33].—Feeling of coolness gave place to an easily endured burning (after two hours),[50].—Irritative fever; dry heat, and then easy perspiration,[63].—Increased sensation of warmth in various parts,[36].—Sensation of warmth in the stomach,[36].—Sensation of heat arising from the nape of the neck into the head,[36].—[**880.**] Sensation of heat in the lobules of the ears,[5].—Sensation of heat in face, with cold hands (after one and a half hours),[2].—Sensation of heat through whole back,[36].—When sitting, a sense of heat, and at the same time an internal quaking, proceeding from the nape of the neck and between the scapulæ, and extending as pressure in the limbs, with heat and perspiration of the forehead,[36].—Heat in the head and face,[36].—Heat of the head, hands, and feet, without thirst,[1].—Heat in the head, and a sensation as if sweat would break out, during shivering of the limbs and abdomen (after three hours),[1].—Heat in the occiput,[36].—Heat in the face, with increased redness (after ten minutes),[30].—Heat in the hands,[36].—[**890.**] Creeping heat in back,[36].—*Sweat.* Moist skin of whole body and face,[3].—After one and a half or two hours, skin began to grow moist. Next morning awoke miserably weak, the sweat having penetrated to the lower side of the featherbed, and shirt and clothes drenched,[47].—Some inclination to perspire, on slight exertion in cool rainy weather,[36].—More perspiration than usual,[32].— Copious perspiration,[33].—Perspiration profuse during the whole day,[28].— General warm perspiration,[36].—Cold perspiration, especially on forehead and chest (after twelve minutes),[38].—Perspires greatly during sleep,[51].— [**900.**] Sweat from smelling camphor,[19].—Profuse sweat (for one and a half hours),[51].—Profuse sweat for several hours after taking,[30].—Profuse sweat for some hours, and awaking weak and exhausted,[51].—Profuse sweat relieved the symptoms (after one and a half hours),[45].—Warm sweat over the whole body,[1].—*Cold sweat*,[1].—Cold sweat when beginning to vomit, especially on the face,[6].—Profuse cold sweat,[20].—Clammy sweat breaking out over body (after two hours),[57].—[**910.**] Cold sweating of head,[68].—Warm sweat on the forehead and palms of the hands,[1].—Warm perspiration on forehead (after one and a half hours),[40].—Perspiration on the forehead when sitting,[36].—Perspiration in the nape of the neck when walking,[36].— Perspiration on the back when sitting,[36].—The hands perspire excessively,[36].

Conditions.—**Aggravation.**—(*Morning*), After rising, headache; on waking, headache in temples; on rising, discharge from nose; odor from mouth; nausea, etc.; stitch in hepatic region; on rising and walking, pain in ankle; on waking, sensation of heat.—(*Forenoon*), Dry cough.—(*Evening*), The pains; headache over eye; when lying down, shivering, etc.; sensitiveness to cold, etc.—(*Night*), All symptoms; fearful, etc.; when alone, attacks of terror; cutting colic.—(*Dark*), All the symptoms were greatly aggravated at night and as it began to grow dark; would often be able to comfortably work through the day, and when night came would be almost raving, wretched, and disconsolate; also aggravation by taking cold; even

---

† See S. 736.

after five years this was more or less the case; never goes into the cellar alone at night, but will go with his little daughter, a child of only eight or nine years of age; would scarcely dare, when at the best, to stay alone in his own house over night,[49].—(*Open air*), Lachrymation.—(*Alcoholic drinks*), Toothache.—(*Coffee*), Toothache; vomiting.—(*Cold air*), Toothache.—(*Holding cold water in mouth*), Toothache.—(*In the dark*), Fear.—(*After eating*), Throbbing of heart.—(*Inspiration*), Pain in side of abdomen.—(*Leaning on the part*), Pressure in right elbow-joint.—(*Light*), The symptoms.—(*Lying down*), Pain at base of brain.—(*After lying down*), Immediately, headache; itching.—(*When lying on left side*), Trembling of left chest; stitches in region of heart, etc.—(*Motion*), Most pains; pain in nape of neck; stitches in neck; drawing in cervical vertebræ; pain in thumb-joint; *pain on the backs of the feet.*—(*Pressure*), Pain at base of brain.—(*During rest*), Pressure, etc., on side of arms; pressure, etc., in legs.—(*When sitting*), Feeling in legs; heaviness, etc., in knees; sensation in knee; pressure in knees.—(*During sleep*), Perspires greatly.—(*During morning sleep*), Headache in temples.—(*When standing*), Pain below ankle-bone.—(*On stooping*), Vertigo, etc.; pain at base of brain.—(*Touch*), Toothache.—(*Walking*), Vertigo, etc.; heaviness, etc., in forehead ; air of room seems cooler in nose; drawing in incisors; discharge of flatulence; *stitches in left chest;* drawing in muscles of upper arm; sensation in right thigh; stitches on sides of tendo Achillis; pressure in ankles; weariness of feet; yawning; internal coldness; coldness in loins, etc.; *heat of body.*—(*After walking*), Pain in thighs.—(*Writing*), Trembling in hands.

Amelioration.—(*Afternoon*), During walk in open air, dull headache.—(*Open air*), All symptoms.—(*Beer*), Toothache.—(*During coition*), Toothache ceases.—(*Drinking cold water*), Toothache.—(*Motion*), Tired feeling in arm.—(*Scratching*), Itching on hands.—(*Profuse sweat*), The symptoms.—(*Tobacco-smoking*), Toothache.

CANCER FLUVIATILIS.

Astacus fluviatilis (Cancer astacus, Linn.).   *Class*, Crustacean ; *Sub Order*, Macroura.   *Common Name*, crawfish.   *Preparation*, Tincture, prepared by pouring alcohol on the pounded living animal.

Authorities. Buchner's provings, Hygea, 17, p. 1; 1 and 2, Two men proved large doses of the tincture, repeated doses; 3, case reported by Buchner, loc. cit., of a man who ate a soup made of crabs; 4, Cloyd, Lond. Med. Gaz., 1833, quoted by Buchner, loc. cit., a man ate heartily of crabs ; 5, Seherin von Prevorst, 1, 124, from Buchner, l. c., a woman ate three spoonfuls of crab soup; 6, Hagedorn, Ephem. Nat. Cur. Ann., 3, Obs., 35, p. 99, effects of eating crabs ; 7, Petrus Rommelius, Ephem. Nat. Cur. Ann., 4, Obs., 25, p. 61, effects of eating crabs; 8, Bonetus, from Buchner, l. c., effects of eating warm crabs; 9, Plenk, Bromatologie, p. 157, from Buchner, l. c., statement of effects ; 10, Menage, Gaz. Med. de Paris, 1840, from Roth. Mat. Med.

Mind.—Slight delirium,[10].—Great apprehensiveness, and anxiety in the chest,[2].

Head.—*Confusion.* Confusion of the head,[10].—Great confusion of the head,[2].—Confusion of the forehead,[2].—Some confusion of the forehead,[1].—*General Head.* Inflammation of the head, neck, and chest, with efflorescence of red serous blotches ("maculis rubicundis serosisque"), relieved after a time by sweating,[6].—Excessive pain in the head, caused by the violent sneezing,[7].—Headache extends towards the occiput, but is especially felt in the right temple and about the ear,[2].—[10.] Headache, with pressure to the eyes,[3].—*Forehead.* Pressure on the forehead,[2].—Pressure, confusion of the forehead, about noon,[1].—Constant pressure in the forehead, with frequent yawning,[2].—*Temples.* Pressure in the temples and forehead, after 10 A.M.,[1].

Eye.—Pressure in the upper part of the right eye,[1].—Eyelids swollen,[10]. —Conjunctiva somewhat injected, and decidedly yellow,[1].—Lachrymation,[3].—Pupils dilated,[3].—[20.] Dimness of vision,[1].

Ear.—Sensation in the right ear as if a foreign body were lodged in the meatus, and caused some deafness,[2].—Dragging in the ears from within outward, about 4 P.M., lasting five minutes,[1].—Sticking in the right internal ear, lasting six hours, which changed to a dull pain (after two hours),[1].

Nose.—Frequent spasmodic sneezing,[7].—Slight and sudden discharge from the nose, as in a slight catarrh,[2].—Nose-bleed, repeated daily for a week,[3].—Bleeding of nose toward morning, with relief,[3].

Face.—Puffy face,[3].—Face red, puffy,[10].—[30.] Redness and increased warmth of the face, the whole afternoon, with burning in the left cheek, heat and redness of the ears,[1].—Burning of the face,[1].

Mouth.—Violent dull toothache in a carious tooth, in the afternoon,[2]. —Drawing pains in the teeth, soon followed by sticking in the right ear,[1].— Pressive pain in the tongue, in the pharynx, and in the region of the stomach,[2].—Sweetish taste in the mouth, after coughing,[1].—Continually dumb until the crabs had been vomited,[8].

Throat.—Scraping sensation in the throat, with constant irritation to cough, and tickling in the larynx, the whole day,[1].—Rawness of the throat caused frequent hawking,[1].

Stomach. Appetite diminished,[2].—[40.] Eructations and increased warmth in the pit of the stomach; nausea,[2].—Nausea,[6].—Vomiting of the contents of the stomach, almost without exertion, without nausea, with good appetite, followed immediately by great longing for food; this vomiting took place at the time when he was passing the fatty substance from the bowels, and it persisted during the last ten mouths of his life,[4].†— Sour vomiting after smoking at 5 P.M.,[1].—Stomach empty and sensitive,[2]. —Great heaviness in the stomach,[5].—Violent pains in the epigastric region, especially in the duodenum,[4].—Burning in the pit of the stomach, followed by urging in the anus,[2].—Great oppression deep in the epigastric region, which extended to the lower portion of the chest,[1].

Abdomen.—Hypochondria. Region of the liver was painful to severe pressure (after two hours),[1].—[50.] Uncomfortable feeling in the region of the spleen,[1].—Pressure in the region of the spleen, followed toward evening by a tension, as though the bowels were contracted,[1].—*Umbilical.* Colicky pains around umbilicus,[3].—Colic-like pains about the umbilicus, quarter of an hour after dinner, so that he was obliged to bend double, followed by a soft, at last, pasty, dark-brown stool,[1].—Colic pains about the navel,[2].—*General Abdomen.* Distension of abdomen,[3].—Abdomen distended and painful,[2].—Flatulence, with urging to stool,[2].—Painful sensation in the abdomen, the whole afternoon,[1].—Pressure in the region of

---

† The post-mortem showed a great constriction of the duodenum, so that the cavity was almost obliterated; the opening of the gall-duct into the duodenum was completely closed.

the duodenum caused constant pain,[4].—[60.] Griping in the abdomen, followed by an unsatisfactory stool, after 7 A.M.,[1].—Gripings in the bowels, with urging to stool, and weariness, about 1 P.M.,[2].—Griping and urging to stool, on every motion; relieved when sitting still,[2].—Colicky pains before and during the stool (second day),[1].—Feeling in the bowels as though he would have a painful colic, followed by griping in the left side of the lower abdomen,[1].—Prickling in the left pelvic bone,[1].— *Hypogastrium.* Griping in the left side of the lower abdomen (after two hours),[1].—Short-continuing twingings in the left side of the lower abdomen, with great weariness, after 8 P.M.,[1].

Stool.—Diarrhœa. A second stool at 10 P.M. (the one in the morning had not afforded him relief),[1].—A pasty stool at 5 A.M.,[1].—[70.] Soft, somewhat slimy stool, after eating, followed by scraping in the rectum,[1].—Stool yellowish, consistent, afterwards pasty and offensive, with relief of the colic,[2].—Stool darker than usual,[1].—After some months, passage of a fatty substance from the bowels, looking like melted fat, and after being cold, of the consistence of butter; this substance floated on water, melted in a moderate warmth, and was extremely inflammable, generally was separated from the fæces, sometimes mixed with them, usually of a dark color, sometimes light, but always yellow; at the time this substance was passed the stool had a dark color, but never the color of healthy bile; after the fatty substance ceased to pass the stool became again as white as before,[4].— *Constipation.* No stool the whole day (fourth day),[1].—Stool unsatisfactory, with much urging,[1].—Stool scanty, crumbly, passed with much urging,[1].

Urinary Organs.—Pressure in the region of the bladder, with sensation of heaviness in it,[1].—Twitching below the right kidney,[1].—Drawings along the right ureter,[1].—[80.] Urine bright yellow, slightly acid,[2].—Urine golden yellow, at first not acid, but afterwards slightly acid; with light flakes floating in it (when boiled it frothed a great deal, and when somewhat evaporated, showed much albumen),[2].†—Urine dark yellow, with sediment,[2].

Respiratory Apparatus.—Larynx and Bronchi. Much hawking of mucus,[2].—Irritation to cough in the larynx,[1].—Tickling in the larynx, low down, which caused coughing,[1].—Accumulation of mucus in the bronchi and larynx, which seemed to be adherent,[2].—Oppression and difficult breathing in the bronchial tubes,[2].— *Cough and Expectoration.* Much coughing, without expectoration, in the forenoon, especially about 11,[1].—Cough followed by hawking, in order to loosen mucus, which was light yellow,[1].—[90.] Cough in the morning, with expectoration of bronchial mucus, which was light yellow, through the day, with rawness of the chest,[1].—Cough worse after 3 P.M., so that the chest became painful, with expectoration like saliva, or like white mucus,[1].—The cough did not trouble him while walking, but as soon as he sat down it returned,[1].—Expectoration had a sweetish flat taste, late in the evening,[1].—Hæmoptysis and consumption,[9].— *Respiration.* Respiration more difficult than usual,[1].

Chest.—Rush of blood to the chest, with difficult breathing and spitting of blood,[2].—Oppression of the chest,[1].—Pressive pain in the whole sternum, on waking in the morning,[2].—Slight sticking in the left side of the breast, beneath the nipple,[2].

---

† Translated literally !—A.

Heart and Pulse.—[100.] Pulse 80 (first day), pulse 50 (second morning), pulse 80 (second day, about 2 P.M.),[2].

Neck and Back.—Sudden tearing from the right lumbar region to the kidney, while sitting,[1].

Extremities in General.—Obliged to move the limbs back and forth involuntarily, for it seemed as though she could only digest while doing so; continued half an hour, till digestion was better,[5].

Superior Extremities.—Jerking in the upper extremities, at 6 P.M.,[1].—Weariness of the arms,[1].—Sensation of trembling in the arm upon which he was resting,[1].—Crawling in the arms, with trembling of the hands,[1].—Pressure and tension in the shoulder-joints and deltoid muscles,[2]. —Pressure and heaviness in the bends of the elbows,[2].—Jerklike drawings in the left forearm,[1].—[110.] Trembling of the left hand, while holding a book,[1].—Tearing and sticking in the middle of the thumb, for a short time, early in the morning, immediately after waking,[1].

Inferior Extremities.—Burning on the anterior surface of the left leg, while walking, as from an acid, so that he was frightened, and examined it with his hand,[1].

General Symptoms.—Languor,[3].—Weariness, prostration (after two hours),[2].—Prostration (in two provers),[3].—Great prostration,[10 7].—Pains in various parts of the body, like rheumatic pains, now in the right clavicle, now in the left arm,[1].—Slight tension, extending from the nose downward to the forepart of the feet,[2].—Sticking pains continued till next evening,[3].

Skin.—[120.] Skin red from severe itching,[3].—Jaundice for several months; the urine, saliva, tears, mucus in the nose, and serum of the blood contained a large quantity of bile, but not the slightest amount passed through the intestines; the stools were constantly as white as pipe-clay,[4].— Violent attack of urticaria, with hepatitis, followed by jaundice,[4].—Red, itching urticaria all over,[10].—Urticaria developed on chest, back, arms, inner surface of thighs, under the knees; the large spots were elevated, with red areolæ; was obliged to scratch, so that, after four hours, these places seemed puffed up,[3].—Itching on the neck, about 6 P.M., with continued heat and redness of the face,[1].—Violent itching on neck,[3].

Sleep and Dreams.—Condition of sopor, in the evening,[2].—At night, restless sleep, frequently interrupted, full of lascivious dreams, with increased temperature of the skin,[1].—Waking in the morning, earlier than usual,[1].—[130.] Waking at night, with sweat, especially on the abdomen,[2].

Fever.—**Chilliness.** Shivering,[1 10].—Chilliness over the whole body, in the evening, especially sensitive below the axillæ,[2].—Creeping coldness of the body twice (after two hours),[1].—Shivering in the upper extremities about 6½ P.M.,[1].—**Heat.** Feverishness,[3].—Increased warmth of the body (after two hours),[1].—Increased warmth over the whole body, in the evening,[2].—Severe orgasm of blood,[5].—Heat and redness of face,[3].—**Sweat.** [140.] Sweating easily,[3].—Sweat breaks out easily, at night,[3].

Conditions.—**Aggravation.**—(*Morning*), Cough; on waking, pain in sternum; early, immediately after waking, tearing, etc., in thumb.—(*Forenoon*), About 11 o'clock, cough.—(*About noon*), Pressure, etc., on forehead. —(*Afternoon*), Redness, etc., of face; toothache; painful sensation in abdomen; after 3 o'clock, cough; about 6 o'clock, itching on neck, etc.; about 6.30 o'clock, shivering in upper extremities.—(*Evening*), Sweetish-flat taste of expectoration; sopor; chilliness; warmth.—(*Night*), Sweat breaks out easily.—(*After coughing*), Sweetish taste in mouth.—(*After eating*), Soft stool.—(*On motion*), Griping, etc.—(*While sitting*), Tearing from loins to kidneys.—(*On sitting down*), Cough returned.—(*After smoking*), Sour vomiting.—(*While walking*), Burning on leg.

Amelioration.—(*Sitting still*), Griping, etc.—(*Sweating*), Inflammation of head, etc.

CANCHALAGUA.

Erythræa chironioides, Griesb.† *Nat. order*, Gentianaceæ. *Common name* (Californian), Canchalagua. *Preparation*, Tincture of the whole plant when in flower.

Authority. Dr. Richter, proving with the tincture, N. Am. J. of Hom., 3, 532.

Head.—Head feels congested.—Pressive pains in forehead.—Fulness, tightness of scalp; it feels as if drawn together by india-rubber.

Eye.—Burning in the eyes, first in the left, and then in the right.

Ear.—Slight pain in the ears.—Piercing or stitches in the ears.—Increased buzzing and roaring.

Mouth.—Spitting of white mucus, with trembling and nervousness.

Stomach.—Increase of appetite.—[10.] Ructus.—Regurgitations.—Waterbrash.

Abdomen.—Flatus.—Slight pain, relieved by pressure.

Stool.—Several loose stools a day.—*Constipation.*—Hard, knotty morning stool.

Chest.—Alleviating a catarrh, produced by influenza.

General Symptoms.—That kind of pain in head and fingers which is concomitant with the attacks of intermittent fever.

Sleep and Dreams.—[20.] Sleeplessness (from 1st trit.).

Fever.—Chills repeatedly, down the spine, and all over, especially in bed, at night.—Heat in whole body; I could bear, after the proving, the cool trade-wind, usually setting in, in San Francisco, in the afternoon, better than before.

Conditions.—Aggravation.—(*Morning*), Hard stool.—(*Night*), In bed, chills.

Amelioration.—(*Pressure*), Pain in abdomen.

CANNA.

Canna glauca, Linn. *Nat. order*, Cannaceæ. *Common* (Brazilian) *name*, Imbiri. *Preparation*, Tincture of the leaves (Mure).

Authority. Mure, Pathogenesie Brasilienne (under the name of Canna "angustifolia").

Vertigo on waking.—Weakness of sight.—Roughness in the throat.—Heat at the anus.—Constipation.—Excited sexual desire.—Too speedy ejaculation of semen, without pleasure.—Whitish expectoration in the morning.—Tired feeling in chest.—[10.] Pain in chest.—Swelling of the fingers.—Lancinations in the feet, legs, and hands.—Numbness at the in-

---

† This plant is figured in the U. S. Report on the Mexican Boundary, Botany, Tab. XLII. The same name is applied in South America to Erythræa Chilensis, but the plant above mentioned was doubtless gathered by our authority, as it is in common use in California as a domestic remedy, and popularly known as "Canchalagua."

step.—Desquamation of the skin.—Itching of the skin.—Dreams about the doctor, treatment.—Heat at the ears.

Conditions.—**Aggravation.**--(*Morning*), Whitish expectoration.— (*On waking*), Vertigo.

CANNABIS INDICA.

The East Indian Cannabis sativa, Linn. *Nat. order*, Cannabineæ. *Common names*, Hashish, or Bhang, or Ganja, or Birmingi. (The best variety is that grown in India at an elevation of 6 to 10,000 feet.) *Preparation*, Tincture of the young leaves and twigs.

Authorities. 1, Provings, published by the American Provers' Union, Philadelphia, 1839, obtained by Drs. Cowley, Coxe, Jr., Dubs, Musgrave, Neidhard, Pfeifer, Shaw, and Wolfe, from the tincture, 1st and 3d dec. dil. (no daybooks nor references to individuals furnished) ; 2, proving of W. A. D. Pierce with 3 grains of "Squire's" extract, reported by Dr. Gardiner, Am. Hom. Rev., 3, 411 (and republished in Am. J. of Hom. M. M., New Series, 1, 11) ; 3, G. M. Pease, M.D., N. E. Med. Gaz., 1, 204, experiments on self and some thirty friends, including two ladies, with 6 to 56 grains of extract ; 4, Lembke, Z. f. Hom. Kl., 4, 155, proving with 15 to 50 drops of the tincture ; 5, Norton's provings, B. J. of Hom., 17, 465, 15 drops of tincture ; 6, Dr. J. S. Linsley (of New York), provings on three persons, MSS. ; 7, symptoms from Mure, Pathogenesie Brasilienne ; 8, E. W. Berridge (seven provings), Hahn. Month., 3, 461, proving with 60 minims of tincture ; 9, ibid., 1 dr., *with* 1 *dr. spts. ammon. aromat.* ; 10, ibid., 5 grains of extract ; 11, ibid., 1 dr. of tincture ; 12, ibid., 1 dr. and 10 minims ; 13, ibid., 1 and 2 drs. of tincture ; 14, ibid., 1 dr. of tincture ; 15, E. W. Berridge, M.D., M. Hom. Rev., 13, 726, proving with 2 grains of extract ; 16, omitted ; 17, effects of Hashish, from " Hashish-Eater ;" detailed extracts from this work are given, and also the very clear and concise notes of Dr. P. P. Wells, in Am. Hom. Rev., vol. 3, in order to exhibit the prominent features of the ever-varying effects of the drug ; 18, Bayard Taylor, extracted from the monograph of the American Provers' Union ; 19, Dr. Daditi, effects of $1\frac{1}{2}$ grains of extract, repeated in half an hour, N. Am. J. of Hom., 14, 136 ; 20, Heinrich, experiments with 10 grains of "Birmingi" (see Z. f. Ver. Oest., 2, 306) ; 21, Bigler, Z. f. Hom. Kl., 1, 116, general statement of effects ; 22, Hirschel's Archiv, 2, 70, effects of 4 grains ; 23, All. Hom. Zeit., 49, 88 (Med. Times, 1854), effects of 20 to 30 drops of tincture ; 24, Sonnenberg, Prag. Med. Monats, general statement ; 25, M. Muquet, L'Art Med., 38, 308, general statement ; 26, Urquhart, in " Pillars of Hercules," N. Am. J. of Hom., 10, 343, effects of preparation called " Majorim " (prepared with spices) ; 27, Carl Bower, Am. Druggists' Circular (B. J. of Hom., 22, 514), effects of 5 grains ; 28, Th. Gautier, effects, quoted in L. and Ed. M. J., 5, 695 ; 29, O'Shaughnessey, general statement, L. and E. M. J., 1, 57, also effects on Hindoos, quoted by Christison, Inaug. Dis. ; 30, Editor of L. and E. M. J., effects on himself ; 31, Williams, L. and E. M. J., 3, 949, general statement ; 32, Perry, L. and E. M. J., 3, 949, effects on self and others ; 33, Christison, Inaug. Dis. (L. and E. M. J., 13, 26), effects on self, 1 to 4 grains ; 34, ibid., effects of 2 grains on a friend ; 35, ibid., effects of 3 grains ; 36, ibid., effects of small doses of tincture on a young lady ; 37, on a porter, L. and E. M. J., 13, 26, effects of 1 grain in chronic asthma ; 38, Dr. J. Gardner, L. and E. M. J., 14, 270, effects of 3 grains of extract on three men; 39, Polli, N. Y. J. of Hom., 2, 362, from Trans. of St. Andrew's Med. Grad.; 40, Dawameski, ibid., effects of 15 grains of extract; 41, Dr. S. A. Jones, N. Y. J. of Hom., 2, 368, effects of 10 grains; 42, Olearius, transferred from Hahnemann's résumé of Cannabis sat.; 43, proving of W. A. D. Pierce with the 30th, Am. J. of Hom. M. M., N. S., 1, 51; 44, ibid., provings with 1, 2, and 3 grains of Squire's extract; 45, ibid., proving with the 5000th of Fincke.

Mind.—Emotional. Excitement,[23].—Very excited; he began dancing about the room; frequently laughing; talked nonsense; knew that he was talking nonsense, but could not stop without an effort of the will, which he did not care to make,[8].—Easily excited and irritated, in the afternoon,[1].—He shouts, leaps into the air, and claps his hands for joy,[17].— He sings, and extemporizes both words and music,[17].—On becoming conscious, he finds himself dancing, laughing, and singing before a looking-glass,[1].—**Incoherent talking**,[1].—Tendency to blaspheme,[1].—Every now and then speaks uncontrollably loud, and then corrects himself (after three hours),[5].—**[10.]** While visiting patients, have great difficulty to refrain from saying or doing unusual things,[5].—Had a distinct sensation that he must keep himself sober till he got to bed, otherwise he might do something foolish,[8].—Accents the last syllable in all his words, and laughs immoderately,[1].—Quickness of ideas and pleasant sensations,[30].—Constant succession of new ideas, each one of which was almost instantly forgotten,[33].—Rapid succession of unassociated ideas, and impossibility to follow a train of thought (after one hour),[33].—The flow of ideas was very rapid; though early, it seemed to him that it was very late in the day; the fantasies continued through the night and prevented sleep,[20].—*His mind is filled with ridiculous speculative ideas*,[1].—**Fixed ideas**,[1].—Thoughts followed one another through my head in most rapid succession; they were very vivid, but were forgotten immediately, at their very beginning,[24].—**[20.]** *Constantly theorizing*,[1].—Falls constantly into reveries,[1].—Delightful reveries came over him,[33].—He seemed to have the one idea that he should die and soon be dissected,[20].—He seemed possessed with the idea that he did not know whether he himself existed, or whether men generally existed, or for what purpose he existed,[20].—He became possessed with the idea that he was about to die, from which he cried out, " I am dying; I shall be carried to my death-chamber,"[20].—The idea that he must die returned several times, and seemed to be particularly connected with the sinking and disappearance of the pulse,[20].—Called the nurse, " for he was about to die" (after one hour),[37].—When in bed, he knew where he was, and yet did not; imagined he was at home, and could hear all the usual sounds; by a strong effort he could recollect the truth, then again relapsed (after one hour),[11]. —Looks under beds and tables, unlocks and relocks doors, for he fancies he hears strange noises, and that thieves are in the house,[1].—**[30.]** When his friends went out of the room, he thought they had left him to his fate, and wrote "cowards" in his notes,[8].—Imagines men are bribed to kill him,[1].—He thinks he can fly through the air like the birds,[17].—Said "he had been transported to heaven," and his language, usually commonplace, became quite enthusiastic (after one hour),[37].—All around and within seems to be a great mystery, and is terrifying,[17].—Despair, and fear of being eternally lost. On hearing the name of God, he cried, "Stop! that name is terrible to me; I cannot bear it. I am dying." Now demoniac shapes clutched at him from the darkness, cloaked from head to foot in inky palls, glaring at him with fiery eyes from beneath their cowls. He seemed to be walking in a vast arena, encircled by tremendous walls. The stars seemed to look upon him with pitying human aspect, and to bewail his condition,[17].—The sun seemed reeling from his place, and the clouds danced around him like a chorus,[17].—"I could trace the circulation of the blood along each inch of its progress. I knew when every valve opened and shut. The beating of my heart was so clearly audible that I wondered it was not heard by others,"[17].—Violent ecstasies of pleasure or agonies of terror and pain are constantly followed by more gentle and quiet forms of delirious excitement or hallucination,[17].—He seems possessed of a dual existence, one of which from a height watches the other, while it passes through the various phases of the Hashish delirium,[17].—[40.] Had a feeling of duality. One of his minds would be thinking of something, while the other would laugh at it. Quick transition of the ideas of one mind to the other,[3].—Felt as if he was a third person, looking at himself and his friend (after one hour),[11].—The soul seemed to be separated from the body, and to look down upon it, and view all the motions of the vital processes, and to be able to pass and repass through the solid walls of the room, and to view the landscape beyond,[17].—Extreme apparent protraction of time (second day),[33].—Extreme exaggerations of the duration of time and extent of space—a few seconds seem ages—the utterance of a word seems as long as a whole drama, and a few rods are a distance which can never be passed, it is so great. The room expands, and those around the centre-table near recede to vast distances, and the ceiling is raised, and he is in a vast hall,[17].—When his friends had gone, he went into the bedroom; stood in a reverie, which seemed to last three or four hours, looking through the half-opened door into the sitting-room. The sitting-room seemed to be of an immense depth below him (it was really on the same floor),[8].—Attention principally occupied by an hallucination that *time was indefinitely prolonged*. Seemed to himself to have sat there for hours, and when he tried to think *why* he did so, nearly lost control over his reason, and a rapid whirl of confused and irrelevant thoughts prevented his fixing attention on any one point for a moment, and it was only the effort of checking himself when falling which recalled him to himself, and then he suddenly recollected "*Cannabis Indica*"—but when did he take it? Surely it was yesterday, last week, days ago. On summoning his servant, it seemed a few weeks before he came,[15].—His calculation of the time he enjoyed the dreams was about three hundred years, the fact being that only a quarter of an hour had elapsed,[28].—When writing these notes, time seemed prolonged; he seemed to dream between each stroke of the pencil,[8].—His friends seemed gone out of the room a long time,[8].—[50.] Among the first effects was noticed that the letter or number which had just been written seemed like something that had long since been accomplished,[24].—Minutes seem to be days,[19].—The length of time occupied in urinating seemed days instead of seconds (after four hours),[3].—Only ten minutes had elapsed, and he thought at least hours had gone by,[3].—Only ten minutes had now elapsed, but it seemed to him to be two hours. His sensations were exalted and magnified; his pulse felt to him to be stronger; ideas flowed more rapidly; the pictures on the wall seemed larger than reality,[8].—He could count his pulse well; it did not seem to him to be beating slowly, though time seemed prolonged,[8].—A friend who was in the same room seemed a long way off (after one hour),[11].—Strange feeling of isolation from all around him, with great sense of loneliness, though surrounded by his friends,[17].—He imagines that he is possessed of infinite knowledge and power of vision, and then that he is Christ come to restore the world to perfect peace,[17].—He believes there is creative power in his own word, and that he has only to speak, and it will be done,[17].—[**60.**] He believes he is Daniel Webster, and omnipotent in argumentative eloquence,[17].—Then he possesses the wealth of the world, and with a benevolence equal to his wealth, showers riches on all the needy around him,[17].—It seemed as though I was transparent; the fire in the grate seemed to shine through me, and to warm the marrow of the bones. I felt the blood course in my veins, and everything within me trembled with the most extreme pleasure,[24].—His body seemed to him to become transparent, and he imagined he saw within his breast the hashish he had eaten in the form of an emerald, from which issued millions of little sparks,[28].—*Imagines he is gradually swelling, his body becoming larger and larger*,[1].—Hallucinations which lead the patient to imagine that he is on horseback, is hunting, that he sees blue water, that he is swimming, or that he is captain of a vessel, that he is travelling, that he has no weight,[25].—Illusion that he was a *pump-log*, through which a stream of hot water was playing, and threatening his friend with a wetting,[41].—Illusion that he was an inkstand, and that, as he lay on the bed, the ink might spill over the white counterpane. In the person of an inkstand he opened and shut his brass cover,—it had a hinge,—shook himself, and both saw and felt the ink splash against his glass sides, and, angry at his friends' incredulity, turned with his face towards the wall, and would not speak a word,[41].—He seems to be the subject of the strangest transformations; now he is a huge saw, and darts up and down, while planks fly off on either side of him in utter completeness; and then he is a bottle of soda-water, running to and fro; then a huge hippopotamus; then a giraffe,[17].—He seems to himself to be transformed into a vegetable existence, as a huge fern, and to be surrounded by clouds of music and perfume,[17].—[**70.**] He laughs immoderately and involuntarily at the impression that his leg was a tin case filled with stair-rods, which he hears rattle as he walks. Then suddenly the other leg seems to extend its length till he is raised some hundreds of feet into the air, and on this he is compelled to hop as he is walking with his friend,[17].—His eyelashes became indefinitely prolonged, and began to roll as gold threads upon small ivory wheels, which revolved with great velocity,[28].—His voice seems strange, as if not his own,[17].—All impressions on the senses are exceedingly exaggerated,[17].—It seemed to him as though he was upon the ridge of a mountain, that he must climb a steep ascent over the naked rock to the top of the mountain,[20].—He imagines, while walking with his friend by a small stream, that it is the Nile, and he the traveller Bruce,[17].—He thought he was in Mr. C.'s room, and recognized the pictures as belonging to him, though they were really Mr. R.'s, in whose room he was,[8].—The walls of the room are suddenly covered with dancing satyrs, and mandarins nod from all its corners,[17].—Fancies, on opening his bedroom door, that he sees numberless diabolical imps, with bloody faces and immense black eyes, which so terrify him that he sinks on his knees, a cold sweat breaks out on his body, his heart beats violently, he thinks he will suffocate, and cries loudly for help; suddenly one of the imps commences playing on a hand-organ and making such grotesque grimaces that he bursts into fits of laughter,[1].—On the wall of the room, at a great distance, a monstrous head was spiked up, which commenced a succession of grimaces of the most startling but ludicrous character. Its ferociously bearded under-jaw extended indefinitely, and then the jaw shooting back, the mouth opened from ear to ear. The nose spun out into absurd enormity, and the eyes winked with the rapidity of lightning,[17].—[**80.**] Thrown into "unbearable horror" by the falling upon him of a "shower of soot from heaven,"[17].—All the events of his past life, even those long forgotten, and those the most trivial, were thrown in symbols from a rapidly revolving wheel, each of which was recognized as an act of his life, and each came in the order of sequence the act it indicated occupied in history,[17].—He has ludicrous visions of old and wrinkled females, who are found to be composed of knit yarn,[17].—Illusions of the senses. He hears voices, and the most sublime music. He sees visions of beauty and glory that can only be equalled in Paradise. Landscapes of sublimest beauty, with profusion of flowers of most brilliant colors, in contrast, to afford the greatest delight. Architecture of magnificent beauty and grandeur, and all giving a consciousness of happiness for the time, without mixture,[17].— Vision of a silent army passed him in the street, in the evening, when walking,[17].—When walking in the open air, the plain is suddenly expanded and covered with a band of Tartars, who rush along in mad haste, their caps streaming with plumes and horsehair,[17].—While walking in the street, the houses suddenly become movable and take to nodding, bowing, and dancing in the most remarkable manner,[17].—His familiar acquaintance is mistaken for a Chinese mandarin,[17].—When walking in the street, he suddenly sees the muffled figure of a man start from the wall. His appearance is such as to excite the utmost horror. "Every lineament of his face was stamped with the records of a life black with damning crime. It glared on me with a ferocious wickedness and a stony despair. I seemed to grow blasphemous in looking at him, and in an agony of fear turned to run away,"[17].—Suddenly awoke, after midnight, and found himself in a realm of the most perfect clarity of view, yet terrible with an infinitude of demoniac shadows. Beside the bed, in the centre of the room, stood a bier, from whose corners drooped the folds of a heavy pall, and on it a fearful corpse, whose livid face was distorted with the pangs of assassination. Every muscle was tense, the finger-nails pierced the dead man's palm by the force of his dying clench. Two tapers at the head and two at the feet made the ghastliness of the bier more luminously unearthly, and a smothered laugh of derision from some invisible watcher mocked the corpse, as if triumphant demons were exulting over their prey,[17].—[**90.**] "Then the walls of the room began slowly to glide together, the ceiling coming down, the floor ascending, like the captive's cell which was doomed to be his tomb. Nearer and nearer I was borne toward the corpse. I shrunk back; I tried to cry out, but speech was paralyzed. The walls came closer and closer. Presently my hand lay on the dead man's forehead. I was stifled in the breathless niche, which was all the space still left to me. The stony eyes stared up into mine, and again the maddening peal of fiendish laughter rang close beside my ear. Now I was touched on all sides by the walls of the terrible press; then came a heavy crush, and I felt all sense blotted out in darkness,"[17].—"I awakened; the corpse was gone, but I had taken its place on the bier. The room had now grown into a gigantic hall, whose roof was framed of iron arches. Pavement, walls, cornice were all iron, and a thrill from them seemed to say this iron is a tearless fiend. I suffered from the vision of that iron as from the presence of a giant assassin. Then there emerged from the sulphurous twilight the most horrible form—a fiend, also of iron, white-hot, and dazzling with the glory of the nether penetralia. A face that was the incarnation of all malice and irony looked on me with a glare, withering from its intense heat, but more from the wickedness it symbolized. Beside him another demon rocked a cradle framed of bars of iron, and candescent with a heat fierce as the fiends. And now a chant of blasphemy, so fearful that no human thought has ever conceived of it, from the demons, till I grew intensely wicked by hearing it. The music accorded with the thought, and with its clangor mixed the maddening creak of the forever oscillating cradle, until I felt driven to a ferocious despair. Suddenly, the nearest fiend thrust a pitchfork of white-hot iron into my side, and hurled me into the fiery cradle. I lay unconsumed, tossing from side to side by rocking of the fiery engine, and still the chant of blasphemy, and the eyes of demoniac sarcasm smiled at me in mockery. 'Let us sing to him,' said one of the fiends, 'the lullaby of hell!'"[17].—"Withered like a leaf in the breath of an oven, after millions of years, I felt myself tossed on the iron floor. Presently, I was in a colossal square, and surrounded by houses a hundred stories high. With bitter thirst, I ran to a fountain carved in iron, every jet of which was sculptured in mockery of water, and yet as dry as the ashes of a furnace. I called for water, when every sash in all the hundred stories of that square flew up, and a maniac stood at every window. They gnashed at me, glared, gibbered, howled, laughed, horribly hissed, and cursed. Then I became insane at the sight, and leaping up and down, mimicked them all,"[17].—From zenith to horizon an awful angel of midnight blackness floated. His face looked unutterable terrors into me, and his dreadful hands half-clenched above my head, as if waiting to take me by the hair. Across the firmament a chariot came like lightning, with wheels like rainbow suns. At its approach, the sable angel turned and rushed down into the horizon, that seemed to smoke as he slid through it, and I was saved,[17].—The scene then became theatrical, and he an actor, who improvised his tragedy and held his immense audience entranced. Suddenly, a look of suspicion came over every face. "I sought relief by turning from the pit to the boxes. The same stony glance met me still. Oh! they knew my secret, and at that instant one maddening chorus broke from the whole theatre, 'Hashish! Hashish! He has eaten Hashish!' I crept from the stage in unutterable shame. I crouched in concealment. I looked at my garments, and beheld them foul and ragged as a beggar's. From head to foot I was the incarnation of squalidity. My asylum proved on the pavement of a great city's principal thoroughfare. Children pointed at me; loungers stood and searched me with inquisitive scorn. The multitude of man and beast all eyed me; the very stones in the street mocked me with a human raillery as I cowered against a side wall in my bemired rags,"[17].—*Imagines some one calls him*,[1].—He hears music of the sweetest and sublimest melody and harmony, and sees venerable bards with their harps, who play as if it were the music of heaven,[17].—In music, a single tone seemed like the most divine harmony,[24].—**Imagines he hears music; shuts his eyes, and is lost for some time in the most delicious thoughts and dreams**,[1].—*He fancies he hears numberless bells ringing most sweetly*,[1].—[100.] For fully two weeks after, when sitting in his office, in quiet summer afternoons, reading desultorily, he would hear most magnificent harmony, as if some master-hand were playing an organ, and using only the softer stops. There was this peculiarity about the hearing of the music, namely, one must be in a state of half reverie, and then the divine strains, soft and marvellously sweet, followed one another in a smoother legato than any human fingering ever accomplished. If one roused the attention and strained the ear, as if to be sure of catching every chord, *silence came at once,*[41].—Heard the noise of colors, green, red, blue, and yellow sounds coming to him in perfectly distinct waves,[28].—After such experience of ecstasy as has already been described, when just emerging from a dense wood, he heard a hissing whisper, "Kill thyself! Kill thyself!" "I turned to see who spoke. No one was visible. The whisper was repeated with intenser earnestness; and now unseen tongues repeated it on all sides and in the air above me, 'The Most High commands thee to kill thyself.' I drew forth my knife, opened it, and placed it at my throat, when I felt the blow of some invisible hand strike my arm; my hand flew back at the force of the shock, and the knife went spinning into the bushes. The whispers ceased,"[17].—In his first experiment, the sensations it produced were those, physically, of exquisite lightness and airiness; mentally, of a wonderfully keen perception of the ludicrous in the most simple and familiar objects,[18].—Objects by which he was surrounded assumed such a strange and whimsical expression, became in themselves so inexpressibly absurd and comical, that he was provoked into a long fit of laughter. The hallucination died away as gradually as it came, leaving him overcome with a soft pleasant drowsiness, from which he sank into a deep refreshing sleep,[18].—In his second experiment, the same fine nervous thrill (that he experienced in his first experiment) suddenly shot through him. But this time it was accompanied by a burning sensation at the pit of the stomach, and instead of growing upon him with a gradual pace of healthy slumber, and resolving him, as before, into air, it came with the intensity of a pang, and shot throbbing along the nerves to the extremities of his body. It seemed to him as if he existed without form throughout a vast extent of space. His whole body seemed to expand, and the arch of his skull to be broader than the vault of heaven. His sensations presented themselves to him in a double form; one physical, and therefore, to a certain extent, tangible, and the other spiritual, and revealing itself in a succession of splendid metaphors. His physical feeling of being was accompanied by an image of an exploding meteor, not subsiding into darkness, but continuing to shoot from its centre or nucleus, which corresponded to the burning spot at the pit of his stomach, incessant coruscations of light, that finally lost themselves in the infinity of space. His mind was crowded with a succession of visions, but all ending in the ludicrous,[18].—While he was most completely under the influence of the drug, he was perfectly conscious that he sat in the tower of Antonio's hotel, in Damascus, knew that he had taken Hashish, and that the strange, gorgeous, and ludicrous fancies which possessed him were the effects of it,[18].—He was conscious of two distinct conditions of being in the same moment, of which neither conflicted with the other. His enjoyment of the visions was complete and absolute, undisturbed by the faintest doubts of their reality; while, in some other chamber of his brain, reason sat coolly watching them, and heaping the liveliest ridicule on their fantastic features,[18].—One set of nerves was thrilled with the bliss of the gods, while another was convulsed with unquenchable laughter at that very bliss. His highest ecstasies could not bear down and silence the weight of his ridicule, which, in its turn, was powerless to prevent him from running into other and more gorgeous absurdities. After awhile the visions became more grotesque than ever, but less agreeable; and there was a painful tension throughout his nervous system. He laughed until his eyes overflowed profusely; every drop that fell immediately became a large loaf of bread, and tumbled upon the shopboard of a baker in the bazaar at Damascus. The more he laughed, the faster the loaves fell, until such a pile was raised about the baker that he could hardly see the top of his head,[18].—A fierce and furious heat radiated from the stomach throughout his system; his mouth and throat were as hard as though made of brass, and his tongue, it seemed to him, was a bar of rusty iron. Although he seized a pitcher of water and drank long and deeply, his palate and throat gave no intelligence of his having drunk at all,[18].—[110.] About midnight his excited blood rushed through his frame with a sound like the roaring of mighty waters. It was projected into his eyes until he could no longer see; it beat thickly on his ears, and so throbbed on his heart, that he feared the ribs would give way under its blows. He tore open his vest, placed his hand over the spot, and tried to count the pulsations; but there were two hearts, one beating at the rate of a thousand beats a minute, and the other with a slow, dull motion. His throat he thought was filled to the brim with blood, and streams of blood were pouring from his ears. After the visions were over, there arose a sensation of distress, which was more severe than pain itself,[18]. —His throat was as dry as a potsherd, and his stiffened tongue cleaved to the roof of his mouth,[18].—About 3 o'clock the next morning, rather more than five hours after the Hashish had been taken, he sunk into a stupor. All the following day and night he lay in a state of blank oblivion, broken only by a single wavering gleam of consciousness,[18].—He arose, attempted to dress himself, drank two cups of coffee, and then fell back into the same deathlike stupor,[18].—On the morning of the second day, after a sleep of thirty hours, he awoke again to the world, with a system utterly prostrate and unstrung, and a brain clouded with the lingering images of his visions,[18]. —There was no taste in what he ate, no refreshment in what he drank, and it required a painful effort to comprehend what was said to him, and return a coherent answer,[18].—After drinking a glass of very acid sherbet, he experienced instant relief of these symptoms. The spell was not wholly broken, and for two or three days he continued subject to frequent involuntary fits of absence of mind,[18].—The ruling hallucination of one of his companions was that he was a locomotive,[18].—In about an hour and a half after taking I perceived a heaviness of the head, wandering of the mind, and apprehension that I was going to faint. I thence passed into a state of half-trance, from which I awoke suddenly and much refreshed. The impression was that of wandering out of myself; I had two beings, and there were two distinct, yet concurrent trains of ideas. Images came floating before me; not the figures of a dream, but those that seem to play before the eye when it is closed; and with those figures were strangely mixed the sounds of a guitar that was being played in an adjoining room; the sounds seemed to cluster in and pass away with the figures in the retina. The music of the wretched performance was heavenly, and seemed to proceed from a full orchestra, and to be reverberated through long halls of mountains. These figures and sounds were again connected with metaphysical reflections, which, also, like the sounds, clustered themselves into trains of thought, which seemed to take form before my eyes, and weave themselves with the colors and sounds. I was following a train of reasoning; new points would occur, and concurrently there was a figure before me throwing out corresponding shoots, like a zinc tree; and then, as the moving figures reappeared, or as the sounds caught my ear, the other classes of figures came out distinctly, and danced through each other. The reasonings were long and elaborate, and though the impression of having gone through them remains, every effort has been in vain to recall them.

The following scene was described by me, and taken down at the time : A general commanding an army, and doubting whether he should engage the enemy, consulted the oracle. The oracle answered : "Go with the fortune of Cæsar." He gave battle, and was beaten. His king ordered his head to be cut off; but the general accused the oracle. The king cried, "The oracle is not in fault; it did not tell you that you were Cæsar. You were twice a fool to mistake its meaning, and your own worth." The general answered, "Then is the fault his who sent a fool to command his armies." "Nay," answered the king, "thou shalt not twist one phrase to thy benefit, and another to my loss." This scene seemed to pass before me, and in the region of Carthage, which was all familiar, though I had never been there. The general was an Abyssinian ; the king a white man with a black beard. The next time I tried it the only effect was to make me lose a night's rest (taken toward evening). The first time (taken in the morning) it had given me a double portion of sleep; on both occasions it enormously increased my appetite. It was followed by no depression. The first time I took it at half past four, and after that a liqueur-glass of caraway spirits, to hasten the effect. I did not feel cold, while those who were walking with me, and wrapped in mantles, were complaining of it. Then came an unsteadiness of gait; not that of one who fears to fall, but of one who tries to keep down, for I felt as if there were springs in my knees, and was reminded of the story of the man with the mechanical leg, that walked away with him. I sat down to dinner at half past 6 o'clock. There was a glass between me and the rest of the company, and an inch or two interposed between me and whatever I touched. What I ate and how much did not matter; the food flowed like a river through me. There was a wind going by, blowing over the table and carrying away the sounds, and I saw the words tumbling over one another over the falls. *There was a dryness of the mouth, which was not thirst.* The dryness radiated from the back of the throat, opposite the nape of the neck. It was a patch of dark-blue color; the food, as it reached this point, pouring down, and taking the color of the patch. I was under the impression that I described all this at the time, but was told that I would not say anything about myself, or describe what I experienced. I should have been relieved if some one present had been under the same influence. The bursts of laughter to which I gave rise were not at all pleasing, except when they were excited by any observation I made which was not connected with myself. I never lost the consciousness of what was going on ; there were always present the real objects, as well as the imaginary ones; but at times I began to doubt which was which, and then I floated in strange uncertainty. It came by fits, with, I thought, hours of intervals, when only minutes could have elapsed,[26] —Their first sensations were of intense astonishment at the circumstance that they found themselves no longer masters of their own acts, while they still remained lucid witnesses of all acts, however foolish. Here the difference between alcoholic inebriation and that from Hashish is strongly marked. They saw themselves committing absurdities of the most grotesque kind ; leaping, beating time to nothing, moving their arms as if receiving electrical shocks, writing ridiculous words, and so forth, without any power on their part to prevent such exhibitions; but yet standing, as it were, independently of them, as though they were merely subjects of observation exhibited from other persons than themselves. At first they had the sensation and appearance of feigning a state of exaltation which they did not feel, and which was even feigned with so much uncertainty and awkward-

ness that any one not aiding in it would for a long time believe in its un-
reality. It is, nevertheless, an irresistible propensity,[39].—[**120.**] At one mo-
ment·the intellect is obscure, and loses itself in forgetfulness of the past;
then it returns clear, and is able to form a judgment for a moment, and
disapprove of any acts it may have before sanctioned, but only to be again
involved in that state of automatic folly which is so peculiar a phenomenon
during Hashish intoxication. During the intervals of confusion or darkness, the lucid moments possess a power and comprehension truly marvellous, so that in a few seconds the most distinct and accurate picture of a
range of life, including as much as forty years, may be recast and sur-
veyed. The alternation from obscurity to lucidity is like the effect of a
sea-wave; a lucid wave is followed by a dark overhanging wave on which
the mind is shipwrecked, and carried with the sensation of a melancholy
floating towards forgetfulness and oblivion, to be roused instantly by the
passage over it once more of the wave of life and light. The dark waves
chase each other so long as they continue, and the mind, unable to continue its thoughts and acts, but bending under a successive series of impressions, the shortest space of time seems to present the duration of an
eternity,[39].—A seeming extraordinary slowness of time, which struck the
observers in so singular a manner, and made them so impatient of delay,
that they were continually recurring to their watches, and observing, with
a kind of awe, how minutes were transformed into epochs. With this apparently interminable length of time, there seemed to occur a kind of forgetfulness, by which an act of the mind, taking place an interval before,
or an impression received some time before, were in a manner forgotten;
but, in a few brief moments they returned, or presented themselves, as it
were, for the first time and in such manner, almost unaccountably repeated
themselves, and reproduced frequently, as now, the impressions they rein-
spired,[39].—There was noticed in the observers, so different themselves ordinarily in general character and temperament, a common docility and absence of susceptibility which was most remarkable. Thus one of them gave
to another with whom he was but slightly acquainted a series of hard blows
on the back, saying that he himself felt nothing of the Hashish, and asking
whether the blows he inflicted were felt. On his part, he who received the
blows took them all in good humor, uttering no complaint, and seeming,
indeed, insusceptible of complaint. Again, one of them, who sat writing,
submitted to receive the infliction of two sharp blows, boxes on the ears,
and to have his pen snatched out of his hand, without any expression of
pain or even annoyance. Reproaches between them for having taken the
drug never passed; but each, laughing all the time, tried often, in lucid
intervals, to produce sickness. Such was the good humor that prevailed
that each one mutually yielded up his own will and obeyed the other; the
whole trio joyfully concurring in all that suggested itself to them, as with-
drawing them from the idea of danger, and fully agreeing in particulars as
to the sensations they experienced,[39].—Was seized with melancholy, from
which he could rouse himself only by imitating the movements and follies
of the others. Then he had a great inclination to laugh, but kept himself
free from the obvious action of the drug by going behind his companions.
Suddenly he perceived a change in his intellectual faculties, which appeared
less obedient to his will, and feeling he should be worse, he began to register
his thoughts of what happened to him. Scarcely had he began, than it
seemed more important to him to record the follies uttered by one of his
companions. He soon felt himself, however, unable to continue, and his

hands with difficulty traced unformed characters. Then becoming preoccupied with a scheme which scribblers might think the act of a madman,
he with great difficulty wrote a short justification of his conduct in Mil-
anese. He next began to feel a pleasing stupor; his head seemed to dilate,
but without strain, gently! gently! He possessed the use of his senses and
mind, but every occupation wearied him. He passively assisted in what
was occurring around him, and unable to give any account of it or reason,
was able to laugh at all or everything,[39].—After about a quarter of an
hour, a weakness of his whole body came on, his legs would not support
him, his arms became heavy, and he was seized with a kind of fainting
similar to that which at times follows loss of blood. He was obliged to
throw himself on the sofa, his limbs became rigid, he entirely lost his sensations, becoming cataleptic, and remained for a long time in this state.
By degrees his senses partially returned, so that he was enabled to understand and retain some directions given to him, but he became insensible
again, and when put to bed a very hot box placed at his feet, which were
very cold, produced no impression. By degrees the insensibility or anæsthesia which had pervaded his whole body relaxed in the left half of his
body, but remained perfect in the right. His consciousness, which had
never entirely left him but for a few brief moments, by degrees returned to
its natural state, so that he could recall what had occurred to him and
reflect upon his condition. Again, anæsthesia extended all over his body,
and now was added an automaton-like and rapid movement of the hands,
one hand being pressed upon the breast, and rubbed actively on the back
with the palm of the other hand; his head also ached, and he had a sensation of weakness. The anæsthesia gradually decreased, but the sensibility
did not return universally, nor steadily, there being frequent relapses. By
turns the right arm or the leg, or the right half of the face, and then all
these parts together, would seem petrified, so that he could not move them,
and would then relax. As time went on these phenomena were more frequently repeated in the head and face, the change being quick enough to
give great pain; when suddenly the mass of his brain, all except a small
portion, seemed changed to marble, and appeared to him to possess all the
properties of such a substitution; his right eye, for a long time, retained the
sensation of marbly hardness. These symptoms, now going, now returning,
lasted more than thirty-six hours. The mind, meantime, had not remained
idle, but during moments of returned consciousness assisted as a spectator;
ideas succeeded each other with such rapidity that they made a short space
of time seem very long. These ideas, although more often scattered, had
at times an intimate and long connection; thus every person who had ever
assisted him he seemed to see for years and years performing all those long
and varied series of acts, which might in reality have been performed
during such a period, so that he felt convinced that all those years had
really passed. He also had a sort of hallucination in which he seemed
transported to a place whimsically made of brass; this, he thought, was
the vestibule of Mohammed's paradise, and that he was denied entrance to
it. On going out he found himself launched into space, and compelled to
describe very rapidly a vast orbit, in a gloomy, painfully breathing, oppressive circle. This painful sensation lasted a long time, and was among
the most disagreeable of the experiment,[39].—Was a prey to extreme loquacity and mobility of ideas; was continually preoccupied with solicitous
impressions as to the fate of his companions, for whom he feared the dose
of Hashish had been excessive, and might even prove poisonous. After he

had taken the drug about six hours he was seized with a sort of gesticulatory convulsions in the arms and legs, and by degrees his symptoms assumed the appearance of those which characterize hydrophobia. He was possessed with outbreaks of fear at the sight of bright objects, at the sensation of every sharp little breath of air, or the approach of any one; but these exhibitions were momentary only, and he then paid no attention to what had been previously exciting influences. He asked for water, and seized the cup with a trembling and convulsive hand, but carried it to his lips only to thrust it away without drinking, being unable even with the greatest effort to swallow a single draught. Upon this there succeeded a feeling of uneasiness, as though from dryness of the throat, or rather a sensation that the tongue and throat were covered with a dry soft body. An urgent desire to be held, to be guided, and to be taken care of altogether, under the involuntary feeling that, if such protection were not bestowed, he should get out of bed (in which he was by this time laid) to commit some foolish act. Sensation of pressure at the back of the head, before the occurrence of convulsive movements, which changed into an unpleasant feeling of heat, then of cold, in consequence of which his hands were carried automatically to that spot, and held there, as though there were a difficulty in detaching them. There was also a sensation of cramps in the calves of the legs, which rendered the movement of the legs impossible, or caused them to be distended, or to take a sudden jump.[39].—Four hours and a half after taking I was sitting with the family, playing the guitar, when one of the tunes, a rather solemn one, seemed suddenly to assume a more melodious character; it gradually increased in grandeur bar after bar, sinking deep in my soul until I was wholly absorbed with it. The words died away and I still went on with the accompaniment; my mind carried the air, and all surrounding objects faded; I lived wholly in the music, and a deep subdued joyous feeling, such as I never before felt, pervaded my whole being. At last I came to myself somewhat, and turned to the others and remarked that it was beautiful, and asked if they did not think so. They were much surprised at the question, and said it possessed very little merit. I was now surprised in my turn and began to argue its merits, offering to play it over. At this moment a strange crawling sensation commenced in my body, it extended to my limbs, down my arms, to my fingers' ends, and up into my brain; it travelled slowly, yet so powerful was it that I was wholly overcome with surprise. I was a little alarmed at the feeling, but immediately the word "Hashish" passed through my mind. Ah! that was it, that was the enchanter that made my music sound so sweet. I was glad to find it had not failed; I was reassured; it was undoubtedly the legitimate effect of the drug. All these things were very nice, but yet the thrill was a thing I had not expected, and another and another following in close succession, I began to wish the last dose had been as ineffectual as the first. I commenced considering what was best to be done. I could not decide whether to sit still or go to my room. I tried to play, but an apparent ebullition in the air prevented me from seeing the notes; the thrills were growing stronger every moment, and I concluded I had best leave the room lest I should do something foolish. I arose abruptly, and with guitar in one hand and music-stand in the other, I sallied forth to go down stairs. No sooner did I commence to move than the thrills increased; stronger and stronger they came, closer and closer they succeeded each other, until one ceased not until an almost overwhelming thrill gave notice of another's birth. In going down stairs my mind ever and anon would wander to other matters and things, and when I recalled my thoughts to what was immediately before me I wondered to find myself still going down stairs. Then a feeling of dread uncertainty seized me, "Shall I ever reach the bottom?" I doubted that I would, yet my reason told me I was going right; so I pressed on. I put my guitar away safely and this reassured me. I say reassured, because I had begun to doubt that any of the things around me had existence, but I reasoned that I had succeeded in finding the guitar-box, and hence some things must exist, and, as I had seen one right, so it was likely all existed. Still I was uncertain that I maintained control of my faculties and motive powers; an intuitive assurance, however, made me depend on them, and I determined to go quietly upstairs to my room; I went up very quietly; indeed, I seemed not to touch the steps; I trod the air as a swimmer treads water; my feet came near the steps but did not strike them. I reached my room, but what to do now; it did not improve my condition. I determined to lie down until the thrills went off, which I thought would certainly be very soon, and then I expected other effects to follow. I threw myself on the bed, but immediately sprang to my feet again, for no sooner did I lie down than I thought of catalepsy being sometimes produced by the use of the drug; no, I must not lie down; I must keep my soul in my body by force of will, or perhaps it would never return, and I felt that it was trying to wing itself away. As the extract was strong and so small an amount had produced so great an effect, I was afraid I had taken too great a dose, and became alarmed lest it should play me foul. The thrills had now become continuous, the commencing of each being only known by an increase in their force; my heart and veins began to throb violently, the blood began to rush to my head, and I feared apoplexy. My tongue became coated with saliva, and I thought my body was dissolving into fluids. I spit from the window. I afterwards thought it was foolish for me to do so as I might jump from the window, for I felt certain I did not possess the full command of my faculties. The uncertain aspect of things now increased, with the whole force of my reason seemingly unimpaired. I could not convince myself the furniture in the room had other than an ideal existence; this feeling was so oppressive that I determined to seek the rest of the family. But how could I reach them? I was in another sphere; I had journeyed to a world whose objects I could not realize, an uncertain world whose paths I did not know. An atmosphere surrounded my little world through which I could not pass; to break through the open doorway seemed as impossible as to wing my way through the ethereal regions to the throne above. This was my station; here I must remain. A feeling of loneliness now overwhelmed me. I must seek the rest of the family. I hurled my body through the seemingly impenetrable though invisible barrier. On, on, I went, pushing my way through a resistant atmosphere, or surrounding, which was a creation of my state. I know not how to express the feeling of this existence; there is no type among natural things to which I can compare it; an ethereal fluid it seemed to be, not dense as water nor rare as air, yet it resisted, and I by force of will overcame it step by step. Here I noticed the two parts of my being acting separately; my will or spiritual existence was separate from my bodily existence, and spurring it onward, pushing it forwards and using it much as an artificer uses a tool; onward it forced my body, seeming to exult in its supremacy. I cannot say whether my feelings at this time were more oppressed or buoyant, for while my mind seemed oppressed by the appearance of the objects along my route, and fear of injury from the effect of the drug, my soul was exultant as though in a more congenial atmosphere, and glad of its partial disenthralment. I at last reached the room I sought; so long a time seemed to have elapsed since I had been last there, that I did not expect to see the family there; it was impossible for me to keep any record of time, but it seemed as though I had been a long time away, and I expected to find the room tenantless; so certain was I that this would be the case that I was surprised to see them seated as I had left them. When I saw them, for an instant I thought they were really there, but it was only for an instant; they immediately assumed the same unreal appearance which other things held. I had determined that I would say nothing about my having taken the drug to the others for fear of frightening them, though I had told them I intended to take it. I did not doubt I could control my tongue, but things about me seemed so unreal, and they were so silent, that I could not restrain myself; I must speak to them, and see if they are really here, but what should I say? I rummaged my brain for a question to ask, but could think of nothing but "Hashish." This I did not wish to speak of, but nothing else would come to my mind; I must say something, for I could bear this feeling no longer. Then my reason told me it was best that they should know I had taken the drug, as they would then know how to treat me if any dangerous symptoms occurred, so I opened my mouth and said, "I have taken Hashish." My voice appeared strange to me; it seemed as though another person spoke; I looked around; my words had made no impression on those around me; is it possible they can sit silent? I had thought they would have all sprang to their feet, so suicidal did it appear to me for one to take the drug. "I have forgotten," thought I; "they do not know the nature of the drug." I explained to them that it was the drug I had spoken to them of shortly before; I told them of its effects; how everything, even themselves, seemed unreal; that I did not feel certain that I was even in the room with them; they all looked up and smiled, and again resumed their former positions without saying a word. This was agonizing; were these only the phantoms of my friends that I had called up? "Speak to me," I cried; "speak to me, or I will go crazy. I think I see you here; I appear to be in the room with you, yet so uncertain does everything look that I cannot convince myself that it is so. Speak to me, that I may be assured that at least I am not deceived in this." Some one answered me; I heard the voice, it seemed familiar, yet it was the phantom that spoke; all was still unreal; I myself was unreal, even my voice did not seem my own. I tried to reassure myself by conversing with them. I saw they knew not how I felt. An irresistible desire to make them know how I felt now seized me; this I felt was impossible; they had now no fellow-feeling with me. I was alone; no earthly being could sympathize with me; I saw the impossibility of making them understand me, yet I must make the attempt; I told them all my feelings; they seemed to think it only imagination, and that I was only using symbols to represent them; my feelings were hurt, and I almost wept; it seemed as if they doubted my word. I now began to think over my past actions while in this state; it seemed to me a dream; I could not believe I had been upstairs, or even out of the room, no, I had fallen asleep with my guitar in my hand, and had dreamed I was upstairs. I looked for my guitar; it was not there; certainly then I must have put it away, or else I was dreaming yet; perhaps I had gone to bed at night and been dreaming all along, making a full day's work of dreaming. I became convinced that this was so, but I immediately thought

of the Hashish, which dispelled the illusion; I then asked how long I had
been absent from the room; I was answered, "About five minutes;" it had
seemed to me as many hours. I asked how I looked; was told, "pale, eyes
half-closed and dull, and my hands were cold and clammy." I now felt a
resinous matter exude from every pore of my body; it lined my mouth and
throat, creating a great thirst. I got a glass of water and drank it; it
seemed to form a continuous stream, and ran down my throat by its own
gravity without any aid from me. I became afraid to drink any more;
immediately on ceasing to drink it seemed to me that the water had formed
itself into one bolus and gone down my throat within an atmosphere of its
own, without touching either side. So everything appeared different after
I had done it from what it did while I was doing. I would sometimes
make a remark which I would think of the greatest importance, and speak
it in a very impressive manner that it might not be lost; immediately it
would be figured to me as that of another, and I would have to smile at the
foolish fellow for making so ridiculous a remark. At one time I felt constrained to let all my thoughts be known. I would think of a thing, digest
it in my mind, and then with a pompous air, would make it known to those
about me, something as follows: I was thinking of my thirst and feelings
together, and suddenly broke forth with, "This drug is acting very
strangely; it is operating upon the fluids of my body; it decomposes my
blood, throwing off the equivalents of water, the oxygen being thrown off
at the + poles, the hydrogen at the — poles, and the electricity produced by the decomposition as well as by the reunion of these gases, as they
escape through the pores in the form of perspiration, acts upon my nerves
and produces this strange feeling; my stomach is the battery, Hashish
the acid, and my nerves the conductors." My tongue seemed to be under
the control of my will, and things I thought best left unsaid I could
generally keep to myself. My ideas of the propriety of things, however,
were at times quite different from what they were in the natural state.
After pacing the room (which I did continually to assure myself I still
could move), I stopped suddenly, and turning to a sister, I told her what I
thought to be a grand discovery, clothed in the choicest language the
English tongue could admit of: "This Hashish," said I, "acts upon the
urinary glands, and I feel that could I pass water I would feel better."
This was not received as reverently as it should have been, which called
forth a lecture on propriety from me, much to the amusement of the rest.
I then began a censorship of my own conduct. I began noting my manner
of walking and talking, at one time asking if I did not look like Mr. C.,
consequential; at another, like Mr. F., a nervous individual; and again, if
I did not act like a Mr. C., a crazy man, remarking that I thought the
last-named had taken Hashish. The others now became alarmed at my
strange actions, and procured for me an emetic. I laughed at them, and
told them it was no use, I had taken the drug early in the morning. They
then brought a mixture of ether, camphor, etc.; I told them it would only
make matters worse; I took it, however, at their persuasion. It put me for
awhile in awful agony without taking away my strange feelings, and when
its first effects passed off left me extremely melancholy. I gave up hope of
coming back to my right state of mind. I asked them to send to the
doctor for an antidote, being satisfied by their answering that they would
if I grew worse. I turned my thoughts to what the doctor would say.
"What," said I, "if the doctor should say I would never recover; minutes
seem years, what an eternity of madness would there be before me then;

to know that I must die in my madness at last, how awful!" I could not bear the thought. At the suggestion of the others I went to the parlor, they thinking it would be more cheerful. As it became dark, I became more melancholy. I said that if God did not will that the antidote should be effective, it would not be effective, but if he willed it to be so, so it would be; suppose we go to God at once, instead of going for the antidote. "There is no use," said I, "of me praying, as I cannot tell whether I am talking or not; besides, God would not hear the prayer of a crazy man; you are in your right senses, one of you pray for me." We knelt down, but the prayer being on the wrong subject, I in disgust turned my thoughts to other matters, and talked of other things until supper-time. As I entered the room the light fell full upon me. How beautiful did that light appear; all my melancholy feelings at once left me; I felt a dark shadow lifted from my soul, and all was light within. The light penetrated through my body. I seemed transparent; I could almost look into my own body and see the various organs thereof, all of which seemed to me to be reflecting from their surface a calm lustre, which filled my whole soul. On turning myself to eat, I thought everything had something hurtful in it. I could not eat meat, because it had chloride of sodium on it, nor eat bread, because the butter was too strong a stimulant. Being persuaded, however, I ate a piece of meat; to do so I had to call to mind the various processes and modus operandi of "feeding." "First," I reasoned, "they put the substance in the mouth, and by moving the under jaw down and up and mixing the saliva with it by motion of the tongue, they masticate it." This was easily accomplished. The spittle seemed to have legs and arms, and I could feel it scrambling through the meat, but when it was thoroughly masticated, I could not remember, or rather could not date back to the time I put the meat in my mouth; chewing seemed to have been my regular business for some time past. It was time now to swallow it; here was a great difficulty. I could move my jaws at will, but to get command of the muscles of my throat wholly baffled all my endeavors. At last I made a sort of compromise. "They throw the bolus back on the tongue, press the tongue on the roof of the mouth, the bolus slides back, irritates the muscles of the pharynx, and down it goes." I tried this, it succeeded admirably, and I applauded myself for my good generalship. A friend called to see me after supper; I determined to keep myself rational while he remained, by force of my will, which I found I could do. At this time the sedative you sent reached me; I took it, and afterwards went to the piano and played until the thrills went off. I had perfect control of my fingers, excepting when I tried to vary a piece I knew well, in which case I could not play anything but the proper notes of the piece, my fingers being drawn to the keys either by force of custom or by tenor of the tune. The full effect of the drug did not go off for a week, and even during the next succeeding week I brought back the thrills strongly by taking hot stimulants, though they lasted but a few seconds and brought no hallucinations,[2]. —A shock, as of some unimagined vital force, shoots without warning through my entire frame, leaping to my fingers' ends, piercing my brain, startling me till I almost spring from my chair,[17].—No pain anywhere, not a twinge in any fibre, yet a cloud of unutterable strangeness was settling upon me, and wrapping me impenetrably in from all that was natural or familiar. Endeared faces, well known to me of old, surrounded me, yet they were not with me in my loneliness. I had entered upon a tremendous life which they could not share. If the disembodied ever return to hover

over the hearthstone which once had a seat for them, they look upon their friends as I then looked upon mine. A nearness of place with an infinite distance of state, a connection which had no possible sympathies for the wants of that hour of revelation, an isolation none the less perfect for seeming companionship,[17].—Yet it was not my voice which spoke; perhaps one which I once had far away in another time and another place. For awhile I knew nothing that was going on externally, and then the remembrance of the last remark which had been made returned slowly and indistinctly, as some trait of a dream will return after many days, puzzling us to say where we have been conscious of it before,[17].—[130.] A fitful wind all the evening had been sighing down the chimney; it now grew into the steady hum of a vast wheel in accelerating motion. For awhile this hum seemed to resound through all space. I was stunned by it, I was absorbed in it. Slowly the revolution of the wheel came to a stop, and its monotonous din was changed for the reverberating peal of a grand cathedral organ. The ebb and flow of its inconceivably solemn tone filled me with a grief that was more than human. I sympathized with the dirge-like cadence, as spirit sympathizes with spirit. And then, in the full conviction that all I heard and felt was real, I looked out of my isolation to see the effect of the music on my friends. Ah! we were in separate worlds indeed. Not a trace of appreciation on any face,[17].—As mechanically as an automaton I began to reply. As I heard once more the alien and unreal tones of my own voice, I became convinced that it was some one else who spoke, and in another world. I sat and listened; still the voice kept speaking. Now, for the first time, I experienced that vast change which Hashish makes in all measurements of time. The first word of the reply occupied a period sufficient for the action of a drama; the last left me in complete ignorance of any point far enough back in the past to date the commencement of the sentence. Its enunciation might have occupied years. I was not in the same life which had held me when I heard it begun. And now with time, space expanded also. At my friend's house one particular arm-chair was always reserved for me. I was sitting in it at a distance of hardly three feet from the centre-table, around which the members of the family were grouped. Rapidly that distance widened. The whole atmosphere seemed ductile, and spun endlessly out into great spaces surrounding me on every side. We were in a vast hall, of which my friends and I occupied opposite extremities. The ceiling and the walls ran upward with a gliding motion, as if vivified by a sudden force of resistless growth. Oh! I could not bear it. I should soon be left alone in the midst of an infinity of space. And now every moment increased the conviction that I was watched. I did not know then, as I learned afterwards, that suspicion of all earthly things and persons was the characteristic of the Hashish delirium,[17].—In the midst of my complicated hallucination, I could perceive that I had a dual existence. One portion of me was whirled unresistingly along the track of this tremendous experience, the other sat looking down from a height upon its double, observing, reasoning, and serenely weighing all the phenomena. This calmer being suffered with the other by sympathy, but did not lose its self-possession. Presently it warned me that I must go home, lest the growing effect of the Hashish should incite me to some act which might frighten my friends. I acknowledged the force of this remark very much as if it had been made by another person, and rose to take my leave. I advanced towards the centre-table. With every step the distance increased. I nerved myself as for a long pedestrian journey,[17].—Still the lights, the faces, the furniture receded. At last, almost unconsciously, I reached them. It would be tedious to attempt to convey the idea of time which my leave-taking consumed, and the attempt, at least, with all minds that have not passed through the same experience would be as impossible as tedious. At last I was in the street. Beyond me the view stretched endlessly away. It was an unconverging vista, whose nearest lamps seemed separated from me by leagues. I was doomed to pass through a merciless stretch of space. A soul just disenthralled, setting out for his flight beyond the farthest visible star, could not be more overwhelmed with his newly acquired conception of the sublimity of distance than I was at that moment. Solemnly I began my infinite journey,[17].—Before long I walked in entire unconsciousness of all around me. I dwelt in a marvellous inner world. I existed by turns in different places and various states of being. Now I swept my gondola through the moonlit lagoons of Venice. Now Alp on Alp towered above my view, and the glory of the coming sun flashed purple light upon the topmost icy pinnacle. Now in the primeval silence of some unexplored tropical forest I spread my feathery leaves, a giant fern, and swayed and nodded in the spice-gales over a river whose waves at once sent up clouds of music and perfume. My soul changed to a vegetable essence, thrilled with a strange and unimagined ecstasy. The palace of Al Haroun could not have brought me back to humanity. I will not detail all the transmutations of that walk. Ever and anon I returned from my dreams into consciousness, as some well-known house seemed to leap out into my path, awaking me with a shock. The whole way homeward was a series of such awakings and relapses into abstraction and delirium until I reached the corner of the street in which I lived,[17].—My sensations began to be terrific, not from any pain that I felt, but from the tremendous mystery of all around me and within me. By an appalling introversion, all the operations of vitality which, in our ordinary state, go on unconsciously, came vividly into my experience. Through every thinnest corporeal tissue and minutest vein I could trace the circulation of the blood along each inch of its progress. I knew when every valve opened and when it shut; every sense was preternaturally awakened; the room was full of a great glory. The beating of my heart was so clearly audible that I wondered to find it unnoticed by those who were sitting by my side. Lo, now, that heart became a great fountain, whose jet played upward with loud vibrations, and, striking upon the roof of my skull as on a gigantic dome, fell back with a splash and echo into its reservoir. Faster and faster came the pulsations, until at last I heard them no more, and the stream became one continuously pouring flood, whose roar resounded through all my frame. I gave myself up for lost, since judgment, which still sat unimpaired above my perverted senses, argued that congestion must take place in a few moments, and close the drama with my death,[17].—But my clutch would not yet relax from hope. The thought struck me, might not this rapidity of circulation be, after all, imaginary? I determined to find out. Going to my own room, I took out my watch, and placed my hand upon my heart. The very effort which I made to ascertain the reality gradually brought perception back to its natural state. In the intensity of my observations, I began to perceive that the circulation was not as rapid as I had thought. From a pulseless flow it gradually came to be apprehended as a hurrying succession of intense throbs, then less swift and less intense, till finally, on comparing it with the second-hand, I found that about 90 a minute was its average rapidity. Greatly comforted, I desisted from the experiment.

Almost instantly the hallucination returned. Again I dreaded apoplexy, congestion, hemorrhage, a multiplicity of nameless deaths, and drew my picture as I might be found on the morrow, stark and cold, by those whose agony would be redoubled by the mystery of my end. I reasoned with myself; I bathed my forehead; it did no good. There was one resource left: I would go to a physician,[17].—With this resolve, I left my room and went to the head of the staircase. The family had all retired for the night, and the gas was turned off from the burner in the hall below. I looked down the stairs: the depth was fathomless; it was a journey of years to reach the bottom! The dim light of the sky shone through the narrow panes at the sides of the front door, and seemed a demon-lamp in the middle darkness of the abyss. I never could get down! I sat me down despairingly upon the topmost step. Suddenly a sublime thought possessed me. It shall be tried. I commenced the descent, wearily, wearily down through my league-long, year-long journey. To record my impressions in that journey would be to repeat what I have said of the time of Hashish. Now stopping to rest, as a traveller would turn aside at a wayside inn, now toiling down through the lonely darkness, I came by and by to the end, and passed out into the street,[17].—On reaching the porch of the physician's house I rang the bell, but immediately forgot whom to ask for. No wonder; I was on the steps of a palace in Milan—no (and I laughed at myself for the blunder), I was on the staircase of the Tower of London. So I should not be puzzled through my ignorance of Italian. But whom to ask for? This question recalled me to the real bearings of the place, but did not suggest its requisite answer. Whom shall I ask for? I began setting the most cunning traps of hypothesis to catch the solution of the difficulty. I looked at the surrounding houses; of whom had I been accustomed to think as living next door to them?- This did not bring it. Whose daughter had been going to school from this house but the very day before? Her name was Julia—Julia—and I thought of every combination which had been made with this name from Julia Domna down to Giulia Grisi. Ah! now I had it, Julia H.; and her father naturally bore the same name. During this intellectual rummage, I had rung the bell half a dozen times, under the impression that I was kept waiting a small eternity. When the servant opened the door she panted as if she had run for her life,[17].—My voice seemed to reverberate like thunder from every recess in the whole building. I was terrified at the noise I had made. I learned in after days that this impression is only one of the many due to the intense sensibility of the sensorium as produced by Hashish. At one time, having asked a friend to check me if I talked loudly or immoderately while in a state of fantasia, among persons from whom I wished to conceal my state, I caught myself singing and shouting from very ecstasy, and reproached him with a neglect of his friendly office. I could not believe him when he assured me that I had not uttered an audible word. The intensity of the inward motion had affected the external through the internal ear,[17].—[140.] All was perfect silence in the room, and had been perfect darkness also, but for the small lamp which I held in my hand to light the preparation of the powder when it should come. And now a still sublimer mystery began to enwrap me. I stood in a remote chamber at the top of a colossal building, and the whole fabric beneath me was steadily growing into the air. Higher than the topmost pinnacle of Bel's Babylonish temple—higher than Ararat—on, on forever into the lonely dome of God's infinite universe we towered ceaselessly. The years flew on; I heard the musical rush of their wings in the abyss outside of me, and from cycle to cycle, from life to life I careered, a mote in eternity and space. Suddenly emerging from the orbit of my transmigrations, I was again at the foot of the doctor's bed, and thrilled with wonder that we were both unchanged by the measureless lapse of time,[17]. —The thought struck me that I would compare my time with other people's. I looked at my watch, found that its minute-hand stood at the quarter mark past eleven, and, returning it to my pocket, abandoned myself to my reflections,[17].—Presently I saw myself a gnome, imprisoned by a most weird enchanter, whose part I assigned to the doctor before me, in the Domdaniel caverns, "under the roots of the ocean." Here, until the dissolution of all things, was I doomed to hold the lamp that lit that abysmal darkness, while my heart, like a giant clock, ticked solemnly the remaining years of time. Now, this hallucination departing, I heard in the solitude of the night outside the sound of a wondrous heaving sea. Its waves, in sublime cadence, rolled forward till they wet the foundations of the building; they smote them with a might which made the topstone quiver, and then fell back, with hiss and hollow murmur, into the broad bosom whence they had risen. Now through the street, with measured tread, an armed host passed by. The heavy beat of their footfalls, and the griding of their brazen corslet-rings alone broke the silence, for among them all there was no more speech nor music than in a battalion of the dead. It was the army of the ages going by into eternity. A godlike sublimity swallowed up my soul. I was overwhelmed in a fathomless barathrum of time, but I leaned on God, and was immortal through all changes,[17].—And now, in another life, I remembered that far back in the cycles I had looked at my watch to measure the time through which I passed. The impulse seized me to look again. The minute-hand stood half way between fifteen and sixteen minutes past eleven. The watch must have stopped; I held it to my ear; no, it was still going. I had travelled through all that immeasurable chain of dreams in thirty seconds. "My God!" I cried, "I am in eternity." In the presence of that first sublime revelation of the soul's own time, and her capacity for an infinite life, I stood trembling with breathless awe. Till I die, that moment of unveiling will stand in clear relief from all the rest of my existence. I hold it still in unimpaired remembrance as one of the unutterable sanctities of my being. The years of all my earthly life to come can never be as long as those thirty seconds,[17].— The moment that I closed my eyes a vision of celestial glory burst upon me. I stood on the strand of a translucent, boundless lake, across whose bosom I seemed to have been just transported. A short way up the beach a temple, modelled like the Parthenon, lifted its spotless and gleaming columns of alabaster sublimely into the rosy air, like the Parthenon, yet as much excelling it as the godlike ideal of architecture must transcend that ideal realized by man. Unblemished in its purity of whiteness, faultless in the unbroken symmetry of every line and angle, its pediment was draped in odorous clouds, whose tints outshone the rainbow. It was the work of an unearthly builder, and my soul stood before it in a trance of ecstasy. Its folded doors were resplendent with the glory of a multitude of eyes of glass, which were inlaid, throughout the marble surfaces, at the corners of diamond figures, from the floor of the porch to the topmost moulding. One of these eyes was golden like the midday sun, another emerald, another sapphire, and thus onward through the whole gamut of hues, all of them set in such collocations as to form most exquisite harmonies, and whirling upon their axes with the rapidity of thought. At the mere vestibule of the temple I could have sat and drunk in ecstasy forever; but lo! I am yet more blessed. On silent hinges the doors swing open, and I pass in. I did not seem to be in the interior of a temple. I beheld myself as truly in the open air as if I had never passed the portals, for whichever way I looked there were no walls, no roof, no pavement. An atmosphere of fathomless and soul-satisfying serenity surrounded and transfused me. I stood upon the bank of a crystal stream, whose waters, as they slid on, discoursed notes of music which tinkled on the ear like the tones of some exquisite bell-glass. The same impression which such tones produce, of music refined to its ultimate ethereal spirit and borne from a far distance, characterized every ripple of those translucent waves. The gently sloping banks of the stream were luxuriant with a velvety cushioning of grass and moss, so living green that the eye and soul reposed on them at the same time, and drank in peace. Through this amaranthine herbage strayed the gnarled, fantastic roots of giant cedars of Lebanon, from whose primeval trunks great branches spread above me, and interlocking, wove a roof of impenetrable shadow; and wandering down the still avenues, below those grand arboreal arches, went glorious bards, whose snowy beards fell on their breasts beneath countenances of ineffable benignity and nobleness. They were all clad in flowing robes like God's high priests, and each one held in his hand a lyre of unearthly workmanship. Presently one stops midway down a shady walk, and, baring his right arm, begins a prelude. While his celestial chords are trembling up into their sublime fulness, another strikes his strings, and now they blend upon my ravished ear in such a symphony as was never heard elsewhere, and such as I shall never hear again out of the Great Presence. A moment more, and three are playing in harmony; now the fourth joins the glorious rapture of his music to their own, and in the completeness of the chord my soul is swallowed up. I can bear no more. But yes, I am sustained, for suddenly the whole throng break forth in a chorus, upon whose wings I am lifted out of the riven walls of sense, and music and spirit thrill in immediate communion. Forever rid of the intervention of pulsing air and vibrating nerve, my soul dilates with the swell of that transcendent harmony, and interprets from it arcana of a meaning which words can never tell. I am borne aloft upon the glory of sound. I float in a trance among the burning choir of the seraphim. But, as I am melting through the purification of that sublime ecstasy into oneness with the Deity himself, one by one those pealing lyres faint away, and as the last throb dies down along the measureless ether, visionless arms swiftly as lightning carry me far into the profound, and set me down before another portal. Its leaves, like the first, are of spotless marble, but ungemmed with wheeling eyes of burning color,[17].—I will make a digression, for the purpose of introducing two laws of the Hashish operation, which, as explicatory, deserve a place here. First: after the completion of any one fantasia has arrived, there almost invariably succeeds a shifting of the action to some other stage entirely different in its surroundings. In this transition the general character of the emotion may remain unchanged. I may be happy in Paradise, and happy at the sources of the Nile, but seldom, either in Paradise or on the Nile, twice in succession. I may writhe in Etna and burn unquenchably in Gehenna, but almost never, in the course of the same delirium, shall Etna or Gehenna witness my torture a second time. Second: after the full storm of a vision of intense sublimity has blown past a Hashish eater, his next vision is generally of a quiet, relaxing, and recreating nature. He comes down from his clouds or up from his abyss into a middle ground of gentle shadows, where he may rest his eyes from the splendor of the seraphim or the flames of fiends. There is a wise philosophy in this arrangement, for otherwise the soul would soon burn out in the excess of its own oxygen. Many a time it seems to me has my own thus been saved from extinction,[17].—Although the last experience of which I had been conscious had seemed to satisfy every human want, physical or spiritual, I smiled on the four plain white walls of my bedchamber, and hailed their familiar unostentatiousness with a pleasure which had no wish to transfer itself to arabesque or rainbows. It was like returning home from an eternity spent in loneliness among the palaces of strangers. Well may I say an eternity, for during the whole day I could not rid myself of the feeling that I was separated from the preceding one by an immeasurable lapse of time. In fact, I never got wholly rid of it,[17]. —Every function had returned to its normal state, with the one exception mentioned; memory could not efface the traces of my having passed through a great mystery,[17].—The phenomenon of the dual existence once more presented itself. One part of me awoke, while the other continued in perfect hallucination. The awakened portion felt the necessity of keeping in side streets on the way home, lest some untimely burst of ecstasy should startle more frequented thoroughfares,[17].—And now that unutterable thirst which characterizes Hashish came upon me. I could have lain me down and lapped dew from the grass. I must drink, wheresoever, howsoever. We soon reached home; soon, because it was not five squares off where we sat down, yet ages, from the thirst which consumed me, and the expansion of time in which I lived. I came into the house as one would approach a fountain in a desert, with a wild bound of exultation, and gazed with miserly eyes at the draught which my friend poured out for me until the glass was brimming. I clutched it; I put it to my lips. Ha! a surprise. It was not water, but the most delicious metheglin in which ever bard of the Cymri drank the health of Howell Dda. It danced and sparkled like some liquid metempsychosis of amber; it gleamed with the spiritual fire of a thousand chrysolites. To sight, to taste it was metheglin, such as never mantled in the cups of Valhalla,[17].—[150.] After the walk which I last recorded, the former passion for travel returned with powerful intensity. I had now a way of gratifying it, which comported both with indolence and economy. The whole East, from Greece to farthest China, lay within the compass of a township. No outlay was necessary for the journey. For the humble sum of six cents I might purchase an excursion ticket over all the earth; ships and dromedaries, tents and hospices, were all contained in a box of Tilden's extract. Hashish I called the "drug of travel," and I had only to direct my thoughts strongly towards a particular part of the world previously to swallowing my bolus, to make my whole fantasia in the strongest possible degree topographical. Or, when the delirium was at its height, let any one suggest to me, however faintly, mountain, wilderness, or market-place, and straightway I was in it, drinking in the novelty of my surroundings in all the ecstasy of a discoverer. I swam up against the current of all time; I walked through Luxor and Palmyra as they were of old; on Babylon the bittern had not built her nest, and I gazed on the unbroken columns of the Parthenon,[17]. There are two facts which I have verified as universal by repeated experiment, which fall into their place here as aptly as they can in the course of my narrative. 1st. At two different times, when body and mind are apparently in precisely analogous states, when all circumstances, exterior and interior, do not differ tangibly in the smallest respect, the same dose of the same preparation of Hashish will frequently produce diametrically opposite effects. Still further, I have taken at one time a pill of thirty grains, which hardly gave a perceptible phenomenon, and at another, when my dose had been but half that quantity, I have suffered the agonies of a martyr, or rejoiced in a perfect frenzy. So exceedingly variable are its results that, long before I abandoned the indulgence, I took each successive bolus with the consciousness that I was daring an uncertainty as tremendous as the equipoise between hell and heaven. Yet the fascination employed Hope as its advocate, and won the suit. 2d. If, during the ecstasy of Hashish delirium, another dose, however small, yes, though it be no larger than half a pea, be employed to prolong the condition, such agony will inevitably ensue as will make the soul shudder at its own possibility of endurance without annihilation. By repeated experiments, which now occupy the most horrible place upon my catalogue of horrible remembrances, have I proved that, among all the variable phenomena of Hashish, this alone stands unvarying. The use of it directly after any other stimulus will produce consequences as appalling,[17]—The effects of the Hashish increased, as it always does, with the excitement of the visions and the exercise of walking. I began to be lifted into that tremendous pride which is so often a characteristic of the fantasia. My powers became superhuman; my knowledge covered the universe; my scope of sight was infinite,[17]— What mattered it that my far-off battlements were the walls of a college, my mighty plain a field, and my wind of balm but an ordinary sunset breeze? To me all joys were real; yes, even with a reality which utterly surpasses the hardest facts of the ordinary world,[17]—Upon William N., Hashish produced none of the effects characteristic of fantasia. There was no hallucination, no volitancy of unusual images before the eye when closed. Circulation, however, grew to a surprising fulness and rapidity, accompanied by the same introversion of faculties and clear perception of all physical processes which startled me in my first experiment upon myself. There was stertorous breathing, dilatation of the pupil, and a drooping appearance of the eyelid, followed at last by a comatose state, lasting for hours, out of which it was almost impossible fully to arouse the energies. These symptoms, together with a peculiar rigidity of the muscular system, and inability to measure the precise compass and volume of the voice when speaking, brought the case nearer in resemblance to those recorded by Dr. O'Shaughnessy, of Calcutta, as occurring under his immediate inspection among the natives of India than any I have witnessed,[17]. —Repeatedly have I wandered past doors and houses which, in my ordinary condition, were as well known as my own, and have at last given up the search for them in utter hopelessness, recognizing not the faintest familiar trace in their aspect. Certainly a Hashish-eater should never be alone,[17].— In William N., I observed, however, one phenomenon which characterizes Hashish-existence in persons of far different constitutions, the expansion of time and space. Walking with him a distance not exceeding a furlong, I have seen him grow weary and assume a look of hopelessness, which he explained by telling me that he could never traverse the immensity before him. Frequently, also, do I remember his asking to know the time thrice in as many minutes, and when answered, he exclaimed, "Is it possible? I supposed it was an hour since I last inquired." His temperament was a mixture of the phlegmatic and nervous, and he was generally rather unsusceptible to stimulus,[17].—Suddenly Bob leaped up from the lounge on which he had been lying, and, with loud peals of laughter, danced wildly over the room. A strange light was in his eyes, and he gesticulated furiously, like a player in a pantomime. Suddenly he stopped dancing, and trembling, as with an indefinable fear, he whispered, "What will become of me?"[17].—Having taken Hashish and felt its influence already for several hours, he still retained enough of conscious self-control to visit the room of a certain excellent pianist without exciting the suspicion of the latter. Fred. threw himself upon a sofa immediately on entering, and asked the artist to play him some piece of music, without naming any one in particular. The prelude began. With its first harmonious rise and fall the dreamer was lifted into the choir of a grand cathedral. Thenceforward it was heard no longer as exterior; but I shall proceed to tell how it was embodied in one of the most wonderful imaginative representations that it has ever been my lot to know. The windows of nave and transept were emblazoned, in the most gorgeous coloring, with incidents culled from saintly lives. Far off in the chancel monks were loading the air with essences that streamed from their golden censers; on the pavement of inimitable mosaic knelt a host of reverent worshippers in silent prayer. Suddenly, behind him, the great organ began a plaintive minor, like the murmur of some bard relieving his heart in threnody. This minor was joined by a gentle treble voice among the choir in which he stood. The low wail rose and fell as with the expression of wholly human emotion. One by one the remaining singers joined in, and now he heard, thrilling to the very roof of the cathedral, a wondrous miserere. But the pathetic delight of hearing was soon supplanted by, or rather mingled with, a new sight in the body of the pile below him. At the farther end of the nave a great door slowly swung open, and a bier entered supported by solemn bearers. Upon it lay a coffin covered by a heavy pall, which, being removed as the bier was set down in the chancel, discovered the face of the sleeper. It was the dead Mendelssohn! The last cadence of the death-chant died away; the bearers, with heavy tread, carried the coffin through an iron door to its place in the vault; one by one the crowd passed out of the cathedral, and at last, in the choir, the dreamer stood alone. He turned himself also to depart, and, awakened to complete consciousness, beheld the pianist just resting from the keys. "What piece have you been playing?" asked Fred. The musician replied it was "Mendelssohn's Funeral March." This piece, Fred. solemnly assured me, he had never heard before. The phenomenon thus appears inexplicable by any hypothesis which would regard it as a mere coincidence. Whether this vision was suggested by an unconscious recognition of Mendelssohn's style in the piece performed, or by the awaking of some unknown intuitional faculty, it was produced as an original creation, I know not, but certainly it is as remarkable an instance of sympathetic clairvoyance as I every knew,[17].—In the broad daylight of a summer afternoon, I was walking in the full possession of delirium. For an hour the expansion of all visible things had been growing towards its height; it now reached it, and to the fullest extent I apprehended what is meant by the infinity of space. Vistas no longer converged; sight met no barrier; the world was horizonless, for earth and sky stretched endlessly onward in parallel planes. Above me the heavens were terrible with the glory of a fathomless depth. I look up, but my eyes, unopposed, every moment penetrated farther and farther into the immensity, and I turned them downward, lest they should presently intrude into the fatal splendors of the Great Presence. Unable to bear visible objects, I shut my eyes. In one moment, a colossal music filled the whole hemisphere above me, and I thrilled upward through its environment on visionless wings. It was not song, it was not instruments, but the inexpressible spirit of sublime sound—like nothing I ever heard—impossible to be symbolized; intense, yet not loud; the ideal of harmony, yet distinguishable into a multiplicity of exquisite parts. I opened my eyes, but it still continued. I sought around me to detect some natural sound which might be exaggerated into such a semblance; but no, it was of unearthly generation, and it thrilled through the universe an inexplicable, a beautiful, yet an awful symphony. Suddenly my mind grew solemn with the consciousness of a quickened perception. And what a solemnity is that which the Hashish-eater feels at such a movement! The very beating of his heart is silenced; he stands with his finger on his lip; his eyes are fixed, and he becomes a very statue of awful veneration. The face of such a man, however little glorified in feature or expression during his ordinary states of mind, I have stood and looked upon with the consciousness that I was beholding more of the embodiment of the truly sublime, than any created being could ever offer me. I looked abroad on fields, and waters, and sky, and read in them a most startling meaning. I wondered how I had ever regarded them in the light of dead matter, at the farthest only *suggesting* lessons. They were now, as in my former vision, grand symbols of the sublimest spiritual truths—truths never before even feebly grasped, and utterly unsuspected. Like a map the arcana of the universe lay bare before me. I saw how every created thing not only typifies, but springs forth from some mighty spiritual law as its offspring, its necessary external development, not the mere clothing of the essence, but the essence incarnate,"—[160.] As I have frequently said, I felt no depression of body. The flames of my vision had not withered a single corporeal tissue nor snapped a single corporeal cord. All the pains induced by the total abandonment of Hashish were spiritual. From the ethereal heights of Olympus I had been dropped into the midst of an Acherontian fog. My soul breathed laboriously, and grew torpid with every hour. I dreaded an advancing night of oblivion. I sat awaiting extinction. The shapes which moved about me in the outer world seemed liked galvanized corpses; the living soul of nature, with which I had so long communed, had gone out like the flame of a candle, and her remaining exterior was as poor and meaningless as those wooden trees with which children play, and the cliffs and chalets carved out of boxwood by some Swiss in his winter leisure. Moreover, actual pain had not ceased with abandonment of the indulgence. In some fiery dreams of night, or some sudden thrill of daylight, the old pangs were reproduced with a vividness only less than amounting to hallucination. I opened my eyes, I rubbed my forehead, I arose and walked; they were then perceived to be merely ideal; but the very necessity of this effort to arouse myself, a necessity which might occur at any time and in any place, became gradually a grievous thraldom,"—Constantly, notwithstanding all my occupation of mind, the cloud of dejection deepened in hue and in density. My troubles were not merely negative, simply regrets for something which was not, but a loathing, a fear, a hate of something which was. The very existence of the outer world seemed a base mockery, a cruel sham of some remembered possibility which had been glorious with a speechless beauty. I hated flowers, for I had seen the enamelled meads of Paradise; I cursed the rocks, because they were mute stone; the sky, because it rang with no music; and earth and sky seemed to throw back my curse,".—An abhorrence of speech or action, except towards the fewest possible persons, possessed me. For the sake of not appearing singular or ascetic, and so crippling my power for whatever little good I might do, I at first mingled with society, forcing myself to laugh and talk conventionalities. At last, associations grew absolutely unbearable; the greatest effort was necessary to speak with any but one or two, to whom I had fully confided my past experience. A footstep on the stairs was sufficient to make me tremble with anticipations of a conversation; every morning brought a resurrection into renewed horrors, as I thought of the advancing necessity of once more coming in contact with men and things,[17].—Gradually it grew the habitual tendency of my dreaming state to bring all its scenes, whether of pleasure or of pain, to a crisis through some catastrophe by water. Earlier in the state which ensued upon my abandonment of Hashish, I had been affrighted particularly by seeing men tumble down the shafts of mines, or, as I have detailed, either dreading or suffering some fall into abysses on my own part; yet now, upon whatever journey I set out, to cross the Atlantic or to travel inland, sooner or later I inevitably come to an end by drowning, or the imminent peril of it,[17].—Gradually my rest began to be broken by tremendous dreams, that mirrored the sights and echoed the voices of the former Hashish life. In them I faithfully lived over my past experience, with many additions, and but this one difference. Out of the reality of the Hashish state there had been no awakening possible; from this hallucination of dreams I awoke when the terrors became too superhuman,[17].—The existing mood is heightened,[21].—All his feelings of pleasure and pain seem exalted,[8].—Feeling of exhilaration (after five hours),[13].—The excitement seemed to increase all his powers. "I was bursting with an uncontrollable life; I strode with the thews of a giant,"[17].—Cannot say he has any decidedly elated feelings, but only a tendency that way, which he repressed (after eight hours),[5].—Elevation of spirits, with a feeling of lightness in the body in the evening,[1].—[170.] Alarming exaltation, with strange hallucinations,[22].—**Exaltation of spirits, with excessive loquacity,**[1].—*Exaltation of spirits, with great gayety and disposition to laugh at the merest trifle,*[1].— For one hour and three-quarters, better humor and lightness of the mind, nearly unmindful of the medicine (after forty-five minutes),[19].—Felt very jolly, bursting into laughter; talked nonsense; knew that he was talking nonsense, but could not stop (after one hour),[11].—*Full of fun and mischief,* and laughs *immoderately,*[1].—Everything that he saw seemed ludicrous (after one hour and a half),[20].—He whistles and wishes to hug every one he meets,[1].—Propensity to caress and chafe the feet of all bystanders,[29].— Slight inclination to laugh,[34].—[180.] Suddenly inclined to laugh; sang alone very joyously; wondered at my own singing,[24].—Desire to laugh at every remark made by his companions, because it was so funny,[41].—Laughed heartily several times,[33].—*Laughs indiscriminately at every word said to him,*[1]. —Laughed long and heartily, but never lost the feeling of intense anxiety with which he awoke,[15].—Frequent involuntary fits of laughter,[6].—**Uncontrollable laughter, till the face became purple and the back and loins ache,**[1].—Uncontrollable laughter, and a succession of vivid and pleasurable ideas,[29].—Laughed at the idea of laughing, and could not control himself,[3]. —Spasmodic laughter, seemingly increased by flatulence rising in his throat, threatening to choke him and to make him vomit; there was, however, no nausea,[1].—[190.] Burst into an immoderate fit of laughter without any cause, and was obliged to retire on account of repeated recurrence of the fits (after two and one-quarter hours),[33].—Perpetual giggling,[29].—*Moaning and crying,*[1].—Involuntary weeping; the tears seem blood,[1].—For a day or two, depression of spirits, and disinclination to study,[8].—Great depression of spirits, with weariness, and a pale face,[1].—Fits of mental depression,[8].— Feels wretched,[1].—Very subdued feeling; marked taciturn tendency (after four hours),[13].—Thinks each one he meets has some secret sorrow, and wishes to sympathize with him,[1].—[200.] No power of will,[8].—His power of will, with regard to the commands of others, seemed intact, but not over himself, except under a strong stimulus. Thus, when Mr. H. came into the room, not wishing to be thought drunk, he lay down on a sofa, and could restrain himself from talking by a great effort, but when he did speak to Mr. H., he slightly wandered. When Mr. H. left, he went on as before,[8].—Loquacity,[29].—Conversed with great volubility; very happy to see them, and begging them to stay with him, "as he was at the point of death" (after one hour),[37].—Taciturnity,[1].—After dinner, the tranquil taciturnity came on. She saw, she observed, she paid attention, but she could not open her mouth to speak,[40].—She talked during the early part of the meal, but afterwards lapsed into a tranquil taciturnity,[40].—Disposition to remain perfectly quiet, without speaking (after four hours),[13].—The anxiety and weakness overcame him to such a degree that he lost all power of will, and his attendants were obliged to hold him up under the arms in order to get him along,[20].— *Great anguish and despair,*[1].—[210.] **Anguish accompanied by great oppression; ameliorated in the open air,**[1].—**He was in constant fear he would become insane,**[1].—Fear of spectres,[1].—*Horror of darkness,*[1].—*Great apprehension of approaching death,*[1].—Dread of "congestion, apoplexy, hemorrhage, and a multiplicity of deaths." Fear of death, which is thought near,[17].—Went upstairs all right; avoided the coal-scuttle, of which he seemed to be somehow afraid,[8].—Did not dare to use his voice, in case he should knock down the walls, or burst himself like a bomb,[28].—Very passionate,[1].—Very sarcastic,[1].—[220.] Felt displeased when his name was called out, at 3 A.M., by a friend, who told him to take care of a coal-scuttle at the foot of the stairs,[8].—Extreme intolerance of contradiction,[17].— He grows suddenly suspicious of all persons and things,[17].—The most delightful ecstasy was converted into deepest horrors, and horrors, when present, were greatly aggravated by darkness,[17].—Some had great fear, at times, of things either real or unreal, and at other times the mind wandered into delightful realms,[3].—Indifference to the world; the mind seems blunted; a reckless indifference to the dictates of conscience (after seven hours),[5].— *Intellectual.* My mind was capable of a greater effort for a while afterwards. During the succeeding week, I read a work on Psychology of ov seven hundred pages, and could for a long while refer to any part of it without my notes. This I could not have done before nor since,[2].—He seemed to examine his own character, though in an incomplete manner,[20].— Tendency to make puns, and talk about grammatical questions,[25].— Thoughts rush so rapidly that it is impossible to write them,[17].—[230.] *Inability to recall any thought or event, on account of different thoughts crowding on his brain,*[1].—On the next day, he was unable to attend to his business on account of his diffused thoughts, which he was unable to collect,[20].—He wished to write down his symptoms, but he had to give up the attempt on account of the wandering of his thoughts,[1].—It was only after repeated trials that he made a memorandum, while persons were conversing in the room, on account of his not being able to attend to more than one thing at a time; new ideas would constantly occur to him, which occupied his mind for a short time, when others would rise; all seemed to come in a misty sort of way, and the time elapsing between one train of thought and another, seemed to him long, although really short,[1].—His brains seemed cataleptic; he commenced to do something; his fingers moved slowly, a new thought presented itself, which he pursued for awhile, then another would suggest itself; in this manner ideas passed through his mind, not quickly, but as though each one stopped there a little while on account of the torpidity of his brain; the slow motion of his fingers seemed to be caused by the cataleptic state of his mind,[1].—**Very absent-minded,**[1].—Occasionally absent-minded and dreamy (second day),[3].—Pays no attention when spoken to,[1].—Answered questions incoherently, and immediately forgot what they were about and what I had answered,[33].—Wanted to refer to something in his MS.; had to stop and think what he wanted to find, and where to look for it; had to think for some seconds before he could bring his mind to the subject (after one and a half hours),[14].—[**240.**] Writes one word for another,[1].—*He could not read, partly on account of dreamy spells, and partly because he had not full power of vision,*[1].—In the morning, some letters were brought for him, but he could not read or understand them properly (second day),[8].—On referring to a MS. index of cases of poisoning, etc., he did not seem to know where to look for what he wanted; when found, he read it over two or three times without seeming to understand it (after one hour),[14].—Stupidity,[21].—Stupidity and forgetfulness, but without reverie,[34]. —Stupid and forgetful (second day),[33].—More stupid (second day),[34].—His usual forgetfulness improved under the proving,[19].—Tales of youth again charmed his existence; pictures and scenes long forgotten were again for an instant as plain as if seen only a day before,[27].—[**250.**] Remembered events that had happened, and ideas that had passed through his mind when a child, as about toys. (Does not now remember them distinctly, but recollects that he could then call them to mind),[8].—All the thoughts and deeds of his childhood returned,[20].—Tried to write down a reference in his MS. Wrote down the first half correctly, though feeling he might write some nonsense in the state he was; on attempting to finish it, did not know what it was he had to write, and could only do so by looking constantly at the passage in the printed book while he wrote it down in the MS., and even then omitted something,[14].—Memory weak (after one hour and three-quarters),[19].—Memory seemed failing him,[5].—His memory seemed gone (afterwards, however, he remembered nearly all that had taken place),[8]. —Great defect and shortness of memory (second day),[33].—Forgetful; was not able to recite the simplest sentence,[24].—His forgetfulness caused those present to smile, upon which he laughed in a very silly manner,[1].—*He forgot his last words and ideas, and spoke in a low tone with a thick voice, as if tired,*[1].—[**260.**] Forgetfulness, then liveliness,[23].—*He begins a sentence, but cannot finish it, because he forgets what he intends to write or speak,*[1].—When repeating some French sentences, forgot the beginnings before he came to the endings (after four hours),[5].—In conversation, cannot recollect of what he was speaking (after forty-five minutes),[19].—Sprang from his bed like a maniac, struck a light, took his watch and began to count his pulse, just one beat at each second; but when the minute had elapsed, could not remember how many he had counted,[3].—The most familiar objects appear strange and are not recognized,[17].—Felt he knew where he was, and yet did not (after one hour),[11].—Cloudiness of internal and external consciousness,[21]. —He seems as if he had lost his consciousness for a time, which gradually returns,[17].—**Every few moments he would lose himself, and then wake up, as it were, to those around him,**[1].—[**270.**] While listening to the piano, he loses consciousness, and is seemingly raised gently through the air to a

great height, when the strains of music become perfectly celestial ; on regaining consciousness, his head is bent forward, his neck is stiff, and there
is a loud ringing in his ears,[1].—At night, unconsciousness, delirium, and
semi-unconsciousness alternate,[19].—He was unconscious of a severe chill,[20].—
Candlelight obliterates all consciousness,[19].—Candlelight produces stupefaction of the senses, compression of the brain, paralytic feeling of the whole
body; everything appears without color,[19].

Head.—Confusion and Vertigo. Forehead confused, heavy
(after one hour),[4].—**Vertigo,**[1 21 23].—Vertigo (after one hour and three-quarters),[19].—*Vertigo on rising,*[1].—*Vertigo on rising, with a stunning pain in
the back part of the head, and he falls,*[1].—**[280.]** Vertigo, with backward inclination of the head (first day),[7].—On walking, slight inclination to vertigo (after five hours),[4].—Head dizzy (second day),[3].—Dizziness in head
(after two hours),[14].—Dizziness as in intoxication (second day),[7].—Dizziness on bending forward, or walking (first day),[7].—Strong coffee relieved
the dizziness (second day),[3].—Giddiness (after one hour),[33].—Giddiness;
everything seemed turning round, for some time (after one hour),[12].—Transient feeling in head as if something were going round in it, from before
backwards, on right side (after one hour and one-sixth),[14].—**[290.]** Peculiar
feeling of moving, or what is called swimming in head, with transient feeling of constriction round head (after one hour and two-thirds),[14].—Scarcely
any effect while sitting quiet, but on beginning to walk, perhaps three hours
afterwards, staggered, and was quite drunk. These symptoms would abate
on sitting down, but would be again reproduced on rising,[32].—*General
Head.* Frequent involuntary shaking of his head,[1].—Dulness of head
(after forty-five minutes),[19].—Felt an opium-like dulness in the head (after
one hour),[5].—Seething or crisping of blood through the brain, quick, like
a flash of sheet lightning,[14].—For several months, in fact for nearly a
year afterwards, I was troubled with a crisping sensation in the brain, just
as I fell asleep or awoke from sleep ; not every night, but probably once a
week,[2].—The head felt light, mind remarkably active, and yet apparently
sluggish,[3].—Head heavy, confused, with vertigo (after one hour and a
half),[4].—*His head feels very heavy; he loses consciousness and falls,*[1].—**[300.]**
Heaviness of the head, wandering of the mind, and apprehension that he
was going to faint,[26].—Pain from bottom of orbit, through brain and in the
ear,[44].—Fulness of the head, with a sharp intermittent pain in the right
side, under the parietal bone,[1].—Gradual expansive feeling of the brain, as
if myself were apart from myself and dwelling in a new world, within the
cavity of the skull,[6].—Fulness in the head, with drowsiness and flushes in
the face,[1].—Curious constrictive feeling in head, with inability to think
(after two hours),[9].—Great constriction in head, as from an iron skull-cap,[8].
—Head feels achy and confused (second day),[5].—On awaking, headache,[21].
—Severe headache, especially at the vertex, with beating (second day),[7].—
[310.] Intermittent headache, in a spot on left side of head, near the an-
terior-inferior angle of parietal bone (after one hour and two-thirds),[13].—
Dull, heavy, throbbing pain through the head, with a sensation like a heavy
blow on the back of the head and neck,[1].—*Heavy insurmountable pressure
on the brain, forcing him to stoop,*[1].—In warm room again compression of
brain, with paralytic feelings,[19].—The head feels bruised, with a pressive
pain,[1].—**On regaining consciousness, violent shocks pass through his
brain,**[1].—Headache while in the sun,[1].—Coffee almost instantly relieved the
headache following,[3].—*Forehead.* Pains in forehead for some time (after
one hour and a half),[12].—Heavy frontal headache (in about thirty prov-

ers),[3].—[320.] Heavy frontal headache in the brain, more to left side,[44].—Heaviness and heat in the forehead, very slight, and short-lasting (after three hours),[4].—Heat in the forehead,[1].—Fulness in the forehead, as if it would burst,[1].—Fulness and heaviness in forehead, with pressure at root of nose and over the eyes; headache over left eye; dull hard pain in top of head; pain in back of head, left side,[44].—*Dull drawing pain in the forehead, especially over the eyes,*[1].—Pressure on his forehead and top of his head, which seemed to cause his slowness of speech and action,[1].—All the afternoon had headache, pressing outwards over the eye,[44].—*Throbbing, aching pain in the forehead,*[1].—*Jerking in the right side of the forehead, towards the interior and back part of the head,*[1].—**Temples.** [330.] Burning pain in both temples,[1].—*Aching in both temples, most severe in the right,*[1].—*Dull, sticking pain in the right temple,*[1].—Darting, throbbing pain in the right temple, and from the back of the head to the forehead,[1].—*Severe stitch in the right temple, gradually changing to a pressive pain,*[1].—**Parietals.** *Pain in the whole right side of the head,*[1].—Sharp pain in right side of head, running from inner canthus of eye up, back, and out (after eleven hours),[44].—11 A.M., boring pain in right parietal protuberance (third day),[44].—**Occiput.** Headache in occiput and temples (first day),[7].—Fulness in the right side of the cerebellum, with a dull pain, worse on shaking the head,[1].—[340.] Sensation of pressure at the back of the head, before the occurrence of convulsive movements, which changed into an unpleasant feeling of heat, then of cold, in consequence of which his hands were carried automatically to that spot, and held there, as though there were a difficulty in detaching them,[39].—Feeling of something surging up from posterior part of head toward forehead (after two hours),[14].—Feeling, for a few seconds, of something surging like waves up the neck into the head, seeming to press it forwards (after one hour and one-sixth),[14].—**External Head.** Scalp and skin of forehead felt as though tightly stretched over skull, as a bladder is stretched over a jar (after one hour and two-thirds),[13].—Soreness of the scalp to touch,[1].—Crawling in the scalp on the top of the head,[1].—Pressing pain on different spots of the cranial bones, in the left wrist and ankle, and violent pain in the muscles below the left shoulder-blade (after three and a half hours),[4].

Eyes.—Objective. Wild-looking eyes (first day),[7].—Seemed to have awakened suddenly, and stared wildly about him (after one hour),[37].—Fixed gaze,[1].—[350.] Eye has an expression of cunning and merriment,[29].—On looking at himself in the mirror was struck with the small drunken appearance of the eyes (after eight hours),[5].—Languid eyes; heaviness of the head (second day),[1].—Eyes swollen and inflamed (second day),[3].—Eyes dull and swollen (in about thirty provers),[3].—**Subjective.** Weakness of the eyes,[1].—Heaviness in the eyes,[1].—Heaviness and pressure over the eyes, with nausea,[1].—Heat in the eyes,[1].—Feeling of burning heat, more marked in the eyes than in the lids, and severe (after three hours),[13].—[360.] Burning and smarting in the eyes,[1].—Great pressure in the right eye,[1].—**Orbit.** Pain as from a blow over the orbit of the right eye,[1].—**Lids.** Bloodvessels of upper eyelids become very full and distended, with feeling of heat (after one hour and one-sixth),[13].—Contraction of the eyelids (second day),[7].—Drooping appearance of the eyelids, followed at last by a comatose state, lasting for hours, out of which it was almost impossible fully to arouse the energies,[17].—Twinkling of the eyes (first day),[7].—His eyelids feel very heavy, and he can only partially open them,[1].—Burning and itching of the edges of the eyelids,[1].—Slight soreness of upper ey 'lids (after one hour and two-thirds),[13].—[370.] A cool burning-stinging in inner corner and canthus of left eye and adjacent side of nose,[44].—*Jerking in the external corner of the eye and eyelid*,[1].—Jerking from the head to the outer canthus of the left eye, from above downwards,[1].—*Lachrymal Apparatus.* Inflammation and swelling of the caruncula lachrymalis of both eyes,[1].—*Conjunctiva.* Conjunctiva congested, without any abnormal sensation there,[12].—Conjunctiva of eyes covered with distended vessels (after three hours),[13].—**Injection of the vessels of the conjunctiva of both eyes**,[1].—*The vessels of the conjunctiva of both eyes are injected in a triangular patch extending from the internal canthus to the cornea; worse in the night*,[1].—*Ball.* Slight pain at back of eyeball,[44].—Feeling of distension of eyeballs, as if starting out of head; they ached when he tried to read (after one hour and a half),[10].—*Pupil.* [380.] Dilatation of the pupil,[17].—Pupils moderately dilated, iris somewhat sensitive to the light, conjunctiva somewhat injected,[20].—Pupils widely dilated,[15].—Pupils contracted (second day),[3].—Clairvoyance (in about thirty provers),[3].—Apparent clairvoyance, that is, I saw or fancied I saw, articles in another room, but the sensation was of short duration (after four hours),[3].—At midnight precisely, awoke suddenly and fully; the room was dark, still the location of every article about him seemed perfectly plain; he could read the titles of books upon a table twelve or fifteen feet off (after four hours),[3].—As soon as he had urinated, the clairvoyant-like vision left him,[3].—Weakness of sight,[21].—Sight rather hazy,[8].—[390.] He cannot see, with the exception of a small spot where he looks,[1].—Sensitiveness of the right eye to the light, with lachrymation,[1].—Ugly faces assume a pleasing expression,[1].—Faces assume such ridiculous appearances that he bursts into fits of laughter,[1].—The room seemed larger (after one hour),[11].—The globe of the lamp appeared of an enormous size,[8].—Whatever he looked at became lost, as it were, in a maze; the lamp appeared to be slowly turning round, and when he lost sight of this, the red lines in the paper of the room appeared to intertwine in a most beautiful manner,[33].—Photopsia,[21].—**While reading, the letters run together**,[1].—*Twinkling, trembling, and glimmering before the eyes*,[1].—[400.] A large spot hovers a little above the vision of the left eye, sinking when he looks down, rising when he looks up,[1].—Violet spots on the paper, while reading,[1].—The flame of a candle seems surrounded by a pea-green circle,[1].

Ear.—Pain and singing in left ear,[44].—Burning in the ears,[1].—Stuffed feeling of the right ear (after forty-five minutes),[19].—*Aching in both ears*,[1].—Boring pain immediately above and back of right ear (after three hours),[44].—Boring pain in right ear,[44].—Tearing pain in the right ear, ameliorated by pressure,[1].—[410.] **Throbbing and fulness in both ears**,[1].—Jerking or electric shocks in the ears,[1].—*Hearing.* Great acuteness of hearing,[17].—Sensitiveness to noise,[1].—Increase in power of hearing, whereby slight noises became as loud as thunder,[28].—Sounds seem unusually loud,[1].—His own voice seems intensely loud. Believes he has been talking indecently loud, when he has not spoken at all,[17].—Music of any kind is intensely agreeable to him,[1].—Difficult hearing,[21].—His own voice sounded to him a long way off (after one hour),[11].—[420.] *Noise in the ears like boiling water*,[1].—Buzzing in ears, lasting some time (after one hour),[12].—Buzzing in right ear,[8].—Buzzing in ears, with slight giddiness (after two hours and a quarter),[35].—Singing in ears (after one hour),[11].—Singing in ears, while lying down, dozing, which went off when he got up (after one hour and two-thirds),[14].—*Periodical singing in the ears, that always ceased* *as soon as he came to himself, and renewed itself when a dreamy spell came on,*[1].—Singing in left ear,[44].—**Ringing and buzzing in the ears,**[1].

Nose.—Sneezing (after one hour and three-quarters),[19].—**[430.]** He blew coagulated blood from his right nostril,[1].—Dry, feverish feeling of left nostril (after three hours),[44].—Pain at the root of the nose,[1].—Fulness and aching at the root of the nose,[1].

Face.—Objective. Thinks his expression must be altered, as people look at him more than usual (after three hours),[5].— *Wearied, exhausted appearance,*[1].—**He looks drowsy and stupid,**[1].—He looks as if thoroughly intoxicated,[1].—Pale face (first day),[7].—Face a little pale (second day),[5].— **[440.]** Face pale and anxious (after one hour),[37].—Paleness of face, as in fainting, ameliorated by fresh air,[19].—Face flushed, from mounting the stairs,[41].—Redness of the face, as during intoxication,[1].—The face and eyes became very red,[20].—By a great exertion moved his hand and felt his face, and it felt hard ; there was no sensation in the face, but to the hand it felt stony,[3].—The skin of his face, especially of his forehead and chin, feels as if it were drawn tight,[1].—Feeling of pressure on both cheeks, in corresponding spots, about posterior border of malar bone. This did not last long (after one hour and one-sixth),[14].—Stinging in right side of face as though stuck with pins; leaves on scratching, but comes again immediately on another part of body,[44].—Drawings in the muscles of mastication,[44].—**[450.]** Sensation as though the muscles of the face were drawn tightly around the jaw,[44].—Pain in right upper jaw, at root of first molar tooth (after four hours),[44].—**His lips are glued together,**[1].—Jerking of the lower lip,[1].—A well-marked burning line from lip to chin, straight down left side, as though it were a cicatrix (after nine hours),[44].—Cold burning (like turpentine) in vermilion border of lip and point of nose, left side,[44].—Before falling to sleep, the lower jaw was very stiff and immovable,[5].—Some had tetanus at the moment water was taken; others had some froth at the mouth,[3].

Mouth.—Teeth. *Gritting and grinding of the teeth while sleeping,*[1].— The teeth of right side of mouth seem to him to be clenched. (This condition was not noticed by his friend, and was probably subjective),[8].—**[460.]** Aching in all the teeth of the upper jaw, which felt as if they were loose,[1].— Pain in lower molar teeth, right side,[44].—Boring pain in right lower molar teeth, better from pressure, worse from grinding them together,[44].—Dull pain in right lower molar teeth (after three hours),[44].—Heavy throbbing at the roots of the teeth,[1].—Soreness at the union of the front teeth and gums, especially on the inside, with sensitiveness to the touch of the tongue,[1].—Cessation of toothache (after one hour),[33].—Felt no pain, while quite conscious that the toothache was present (after one hour),[33].— ***Tongue.*** White-coated tongue (second day),[7].—Tongue white and sickly-looking (second day),[5].—**[470.]** In morning, tongue white and foul, with a bad taste, as if he had been intoxicated over night (second day),[5].—6 A.M. Before rising, a considerable collection of thick mucus on tongue (second day),[44].—Tongue feels dry, as if scalded (second day),[44].—Tongue and throat have a dry feeling, but no particular desire for water,[44].—Peculiar, somewhat metallic sensation on right half of tongue,[8].—Tongue as if covered with pepper (after forty-five minutes),[19].—Stinging-burning, as of a blister, on back part of tongue, right side, at anterior pillar of fauces (after three hours),[44].—***General Mouth.*** Some dryness of mouth, without thirst (after one hour and a half),[10].—**Dryness of the mouth and lips,**[1].—*Dryness of the mouth, which was not thirst.* The dryness radiated from the back of the throat, opposite the nape of the neck,[26].—[**480.**] Dryness of mouth, with thirst, for some time (after half an hour),[12].—Dryness of mouth, with thirst, all day (second day),[6].—When in bed, had dryness of mouth lasting until next morning, with thirst (after one hour),[11].—Very dry mouth and fauces, so that he could hardly speak or swallow (after half an hour),[27].—Mouth dry and frothy (after four hours),[3].—*Saliva.* Foaming at the mouth,[1].—Increased flow of thick, tasteless saliva,[44].—Slight exudation of resinous saliva, or rather mucus, from tongue,[43].—Viscid mucus from tongue, over its whole upper surface,[44].—**White, thick, frothy, and sticky saliva,**[1].—*Taste.* [**490.**] *Every article of food is extremely palatable,*[1].—Bitter mouth (second day),[7].—Taste of copper in the mouth,[17].—Metallic taste on tongue,[43].—Metallic taste on tongue, with dry sensation and exudation of gummy mucus,[45].—*Speech.* *Stammering and stuttering,*[1].—His lips failed of utterance as if paralyzed,[17].

Throat. The carotid and temporal arteries beat slower and weaker than usual,[20].—Hawks up in the morning glairy lumps with a spot of blood in each,[1].—Dryness and roughness in the throat,[1].—[**500.**] A dryness in the throat led to a request for water,[41].—Feeling of uneasiness, as though from dryness of the throat, or rather a sensation that the tongue and throat were covered with a dry, soft body,[39].—The attempt to smoke a cigar in the open air had to be abandoned on account of the dryness and rawness of the throat,[20].—**The throat is parched, accompanied by intense thirst for cold water,**[1].—Sensation as of a fleshy body at the pit of the throat, impeding deglutition,[1].—Sensation of a plug rising in his throat, causing him to choke,[1].—Burning sensation in throat,[27].—Pressure in tonsils (after one hour and three-quarters),[19].—Scraping of the pharynx, eructations, and slight nausea (soon),[20].

Stomach.—Appetite. Appetite increased,[21].—[**510.**] Increased appetite,[1].—Enormously increased the appetite,[26].—Increased appetite at dinner (second day),[8].—1.30 P.M., increased appetite; had a good lunch (had had no breakfast), (second day),[8].—One effect to which all patients testified, and without being interrogated, was that it improved their appetite and general health, and seemed to improve all their secretions,[31].—Appetite strong (second day),[34].—Great appetite,[12].—Excellent appetite for supper at 6, but mouth still very dry,[27].—Great hunger for several days (second day),[7].—**Ravenous hunger,**[1].—[**520.**] *Ravenous hunger, which is not decreased by eating enormously; he ceases eating only from fear of injuring himself,*[1].—Bulimia,[29].—At tea, ate voraciously,[33].—At tea, ate ravenously, without feeling satisfied,[33].—Pastry and fat food, which previously he never ate without suffering from rancid risings and headache, are now digested easily,[1].—He eats large quantities of bread, declaring it to be delicious,[1].—Little appetite (first day),[7].—Loss of appetite (in about thirty provers),[3].—Loss of appetite (second day),[7].—He has intense thirst, and yet he fears to drink, for he will be suffocated by the magnitude of the stream as it passes down his throat; and again it is not water, but the most delicious metheglin that he swallows with superhuman delight,[17].—[**530.**] Desire for and dread of water (in about thirty provers),[3].—Had a great craving for water, but a single swallow passing down the throat gave the sensation as of holding his mouth under a cataract; a spasm came upon him, with a sensation of fear or dread, but this was only for an instant (after four hours),[3].—*Eructations.* Eructations reminding him of the extract (after forty-five minutes),[19].—Eructations when moving (after one hour and three-quarters),[19].—Eructations of tasteless wind, which relieve a dull pain in the epigastric region,[1].—Slight but continual eructations of wind, tasteless,[44].—For one hour, frequent empty eructations of wind, flavored with *Cannabis* (after two hours),[44].—*Nausea.* Nausea,[1].—Slight nausea (after four hours),[5].—*Stomach.* Sinking at the stomach,[1].— [540.] Cold feeling in stomach, very disagreeable, as though he had drunk cold water (soon after),[44].—Sensation of warmth in the stomach, changing to an aching pain, accompanied by oppression of the chest,[1].—Burning sensation in stomach, for some time (within one hour),[12].—*While eating, his stomach felt so swelled and his chest so oppressed, as if he would suffocate, that he was forced to loosen his clothes,*[1].—Crampy pain in the stomach,[1].— Agonizing clutching in the stomach,[1].—Sensation of weight at stomach,[40].— Cutting-griping pain in the stomach,[1].—Pain in pit of stomach; nervous grumbling sensation in stomach, coming on every few moments, and extending up into the thorax,[44].—Slight pain at pit of stomach, followed by a very marked pricking sensation; these pains cease after a meal (first day),[7].—[550.] **Pain in the cardiac orifice,** relieved by pressure,[1].

Abdomen.—Stitches in right hypochondrium, when breathing (after one hour and three-quarters),[19].—Immediately on lying down again, a disagreeable rumbling in the abdomen, as though a looseness was coming on (immediately),[44].—Disagreeable flatulent rumbling in the bowels, at night, when lying down,[44].—The abdomen feels swelled; relieved by belching up a considerable quantity of wind,[1].—Stitches above the symphysis pubis,[1].

Rectum and Anus.—Tenesmus,[21].—*Sensation in the anus as if he were sitting on a ball; as if the anus and a part of the urethra were filled up by a hard round body,*[1].

Stool.—Painless yellow diarrhœa was present in *every* case (in about thirty provers),[3].—Two liquid stools, besides frequent ineffectual urging (first and second days),[4].—[560.] Had a discharge from the bowels (after five hours), and in half an hour had another. They were thin, yellow, and painless. The diarrhœa increased, and heat pervaded the abdomen internally, and frequent discharges of this kind followed, but entirely without pain,[3].—Constipation,[21].—Constipation followed the proving,[20].—In one or two cases, a little constipation for a few days,[3].—Costiveness,[1].

Urinary Organs.—Kidneys. Pain in the kidneys, when laughing,[1].—[570.] Burning in the kidneys,[1].—Aching in the kidneys, keeping him awake at night,[1].—Sharp stitches in both kidneys,[1].—*Urethra.* Slight inflammation of the orifice of the urethra,[1].—**On squeezing the glans penis, a white glairy mucus oozes out,**[1].—Uneasiness in the urethra,[1].—*Feelings in the urethra as if there were a gonorrhœal discharge,*[1].—*Pain and burning during urination,*[1].—Burning pains in the urethra, worse in the evening,[1]. —**Burning and scalding before, during, and after urination,**[1].—[580.] *Intense burning at the orifice of the urethra, during urination and afterwards,*[1].—Stitching in urethra,[4].—Stitches in urethra (second day),[4].— Stitching pains in urethra and anus for one minute (after one hour and three-quarters),[19].—Stitching in the end of the urethra (after eleven hours),[4].—Stitching in end of urethra (evening and night), (second day),[4]. —[590.] **Stinging pain before, during, and after urination,**[1].—*Sharp prickings, like needles, in the urethra, so severe as to send a thrill to the cheeks and hands,*[1].—Constant inclination to urinate (after one hour and three-quarters),[19].—Continual desire to urinate (second day),[44].—Although the urine had been voided on retiring, a great desire was felt to pass more, which he essayed to do, but could scarcely retain it until the vessel could be got ready (after four hours),[3].—No desire to urinate (first day),[44].—*Urging to* *urinate, but he cannot pass a drop*,[1].—*Urging to urinate, with much straining*,[1].—*The urging continues after urination*,[1].—**Micturition.** Frequent micturition of much urine,[12].—Frequent micturition in night, much in quantity,[11].—*Urinating frequently, but in a small quantity*,[1].—*Frequent urination, with burning pain, in the evening*,[1].—At night, frequent urinating; urine dark,[4].—Urinating every hour,[1].—Was obliged to urinate several times; at the beginning, with difficulty,[20].—Could not voluntarily retain the urine,[20].—**Profuse colorless urine,**[1].—**[600.]** *Copious discharge of clear, light-colored urine*,[1].—*Immense flow of urine in a full, clear stream*,[1].—As much urine was passed as is usually collected during the whole night (after four hours),[3].—*He has to wait some time before the urine flows*,[1].—*He has to force out the last few drops with his hand*,[1].—For several days, incomplete passage of urine, which could only be finished by violent pressure,[4].—**The urine dribbles out after the stream ceases,**[1].—The stream suddenly stops, and then flows on,[1].—The urine passes freely at times, then again in small quantities, with burning and biting,[1].—**Urine.** Urine clear, and in great quantity (third day),[7].—**[610.]** Thick red urine (second day),[7].—Urine darker, but without sediment and more scanty,[4].

Sexual Organs.—Male. Excitement of the genitals,[21].—**Satyriasis,**[1].—*Erections while riding, walking, and also while sitting still; not caused by amorous thoughts*,[1].—After coition, the erection continues so long and becomes so painful that he has to apply cold water to the penis,[1].—*Violent erections*,[1].—*Priapism*,[1].—*Chordee*,[1].—*Penis relaxed and shrunken* (after one hour and three-quarters),[19].—**[620.]** *Uneasiness, with burning sensation in the penis and urethra, accompanied by frequent calls to urinate*,[1].—The sexual thrill is very much prolonged, with more than a dozen ejaculations of semen,[1].—In the night, during coitus, little or no sensation. Scarcely any emission or sensation, but soon after a rather acute pain in the loins, which lasted a short time (quite unusual), (second day),[5].—The sexual thrill consists merely of an intense burning, with no ejaculation of semen,[1].—Sticking-burning soreness in the glans penis,[1].—*Itching of the glans penis*,[1].—Itching and burning of the scrotum,[1].—Aphrodisia,[29].—Aphrodisiac feeling to an unusual degree (after seven hours),[5].—*Excessive venereal appetite, with frequent erections during the day*,[1].—**[630.]** Excessive discharge of prostatic fluid, at night, during a hard evacuation,[1].—***Female.*** *Very profuse menstruation, which lasted five days* (in two women, after 10 grains, on two occasions),[3].—Nymphomania,[1].—Excites sexual desire, but causes sterility,[42].

Respiratory Organs.—Voice. The pitch of the voice is much higher,[1].—Talks in so low a tone as not to be heard, and laughs excessively when told of it,[1].—Inability to measure the compass and volume of the voice when speaking,[17].—**Cough.** Rough cough, scratching the breast immediately under the sternum,[1].—Slight dry cough (after four hours), afterward becoming harder, but still dry, almost like a bark,[3].—Hard, dry cough (in about thirty provers),[3].—**Respiration.** **[640.]** Hot breath,[1].—Stertorous breathing,[17].—Difficult respiration,[21].—*It requires great effort to take a deep inspiration*,[1].—The least pressure on the stomach brings on a fit of suffocation,[1].—Desire for open air,[23].

Chest.—Pains in thorax (after forty-five minutes),[19].—Anxious sensation in chest, and rapid, irregular, small beats of the heart, almost all day (second day),[4].—Heaviness of chest in walking (after forty-five minutes),[19].—Burning in chest,[21].—**[650.]** On ascending some steps quickly, felt a constricted pain across the chest on a line with the heart; it only lasted a moment or two; never felt such a pain before (second day),[5].—Pains pressing, stitching, in thorax and extremities (after one hour and three-quarters),[19].—Oppression on chest,[8].—Oppression of the chest with a pressive and tightened sensation in the pit of the stomach,[20].—*Oppression of the chest, with deep, labored breathing. He feels as if suffocated, and has to be fanned,*[1].—Considerable oppression of chest, as if suffocation would surely supervene; increased by mounting the stairs,[41].—Stitches extending from both nipples through the chest,[1].—Sharp, cutting pain behind the sternum, aggravated by swallowing,[1].

Heart and Pulse.—Præcordium. Oppression in præcordium,[23]. —Sense of weight in region of heart (soon after),[36].—[660.] Indescribable sensation of oppression about heart; feeling of sickness at heart; heart's beating seemed to him to be very much embarrassed, sharp and quick, weak and small; its contractions seemed jerky. This condition of heart lasted until he went to bed, about 3 A.M.,[8].—For a long time after, annoyed and alarmed by pains about the heart,[41].—Pricking pains, apparently on surface of heart, off and on,[13].—On breathing, the heart feels as if it rubbed against the ribs,[1].—Felt sick at the heart. (The last word really refers to the heart, and not to any other part),[8].—Anguish at the heart,[1].—Pain in the heart, with palpitation of the heart,[1].—*Pressing pain in the heart, with dyspnœa the whole night,*[1].—Sticking pains in small circumscribed places in the heart,[1].—*Painful sticking as with the prongs of a fork in the heart,*[1].— [670.] *Stitches in the heart, accompanied by great oppression; the latter relieved by deep breathing,*[1].—*Heart's Action.* Impulse of the heart very weak, at times scarcely perceptible,[20].—Intense and rapid beating of heart, and widely dilated pupils (after half an hour),[27].—Small, uneven, anxious beats of the heart, when sitting or stooping (after three hours),[4].— *Palpitation of the heart, awakening him from sleep,*[1].—Painful palpitation of the heart,[1].—*Pulse.* Slight increase in the force of the pulse (after one hour),[33].—His pulse seemed to him to be full and bounding,[8].—His pulse began to throb heavily, and his head to be dizzy,[3].—Increased quickness of pulse,[29].—[680.] Pulse quickened,[21].—Slight increase of pulse,[36].—Pulse beating at a tremendous rate, but so feebly that he could not feel the impulse of the heart against the chest,[15].—Pulse, as counted by a friend, 120, full and bounding. It is usually about 84 at this time,[8].—His pulse he counted to be 130,[6].—Pulse 150–160 (after half an hour),[27].—Pulse very feeble (soon after),[36].—**Pulse below the natural standard, as low as 46,**[1].— Pulse very small and slow, with long intermissions,[20].—Pulse at the wrist frequently intermitting, often not noticed for a minute, and when it returned it was remarkably weak, and only felt with great care; afterwards it became more decided and more frequent and rose eighteen beats above the normal,[20].

Neck and Back.—Neck. [690.] Aching in the nape of the neck, in the right shoulder, and in the right ear,[1].—*Back.* Peculiar feeling like a stream of warm water, which gradually stole up the back, and made its way to the brain (after half an hour),[27].—Sensation as though a red-hot iron rod was passed from sacrum up the spine to the atlas, around the occiput, over the eyes from right side stopping at left ear, leaving a feeling as if charred, taking six hours to perform the passage,[44].—Stunning pain between the shoulder-blades,[1].—**Pain across the shoulders and spine, forcing him to stoop, and preventing him from walking erect,**[1].—4 P.M. Pain very severe on the outer edge of trapezius muscle (second day),[44].—Reflex movements of spinal column; a wavelike motion beginning at dorsal region, and extending to pelvis, alternately raising and depressing first the dorsum, afterwards the pelvis, slowly and involuntarily. While the dorsum and shoulder were pressed against the bed, the lumbar and pelvic regions were slowly elevated, and then slowly but firmly depressed while the dorsum was slowly elevated,[6].—Cold feeling in small of back and between the shoulders,[14].

Extremities in General.—Objective. Seized with a sort of gesticulatory convulsions in the arms and legs, and by degrees his symptoms assumed the appearance of those which characterize hydrophobia,[39].— **Paralysis of the lower extremities and right arm,**[1].—*Subjective.* [700.] Pleasant numbness in the limbs (after one hour),[33].—Unpleasant shuddering through all the limbs, with a painful feeling of weight in the occiput, and a tetanic intermittent contraction of the muscles of the nape of the neck,[22].—Leaden feeling in the limbs, as though he could not move them, for some time (after two and a half hours),[12].—Tired feeling in the limbs, with disposition to retire to bed,[1].—Pains in wrists and ankles (second day),[4].—Pains in the joints (second day),[7].

Upper Extremities.—Objective. Trembling of the arms and hands,[1].—Inability to raise the right arm, with coldness of the right hand,[1].—*Subjective.* Curious shooting pain in left arm, from shoulder to tip of middle finger, producing in the finger a feeling of internal soreness, the same as is felt in neuralgic pains. The pain at one time concentrated itself in the pulpy part of the ungual phalanx, and at another at the upper part of the axillary border of the scapula, whence it seemed to radiate, like the spokes of a wheel, for a distance of two inches (after one hour and two-thirds),[13].—**Agreeable thrilling through the arms and hands,**[1].—*Shoulders.* [710.] Lameness of the shoulders,[1].—Feeling in the shoulders as if beaten, particularly in the left shoulder,[1].—*Arm.* Pain in front of the arm and back of the elbow,[44].—*Elbow.* Pain as from fatigue in the bend of the right elbow (at 7 A.M., first day),[7].—*Forearm.* Unable to raise his hands, the feeling being as if a weight was upon the forearm,[3].—Heaviness of forearm and feet (in about thirty provers),[3].— *Wrist.* Pains in left wrist (second day),[4].—*Hands.* Constant rubbing of hands,[29].—Shaking of the hands so that he cannot write,[17].—The hands feel monstrously large,[1].—*Fingers.* [720.] Sudden appearance of redness in all the fingers, with burning and pricking in the joints,[1].—Sharp sticking pain in the fingers,[1].—Aching in the finger-joints,[1].

Lower Extremities.—Objective. Unsteadiness of gait; not that of one who fears to fall, but of one who tries to keep down, for he felt as if there were springs in his knees, and was reminded of the story of the man with the mechanical leg, that walked away with him,[26].—While going along a plank walk, just one board wide, every now and then, and suddenly, the right leg would shoot to the left, missing the plank. After observing this muscular freak a few times, the attention was centred upon locomotion, with a view of preventing a repetition of the erratic misstep. Out shot the leg again and again, defying volition, and invariably going over to the left,[41].—**Entire paralysis of the lower extremities,**[1].—*He is unable to walk upstairs, on account of an almost entire paralysis of the limbs, with stiffness and tired aching in both knees,*[1].—Limbs unable to support him (after two hours and a quarter),[35].—Legs hardly able to support body,[27].— The right limb suddenly gives way and he falls,[1].—[730.] About 3 A.M., having roused himself to sobriety, he went to bed. Stumbled down the steps on leaving his friend's room,[8].—Lameness of the right limb, with drawings in the calves,[1].—Great weakness of the left leg,[1].—*Weariness in both limbs, almost amounting to paralysis; worse in the left*,[1].—**Subjective.** His limbs feel very large,[1].—**Agreeable thrilling in both limbs from the knees down, with a sensation as if a bird's claws were clasping the knees,**[1].—*The right limb feels paralyzed when walking*,[1].—Tired feeling in the left limb,[1].—Numbness of the left limb and foot,[1].—**Hip.** Pain in the right hip. Pain in the left thigh-bone,[1].—**Thigh.** [740.] Pain and itching in left leg just above the knee,[44].—**Knee.** Laming pain, with drawing and aching in the right knee,[1].—Tearing pain in left knee (after fifteen hours),[4].—The patellæ feel as if forcibly dragged down,[1].—**Leg.** A strange, painful lassitude in both legs (after fourteen hours),[4].—Aching pain in leg, near left external malleolus, while lying on back, not when lying on side,[44]. —Sensation of cramps in the calves of the legs, which rendered the movement of the legs impossible, or caused them to be distended, or to take a sudden jump,[39].—**Ankle.** Pain in right ankle (evening),[4].—**Foot.** He drags his feet when walking,[1].—His feet repeatedly go to sleep,[1].—[750.] On attempting to walk, his feet felt heavy; his hands were with difficulty raised, as the forearm felt as if kept down by weights (after four hours),[3]. —*On attempting to walk, he experienced intensely violent pains, as if he trod on a number of spikes, which penetrated the soles of his feet and ran upward through his limbs to his hips; worse in the right limb, and accompanied by drawing pains in both calves;* these pains forced him to limp and cry out in agony,[1].—*Numb feeling of the sole of the left foot, then the foot, increasing to a numbness of the whole limb*,[1].—Burning in the soles of the feet,[1].—Sticking in the soles of the feet,[1].—Numbness in the joints of both feet,[1].—Bone-pain in metatarso-phalangeal joint of right foot,[44].—**Toes.** *Shooting pains in the joints of the toes of the left foot, worse in the great toe*,[1].—Violent pains in the joints of right great toe (forenoon and evening), (third day),[4].— *Aching and stitching pain in the ball of the left big toe*,[1].—[760.] *Pricking and aching in the joints of the big toes of the left foot*,[1].

General Symptoms.—Objective. Determination of blood to surface,[29].—Great excitation of the whole system, as if the blood were circulating very quickly; as if streams of it were poured from below towards the head, which felt dull, while his eyes were glistening; on walking, he could scarcely find his way; everything seemed dark and perverted; on reaching home great cheerfulness and serenity, as though an unseen power lifted him up into other and higher regions; everything appeared too small and too dark; frequent protestations that he saw something unearthly, and could accomplish great things; he saw spirits dancing around him as happy as himself; his hearing was very acute; the slightest noise, as the beating of his own heart, seemed too loud; violent thirst; cataleptic and epileptic attacks,[22].—Strange, balancing gait,[29].—From time to time shaking of the whole body,[1].—Catalepsy,[21].—Sometimes catalepsy,[29].—He did things automatically,[1].—Cannot avoid running against people in the street,[1].—Unconsciously walks sidewise in the street,[1].—[770.] Creeps on hands or knees in open air,[23].—During the intoxication, when the spells of laughter came on, he stamped with his feet, and raised his body up and down on the sofa in a violent manner,[1].—Closed his eyes and tried to think of something solemn. Suddenly felt as if he were a marble statue, had no ability to move, and a chill all over him,[3].—Feels as if under the sedative influence of an opiate (after three hours),[5].—Disinclination to physical labor,[1].—Felt idle in morning (second day),[5].—Luxurious indolence and erotic delirium,[22].— *Great desire to lie down in the daytime*,[1].—Much torpidity (second day),[33].—

Feels greatly fatigued,[1].—[780.] Relaxation of muscular power (after four and a quarter hours),[13].—Felt very weak (second day),[20].—Felt as if weak, chiefly about the knees (after two and a quarter hours),[34].—Great muscular weakness,[21].—Too weak and nervous to work,[27].—*He felt so weak that he could scarcely speak, and soon fell into a deep sleep*,[1].—**Thoroughly exhausted from a short walk**,[1].—Prostration (soon after),[36].—State of collapse (nearly ending in death),[38].—As soon as he closed his eyes he fell into a state of syncope,[22].—[790.] Sense of vague uneasiness,[41].—Felt in the highest degree nervous,[27].—Nervous, restless feeling over the whole body,[44].—Impulse to change about from place to place,[22].—After experiencing peculiar visions and sensations a necessity for exercise came on; he raised himself as if by some elastic power, struck himself on the breast, and began to sing and dance in the most extravagant manner,[22].—Feeling of numbness,[28].—Felt a peculiar numbness creeping through body and limbs,[33].—Skin insensible to irritation, for example, to mustard, brushes, etc.,[20].—Was unconscious that mustard has been placed to his feet, and that they had been rubbed with brushes; the sensitiveness of the skin seemed to be completely blunted,[20].—Gradually total anæsthesia,[21].—[800.] Anæsthesia extended all over his body. It gradually decreased, but the sensibility did not return universally, nor steadily, there being frequent relapses,[39].—*Subjective.* An indescribably "queer" feeling pervaded the whole body (after one hour),[41].—There was also a curious sensation connected with the air, but he cannot recollect it,[8].—Feeling of lightness on motion was very marked,[20].—Feeling of lightness or buoyancy, as though he could fall like a cork, without sustaining harm (after four and a quarter hours),[13].—Especially characteristic was the sensation as if his body were raised up from the ground, and as if he could fly away,[20].—Felt as if under influence of intoxicating drink (after half an hour),[27].—Felt drunk (after one hour),[12].—Felt drunk (after one hour and a half),[10].—Woke in morning not quite sober (second day),[8].—[810.] Felt very badly,[8].—After going to bed, sensation of heaviness or drowsiness; could not lift his arms or legs (after one hour),[11].—Rigidity of the muscular system,[17].—Felt the characteristic *thrill* produced by the drug (after exactly four hours),[3].—Agreeable thrilling through the body and extremities,[1].—All agree that the first symptom is experienced after the lapse of some hours, and is uniformly a thrill through the whole frame to the finger-ends, and through the brain, followed by great terror,[17].—Had a *real* Hashish thrill, so violent that I took hold of a counter to prevent myself from reeling, experiencing the same want of confidence in myself and anxious terror I had felt on taking the larger dose (after one hour),[43].—The right side of the body seemed to him to be greatly enlarged, so that he thought if he thus continued to grow he must bend over to opposite side,[8].—Sensation as if single parts had become larger and thicker, *e. g.*, the lower lip seems swollen to the level of the nose, or the nose so large as to obstruct vision,[21].—Sudden, dull, aching pain and constriction, mixed with numbness and tingling, as if he had been electrified. It began in right upper arm, extending down the arm and up to the axilla, gradually passing down to the feet, and then up to the head. It was chiefly felt in arm and axilla. This feeling came on and off like a wave of sensation; it was confined entirely to the right side, and seemed to stop at the mesial line. (The prover's right side was next the fire), (after forty minutes),[8].—[820.] Suddenly a great degree of oppression; everything seemed too narrow to him; features became distorted; he became pale; the oppression increased to anxiety, with a feeling as though his blood mounted to his head in a boiling condition,[20].

—The symptoms develop themselves mostly on the right side,[1].—It affects persons of the highest nervous and sanguine temperament with the strongest effect; the bilious nearly as much; the lymphatic but slightly, with such symptoms as vertigo, nausea, coma, or muscular rigidity,[17].

Skin.—Formication,[21].—Itching in face, shoulder, abdomen, and feet, relieved by scratching,[44].—Itching of nose continually,[44].—Itching of the sole of the foot,[44].

Sleep and Dreams.—Sleepiness. Sleepiness (after one hour),[11].—Sleepiness, drowsiness,[44].—*Day sleepiness*,[1].—[**830.**] **Excessive sleepiness**,[1].—Great sleepiness in the afternoon,[1].—Became sleepy without any previous excitement or exhilaration; it is a muddled state (after four hours),[5].——More than usually sleepy in the evening (after fourteen hours),[5].—Felt sleepy, for some time (after two and a half hours),[12].—Drowsiness, with cold feeling of back of head and neck, as though air blew thereon,[44].—Great drowsiness, even in daytime (second day),[7].—Species of interrupted drowsiness,[40].—Felt drowsy, and fell asleep in arm-chair (after two hours),[14].—In morning felt drowsy, and still under the influence of the drug; the drowsiness lasted till 1.30 P.M., with alternate waking and sleeping, but the waking was a pleasant dreamy state (second day),[8].—[**840.**] On going to bed fell into a drowsy state, in which he imagined that the finger-nails of both hands were about the size of plates, very curved, but otherwise of natural shape; on opening and shutting the fingers (subjective or objective?) they seemed to slide over one another like a fan; and on tapping them against a hard surface (subjective or objective?) a delicious sensation was produced,[8].—Feeling of sleep; could easily sleep if he were to lie down and give way to the feeling; but when necessary he could always rouse himself (after four hours),[13].—Strong inclination to sleep, and therefore hurried to bed, without undressing,[27].—Stronger disposition to sleep, which continued for half an hour (after six and two-thirds hours),[13].—Was obliged to yield himself to sleep (after four hours),[5].—Indisposition to rise in the morning,[1].—Frequent intervals of sleep (after one hour),[33].—Seemed to go to sleep now and then for a few moments, which, however, appeared very much prolonged, with pleasant dreams; then woke up, and wrote down these notes,[8].—Gave him a double portion of sleep,[26].—After a full night's rest he slept soundly the whole of the next day,[1].—[**850.**] Prolonged and tranquil sleep,[1].—Slept three days and three nights, with the exception of those times he was awakened to eat his meals,[1].—**Sound sleep**,[1].—*Sound sleep with melancholy dreams*,[1].—Slept soundly,[35].—Slept soundly at night,[33].—Sleep, like that of one "dead drunk,"[41].—At night, slept profoundly, no dreams,[5].—Slept very quietly, without dreams,[27].—When asleep, looked stiff, as if dead, with the lower jaw down,[5].—[**860.**] *Starting of the limbs while sleeping, which awoke him, when he feared he would have a fit*,[1].—Screaming while sleeping,[1].—*Talking during sleep*,[1].—Dozed a little on a sofa, in a friend's room; was heard chuckling to himself; woke up every five minutes, when it seemed to him as if hours had elapsed. After his friend had gone to bed, kept waking up, thinking he was still in the room, but on rousing himself, recollected all; then relapsed (after two hours),[9].—All the afternoon, alternate dozing and waking; the same pleasant dreamy state when waking (second day),[8].—After dinner, dozing and waking as before. Took coffee, which removed it (second day),[8].—*Sleeplessness.* Woke once in night, which is unusual,[13].—Woke at 4 A.M. and at 7 A.M., which is very unusual,[13].—He wakes at 6 o'clock in the morning, with fulness of the head and heaviness of the body,[1].—He wakes soon after midnight, with intense thirst,[1].—[**870.**] He wakes before midnight in a state of semi-consciousness; with inability to move; palpitation of the heart, slow, deep, labored, and intermittent breathing, and a feeling as if he were dying,[1].—He wakes before midnight, overcome with dreadful sensations; imagines that he is going to be choked, cries and moans for some time, when all the objects in the room appear their respective sizes, and he falls asleep again,[1].—Wakeful all night; mild, pleasant dreams; cat-naps (second day),[44].—The only effect was to make him lose a night's rest,[26].—When in bed, not able to go to sleep; mind wandered rapidly from one subject to another; he seemed to be dreaming with open eyes, for he saw, heard, and noticed everything around him,[27].—*Dreams.* She seemed to dream with open eyes, and the time appeared to her very long,[40].—When he ceases to exercise his will, he falls into a kind of dream; the period of this dreamy state seems painfully prolonged; he feels as if he never would get through the night,[8].—*In the daytime, dreams, returning periodically, or dreamy attacks,*[1].—The dreams lasted about an hour, and then changed to a slight headache, which he felt till late at night,[27].—Vivid dreams, sometimes ecstatic (second day),[7].—[**880.**] A variety of delightful dreams came over him (after two hours and a quarter),[35].—Very delicious dreams; cannot remember much of them now,[8].—*Voluptuous dreams, with erections and profuse seminal emissions,*[1].—*Prophetic dreams,*[1].—*Vexatious dreams,*[1].—Slept well, with the exception of an ugly dream,[5].—Woke in the midst of a wild, shapeless dream, in a state of extraordinary agitation, and bathed in perspiration,[15].—*Dreams of danger, and of perils encountered,*[1].—*Dreams of dead bodies,*[1].—*Nightmare every night, as soon as he falls asleep,*[1].—[**890.**] Sleep, which before the habit of taking Hashish, was always with dreams more or less vivid, was during the whole period of the indulgence entirely dreamless,[17].

Fever.—*Chilliness.* *Loss of animal heat,*[1].—Coldness of surface (soon after),[36]. Shivering (first day),[7].—A pleasant cooling seemed suddenly to affect the whole body,[24].—Coldness and shivering, with external heat (second day),[7].—*General chilliness,*[1].—Hard shaking chill, with the following symptoms: loud chattering of the teeth; coldness of the body and extremities; profuse cold sweat; tired feeling in the limbs, with aching in the joints; dry mouth, with thick white sticky saliva; intense thirst; drinking of large quantities of water; staggering and falling on attempting to walk; thumping in the head and heart; inability to rise from a stooping position on account of a crushing weight on the cerebellum, neck, and shoulder; blindness, with the exception of a small point immediately where he looks; extremely slow and full pulse; seeming descent of the ceiling to crush him; earnest belief that he is dying, but cannot cry for help; falling to the floor and lying for some time unconscious; sleeping for three nights and three days afterwards,[1].—9 A.M., an icy coldness across the root of nose, comes on when leaning forward writing, goes away when moving about (third day),[44].—*Coldness of the face, nose, and hands, after dinner,*[1].—[**900.**] *Coldness of the right hand,* with stiffness and numbness of the right thumb,[1].—Coldness of the hands, feet, and especially of the nose, after dinner, with shivering, shaking, and inability to get warm,[1].—Extremities, upper and lower, cold, at times trembling,[20].—*Heat.* The heat of the body was increased,[20].—In the cold, 2° F. below zero, he does not feel cold, although nearly undressed,[19].—Did not feel cold, while those who were walking with him, and wrapped in mantles, were complaining of it,[26].—Sensation of heat,[21].—Pleasant sensation of warmth, beginning in the spine and extending all through the body (after one hour),[11].—While lying down, sensation of glow and warmth,[6].—Pleasant burning heat all over body,[8].—[910.] Burning in the skin of the body and extremities,[1].—Intense fever boiled in my blood, and every heart-beat was like the stroke of a colossal engine,[17].—Forehead and head only moderately warm, never hot,[20].—Warm tingling sensation, over the whole left side of face,[44].—Moist warmth of palms of hands,[44].—Feeling of warmth over front of body and arms,[44].—*Sweat.* Slight sweat,[21]. —Sweat on front of limbs, and moist feeling of whole body, especially the front,[44].—**Profuse sticky sweat, standing out in drops on his forehead,**[1].—No sweat for several days,[20].

Conditions.—Aggravation.—(*Morning*), Tongue white, etc.; before rising, mucus on tongue; hawks up lumps.—(*Afternoon*), Easily excited, etc.; sleepiness.—(*Evening*), Pains in urethra.—(*Night*), *Injection of the conjunctiva;* when lying down, rumbling in bowels; frequent micturition.—(*Ascending stairs*), Oppression of chest.—(*When in bed*), Dryness of mouth, etc.—(*When breathing*), Stitches in hypochondrium.—(*Candlelight*), Obliterates consciousness.—(*Coffee*), The symptoms, especially those of the brain. —(*After dinner*), *Coldness of face*, etc.; coldness of hands, etc.—(*While eating*), *Stomach feels swollen, etc.*—(*Grinding teeth*), Pain in teeth.—(*When laughing*), *Pain in kidneys.*—(*When lying down*), Singing in ears.—(*While lying on back*), Pain in leg.—(*On motion*), Eructations.—(*On rising*), *Vertigo, etc.*—(*Shaking head*), Fulness in cerebellum, etc.—(*When sitting*), Small, etc., beats of the heart.—(*On falling asleep*), Sensation in brain.—(*Spirituous liquors*), The symptoms, especially of the brain.—(*On stooping*), Dizziness; small, etc., beats of heart.—(*In the sun*), Headache.—(*Swallowing*), Pain behind sternum.—(*Tobacco smoking*), The symptoms, especially of the brain.—(*Before, during, and after urination*), **Stinging pain; burning,** etc.—(*On waking*), Sensation in brain; headache.—(*On walking*), Inclination to vertigo; dizziness; heaviness of chest.—(*In warm room*), Compression of brain, etc.

Amelioration.—(*Fresh air*), Paleness of face.—(*Deep breathing*), Stitches in heart, etc.—(*Coffee*), Dizziness; headache.—(*Washing in cold water*), The symptoms.—(*Eructation*), Pain in epigastric region; swelling of abdomen.—(*Pressure*), Pain in right ear; pain in teeth; **pain in cardiac orifice.**—(*Rest*), The symptoms.

APPENDIX.

THE editor has deemed it expedient to retain the natural grouping and sequence of the following effects, recorded by Dr. Edgar Holden in his work on the sphygmograph (Philadelphia, 1874), thus preserving the association of some general symptoms with the condition of the pulse.

9.15 P.M. Feeling vigorous and well. First tracing normal, smooth, and even (not recorded), 5 grains taken.

9.35. A feeling of lightness perceptible. (Tracing 181.) Two records, at 0° and 2½°.* Diminished frequency.

10 P.M. Nervous and excited. (Tracing 182.) Two records at 4½°.

---

* These degrees refer to the pressure of the instrument on the artery, regulated at will; 0° equals 100 grammes; 2½° equals 186 grammes; 5° equals 690 grammes.

Oscillation singularly marked; tension increased; amplitude and frequency diminished.

10.05 P.M. Sudden freedom from any unusual feeling. (Tracing 183.) Two records showing a sudden return of, or rather approach to, a normal condition.

10.15 P.M. 7 grains more.

10.40 P.M. Excited. (Tracing 184.) Record at 2½° shows capillary resistance and wave of recoil.

11.45 P.M. (Tracing 185.) Two records at 2½° and 0° gave similar results, indicating venous impletion. Frequency increased.

11.50 P.M. Drowsy and calm. (Tracing 186.) Record at 2½°.

11.55 P.M. (Tracing 187.) Record at 2½°, both the latter exhibit impaired propulsive power of the heart.

Total amount, 12 grains within two hours.

November 2d, 1872, 9.15 P.M. 30 drops.

9.45 P.M. Beginning to feel an indefinable sensation of comfort. 9.20, 9.25, and 9.45 P.M. (Tracing 188.) Records all taken at the same pressure. At the latter hour the amplitude began to show increase of tension.

9.45 P.M. 40 drops more.

10 P.M. Slightly exhilarated. 10.15. Somewhat drowsy. Tracings at 9.50, 10 (tracing 189), and 10.15 P.M. (tracing 190) exhibit only increase of tension, with, at the latter hour, diminished frequency equal to ten beats.

10.20 and 10.25 P.M. (Tracing 191.) Tension and frequency variable.

10.25 P.M. All effects apparently gone. 40 drops more.

10.45 P.M. Again exhilarated. (Tracing 192.) Records exhibit great increase of arterial tension.

11 P.M. Drowsy, but not pleasantly so, nor as if from desire to sleep. (Tracing 193.) Frequency greatly increased, equal to thirty beats and falling in five minutes as many; tension less.

11.05 P.M. (Tracing 194.) Record shows increased cardiac excitement at beginning of systole, with some obstruction, either proximate or distal.

Total amount, 110 drops.

November 5th, 1872, 9 P.M. Feeling well. 100 drops. Tracing normal.

9.10 P.M. (Tracing 195.) Amplitude, and therefore tension increased, frequency steadily diminishing till 9.45. Tracings at 9.30, 9.45.

10 P.M. No effects experienced. 120 drops more.

10.10 P.M. (Tracing 196.) Diminished tension and the oscillation of cerebro-spinal implication. This tracing, by accident in transfer, fails to show this except in the first wave.

10.15 P.M. Same.

10.35 P.M. (Tracing 197.) Obstruction either proximate or remote.

10.40. (Similar to tracing 195.) Diminishing obstruction.

10.45 P.M. Very little effect. 200 drops more.

11.15 P.M. (Tracing 198.) Diminished tension and evident sedation, but frequency slightly increased.

11.18 P.M. No effect whatever. Same.

Total amount taken, 420 drops!

November 9th, 1872, 9.50 P.M. Feeling not well as usual, owing to overwork; otherwise all right. 12 grains of fresh extract taken.

10.15 P.M. A little nauseated and eyes heavy.

10 and 10.15 P.M. Tracings showed diminishing frequency and tension, and not feeling well a pressure of 0° was found to be the best for observation, instead of 2½° as heretofore.

10.30 P.M. Feeling comfortable and well. (Tracing 199.) Frequency still less; pulse small, but normal, showing sedation.

10.45. Effect passing off; pulse somewhat excited. 14 grains more taken.

11.25. A few minutes exhilarated, then very drowsy, but no impairment of will.

11.25 and 11.40 P.M. (Tracings 200 and 201.) Records exhibited great weakness of cardiac power, it being difficult to obtain them even at 0°.

11.45 P.M. Drowsiness gone, and feel free from any effect. 11.45, 11.48, and 11.50 P.M. (Tracing 202.) The records taken showed a sudden decrease of frequency and tension, and equally sudden increase.

12.30 M. Terrific excitement, twitchings, dreams, etc.; sensations as of swelling of the head, painful insomnia and feeling of desperate recklessness.

November 10th. (Tracings taken the day following the use of the drug.)

7.50 A.M. Peculiar action of medicine still evident, head swollen, confusion of ideas, etc. Tracings small, and showing weak heart.

12.30 M. Have been asleep and feel better; influence passing off. (Tracing 203.) Same, but showing also the slight dicrotism of capillary dilatation.

Total amount taken, 26 grains. Time, two hours and forty minutes.

SYNOPSIS OF EFFECTS.

First Experiment.—5 grains, 9.15. After twenty minutes, diminished frequency; after forty-five minutes, marked cerebral disturbance, exhibited in oscillation and minimum amplitude and frequency, with increased tension. *Maximum effect of first dose in forty-five minutes.* In fifty minutes sudden cessation of effect.

Seven grains, 10.15. *Maximum effect of second dose in thirty minutes.* In thirty-five minutes, capillary disturbance and increased tension, with increased frequency. In forty minutes, beginning of impairment of cardiac impulse, continuing two hours from administration of remedy.

Second Experiment.—30 drops of tr., 9.15 P.M. In thirty minutes increased tension.

Forty drops more, 9.45. In sixty minutes from first dose, diminished frequency; arterial tension great. In one hour and ten minutes, irregularity in tension and frequency, with increase in prominence of waves, showing cerebro-spinal stimulation.

Forty drops more, 10.25. In one hour and forty-five minutes, great increase of frequency, equal to thirty beats; falling as many in five minutes more, with reduced tension. In one hour and fifty minutes from first dose, evidences of increased irritability of the heart, with some obstruction, either proximate or remote. *Maximum effect of tension* in thirty-five minutes; *of irritation* in thirty-five minutes; *of frequency* in one hour forty-five minutes; *of diminished power,* one hour five minutes; *of some obstruction* to circulation, one hour forty-five minutes.

First Experiment.—5 grains, 9.15. In twenty minutes, lightness. In forty-five minutes, nervousness and excitement. In fifty minutes, sudden freedom from any effect.

Seven grains, 10.15. In twenty-five minutes, excitement. In ninety-five minutes, drowsiness and calm. *Maximum effect,* from first dose, maximum of excitement in forty-five minutes; from second, maximum of excitement in twenty-five minutes; maximum of sedative effect in twelve minutes.

Second Experiment.—30 drops of tr., 9.15 P.M. In thirty minutes quiet. In forty-five minutes, exhilaration. In one hour, drowsiness.

Forty drops more, 9.45. In twenty minutes after *second* dose, new excitement.

Forty drops again, at 10.25. In thirty-five minutes, drowsiness. *Maximum effect* of exhilaration in this experiment, forty-five minutes from first dose; maximum of drowsiness, in one hour; of exhilaration after second dose, in twenty minutes; of drowsiness, in thirty-five minutes.

Synopsis of the two later experiments with Cannabis Indica need not be given. It may be briefly said of them that the doses were large and repeated at nearly one hour intervals. The effect was in the first of these apparent in the tracing in ten minutes, and a steady diminution of frequency resulted, until in forty-five minutes there occurred evidence of implication of the nervous system. In thirty-five minutes after the second dose there appeared evidence of some obstruction to circulation, either near the heart or in the capillaries, and after 420 drops had been taken, the arterial tension was greatly reduced, with corresponding increase of the venous pressure, and marked sedation, just two hours and fifteen minutes from the first dose, and thirty from the last and largest.

Finally, sudden cessation of effect.

In the last experiment detailed, in which a fresh alcoholic extract was again used, the following facts were noticed.

First. Tracings abnormal from malaise at the beginning became normal in forty minutes, with marked sedation and diminished frequency. In fifty-five minutes began the stage of exhilaration, at which time a larger dose was taken. After fifty-five minutes the heart's impulsive power was evidently weakened, and shortly after began a vacillation, alike of equilibrium, of pressure, and of weakness.

In one hour and forty-five minutes the nervous system was broken down by the excitement of reaction, a state lasting three hours.

CANNABIS SATIVA.

C. sativa, Linn. *Nat. order* (Cannabineæ), Urticaceæ. *Preparation,* Tincture of the twigs and young leaves of the fresh *European* (or *American*) plant, collected when in flower.

Authorities. 1, Hahnemann, R. A. M. L., 1, 139; 2, Franz, ibid.; 3, Gross, ibid.; 4, Fried. H——n, ibid.; 5, Hempel, ibid.; 6, Hugo, ibid.; 7, Stapf, ibid.; 8, Hartlaub and Trinks, ibid.; 9, Wahle, ibid.; 10, Haller, in Vicat's Mat. Med., a general statement, ibid.; 11, Morgagni, de sed. et causis morb., Ep. 7, 10, 15, 25, cases of disease occurring in adult male hemp-dressers, but not adduced as results of this occupation, ibid.; 12, Neubold, Acta nat. cur., III, 150, effects of effluvia of hemp before being dried, therefore not mere local irritation, ibid.; 13, Olearius, Orient. Reischeschreib., p. 529, general statement, but Cann. indica must be meant, ibid.;† 14, Ramazzini, De morbis artif., cap. 26, affections of workers in hemp and linseed, therefore mere local irritation, ibid.; 15, Dr. Schreter, proving with the tincture, N. Archiv., 3, 1, 172; 15*a*, Dr. Schreter's wife, proving with the tincture, ibid.; 16, Dr. Knorre, effects of an infusion of the fresh herb, A. H. Z., 6, 34; 17, Wibmer, effects of 5 to 50 drops of the tincture, Wirk.

---

† Transferred to Cann. Ind.—A.

der Arzneimittel, 1, 23; 18, Lembke, Z. f. H. Kl., 4, 155, proving with 10 to 70 drops of the tincture.

Mind.—Emotional. [At times raging delirium, so that he spits into people's faces],[11].†—[In part joyous, in part earnest delirium],[11].‡—State of mind cheerful, serenely self-contented. (Curative reaction from the opposite condition),[15].—Gayety, as from intoxication (after one hour),[6].—*Sadness*,[1].—Depressed, out of humor,[15].—For several days, especially at dinner, he has a desire for wine to enliven his depressed mood,[15].—After taking wine and water he grew more excited, cheerful, but only while the effect of the wine lasted; after that the former nausea and discomfort returned,[15].—Anxious mood,[1].—[10.] *He became anxious and apprehensive in the pit of the stomach, with oppression of the breath and palpitation;* rising of something warm into the throat, with arrest of breathing; soon something became lodged in the trachea, with flushes of heat,[3].—(Extreme fear of the bed, in which, however, he afterwards lay down),[2].—Frightened at the slightest noise (after one and a quarter hours),[6].—Fretful, especially in the afternoon,[4].—He is very much angered and frenzied by trifles,[7].—Unsteadiness and oscillation of mood,[5].—Despondent in the forenoon, lively in the afternoon,[1].—Mind calm,[15a].—Nothing pleases him; he is indifferent to everything,[2].—**Intellectual.** Afternoon and evening, his thoughts are confused, so that he can no longer distinguish truth from imagination, with a kind of forgetfulness. Thus, he does not know all the evening what remedy he has taken, and is not certain the following day that it was *Cannabis.* He writes something in an entirely wrong place, and is not conscious of it till the next day. At the same time heat and congestion to the head, but he is cold as soon as he goes into the open air,[15].—[20.] Wavering and uncertainty of the mind; the ideas became overwhelmingly vivid,[5].—He is very absentminded, cannot comprehend anything properly, often does not know exactly what to write, and says one thing for another when speaking,[15].—The ideas seem to stand still; he stares in front of him; he is absorbed in higher thoughts, but is unconscious of them, with slight sensation of pressive headache in the parietal bone,[2].—He makes frequent mistakes in writing,[7].—He was able to recollect different things; the ideas remained fixed, stationary, after fixing his mind a long time upon the subject he was preparing,[2].—Loss of mind, senseless, without fantasies,[7].

Head.—Confusion and Vertigo. Confusion of head,[16].—Confusion, obscuration of the head,[7].—Confused head; it feels heavy, and she feels a painful pressure in the forehead and on the eyelids, so that they threaten to close,[3].—Vertigo,[16].—[30.] Attacks of vertigo,[12].—*Vertigo when standing, with dizziness,*[3].—*Vertigo when walking, with tendency to fall sideways* (after one hour),[6].—Dizziness and confusion of the head,[9].—She is always dizzy, as if everything would turn around with her,[15a].—Head always as if dizzy, and it seems to her as if it moved from one side to the other,[15a].—**General Head.** Congestion to the head when writing (first hour),[15].—Rush of blood to the head, which causes a pleasant warmth in it, though with a pressive headache in the temples,[2].—Great rush of blood to the head,[1].—*Blood often rushes to the head, causing heat and flushes,*[15].—[40.] Pleasant warmth in the brain,[2].—Dulness and whirling in the head

---

† After an application to the head, convulsions, subsultus tendinum, death. The post-mortem showed tubercles and pus in the lungs, inflammation of the pleura and diaphragm, firm polypi in the cavities of the heart.—H. Subject of S 304.

‡ Subject of S. 304.

(immediately),[3].—A painful sensation in the head and neck on moving the head,[7].—Headache,[16].—Violent headache,[12].—A very piercing headache,[12].†—Violent throbbing, *with heat of the head* and fever, with which he was obliged to lie down,[17].—Uninterrupted headache the whole day,[2].—Throbbing and pressure in the head (after ten minutes),[17].—Jerking, as if in the blood of the head, chest, and stomach,[1].—*Forehead.* [50.] Slight headache in the forehead (after five minutes),[17].—Painful constriction in the forehead,[3].—*The forehead feels compressed from the margin of the orbits as far as the temples; not relieved by stooping,*[3].—Drawing pain through the forehead (seven minutes after 50 drops),[17].—*Pressure beneath the frontal eminence, extending deep through the brain to the occiput,*[3].—Throbbing from within outward beneath the left frontal eminence; soon afterwards a stupefying pressure in this place,[3].—*Temples.* In the morning, palpable and visible throbbing of the right temporal artery,[15].—A kind of tickling cramp in the temples (after three-quarters of an hour),[6].—*Pressure in the temples,*[6].—Throbbing headache, extending forward into the right temple, together with warmth about the head, red and hot cheeks; the nausea was increased in the warmth,[6].—*Vertex.* [60.] Continual headache in the top of the head, as though a stone were lying upon it,[2].—*Parietals. *A cold sensation in a small spot on the parietal bone (afterwards also in other places on the head), as if a drop of cold water had been dropped upon it,*[3].—When leaning the head against a wall, a pressure internally in the other side of the head,[3].—Violent tearing and boring in the right cranial bones (a symptom which formerly I have often noticed when not proving),[18].—*Occiput.* Heaviness and heat in the occiput, last till evening,[18].—Tension, first in the occiput, then also in the forehead, *lastly in the temples* (after half an hour),[6].—Drawing pain in the occiput, extending to the ears,[7].—Pressive pain in the right side of the occiput,[9].—*External Head.* On the hairy scalp, in the nape of the neck, and behind the ears, painful pimples that heal after several days, without making scabs, and are painfully sensitive to the touch,[15].—Crawling in scalp,[1].

Eye.—[70.] Sensation of weakness in the eyes, with weakness of vision; both far and near objects are indistinct (after one and a half hours),[6].—Sensation in the right eye as if a grain of sand were in it; he must rub it,[15].—Burning in the eyes, evenings,[15].—*Sensation of spasmodic drawing in the eyes* (after three-quarters of an hour),[6].—*Pressure from behind the eyes forward* (after three-quarters of an hour),[6].—*Orbit.* Sensation as if the eyebrows were pressed down,[3].—*Lids.* Pressure in the eyelids that made it difficult to open them, and sticking in the orbits,[15a].—Tearing pressure in the upper lid,[3].—*Ball.* The cornea becomes obscured; (film over the eye),[1].—[Gray cataract],[12].‡—[80.] Pressing and itching in the eyeballs; scratching and burning in the throat for several days, he is compelled to hawk, and cough hackingly and dry; later much mucus is loosened in the morning, and he ejects a good deal without exertion (curative effect),[15].—*Pupils.* Alternating dilatation and contraction of the pupils in the same light (after one hour),[6].—*Vision.* A circle of white flaming rays on the right side near the field of vision, so that only a portion of objects is indistinctly seen,[3].—Mornings on waking, nothing but vertical, shining, white points

---

† See S. 284.

‡ "The original is *suffusiones oculorum*, and occurs in a list of observed effects of hemp. Though assuredly this phrase may mean cataract (Celsus VII, 7, 14), yet it seems very unlikely that the author means to hazard in this maner so startling an assertion as that hemp can cause it."—*Hughes.*

that move in lines from one eye to the other; they did not cease until some time after he was up; later, occasionally flickering before the eyes; light and dark dots float in different directions before the vision,[15].

Ear.—Pain behind the right ear, as if one pushed forcibly with a blunt point,[3].—Coarse sharp stitches in the mastoid process,[3].—Smarting pain in the external cartilage of the ear, which may have been pressed upon while lying at night in bed,[3].—Sensation as though a membrane were stretched before the ears,[9].—A throbbing dragging in the ear, which extends almost to the cheeks, disappearing immediately on stooping, and again returning on becoming erect (after three hours),[7].—Momentary pain, as if the external ear were drawn out of the head,[3].—[90.] Sticking in the ears and pain in the throat, three hours after, at ten in the morning; then cold and heat alternating with dull headache, increased by motion or stooping, and as if everything in the head were shaken; she was obliged to hold herself perfectly straight when walking or to sit still and lean back; supporting herself on the right side was easier; besides she often had stitches in the head, on the left side, near the skull and opposite to it; behind the right ear the stitches were so violent that she involuntarily started; this lasted even at night during sleep, so that she constantly moaned and groaned and complained, and was frequently awakened,[15a].—Stitches in the external meatus while chewing,[3].—Fine stitches in the left ear from within outward,[9].—Throbbing in the ears,[7].—A sensitive jerking pain in the right tympanum, extending thence to the shoulder,[9].—*Hearing.* Ringing in ears,[16].—Tinnitus aurium,[12].—Roaring in the ears,[1].—A sound in the left ear, as if the string of an instrument were struck, and reverberates a long time (after four days),[15].

Nose.—Objective. Itching-swelling in the wing of the nose (after a few hours),[1].—[100.] Sneezing and sensation of stopped coryza, although air passed through the nose,[9].—Bleeding of the nose,[1].—Blood spurts from the nose until one faints,[12].†—Dryness and dry sensation in the nose (after five days),[1].—*Subjective. Dryness of the nose,*[1].—Dryness and heat in the nose,[1].—Feeling of warmth in the nose, as though it would bleed,[2].—Stupefying pressure, as with a dull point, on the root of the nose,[3].

Face.—Pale face,[16].—Paleness of the face,[17].—[110.] (Paleness of the face),[11].†—Very decided paleness and sunkenness of the face for a long time,[17].—Slight palpitations in various portions of the face, especially in the left buccinator,[3].—*Cheeks.* Her left cheek is red and the right one pale, with some pain in a right tooth; the left cheek is not hot to the touch; in spite of the redness, she experiences no internal heat,[15a].—Drawing-pressure in the left malar bone,[3].—The right upper jaw swelled on the gum with a painful bunch on it, as if from an ulcerated tooth,[15].—*Chin.* Stupefying compressive pain in the left side of the chin, which affects the teeth of the same side,[3].—Fine pricking in the left ramus of the lower jaw; when this ceases it is always followed by drawing,[3].

Mouth.—Teeth and Gums. A hollow tooth crumbled away, and the pieces are like hard leather,[15a].—Teeth dull, as if after acid,[15].—[120.] Cramplike pain in the teeth of the left lower jaw,[2].—Drawing pain in a hollow tooth, with swelling of the gums; worse evenings,[15].—Slight drawing in a hollow tooth, especially if something acid touches it,[15].—Toothache; drawing in a hollow tooth after some vexation; after trying to suck the air

---

† From the odor alone.
‡ Merely a statement that the man was pale, but otherwise in good health.

from it with his tongue it changes to violent sticking,[15].—Shooting in several teeth at the same time, with fine pricking in them,[9].—The gums around hollow broken tooth inflamed, swelled, and painful; even a slight drawing in the root,[15a].—*Tongue.* Thickly coated tongue,[17].—*General Mouth.* A bitter sour liquid rises into the mouth, with eructations,[3].—Dryness of the mouth, throat, and lips,[17].—Dryness of the mouth; the saliva is sticky, with loss of thirst, especially in the evening, and hot hands,[7].—[130.] In the morning, burning dryness of the palate,[1].—*Taste.* Loss of taste,[16].—*Speech.* [Speech difficult],[11].†—He was utterly unable to speak as usual; at one time he missed a word, at another he lost the voice (for four hours); towards evening these attacks were repeated; there was at one time a torrent of words, as if one were driving him; at another time he faltered in his speech, so that he sometimes spoke the same word ten times in succession in the same breath; at times his whole idea was anxiously repeated, and it angered him if he was unable to repeat it in the same words,[2].

Throat.—Tasteless water rises into the throat and gets into the trachea, so that he is obliged to swallow, without nausea or retching,[3].—Hawking of mucus; it is raised with difficulty, and irritates his throat,[15].—[Burning in the throat],[11].‡—Pain in the throat, as if sore, with great sensation of dryness, worse mornings in bed; after rising a small lump of mucus is discharged from the throat, which afforded much relief (second day),[15].

Stomach.—Appetite. For several days he has a great deal of appetite, evenings; eats more than he ought to, and feels uncomfortable in consequence,[15].—Loss of appetite,[16].—[140.] Complete loss of appetite,[17].—On taking food which he relished he soon became satisfied, with transient nausea rising into the throat,[3].—His breakfast-cocoa relishes tolerably, but he can take very little, and feels neither hungry nor satisfied; growling and rumbling in the abdomen, in the stomach like a slight cramp; when he thinks of what he could eat he has no desire for anything, and yet he feels as if his stomach were empty,[15].—*Eructations and Hiccough.* Eructations,[16].—*Eructations of air*,[3].—*Eructations of a bitter acrid fluid*,[3].—Eructation, with taste of bread, after breakfast; later empty eructation,[15].—Violent hiccough in the morning,[15a].—Heartburn,[15].—*Nausea and Vomiting.* Nausea, causing a desire to vomit,[8].—[150.] Nausea and inclination to hawk mucus, and vomiting, lessened after drinking coffee,[15].—Nausea, discomfort, and prostration all day; frequent empty eructations, with fulness in the abdomen, no appetite with it, but tolerable relish when he eats,[15].—Waked December 12th with nausea and inclination to vomit, as the day before, although he had eaten little the evening before and only drank water; uncomfortable all the morning; yawns sleepily, indolent, not inclined to anything,[15].—When waking later he still feels nausea, which is increased by thinking of food he has eaten,[15].—December 11th, in the morning he awakes with great nausea and inclination to vomit, especially when lying on the right side; lying on the left relieved it; finally the excessive inclination to vomit ceased, and allowed him to sleep again,[15].—Gagging, with inclination to vomit,[15].—A retching sensation suddenly rises up into the throat, as from acidity of the stomach,[3].—A retching in the pit of the stomach rises thence into the throat,[3].—Excessive inclination to vomit, and vomiting, with great exertion, of mucus, bitterish at first, then flat, which left the teeth dull, directly after taking; immediately afterwards hunger; he eat something with relish,[15].—Vomiting of slimy, bitter water;

---

† In subjects, S. 311, q. v.   ‡ As S. 132.

with scraping in the throat, followed by dulness and confusion of the head in the occiput,[8].—[160.] Vomiting, directly after coffee, of tough acid mucus (after twelve days),[15].—[Green bilious vomiting],[11].†—*Stomach.* —It seems in the stomach as if he had taken cold, especially in the fore-noon, with movings in the abdomen and gripings, though without diar-rhœa,[1].—Several attacks of most violent pain in the stomach at various times, with paleness of the face and sweat on the face; almost pulseless, with rattling breathing, as if dying,[11].‡—Cutting across the upper part of the stomach, after stooping,[2].—Cramp in the stomach,[15].—Cramplike pres-sure in the stomach during several mornings,[15].—The stomach is extremely painful to touch, as if ulcerating; this disappears on eating,[2].—Pinching in the pit of the stomach,[3].—[170.] Pressure in the pit of the stomach,[12].—Cutting in the pit of the stomach,[3].—*Uninterrupted dull stitches in front near the pit of the stomach, just below the ribs, which varied in intensity; they were momentarily relieved by bending the trunk forward or backward, but soon returned,[3].*

Abdomen.—*Hypochondria.* Painful hard swelling of the right hypochondrium,[11].§—*Dull sticking in the left side, just below the ribs, when breathing and when not,[3].*—Beating as with a hammer in the left side below the lowest ribs, extending towards the back,[3].—*Umbilical.* Several mornings, from eight to ten, sensation below the navel as if he had taken cold, with movings in the abdomen, though without diarrhœa,[1].—Pain on the left side near the navel, and also posteriorly near the spine, as if the parts were pinched and compressed by pincers,[3].—Griping just above the navel (after eating),[3].—Pain in the right side near the navel like a beating from within outward,[3].—*General Abdomen.* [180.] [Sacklike swell-ing of the abdomen without swelling of the legs or feet],[11].‖—Complete loss of tone of the intestines; even the strongest cathartics in the largest doses did not suffice to overcome it,[17].—Shaking of the intestines in the abdomen, on violent motion of the arms, as if the intestines were quite loose,[2].—Movings in the abdomen, followed by dull stitches in the left side extending to the ear,[3].—Incarcerated flatus in the upper and lower abdomen, lasting until evening, with colic pains,[9].—Noisy passage of flatus in the morning,[15].—Pain in the abdomen, cutting; did not stop after rubbing, and only diminished after drinking cold water,[15a].—Slight pain always before stool, as if before the menses,[15a].—Fulness of the abdomen, which compelled deep breathing,[1].—Pinching in the abdomen as if to stool (after half an hour),[15].—[190.] Griping in the whole abdomen,[3].—Colic-like pains in the upper abdomen, followed by diarrhœa-like stool and smarting pain in the anus,[9].—A stitch from within outward in the sides of the abdomen,[2].—Dull stitches in both sides of the abdomen in the evening, in bed, they then ex-tend up the back and stitch in like manner between the shoulder-blades, and again extend downward along the sides of the abdomen,[3].—Transient pinching stitches in the abdomen,[3].—All the intestines pain as if bruised,[2]. —[The abdomen and chest are painful externally],[11].¶—Anxious throbbing in the upper abdomen like a strong pulsation,[3].—Shivering in the abdomen as from the moving of cold water in it (after eight minutes),[6].—Sharp

† Local effect, see S. 314.
‡ Subject of S. 332, 333, 310, 336; heart found much enlarged, post-mortem.
§ Liver found diseased, post-mortem.
‖ Subject of S. 322, found on post-mortem to be due to spinal incurvation; this occurred eight days before death.
¶ As S. 132.

shocks in the sides of the abdomen just below the ribs,[3].—[**200.**] *Painful
jerks in the abdomen, moving from one place to another, *as if something
living were in it,* accompanied by drawing from the left hip-bone across to
the right and thence into the knee; still however the pain remained in the
hip, where it seemed like a tearing, pushing pain,[3].—***Hypogastrium
and Iliac Regions.*** Griping in the lower abdomen and cutting in
the loins,[3].—Tickling sensation in the parietes of the lower abdomen (after
half an hour),[6].—Sensitive shocks above the left groin,[3].—Pain and pressing
outward in the abdominal ring as if the parts would suppurate,[2].

Rectum and Anus.—**A pressing in the rectum and sacral region
as if the intestines were sinking down and would be pressed out while
sitting,*[2].—Sticking in the rectum, with a kind of contraction of the
sphincter; often during the day, especially when walking (first day),[15].—
**Constrictive pain in the anus, together with a sensation as if the thighs were
drawn together, so that she was obliged to close them,*[3].—Sensation in the anus
as if something trickled out on to the skin which was cold,[2].—Urgency to
stool after dinner; later, itching in the rectum with slight stitches in it,[15].—
[**210.**] Woke up at 6 with desire to stool; went twice but only passed very
much noisy flatus; urgency to stool continued. After taking a cup of
coffee and smoking a pipe the sensation of disagreeable urgency ceased, and
a somewhat hard stool succeeded; but nausea and inclination to vomit set
in, that was only allayed by keeping quiet,[15].—Urgency to stool; tenesmus
and urinating continued, so that he could hardly walk. After coffee and a
pipe of tobacco some evacuation of crumbling stool, and decrease of the
symptoms, but he was soon obliged to vomit up the coffee, which was
strongly mixed with mucus,[15].

Stool. — The usually regular stool appears irregularly, sometimes
mornings, sometimes afternoons, sometimes evenings, usually with a kind
of tenesmus; only a little is evacuated by straining, and a sensation of
tenesmus remains after it. Sometimes he is suddenly urged to stool, and
forcibly evacuates a pappy or rather liquid substance with relief,[15].—Stool
sometimes like diarrhœa, sometimes hard,[15a].—Stool quite thin and yellowish;
she thought it was flatus, but passed this stool,[15a].—Stool scanty, crumbling,
with passage of flatus,[15].—The usual stool for the first five days; for the
next two days it was completely suppressed,[3].

Urinary Organs.—*Kidneys.* **Drawing pain in the region of
the kidney extending into the inguinal glands, with anxious nauseous sensation in the pit of the stomach,*[1].—Pain in the region of the kidneys as if
ulcerated, when touched and when not,[2].—***Urethra.*** Orifice of the
urethra somewhat inflamed, painful, and somewhat hard to the touch,[15].
—[**220.**] Painless mucous discharge from the urethra (a beginning of
gonorrhœa?),[1].—Painless discharge of clear, transparent mucus from the
urethra, without erections,[2].—Watery mucous discharge from the urethra,[4].
—The orifice of the urethra was agglutinated by moisture, which could be
seen by pressing it out,[5].—***Pain extending from the orifice of the
urethra backward, burning-biting, posteriorly more sticking, while
urinating,**[1].—***The urethra feels inflamed and sore to touch along its
whole length; during erections, tensive pain,**[1].—*Burning while urinating,
but especially just after urinating,**[1].—Burning while urinating, but especially afterward; worse in the evening,[1].—**Burning along the whole urethra,
though only at the commencement and end of urinating,*[4].—While urinating,
at first burning from the glans backward; after urinating, a biting pain,[1].—
[**230.**] Simple, but violent burning in the forepart of the urethra, while

passing urine,[1].—* *When not urinating, some burning pain in the forepart of the urethra, which compels him to urinate almost constantly, even when there is no more urine to pass,*[1].—Burning in the orifice of the urethra, while urinating,[1].—**Pressure as if to urinate, especially in the forepart of the urethra, when not urinating,*[1].—Cutting pain in the forepart of the urethra, when urinating,[2].—**Stitches along the urethra, when not urinating,*[1].— Stitching in the end of the urethra, which is repeated several times, but not on urinating,[18].—Burning stitches in the posterior portion of the urethra, while urinating (after ten hours),[6].—**Jerking stitches in the posterior portion of the urethra, when standing,*[1].—Itching-tickling stitches in the forepart of the urethra,[9].—[240.] * *Tearing as if in the fibres of the urethra in the form of a zigzag,*[5].—Sticking-biting pain on urinating; biting when not urinating,[1].—Very fine sticking-pricking in the forepart of the orifice of the urethra, when not urinating,[2].—Itching in the urethra,[15].— * *Urging to urinate with pressive pain,*[1].—Frequent desire to urinate, with pressure and urgency, occasionally some burning; with the urine, especially mornings, quite whey-like and turbid,[15].—*Micturition.* * *The stream of urine was forked,*[1].—Less passage of urine than usual,[15a].—Enuresis; he is obliged to urinate frequently at short intervals, and passes a large quantity of watery urine (immediately),[3].—[Difficulty in urinating; paralysis of the bladder (the urethra had at first to be evacuated by the catheter, but afterwards this could not be done, because it became clogged by mucus and pus)],[11].†—*Urine.* [250.] White turbid urine,[1].—Urine red and turbid,[1].— Urine full of fibres, as of mucus, with pus,[4].

Sexual Organs.—Male. Coldness in the genitals, with warmth in the rest of the body (on the same day, and lasting three days),[5].—* *The whole penis was swollen, without marked erections,*[4].—Erections while coughing, followed by pain in the urethra,[1].—Frequent erections during the day, only when sitting, not when walking,[1].—**Frequent erections, followed by stitches in the urethra,*[1].—Mornings, in bed, excessive erections without desire, and a cutting-sticking in the orifice of the urethra,[15].—He had an embrace in the evening without desire, followed at night by excessive and painful erections that roused him from sleep,[15].—[260.] Pain on the right side near the penis, like piercing shocks, during rest and motion,[3].—Very indifferent to sexual intercourse during the day, but after an embrace in the evening excessive erections followed in the morning, and again frequently during the day, especially during the forenoon,[15].—No proper erection during an embrace in the morning, especially towards the last; scarcely perceives the ejaculation,[15].—* *The whole penis is painful, as if sore or burnt, when walking (he was obliged to have it suspended),*[4].—Swelling of the prostate gland,[1]. —Moisture about the corona glandis,[4].—The skin of the glans is covered with bright red spots of the size of a pea, brighter than the glans itself,[4]. —* *The glans itself is dark-red, as dark as the prepuce,*[4].—Swelling of the glans and penis; a kind of insensible erection,[2].—Swelling of the frænum and the prepuce, especially where it unites with the frænum,[5].—[270.] The whole prepuce is dark-red, hot, and inflamed,[4].—Swelling of the right side and lower portion of the prepuce,[4].—Constant burning of the whole prepuce and glans for four days; applications of cold water caused smarting,[4]. —Corrosive burning and sticking in the outer parts of the prepuce and the urethra, in the region of the corona glandis,[2].—Smarting on the border and inner side of the prepuce,[4].—The margin of the prepuce is sore,[4].—An

† In subject S. 180, eight days before death, after paraplegia had lasted some time.

itching beneath the prepuce and on the frænum, with some redness and moisture behind the corona glandis,[5].—Agreeable itching on the border of the prepuce and in the orifice of the urethra,[9].—Disagreeable itching on the right side of the prepuce near the anterior margin, more internally, but becoming agreeable during and after scratching,[4].—*A pressive sensation in the testicles when standing, a dragging in them,[1].—[280.] A worrying sensation in the left testicle; the epididymis and spermatic cord seem to swell and divide into various small lumps like soft beans, and to fill out the somewhat drooping scrotum. This worrying pain is felt only when walking (first day, afternoon),[15].—A tensive pain in the spermatic cord, and contraction of the scrotum, with a contractive sensation in it when standing,[1].—*It excites sexual desire in men and animals,[10].—Aversion to coition,[4].—*Female.* Miscarriage at the eighth month, with frightful convulsions,[12].†—Needle-like stitches in the right side of the mons veneris,[9].—Leucorrhœa, as usual, before the menses,[15a].—She experiences much pleasure during an embrace,[15a].—An itching-sticking in the vagina, and a good deal of leucorrhœa after an embrace,[15a].—Very profuse menstruation (from external applications),[12].—[290.] [The sexual desire was excited but sterility caused],[13].‡—Some desire during the morning sleep, but no pleasure during an embrace,[15a].—Sexual excitement without desire; afterwards very much out of sorts, with aversion to sexual intercourse,[15a].

Respiratory Organs.—Trachea. *In the morning, tough mucus in the lower portion of the trachea, which cannot be dislodged by coughing and hawking; he makes great exertions, but only loosens a little, and even this does not come into the mouth, but he is obliged to swallow it; after hawking and coughing a scraping sensation remains in the trachea, as if it were raw and sore; finally the mucus loosens itself, and he is obliged to hawk it up repeatedly,[3].—Towards the seventh day, the previously tenacious mucus is easily loosened in the morning, and the difficulty of breathing, which she had felt up to this time (as if a load were lying upon the chest), was immediately relieved,[3].—*Voice.* The voice is raised, with unusual anxiety and complaint of pain in the back,[2].—[Voice changed, more like a clangor than the human voice],[11].§—Voice frequently inaudible,[16].—*Cough.* Cough,[16]. —[Constant cough],[14].§—[300.] Dry, very violent cough,[12].—*A hacking cough arises at times from the pit of the throat, with which a cold salty fluid is felt deep down in the throat,[7].—[Expiration causes cough],[11].||—*Respiration.* [Respiration very much impeded],[11].¶—[Difficult inspiration, without expectoration],[11].††—[Dyspnœa],[14].—Oppression of breathing, and pressive pain over whole chest,[16].—*Oppression of breathing, from tensive-pressive pains in the middle of the sternum, which was also sore to touch, together with sleepiness,[1].—Oppressed breathing; he feels anxiety in the chest, with stitches between the shoulder-blades; is obliged to sit down, which relieves it; increased after dinner (after ten days),[15].—Breathing was difficult; a weight seemed to lie upon her chest,[3].—[310.] [Difficult breathing on lying down],[11].‡‡—[Orthopnœa; he was only able to breathe with the

---

† From lying all day on fresh hemp, preceded by S. 45.
‡ See "Authorities."   § Local effect.
|| See note to S. 311.   ¶ Part of S. 311.
†† Subject of S. 312; being tired with carrying a burden, he had S3. 321, 449, and came into the hospital with this dyspnœa; died of phrenitis; see Hahnemann's note to S. 1.
‡‡ See note to S. 163.

neck stretched upward, with whistling in the trachea and with great distension of the abdomen],[11].†

Chest.—[Inflammation of the chest and lungs six or seven times],[11].‡ —[Inflammation of the lungs, with delirium],[11].§—[Inflammation of the lungs, with vomiting of green, bilious substances],[11].§—* *The chest feels oppressed, with a sensation of apprehension in the throat; she is obliged to breathe deeply,*[3].—Cutting across the external parietes of the chest,[2].—Stitches in the external parietes of the chest,[2].—Chest rough, scratchy, and dry,[15].— Early in the morning, a sensation of scraping in the chest as from salt; she is obliged to hawk to loosen something, which she swallows, because it is not raised into the mouth,[3].—[**320.**] The male nipple becomes inflamed, itches, and is painful to the ·touch; beside the nipple a mattery pimple, that heals without opening, with the nipple,[15].—[Pain like needle stitches in the left nipple],[11].‖—*Front.* [An elevation and a nodule on the ensiform cartilage, which for two years had remained painless, afterwards caused difficulty in breathing],[11].¶—Violent pinching under the sternum in the lower portion of the chest, which does not hinder breathing; it was relieved on bending backward, and was most violent on bending forward, when it was worse on inspiration,[3].—*A digging beneath the upper part of the sternum, without oppression of the breath,*[3].—A sensation of hammering beneath one of the cartilages of the ribs, near the sternum,[3].—*Sides.* A tensive confusion of the left half of the chest, with slight jerkings, palpitation, and anxiety,[3].—Drawing pain in the left lowest ribs,[2].—A pushing, as with intermitting dull stitches, a kind of pressing inward in the left side of the chest, without oppression of breathing,[3].—Pushings or beatings in both sides of the chest, which frequently return and arrest the breathing; they are most painful in the region of the heart,[1].—[**330.**] Burning-sticking pain in the left side near the ensiform cartilage,[9].—Throbbing against the ribs in the left side,[3].

Heart and Pulse.—Præcordium. Pain in the region of the heart,[11].††—*Heart's Action.* Pulsations of the heart felt below the natural limits,[11].††—* *On moving the body and on stooping, a few violent beatings at the heart, as if it would fall out, together with a warm sensation about the heart* (after forty-eight hours),[1].—Sudden, violent palpitation,[16].—*Pulse.* Very small pulse,[11].††—Slow, scarcely perceptible pulse,[6].

Neck and Back.—Neck. Drawing in the neck, extending upward into the cervical vertebræ,[2].—Drawing from the neck to the ear, more like a pinching, externally,[3].—[**340.**] Painful pressure in the cervical muscles above the throat,[3].—Stitches in the lowest portion of the neck, as with a knife,[2].—*Back.* The pain in the back frequently arrested breathing,[2].— *Dorsal.* Burning beneath the right shoulder-blade,[2].—An itching fine stitch in the right side near the shoulder-blade, which disappears after scratching,[3].—[In the lower dorsal vertebræ a heavy pressure and fine sticking pain (lasting fifty days), which sometimes extended down to the loins or towards the shoulder-blades],[11].‡‡—*Lumbar.* Pain in the middle of the back, as if one were pinched with pincers, which extends towards the abdomen,[2].—Slow, intermitting, dull stitches in the left side of the back, beneath the lowest ribs,[3].—Severe pain in the small of the back, especially

---

† A man convalescing from an acute fever, after irregularities in food and drink and long handling of hemp, had this with Ss. 303, 132, 137, 196, and 302.

‡ Local effect.   § As S. 312.   ‖ See note to S. 304.
¶ See note to S. 180.   †† See note to S. 163.   ‡‡ See note to S. 180.

aggravated after the slightest exertion, and obliging him to sit down and rest,[17].—*Sacral.* Pressure on the coccyx, as with a dull point,[3].—[350.] Pain on the left side near the coccyx in the bone, as if some hard body pressed forcibly against this part,[3].

Extremities in General.—The weariness of the limbs lasted several weeks,[17].—Immediately after eating, all the limbs are tired, with tearing pressure in the left side, beneath the short ribs; the spot is painful to pressure,[3].—Rheumatic drawing in the periosteum of the long bones of all the limbs, on motion, as if they were bruised,[2].

Superior Extremities.—Shoulder. A severe pain on pressing between the end of the clavicle and the head of the humerus, which extends into the fingers,[3].—Tearing pressure upon the top of the shoulder, intermitting,[3].—Sensation in the shoulder, as if it were bruised, on stretching out the arm,[2].—*Arm.* Sticking in the upper arm and bones of the little finger; this condition lasted three days, diminishing daily,[15a].— *Wrist.* (The wrist feels dead; he is unable to move it),[1].—*Hand.* Heaviness and going to sleep of the right hand; relieved by motion, writing, for instance,[15].—[360.] Sudden lameness of the hand; he was unable to hold the fork with the fingers while eating; the whole hand trembled on taking hold of anything; it seemed helpless, with painful loss of power in it,[7].—Cramplike intermitting contraction of the right hand,[3].—Cramplike contraction of the metacarpal bones,[3].—A dull stitch in the hollow of the hand, over the carpal bones,[3].—*Fingers.* Cramp in the joints of the thumb, while writing,[2].—Stitches in the third finger of the right hand, as if with a needle (after three hours),[15].—Crawling in the tips of the fingers, as if they had begun to go to sleep and were numb (immediately after taking),[5].—Later in the afternoon, sensation as when severe cold causes tingling under the nails,[15].

Inferior Extremities.—Weariness in the limbs, which disappeared when walking (after 40 drops),[17].—He feared that he should sink down, such sudden weariness attacked the lower limbs especially; he staggered on the slightest motion of the body, though when walking he seemed to be more steady (after three hours),[2].—[370.] [The right leg is very difficult to move; afterwards paralyzed, with greater loss of motion than of sensation],[11].†—*Hip.* A pinching jerking-digging pain in the right hip, which almost makes one cry out,[1].—*Thigh.* When stooping, cramp in the buttocks; must stand erect at once; on repeated stooping, repeated cramp in the same place (after 10 drops),[15].—Sitting causes a pain in the right buttock, as if from strong pressure, with going to sleep of the right foot,[15].—Painless cramplike sensation in the posterior portion of the right thigh, as if a muscle would begin to twitch,[2].—Continued pressure in the middle of the forepart of the thigh, when sitting,[3].—In the flesh of the upper part of the thigh, near the groin, sensitive, sharp, needle-like stitches,[3].—In the bend of the thigh, at first some jerking shocks, followed by a sensation in the region of the abdominal ring as of distension, and a sensation as if the ring itself were pressed outward,[2].—*Knee.* When going upstairs, the patella snaps sideways,[2].—Prickling-burning in the left knee, intermitting,[3].—[380.] When walking, a drawing-like cramp in the hollow of the knee, which extends along the inner muscles of the thigh,[2].—Tearing constrictive pressure in the left knee, in the forehead, and over all parts of the body,[3].—*Legs.* A burning in the right tibia, when standing,[2].

---

† See note to S. 180.

—Beside the left tibia, in the flesh, a pain from within outward, as if after a severe bruise, and then sticking in the whole left extremity,[15a].—Cramp in the calves, when walking,[1].—*Ankle.* Sticking and sore pain in the left ankle-joint, relieved by washing with cold water,[15a].—*Foot.* Heaviness in the feet when ascending stairs, so that he feels them as he lifts them,[15].—After eating, the feet felt very heavy,[3].—Drawing to and fro in the left foot, from the toes to the ankle,[3].—Painful throbbing on the back of the feet,[3].—[390.] Painless tensive stretching in the instep,[3].—Drawing and pressure in the heel, when sitting,[2].—*Toes.* Like a cramp in the right toe,[15].—A prickling sensation under the left great toe, as when severe cold settles, so to speak, under the nails,[15].—Drawing in the ball of the right great toe,[2].—Stinging-itching in the ball of the left great toe,[2].—A sticking-pressing pain in the little toe of the left foot, where he formerly had a corn,[15].

General Symptoms.—Secretions generally increased,[17].—[Hysterical attacks],[12].†—[Cataleptic spasms of the upper limbs and trunk from time to time, which lasted a quarter of an hour, during which he vomited a yellow fluid, which was followed by some delirium],[11].‡—[400.] Indolence and weariness in the whole body,[4].—He is indolent and weary, yawns much, and stretches as if he desired to sleep,[3].—Weariness, tottering of the knees, and a dull pain in them (after one hour),[6].—Great weariness after a slight motion; after going upstairs he lay upon the sofa quite exhausted and unable to move or talk freely,[7].—He is more weary in the morning, after waking from an almost unbroken sleep, than he was the evening previous, on lying down,[3].—After eating, he was weary and indolent; everything affected him, even talking and writing,[3].—Weakness,[16].—[Loss of power of the body],[11].§—He felt very uneasy directly after taking; what he wished to write was suddenly effaced from his memory,[15].—*Subjective.* She felt sick in her whole body, could not endure it, must lie down on account of weariness and heaviness of the limbs,[8].—[410.] An hour after breakfast, discomfort in the whole body, especially in the abdomen, as if inflated, with sticking-cutting pains there, chilliness all over at the same time,[15].—Superficial pinching here and there in the flesh, as if the parts were pinched with the finger,[3].—Tearing pushes and tearing deeply penetrating stitches in many parts, especially in the limbs,[3].

Skin.—Eruptions, Dry. Large pimples on the nose, surrounded by red swelling, like acne rosacea,[1].—Eruption on the red portion of the lips and in the corner of the mouth,[1].—Pimply eruption, that itches and pains, on breast and back,[15].—Itching pimples on the neck, nape of the neck, and breast,[15a].—Itching pimples (urticaria?) rise on the arms and nape of the neck, that, however, soon pass away (evening),[15].—*Eruptions, Moist.* Eruptions on head and chest of vesicles filled with white serum, surrounded by a red areola; vesicles burn on touch,[16].—Papulous eruption on the nates and thighs; small white vesicles, with a large, red, smooth border, which burned like fire, especially when lying upon them or touching them; they left brownish-red spots after two days, which were very painful to touch,[2].—*Eruptions, Pustular.* [420.] An inflamed

---

† In those predisposed to them.
‡ Paralysis and death followed this; the post-mortem showed pus in the kidneys, thickened mucous membranes in the bladder, congestion of the bloodvessels of the diaphragm, water in the convolutions, but none in the ventricles of the brain. See note to S. 180.
§ See note to S. 180.

pimple in the right ear, very painful to the touch, with swelling of the inner ear; matter gradually forms that discharges after four days, mixed with blood, and it heals (after four days),[15].—A mattery pimple on the nape of the neck, painful at night (sixth day),[15].—*Sensations.* A very obstinate fine sticking, as with a thousand needle-points, over the whole body, so that he is unable to endure it, at night, in bed, when he became sweaty from warm coverings; at first it began in a few places, and when he scratched them it suddenly changed, and extended to several other places; with this he had great anxiety of the heart, and a sensation as if hot water were thrown repeatedly over him; this was relieved on uncovering himself,[3].—Crawling itching-biting, as from salt, on the face,[1].—Itching here and there on the face,[1].—Itching on the chin and tip of the nose,[15].—Almost sore, painful itching about the navel, for several hours, which pained as if sore, and was sensitive after rubbing,[1].—Itching in the perineum,[1].—Itching on the hands and fingers, without visible eruption,[15].—Itching around the knee,[1].

Sleep and Dreams.—Sleepiness. [430.] Constant frequent yawning for a quarter of an hour (after one and a half hours),[6].—Sleepiness,[17].—Sleepiness during the day,[7].—Sleepiness the whole day,[2].—Overpowering sleepiness during the forenoon,[1].—Sleepy after dinner for a quarter of an hour; after the sleepiness passed off he began to yawn and grew sleepy again,[15].—*Sleeplessness.* Sleeplessness after midnight,[1].—(Loss of sleep),[11].†—Uneasy sleep,[1].—Uneasy sleep at night, frequent waking; confused, and at times anxious dreams; emissions, followed by light sleep,[2].—*Dreams.* [440.] Dreamy in the head for several days, as if the room were turning round with her,[15a].—Very vivid dreams, of a rather agreeable kind,[15].—He had confused dreams every night, which continued even after waking, and were recollected,[3].—Dreams of mishaps to others,[1].—*Disagreeable and frightful dreams; he is disappointed in everything, and is filled with great anxiety,[3].—*He awoke at night from slumber with frightful dreams, without knowing where he was,[1].—Very vivid, horrid dreams, which, however, did not make him anxious, but he always retained a kind of presence of mind,[3].

Fever.—Shivering frequently creeps upward from the soles of the feet,[3].—Shivering creeps over the whole body, but also reaches the head, and seems to draw the hairs together,[3].—[Febrile chill],[11].‡—[450.] Chill, with thirst, without subsequent heat and without sweat, in the afternoon (after fifty-two hours),[1].—Chilly for several hours (immediately),[9].—Evenings, chilliness, yawning, stretching of the limbs, and indolence; goes to bed early without being exactly sleepy,[15].—Fever, shaking chill, with excessive thirst and shuddering after drinking, together with cold hands, knees, and feet; accompanied by hurriedness, trembling, distortion of the face; at one time weeping, at another joyous, at another raging mood; everything angered him so that he got into a rage about it; during the chill some warmth in the back and in the feet, which perspired, but were not warm to touch,[2].—Shivering in the right thigh, as if goose-flesh would form,[2].—Creeping shivering in the thighs (immediately),[3].—Creeping shivers over the trunk, with a sensation of a kind of discomfort, at short intervals,[3].—The whole body is cold, but the face becomes constantly warmer and warmer,[6].—The limbs are cold to the touch, and he trembles from chilli-

---

† In subject of S. 311. Much serum found in the brain, post-mortem.
‡ See note to S. 304.

ness,[3].—Coldness and cold sensation of the hands,[6].—***Heat.*** [460.] Warmth, with warm sensation in the face,[6].—Excessive heat and fever; she glowed in the face, but was cold at every motion, with violent pains in the throat; throat swollen inside and out, with difficulty in swallowing; very much prostrated; she was obliged to lie down all day, and the stitches in the head continued,[15a].—He is very hot during the night, and begins to perspire slightly towards morning,[15].—Violent burning of the whole skin, especially feet, hands, abdomen, also in the palms; afterwards itching, that compels him to scratch all night, also early the following day (six days),[15]. —Orgasm of blood,[12].—***Sweat.*** Sweat on the forehead and neck, at night,[1].

Conditions. — **Aggravation.** — (*Morning*), Throbbing of temporal artery; on waking, white points before eyes; dryness of palate; in bed, pain in throat; hiccough; pressure in stomach; from 8 to 10 o'clock, sensation below navel; passage of flatus; urine whey-like, etc.; in bed, erections, etc.; early, sensation in chest.—(*Forenoon*), Despondent; feeling in stomach; sleepiness.—(*Afternoon*), Fretful.—(*Evening*), Burning in eyes; pain in hollow tooth; dryness of mouth, etc.; excessive appetite; in bed, stitches in sides of abdomen; burning while urinating.—(*Night*), Heat; sweat on forehead, etc.—(*After midnight*), Sleeplessness.—(*Towards morning*), Perspiration.—(*Contact with acids*), Drawing in hollow tooth.—(*When ascending stairs*), Heaviness in feet.—(*After breakfast*), Eructations, etc.—(*While chewing*), Stitches in external meatus.—(*At dinner*), Desire for wine.— (*After eating*), Feet feel heavy; weary, etc.—(*After an embrace*), Itching, stinging in vagina, etc.—(*During erections*), Tensive pain.—(*Exertion*), Pain in small of back.—(*Inspiration*), While bending forward, pinching under sternum.—(*On lying down*), Difficult breathing.—(*Lying on right side*), Nausea, etc.—(*On motion*), Beating at heart; drawing in periosteum of long bones.—(*While sitting*), Pressing in rectum, etc.; erections; pain in buttock, etc.; pressure in thigh; drawing, etc., in heel.—(*When standing*), Vertigo, etc.; stitches in urethra; pressive sensation in testicles; pain in spermatic cord; burning in tibia.—(*Before stool*), Slight pain.—(*After stooping*), Cutting across stomach.—(*Walking*), Sticking in rectum, etc.; penis painful; pain in testicle; cramp in hollow of knee; cramp in calves.— (*Warmth*), Nausea.—(*When writing*), Congestion to head; cramp in joints of thumb.

Amelioration. —(*Afternoon*), Lively.—(*Bending backward*), Pinching under sternum.—(*Bending trunk backward or forward*), Stitches near pit of stomach.—(*Coffee*), Nausea.—(*Drinking cold water*), Pain in abdomen.—(*After eating*), Pain in stomach disappears.—(*Lying on left side*), Nausea, etc.—(*Moving the part*), Heaviness, etc., of hand.—(*Keeping quiet*), Nausea, etc.—(*After scratching*), Stitch in side disappears.—(*Sitting down*), Oppressed breathing.—(*On stooping*), Dragging in ear disappears; beatings at the heart, etc.; cramp in buttocks.—(*When walking*), Weariness in limbs disappears.—(*Washing with cold water*), Sticking, etc., in ankle-joint. —(*After wine*), More excited, etc.

CANTHARIS.

Cantharis vesicatoria, Geoff. (Meloe vesicator, Linn.; Lytta vesicator, Fabr.), Insecta, *class,* Coleoptera. *Common name,* Spanish Fly. *Preparation.* Tincture (or triturations, used for some of the provings) of the imported dried beetles.

Authorities. 1, Hahnemann, Fragmenta de viribus med., p. 57; 1a, Hahnemann, additional, from Archiv. 13, 1, 157; 2, Baudis, Hartlaub and Trinks, R. A. M. L., 1; 3, Bethmann, ibid.; 4, Giacomini, Farmacologia 11, 152, experiments of students with repeated doses of from ⅝ of a grain to 4 grains; detailed account in Revue Crit. et. Retrospect, 5, 265; 5, Hering, H. and T., R. A. M. L.; 6, N—g, ibid.; 7, Ruckert, ibid.; 8, Hartlaub, ibid. (vol. 1 and vol. 2); 9, Schreter, ibid. (vol. 2); 10, Baccius in Schenk, Obs., 126 (from H. and T., vol. 1); 11, Baglivi, diss. de vesicant. op., p. 654 (ibid.); 12, Bernt, Rettungsmettel, p. 181 (ibid.); 13, Barrichius, Act. Hafn. IV. (ibid.); 14, Brassavolus de Med., 1555 (ibid.); 15, Joach. Camerarius, in Schenk (ibid.); 16, Cardanus, de Subtilit., lib. ix (ibid.); 17, Cullen, Arzneimittell. II (ibid.); 18, De Forell, diss. sist. hyperdruresin ex pervers, Canth. usu Externo ort. (ibid.); 19, Dioscorides (ibid.); 20, Fabric v. Hilden, Cent VI (ibid.); 21, Forestus, Obs. (ibid.); 22, Gmelin, All. Geschichte d. Gifte (ibid.); 23, Greenfield, Treatise on Canth. (ibid.); 24, Guldenklee, Cas. Med. et Observ., etc. (ibid.); 25, Hecker, Arzneim. 1 (ibid.); 26, Horn, Archiv. fur die Med. Erf., 1815 (ibid.); 27, J. L. Hoffmann, in Forsten, Hist. Canth., effects of half a drachm of tinct. on a woman (ibid.); 28, Home, Clinical Experiments, p. 405 (ibid.); 29, Jahn. Arzneim. (ibid.); 30, Lanzoni, opera, tom. iii (ibid.); 31, Lange, in Schenk, lib. vii (ibid.); 32, Lindestolpe, de venenis, effects of external use (ibid.); 33, Ledelius, in Misc. Nat. Cur. Dec. I (ibid.); 34, Ludovici, in Forsten, Hist. Canth., effects of external use (ibid.); 35, Misc. Nat. Cur. Dec., II (ibid.); 36, Pallas, in Froriep Notizen (ibid.); 37, Parmentier, Annal. de Chim., effects of the dust from bruising the beetles (ibid.); 38, Paschalius and Occo, in Schenck, Obs., 125 (one symptom) (ibid.); 39, Stalpaart van der Wiel, effects of external use (ibid.); 40, Spielmann, Mat. Med. (ibid.); 41, Stockar a Neufarn, Diss. de Canth., 1781, effects of 12 "Spanish flies" (ibid.); 42, Tarrie, from Lond. Med., and Phys. Journ., 1825, effects of poisoning in a man of 40 (ibid.); 43, Tralles, de usu vesicant, 1795 (ibid.); 44, Wierus, de præstig. dæm. III., c. 35 (ibid.); 45, Wendt, in Hufeland's Journ., effects of an electuary of pulv. Canth., and of 90 drops of the tincture (ibid.); 46, Werlhoff, opera (ibid.), also in Christison; 47, Wilbrecht, Geschichte und Versuche, Copenhagen, 1774, effects of a drachm of pulv. Canth., taken in one dose, on a woman aged 35 (ibid.); 48, Leviani, Mem. di. Matem., etc., 1803 (ibid.); 49, William Batt, Mem. de la Soc. Med. de Genes. (detailed in Revue Crit. et Retrospect, 5, 256), effects of five flies; 50, Biett, from Orfila Tox., 228, effects of 1 dr. of powder on a young man; 51, Gaz. de Santé, 1819, effects of two doses, each of 24 grains, with an interval of a day (from Christison); 52, Giulio, Mem. de l'Acad. de Turin, 1802, tetanus and hydrophobic symptoms produced by Canth., detailed in Rev. Crit. et Retrospect, 5, 250; 53, Dr. Maxwell, Lancette Franc., 1838, effects of the powder in rum, in three cases, from Revue Crit. et Retrospect, 5, 257; 54, Ambroise Paré, "Des Venen," effects of fly-blister, Rev. Crit. et Retrosp.; 55, as last, an abbé took Canth. in sweetmeats; 56, Piquet d. l. Houssiette, detailed in Rev. Crit. et Retrosp., 5, 249, effects of 8 grs. of powder; 57, Recueil, Period, etc. (in Rev. Crit. et. Retrosp., 5, 256), effects of powder in chocolate : 58, Graaf, Hufeland's Journ., 1821 (Rev. Crit. et Retrosp., 5), effects of the tincture drank from a flask; 59, Seiler, Horn's Archiv., 27 (from Roth's Mat. Med., article Cantharides); 60, Champy, Diss. sur Canth., 1809, effects of the fumes (ibid.); 61, Montagnana, Schenk a Graffenberg, Obs. Med. de

Venenis (ibid.); 62, Occo, Medicament., effects of carrying Canth. in the hand (ibid.); 63, Rust, Salz. Med. Zeit., 1811 (ibid.); 64, Pareus, in Schenk, Obs. Med. (Hartlaub and Trinks); 65, omitted; 66, Weisse, Petersburger Abhandl., 5, 427, effects of a blister applied by mistake over swollen cervical ganglia. (from Roth's Mat. Med.); 67, Harder. Petersb. Abhand., 4, 166, effects of a blister (ibid.); 68, Robertson, Ed. Med. Journ., 1806, effects of a blister (ibid.); 69, Hartte, Ed. Med. Journ., 1806 (ibid.); 70, Benedictus, De Curand Morbis, 24 (ibid.); 71, Grainger, Hist. Febris anom., Edinburg, 1753 (ibid.); 72, Clinch, Diss., London, 1726 (ibid.); 73, Schrœder, Pharmacop. (ibid.); 74, Lafitte, Rev. Therap. du Midi., 1858 (ibid.); 75, Rouquaryrol, Annales de la Med. phys., 1829 (from Christison); 76, Dr. Ives, Am. J. of Med. Sc., 1833, a boy of 17 took one ounce of tincture (from Christison and Taylor); 77, Werlhof, Mem. della Soc. Med. di Genoa (Christison); 78, Lond. Med. Gaz., 1841, a woman took 1 oz. of tinct. (ibid.); 79 (same as 77); 80, Report of inquest, girl anointed whole body with ung. Canth. for scabies (Christison); 81, Fisher, Med. Gaz., 39, p. 855, a man took 60 grs. of powdered Canth. (Taylor on Poisons); 82, Ed. M. and S. Journ., 1844, some plaster containing two drachms of powdered Canth. was taken by a lunatic (ibid.); 83, Journ. de Chim. Med., 1847, six students took powdered Canth., by mistake, instead of pepper, with their food, for six months (ibid.); 84, Schlegel, Material, 1819, effects of a teaspoonful of tinct. on a child nine years old (Frank's Mag., 3, 465); 85, Duprest Rony, Diss. sur Satyriasis, 1570, two men took each two drs. of pulv. Canth. for ague (Wibmer); 86, Oest. Zeit., 3, 629 (Gaz. Med. di Milan), a priest of 80 years and a sexton of 60 years, took a mixture of half an ounce of tinct. Canth. in six ounces of alcohol; 87, Podrecca, Omod. Ann., 1843 (Schmidt's Jahrbucher, 42, 290), a dancing-master aged 32 was given twenty grs. of pulv. Canth.; 88, La Fitte, Rev. Ther. chemichi, 1853 (Schmidt's Jahrb., 78, p. 167), a man aged 25 took one gramme of pulv. Canth. in two doses;[†] 89, Jaffe, Schm. Jahrb., 91, p. 297, two flies in brandy for loss of sexual desire; 90, Pallé, Journ. de Brux., 1870 (Schm. Jahrb., 148, p. 276), poisoning of ten soldiers by a solution of Canth. in coffee; 91, Morel, A. H. Z., 33, effect of blisters; 92, Zeit. f. v. Oest., 1857, 1, 561, effect of eight "flies" taken internally; 93, Lond. Med. Gaz., 1847 (from A. H. Z., 73, 189), a man took two teaspoonfuls of pulv. Canth.; 94, La Lancette, 1843 (from Oest. Zeit.), 3, 629, effects on a man of a gramme of pulv. Canth. mixed with food; 95, Radecki, Inaug. dis. on Canth., Dorpat, 1866, effects on a man suffering from chronic rheumatism, of Canth. ointment rubbed into a blister; 96, Cattell, fragments from various sources, B. J. of Hom., 11, 159; 97, Med. Times and Gaz., 1864 (in B. J. of H., 23, 131, a girl of 13 ate a Spanish fly in a jam tart); 98, Dr. H. G. Dunnell, Hom. Exam., 3, 145, effects on a boy of 12 of a Spanish fly in an apple; 99, Am. J. of Med. Sc., 1, 368, a lad swallowed one ounce of the tincture; 100, Kline, Phil. Med. and Surg. Rep., 1872, a woman took more than 50 grains; 101, Chalvigirac, de l'empoison. par la teint. de Canth., effects of about 100 grammes (from Tardieu, L. empoisonnement, 2d ed., 1875); 102, Same author and source as the last (the six victims of 101 recovered), this one died (ibid.); 103, Schwerin, Rev. des. Sc. Med. de Hayem, 1874, an hysterical woman took 15 drops of Canth. collodion (ibid.); 104, Dominico Nardo, Antolog. Med., 1836

† This is probably the same case as No. 74, but differently reported.

(from Am. J. of M. S., 1837), proving with two grs. of Cantharidin taken in two doses, and after a fortnight two grains in four doses; 105, Gaz. des Tribunaux (from Am. J. of M., 3, 1847), man poisoned by Canth. in soup; 106, Dr. Baehr, Zeit. f. H. Kl., 4, 125, provings, effects of repeated doses of the 6th, 3d, 2d, and 1st dils.; 107, ibid., proving with the tinct.; 108, ibid., with the 1st and 2d trits.; 109, ibid., with one grain of pulv. Canth.; 110, Dr. M. Macfarlan, Am. J. H. M. M., 4 and 5, effects of the 400th, Fincke, given in water three times a day for two weeks; 111, W. M. Williamson, Proc. Hom. Med. Soc. Penn., 1873, effects when used to relieve chilblains; 112, Thos. Souttell, Pharm. Journ., 2, 655, effects of fumes inhaled while preparing ung. Canth.

Mind.—Emotional. Apparently intoxicated (first day),[78].—Appears intoxicated and crazy,[96].—Excited mood,[2].—General excitement; they rose from bed and ran about the room, racked by vomiting and copious stools,[101].—Frenzy,[31].—Raging frenzy,[16].—Violent frenzy of three days' continuance (during convalescence), (one case),[58].—Delirium (after two days),[78].—Delirium in evening,[76].—[10.] Delirious at night (second day),[78].—Delirium and convulsions,[96].—*Furious delirium,*[96].—*Constant, complete, furious, almost frenzied delirium,*[52].—He talked deliriously when lying, sitting, and walking, disconnectedly of his business and of people who had long since been dead,[1a].—Senseless talking,[12].—Visions at night, when half awake; she heard soft steps in the room, then knocking under the bed, and the bed was raised up (midnight),[6].—Visions at midnight, while awake, lying with the right hand on the left shoulder; something took hold of her hand, and bent it several times up and down, then it seemed as if some one took her by the throat with ice-cold hands (fourteenth night),[6].—Everything affects him more profoundly than usual, so that he is obliged to cry very much (second day),[3].—Screaming, with legs drawn upon thighs,[81].— [20.] Piercing screams and frequent loss of consciousness,[56].—Incessant groaning (second day),[53].—Very active, happy; she feels as if newly born; the room and all the objects appear clearer to her and more pleasant (sixth day),[6].—Great depression, incessant moaning (third day),[96].—Extreme despondency and faintheartedness; she says she must die,[6].—Melancholy and anxious after dinner, soon disappearing,[6].—Distrust of himself, like a hypochondriac (in the afternoon),[1a].—Anxiety,[87].—Anxiety, which increases from moment to moment,[45].—Anxiety in the morning, as if he expected something very important (after twenty hours),[1a].—[30.] Great anxiety,[15].—Great anxiety,[84][93].—Extreme anxiety,[4].—Increasing anxiety, with trembling over the whole body; the trembling continues while walking in the open air (after two hours),[8].—Internal anxiety,[1a].—She is anxious, without knowing why (after a quarter of an hour),[6].—He is as anxious as if he had committed a murder; it seems to arise from the stomach (after half an hour),[8].—Easily irritated by offenses,[1a].—Ill-humor,[1a].— Fretful only in the morning, when rising,[1a].—[40.] Discontented, talkative (after three hours),[6].—Discontented, morose, peevish (after two hours),[6].— Discontented, absorbed in thought (after two hours),[6].—Very peevish, irritable during the pains, in the evening,[6].—Very peevish, brawling; nobody does anything to suit her (second day),[6].—Extremely passionate and angry,[6].—Churlish mood (second day),[92].— Morose disposition,[1].—Very morose, anxious, lachrymose (third day, forenoon),[6].—Very morose, lazy, sleepy, melancholy, peevish,[9].—[50.] *An insolent and contradictory mood, in the afternoon,*[1a].—Alarmed and agitated (after three weeks),[98].—Fright and dreams of falling (ninth and tenth nights),[96].—Instability,[31].—*Intel-*

lectual. In the morning, great depression of the mental powers (second day),[3].—Mental confusion,[11].—In the morning, some hours after rising, very distracted in mind, and many ideas of various kinds run through his mind, which he cannot keep away,[1a].—When he wishes to think of anything, he immediately loses his thoughts; his gaze remains fixed in silence on one object (which, however, he scarcely notices), and he has trouble in recollecting himself in order to express a few words coherently (second day),[3].—Dulness of perception, followed by stupidity and a loss of the reflecting faculty,[4].—Very forgetful,[9].—[60.] Loss of consciousness (second day),[76].—Completely unconscious (fourth day),[99].—Coma (after fourteen days),[76].—After a sudden attack of severe pain in head, pain in right side, chilliness, trembling, and universal spasms, he again sunk into a comatose state; then, until death, alternately lethargic, comatose, rational, or convulsed,[99].

Head. — Confusion and Vertigo. Confused head (second day),[92 9].—Confusion of the head, and especially a sort of heaviness in the vertex (after half an hour),[8].—*In the morning, confusion of the head, with pulsation in the forehead, for several hours,[1a].—Head very much confused and dull,[9].—Confusion of the forehead, as well as a slight pressing and drawing in it (after twelve hours),[3].—*Vertigo,*[4 55 104].—[70.] Vertigo and staggering,[4].—Vertigo and fainting,[25].—On walking in the open air, vertigo, with very transient attack of unconsciousness, during which there seemed to be a fog before his eyes, returning several times in half an hour (first day),[3].—Dizzy and weak in the head,[1a].—Giddiness (after half an hour),[97].—Tottering about, as if dizzy (tenth, eleventh, and twelfth days),[6].—*General Head.* Brain congested,[96].—Heaviness of the head,[49].—Head heavy, with dull pressing, worse on motion,[9].—Head and hair feel stiff to him (after three weeks),[98].—[80.] Pain in the head, trembling, and universal spasms, followed by coma (seventh day),[76].—Dull pain in the head,[104].—His head is heavy and confused,[8].—Headache,[68].—Headache,[2].—Headache, the whole day,[9].—Headache, disappearing after breakfast (one hour),[6].—Headache, sometimes with delirium,[79].—Headache and shivering (after fourteen days),[76].—Headache, boring, drawing, tearing, throbbing, and pressing, all together,[9].—[90.] Headache, with heat in the forehead, which is also perceptible externally (after three-quarters of an hour),[6].—Headache, with dizziness (after three weeks),[98].—Headache, dragging and tearing only on motion; on stooping and turning the head, immediately, a sensation starting from the neck and pressing the head forward, with a feeling as if everything would press out at the forehead,[1a].—Headache, very severe, like a pressure in the vertex, alternating with sensitive throbbing, aggravated by every motion, at 8 P.M. (third day),[107].—Increased headache, with, at intervals, slight delirium,[49].—Violent headache (eleventh day, forenoon),[6].—Pressing-sticking headache in the forenoon and evening, which disappears on walking,[9].—Head oppressed,[104].—Sticking-pressing and pain as if sore in the whole head, with sensation as if the pains would extend through the eyes,[9].—Cutting stitches in the head, which wake him from sleep,[1a].—[100.] Violent pain, as if sore, internally in the head,[9].—*Forehead.* Heaviness and dulness in the forehead, deep in the brain, with a sensation as if her head were being pressed forward (after two hours),[6].—Headache, like a heaviness, in the forehead (fourth morning),[6].—Dull pain in forehead (second day),[92].—Headache in the forehead, extending to both temples,[8].—Slight aching in the forehead, like a tearing (after one hour),[6].—Slight headache in the frontal and suborbital regions,[102].—He was wakened at night by headache, a pressing-out in the forehead, which disappeared on sitting up in bed,[1a].—Stitching in the right frontal region (after two hours and a half),[6].—Tearing in the forehead,[3].—[110.] Tearing in the forehead and in the nape of the neck,[6].—Tearing, first in the forehead, next in the region of the right ear, then in the lower jaw, and finally on the ear again, where it disappeared (seventeenth day),[6].—A stitch in the left frontal eminence, on standing,[6].—Pressive headache in the region above the nose,[8].—*Temple.* Compression of both temples towards each other,[9].—A pain in the right temple, as if it would be forced out, whence the sensation passes down toward the teeth,[9].—Gnawing in the periosteum of the right temporal bone (after one hour),[6].—Stitching in the left temple (after two hours and a half),[6].—Fine stitching in the right temple, which becomes a painful throbbing, disappearing on rubbing,[6].—Several small stitches in the right temple, in the afternoon,[6].—[120.] Tearing in both temples (second day),[3].—Tearing in the right temple (after a meal),[6].—A tearing in the right temple (after four hours),[6].—A couple of tearings in the right temple (after three hours),[6].—Throbbing externally in the right temple, and a painful drawing in the bone at the same place (after two hours and a quarter),[6].—*Vertex.* Pressing on the vertex and in the temples, with stitching in the temples, especially the right,[9].—Painful tearings on the vertex, with sensation as if a lock of hair were being drawn upward (fourth forenoon),[6].—*Parietals.* Drawing pain in the left side of the head and in the forehead,[3].—Stitching in the left side of the head (second morning),[6].—Stitching in the right side of the head, in the afternoon,[6].—[130.] Tearing and stitching in the right side of the head,[6].—Dull headache in the left half of the head,[9].—Stitching in the left parietal bone, and at the same time tearing in the same jaw, while speaking (one hour after dinner),[6].—Stitching in the upper part of the right parietal bone (after seven hours and a half),[6].—Very violent, painful stitching in the left parietal bone, then boring in the left ear (after seven hours),[6].—Very acute stitches in the right side of the head, with throbbing, in the evening, when sitting and when standing,[6].—Tearing in the right parietal bone, disappearing of its own accord (after two hours),[6].—Painful throbbing in the right side of the head, deep internally (after two hours and a half),[6].—*Occiput.* Painful twitching in the right occipital bone, externally (after two hours and a half),[6].—In the evening, on lying down, a sticking-pressing pain in the occiput,[9].—[140.] Stitching in the left occiput, after dinner,[6].—In the upper part of the occiput, intolerable stitching and tearing from both sides inward (after three hours and a half),[6].—Stitches deep into the brain on the right occipital bone, more in the upper part, in the afternoon,[6].—Many dull violent stitches in succession in the occiput, so that the pain extended into the forehead, deep internally, in the afternoon,[6].—Tearing from the left side of the occiput into the forehead on the left side, with vertigo, which lasted longer than the pain (after half an hour),[6].—*External Head.* The hair falls out very much on combing,[9].—On the right occipital bone, several fine stitches in the skin (after two hours and three-quarters), then several tearings as if in the left parietal bone,[6].

Eye.—Objective. Inflammation of the eyes,[37].—Inflammation of the eyes, so severe that he was blind for several days (after several hours),[112].—Protruding eyes,[45].—[150.] The eyes protrude,[25].—Sunken eyes,[87].—Eyes sunken, surrounded by blue rings (second day),[94].—Lustreless eyes,[4].—Redness of eyes (soon after),[76].—Eyes red,[96].—Eyes red and suffused with tears (after one hour),[99].—*Subjective.* His eyes give out, and pain on writing as usual,[9].—The eyes pain on exertion,[9].—The eyes pain, as after excessive weeping,[9].—[160.] Glowing heat of the eyes, as from coals,[9].—Burning of the eyes,[2].—The eyes burn,[6].—Pressing in the eyes,[3].—Pressing in the eyes, so that the lids close, in the afternoon,[9].—Biting sensation in the eyes, as if salt were in them,[1a].—Cutting in the eye, while writing,[9].—Sticking and itching in the left eye,[9].—Tearing in the right eye (after one hour),[3].—Smarting in the right eye, in the afternoon,[6].—[170.] Smarting in the eyes, as if salt were in them,[1].—Itching in the right eye, in the afternoon,[6]. —*Orbit.* Pain in the left orbital arch, as if it was pressed violently with a blunt instrument,[3].—*Lids.* The lids more closed than usual; the eyes look small,[9].—Quivering and stitching on the right lower lid,[6].—Twitching in the left lower lid (after two hours),[6].—Twitching in the right upper lid, in the afternoon at 2 o'clock,[6].—*Lachrymal Apparatus.* Lachrymation,[96].—Lachrymation (soon after),[76].—Lachrymation and tension in the upper lids (from the vapor),[5].—Lachrymation in the open air; was obliged to close the eyes; if he opened them the margins of the lids pained as if sore, like raw flesh,[1a].—*Conjunctiva.* [180.] Conjunctiva slightly suffused (after three weeks),[98].—Sudden cure of a chronic conjunctivitis (second day),[4].—*Ball.* Painful drawing in the right eyeball, before dinner,[6].—*Pupil.* Dilated pupils,[51].—Dilated pupils, with dim vision,[8].—Remarkably contracted pupils (after three hours),[9].—*Vision.* Dimness of vision; was obliged to make great exertion in order to see clearly either near or distant objects,[1a].—(Dimness of vision on writing; he could not see the places at which he looked; followed by headache),[1a].—Cannot distinguish an object till he nearly closes the lids and shakes the head two or three times (after three weeks),[98].—Everything at which she looks is yellow (for an hour in the morning), (second day),[6].—[190.] Eyes weak and watery, to which he is subject; but now the letters on the paper are green and yellow (after three weeks),[98].

Ear.—A hot vapor frequently issues from either ear, alternately,[6].—Pressing behind the right ear,[3].—Sticking in the ears (after one hour),[9].—Stitching in the left ear (after seven hours),[6].—Tearing deep in the right ear, and at the same time tickling in the left ear,[6].—Tearing externally in the right meatus auditorius, then the left shoulder,[6].—Tearing and stitching in the right mastoid process, so that she believed that it must tear the bone out; she had to cry out (in the evening for one hour),[6].—Single tearing in the right mastoid process, very painful and frequently repeated,[6].—Painful tearing in the right mastoid process below the ear, as if with a knife, not disappearing on rubbing; at the same time headache in the forehead, like a heaviness; frequently, even at night (after half an hour),[6].—[200.] Violent, painful, sudden tearing in the right mastoid process, extending into the lobule of the ear, and at the same time stitching in the ear, frequently disappearing on rubbing (after three-quarters of an hour),[6].—*Hearing.* Incessant drumming in the ears (after three weeks),[95].—Ringing and humming before both ears,[8].—Roaring in the ears, after supper,[6].

Nose.—Objective. Inflammation of the tip of the nose,[9].—Inflammation on the edge of the right wing of the nose, especially toward the end, appearing at irregular intervals red and shining, with a little swelling and some pain (after several hours); disappeared only on the second day,[5]. —Inflamed, spotted nose, with pain, as if sore; several crusts form, which fall off after three days,[9].—Red, swollen nose, with sensation as if it would fester, especially internally; on touch and on talking the pain is increased,[9]. —The nose red and hot, with a festering pustule,[9].—Nose swollen; red and sore in the interior (after three weeks),[98].—[210.] He has a violent catarrh, which makes itself apparent by the secretion of much tenacious mucus from the nose, without sneezing; by hoarseness and hawking of tough mucus from the chest, and (which was never the case in catarrh with him) by nightly dry, cutting-stitching along the trachea externally (second day),[8]. —Sneezing (after three hours),[6].—Sneezing, followed by sticking in the left wing of the nose,[9].—Violent sneezing (second morning),[6].—Bleeding of the nose,[9].—Bleeding of the nose (ninth day, A.M.),[6].—The nasal mucus is mixed with blood,[9].—The mucus from the nose in an old catarrh becomes bloody,[1a].—Pain and tension in the nose and throbbing, with sensation as if it were swollen; it is also painful to the touch (fourth and fifth days),[7]. —Pain at 3 A.M. above on the top of the nose, so that he thought he had pressed it, followed by tension and erysipelatous inflammation and swelling from the back of the nose down both sides into the cheeks, especially on the right, like great redness of the cheeks, becoming white under the pressure of the finger, then rapidly again red; hard to the touch. It continued to increase on the following days and decreased on the third day, followed by slight desquamation (thirtieth day). After several weeks, without marked cause, a similar inflammation, especially on the right upper lip, the sides and tip of nose,[5].—[220.] Transient, stitchlike pain above the root of the nose,[8].—Several stitches in the left wing of the nose, from within outward,[9].—Drawing and tickling, with ineffectual irritation to sneeze, in the right nostril (after three and a half hours),[6].—Stitches in the nostrils,[9]. —Nostrils sore,[81].—Itching of the nostrils, uvula, and throat,[60].—*Smell.* Constant stench before the nose, that passes down his throat (after three weeks),[98].

Face.—Objective. Animated expression,[60].—*Expression of extreme suffering,*[6].—*Very suffering, pale look (fourth, fifth, sixth, etc., days),*[6].— [230.] Sickly look, sunken, pale face,[3].—Sickly look, with dim eyes, surrounded by dark rings (second day),[107].—*Deathlike look, during and after the pains* (second day, afternoon),[6].—Countenance anxious,[81].—Very anxious countenance,[96].—Hippocratic countenance,[4].—On stooping he immediately becomes very red in the face, the blood shoots forcibly into the head; even when sitting the head becomes very hot, not when walking,[1a].—Red spots in the face, which glow like fire (after three hours),[9].—Flushed face (soon after),[76].—Flushed face (after one hour),[99].—[240.] Face flushed, anxious expression,[96].—Flushed, anxious countenance (second day),[18].—Glowing of the whole face,[9].—The right side of the face glows, while the left is a waxy yellow,[9].—Face cyanotic,[94].—Cyanotic color of the face,[87].—Yellow color of the face and eyes (tenth day),[8].—Earthy color of the face,[28].—Pale looks (after one and a half hours),[6].—Paleness of the face,[6].—[250.] Faces pale, sunken, expressive of terror,[101].—Face pale, sunken, haggard, expressive of anxiety,[102].—Face pale as plaster, and covered with sweat,[4].—During the chill very pale,[6].—Pale face, with red flushes (second day),[92].—Pale in the face, with internal sensation of coldness,[6].—Deathlike pallor,[4].—Face disfigured,[4].—Swollen face,[45].—*Face very much swollen and puffy (after three months),*[97].—[260.] Face, neck, and abdomen swell,[25].—Right half of face quite swollen (after three weeks),[98].—The right side of the face swollen, with tension without redness or heat (eighth, ninth, tenth, and eleventh days),[6].—Sunken, hippocratic face,[6].—*Subjective.* Spasmodic stitches, drawing downward, from the eyebrows to the chin, with a hot sensation in the palate, as if he had eaten something burning (first day),[7]. —Pain, as if sore, in the facial bones, which extends into the ear, more on the right side,[9].—*Cheek.* The right cheek is swollen and inflamed, with drawing toothache in the upper jaw,[9].—*Lips.* Lips much swollen (second day),[92].—Desquamation of the lips, with moderate thirst (nineteenth day),[6]. —*Dry lips, without thirst* (after eight days),[6].—[**270.**] Dryness of the lips and thirst during and after the pains,[6].—A cutting pain in the middle of the margin of the lower lip, which passes toward the right ear and ceases behind it (after four hours),[6].—*Chin.* Twitching in the middle of the left lower jaw while speaking (after two and a half hours),[6].—Stitching in the external chin, somewhat on the right side, in the afternoon,[6].—Gnawing in the middle of the right lower jaw (after two hours),[6].—Painful gnawing in the centre of the lower jaw, spreading to the teeth (after three-quarters of an hour),[6].—Tearing in the right lower jaw (second morning), on walking,[6]. —Tearing in the left lower jaw, extending backward, in the afternoon,[6].— Violent tearing in the centre of the right lower jaw, and in a tooth there,[6].— Pain as if sore on the inner margin of the lower jaw, where there is also an eruption of tetter, which itches somewhat; on speaking and touch, the bone aches still more,[9].

Mouth.—Teeth. [**280.**] Drawing, followed by sticking, in the teeth, especially in the evening, after lying down, so that it is an hour before she falls asleep,[9].—In the upper teeth a drawing pain, worse on eating, in the afternoon,[9].—Tearing in the right lower molars (ninth day),[6].—A few tearings in a carious molar, on the lower right side,[6].—A root of a tooth on the right lower side rises up and can easily be drawn out, without the tearing ceasing (ninth day),[6].—*Gums.* Gums red and swollen,[96].—Gums red and swollen (one case), (third day),[53].—On the gum above the left upper incisor there appears a red, somewhat painful spot, which constantly grows more painful, and finally becomes a small, round, elevated, inflamed spot, of a yellow-reddish appearance, which is sore and also painful to more severe pressure externally; the whole upper lip is swollen,[5].—On the gum there appears, after six hours, a small blister, with red points; after fifteen hours the blister disappears, and leaves only a red spot; at the same time the upper lip is remarkably swollen, but little painful,[5].—After several weeks a dental fistula, lasting many weeks; a red spot above the carious root of an upper incisor, somewhat painful, of the size of a pin's head, with a small opening in the centre, from which, if it is pressed, pus discharges,[5].—[**290.**] Gums and mucous membrane of cheeks swollen (second day),[92].—Pains in the gums,[2].—A quivering in the gum of the left upper eye tooth,[8].—Painful drawing in the right gum extending outward on the right upper incisor, with sensation as if something were drawing across the lip (after four hours),[6].—A sudden painful tearing in the gum and left lower incisor (after three hours),[6].—*Tongue.* Tongue red at the edges, with a thick yellow coating on its anterior two-thirds,[102].—Tongue bluish-red, covered with white blisters containing bile-like fluid (second day),[92].—Tongue rather pale and dry,[96].—Tongue coated white,[89].—Tongue coated white during the attack,[6].—[**300.**] The tongue white, taste bitter, with nausea and aversion to everything,[6].—*Tongue highly furred, red at the edges* (third day),[96].— Tongue much coated, with red edges (one case), (third day),[53].—*Tongue swollen and thickly coated,*[81] [93] etc.—*Sublingual glands swollen and red,*[96].— Tongue, throat, and gum were festering,[42].—*Tongue and back of mouth in part excoriated, in part covered with blisters,*[49].—A large blister along centre of tongue reaching far back, painful (second day),[92].—Trembling of tongue,[93]. —Dry, pale tongue (second day),[78].—[**310.**] Tongue dry and coated with mucus, in the morning,[6].—Long-lasting burning on the tongue and palate (after quarter of an hour),[8].—Stitch on the tip of the tongue, as if she had bitten it (first day),[17].—Tickling on the tip of the tongue,[9].—*General Mouth.* Inflammation and considerable swelling of the buccal mucous membrane, with very profuse salivation (after a few hours),[52].—Inside of mouth inflamed and ulcerated (third day),[96].—The lips, tongue, palate, and pharynx, as far as could be seen, inflamed and full of blisters,[45].—*Mucous membrane of the mouth red and covered with small blisters* (after two hours),[82]. —Mucous membrane of lips and mouth peels off in large flakes (after one hour),[103].—Mouth excoriated,[93].—[320.] Back of mouth swollen and red, as if from erysipelas; the tissues crossed by enlarged veins (second day),[58].—A swelling, large as a hazel-nut, of a purple color, on the inside of the mouth near the last lower molar, painless (ninth day); on the third day it breaks, and clotted blood is discharged, without pain,[6].—Aphthæ in the mouth,[35]. —Blisters in the mouth and pharynx,[25].—*Lining of mouth and throat covered with white blisters from the size of a pin's head to that of a bean,*[84].—Toward morning a piece of clotted blood comes into the mouth (fourteenth day),[6]. —Early in the morning, in bed, a clot of blood comes into her mouth (eleventh day),[6].—From the mouth, breath like cedar pitch,[21].—Very nauseous odor from the mouth, many days,[6].—*Dryness in the mouth* (second evening),[6].—[330.] Dryness in the mouth, with violent thirst,[25].—Remarkable dryness in the mouth and nose (first hour),[8].—Mouth slimy, bitter (fourth day, A.M.),[6].—Mouth slimy, tongue white (fourth day, A.M.),[6].—At night, on waking, slimy mouth,[6].—Painful heat of the mouth (soon after),[49].— Burning heat in mouth and œsophagus (after one hour),[103].—*Burning pain in the mouth, throat, and stomach,*[81].—Burning of whole mouth and throat, which are hot, obliging him to drink often without quenching the thirst (second day),[92].—*Burning in the mouth, pharynx, and stomach,*[25][29], etc.— [340.] Burning of the lips, tongue, and palate (immediately),[52].—Exceedingly violent burning in the mouth, pharynx, and œsophagus,[45].—Mouth and tongue seem deprived of their mucous membrane,[96].—On the right side of the mouth sensation as if the membrane were being raised with a needle (after one hour and a half),[6].—Biting pain in the palate (especially after eating), (after six hours),[18].—*Saliva.* Flow of saliva,[29].—Profuse flow of saliva, so that the patient constantly had to lie on his side,[45].—Much secretion of saliva,[2].—Much saliva accumulates in the mouth,[9].—[350.] A disgusting sweet saliva accumulates in large quantities and constantly fills the mouth, on account of which he must spit incessantly for a quarter of an hour (after half an hour),[8].—Much expectoration of saliva,[42].—*Salivation,*[93][96].—Salivation, *without coppery taste* (third day),[96].—Salivation and mucus from mouth,[54].—Salivation; constant spitting of mingled mucus and saliva, of a dark color (second day),[53].—Much salivation,[75].—Salivation profuse,[76].— Profuse salivation; margin of tongue and gums covered with aphthæ; teeth loosened (increasing for two days, lasting seven days), (after five hours),[96].— Copious salivation, gums red (third day),[96].—[360.] Flow of water into the mouth (eighth day, A.M.),[6].—Mouth constantly full of tasteless water (after a quarter of an hour),[6].—Frequent accumulation and spitting of tasteless water (after one hour and a half),[6].—Mucus and blood from mouth and nose,[84].—*Taste.* Insipid taste, as of sweet cheese (immediately after 6 drops),[107].—(Bitter taste),[18].—Bitter taste in the mouth (ninth day),[6].—Sour taste,[9].—Taste nauseous, bitter (second day),[92].—Nauseous taste and much saliva (after three hours),[9].—[370.] Foul taste in the mouth, on rising,[18].— Filthy, disgusting taste in the mouth, several afternoons in succession,[7].— Taste as of cedar pitch,[31].—Bloody taste in the mouth (tenth day),[6].—Loss of taste during the attack,[6].—The food seems unsalted to her,[6].

Throat.—*Throat inflamed, and covered with plastic lymph* (one case) (third day),[53].—He draws much tough mucus into the mouth through the posterior nares (in the first hour),[8].—The throat dry, without thirst, in the afternoon,[9].—Roughness and hoarseness in the throat (third forenoon),[6].— [380.] Burning heat in the throat soon after,[53].—*Burning sensation in throat* (after half an hour),[97].—Sense of burning in throat and stomach (soon after),[50].—Burning sensation in the throat, especially at the entrance of the œsophagus, extending to the epigastrium (second day),[53].—Burning sensation in throat and pit of stomach, increased by pressure,[98].—Sense of constant burning in throat, most intense at top of œsophagus, and descending down towards stomach (third day),[96].—*Throat feels "on fire"* (third day),[96].—*Throat swollen* (third day),[96].—*Constriction and intense pain at the back of the throat,*[102].—*Burning soreness of the throat, which is inflamed* (after three weeks),[98].—[390.] Intolerable scraping in the throat, with necessity for hawking up mucus after meals,[9].—*Uvula.* Uvula relaxed,[96].— *Tonsils.* The tonsils are somewhat inflamed,[2].—Tonsils swollen,[96].— *Fauces, Pharynx, and Œsophagus.* Erysipelatous blush of inflammation and turgid veins run across fauces (third day),[96].—The fauces red, painful, with a pressing sensation, which on swallowing changes to a sticking,[9].—Fauces abraded and blistered,[96].—*Aphthous ulcer at back part of fauces, size of a sixpence, covered with a whitish adherent crust; a similar one on side of right tonsil* (third day),[96].—Dryness in the pharynx, with occasional sticking,[8].—With hunger, a sort of pain in the pharynx (the fourth day),[5].—[400.] Burning in pharynx and mouth (first day),[92].— Burning in the pharynx on swallowing,[2].—Burning and constriction in the pharynx,[87 90].—Œsophagus felt as if on fire (second day),[53].—Constrictive pain in the pharynx (after seven hours), (sexton),[56].—Contractive sensation in the pharynx,[1a].—Burning-scraping sensation in the pharynx, and sweetish, disgusting taste on the tongue and in the whole mouth as far as the pharynx,[8].—A large cylindrical mass, apparently the inner membrane of the gullet, was discharged by vomiting (second day),[75].—Burning sensation along œsophagus, intolerable while drinking,[96].—Burning and constriction of the œsophagus,[101].—*Swallowing.* [410.] *Dysphagia* (second day),[53]. —Difficulty of swallowing, for several months,[50].—*Swallowing very difficult* (third day),[96].—Difficult, or rather impossible, deglutition,[58].—Painful and difficult deglutition,[102].

Stomach.—Increased appetite (some provers),[4].—More appetite than usual,[6].—Appetite not diminished during the whole action of the medicine,[6]. —Hunger immediately after relief of the pains (seventeenth day),[6].— Awakened at night by sensation of hunger (which had never happened before), (second night),[106].—[420.] Without feeling hungry, he would eat now this, now that (first day),[3].—*Diminished appetite,*[4].—Loss of appetite,[4]. —Loss of appetite (after three weeks),[98].—Loss of appetite, evening and morning; he relished nothing,[1a].—Loss of appetite for food,[1a].—Appetite lost; weakness; she becomes bedridden (eighth day),[6].—The appetite, which had been somewhat excited, disappeared after coffee,[6].—No appetite (second day),[92].—No appetite for supper (third day),[107].—[430.] No desire for food,[1].—*Disgust for food* (second day),[1 92].—Disgust for everything; she cannot bear to see or hear about food; in the evening during the paroxysm,[6]. —Disgust and ill humor,[21]—Disgust, with frequent gathering of water in the mouth,[6].—Constant disgust and nausea,[47].—Aversion to tobacco,[1a].— *Thirst.* Thirst (first day),[92].—Thirst (fifteenth day, A.M.),[6].—Thirst when not in pain (ninth and tenth days),[6].—[440.] Thirst during dinner (unusual),[6].—Thirst after the shaking chill, 8 P.M.,[6].—Thirst after the chill.

After the chill neither heat nor sweat (second day, 5 P.M.),[6].—Thirst is very trifling, and appears to come only from dryness of the lips; drink easily dispensed with,[6].—Some thirst during the coldness (ninth day),[6].— Increased thirst (after six hours),[3].—Increased thirst, with much drinking; the urinary secretion does not compare with the quantity of liquids taken; the secretion of quite scanty thin urine occurs first in the evening, four hours after the drinking, and without any unpleasant sensation in the urethra; the prover was usually obliged to urinate immediately, however little she had drank,[6].—Much thirst during the day,[9].—*Great thirst*,[84].—Great thirst (one case), (third day),[53].—[450.] *Great thirst, constant*,[96].—*Urgent thirst, with burning pain in throat and stomach*,[96].—Intense thirst,[81].—Intense thirst, but liquids can hardly be swallowed, and are at once vomited up again,[102].—At night, intense thirst and fever,[96].—Excessive thirst, but could not swallow any liquid without unutterable anguish,[50].—Violent thirst,[12]. —Violent thirst (first day),[92].—Unquenchable thirst,[27 29], etc.—Burning thirst,[101].—[460.] Loss of thirst during the whole action,[6].—No thirst; water does not taste good to her,[9].—No thirst during the chill, or heat,[6].—*Eructations and Hiccough.* Eructation (after half an hour),[8].—Eructatious becoming daily more frequent and violent (eighth and ninth days, afternoon),[6].—Eructation, with taste of the food, after dinner,[6].—Frequent empty eructation (after three-quarters of an hour),[6].—Eructation of air, with relief (fourteenth day),[6].—Eructations of air, even on the third day, with relief of the chest symptoms,[6].—*Eructations of sour, frothy mucus, tinged bright-red*,[96].—[470.] Frothy and acid eructations (two cases), (third day),[53].—Hot eructation; heartburn; she has no thirst, and the burning sensation in the pharynx is increased by drinking water,[9].—A sort of incomplete eructation, almost like hiccough, which passes backward from the pharynx toward the stomach, before dinner (after three hours),[5].—Frequent hiccough (second day),[92].—Hiccough in the afternoon,[6].—*Nausea and Vomiting.* Nausea,[86 93].—Nausea (one prover), (after two hours),[6].— Nausea (soon after),[53].—Nausea (second day),[3].—Nausea toward evening,[9]. —[480.] Nausea in the stomach, on walking and standing (after one hour),[6]. —Nausea, like a weakness in the stomach (after fourteen days), after coffee in the forenoon,[6].—Nausea and inclination to vomit,[87].—Nausea, increasing to vomiting (second day),[95].—Nausea and disgust, when eating,[18].— Nausea and disgust for everything (fifth day),[6].—Nausea and disgust for all food (eighth day),[6].—*Nausea and vomiting* (first day),[92].—Nausea, and vomiting of bloody mucus,[96].—Nausea and repeated vomiting without exertion; the matter vomited consisted of mucus and ingesta,[83].—[490.] Nausea, with trembling of the feet (fourth day),[6].—In the morning, nausea with coldness, without thirst; in the afternoon heat, without thirst, and without subsequent sweat,[9].—Slight nausea, with insipid taste and dryness of the throat (seventh day),[106].—Much nausea, soon followed by vomiting of blood to the extent of half a pint (second day),[97].—In the morning, great nausea, almost to vomiting,[9].—Violent nausea,[96].—She feels remarkably nauseated, as if she would vomit (after five minutes),[8].—Qualmishness in the stomach, frequently disappearing and returning (after two hours),[6].—Qualmishness and vomiting,[12].—Frequent inclination to vomit (eighth day),[6].—[500.] Great efforts to vomit and excessive gagging,[84].— Retching and vomiting,[25].—Violent retching, and vomiting of the contents of the stomach and bilious mucus,[45].—*Vomiting*,[86].—Vomiting, nausea in the stomach, with pressing, followed by cutting,[6].—Vomiting, with strangury, followed by inflammation of the kidney,[96].—Vomited and urinated incessantly,[54].—Vomiting of ingesta,[4].—He could not retain anything, vomited everything,[45].—Takes a glass of water, which is returned again,[96].—[510.] Vomits the water he drinks, with a considerable quantity of blood,[96].—Vomiting of greenish, offensive matter,[96].—Vomited greenish and peculiarly offensive matter,[81].—What was vomited was of a greenish color and an unpleasant smell,[93].—Vomits membrane,[84].—Vomiting of membranous flakes (a morbid secretion of the alimentary canal),[79].—After an emetic, vomited membrane-like fragments, looking as if detached from the walls of the stomach and œsophagus,[49].—Vomiting of tenacious mucus, taking the form of the gullet, or often of the mucous membrane itself,[96].—Vomiting of bile and ingesta,[90].—Vomits frothy mucus, tinged bright-red (bloody), (third day),[96].—[520.] Vomits, sometimes with, sometimes without, blood,[96].—Bloody vomiting (four cases),[58].—Vomiting of blood, with strangulation,[58].—Frequent vomiting,[101].—Repeated vomiting,[90].—Constant vomiting,[64].—Incessant vomiting,[81].—Copious vomiting of bile (after one hour),[103].—Severe vomiting,[87].—Violent vomiting of bloody and frothy mucus (soon after),[53].—*Stomach.* [530.] Inflammation of the stomach,[23].—Acute inflammation of the stomach,[96].—Weakness of the stomach (third and fourth days),[6].—Sensation of weakness in the stomach (second day),[3].—An indescribable sensation in the epigastric region; she feels hungry without being really so,[6].—On stooping, or on inspiration, a sensation of resistance in the epigastric region,[6].—Had scarcely journeyed half a mile, when obliged to dismount from distressing sensation in stomach and strong desire to vomit,[96].—Pain in the stomach,[88].—Pain in the stomach (sexton),[86].—Pains in the epigastrium,[90].—[540.] Sharp pain in stomach and bladder,[55].—Acute pain in stomach and bladder (after one hour),[99].—*Acute pain in the region of the stomach and bladder, with such exquisite sensibility that the slightest pressure produces convulsions,*[76].—Severe epigastric pain (cramps in the stomach), (after one hour),[103].—Violent pain in stomach and bowels (soon),[105].—Violent pains in the epigastric region and in the groins,[12].—Such violent pains in the region of the stomach and kidneys that the patient tossed about in his bed, beat the walls with his hands, and scratched off the lime,[26].—The most violent pains in the stomach, in the whole abdomen, in the kidneys, in the whole body,[20].—Excessive pain at the epigastrium and umbilicus, aggravated by pressure,[101].—Cardialgia and sour eructations, especially after drinking,[98].—[550.] Heat and pain in the epigastric region,[42].—Sensation of burning heat in the stomach, and, in a less degree, in the œsophagus,[49].—Burning in the stomach,[2] [86].—Burning at the orifice of the stomach,[2].—Burning pain in gastric region (second day),[53].—Violent burning in the stomach,[27].—Violent, but not painful, burning in the stomach, with taste of wine in the mouth; the whole forenoon (first days),[6].—Fulness, with pressure in the stomach, as if he would eructate, without its amounting to anything (after three-quarters of an hour),[8].—An uncommon sensation of fulness in the epigastric region, together with anxiety and restlessness (after one hour),[8].—Sensation in the stomach as if screwed together, very painful; before dinner,[6].—[560.] Violent spasmodic pains in stomach, accompanied by free emesis,[100].—Pinching and stitching in the right epigastric region (second morning),[6].—Sense of heaviness, heat, and slight smarting at the epigastrium and umbilicus,[101].—Violent pressing in the stomach, most when it was empty (second day),[6].—Painful pressing in the stomach, extending backward from both sides into the spinal column, where it seems to her as if screwed together; continuing for a long time in all positions (after two hours),[6].—Pressure in the pit of the stomach, in the afternoon,⁹.—A crushing in the pit of the stomach, which diminishes as soon as she takes anything warm or drinks anything cold.⁹.—Cutting pain in the stomach (after half an hour),³.—Drawing pain in the stomach,³.—Cutting pains at intervals in the pit of the stomach and about the umbilicus,⁵².—Sharp lancinating pains in the stomach (soon after),⁵³.—[570.] The epigastric region is sensitive, internally and externally (second day),⁶.—The stomach internally sensitive, with good appetite (second forenoon),⁶.

Abdomen.—Hypochondria. Incarceration of flatus under the short ribs (as of offensive flatus), (after two hours),¹ᵃ.—(Inflammation of the liver and erosion of the intestines),¹¹.—Sensation as if something held her together below the right false ribs (after two hours),¹⁶.—*Umbilical and Sides.* Burning pain above the navel on coughing, sneezing, and blowing the nose, whereby the abdomen seems very hot; in the region of this pain externally are several yellow spots, which when touched are more stinging than burning,¹ᵃ.—Pinching about the navel (one hour after dinner),⁶.—Before and during the stool, griping in the abdomen, below the navel,⁶.—Pinching in the left side of the abdomen (after four hours),⁶.—Pressing pain in both sides below the ribs (after two hours),³.—[580.] On both sides of the lower abdomen, sensation as if something were compressing them there, but in the left side farther downward (four hours),⁶.—Cutting in the right side of the abdomen (three hours),⁶.—Stitching in the left side of the upper abdomen, and in the centre of the sternum,⁶.—*General Abdomen.* Inflammation of whole alimentary canal, ureters, kidneys, and internal organs of generation,⁹⁶.—Violent intestinal inflammation,¹².—The pains in the intestinal canal change to inflammation and gangrene,²⁹.—Erosion of the intestines,¹¹.—The abdomen was prominent,⁴⁵.—*Abdomen swollen and tympanitic,*⁷⁸.—Abdomen swollen to the size at full period of utero-gestation, tense and tympanitic,⁹⁶.—[590.] Diffusive swelling, extending over the whole abdomen,⁹⁶.—*Abdomen distended,*⁸⁴.—*Abdomen much distended* (second day),⁹⁷.—The abdomen is very much distended, with much moving about in it, as if flatulence would pass,⁸.—Distension and constant pain in the abdominal region,⁵⁸.—Distension of the whole abdomen, with the pains,⁶.—*Great distension and tenderness of the belly* (second day),⁷⁸.—Movings in the abdomen and yawning,⁶.—The flatulence moves about the whole abdomen, with violent pinching; the pain extends into the chest (first evening),⁶.—Flatulence moves about in the abdomen, and gives rise to lumps, as if a child were there (fourteenth day),⁶.—[600.] Rolling in the abdomen, with sensation as if diarrhœa would appear,⁶.—Rumbling and rattling in the abdomen (after one hour and a quarter),⁸.—Audible rumbling in the abdomen while sitting (after half an hour),⁶.—Growling, audible rumbling, and gurgling in the bowels (third day),⁶.—Very loud growling, more on the right side of the lower abdomen, passing backward (after three-quarters of an hour),⁶.—Much flatulence,⁹.—A very large amount of flatulence (first day),¹⁰⁸.—Discharge of much flatulence,³.—Profuse discharge of flatulence (eighth day, evening), with noise,⁸.—Passage of very much flatulence,⁸.—[610.] After frequent urging, some flatulence, with relief,⁶.—Sensation in the abdomen as if the menses would appear, after midnight,⁶.—Pain in the upper part of the abdomen (second day),⁹⁴.—Pain in the abdomen,¹ ¹⁵.—Severe pain in the abdomen, increased by pressure,⁷⁸.—Violent pain in the abdomen,¹⁷.—Renewal of the violent abdominal pains after coffee (fourteenth day),⁶.—Excruciating pain over abdomen, worse over hypogastric region and scrobiculus cordis; increased by pressure,⁹⁶.—Excessive abdominal pain until death (from 4 grains),⁴¹.—

Pains in the bowels (some provers),[4].—Pain in the bowels,[2].—[620.] Excruciating pain in bowels (second day),[78].—Pains in the intestinal canal and in the anus, especially with the stool, which is increased thereby,[25].—Severe pains in the intestines,[86].—In the intestines, a sensation of warmth, as if he had drank strong wine,[9].—*Great heat along the whole course of the alimentary canal,*[50].—*Burning sensation along the alimentary canal,*[58].—Burning and twisting in the abdomen, until he had been to stool a few times, especially in the morning,[1a].—In the abdomen, sensation of fulness and flatulence,[6].—Griping in the abdomen, which extended upward, and became stitching; then stitching backwards on both sides, so that it hindered her respiration (eighth day),[6].—Griping in the abdomen, followed by liquid stool, without pain,[6].—[630.] Violent griping pain in abdomen,[96].—Violent griping in the abdomen, at 3 A.M. (eighth day),[6].—With the stool, pinching in the abdomen; after the stool, shivering, in the afternoon,[6].—Sensation in the abdomen as after a drastic purge,[6].—*Cutting in the abdomen,*[1].—Cutting in the abdomen, the whole day,[9].—*With the stool, cutting in the abdomen; towards evening, and after the stool, shivering,*[6].—Slight cutting in the upper abdomen (fourth day),[6].—Violent cutting in the abdomen,[15].—Violent cutting pain in the abdomen and boring pains in the knees, so that she cried aloud: Camphor brought no relief; after coffee she vomited bitter stuff, after which it remained bitter in her mouth; after repeated doses of Camphor, there at last came relief of the intolerable pains,[6].—[640.] Fearful cutting pains from 5 P.M. till morning; she had to roll about (third night),[6].—Colic; some sudden gripings in the sides of the abdomen, rather external, when standing,[1a].—Violent colic, nausea, and abundant vomiting of ingesta,[101].—Colic, followed by ten diarrhœic stools,[70].—Since taking the medicine, daily colic, followed by diarrhœa,[9].—Tearing and pinching in the abdomen,[9].—Tearing in the abdomen, with diarrhœa and pain in the anus,[9].—Most extreme sensitiveness of the abdomen to touch (tenth day),[6].—*Hypogastrium.* Fermenting in the intestines of the lower abdomen (after a quarter of an hour),[3].—Pain in the hypogastrium,[102].—[650.] Slight pains in the hypogastrium and in the lumbar region,[101].—Excessive pains in the hypogastrium,[11].—Excessive pains in the hypogastrium, followed by mental confusion and death,[11].—Pain in hypogastric and lumbar regions,[59].—Severe pain in the hypogastric region,[56].—Violent pain in the lower belly (after one hour),[50].—Gnawing pain in the lower abdomen,[10].—Griping in the lower abdomen, with pressing towards the genitals (fourth day, in the morning, till 1 P.M.),[6].—Excessive cutting pains in the lower abdomen, which constantly wander about and intermit but a short time,[6].—Slight pains above the symphysis pubis, and downward along the ureters, which constantly become worse (after five hours),[5].—[660.] Drawing and tearing in the pubic region,[3].—Bearing-down pains (second day),[97].—Painful tension along the inguinal canal and the testicles, around the pelvic region (after three weeks),[98].—Cutting pains in the groin all day, less when sitting and standing, but more when walking,[9].—Cutting-sticking and burning in the groin; on urinating, violent cutting,[9].—Stitching in the left groin, extending downward (fifteenth day),[6].—Acute stitching in the right groin (third day),[6].

Rectum and Anus. —Tenesmus (some provers),[4].—Very great tenesmus,[30].—A violent cutting pain attacked her in the rectum, such as she had never experienced in her life before; on standing and walking, discharge of flatulence with relief, but immediately afterwards the same pain, with urging to stool, followed by soft stool, with cessation of the pain, at 8 P.M.,[6].—[670.] Crawling in the rectum,[9].—*Burning, like fire, in the anus, after the diarrhœa* (tenth day),[6].—After the stool, burning and stitching, as with needles, in the anus (first day),[6].—*Pain in the perineum, seemingly arising from the neck of the bladder rather than from the root of the penis*,[49].—Pressure in perineum,[91].—Frequent desire for stool,[1a].—Urging to stool,[2].—Urging, without stool (fourth day),[6].—Urging to stool, and then copious discharge of soft fæces,[6].—Increased painful urging to stool,[29].—[680.] Frequent urging to stool, with scanty discharge of fæces,[1a].—Constant as well as ineffectual urging to stool,[6].—Ineffectual urging to stool (after two hours),[6].—Ineffectual urging to stool, soon after the first stool,[6].—When he passed water, was obliged at the same time to go to stool, though nothing passed; this desire for stool ceased after the bladder became empty,[1a].

Stool.—*Diarrhœa*. Diarrhœa,[59].—Diarrhœa, without colic,[1].—Diarrhœa, by which the colic was somewhat relieved (after thirteen hours),[26].—*Diarrhœa, with burning in the anus*,[86].—Diarrhœa three times a day, with very violent colic,[9].—[690.] Diarrhœa, without any pain, several times during the day,[8].—Diarrhœa of frothy fæces (twenty-second day),[6].—Watery diarrhœa,[8].—Mucous diarrhœa,[84].—Diarrhœa of green mucus (tenth day), after constipation for three days,[6].—*Diarrhœa, consisting of blood and mucus*,[95].—*Violent diarrhœa, with intolerable burning in the anus*,[45].—Diarrhœa-like stool of brown liquid fæces, twice (nineteenth day),[6].—In the morning, usual stool, and at 6 P.M. two diarrhœic stools (third day); also one diarrhœic stool (fourth day),[6].—Two morning stools, with some tenesmus,[9].—[700.] In forenoon, two natural stools,[6].—Two natural stools in quick succession (after four hours), in the afternoon,[6].—A natural stool four times in the day,[1a].—Two liquid yellow stools during the day, with cutting in the abdomen after every stool, biting pain in the anus, without tenesmus,[1a].—*Copious stools* (some provers),[4].—Stool thin, pasty (third day),[106].—Thin stool, with much irritability in the rectum,[1a].—Slight, somewhat hard stool, passing with difficulty, with cutting pains in the rectum (first day),[8].—Stool hard, and only passed by pressing, so that she could have screamed (first day),[6].—Discharge of hard fæces, with protrusion of the rectum,[2].—[710.] In the morning, hard stool, but afterward soft, with colic,[9].—Urging to stool, which consisted of hardened fæces; soon afterward, liquid stool, preceded by colic, in the afternoon,[6].—After constipation for five days, two very hard stools, with pressing; after the second, twinging in the anus (eighteenth day),[6].—Difficult evacuation of stool; he must press much more violently than usual, and still does not pass a sufficient stool (third day),[3].—Stool, with vomiting of herby-tasting food (first day),[92].—*Fæces red, slimy*,[90].—*Evacuation of red, mucous, fecal masses*,[90].—*Passage of white tough mucus with the stool, like scrapings from the intestines, with streaks of blood*, seven times in one night,[1a].—*Slimy and bloody stool* (after six days),[1a].—*Passage of pure blood from the anus and urethra*,[55].—[720.] After violent efforts, he succeeded in passing by the anus and urethra only a few drops of blood,[50].—Looseness of the bowels, like dysentery,[55].—Fatal dysentery,[57].—*Constipation.* The primary action of Cantharides is to retard and harden the stool,[6].—No stool, but passage of flatulence (second day),[6].—The whole first forenoon, neither stool nor urine,[6].

Urinary Organs.—*Bladder and Kidneys*. Inflammation of the uropoïetic organs,[25].—Inflammation of the urinary organs, and bleeding from them,[29].—Great irritability and severe pain of the urinary organs, attended by frequent micturition,[100].—*Cutting and contracting pains* *from .he ureters down toward the penis; at times the pains pass from without inward; pressure on the glans relieves the pain somewhat,*[5].—[**730.**] Kidneys inflamed,[96].—Inflammation of the kidneys,[40].—Inflammation of the kidneys, the bladder, and the penis, which becomes gangrenous,[41].—Inflammation of the kidneys, the ureters, the bladder, and the urethra,[22].—Renal congestion,[97].—Pain in kidneys,[29] [78].—**Dull pressing pains in both kidneys* (second day),[92].—**Pains in the region of the kidneys,*[95].—**Pains in the region of the kidneys and urging to urinate* (after three hours), *steadily increasing in severity,*[89].—Pain in region of kidneys and bladder,[96].—[**740.**] Severe pain in the region of the kidneys and bladder (after two days),[78].—**The region of the kidneys is affected by a continued dull painful sensation, late in the evening,*[8].—Pains in the kidneys and whole tract of the ureters, extending to the bladder,[4].—Pains in kidneys and bladder,[33].—Violent paroxysmal cutting and burning pains in both kidneys; *the region was very sensitive to the slightest touch;* this alternated with equally severe pain and burning in the tip of the penis, urging to urinate, and extremely painful evacuation, by drops, of bloody urine; at times also he passed pure blood with some clots,[89].—Pain in right kidney (soon after),[4].—A couple of very violent stitches in the region of the right kidney, so that she could have screamed (after two and a half hours),[6].—A twitching and throbbing sensation in the region of the right kidney (after nine hours),[6].—Inflammation of the bladder,[48].—Inflammation of the bladder; burning on urinating, finally bloody urine (in a woman, from the application of a fly-blister to the nape of the neck),[41].—[**750.**] Ulceration of the bladder,[96].—(At the post-mortem, the bladder, urethra, and kidneys were found ulcerated),[30].—Exulceration of the bladder and the urethra,[11].—Gangrene of the lining of the bladder,[12] —Discharge of much dirty, purulent matter from the bladder,[23].—**Irritation of the urinary organs, so that he can bear scarcely more than a spoonful of urine in the bladder, without urging to urinate the whole day,*[3].—Pain in the bladder,[37] [87].—***Violent pains in the bladder, with frequent urging to urinate; intolerable tenesmus,**[94].—**Fearful pains in the bladder,*[44].—Great heat in the bladder,[96].—[**760.**] Extraordinary heat at the bladder (after four hours),[54].—Burning of the bladder,[15].—Tenesmus vesicæ,[48].—**Intense vesical spasm* (after one hour),[103].—***Tenesmus of the bladder,**[86].—*Tenesmus and strangury,*[50].—**Most excessive tenesmus of the bladder and rectum,*[90].—Painful pressure downward toward the bladder,[6].—A sort of paralysis of the neck of the bladder; the urine passes without the slightest power to force; this attack lasted for some time, and gradually increased to such an extent that the urine could scarcely be retained without effort (first days),[8]. —Great pain in the neck of the bladder,[23].—[**770.**] Violent pain in the neck of the bladder,[25].—***Violent burning, cutting pains in neck of bladder,** *extending to the navicular fossa of urethra, especially worse before and after urinating* (second day),[92].—**When there is urgency to urinate there is a sticking pain in the forepart of the neck of the bladder, and on continued urging to urinate only a few drops of urine are passed,*[1a].—Pressing-stitching pain in the neck of the bladder,[1].—Pressing-tearing pain in the neck of the bladder,[1].—*Urethra.* Mouth of urethra inflamed,[84] [1a] [45] [2].— The urethra is swollen internally,[1a].—Urinary flatulence,[22].—White, watery discharge, like gleet,[110].—Discharge from the urethra of a small quantity of pasty, colorless liquid (fourth to fifth day),[109].—[**780.**] Discharge from the urethra like gleet, accompanied by constant desire to urinate,[110].— Yellow-colored gonorrhœa, which stains the linen yellow,[1a]. — Bloody gonorrhœa (after four days),[1a].—**Passage of blood from the urethra,*[62].—

Flow of blood from the urethra; in a short time five drops of blood ᵖ ssed, (from external use),³².—*Passage of bright-red blood, with the most violent urging to urinate, and cutting, burning pains through the whole urethra* (after nine hours),⁶.—He passes five pounds of blood from the urethra,⁶¹.—(Removes the urgent, inflammatory symptoms of incipient gonorrhœa),ᶜ¹.—Every time on urinating there is a sensation in the forepart of the urethra, at the tip of the glans, as if the urine was retained at that point and could not come out, with a pressive pain there; the urine, however, passes freely,¹ᵃ.—Painful sensation along urethra,⁹⁶.—[790.] Pain in urethra,⁹¹.—On urinating, he has pain only toward the close; if much urine has collected, this pain is much less than with little urine,⁵.—A few pains on urinating, with continual urging to urinate (after four and five hours),⁵.—A peculiar pain on urinating, as if it were impossible to evacuate the urine, with an unpleasant pressure in the region of the bladder (first day),¹⁰⁹.—*Could not pass urine without extreme pain; the quantity discharged was small and bloody,*¹⁰⁵.—Violent pain, with continual urinating (from external use), (after a few hours),³⁹.—*The most violent pain on urinating; it seems to her as if one were cutting with knives, with frequent urging, and yet she always passes but a few drops,*⁹.—Slight heat in urethra (soon after),⁴.—Feeling of heat in urethra, with slight constriction at the prostate (after two hours),⁴.—Burning in the forepart of the urethra, as if a drop of urine remained there (sixth day),¹⁰⁶.—[800.] (Burning before and during urinating),¹ᵃ.—*Ardor urinæ,⁶⁰ ⁶³, etc.—*Burning, when urinating, and when not* (after two hours),⁶.—Burning when urinating, and a white sediment in the urine, before the menses,¹ᵃ.—*Burning while urinating,*¹⁰ ²⁷, etc.—In the morning on urinating, he had a tensive sensation along the urethra, as if the urine were checked in its course (second day),³.—Pressive pain in the urethra with the gonorrhœal discharge,¹ᵃ.—Cutting pain, extending from the back and the abdomen out through the urethra,¹ᵃ.—Violent cutting before, during, and after urination (after six hours),⁶.—*Before, during, and after urinating fearful cutting pains in the urethra; she must double herself and scream from pains;* in the afternoon,⁶.—[810.] At times, an unlooked for sticking in the urethra, and burning, during the passage of urine,¹ᵃ.—Coarse stitches in the orifice of the urethra, extending to the anus, in the evening and night (after ten hours),¹ᵃ.—Biting pain in the urethra, while urinating,¹ᵃ.—Twitching and burning pain on urinating,²⁹.—Smarting in the urethra during urination,¹.—The urethra is painfully sensitive (after twelve hours),¹ᵃ.—Great soreness on urinating (after three weeks),⁹⁸.—A crawling and itching in the urethra, after urinating,¹ᵃ.—Unpleasant tickling and voluptuous warmth in the urethra,⁶⁷.—Burning while urinating; urine yellow (fifth day),⁶.—[820.] *Violent burning on urinating,*² ⁴⁷.—*Burning on urinating, so violent that he could not pass a drop of urine without tears and blood* (from the application of Cantharis powder, with yeast, to a cold swelling),²⁰.—Urine burns severely in passing (this symptom was very troublesome in the case of two or three provers who had drank very little at dinner),⁴.—Continual burning of the urine,³¹.—*Urine scalds him; it is passed drop by drop* (third day),⁹⁶.—*Burning along the urethra, after urinating,*² ²⁵.—Slight burning in the urethra,⁶⁷.—Troublesome burning in the urethra, at night, with passage of a few drops of blood (one prover),⁴.—Constant burning sensation in the urethra, even when not urinating (after ten hours),⁶.—Itching in the urethra,²⁵.—[830.] Itching sensation in the external meatus urinarius, which at times is almost a cutting sensation, but without voluptuous sensation,⁸.—Urging to urinate,¹.—Urging to urinate, with great pain at every attempt,[42].—*Urging to urinate, with burning sensation in the urethra,[95].—Urging to urinate, immediately; if the urine is passed at all, some of it passes in small quantities, at several times (from the vapor),[5].—*Every moment urging to urinate, and always but one teaspoonful passes (after four hours),[6].—Urging to urinate, without being able to pass any (first hour); later, there passed several drops, with bloody streaks, and the most violent pains (after five and six hours),[26].—*Urging to urinate, with strangury and ischuria,[29].—Urging to urinate, with increased secretion of urine, priapism, pain in stomach, and dysuria,[74].—Awakened at 3½ A.M. by urging to urinate; after the discharge of some urine, an extremely tormenting burning in the urethra. I could not remain in bed; on sitting, the trouble was somewhat relieved; was obliged to pass urine every three or four minutes, with almost unendurable pains. I drank three glasses of cold water in rapid succession, and after thirty minutes, passed a large amount of urine, with relief of the pain,[109].—[840.] *He has far greater urging to urinate when standing, and still more when walking, than when sitting (after five hours),[5].—*Frequent urging to urinate,[19], etc.—Frequent urgent need to urinate, always preceded by severe pain at the end of the penis; the passage of urine is always attended by severe scalding; urine turbid, and slightly tinged with blood,[81].—Frequent urging to urinate, renewed every two or three minutes,[101].—Frequent urging to urinate, with scanty urine, without pains; only toward the end of micturition, pressing pain in the base of the urethra, extending to the external meatus (after eight hours),[6].—Excessive urging to urinate,[88].—Violent urging to urinate (after two hours),[6].—Violent urging to urinate, whereby two spoonfuls, at the most, of dirty, tenacious mucus pass, with violent cutting,[23].—*Every three to four minutes the most violent urging to urinate, but at the most only a teaspoonful passes, and at the end of this scanty micturition, most intolerable burning-cutting pains in the urethra (after nine and a half hours),[6].—Constant urging to urinate, with intolerable pain,[35].—[850.] *Constant urging to urinate; only a small amount passed, with frightful pains (first day),[92].—*Constant urging to urinate; urine was passed drop by drop, with extreme pain,[56].—*Constant urging, and always but one spoonful of urine, with great pain, in the morning,[6].—*Constant urging to urinate, with which but a few drops pass, with such violent pain that she is forced to cry out,[9].—Constant urging to urinate, with passage of a few drops, causing severe smarting and burning along the urethra, especially in the neighborhood of the fossa navicularis. Finally, after long and painful straining to pass a few drops of bloody and albuminous urine, a convulsive tremor attacks all the limbs, the forehead and chest are covered with cold sweat, and he sinks on his bed half-exhausted; he cannot get a moment's rest, on account of the immediate return of these sufferings,[102].—*Constant painful urging to urinate, with dribbling discharge, reddish, sometimes mixed with blood (second day),[92].—Pressure and urging to urinate,[9].—*Frequent desire to urinate,[13].—Violent desire to urinate,[22].—Very urgent desire to urinate, which must be attended to (fifth day),[106].—[860.] *Painful efforts to pass urine and fæces,[90].—Every now and then she strains most painfully, and with all her might, only to pass a few drops of urine (after four hours),[103].—*Fruitless efforts to urinate,[93].—At noon, ineffectual urging to urinate; at one o'clock, a few drops of blood-streaked urine,[59].—Increased secretion of urine,[88].—Urine increased (fifth day),[6].—Urine increased (fifteenth and sixteenth days), becoming cloudy immediately after passing (fifteenth day),[6].—Increased urine, which at times passes with difficulty (from small doses),[28].—The first hours, increased urination, without difficulty,[5].—Urine increased in quantity, containing organized lymph, and a substance resembling mother of vinegar,[96].—[870.] Urine more seldom, but increased (sixth day),[6].—Urination is increased; at times restrained,[29].—Urine, in an hour and a half, scarcely a pint and a half, with coagulated blood,[8].—The amount of urine passed varied between 31¼ ounces and 37¾ ounces,[108].—The urine amounted to 59 ounces in five discharges (first day), (probably the effect of the tincture taken the previous days); 32¼ ounces (second day); 35½ ounces (third day.); 35 ounces (fourth day); 38 ounces, 1 dose of 1st. trit.; 34 ounces (second day); 37 ounces (third day),[108].—42 ounces of urine (third day); 33 ounces of urine (fourth day); 43½ ounces in only three passages (fourth day); 35 ounces of urine in three passages (fifth day); 35 ounces in three passages (sixth day),[107].—24½ ounces of urine (first day), (from 4 doses of 6th dil.); 29 ounces (second day); 28¼ ounces (third day), (from 4 doses of 3d dil.); 33½ ounces (fourth day),[106].—33¼ ounces (sixth day) (from 4 doses of 2d dil.); 34½ ounces (second day), (from 2 drops of 2d dil.); 35¼ ounces (fourth day), (from 25 drops of 6th dil.); 48 ounces (fifth day), (from 30 drops twice, and 5 drops once of the 1st. dil.); the quantity passed at each time this day was as follows: 13, 10, 9, and twice 7 ounces; 39½ ounces (sixth day), (from 50 drops of 1st dil., morning and evening); 34¼ ounces (seventh day), (from 50 drops of 1st dil. three times),[106].—The daily quantity of urine, while taking the tincture, varied between 33¼ and 43½ ounces; in order to obtain the average amount, I included the quantity passed on the day after this proving (the first day of taking the 2d trituration), which amounted to 59 ounces, because it seemed to be the effect of the tincture, and not that of the trituration taken that day; the average thus amounted to 41¼ ounces,[107].—Copious urination (after two hours),[4].—[880.] Copious, painful, and even bloody flow of urine,[41].—Very copious urination,[4].—Urine copious (after quarter of an hour),[104].—Urine copious and scalding, though but little fluid had been taken,[104].—Immoderate flow of urine,[18].—Frequent urinating,[6].—*Frequent and copious urinating* (fifth day),[6].—*Urination more frequent and more copious than usual* (five provers), (after two hours),[4].—Urine more frequent, but not increased (sixth day),[6].—Frequent urination, always with a small discharge,[109].—[890.] Frequent bloody urine,[31 44].—The bloody urine was passed more frequently, but always in smaller quantity (eight to ten hours),[26].—Frequent discharge of scanty, watery urine; at first it passes with pain, and, towards the end, with violent cutting pain; at last some passes by drops, or in a weak, intermitting stream,[5].—Micturition frequent and painful,[96].—*Frequent, painful urination, constantly preceded by violent pain in the glans*,[93].—Very frequent urinating (soon after),[23].—Makes water continually during the day, especially when walking; not at night; (urinated one day about forty times),[110].—Must rise twice at night to urinate,[12].—As many as sixty urinations in one hour,[6].—Fatal flow of urine (from external use on the nape of the neck),[36].—[900.] Dysuria,[43 86].—Dysuria (from a blister on the nape of the neck),[13].—Ischuria,[10 21], etc.—Difficult and painful micturition (ischuria),[29].—Urinating difficult and seldom.[84].—Difficult evacuation of clear, bloody urine,[90].—*Strangury,[65 71 87] etc.—Strangury (in a woman),[68].—Drops of bloody urine; strangury,[31].—Strangury; ischuria,[41]. — [910.] Strangury with burning sensation,[43].—Strangury, very painful and distressing, accompanied by a strong and disagreeable smell in the nostrils (third day),[97].—Frequent strangury, and pain in the back (from large doses),[23].—Severe strangury,[23].—*Intense* *strangury; urine passed in small quantities* (third day),[53].—Very obstinate strangury (two cases),[48].—*Painful urination the whole day, with pain in the kidneys* (third day),[109].—Extremely painful urination,[24].—*Extremely painful urination of blood* (from twelve Spanish flies),[41].—[920.] *Painful discharge of a few drops of bloody urine, causing very severe sharp pain, as if a red-hot iron were passed along the urethra;* this pain was most acutely felt at the membranous portion of the canal, and in the meatus urinarius,[101].—Painful dribbling discharge of albuminous urine, with membranous pieces, which are rolled up, grayish-red, covered on both sides with blood-streaked mucus, and some large pieces, white on one side, red on the other, firm and elastic,[91].—*The urethra is contracted internally, hence the urine passed in a thin stream* (after twenty-four hours),[1a].—*The urine passed in a thin and divided stream, and with difficulty,* especially at 9 A.M.,[1a].—The urine is passed in drops,[1].—*Urine is passed only in drops,*[1a].—*The urine passes only in drops, with cutting pains* (after seven hours),[6].—While he is going to pass urine, he can only with difficulty prevent some from passing,[5].—Incontinence of urine (after six to eight days),[90].—Involuntary dribbling of urine (after seven hours),[6].—[930.] A few drops of watery blood followed the urine,[1a].—Urine rather diminished than increased,[6].—Urine scanty and high-colored (second day),[97].—Very scanty urine, with violent cutting pains in the urethra, especially in the front part,[6].—Very scanty emission of bloody urine,[59].—He passes less urine in the morning than usual (second day),[3]. — *Inability to urinate,*[78] [94]. — *Retention of urine,*[19].—*Retention of urine* (second day),[78].—Retention of urine, the urine was discharged every time by means of a catheter,[78].—[940.] Retention of urine (removed by local application of ice),[96].—Retention of the urine, without priapism (sexton),[86].—*Retention of the urine, causing pain.*[35].—Retention of the urine; only a few drops are infrequently discharged after violent exertion,[45]. —Retention of urine, on account of too great fulness of the bladder, and consequent inability to pass the urine,[41].—Retention of urine; even the smallest and most flexible catheter could not be passed further than an inch,[45].—Urine and stool retained (first day),[6].—Suppression of urine,[4].—Urine suppressed for thirty-six hours,[94].—Suppression of urine on one occasion for four days,[97].—*Urine.* [950.] Hot and bloody urine,[23].—The urine seemed acrid,[1a].—Discharge of white urine,[2].—Urine light and clear in the afternoon and evening, very light-colored in the morning (third day); somewhat darker (fifth day); very colorless, turbid when discharged (sixth day),[107].—Urine pale yellow, during the chill, with pain in the evening,[6].—Very pale yellow urine (second day, A.M.),[6].—Reddish urine (soon after taking),[6].—Urine red (second day),[6].—Urine red, bloody,[93].—*Red-colored urine, as if mixed with blood* (after eight hours),[6].—[960.] *Urine dark,*[84].—*The urine was dark-colored,*[108].—The urine is again colored darker, and the pain on urinating is less (after twenty-four hours),[5].—*Bloody urine,*[10] [15] [21], etc.— *Bloody urine* (from external use),[38].—Bloody urine, which is passed with great pain, and only in drops,[41].—Bloody urine, with great pain,[20].—Bloody urine, convulsions, and death (in a girl, from the application of a salve containing Cantharides),[41].—Bloody urine till death,[34].—Urine mixed with blood,[82].—[970.] Urine mixed with blood and mucus, with great pain (even after the use of Camphor),[6].—Urine mixed with blood; somewhat gravelly,[48]. —Discharge of blood and urine,[19].—He passes blood, or bloody urine,[96].— *Urine turbid and scanty,*[96].—Urine turbid and slightly bloody,[93].—*Urine during the night cloudy like mealy water, with white sediment* (second day), —The urine was always very cloudy, from mucus,[109].—The urine frequently became cloudy immediately after passing, *and frequently deposited a fine white sediment, which adhered to the glass* (something I had never noticed before) ; an iridescent film was at times noticed on the surface of the urine, a short time after it was passed,[106].—Mucous urine,[48].—[**980.**] In the urine passed during the first hours, there was floating, after it had stood, some thready mucus,[5].—Mucus and sand at times discharged with the bloody urine,[23].—Albuminuria (after six to eight days),[90].—*Urine deposits albumen, or contains it in solution,*[96].—With the urine there passed at first bloody filaments, then blackish, coagulated masses of blood, and at last much mucus,[27].—Urine loaded with sediment and fibrinous matter (second day),[75].—Reaction of urine on the whole about normal ; in the morning decidedly acid ; in the evening slightly acid ; and in the afternoon, neutral ; twice it was slightly alkaline,[108].—The reaction of urine during the proving with the dilutions was slightly alkaline ; neutral, however, always after meals, and often at other times, especially in the morning and late in the evening,[106].—Reaction of urine, three times alkaline, eight times neutral, at other times slightly acid,[107].—The sp. gr. was very high, varying between 10.18 and 10.29,[108].—[**990.**] The sp. gr. was very high for the amount of colorless urine ; it varied from 10.09 to 10.28 ; in general the amount seemed to be higher than the normal sp. gr.,[107].—Sp. gr. 10.14, 10.05, in the morning ; 10.26, 10.23, in the evening (third day) ; sp. gr. high (fourth day) ; 10.20, 10.28 (fifth day),[107].—Sp. gr. of the urine while taking the dilutions varied between 10.05 and 10.34 ; it increased, especially during the first and second days, when 10.05 was the lowest point marked,[106];—On the appearance of the urinary difficulties, all the other symptoms cease ; in the evening,[6].—The urinary symptoms are permanently removed by Camphor (fourth day),[6].

Sexual Organs.—*Male.* Genitals inflamed,[96].—Feeling of weakness in the genitals (first hours),[1a].—Burning heat and itching of the genitals,[56].—Pressing pain from the lower abdomen toward the genitals, in the afternoon,[6].—*Fatal gangrene of the penis,*[55].—[**1000.**] The penis is swollen,[1a]. Swelling and heat of the penis, without erection, and without sexual desire,[90].—*Swelling of the glans, which is very painful, even to external pressure,*[6].—About the corona glandis, a brown, cheesy mass accumulates, without any special sensation, in the morning,[9].—A tumefaction of the prepuce, of a red, hot, and diaphanous nature, with phimosis ; there issues from beneath it a purulent secretion (after three weeks),[98].—Swelling of the frænum of the prepuce,[1a].—Total absence of the usual smegma preputii,[109].—Blood passes out of the rigid penis and from the anus,[41].—Instead of semen, blood flows,[35].—Erections,[67].—[**1010.**] Erection and involuntary emission (from smelling the powder),[77].—*A strong and persistent erection of the penis, painless, and without voluptuous sensation,*[49].—Very persistent erection every morning, immediately on rising,[109].—Continued erection of the penis, with some painful sensation, for three hours,[2].—Difficult erection of the penis,[41]. —*Severe erections at night, during which there is contraction and sore pain in the whole of the urethra,*[1a].—Painful erections,[25 26 29].—Painful erection, lasting fifteen minutes (one case),[101].—Very painful erections,[59].—Nightly erections,[1a].—[**1020.**] ***Priapism,**[35 50] etc.—Priapism occasionally,[51 87].—Traces of priapism at times,[94].—Priapism, with pain about bladder, and wild delirium (third day),[99].—Severe priapism, with swollen genitals,[96].—*Painful priapism,*[86].—Painful, obstinate priapism,[96].—Most violent priapism, with fearful pains,[34].—Penis lax (second day),[92].—Penis lax and drooping, with total absence of erections,[102].—[**1030.**] Constant pain in the penis,[102].—

Severe burning pain in the penis, especially at the tip of the glans, with frequent urging to urinate,[101].—A drawing pain in the penis, and in the back and thighs, relieved by passing flatus upward and downward (after seventy-two hours),[1a].—Pruritus of glans penis,[96].—Pruritus of the glans penis, with desire to urinate and ardor urinæ (three hours after a meal); the desire for micturition continued two to four hours, and then gradually ceased, leaving some irritation in the urethra,[83].—*Burning in the excretory ducts of the vesiculæ seminales in the urethra, during and after coition* (after twenty-four hours),[1a].—*A drawing pain in the spermatic cord while urinating* (after three to six hours),[1a].—Painful swelling of the right testicle (after nine hours),[6].—Excitement of the genital organs,[60].—*Sexual desire disturbed sleep at night,*[67].—[1040.] Satyriasis,[96].—Satyriasis, and desire for coition, so that he forgot all modesty and reason,[85].—Violent satyriasis, with overpowering, insatiable desire for coition, making him furious,[85].†—Sexual desire entirely absent (second day),[92].—Emission of semen; in the morning while lying in bed awake, discharged from the relaxed penis, and almost without sensation, a considerable quantity of semen, of natural character (in a strong young man); this attack was repeated, after twenty-four hours, exactly in the same manner,[8].—A slight emission in the night (third night),[109].—Nightly emissions,[1a].—Emission very profuse, without dreams and without waking (fourth night),[109].—A copious emission seemed to have taken place during the second night, although one had happened but two nights previously; the next morning an uncommon weariness, so that I lay down again immediately after rising, and fell into a restless, unrefreshing slumber,[106].—**Female.** Swelling of the neck of the uterus; burning in the bladder; abdominal pains; continued vomiting, and hot fever (in a woman from a fly-blister),[4].—[1050.] Great swelling of the neck of the womb, with much tenesmus,[54].—A woman, who had not conceived in fourteen years, became pregnant within four months after the use of an essence, which consisted mainly of Cantharides,[23].—Miscarriage, after symptoms of irritation in bowels and urinary organs,[51].—Abortion,[73 96].—*Swelling and irritation of vulva* (second day),[97].—Burning in the female genitals,[6].—Bloody, mucous discharge from the vagina, for three days after the menses,[1a].—Burning in the vagina, with a thick, white discharge,[68].—Intolerable itching in the vagina,[27].—Menstruation appears four days too soon, with great nausea and colic (she usually had colic),[9].—[1060.] The menses appear three days later than usual (eighth day),[6].—Menstruation, which had ceased one day, reappeared, with pain (in the forenoon), and lasted till noon (fourth day),[6].—Menstruation somewhat increased and painful (ninth day),[6].—More profuse flow of the menses,[6].—Menstruation, which appeared the night before taking Cantharis, is more profuse than usual, but without pain (after one hour and a half),[6].—Menstruation appears too early, but scanty (third day),[6].—Black blood with the menses (this was often the case),[6].—Menstruation ceased almost altogether on the second day (it usually lasted three to four days),[6].—Menstruation ceased on the third day,[6].—Menstruation entirely ceased during the illness, although it had occurred on three occasions previously. It was not re-established till seven months,[97].

Respiratory Organs.—Larynx and Trachea. [1070.] Hawking of tenacious mucus from the larynx (after half an hour),[8].—Intense pain in larynx (one case), (third day),[53].—Burning in the larynx and stomach,[27].—Tickling, provoking cough,[8].—Contraction of the trachea,[2].—

† Followed by death.

Voice. Rough voice (second day),[94].—Hoarse voice,[87].—Hoarseness in the chest,[1a].—Voice feeble,[50].—*Speech very low, with sensation of weakness of the vocal organs* (twelfth day),[6].—[1080.] On deep respiration, and on speaking, she feels as if she dare not exert herself, on account of extraordinary weakness of the respiratory organs; she therefore speaks only in a weak and frightened tone,[6].—Inability to speak (sexton),[86].—*Cough and Expectoration.* Cough, with pain in the abdomen,[1a].—Hacking cough, frequently (second day),[6].—Frequent dry hacking cough (fifteenth day),[6].—Several short paroxysms of dry-cough, caused by irritation in the larynx, with more rapid respiration and a sort of tightness in the chest (immediately after taking),[2].—Cough in the morning on rising, with difficult expectoration,[1a].—Sputa frothy and bloody,[96].—Bloody expectoration, after short cough (eighth day),[6].—*Respiration.* Hurried breathing (soon after),[76].—[1090.] Respiration hurried,[76].—Hurried respiration (after one hour),[99].—Hurried and difficult respiration,[60].—Difficult respiration,[25].—Respiration becomes difficult,[29].—Difficult and oppressed respiration, partly, as it appears, on account of contraction of the larynx and the trachea, partly also on account of dryness of the nose (soon after),[8].—Respiration labored,[96].—Breathing laborious,[50].—Gasps for breath,[96].—On ascending a mountain he gets out of breath; it catches him in the chest; he becomes nauseated (third day),[14].—[1100.] Oppression of breathing (second day),[6].—Threatening suffocation (sexton),[86].

Chest.—Pneumonia,[96].—(Is drawn together at times when coughing; the lungs themselves are contracted),[1a].—The side of the diaphragm is inflamed,[21].—Feeling of dryness in the chest, for several days,[1a].—Burning in the chest,[2].—Burning on the chest like fire; and again a small clot of blood in the mouth, in the morning (seventeenth day),[6].—Hot burning on the chest, and pinching in the abdomen, with constipation (fifteenth afternoon),[6].—Violent burning, with stitches over the whole chest, externally and internally, as if in the bones,[6].—[1110.] Sensation of fulness in the chest, stomach, and abdomen, after coffee (fourteenth day),[6].—Pressure on the chest for a long time,[6].—*Sticking in the chest, from one side to the other,*[9].—Slight stitches in the chest, which do not affect respiration (after three hours),[5].—*A fine stitch extending from the right axilla into the chest* (after one hour),[6].—Several fine needlelike stitches, deep in the left lower ribs, in the afternoon,[6].—Tearing in the thorax, especially in the region of the heart (after half an hour),[3].—Extreme sensitiveness of the chest to touch (tenth, eleventh, and twelfth days),[6].—Relief of habitual oppression of chest (one prover),[4].—*Front.* Burning on the sternum (after eight hours),[9].—[1120.] Squeezing and contraction in the forepart of the chest, with impeded respiration, and stitching in the whole chest, from 11 A.M. till 8 P.M.; relieved on lying, but returning again (third day),[6].—Pressure on the sternum,[9].—Pressure from the heart toward the sternum, toward evening, increased by speaking and deep respiration,[9].—On the right side of the sternum, deep internally, a pressing, with stitching from within outward (after four hours),[6].—Stitching in the centre of the sternum (third evening),[6].—Frequent stitching in the forepart of the chest, especially on inspiration,[6].—Several acute stitches in succession in the sternum, so that she screamed with pain, in the afternoon,[6].—Many fine needlelike stitches in succession, in the lower part of the sternum (after three-quarters of an hour),[6].—*Pain in the chest, like a shooting, from the front toward the back, which impedes respiration,*[9].—*Sides.* In the morning in bed, a violent pressure in the side of the chest, which disappears on rising,[9].—[1130.]

*Stitching pain in the forepart of the right chest; it then passes downward into the right lower ribs (after one hour and a half),[6].—*Stitching in the right side of the thorax,[3].—*Stitching in the right side of the chest (after two hours and a half),[6].—*Stitching in the lower part of the right chest, extending toward the middle of the sternum (after eight hours),[6].—Stitching in the right side of the chest, on each inspiration, after midnight, and also on the following day,[6].—Stitching in the right costal region, after dinner,[6].— Stitching in the right false ribs (after seven hours),[6].—Very fine stitching in the right chest, more in the upper part; immediately afterward in the left side; three-quarters of an hour after dinner,[6].—Stitching in the left chest (after two hours and a half),[6].—Stitching in the left side of the chest, more externally on the ribs (after ten hours),[6].—[1140.] Stitching in the left chest, after dinner,[6].—Stitching, inward, below the left breast, extending up under the axilla (after half an hour),[6].—Stitching in the lowest left ribs, extending toward the back,[6].—She cannot lie on the left side, on account of stitching on inspiration (midnight), (third night),[6].—Acute stitching in the left side of the chest under the arm, extending to the middle of the sternum,[6].—Acute stitching in the left lower ribs, followed by a tearing near the right wrist, and then acute stitching in the left upper arm,[6].— Very painful stitching in the left chest, and immediately afterward below the right breast,[6].—During slight, somewhat sudden, turning of the body, violent stitching in the left side, below the arm, on inspiration, extending through the whole body, just as if some one violently pierced him with a fine spear, with a jerk, so that it arrested the breathing for a moment; it occurred but once on the other side with the same violence, and less violently during rest, but not at all on respiration or motion (second day),[7].— (Stitches in the sides, during motion and rest),[1a].—A violent, stitchlike pain in the left side of the chest in the region of the heart, or in the heart itself (after five hours),[8].—[1150.] After the stitching in the sternum, several similar stitches in the last right false rib,[6].—Fine stitches in the left side of the chest, below the axilla (after four hours),[6].—A few fine stitches in the middle of the right clavicle (after four hours),[6].—Several fine stitches in the right lower ribs, in the afternoon,[8].—Many fine stitches in the region of the left axilla on the side of the chest (second morning),[6].—Painful, acute stitches in the right costal region below the arm, frequently repeated, in the afternoon,[6].—A stitch under the right arm extending into the chest,[9]. —In the right lower false ribs a painful stitch, while yawning (after four hours),[6].—A pointed stitch in the right side of the chest; then tearing between the shoulder-blades; then acute stitching in the right shoulder; then stitching in the right hypochondriac region; then in the right shoulder-blade, whence it then passes into the right hypochondriac region, in the afternoon,[6].

Heart and Pulse.—Anxiety in the præcordium,[21].—[1160.] Extreme præcordial anxiety,[94].—Anxiety about the heart in the afternoon,[6].— Pain in the heart,[85].—Drawing pain in the region of the heart,[8].—Stitch in the heart, followed by a crawling sensation,[9].—**Heart's Action.** Violent jerking of the heart, that runs quite to the head (after three weeks),[94].— Palpitation of the heart,[4].—Violent palpitation, toward evening,[9].—Violent palpitation of the heart, for several minutes (soon after taking),[8].—Habitual palpitation of the heart entirely ceased (one prover),[4].—**Pulse.** [1170.] Uneasy beating of the pulse in the whole body, so that the limbs tremble, several days,[7].—Hard full pulse, as in inflammatory fevers,[45].—Pulse contracted,[50].—Pulse thready (second day),[94].—Weak pulse,[2].—Pulse feeble, and scarcely perceptible (after two days),[78].—Pulse scarcely perceptible,[87]. —Scarcely perceptible pulse (second day),[78].—Pulse imperceptible,[96].— Pulse scarcely changed during the chill,[6].—[**1180.**] Rapid pulse,[41].—Hard, rapid pulse,[27].—Pulse full, hard and rapid, as in inflammatory fever,[84].— Pulse rapid, full, tense (second day),[92].—Pulse weak, trembling, rapid,[93].— Pulse quick and hard,[96].—Small, quick pulse (after one hour),[99].—Pulse quickened by two beats (two provers),[4].—Pulse quickened by two beats, but evidently softer (two provers),[4].—Pulse increased, fuller, after disappear- ance of the pains, in the morning (fourth day),[6].—[**1190.**] Pulse acceler- ated, full (third day),[107].—Pulse accelerated twenty beats per minute (third day),[96].—Frequent and small pulse,[58].—Frequent, small, and weak pulse,[101]. —Small, frequent pulse,[93].—Pulse weak, compressible, frequent (110),[102].— Pulse full, 80,[89].—Pulse 98, full and soft (third day),[96].—Pulse 100 (two cases), 80 (one case), (second day),[53].—Pulse more than 100 to the min- ute,[42].—[**1200.**] Pulse 104, full and regular (third day),[53 96].—Pulse 130, weak and tremulous,[96].—Pulse slightly diminished (in some), (after two hours),[4].—Progressive diminution of the pulse; the maximum of this dimi- nution was twenty-two beats,[4].—Pulse remarkably diminished (after three hours),[4].—Remarkable *diminution of pulse* (five to sixteen beats), (after two hours),[4].—Pulse slow and full (after two hours),[6].—Pulse slower, by from two to forty beats (eight provers), (after two hours),[4].—Pulse fell five beats,[104].—The pulse, after violent action, lost seven beats in a minute,[101].— [**1210.**] Pulse fell to about fifty per minute,[100].—Pulse 45 (after vomit- ing),[4].—Pulse 35, small and intermittent,[4].—Pulse 20 and small (second day),[53].—Pulse irregular and intermittent,[49].—Small, hard, intermitting pulse,[47].—Pulse 130, weak and paroxysmal,[81].

Neck and Back.—Neck. Thick neck,[45].—Twitching in the left cervical muscles,[6].—Stiffness in the neck, with tensive pain on stooping,[1a].— [**1220.**] Fine but sharply drawing pain in a narrow line extending downward, deep in the right cervical muscles (after two hours),[8].—Several dull stitches in the left cervical muscles, in the afternoon,[6].—Tearing in the left cervical muscles, with headache, like a heaviness, on walking (second day),[6].— Tearing in the nape of the neck, extending upward toward the vertex (sixth day, A.M.),[6].—Tearing in the nape of the neck and stitching in the right cervical muscles, on moving the head, whence it extends into the upper part of the head (after six hours),[6].—Swollen cervical glands painful to touch,[9]. —*Back.* Pain in the back, in the vertebral column,[87].—Pains in the back and limbs,[29].—Violent pain in the back,[23].—Dragging in the back, as if about to be "unwell," which period she had passed about ten days before; slight show, but the pains the same,[111].—[**1230.**] Sticking-cutting pain through the back and abdomen, which speedily passes off (after nine hours),[8].—Tear- ing pain in the back,[1].—*Tearing pain in the back*, especially in the morn- ing,[1a].—*Dorsal.* A stitch inward, below the right shoulder-blade (after four hours),[6].—Several violent dull stitches in the upper part of the right shoulder-blade, with burning on the skin in the same place, in the after- noon,[6].—Extremely violent acute stitches in the right shoulder-blade, in the evening,[6].—Tearing in the shoulder-blade (after one hour),[3].—Tearing and stitching in the right shoulder-blade, in the upper part (after three hours),[6].—Pain between shoulders (after half an hour),[97].—Continued stitching between the shoulders on every motion, as if the parts were sprained,[1a].—[**1240.**] Tearing between the shoulder-blades (after two hours and on the third day),[6].—A throbbing sensation on the right side of the spine, near the eleventh and twelfth dorsal vertebræ, disappearing for a few moments, and returning again, increased by every motion, extending by single jerks downward to the right thigh, at 11 P.M. (sixth day),[106].—*Lumbar.* Pain in lumbar region,[96].—Dull pain in the lumbar region and hypochondria, increased by pressure,[93].—Dull heavy pain in the lumbar region, increased by pressure,[81].—Large pointed stitches in the left lumbar region, with the cutting in the abdomen,[6].—A stitch extending into the right lumbar region (after four hours and a half),[6].—In the right lumbar region painful stitching, then tearing in the left hypochondriac region internally, unchanged on rubbing (after a quarter of an hour),[6].—Pains in the region of the loins and the lower abdomen,[26].—*Pain in the loins, kidneys, and in the whole abdomen, with such pain on urinating that he could not pass a single drop without moaning and screaming* (from a fly-blister on the knee-joint),[41].—[1250.] *Pain in the loins, with incessant desire to urinate; he passes only a small quantity,*[96].—Intolerable pains in the loins, kidneys, and the whole abdomen,[20].—Boring pains in the loins (after one hour),[103].—Cutting pain in both loins, which extends to beneath the shoulders, where it becomes stitching (third afternoon),[6].—Great weariness in the small of the back, with a peculiar pressing pain in the region of the last rib, in the back, while sitting (second day),[108].—Pain across the small of the back, on motion, as if he had injured himself (first days),[1a].—Pressing pain in the small of the back for two days,[3].—Almost constant cutting pain in the small of the back, especially on sitting (first day),[7].—Stitching in the small of the back, after rising from sitting or on walking,[6].—Pain like biting in the small of the back (the whole second day),[6].—[1260.] Biting and gnawing in the small of the back (third day),[6].—Tearing, with stitching, in the small of the back (after one hour),[6].—*Sacral.* Gnawing in the sacrum, in the evening (second day),[6].—Stitching and gnawing on the right side of the sacrum, as if in the bone (after two hours and a half),[6].—A stitch and a tearing in the coccyx, so that she was frightened; frequently repeated,[6].

Extremities in General.—Objective. Great weakness of limbs (second day),[92].—In the morning, laxness and lassitude in all the limbs, so that he remains in bed much longer than usual (second day),[3].—Weariness in the hands and feet (fourth day),[6].—Collapse of limbs,[4].—Trembling of the limbs,[4][87].—[1270.] Trembling of the limbs,[87].—Trembling and weakness of the limbs, lasting a long time,[94].—Trembling of the hands and feet, during the chill, in the evening,[6].—Unconscious tossing about of the limbs,[64].—Convulsions in all the limbs,[93].—Numbness of arms and legs (after three weeks),[98].—*Subjective.* A feeling of dryness in the joints of the arms and limbs, for twelve days,[1a].—Pain and stiffness of limbs (after three weeks),[98].—Contracting, almost paralytic, pain in the limbs,[1].—Drawings in the extremities,[87].—[1280.] Drawing, almost paralytic, pain in the limbs,[1a].—The forearms and lower legs feel bruised (third, fourth, fifth, and sixth days),[6].

Superior Extremities.—Shoulder. Drawing pain in the left shoulder-joint,[3].—Stitching below the right chest, extending into the right shoulder, on inspiration,[6].—Stitching-tingling in the axillæ.[1a].—Tearing in the axilla,[3].—*Arm.* Boring pain in the middle of the upper arm,[6].—Drawing and stitching in the right upper arm, as if in the bone, after dinner,[6].—Gnawing in the right humerus in the middle, and at the same time stitching farther above,[6].—Gnawing in the middle of the upper arm, on the external surface (after four hours),[6].—[1290.] In the middle of the right upper arm, a painful gnawing (after one hour and three-quarters), then stitching in the left knee, on the inner surface,[6].—Tearing on the inner surface of the right humerus, disappearing on pressure, during breakfast (one hour),[6].—Tearing in the middle of the right upper arm, in the afternoon,[6].—Tearing from the bend of the right elbow into the shoulder,[6].—Pain, as if bruised, in the right upper arm (after two hours and a half),[6].—*Elbow.* Sensation in the right elbow as if something were holding her fast there,[6].—A drawing pain in the right elbow,[9].—Tearing in the bend of the elbow; on rubbing, it passes into the outer side of the upper arm, after dinner,[6].—Tearing in the bend of the right elbow,[6].—*Forearm.* Tearing from the middle of the left forearm to the middle of the upper arm,[6].— [1300.] Painful tearing from the middle of the right upper arm to the middle of the forearm, relieved by rubbing (after one hour and a half),[6].— Violent tearing in the middle of the right forearm, and at the same time in both calves (in the evening and also the second day, frequently repeated),[6].—*Wrist.* Stitching from the right wrist up toward the elbow, and with each stitch a throb, in the afternoon,[6].—*Hand.* Drawing pain in the bones of the hands and forearm (after eighteen hours),[1a].—Tearing in the left hand (second day),[3].—Tearing on the inner margin of the right hand, toward the little finger, disappearing on rubbing (after two hours),[6].—Tearing on the back of the right hand, together with stitching extending into the left upper arm,[6].—*Fingers.* Pain and tension in the little finger for several days,[7].—Burning in the tips of the fingers,[9].—Painful drawing and tension from the right hand into the fingers (after three hours and a half),[6].— [1310.] Stitch in the bones of the right shoulder, through and through, repeatedly during the first afternoon, then not again,[7].—Tearing in the left little finger, in the afternoon,[6].

Inferior Extremities.—Inability to stand or walk,[87].—Paralysis of the lower extremities,[87].—Paralysis of the lower limbs,[94].—Paralysis of lower extremities and weak arm, without apparent spinal tenderness,[96].— The pains on the legs become ameliorated on violent rubbing,[6].—*Hip.* Large stitches in the right hip, in the afternoon,[6].—*Thigh.* Falling asleep now of one, now of the other thigh,[6].—Feeling of weight in the muscles of the thighs,[4].—[1320.] Tearing and stitching in the posterior portion of the left thigh,[6].—Tearing from the left hip-bone into the knee, followed by a very painful drawing in the right mastoid process, frequently (after one hour),[6].—Tearing from the right hip to the knee, down along the posterior surface, not disappearing on rubbing (after a quarter of an hour),[6].— Painful tearing from the right nates down to the knee on the posterior surface, not disappearing on rubbing (after half an hour),[6].—In the flesh of the middle of the thigh, posteriorly, a fine twitching, together with itching in it, in the afternoon,[6].—*Knee.* On ascending steps, the knees totter,[1a].—Painful feeling of extreme weariness in the knees and legs,[102].—Lamenting and whining on account of fearful pains in the knees (the whole day), (ninth day),[6].—Tension on the right knee,[6].—Pain in the knee, as if it were swollen, which impedes walking; in the left it is transient, in the right remaining several days,[7].—[1330.] Boring pain in both knees, so violent that it contracted both her lower legs (third day),[6].—Drawing pain in the hollows of the knees,[1a].—(Cutting in the knees, when walking),[1a].—Frequent painful stitches deep into the right knee (after three hours and a half),[6].—Tearing about the right knee (after nine hours),[6].—Tearing in the right knee, disappearing on rubbing (after a quarter of an hour),[6].—Tearing in the right knee, extending to the middle of the lower leg (after three hours),[6].—Tearing on the external surface of the left knee, and sensation like falling asleep, after sitting down (after one hour and a half),[6].—Tearing from the middle of the right thigh into the hollow of the knee, in the afternoon,[6].—Boring-tearing pains, with sticking, now in both knees, now in the right only; the pain extends backward and downward into the feet, upward into the right hip, and thence into the left hip; only warm dry applications somewhat relieve the pains; Camphor gave no relief on this day (eighth day),[6].—[1340.] The knee and lower leg can scarcely bear to be touched (ninth day),[6].—She dare not bend the knees, on account of great pain and sensitiveness,[6].—*Leg.* Trembling of the legs on motion,[6].—Weariness in the lower legs,[6].—Painful drawing on the external surface of the left leg, a hand's breadth above the knee, as far below the knee, and also from the right elbow to the middle of the forearm, on the inner surface (after two hours and a half),[6].—Gnawing in the bone on the external surface from the middle of the right thigh into the calves (after two hours),[6].—Tearing and stitching from the right instep up to the middle of the thigh; when this ceased a tearing in the left side of the head, renewed, after it had ceased, by touching the spot,[6].—A feeling as if the flesh and skin were loosened from the bone on the tibia, just above the ankle, not noticed on touching it, for fourteen days,[1a].—Renewal of the pain in the calves; it disappeared on walking violently till she sweated (at 2 P.M.), (third day),[6].—Tension in the right calf, one hour after dinner,[6].—[1350.] Tearing in the left calf, one hour after dinner,[6].—Painful tearing in both calves, worse walking than while sitting,[6].—Intolerable tearing, so violent that it seems to her as if the flesh were being forcibly torn from both calves, not disappearing on rubbing, lasting a long time, at 10 A.M. (second day),[6].—The legs feel bruised when walking (fourth forenoon),[6].—*Foot.* Lassitude in the feet, so that she can scarcely go upstairs,[9].—Drawing in the right foot, inner surface (after three hours and a half),[6].—In the right foot, at first a feeling of formication, then it feels completely dead, like a piece of wood,[9].—On the back of the left foot a swelling which burns; the burning ceases on rubbing,[9].—Tearing on the back of the right foot (the seventh afternoon),[6].—*Fearful pain in the soles of the feet, like an ulcer; she could not step for four days* (ninth day),[6].—*Toes.* [1360.] A tearing and stitching in the second left toe (after two hours),[6].—Tearing in the right toes toward the tips, disappearing on rubbing; it then appears in the right external malleolus, disappearing on rubbing (after three-quarters of an hour),[6].

General Symptoms.—*Marasmus*,[96].—Complete emaciation; she can scarcely sit any more, because the tuberosities protrude,[6].—The body is bent almost double, and the arms are folded across the hypogastrium (after four hours),[103].—The plasticity of the blood drawn from the veins is increased,[25].—Increased discharge from the diseased part, in the ulcer on the feet, from the nose in chronic catarrh, from the urethra in gonorrhœa,[1].—Erosion of the mucous membrane from the mouth to the anus,[21].—Twitchings of tendons,[93].—Convulsive motions,[93].—[1370.] Convulsive motions,[51].—Convulsive agitation and trembling (after one hour),[99].—Convulsions (after fourteen days) gradually increasing, till death,[76].—Convulsions, which returned at short intervals,[47].—Convulsions in paroxysms, accompanied by painful priapism,[76].—Convulsions, followed by severe pain in head and coma (fourth day),[99].—Convulsions, with horror of liquids,[96]. Violent convulsions,[12].—Violent convulsions, followed by insensibility and death (fourteenth day),[76].—Frightful convulsions, and death on the second day,[60].—[1380.] Horrible convulsions, with writhing of the limbs,[56].—Terrible convulsions; sometimes he tossed about and rolled on his bed in despair; sometimes he got up and rushed like a madman to a friend's bed in an alcove of the same room, seized the iron curtain rods and bent them like reeds, screaming and howling dreadfully; eight strong men could scarcely hold him; the convulsions succeeded each other almost uninterruptedly, and lasted for hours at a time, with a few minutes' quiet interval; sometimes they took the form of emprosthotonos, sometimes of opisthotonos; sometimes he opened his mouth, and sometimes the violent trismus closed it tightly, with very hard grinding of the teeth, and running of frothy, at times blood-streaked saliva; his face was expressive of fright and despair. In the convulsions, his hair was seen to stand on end; his gaze was fixed, his eyes sparkled and flashed, and as their muscles were successively thrown into spasmodic movements they rolled frightfully. The temperature of the skin was natural, the pulse full and slow, 55 per minute. When a hand was pressed upon the umbilical region, the abdominal muscles entered into contraction, and that portion of the abdomen seemed glued to the spine, especially the recti, which were like tightened cords; suddenly the disturbance extended all over the body, the spasms became general, and the head was thrown backward in a manner fearful to behold. When we sought to apply a sponge, dipped in a warm and oily embrocation, to the most painful part of the abdomen, the patient instantly broke away like a madman; he frothed at the mouth more than ever; his eyes became fiercer; the constriction of the throat almost choked him; *he howled frightfully, like the barking of a dog; and immediately after these symptoms fell into general convulsions, which ended in fainting and profound sopor.* These attacks were renewed frequently; pressure upon painful places in the hypogastrium, or the mere sight of liquids, was sufficient to produce them,[52].—Sudden attack of epilepsy, which lasted a very long time and was very severe (after seventeen days); a second fit, eight hours after, complicated with hysterical symptoms; and during the following two days fits came in quick succession,[97].—Falls at intervals into a cataleptic state (after four hours),[103].—Sluggish, dejected (after three hours),[6].—Indolent, indifferent, pensive,[6].—Great lassitude in the whole body,[9].—Great lassitude, especially of the legs (second day),[3].—Such lassitude that she could hold nothing in her hands,[6].—Continually tired, more especially on right side of body (after three weeks),[98].—[1390.] Very weary, as after much physical exertion,[8].—* *Weakness*,[87].—Weakness of whole body (first day),[92].—* *Weakness and sinking of strength*,[1].—Such weakness that she could not leave the bed,[6].—*Extreme weakness* (second day),[78].—Extreme weakness and wasting,[6].—General debility,[4].—Extreme debility (one prover was unable to leave his room),[4].—Loss of strength,[64].—[1400.] Sinking of strength,[94].—The strength is very much exhausted,[26].—General prostration of strength,[102].—Considerable prostration (second day),[53].—Considerable *prostration of strength*, a sort of progressive languor (*relieved by drinking freely of alcoholic liquors, which produced no symptoms of intoxication*),[4].—Extreme prostration; muscles almost unable to contract,[4].—A kind of restless prostration, at night (one prover),[4].—Felt as if dying (second day),[53].—Threatened syncope,[4].—*Faintness*,[21 41], etc.—[1410.] Paraplegia more or less decided, with cramps and itching of the skin,[90].—Restlessness,[2].—Great restlessness,[83 96].—Great general restlessness,[89].—Very great restlessness; walks the room screaming (after four hours),[103].—Anxious restlessness, so that he cannot lie in bed (second day),[92].—Extreme restlessness while sitting or lying; she must constantly move up and down, here and there, day and night (for eight days),[6].—At all times, restless and uncomfortable,[97].—Extremely restless at night;

falls asleep late on account of unusually anxious thoughts; afterwards nightmare after a short sleep (seventh night),[106].—He has no rest, constantly seeks another place, together with internal heat in the head,[1a].—[1420.] General uneasiness, seeming to originate in the stomach, soon increasing, and accompanied by prostration, slight shiverings, restlessness, and desire to vomit (after half an hour),[96].—Threw herself about, as if in a fire,[54].—Sensation of weakness in the whole body, as in the beginning of a nervous fever,[3].—Sense of prostration of strength, with feeling of emptiness in stomach, and irresistible desire for food (third day),[96].—The whole body feels as without joints and heavy; ascending steps is very troublesome, the legs then feel as if filled with lead. This condition continued almost eight days,[7].—General discomfort in the whole body (fourteenth day),[6].—*Raw and sore pain over the whole body, internally and externally,[6].—Violent pains,[35]. —Violent pains generally,[90].—Most violent pains in the stomach, the abdomen, the kidneys, in fact every portion of the body (from twelve Spanish flies),[41].—[1430.] All the cavities of the body burn as if raw and sore,[6].—General tense condition, with dryness in the mouth, thirst, anxiety, and pains in the limbs,[29].—*The whole body feels crushed to pieces; every part is sensitive, internally and externally, with such weakness that she can scarcely rise from bed,[6].—Stitching and tearing, now here, now there (fifth day),[6].—Stitching, now here, now there, in the trunk (tenth day, afternoon),[6].—The stitching pains are generally combined with tearing,[6].—The stitching pains all extend inward,[6].—Stitches over the whole body,[31].—Intermitting, painful twitching, now on the right side of the occiput, now on the external surface of the left knee, continuing for a long time, always alternating, not disappearing on rubbing (after two and a half hours),[6].—Tearing pain in the affected parts; for example, ulcers,[1 1a].—[1440.] The attacks, except the urinary symptoms, reappear every seven days,[6].—Most of the symptoms appear on the right side,[6].—Camphor first relieves the icy coldness; after frequent doses the pains in the abdomen are relieved, while the terrible cutting urinary symptoms are relieved later,[6].—Oil seems to dissolve the active principle of Cantharides, and hence to increase its action, on which account oil should not be given as an antidote in cases of poisoning by large doses of Cantharides,[36].

Skin.—Eruptions, Dry. Skin pale,[104].—Goose-flesh during the chill,[6].—Yellow spot the size of a two-shilling piece on the abdomen near the umbilicus, and another on the inside of the left thigh (after three weeks),[98].—An itching swelling on the last phalanx of the finger,[1a].—On the first phalanx of the left thumb two small red spots, without sensation, as if a pimple would form, at 2 P.M.,[6].—Psoriasis,[96].—[1450.] Eruption in the corners of the mouth,[9].—Eruption on the breast-bone, which pains on touch like an ulcer,[1a].—A burning eruption on the left buttock,[9].—An eruption on the knee, which pains, especially on touch, and impedes free motion,[9].—A papulous eruption on the side of the neck; burning pain in it,[1a].—Eruption of pimples on the forehead and cheeks, burning only on touch (sixth day),[6].—A pimple on the right upper lid (after seven days),[6].—Two pimples on the right mastoid process burning on touch (after one hour),[6].—In the left nostril a small pimple, burning on touch (third day),[6]. —A pimple seated deep in the cheek, which itched when touched,[1a].—[1460.] A pimple upon the cheek near the corner of the mouth, which felt tense, but when touched caused burning pain,[1a].—Pimples on the margin of the upper lip (second evening),[6].—Pellucid pimples between the chin and lip, from one angle of the mouth to the other, without sensation; in

the afternoon,[6].—A large pimple on the nates, painful to touch (burning),[1a].
—The inner surface of the arms and the middle of the chest are full of
itching pimples, which burn after scratching (eighth and ninth days),[6].—
Pimples on the back of the hands (sixth day),[6].—Pimples on the back of
the right hand between the fourth and fifth fingers (second day),[6].—A
small pimple on the right hand between the thumb and index finger (preceded by tickling in this place), burning on touch; one hour after dinner,[6].
—A pimple, with red areola, between the right thumb and index finger,
after dinner, disappearing after twenty-four hours,[6].—A pimple on the
right little finger, on the external surface, sticking on pressure,[6].—*Eruptions. Moist.* [1470.] Vesication,[80].—Redness, inflammation on the skin,
and collection of serous fluids below the epidermis, which is raised in blisters therefrom (from external use),[25].—Several itching-burning vesicles
upon nose (after three weeks),[96].—Small blisters on the right cheek, itching, burning after scratching, in the evening,[6].—Blisters between the chin
and lips, and on the forehead, lasting twenty-four hours, *burning on touch*
(fourth day),[6].—A blister on the palm of the right hand (sixth day),[6].—
Eruptions, Pustular. Eczema,[98].—A pustule on the chin, which
burned on touch,[1a].—Ulcers on the leg,[14].—Increased discharge from an
ulcer on the foot, from the nose, in an old catarrh, and of the mucus of an
old gonorrhœa,[1a].—*Sensations.* [1480.] Dryness of the skin,[2].—Burning and some itching-tearing here and there in the skin,[1a].—Violent burning pain of the integuments,[80].—If he bruises himself anywhere, the spot
burns for some time,[6].—Itching,[37].—Itching of the skin,[1].—Itching in the
skin,[1a].—Itching, now here, now there, as if from lice (tenth, eleventh, and
twelfth days),[6].—Violent itching and sticking in the skin,[23].—Stitches in
the skin of the abdomen,[31].—[1490.] A few fine needle stitches on the skin
below the right breast (after three-quarters of an hour),[6].—Fine stitching
in the skin of the neck,[5].—Twitching in the skin of the left knee, inner
surface (after two hours),[6].—Itching and tearing in an ulcer,[1a].—Itching in
the forehead, obliging him to rub,[1a].—Itching at the perineum, with a sort
of tenesmus at the anus (some provers),[4].—Itching about the genitals,[31].—
Itching on the genitals,[41].—Violent itching on the right side of the chest
under the right arm, in the afternoon,[6].—Itching on the coccyx above the
anus,[1a].—[1500.] A painless itching and twitching at night, now in the
hands, now in the feet (after four hours),[1a].—Tickling and biting in the
skin, on the outer side of the left upper arm, disappearing on rubbing
(after two hours),[6].—Crawling itching in the bends of both elbows,[1a].

Sleep and Dreams.—Sleepiness. Stretching and yawning (after
two hours),[6].—Much stretching and yawning (soon after),[6].—Yawning,
without sleepiness (after one hour and a half),[6].—Repeated yawning (after
one hour and three-quarters),[6].—Constant yawning, after dinner,[6].—Great
sleepiness, with lassitude; she could hardly help falling asleep; without
yawning, in the afternoon,[6].—Almost unconquerable sleepiness, for three
days,[2].—[1510.] She can scarcely keep up on account of sleepiness, two
hours after dinner,[6].—Sleepy the whole day, especially after meals,[2].—
Sleepy after dinner,[6].—Very sleepy and depressed in the morning,[1a].—She
fell asleep while spinning; her eyes closed involuntarily, followed by smarting in the eyes (after three hours),[6].—Very good, sound sleep (first night),[6].
—*Sleeplessness.* Sleep bad,[57].—Half sleep (seventeenth night),[6].—
Before midnight, only light sleep (third night),[6].—Little sleep,[2].—[1520.]
Little sleep at night,[4].—Restlessness (first day),[92].—Passed a restless night,[57].
—At night very restless, frequent waking (first night),[6].—Extremely rest-

less nights (fifth, sixth, and seventh days),⁶.—Starting up in sleep (ninth day, A.M.),⁶.—Frequent waking, at night,⁶.—Slumbering sleep, from which she constantly woke (ninth day),⁶.—Waking after midnight, and remaining awake till morning,⁶.—Cannot fall asleep for a long time in the evening,⁶.—[1530.] *Loss of sleep,*ᵃ.—Sleeplessness,¹.—Sleeplessness in the evening on account of excitement, followed by remarkably vivid, confused dreams (fifth night),¹⁰⁶.—Total sleeplessness for several nights,⁶. —Sleepless (seven nights),⁶.—Night restless, sleepless (first day),⁹².—No sleep after midnight; constant tossing about, without real pain (third night),⁶.—

Dreams. Dreams during the night, active, confused, not anxious (second night),¹⁰⁶.—Vivid dreams of deer, walks in the woods (second night),⁶. —Many confused dreams (fourth night),¹⁰⁷.—[1540.] Frequent, confused dreams (ninth day, A.M.),⁶.—Voluptuous dreams,².—Anxious dreams (third night),⁶.—*Very anxious dreams during the whole night,*⁸.—Unremembered dreams (first night),⁶.—Dreams of business,⁶.—Dreams of quarrels (twelfth night),⁶.

Fever.—Chilliness. Great coldness of the surface,⁹⁶.—Skin cold and clammy,¹⁰⁴.—Skin cold and covered with sweat,¹⁰².—[1550.] Great coldness of the surface, with imperceptible pulse (after seven hours),⁸².—Cool, moist skin,¹⁰¹.—Temperature averaging two degrees less than normal,¹⁰⁷.—General coldness of the body,⁸⁷.—Coldness of the whole body, especially of the limbs (second day),⁹⁴.—Coldness and chill from 5 to 7 P.M.; she could not even get warm in bed for a long time (seventeenth day),⁶.—As soon as the icy coldness had ceased, there always appeared coldness on rising from bed, which was always followed by transient heat,⁶.—After she has gradually become warm in bed the coldness immediately attacks her again as soon as she puts but one limb out or rises,⁶.—Fever, consisting only of coldness, three days in succession, at 1 P.M., somewhat later each day,⁶.—Constantly cold; cannot sleep at night on account of the cold, although quite sleepy (after three weeks),⁹⁸.—[1560.] Shivering and shaking chill, beginning in the back, the whole afternoon, from 2 till 8 P.M., followed by heat, after which shivering again follows,⁹.—Universal shivering and chill down the spine,¹⁰⁴.—At first shivering and great weakness,⁹⁴.—Chilliness,⁸⁷.—The chilliness awakes him at two in the morning, and he cannot sleep any more (after three weeks),⁹⁸.—Chilliness, irregularly alternating with heat and sweat (second day),⁹².—General chilliness,⁹⁶.—Slight chilliness till toward 1½ P.M., when a violent shaking chill appeared, with creeping in the hands and feet, for half an hour, disappearing by a very warm stove, without subsequent heat, at 11 A.M. (fourth day),⁶.—Frequent chills (first day),⁹².—Chill in bed at 10 o'clock for half an hour, followed by natural warmth (sixteenth day),⁶.—[1570.] Chill immediately on getting out of bed (eighth day),⁶.—Chill and shivering from 11 till 1 o'clock, without subsequent heat (fifteenth day),⁶.—Chill and shivering, at 3 P.M., for an hour; relieved by warming with cloths (after seven hours),⁶.—Chill and shivering, for half an hour, at 4 P.M. (second day),⁶.—Shaking chill from 3 P.M. till 3 A.M., followed by warmth, without thirst (fourteenth day),⁶.—Short shaking chill and tossing, as if from electricity; immediately after sticking in the shoulder-blade, without perceptible coldness, about 6½ P.M.,⁶.—Severe chill at night in spite of increased covering (one prover),⁴.—Violent chill after rising at 3 A.M., disappearing on lying down (seventh day),⁶.—Violent chill after stool, with sensation as if she were dashed with icy-cold water, with internal warmth; toward evening,⁶.—Violent chill from 11 till 3 P.M., when she took Camphor, with the most violent pains in the

knees and calves, which continued till lying down (seventh day),⁶.—[1580.]
The chill can be relieved neither by the warmth of the stove nor by covering during the severest paroxysm, lasting three hours in the evening,⁶.—
Cold face,⁴⁷.—Shivering runs up her back, in the afternoon,³.—Feeling of
coldness in the vertebral column,⁹⁵.—A sensation of coldness on the left
side of the lumbar vertebræ, in a spot as large as the hand, together with
a feeling of formication, which was often very violent and unpleasant;
especially worse in the evening while sitting,¹⁰⁹.—*Cold extremities* (second
day),⁷⁸.—*Coldness of the limbs*,¹⁵ ⁵⁸.—Limbs cold and covered with cold
sweat,⁴.—Very cold hands, which look yellowish,⁹.—Icy coldness of the
hands and feet, with fearful pains in the urethra,⁶.—[1590.] **Heat.** Temperature increased,⁸⁹.—After the coldness a transient warmth,⁶.—Warmth
and slight sweat over the whole body (after seven hours),⁶.—External heat
from 10 to 3 P.M., three days in succession (eleventh day),⁶.—Skin hot
(second day),*².—Heat of the skin, which she herself does not feel, with
some thirst (tenth night),⁶.—Heat, with some thirst (eleventh day),⁶.—
Heat in the whole body,⁷.—Heat in the whole body, with accelerated
pulse,⁶.—Heat in the whole body at night, especially in the anus and genitals (after a few hours),¹ᵃ.—[1600.] After every somewhat violent or continued motion the whole body is very much heated, also at other times
very hot, especially in the afternoon,⁷.—The whole afternoon heated, as
after much walking on a hot day, together with red face and increased
perspiration (after eight hours),⁸.—Suddenly rising heat, with redness in
the face and thirst (third evening),⁶.—Transient heat,⁹.—Great heat, with
thirst and redness all over the body,¹ᵃ.—Burning heat at night, which she
does not feel; three nights,⁶.—Very unpleasant heat,¹².—Fever,¹⁷.—(Fever,
a mixture of heat and chill; heaviness of the feet; a paralytic immobility
of the limbs; loss of appetite; pain in the eyes; must lie in bed) (after five
days),¹ᵃ.—Fever, at first scanty and very painful; emission of blackish
urine; then secretion of urine increased to fourfold the amount of liquid
taken, with great thirst and much desire for meat; after a few hours the
urine lost its blackish color, and tasted like rather salt water,⁶⁶.—[1610.]
General fever (with the usual urinary symptoms),⁸⁰.—Burning fever,⁵⁵.—
Violent fever,⁵⁶.—Extremely violent fever,⁶⁴.—Feverish condition (from
small doses),²⁵.—Feverish condition, with dryness in the mouth and thirst,
anxiety, restlessness, and pains in the limbs (from external use),²⁵.—More or
less marked febrile condition,²⁹.—Feverish and beside herself,⁵⁴.—Head burning hot (third day),¹⁰⁷.—Rising of heat into the head; sweaty hands, with
burning in them (one hour after dinner),⁶.—[1620.] Anxious rising of heat
into the head,⁶.—Warm forehead, with sensation of coldness in the body,
in the evening,⁶.—During the coldness very warm forehead, without internal sensation of warmth (ninth day),⁶.—Glowing of the ears and chin for
one hour (after eight hours),⁹.—Heat in the face,⁷.—Burning in the face,
with normal warmth to touch (fourth afternoon),⁶.—Abdomen hot,⁹³.—Sensation of heat on and in the abdomen (fourth morning),⁶.—The palms of
the hands burn like fire,⁶.—Burning in the soles of the feet, in bed (the
whole fourth day),⁶.—[1630.] Burning on the soles of the feet, while the
hands are icy cold,⁹.—*Sweat.* Sweat,²⁵.—Some sweat on waking before
midnight,⁶.—In the beginning, when lying, violent motion caused sweat,
but especially warmth relieved the fearful pains,⁶.— Slight sweat a
night,¹ᵃ ¹.—Much sweat for two nights in succession, followed by wear-
ness in the morning,⁹.—Copious sweat,⁴.—Profuse sweat,⁹⁰.—Profuse sweat
on waking at night,¹⁰⁹.—[1640.] Profuse sweat when walking (after three

days),^{1a}.—Cold sweat,^{4 84}.—Co.1 sweat (second day),⁹⁴.—Surface covered with cold and viscid sweat (second day),⁵³.—Surface covered with cold clammy sweat (third day),⁹⁶.—Very profuse perspiration, on a cool day,⁴.—Profuse perspiration towards morning,⁴.—Forehead covered with cold sweat,⁴⁹.—Profuse sweat on the external pelvic region and in the groins, in the morning (second day),³.—Sweat on the genitals,^{1a}.—[**1650.**] Sweat on the chest, on waking at night (tenth and eleventh days),⁶.—* *Cold sweat of the hands and feet,*⁴⁷.

Conditions.—**Aggravation.**—(*Morning*), Anxiety; when rising, fretful; mental depression; some hours after rising, distracted in mind, etc.; confusion of head; tongue dry, etc.; on rising, foul taste; nausea, etc.; burning, etc., in abdomen; at 9 o'clock, *urine passed in a thin stream, etc.;* immediately on rising, persistent erection; while lying in bed, awake, emission of semen; on rising, cough; clot of blood in mouth; in bed, pressure in side of chest; after disappearance of the pains, pulse increased, etc.; *pain in back;* laxness, etc., in limbs; sleepy, etc.; on rising, at 3 o'clock, chilly; sweat on the pelvic region, etc.—(*Forenoon*), After coffee, nausea; from 11 till 1 o'clock, chilly, etc.—(*Afternoon*), *Insolent; stitches in right temple; stitches in side of head; stitches in occiput;* pressing in eyes; itching in eye; stitching in chin; tearing in lower jaw; on eating, pain in teeth; filthy taste; pressure in pit of stomach; pain from abdomen toward genitals; stitches in lower ribs; from 11 to 8 o'clock, squeezing, etc., in front chest; stitches in sternum; stitches in ribs; anxiety about heart; stitches in shoulder-blade; tearing in upper arm; stitching in arm; tearing in little finger; twitching in thigh, etc.; tearing in hollow of knee; shivering, etc.; at 3 o'clock, chill, etc.; at 4 o'clock, chill, etc.; at 6.30 o'clock, short chill, etc.; from 11 to 3 o'clock, violent chill; shivering up the back; from 10 to 3 o'clock, external heat.—(*Toward evening*), Nausea; pressure toward sternum; palpitation; after stool, violent chill, etc.—(*Evening*), On sitting and standing, stitches in side of head; after lying down, drawing, etc., in teeth; during paroxysm, disgust for everything; stitches in orifice of urethra; stitches in shoulder-blade; gnawing in sacrum; tearing in forearm, etc.; while sitting, sensation on side of lumbar vertebræ; warm forehead, etc.—(*Night*), Delirium; on waking, slimy mouth; thirst; stitches in orifice of urethra; burning in urethra; erections; chill; restless prostration; restless; from 3 P.M. to 3 A.M., shaking chill; heat of body; *sweat;* sweat on chest.—(*Before midnight*), Sweat.—(*Midnight*), Cannot lie on left side.—(*Toward morning*), Perspiration.—(*In air*), Worse.—(*In open air*), Lachrymation.—(*On ascending steps*), Knees totter.—(*In bed*), Burning of soles of feet.—(*Coffee*), The symptoms; abdominal pain; sense of fulness in chest, etc.—(*During and after coition*), Burning in ducts of vesiculæ seminales.—(*During the coldness*), Thirst.—(*During dinner*), Thirst.—(*After dinner*), Eructations, etc.; stitches in costal region; drawing, etc., in upper arm; tearing in bend of elbow; tension in calf; tearing in calf; yawning; sleepy.—(*After drinking*), Cardialgia, etc.—(*When eating*), Nausea, etc.—(*After eating*), Pain in palate.—(*Inspiration*), Sensation in epigastric region; stitching in chest; stitching in left side; stitching below right chest.—(*Liquids, sight or contact of*), Convulsive attacks.—(*After meals*), Scraping in throat; sleepy.—(*Motion*), Head heavy, etc.; *headache;* throbbing in side of spine; pain across small of back.—(*Moving head*), Tearing in nape of neck, etc.—(*Pressure*), Pain at the epigastrium, etc.; *pain in abdomen; pain in lumbar region, etc.*—(*Deep respiration*), Pressure towards sternum.—(*Sitting*), Rumbling in abdomen; weariness in small of back, etc.; pain in small of back.—(*After sitting down*), Tearing on surface of knee, etc.—(*Speaking*), Pressure toward sternum.— (*Standing*), Nausea; urging to urinate.—(*After stool*), Burning, etc., in anus.—(*On stooping*), Sensation in epigastric region; tensive pain in neck. —(*Talking*), Sensation in nose.—(*Touch*), Sensation in nose.—(*While urinating*), *Pains in urethra;* pain in spermatic cord.—(*After urinating*), Crawling, etc., in urethra; burning along urethra.—(*Walking*), Tearing in lower jaw; nausea; pain in groin; urging to urinate; headache; after rising from sitting, stitch in small of back; cutting in knees; tearing in calves; legs feel bruised; sweat.—(*Writing*), Cutting in the eye; dimness of vision. (*While yawning*), Stitch in ribs.

Amelioration.—(*Morning*), In bed, the pains.—(*Evening*), On the appearance of the urinary difficulties, the other difficulties cease.—(*Night*), In the beginning, pains, except those of the abdomen, cease.—(*Alcoholic liquors*), Prostration of strength.—(*After breakfast*), Headache disappears.— (*Camphor*), Pains in abdomen disappear; urging to stool; coldness; *urinary symptoms.*—(*Lying*), The symptoms; squeezing, etc., in chest.—(*On lying down*), Morning chill disappears.—(*Pressure on glans penis*), Pains from ureters downward.—(*On rising*), Pressure in side of chest disappears. —(*Rubbing*), Stitch in temple; stitching in ear; tearing in arm; tearing in hand; pain in legs; tearing in knee; burning in swelling on foot; tearing in toes.—(*Sitting*), Pain in groin.—(*On sitting up in bed*), Headache disappeared.—(*Standing*), Stitch in frontal eminence.—(*On walking*), Headache disappears; pain in calves disappears.—(*Warm applications*), Relieve; pains in knees, etc.—(*Wine*), Refreshes.

CAPSICUM.

Capsicum annuum, Linn. *Nat. order*, Solanaceæ. *Common name,* Cayenne, or red pepper. *Preparation,* Tincture of the powdered ripe pods, with the seeds; in the proportion of 20 grains of the powder to 400 drops of alcohol. (Hahnemann.)

Authorities. 1, Hahnemann, R. A. M. L., 6; 2, Ahner, ibid.; 3, Hartung, ibid.; 4, Mossdorf, ibid.; 5, Wislicenus, ibid.; 6, Browne, in Murray's App. Med., general statement, ibid.; 7, Fordyce, in Murray's App. Med., ibid.; 8, Pelargus, Observ., ii, 206, case of poisoning, ibid.; 8*a*, A few symptoms from Hartlaub and Trinks, R. A. M. L., 1, 303; 9, Baron Larrey, "Observ. on maladies of troops in Egypt," the results of large quantities of Capsicum (taken from Hempel's M. M., vol. 2); 10, Dr. David Hunt, poisoning of a lady by repeated teaspoonfuls of a solution of Caps., taken for a slight cold, N. E. Med. Gaz., 4, 43; 11, Dr. Farrington, Am. J. Hom. M. M., 4, 96, effects of preparing some red peppers for "chow chow."

Mind.—He makes reproaches and becomes angry at the faults of others; he becomes offended at trifles and finds fault,[1].—Even in the midst of joking he becomes offended at the slightest trifles,[1].—Obstinate, with outcries (after three hours),[1].—Indisposition to work or think,[3].—Repugnance and fretfulness,[1].—Anxiety and apprehensiveness; he imagines that he will die,[8].—The aversion to everything and the fretfulness were dissipated by sleep (curative action. H.),[1].—Anxiety, which compels him to take a deep breath,[1].—*Fearfulness* (after two hours),[1].—[10.] He is very easily irritated,[1]. —Capricious; at one time constantly laughing, soon again crying,[1].—An excessively busy uneasy mood,[1].—Indifferent to everything,[1].—*He is taciturn, peevish, and obstinate,[1].—*He is taciturn, absorbed in himself,[1].—Quiet mood (curative action),[3].—Contentment (curative action),[1].—Firmness, happy mood (curative action),[1].—He is in a contented mood, is jocose, and sings, and still he becomes angry from the slightest causes (after four hours),[1]. —[20.] He makes jokes and utters witticisms,[1].

Head.—Confusion and Vertigo. Intoxication,[1].—Confusion of the head,[3].—Confused on first waking from sleep (fourth day),[10].—Obscuration and confusion of the head,[2].—Dizziness and dulness in the head, like a heedlessness and awkwardness, so that she knocked against everything; with a febrile chill and coldness, together with anxiety,[1].—Dizziness in the morning on waking,[1].—Vertigo, staggering from one side to the other,[1].— *General Head.* *A bursting headache, or a feeling as if the brain were too full,[1].—*Headache on coughing, as if the skull would burst,[1].—[30.] Emptiness and dulness of the head (after twelve hours),[2].—When he awoke from sleep his head was so dull that he did not even recognize himself,[1].— *Headache, as if the skull were bruised, on moving the head and on walking,[1].— (Tearing headache),[1].—A headache, more sticking than tearing, which was worse during rest, but relieved on motion,[1].—A sticking headache,[1].—*Throbbing, beating headache in one or the other temple,[1].—Throbbing, beating headache,[1].—*Forehead.* Bursting headache in the forehead,[1].—*Constant pressive headache in the forehead, above the root of the nose, together with some stitches through the ear and over the eye,[1].—[40.] Pressive headache in the forehead, as if it pressed from the occiput outward to the forehead, with a cutting from the occiput to the forehead (immediately),[1].—Throbbing headache in the forehead,[1].—Tearing headache in the forehead,[1].—Drawing-tearing pain in the frontal bone, more on the right side (after six and seven hours, and after third day),[2].—*Temples.* Pressive headache in the temples,[1].— Pressive pain in the temporal region,[3].—*Vertex.* Severe, deeply penetrating stitches in the vertex,[2].—Two sudden, violent stitches from the vertex to the forehead (after one hour),[*a].—*Sides.* Drawing-tearing in the left side of the head (after seventeen and forty-eight hours),[2].—A one-sided, pressive-sticking headache, like an hysterical migraine, which was increased by raising the eyes and the head, or by stooping, and was accompanied by forgetfulness and nausea,[1].—*External Head.* [50.] Slight shivering over the hairy portion of the head, followed by burning-itching on the scalp, which was relieved after scratching, but returned with increased severity (after two hours),[3].

Eyes.—The eyes protrude from the head, with paleness of the face (after sixteen hours),[1].—Inflammation of the eyes,[1].—Painful twitching beneath the right eyelid (after half an hour),[*a].—Pressure on the eyes, so that he was unable to open them sufficiently wide,[2].—A pressive pain in the eye, as from a foreign body,[1].—A burning in the eyes, which become red and watery, in the morning,[1].—*Pupil.* Fine stinging pain in the eyes (from the dust),[1].—Much dilated pupils,[1].—Great dilatation of the pupils,[2].— *Vision.* [60.] Dim vision in the morning, as if a foreign body floated over the cornea and obscured it, so that one saw clearly again for a moment on rubbing the eye,[1].—All objects seem black,[1].—Visual power almost lost, like blindness,[1].

Ears.—*A swelling on the bone behind the ear, painful to touch,[1].— *Tearing pain behind the left ear (after six hours),[2].—Pain beneath the ear,[1]. —*A pressive pain in the ear with every cough, as if an ulcer would open,[1].— *A pressive pain very deep in the ears (after one and eight hours),[1].—Itch-

ing pain very deep in the ear (after sixteen hours),[1].—*Tearing in the concha of the ear*,[1].

Nose.—Objective. [70.] Painful pimples beneath the nostrils,[1].—*Stopped coryza*,[1].—Violent racking sneezing, with discharge of thin mucus from the nose (immediately),[4].—Bloody mucus from the nose,[1].—*Nose-bleed*, in the morning, in bed, and blowing of blood from the nose, several times,[1].—**Subjective.** Burning-crawling in the nose, with violent sneezing and discharge of mucus (immediately, from the dust),[5].—Burning-tensive sensation in the left nostril, as if a pimple would form,[4].—Constrictive jerking pain on the left side of the nose, extending to above the left eye (after five hours),[2].—*Crawling-tickling in the nose, as in stopped coryza*,[1].

Face.—Objective. Heat and redness of the face, with trembling of the limbs (immediately),[1].—[80.] Unusual redness of the face, always followed, after half an hour, by a pale suffering expression (after three hours),[3]. —The face was at one time pale, at another red, with red lobules of the ears, with sensation of burning, without, however, special heat being felt by the hand,[1].—Red cheeks,[1].—**Subjective.** *Pain in the face, partly like bone-pains, excited by external touch, partly like fine pains piercing the nerves, which are tormenting when falling asleep*,[1].—Pain in the left side of the lower jaw, as from a boil or ulcer, lasting three-quarters of an hour,[2].—**Lips.** Ulcerating eruption on the lips (not in the corners), which only pain on motion,[1].—*Swollen lips*,[1].—Scaly lips,[1].—*Cracking of the lips; smarting of the lips*,[1].—Burning lips,[4].

Mouth.—Teeth and Gums. [90.] Drawing pain in the teeth, which was neither increased on touching the teeth nor on eating,[1].—A tooth seems to him too long and raised up, and feels blunt,[1].—Swelling of the gum,[1].—Drawing pain in the gum,[1].—**Tongue.** Pimples on the tip of the tongue, which sting and pain when touched,[1].—Dry sensation on the forepart of the tongue, without thirst, in the morning (after eight hours),[1].—**General Mouth.** Dryness of the mouth,[1].—**Saliva.** Tough *mucus in the mouth* (after two hours),[1].—Salivation,[1].—**Taste.** Sour taste of broth (after two hours),[1].—[100.] Acid taste in the mouth,[1].—A pungent acid taste in the mouth,[1].—Taste as of bad water,[1].—Flat, insipid, earthy taste (for example, of butter),[1].—*Watery, flat taste in the mouth, followed by heartburn*,[1].

Throat. Pain in the palate, as if it was pressed or pinched by something hard, at first more when not swallowing, afterwards worse when swallowing (after one hour and a half),[1].—Pain in the upper part of the throat, when not swallowing, as if the parts were sore; and spasmodic contraction, as in waterbrash,[1].—*Pain on swallowing, as in inflammation of the throat, but when not swallowing, drawing pain in the throat*,[1].—*Pressive pain in the throat, as if an ulcer would break, during a paroxysm of coughing*,[1].—*Pain in the throat, only when coughing, as from a simple painful swelling*,[1].—[110.] A simple pain in the fauces, only when coughing,[1].—Sensation of rawness in the throat, for nearly two days,[4].—*Continued stitching in the throat, in the region of the epiglottis, which caused a dry coughing, without being relieved by coughing*,[4].—*Spasmodic contraction of the throat*,[1].—Pain externally on the throat,[1].

Stomach.—Appetite. Want of hunger, loss of appetite,[1].—He was obliged to force himself to eat; he had no real appetite, although food had a natural taste,[1].—**Thirst.** Desire for coffee (after eight hours),[1].—Loss of thirst,[1].—**Eructations.** Eructations from the stomach only when walking, and with every eructation a stitch in the side; when sitting, no eructations, and so no stitches,[1].—[120.] After eating, fulness and anxiety in the chest followed by sour eructations or heartburn; at last, thin stool,[1]. —*Nausea and Vomiting.* Qualmishness of the stomach (after one hour),[1].—*Nausea,*[1].—Qualmishness and nausea in the pit of the stomach, in the morning and afternoon (after twenty-four hours),[1].—Nausea and spitting of saliva, after drinking coffee,[1].—Cough excites nausea,[1].—Vomiting and purging (immediately),[10].—Heartburn,[1].—*Stomach.* Pressure in the pit of the stomach, with nausea,[1].—Pressive pain in the pit of the stomach,[2].—[130.] Pressure in the pit of the stomach, with nausea, during menstruation,[1].—Pressure beneath the short ribs and the pit of the stomach,[1].—Severe pressure in the pit of the stomach, increased by pressure (after half an hour),[8a].—A pinching, boring-outward pain in the pit of the stomach, especially when sitting bent, lasting severely for eight minutes (after one hour and a half),[2].—Fine sudden stitches in the pit of the stomach (after a few minutes),[5].—Stitches in the pit of the stomach, when breathing deeply and suddenly, talking, or on touch,[6a].—Coldness in the stomach; a feeling as if cold water were in it, followed by a sensation as if he were trembling,[1].—A burning above the pit of the stomach, immediately after eating, at noon and evening,[1].—A burning in the stomach, extending up into the mouth, after breakfast,[1].

Abdomen.—Pinching in the upper part of the abdomen,[1].—[140.] *A pressive tension in the abdomen, especially in the epigastric region, between the pit of the stomach and the navel, which is specially increased by motion, together with a pressive tension in the lower portion of the back,*[1].—*Colic, with cutting-twisting pain about the navel, and passage of tough mucus, like diarrhœa, at times, mixed with black blood;* after every stool, thirst, and after every drink, shivering,[1].—Pain deep in the abdomen, rather burning than sticking, together with cutting in the umbilical region, on motion, especially on stooping and walking, with ill-humor about the pain and discontent and whining about inanimate objects (not about men or moral subjects), with fretfulness, a kind of apprehensiveness, with sweat in the face,[1]. —*Drawing and twisting in the abdomen,* with and without diarrhœa,[1].— Much flatulence,[2].—Rumbling of flatus in the abdomen (after one hour),[1]. Flatus moves painfully about the abdomen,[1].—Painless rumbling in the abdomen,[3].—A rumbling extending upward and downward in the abdomen,[1].—Pressure here and there in the abdomen,[1].—[150.] Pressive-pinching pain in the abdomen, immediately after eating, with incarcerated flatus,[1].—Unusually strong pulsations of the bloodvessels of the abdomen,[3]. —Increased internal warmth in the intestinal canal,[3].—*A tensive pain, extending from the abdomen to the chest, as from distension in the abdomen,*[1].— Distension and hardness of the abdomen, which would not endure tight clothes,[1].—Distension in the abdomen, two hours after eating, followed by shooting headache towards the occiput and profuse sweat,[1].—*A feeling as if the abdomen were distended even to bursting, on which account breathing was impeded, even to suffocation,*[1].—A hernia, consisting of wind, forcibly and painfully protrudes from the abdominal ring,[1].—Colic, as from flatus in the lower abdomen,[1].—Hard, pressive, almost sticking pain in a small spot on the left side of the lower abdomen (after one hour),[1].

Rectum and Anus.—[160.] Urging to stool, with pressive pain in the intestines, but he was constipated,[2].—*Tenesmus,*[1 6].—*Hæmorrhoids in the anus, which itch at times,*[1].—Blind hæmorrhoids; hæmorrhoids in the anus, which pain severely during stool,[1].—Flow of blood from the anus, for four days,[1].—*Burning in the anus,*[6].—*Burning pain in the anus (after three, four, and eight hours),[1].—*Biting-stinging pain in the anus, with diarrhœa-like stool,[1].—Itching in the anus (after three, four, and eight hours),[1].

Stool.—*Mucous diarrhœa, with tenesmus,[1].—[170.] *Diarrhœa, immediately, at once followed by an empty tenesmus,[1].—Stool immediately after eating (at noon), with redness of the cheeks (after six hours),[1].—*After drinking, he was obliged to go to stool, but was constipated; only a little mucus passed,[2].—*As soon as he drank anything, he felt as though he would have diarrhœa, but only a little passed every time,[2].—*Small stool, consisting of bloody mucus,[1].—*Small passages, which consist of only mucus,[1].—*Small frequent passages, consisting of mucus, at times mingled with blood, and causing tenesmus, preceded by flatulent colic in the lower portion of the abdomen,[1].—Constipation, as from too much heat in the abdomen,[1].

Urinary Organs.—Bladder. Tenesmus of the bladder, strangury; he is obliged to urinate frequently, with at times ineffectual urging to urinate (after four to eight hours),[1].—*Pressure towards the bladder, and some stitches extending from within outward in the region of the neck of the bladder, while coughing, and for some time afterwards,[4].—[180.] Spasmodic contraction, with cutting pains in the neck of the bladder, without urging to urinate, at times intermitting, at times returning, in the morning, in bed; it seems to be somewhat relieved by passing urine (after twenty-four hours),[5].—*Urethra.* Frequent desire to urinate, mostly when sitting, not when walking (after forty-two hours),[1].—Purulent discharge from the urethra, a kind of gonorrhœa,[1].—Gonorrhœa,[7].†—(The gonorrhœa became yellow and thick), (after seven days),[1].—The urethra is painful to touch (after seven days),[1].—Pain in the urethra, especially in the forenoon,[1].—*A burning in the orifice of the urethra, immediately before, during, and for a minute after urinating,[1].—A cutting pain in the urethra, extending backward, when not urinating (after six hours),[1].—*Stitches, as with needles, in the forepart of the urethra, when not urinating (after eight hours),[1].—[190.] *Severe stitches in the orifice of the urethra, when not urinating,[1].—Fine sticking in the urethra, immediately after urinating,[1].—*A burning-biting pain in the urethra, after urinating (after seven days),[1].—*Micturition.* The urine passes by drops, and with great difficulty (immediately, and for a long time),[1].—Burning urine,[1].—Passage of a great quantity of urine, which she could not wholly control,[10].—*Urine.* Urine scanty, light-colored (fifth day),[10].—The urine deposits a white sediment,[1].

Sexual Organs.—Erections in the morning, in bed, without sexual thoughts,[1].—Erections in the forenoon, afternoon, and evening,[1].—[200.] Violent erections in the morning, on rising, only relieved by cold water,[1].—A constant pressure and bruised sensation in the glans, especially in the morning and evening,[1].—Fine itching-sticking on the glans, like the stings of an insect,[2].—*Coldness of the scrotum, in the morning, on waking,[1].—Coldness of the scrotum, with impotency,[1].—Loss of sensibility in the testicles, softening and gradual dwindling of these parts; at first this was not noticed by the patient, until the testicles were reduced to the size of a bean, insensible, hard, and drawn up close to the abdominal ring, and suspended by a shrivelled spermatic cord,[9].—Drawing pain in the spermatic cord and a pinching pain in the testicle, while urinating and for some time afterwards (after forty-eight hours),[1].—Emission at night,[1].

---

† From carrying a linen bag filled with the powdered seeds of Capsicum baccatum on the naked abdomen.

Respiratory Organs.—Larynx and Trachea. *A crawling and tickling in the larynx and trachea, with a dry hacking cough, in the evening, after lying down,[1].—Mucus in the upper part of the trachea, which is expectorated from time to time by hawking and voluntary hacking cough (after three hours),[1].—[210.] Tickling sensation in the trachea, so that he was obliged to sneeze violently several times,[2].—*The exhalation from the lungs, on coughing, causes a strong offensive taste in the mouth,[1].—*The cough expels an offensive breath from the lung,[1].—*Voice.* Hoarseness,[1].—*Cough.* *Cough, especially towards evening, from 5 to 9,[1].—Cough, especially after drinking coffee,[1].—*Painful cough,[1].—Paroxysm of cough in the afternoon (about 5 o'clock), which causes nausea and vomiting,[1].—*Frequent dry, hacking cough,[1].—Very frequent hacking,[1].—*Respiration.*—[220.] Freer breathing from day to day,[1].†—Deep breathing, almost like sighing,[1].—He was frequently obliged to take several very deep inspirations, whereby he was relieved of all his troubles,[1].—An involuntary strong expiration,[1].—Asthma; feeling of fulness in the chest,[1].—*Dyspnœa, which seems to rise from the stomach,[1].—Dyspnœa during rest and motion,[1].—Dyspnœa, even during rest, with stiffness of the back, which hurt when stooping, together with deep sighing breathing, from time to time, and dry cough,[1].—Dyspnœa, with redness of the face, eructations, and sensation as if the chest were distended,[1].—Dyspnœa when walking,[1].—[230.] He was only able to inspire with the body outstretched; orthopnœa,[1].

Chest.—*Pain in the chest, when sitting, as if the chest was too full and there was not room enough in it,[1].—*Pain as if the chest were constricted, which arrests the breathing and is increased even on slight motion,[1].—Pain like a pressure on the chest, on deep breathing and on turning the body,[1].—*Throbbing pain in the chest,[i].—*Front.* Pain on the ribs and sternum, on inspiration,[1].—*Sides.* Pain in the chest, beneath the right arm, if he feels the spot or raises the arm,[1].—(Simple pain in one rib, in a small spot, which is most painful when touching it, but is neither excited by breathing nor by coughing),[1].—A pressive pain on the side of the chest on which she lies,[1].—Drawing pain in the side of the chest, extending up to the throat, on coughing,[1].—[240.] Pain, like stitches, in the side of the chest and back, when coughing,[1].—A single stitch in the left side of the chest, between the third and fourth ribs, as with a dull needle,[2].—A stitch in the side of the chest, when breathing or walking, not when sitting,[1].—Some stitches in the left side of the chest, between the second and third ribs (after five hours),[2].—Stitches in the left side, near the fifth and sixth ribs (after one hour),[2].—Stitches in the left side of the chest, arresting breathing (after ten hours),[2].—Stitches in the left side of the chest, on inspiration, between the third and fourth ribs,[2].

Heart. Very severe stitches in the region of the heart, so that he cried out,[1].

Neck and Back.—Neck. Sensation of weakness over the whole neck, as if he were loaded (after four hours),[3].—Stiffness of the neck relieved by motion,[1].—[250.] Painful stiffness of the neck, only noticed on moving it,[1].—A jerking pain in the neck,[1].—*Jerking-tearing pain in the right cervical glands,[2].—*Back.* Pain in the back, on stooping,[1].—Drawing pain in the back,[1].—Drawing-pressive pain in the back,[1].—*Drawing-tearing pain in and near the spine,[2].—Sudden drawing-sticking pain in the middle

---

† Reaction of the organism, secondary action, curative action.—H.

of the spine,[2].—-A pain, drawing downward in the small of the back when standing and moving, together with a bruised pain,[1].

Extremities in General.—Convulsive jerks and twitches, now in the thigh, now in the forearm,[3].—[260.] Weariness and heaviness of the limbs, followed by trembling of the thighs and knees; the hands refused their service when writing (after seven hours),[3].—Sensation of lassitude in the limbs, more during rest and while sitting,[1].—Extreme weariness in all the limbs, as if bruised; all the limbs are affected,[8a].—A pain shoots into one or the other limbs on coughing and sneezing,[1].—Crawling sensation in the arms and legs, from the feet upward as far as the throat,[1].—Cracking and creaking in the joints of the knees and fingers,[1].—After he has lain down, all the joints become stiff, and on rising from bed in the morning, all the joints feel crushed, especially the lameness in the knees and ankles is more severe after rising than during motion,[1].—Sensation of stiffness and simple pain in all the joints, worse when beginning to move, but relieved on continued motion, with catarrh and tough mucus in the trachea,[1].—All the joints pain as if dislocated, with a sensation as if they were swollen,[1].—All the joints felt crushed in the morning on rising; a paralytic stiff pain on beginning to move, especially in the knees and ankles, relieved by continued motion (after ten hours),[1].

Superior Extremities.—[270.] Drawing-tearing pain, extending from the right clavicle along the whole arm to the tips of the fingers, lasting three minutes,[2].—*Shoulder.* Pain in the shoulder-joint, as if dislocated,[1].—(Drawing paralytic pain above and below the shoulder-joint),[1].—*Elbow.* Stitches in the left elbow-joint, which extend into the hand, with flushes of heat, from which the arm felt as if asleep,[2].—*Forearm.* Tingling pain in the left forearm,[2].—*Hands.* Heat in the hands, but not in other portions of the body,[2].—My hands burned and stung so, I washed them in water and then in sweet oil; I felt no more burning, but on washing my hands the next *morning in cold water, the burning returned worse than ever,*[11].—Twitching-jerking, painful sensation in the hollow of the left hand (after eight hours),[2].—*Fingers.* A contractive pain in the left index finger,[2].—Violent, deep stitches in the ball of the left little finger,[3].

Inferior Extremities.—[280.] *A sticking-tearing pain from the hip-joints to the feet, especially on coughing,*[1].—*Hip. *Drawing pain in the hip-joint (pain like a stiff neck), which was aggravated by touch and by bending the trunk backwards,*[1].—*Thigh.* Pain in the muscles of the thighs, like a pressure and a sprain,[1].—A deep pressive pain in the side of the thigh, extending into the knee, on coughing,[1].—Pain as if sprained in the right thigh; the pain became more violent if the thigh was stretched out, but not otherwise,[2].—Drawing digging-sticking pain in the middle of the posterior surface of the left thigh, disappearing on motion,[2].—Tearing pain on the inner side of the left thigh,[2].—Bruised pain in the right thigh, disappearing on walking, but returning during rest,[2].—*Knee. Tensive pain in the knee,*[1].—*Leg.* An internal pain, consisting of a drawing-sticking, in the left lower leg,[3].—[290.] Tension in the calves, when walking,[1].—*Foot.* Trembling weakness of the feet,[1].—(Bruised pain in the bones of the heels, as if the heels had been benumbed and bruised by a long leap, at times becoming tearing, paroxysmal), (after two hours),[1].—*Toes.* Some stitches in the right great toe, ceasing on stamping the foot,[2].—Stitches extending to the tips of the toes,[1].

General Symptoms.—Objective. While caressing, an uncontrollable trembling of the whole body (after twenty-four hours),[1].—*He shuns all motion*,[1].—Weariness, more in the morning than in the evening,[1].—Great weariness, though not enforcing sleep (after two hours),[1].—Complete exhaustion of the strength,[1].—[**300.**] *All the senses are more acute,*[1].†—**Subjective.** A painless sensation in the body, moving upward and downward, with redness of the cheeks,[1].—Sensation over the whole body, as if all parts were asleep (the inspiration of sulphur-fumes speedily relieves),[1].—Cramp, first in the left arm, then in the whole body; the arms were stiff, so that she could not straighten them out; the feet also were stiff, on rising after sitting, with crawling as if asleep,[1].—Drawing pain here and there in the limbs, back, nape of the neck, shoulder-blades, and in the hands, lasting several hours, and were excited by motion,[1].—Transient pressive pain now in one, now in another portion of the body,[1].—When breathing, a sticking pain between the shoulder-blades and in the epigastric region, and single stitches in the side of the abdomen, the ensiform cartilage, and sternum; these pains do not penetrate, but seem to be superficial,[1].—Bubbling sensation; sudden throbbing in some large veins (after twenty-four hours),[5].

Skin.—*Eruptions, Dry.* The eruption spread upward to the scalp, and downward to the soles of the feet; was accompanied by considerable swelling, but the features were not much disfigured; the swelling consisted more of a bagging of the cheeks and neck; the left side of the face was more affected than the right, and the left ear twice the size of the right, which was but slightly enlarged; there was no peculiarity of position to account for this, and it did not hold true of the body (fifth day),[10].—Red points on the face and on the forehead, a tetter, with corrosive itching (after two and twenty-four hours),[1].—[**310.**] (Red round spots on the abdomen and thighs),[1].—(Pimples, with a biting sensation, as from salt, on the left side of the face),[1].—Skin from the neck to the knees covered with a papular eruption; accompanied by intense itching and burning, worse at night, but towards morning she grew quiet and slept from five till eight or nine, and continued more comfortable all day till the nightly aggravation (fourth day),[10].—Papulous eruption on the inner surface of the cheeks,[1].—***Eruptions, Moist.*** The eruption appeared at first as distinctly papular, and the papules were filled in with the erythematous redness; then vesicles appeared, which did not change their character, excepting that where the perspiration was confined the skin was raised and broken, as if the parts had been scalded,[10].—The papular eruption became filled with a bright erythematous redness, and in the afternoon vesicles commenced to form; they were most abundant wherever the perspiration was most confined, as in the folds of the axillary region, where the bindings of the skirts came, etc. (fifth day),[10].—**Sensations.** Burning and itching of the skin (second morning),[10].—Corrosive burning on several tender portions (the lips, mouth, nose, tip of the nose, wings of the nose, eyelids, etc.), (from the dust),[5].—Crawling here and there in the skin, as from an insect,[1].—(Itching, even after rubbing the part),[1].—[**320.**] Itching here and there in the skin, mostly in the face and nose,[1].—Sticking burning-itching on the whole body, but mostly on the chest and face,[3].—Fine sticking pain in the skin of the wrist (from the dust),[1].—Corrosive itching on the scalp as from vermin, which obliges her to scratch; after scratching the roots of the hairs and the scalp become as sore as if the hairs had been pulled out,[1].—Itching in the hair of the head, and in small

---

† Reaction of the organism, secondary action, curative action —H.

spots on the rest of the body, which was relieved by scratching,[1].—(Itching on the nose mingled with stitches),[1].

Sleep and Dreams. Sleepiness.—*Yawning* almost uninterruptedly (after half an hour),[1].—Frequent yawning after eating,[1].—Drowsy all day (eighth day); comatose all day (ninth day),[10].—Great sleepiness after the heat; she could scarcely keep awake, especially after eating (after five hours),[8a].—[330.] During sleep he snores, on inspiring through the nose, as if he could not get any air through it, and it would impede respiration (after one hour),[1].—Sleep interrupted by crying and starting up as if he fell down from a high place,[1].—**Sleeplessness.** He wakes several times after midnight,[1].—*He becomes wide awake in the night and cannot sleep again* (after fifth and ninth hours),[1].—He becomes wide awake after midnight, and also later,[1].—**Dreams.** *Sleep full of dreams,*[1].—Dreams full of difficulties,[1].—Dreams, of a sad character, of past experience; on waking he did not know whether it was real or not,[1].

Fever.—Chilliness. Trembling on account of shivering,[1].—*Shivering and chilliness after every drink,*[1].—[340.] Gradual diminution of the warmth of the body,[1].—* *Coldness over the whole body; the limbs are cold without shivering,*[1].—General coldness in the evening after lying down, followed by coryza (after seventy-two hours),[1].—As the coldness of the body increases,† so also the ill-humor and the contraction of the pupils increase,[1].—He becomes chilly from a little air in bed,[1].—Chill in the evening,[1].—Chill and coldness the first night; the following nights sweat all over,[1].—Chill in the afternoon, lasting some time (half an hour or an hour); during which she lay warmly covered; after the chill the skin burned and itched more than before (fifth day),[10].—(Febrile chill in the evening, with thirst (without heat and without yawning or stretching), with great weariness, short breath, sleepiness, and fretfulness; shivering on the slightest motion, without cold sensation and without being cold; he did not feel too warm, though he was in a hot room),[1].—He is averse to the cold air, especially to a draught; he cannot endure it (after twelve hours),[1].—[350.] Shivering and coldness of the back in the evening, without subsequent heat or thirst, but followed by slight sweat,[1].—Sensation in the thighs as though they were covered with cold sweat, when walking in the open air (as if cold air blew against the sweaty parts); the thighs, however, did not sweat,[1]. —The feet are cold as far as above the ankles and cannot be warmed, with general warmth of the rest of the body, in the morning (after twelve hours),[5].—**Heat.** General heat and sweat without thirst, which lasted some hours, followed by shivering at 6 P.M., with shaking and chattering of the teeth, during which he was thirsty and cold all over, with anxiety, uneasiness, loss of the senses, and intolerance of noise; the next evening at seven a similar shuddering, shivering, and coldness, with thirst,[1].—Heat over the whole body follows the disappearance of the pressure in the stomach, with increased redness of the face (after four hours),[8a].—(Internal heat, with cold sweat on the forehead),[1].—Heat, with shivering and thirst,[1]. —*Heat of the ears, and hot, red tip of the nose, towards evening,*[1].—Glowing hot cheeks, with cold hands and feet, without shivering, at noon, after eating, recurring at the same time for two days,[1].—(Burning hands, feet, and cheeks; the latter are swollen),[1].—**Sweat.** [360.] Sweat all over in the morning,[1].—The perspiration was so acrid that it caused the hands of any

---

† I have seen this increase speedily for twelve hours from Capsicum, and again decrease for twelve hours to complete disappearance.—H.

person brought in contact with the skin of the patient to burn and tingle,[10].—Sweat on the forehead,[2].—Sweat under the arms (after eight hours),[1].—Sweat on the hands (after three hours),[1].

Conditions. — **Aggravation.** — (*Morning*), On waking, dizziness; burning in the eyes; dim vision; *in bed, nose-bleed;* dry sensation on tongue; in bed, contraction, etc., in neck of bladder; in bed, erections; violent erections; on waking, coldness of the scrotum; on rising from bed, joints feel crushed; weariness; feet cold, etc.; sweat all over.—(*Forenoon*), Pain in urethra; pain in testicle.—(*Noon*), After eating, hot cheeks, etc.—(*Afternoon*), About 5 o'clock, paroxysms of cough; chill.—(*Towards evening*), From 5 to 9 o'clock, cough.—(*Evening*), After lying down, crawling, etc., in larynx, etc.; after lying down, coldness; chill; febrile chill; shivering, etc.; about 6 o'clock, general heat, etc.—(*Night*), Eruption on skin.—(*After midnight*), Wakes several times; becomes wide awake.—(*When walking in open air*), Sensation in thighs.—(*Bending trunk backward*), Pain in hip-joint.—(*Sitting bent*), Pain in pit of stomach.—(*After breakfast*), Burning in stomach.—(*When breathing*), Stitch in side of chest.—(*Deep breathing*), Pain in chest.—(*After coffee*), Nausea, etc.; cough.—(*Draught of cold air*), Is intolerable.—(*On coughing*), Headache; pain in throat; nausea; pressure towards the bladder; pain in side of chest, etc.; pain shooting into limbs; pain from hip to feet; pain in thigh; trembling of body.—(*After drinking*), **Shivering**; *urging to stool;* diarrhœic feeling.—(*After eating*), Fulness, etc., in chest; burning above pit of stomach; immediately, pain in abdomen; in two hours, distension of abdomen; immediately, stool.—(*On inspiration*), Pain in ribs, etc.—(*Lying down*), Stiffness of joints.—(*During menstruation*), Pressure in pit of stomach.—(*Motion*), Headache; *tension in abdomen*, etc.; especially stepping and walking, pain in abdomen, etc.; *pain in chest;* stiffness of neck; pain in small of back; pain in limbs, etc.—(*Beginning to move*), Stiffness, etc., in all joints.—(*Raising eyes*), Headache.—(*Raising head*), Headache.—(*Rest*), Headache; lassitude in limbs; pain in thigh returns.—(*After rising*), Lameness in knees, etc.; stiffness of feet.—(*When sitting*), Desire to urinate; pain in chest; lassitude in limbs.—(*On sneezing*), Pain shooting into limbs.—(*After every stool*), *Thirst.*—(*Stooping head*), Headache.—(*When standing*), Pain in small of back.—(*On stooping*), Pain in back.—(*Stretching out part*), Pain in right thigh.—(*Touch*), Pain in hip-joint.—(*On turning body*), Pain in chest.—(*After urination*), Immediately, sticking in urethra; pain in urethra.—(*On walking*), Headache; erections; stitch in side of chest; tension in calves.—(*Washing in cold water*), Burning in hands returns worse.

Amelioration.—(*Very deep inspiration*), All troubles.—(*Motion*), Headache; stiff neck; pain in thigh.—(*Continued motion*), Crushed feeling in joints.—(*Washing in sweet oil*), Burning, etc., in hands.—(*Sleep*), Aversion to everything.—(*On stamping foot*), Stitches in great toe.—(*Walking*), Pain in thigh.

CARBO ANIMALIS.

Preparation, Place a thick piece of ox-hide between red hot coals, where it must remain as long as it burns with a flame, then quickly put the glowing piece between plates of stone, to put a stop to the combustion (if allowed to cool gradually in the air most of the carbon would be consumed). *Triturate.*

Authorities. 1, Hahnemann, Chr. Kn., 3; 2, Adams, ibid.; 3, Hartlaub and Trinks, ibid.; 4, Wahle, ibid.; 5, Rust's Magazine, xxii, ibid.

Mind.—Emotional. *Desire to be alone; she is sad and reflective; avoids all conversation (first four and after eight days),[3].—Involuntary jolly whistling,[1].—Excessively jovial,[2].—Weeping mood,[1].—He cannot seem to weep enough,[1].—Great tendency to sadness,[1].—Extremely melancholy mood, with feeling as of being abandoned,[1].—Melancholy and anxious, in the morning on waking,[1].—Depressed, apprehensive, melancholy, especially in the afternoon,[3].—[10.] Discouraged and sad; everything seems so sad and lonely that she desires to weep (third day),[3].—In the morning, he felt abandoned and homesick,[1].—Homesick,[1].—Thoughts of death,[1].—*Anxiety and orgasm of blood at night, so severe that she was obliged to sit up,[1].—Anxiety and uneasiness in the back, without pain, soon after eating,[1].—Very anxious and depressed, especially in the evening and at night; she was unable to sleep quietly on account of internal anxiety; she felt best in the morning,[1].—Hopelessness,[1].—Shy and fearful mood,[1].—Fearful and frightened the whole day,[1].—[20.] Such great apprehension and heaviness in the body, in the afternoon, that walking was very difficult,[1].—In the evening, he was frightened, even to shuddering and weeping,[1].—Obstinate; no one could do anything to suit him,[4].—Great inclination to get angry,[1].—Angry and wrathful,[4].—Ill-humor,[2].—Fretful, in the morning on waking (first days),[1].—Fretful; she was averse to talking (first day),[3].—Sullen mood and ill-humor about present and past events; this cannot be overcome; it even amounts to weeping,[1].—Unsettled mood day and night,[1].—[30.] At times lachrymose, at times foolishly jovial,[1].—Indifferent at first, afterward increased irritability for passionate impressions,[1].

—Intellectual. Stupid and drowsy in the forenoon, much worse after dinner,[3].—He was unable to write a letter, and could not express his thoughts,[1].—Weakness of memory; he forgot the word that he was about to speak,[3].—Sudden stupefaction, several times; he did not hear, did not see, and had no thoughts,[1].—Sudden stupefaction, when moving the head and on walking,[1].—Great stupefaction, while sitting at a table, with great lightness in the head, and anxious dread that he would fall down unconscious at any moment,[1].

Head.—Confusion and Vertigo. Confusion in the morning, and feeling as in a confused dream,[1].—*In the morning, his head was very much confused; did not know whether he had been asleep or awake,[1].—[40.] Confusion in the head in the morning, and she was vexed with everything that she looked at,[3].—She feels very uncomfortable from 10 A.M. till 4 P.M., as if confused in the head and uncertain on her feet, with paleness of the face, nausea, and blue rings around the eyes,[1].—Vertigo to the right side,[3].—Vertigo, as from moving the head back and forth,[1].—Vertigo, with blackness before the eyes,[1].—*Vertigo, with nausea, on rising up after stooping,[1].—Vertigo, when sitting, as if she would fall backward from her chair, with chilliness,[3].—Vertigo, and a feeling as though he had not slept enough, in the morning,[3].—Vertigo about 7 P.M.; if she raised the head everything seemed to turn around; she was obliged to sit bent constantly, and on rising up she struggled hither and thither, together with confusion in the head and a feeling as if all objects moved; on lying down, she felt nothing the whole night; only in the morning on rising, this returned,[1].—Heaviness in the head,[3].—[50.] *Heaviness in the head in the morning, with dim vision and watery eyes,[3].—*Heaviness in the head at night, with weariness in the feet, which she could scarcely lift (second day),[3].—Heaviness of the head, espe-

cially in the occiput, and of the left temple, with confusion,[1].—*General Head.* *Rush of blood to the head, with confusion in it,[1].—A feeling of painful looseness of the brain, on motion,[3].—Pain in the head and neck at night, as if they were asleep, and had been sprained,[1].—Headache, in the morning on waking, as after intoxication,[1].—Heat in the head, with anxiety, in the evening, in bed; she was obliged to rise, when it became better,[3].—Tension in the head, almost daily,[1].—Drawing-boring pain in the head, together with tearings; when the head became cool it was worse, especially towards the ears (after seven days),[1].—[60.] Headache, which presses down the eyebrows,[1].—Everything which was on the head pressed upon it, even the neckcloth was uncomfortable (after eighteen days),[1].— Pressure and confusion in the whole head after dinner, lasting till evening,[3]. —Sticking in the head, especially in the temples.[1].—Tearing and throbbing in the whole head, in the orbits, in the ears, left side of the face, cheek-bones, and in the lower jaw, coming on immediately after dinner, relieved by pressure with the hands, and suddenly ceasing, when the cheek was somewhat swollen (after twenty-eight hours),[1].—*Forehead.* Stupefying headache in the forehead while spinning, disappearing after dinner,[3].— **Heaviness in the forehead on stooping, with sensation as if the brain would fall forward; vertigo on rising, so that she soon fell down,*[3].—Heat and feeling of heaviness in the forehead, which, however, felt cold externally, in the forenoon,[3].—**Sensation in the forehead as if something lay above the eyes, on account of which she could not look up,*[1].—Sensation in the head, as of something heavy in the forehead, or as if a board pressed upon it; sensation like going from very cold air into a warm room, in front of a hot stove,[1].—[70.] Drawing in the forehead above the eyebrows,[1].—Pricking headache on the left side of the forehead, in the morning after rising, better in the open air,[3].—*Temples.* Pinching pain in the lower portion of the temples,[2].—Boring pain in the temporal bone, extending into the zygoma,[2]. —Pressive headache in both temples,[1].—Stitches in the temples, with a contractive pain or twinges,[3].—*Vertex.* Pain in the top of the head, where there is a sensitive spot externally on stooping; it changes to the forehead,[3]. —Sharp stitches in the vertex, in the evening (second day),[3].—**Pain in the vertex, as if the skull had been split or torn asunder, so that she was obliged to hold the head with the hands from fear lest it should fall asunder, also at night, and especially in wet weather,*[3].—Unendurable throbbing pain and sticking in the vertex, as if the head would crack, when walking,[1].—*Parietals.* [80.] Tearing in the right side of the head,[1].—Frequent tearing in the right side of the head during the day,[1].—Painful heavy sensation in the whole occiput,[3].—Dull pressure in both parietal bones, near the vertex, in a small spot daily, incessant for several hours, mostly in the forenoon, especially caused by dust from dusty clothes, and much relieved in the open air,[1].—*Occiput.* Pressive headache in the occiput,[2].—Pressive pain in a small spot on the occiput,[1].—Pressure in the left side of the occiput, during rest and motion, frequently intermitting,[3].—Pressive headache in the neck, when writing,[1].—Stitches and *throbbing in the occiput,*[3].—Twitching tearings shoot back and forth in the left side of the occiput, in the evening,[3].—[90.] Painful tearing and sticking on the right side of the occiput, during rest and motion, in the evening,[3].—Splashing in the left half of the brain, when walking rapidly,[1].—Falling off of the hair (after eighteen days),[1].—Involuntary anxious tension and drawing up in the skin of the vertex,[1].—Severe tearing on the external parts of the head,[1].—The left side of the head externally is painful, as if suppurating,[1].—Severe itch-

ing in the scalp, so that she was obliged to scratch it till it bled, which,
however, did not relieve it,[3].

Eye.—Twitching of the right eye, with a feeling as if something were
moving in it which blinded her, with drawing downward in the upper lid;
after rubbing, it disappeared, but soon returned, leaving a sensitiveness to
touch in the margin of the upper lid,[3].—The eyes seem quite loose in their
sockets, and he does not have the power, with any exertion, to see distinctly, which makes him anxious,[1].—Weakness of the eyes,[1].—[100.]
Great weakness of the eyes, in the evening; she was unable to do anything
which employed vision,[1].—Unpleasant sensation in the left eye, as if something was in it which prevented vision; he was constantly obliged to wipe
it; together with extreme dilatation of the pupil and great farsightedness,
so that he was unable to see near objects distinctly,[1].—Sticking-burning
and watering of the eyes, after itching and rubbing them,[3].—Pressive pain
in the eyes, in the evening, by a light,[1].—Pressure and sensation of heaviness in the eyes, whence it extends to the forehead, to the vertex, and down
into the left ear (during menstruation),[3].—Stitching in the eyes,[1].—Itching
and pressure in the eyes, during the day,[1].—Biting-itching in the eyes, with
burning after rubbing,[3].—*Lids.* Twitching of the upper lid,[1].—Agglutination of the left eye, the whole forenoon,[3].—[110.] Smarting-burning in
the external canthus,[1].—Pressure in the external canthus (after seventy-
two hours),[1].—Pressive-sticking pain, extending from above downward,
over the left eye into the lid and upper half of the eyeball,[2].—Sticking and
biting in the left inner canthus, in the morning, after rising, relieved by
rubbing,[3].—Lachrymation, in the morning, on rising,[3].—*Vision.* Dimness before the eyes, as if she saw through a mist,[3].—The sight continued
obscure the whole day,[1].—Photophobia, in the evening,[1].—Objects upon
the street seem altered, for example, farther apart and brighter than usual,
as if the city were empty and deserted,[1].—Many small black and yellow
points are seen by candlelight, in regular rows, before the eyes,[1].—[120.]
A net seems to swim before the eyes,[1].—He saw frightful images, in the
evening, before going to sleep,[1].

Ears.—A kind of swelling of the periosteum behind the right ear, with
sticking in it, every evening after 7 o'clock,[1].—Burning in the right lobule
of the ear, like fire,[3].—Pinching in the ear, extending down into the pharynx,
on the left side, which makes swallowing difficult,[2].—Pinching pain within
the left ear,[2].—Drawing in the ear,[1].—Drawing in the external ear and in
the left cheek-bone,[1].—Stitches in the ears,[3].—Tearing in the right lobule of
the ear, and boring in the ear,[3].—[130.] Transient tearing in the left ear,[3].
—*Hearing.* The hearing is weak and dull,[1].—*The hearing is weak
and confused; the tones become commingled; he cannot tell from which side
they come, and it seems as though they came from another world,*[1].—Whistling
in the ear, on blowing the nose,[1].—Ringing in the ears, the whole night,[1].
—Ringing in the right ear, on going into the open air,[3].

Nose.—*Objective.* *The tip of the nose became red and painful to
touch,[1].—Red, cracked, burning, and tensive painful tip of the nose (during menses),[3].—Redness and swelling of the nose, which is internally sore,[1].
—Swelling of the nose, with pimples internally and externally, which form
a scurf that lasts a long time,[1].—[140.] Swelling of the nose and mouth,[1].
—Blisters in the right nostril,[3].—A tensive boil in the nostril,[3].—Stoppage
in the left nostril, in the forenoon (second and third days),[3].—Stopped
coryza; can get no air through the nose,[1].—Stopped coryza, in the forenoon,
lasting till evening (first day),[3].—Stopped coryza, in the morning, on wak-

ing, which disappears after rising,[3].—Frequent passage of mucus from the nose, with stopped coryza,[1].—Coryza, with rawness of the throat,[1].—*Coryza, catarrh, and scraping in the throat, especially in the evening and night, particularly when swallowing,[1].—[150.] Fluent coryza (tenth day),[1].—Fluent coryza of much watery mucus,[3].—*Fluent coryza, with loss of smell, yawning, and much sneezing,[3].—Excessive fluent coryza, for several hours, in the evening,[1].—*Nose-bleed, in the morning, when sitting, and in the afternoon,[1].—*Nose-bleed, preceded by pressure and confusion of the head,[4].—*Nose-bleed, in the morning, for several mornings, preceded by vertigo,[1].—Nose-bleed; a whole cupful of bright red blood,[4].—Nose-bleed, for a quarter of an hour, at night,[1].—Frequent blowing of blood from the nose,[1].—*Subjective.* [160.] A sensation in the nose as of commencing coryza, after eating, increased in the evening,[2].—Fine stitching in the side of the nose,[3].—Bruised pain above and in the root of the nose, also when touched,[3].

Face.—Yellowness of the face,[1].—Much heat and sweat in the face, during dinner,[1].—Transient tearing in the left malar bone, extending towards the temple,[3].—Tearing, frequently repeated, now in the upper, now in the lower jaw, on the right side of the face,[3].—The mouth is swollen,[1].—Swelling of both lips, with burning in them,[3].—The corners of the mouth are ulcerated, with burning pain,[1].—[170.] The lips are cracked,[1].—The lips bleed,[1].—Dryness of the lip, as from too great heat, in the morning,[3].

Mouth.—Teeth and Gums. Great looseness of the teeth, so that she is not able to chew the softest food without pain,[1].—Looseness of the teeth, with tearing in them, most severe in the evening, in bed,[1].—Looseness of the lower teeth, with pain in the gum,[1].—The upper and lower teeth are too long and loose,[1].—The teeth in the right upper row feel too long and loose, without pain, for several days,[3].—She frequently bites the inside of the cheek,[3].—Painful griping in the teeth of the left side, aggravated in the open air,[3].—[180.] Drawing back and forth in the teeth, even in the front teeth,[1].—Drawing in a left lower back tooth, at night, as often as she woke,[3].—Drawing in the teeth, with flushes of heat in the face,[1].—Suddenly, while eating bread, drawing and sticking pains in the nerves of the back teeth,[1].—Constant drawing in the left back teeth, especially in the afternoon,[1].—Tearing toothache, especially in the hollow teeth, even at night, disturbing sleep,[3].—Throbbing in the teeth, worse on pressing upon them and in the evening,[3].—Throbbing toothache from cold drinks, followed by looseness of the teeth,[1].—The nerves of the teeth are sensitive to touching the crowns of the teeth,[1].—A hollow tooth becomes sensitive, and feels prominent; it pains on biting, and still more in the evening, in bed, with much saliva in the mouth,[1].—[190.] The gum is pale and painful, as if suppurating,[3].—*The gum is red, swollen, and very painful,[1].—*Tongue.* Blisters on the tongue, which pain as if burnt,[1].—Small blisters on the margin of the tongue,[3].—Burning on the side of the tongue, as if it were sore,[3].—*Burning on the tip of the tongue, and rawness of the mouth,[3].—*General Mouth.* Blisters in the mouth, which cause burning,[1].—Mucus in the mouth, in the morning, disappearing after rising,[3].—Offensive breath, without noticing it himself,[1].—Offensive smell in the mouth,[1].—[200.] Dryness of the mouth and throat, without thirst, nearly the whole day (second and third days),[3].—The mouth and tongue seem immovable, with difficult stammering or very low speech (after few hours),[1].—*Saliva.* Flow of saliva during sleep,[1].—Frothy saliva,[1].—*Taste.* Sour taste in the mouth,[1].—Slimy sour taste, in the morning, after waking,[3].—Bitter sour taste in the mouth,[1].—*Bitterness in the mouth at times, also in the morning,[1]*

—*Bitter taste every morning,[1].—Bitter taste in the morning, disappearing after rising,[3].—[210.] Bitter foul taste in the mouth,[1].—Foul taste in the mouth, in the morning,[1].—Nauseous taste in the mouth,[3].

Throat.—*Much mucus in the throat, with frequent hawking and raising (after twenty-four hours),[1].—A feeling of mucus in the throat, in the morning, on waking, which compelled her to hawk a long time; it disappeared at noon,[3].—Acidity in the throat, not in the mouth,[1].—Pains in the throat, on swallowing, as if a blister were in it,[3].—*Burning sensation in the throat,[1].—Pressure in the throat, only when swallowing,[1].—Pressure in the throat, extending to the stomach,[1].—[220.] Pressure in the throat, with dryness of the tongue,[1].—Scraping-sticking in the throat,[1].—Sore throat, with ulcerative pain, when swallowing,[1].—Sore pain and burning, like heartburn, in the throat, extending to the stomach, worse towards evening, night, and morning, better after rising and after eating and drinking,[3].— *Raw sensation in the whole throat and œsophagus, extending to the pit of the stomach, not increased by swallowing,[1].—*Rawness of the throat, almost every morning, which disappears after breakfast,[3].—Scraping in the throat, with accumulation of saliva,[1].—Rising up into the œsophagus and into the throat, where it chokes and presses, with a raw sensation,[3].—Swelling of the parotid,[5].—The right parotid gland is swollen (second day),[1].

Stomach.—Appetite. [230.] Increased appetite (first, second, and ninth days,[1].—Unnatural hunger,[1].—After a large dinner, appetite returns in two hours, and again hunger towards evening, followed by thirst,[1].— Very great hunger, in the morning,[1].—Hunger indeed, but he does not relish his food,[1].—Longing for sour and refreshing things,[1].—Appetite for raw sauerkraut, loss of appetite for other things,[1].—Little appetite, but while eating, the appetite returns,[1].—The appetite soon disappears, while eating,[1]. —*No appetite, aversion to food,[4].—[240.] *Aversion to fat,[1].—Fat meat completely spoils his appetite,[1].—**Thirst.** Thirst, even in the morning, quite unusual (sixth day),[3].—Great thirst, especially for cold water, with dryness and heat in the throat,[1].—Aversion to cold drinks,[1].—**Eructations and Hiccough.** Frequent eructations,[2].—*Many eructations from the stomach,[1].—Empty eructations, every time after eating,[3].—Frequent empty eructations, which change to hiccough,[1].—Eructations like hiccough, during dinner,[3].—[250.] *Eructations tasting of food eaten a long time previous,[1].—Almost constant foul eructations,[3].—Foul fishy eructations,[1].—Inclination to waterbrash, with nausea in the stomach, at night,[3]. —An attack of waterbrash, with which salty water rises from the stomach and runs out of the mouth, with retching and a spasmodic sensation in the jaws, followed by violent empty eructations, with cold feet, and at last hiccough, lasting half an hour,[1].—*Heartburn rises up from the stomach,[1].— A scraping heartburn,[1].—**Nausea.** *Long-continued nausea, after eating meat, with qualmishness and many empty eructations,[1].—Nausea, and qualmishness in the stomach, in the morning, after rising, with heat, anxiety, and eructations of water in the mouth, with general weariness,[3].— Nausea, when he sits down, after walking much,[1].—[260.] With the dizzy feeling in the head, he was attacked by nausea, and a watery mist seemed to come suddenly before his eyes, twice repeated,[1].—Nausea and aversion to tobacco-smoking,[1].—**Stomach.** Gurgling in the stomach,[2].—Audible gurgling in the stomach, in the morning, on waking,[2].—Fulness in the stomach, soon after eating a little with good appetite,[1].—Constrictive cramp in the stomach,[1].—Boring pain in the stomach, as after fasting, which extends to the abdomen,[3].—Pressure in the stomach, even when fasting,[1].—

Pressure in the stomach, after eating,[1].—Severe pressure in the stomach, in the evening, after lying down in bed; she was obliged to press upon the epigastric region in order to relieve it (after sixteen hours),[1].—[**270.**] Short sudden pressive pain in the pit of the stomach, on deep inspiration,[1]. —Pressure in the stomach, chest, and sometimes in the abdomen,[1].—Pressure in the stomach, with heaviness and fulness, with inclination to water-brash,[3].—Frequent stitches in the stomach,[3].—Sharp stitches in the right side, near the pit of the stomach, even on inspiration, better when walking,[3]. —A bruised feeling in the pit of the stomach, as after a violent cough (after six days),[1].

Abdomen.—Hypochondria. Pressure in the liver, even when lying,[1].—Severe pressive pain in the liver, almost like cutting; the region is sore externally to touch,[1].—*Umbilicus and Flanks.* Griping in the umbilical region,[1].—A stitching-like pinching above the navel and in the pit of the stomach, every morning in bed, as from accumulation of flatulence; the passage of flatus, of stool, and of urine relieved it, though it also disappeared of itself and was less noticed when walking,[1].—[**280.**] Cutting in the right flank, when sitting, better when walking and on deep breathing,[3].—*General Abdomen.* * *Great distension in the abdomen,*[1]. —*The abdomen is always very much distended,*[1].—Great distension of the abdomen after a moderate dinner,[3].—Abdomen much distended during menstruation,[1].—Protrusion of the abdomen, here and there, like a hernia,[3]. —Fermenting in the intestines,[1].—Fermenting and gurgling in the abdomen,[1].—Motions in the abdomen, with ineffectual urging to stool,[3].—**Mo-tions in the distended abdomen, with passage of offensive flatus,**[3].—[**290.**] Moving of flatus, with a sensation as if something was moving about in the abdomen, as if it were torn and bruised,[1].—Audible rumbling in the abdomen,[2].—Audible rumbling, as from incarcerated flatus, which could find no outlet,[3].—Audible rumbling and grumbling in the colon, which rises up under the stomach and then passes down again,[2].—Frequent passage of offensive flatus, in the forenoon,[3].—Passage of much offensive flatus when walking after supper,[2].—* *Much trouble from flatulence,*[1].—Great weakness and pain in the intestines, as if they would be screwed together, after a stool (the second one in the same day),[1].—Qualmishness (in the abdomen) towards evening, with flushes of heat (tenth day),[1].—A heaviness which lies like a lump in the abdomen, even when fasting (for several days),[1].— [**300.**] Pain in the abdomen, as if diarrhœa would come on,[1].—Heat in the abdomen,[1].—Burning in the abdomen, when walking,[1].—Painful tension in the abdomen, with pain beneath the ribs on touch, as if there was a sore in it and the place was suppurating,[1].—Pinching in the right side of the upper abdomen, with stitches, when sitting,[3].—Sticking-pinching in the upper part of the abdomen every morning, mostly early, in bed,[1].—Severe griping in the abdomen, after a stool,[1].—Griping and uneasiness in the abdomen,[1].—Griping in the abdomen, about the navel, with a feeling as if a stool would follow,[3].—Feeling of constriction in the abdomen, when fasting, with a great sensation of emptiness, though without hunger and without appetite,[1].—[**310.**] Boring in the right side of the abdomen, immediately after eating,[1].—Digging and twisting in the upper part of the abdomen,[1].—Pressive pain in the left side of the abdomen,[1].—Cutting in the abdomen, in the forenoon,[1].—Partly cutting, partly sticking, in the abdomen; very sensitive, every day, and frequently returning through the day,[1]. —Severe cutting in the abdomen, with frequent urging to stool, and even tenesmus, without passing anything more than wind; from morning till noon,[3].—Tearing from the pudenda up into the abdomen, with the stool (twenty-second day),[1].—Pain as if ulcerating in the abdomen,[1].—*Hypogastrium and Iliac Regions.* Rumbling and grumbling in the right side of the lower abdomen, after drinking warm milk, now in the upper, now in the lower part, with ineffectual effort to pass flatus,[2].—Constriction deep in the lower abdomen,[1].—[320.] *Painful sensation in the right side of the lower abdomen, as if something would be squeezed through at that place,*[1].—Short cutting in the lower abdomen,[2].—*Tearing, transversely across the pubes, and then through the pudenda, as far as the anus* (after fourteen days),[1].—Pain in the lower portion of the abdomen, as if sore from coughing,[1].—*A feeling in the left groin, on sitting down, as if a large heavy body were lying there, relieved after pressure by passage of flatus,*[3].—Dragging in the groins at times, like a burning in strangury,[3].—Violent pressing in the groin, in the small of the back and in the legs, with ineffectual attempts at eructations, during menstruation, chilliness, and yawning,[4].—*Sticking in the groin, also at night, disturbing sleep and waking her,*[3].—Stitching pain in the groin, as from flatus, with a hard stool,[3].—Bruised pain and pressure in the crest of the left ilium, worse in the evening, so that she was obliged to bend double; on external pressure the part pained as if ulcerated,[3].

Rectum and Anus.—[330.] Gurgling in the rectum,[2].—*Severe burning in the rectum,* in the evening,[1].—Frequent pressing on the rectum, as for stool, but only flatus passed, and the pressure returned again immediately,[1].—Large hæmorrhoids appear with burning pain,[1].—*The hæmorrhoids swell very much, with a burning pain on walking,*[4].—*Sticky, odorless moisture oozes from the anus,*[1].—Painful contraction of the anus,[1].—*Burning in the anus,*[1].—Severe cutting in the hæmorrhoids during stool,[1].—A bowel protruded, and was painful on walking, on motion, and on touch,[1].— [340.] Sticking in the anus, as with needles, during stool,[2].—*Stitches in the anus, which is sore,*[1].—*Soreness of the anus, with moisture in it, the whole evening,*[1].—*Sticky, odorless moisture on the perineum, behind the scrotum,*[1].—Pinching-biting pain on the perineum,[1].—Frequent but ineffectual urging to stool, like oppression of the rectum,[2].—Frequent urging to stool, which is passed with great difficulty; is hard and streaked with blood,[3].— Much urging to stool; every time some stool is passed, though with great difficulty,[1].

Stool.—Diarrhœa, preceded by griping in the abdomen, with burning in the anus,[3].—Four stools during the day, preceded by pain in the abdomen,[1].—[350.] Stool at night, after midnight,[3].—Soft stool, with mucus like coagulated albumen,[1].—*Soft stool,* preceded by dragging in the pubis (after twenty-seven days),[3].—Soft, green stool, preceded and accompanied by pains in the abdomen,[3].—Liquid stools, followed by straining (seventh day),[3].—Scanty stool, hard and in small pieces (after twenty-four hours),[1].— Stool scanty and light-colored (at first),[3].—*Scanty, delayed stool,* for several days,[1].—Very hard stool, preceded by shivering in the head, as though dashed with cold water,[3].—The first part of the stool was hard and difficult to pass, with a feeling as though it were too little and there would be a little more, which the rectum had not power enough to evacuate,[1].—[360.] Hard crumbling stool, which is passed only with great exertion, as from an inactivity of the abdominal muscles, with oppression of the breath, in the evening,[3].—At first a hard, then a soft stool, with burning in the anus,[3].— *Passage of blood during the stool,*[1].—A portion of a tape-worm passed with a hard stool,[3].

Urinary Organs.—Bladder. Pain in the region of the kidneys, when walking,[3].—Severe pressive pain in the bladder, at night,[1].—Repeated sticking-picking in the region of the kidneys,[3].—*Urethra.* Burning in the urethra, after urinating,[1].—*Urine burns in the urethra, on urinating,[1]. —A spasmodic pain along the urethra, especially in its posterior portion, in the morning on waking, after an emission,[2].—*Micturition.* [370.] *While urinating, a burning sore pain in the urethra,[1].*—Sudden desire to urinate,[2].—Excessive desire to urinate; she is often obliged to hurry to pass water, and after urinating feels a voluptuous tickling in the urethra,[1]. —Urging to urinate after stool (the urine was very red), followed by weariness and early sleepiness without being able to sleep; after lying down she immediately jumped up again, had ringing in the ears, felt as if she would faint, and had a shaking chill,[1].—She urinates frequently without drinking much (first day),[3].—*Frequent passage of urine at night,[1].*—The urine passes on slight pressure, almost against his will (after sixteen days),[1].—Very profuse urinating; she was obliged to rise three times at night to urinate,[1].—Profuse discharge of urine, after a night-fever,[1].—Very profuse discharge of urine, after walking,[1].—[380.] Increased passage of urine, *with frequent urinating at night,* when she passed very much more than she had drunk,[3].—The passage of urine is much more forcible,[1]. —Diminished urine (after four days),[3].—Urine scanty,[1].—Urine scanty and hot at night; it burns on passing,[1].—The stream of urine is interrupted,[3].—*Urine.* Yellow urine with a speedy loose sediment (first day),[3]. —Turbid orange-colored urine,[1].—The urine is turbid even when passed, and soon deposits a turbid sediment (fourth day),[3].

Sexual Organs.—Male. The usual morning erection was wanting (second day),[3].—[390.] Complete relaxation of the genitals, and feeling of weakness in them,[1].—Itching on the genitals,[1].—Sticking on both sides of the scrotum,[1].—The sexual desire is wanting for a long time, even on provocation,[1].—Frequent emissions (the first days),[1].—Profuse emissions for three nights in succession; the like had not happened for years,[1].— Emission at 4 P.M. (fifth day),[3].—An emission (*the first after a very long time*), with a voluptuous dream, without an erection,[2].—*Female.* Leucorrhœa (after fourteen days),[1].—*Leucorrhœa which colors the linen yellow* (twenty-first day),[1].—[400.] Watery leucorrhœa when standing and walking,[3].—Drawing from the anus through the pudenda before the stool,[1].— Menstruation four days too early, preceded by headache,[1].—Menstruation four days too early, with pain in the sacrum and groins,[3].—*Menstruation more profuse than usual,[3].—*Menstruation scanty the first day, more copious than usual the second, the blood dark-colored* (eighth day),[1].—Menstruation not profuse, but lasting longer than usual, and only flowing in the morning,[1].—Menstruation shorter than usual and five days too late,[1].

Respiratory Organs.—Larynx, Trachea, and Bronchi. Pain in the air-passages, as after much coughing,[1].—*Rawness and hoarseness in the morning after rising,* with dry cough,[3].—[410.] Tickling in the trachea with cough, which was relieved after eating,[3].—*Voice.* *Hoarseness, worse in the evening,[1].*—After hoarseness during the day, she had loss of voice at night; awoke with coldness, swelling of the pit of the stomach, cough, difficult expiration, and anxious sweat; she was unable to get her breath,[1]. —*Cough and Expectoration.* Tickling cough,[1].—*Tickling cough, with constriction of the larynx and chest,[1].*—Hacking cough in the evening, especially in bed,[1].—Short hacking cough frequently from tickling in the larynx (first day),[3].—Cough, from dryness in the throat, in the morning;

as soon as mucus is expectorated it disappears,[1].—Suffocative cough in the evening an hour after going to sleep,[1].—Rough cough, with pain in the throat as if sore,[1].—[420.] Cough which impedes the breath,[1].—Dry cough day and night,[1].—*Severe dry cough in the morning on rising and nearly the whole day; it shakes the abdomen, as if everything would fall out; she is obliged to hold the bowels with the hands and sit down; loose râles in the chest until something is coughed up,[1].—Cough without expectoration, from tickling in the larynx, in the evening for three days,[3].—Dry cough only at night, when lying on the right side, for several nights,[3].—Cough, with greenish, purulent expectoration, arising from a small spot, an inch in size, in the right side of the chest,[4].—Cough with expectoration,[1].—Cough with purulent expectoration (after fourteen days),[4].—The former dry cough became loose (second day),[3].—Whitish-yellow mucous expectoration,[4].—[430.] Greenish purulent expectoration after dry cough,[4].—Thick greenish expectoration from a vomica, which formed in the right thorax,[4].—*Respiration.* Catching of the breath on inspiration, with oppression of the chest,[1].—Dyspnœa after eating,[1].—It seems as if the breath remained arrested in the chest,[4].—Fear of suffocation, in the evening, in bed, before going to sleep, lying with closed eyes; this only disappears after sitting up and opening the eyes; it prevented sleep the whole night, with mucus in throat,[1].

Chest.—Rattling and piping in the chest for an hour at a time, in the evening, in bed,[1].—Trembling in the chest, like crying,[1].—Anxiety in the chest, in the morning,[1].—Anxiety in the chest, after eating,[1].—[440.] Speedy fatigue in the chest and organs of mastication, while eating,[1].—Cold feeling in the chest (seventh day),[1].—Burning in the chest, more on the right side.[1].—*Burning in the chest, with pressive pain,[1].—Violent pain in the whole chest, as if it would burst, with sore pain in it,[3].—Constriction of the chest; the whole chest seems oppressed, or over-fatigued,[1].—Sudden constriction of the chest, as if she should breathe deeply,[3].—The chest seems contracted,[1].—Contraction of the chest, with suffocation, in the morning, in bed; she thought she would die, with stitches in the heart on speaking, and a sensation on moving the arm as though the heart and chest would be torn to pieces,[1].—Digging-pinching and tension in the upper part of the chest,[1].—[450.] Violent compression of the chest, with arrest of breathing, when sitting, in the morning,[3].—Oppression of the middle of the chest,[3].—Pain as of oppression in the middle of the chest, when touched and when not, with oppression of breathing, for quarter of an hour,[3].—Painful twisting in and beneath the chest,[1].—Tearing stitches from the pit of the stomach into the chest, on rising after stooping,[3].—Painful nodules in the breasts,[5].—Sticking pain in the lower portion of the female breast, which was aggravated by pressing upon it, and which arrested breathing,[3]. —*Front.* Stitches in the sternum, as with knives, during motion,[1].— *Sides.* Stitches in the side from coughing,[4].—The pain in the side ceases after a dry cough, and afterwards she is obliged to cough frequently without its recurring,[4].—[460.] Stitches in the right cavity of the chest,[4].— Stitches in the right side of the chest on every breath, as if something sore was there,[4].—Stitching below the right breast, so that she could not sit still, when sitting and writing; it disappeared after rising,[1].—Stitches in the lower portion of the right side of the chest, extending into the axilla,[3].— Stitches, with oppression of breathing, now in the lower portion of the left chest, now in the right shoulder-joint, now in the right flank, with some dry cough, which increased the pain, in the morning,[3].—Stitches in the upper part of the left side of the chest, and sometimes also in the right side,[4].—Sharp (burning) stitches in the left side of the chest, even when sitting,[3].—Pressive stitches under the left ribs,[1].

Heart and Pulse.—Pressure of the heart, almost like pinching,[1].—Great palpitation; every beat is felt in the head,[1].—[470.] Great palpitation, in the morning on waking; she was obliged to lie quite still without opening the eyes and without speaking,[1].—Palpitation of the heart in the evening, without anxiety (after twenty-four days),[1].—Palpitation after breakfast, at other times after eating,[1].—Great palpitation, when singing in church,[1].

Neck and Back.—Neck. A feeling in the neck as if the skin on a small spot were raised up,[3].—Stiffness in the neck,[1].—Stiffness in the left side of the neck,[1].—Tension in the neck,[1].—Swelling of the cervical glands,[1].—*Back.* The back is painful on the left side, so that she cannot lie upon it, for three nights in succession,[3].—*Dorsal.* [480.] Sticking tension in the right shoulder-blade,[3].—Painful tension between the shoulder-blades, relieved by rubbing,[3].—Pressing pain in the back between the shoulder-blades, as if she had been hurt or sprained, with a similar pain in the forepart of the chest on moving the arm,[1].—Stitches between the shoulder-blades,[3].—*Lumbar.* Alternating stitches in the back above the right hip,[1].—Stiffness in the small of the back,[1].—Pain in the small of the back when sitting, as if menstruation would appear,[3].—*Drawing pain in the small of the back, and a feeling as if it were broken, when walking, standing, and lying,[1].—*Sharp drawing across the small of the back, very sensitive to every step,[1].—*Pressive pain in the small of the back,[1].—[490.] Severe pains in the small of the back,[1].—Stitches just above the small of the back on deep breathing,[1].—A stitch in the small of the back, extending down into the thigh with every breath,[1].—Violent pain in the loins if she rises after sitting some time,[1].—*Sacral.* Pain in the lower portion of the back,[1].—Pain as from an ulcer under the skin, on the lowest end of the spine, for the most part only when sitting and lying,[1].—*Pain in the sacrum during stool,* with distension of the abdomen, extending up into the chest,[3].—A sharp stitch in the sacrum,[1].—*Pain in the coccyx; on touching the part it became burning,[1].—[500.] Cutting-drawing from the anus through the coccyx between the stools,[1].—*Dragging bruised pain in the coccyx,[1].—Single jerks in the coccyx towards the bladder, which compelled her to urinate,[1].

Extremities in General.—An internal trembling of the limbs, and involuntary twitching of the knees, legs, and feet, on going to sleep in the evening; they moved visibly, and he was obliged to draw them up,[1].—Cracking in the joints,[1].—Much pain in the joints at night,[1].—The joints feel as if broken,[1].—The joints are easily sprained,[1].—Frequent heaviness of all the limbs,[1].—Heaviness in all the limbs in the morning,[1].—[510.] Heaviness, and trembling of the legs and arms,[1].—Frequent sensation as if the hands and feet would go to sleep,[3].—At one time the right arm goes to sleep, at another the right foot, in the evening, in bed,[3].—Numb sensation in all the limbs, especially also in the head,[1].—Pain, when lying, in the ligaments of the elbows and knees,[1].—Pinching pain here and there in the limbs,[1].—Tearing-drawing pain in the fingers and toes,[1].—Pain, as from the pressure of a finger on the arms and limbs,[1].—*Bruised sensation in all the limbs,* especially on motion,[1].

Superior Extremities.—The arm goes to sleep, when resting upon it, and the leg when riding it over the other,[1].—[520.] A digging, extending down the arms, as if it were burrowing in the bone, less perceptible if she lies upon the arm,[1].—Drawing pain in the arms and hands,[1].—*Shoulder.* The shoulders are heavy and tired,[1].—On walking, the shoulders and chest seem oppressed and loaded,[1].—Tearing in the shoulder (disappearing on motion and rubbing),[3].—Much moisture in the axillæ,[1].—*Arm.* Tearing pain in the bone of the right upper arm, towards the elbow,[3].—Tearing in the middle of the right upper arm, after midnight, when lying upon that side; she was unable to sleep on account of the pain,[3].—Severe tearing in the right upper arm, on raising the arm,[1].—*Elbow.* Burning and twing-ing pain in the right elbow, in the evening,[3].—[530.] Sticking pain below the bend of the left elbow, extending to the palm,[3].—Drawing-sticking in the tip of the elbow; the skin is painful, as if sore on slight touch, but not at all when grasped tightly,[1].—*Forearm.* Burning and stinging in the left forearm, frequently repeated, and sometimes extending into the shoulder, only transiently relieved by rubbing,[3].—Tensive pain in the wrist on mov-ing it,[1].—Frequent painful boring in the condyles of the wrists,[1].—*The wrist pains as if sprained,*[1].—*Hand.* The hands go to sleep, daily,[1].—The hands go to sleep during rest,[1].—Numbness in the left hand, in the morn-ing, in bed; it disappears after rising,[1].—Stitches, as with needles, in the left palm and also in the ball of the right hand,[3].—[540.] Drawing stitches in the outer margin of the hand, where the skin is painful on slight touch as if sore, but not at all on pinching it,[1].—Tearing in the hands,[1].—*Fingers.* Chilblains on the little finger,[1].—The fingers go to sleep, after-wards the whole hand goes to sleep,[1].—The middle finger-joints are painful on motion,[1].—Tension in the first joint of the middle finger, on motion,[1].—Stitches in the fingers,[3].—Stitches in the tips of the fingers,[3].—Tearing on the back of the fingers, and in the bones, disappearing on rubbing,[3].

Inferior Extremities.—[550.] The gait is tottering, as if caused by some external power,[1].—The limbs cannot be stretched out on account of tension and contraction in the groin,[1].—The right leg as far as the toes goes to sleep at night, after lying down, on lying on that side, with a feel-ing as if the leg were longer than natural,[3].—Stiffness of the limbs, after sitting,[1].—*Hip.* Pinching in the right hip, when walking,[1].—*Stitches in the left hip, when sitting,*[1].—*Thigh.* Great weariness in the thighs, before and during menstruation,[3].—Boring and drawing in the upper part of the right thigh-bone, after a restless night,[1].—Cramp in the thighs and legs at night,[1].—Drawing and tearing in the muscles of the thighs,[1].—[560.] Fine, burning, transient stitches, here and there, in the thighs and small of the back, the whole day,[3].—Severe tearing stitches in the middle of the right thigh on the inner side, when standing, in the evening,[3].—Tearing in the thighs below both hips from morning till evening, though worse in the fore-noon and when sitting,[3].—Tearing in the outer side of the thigh at night; it disappeared on rising,[1].—Painful tearing while standing, as if in the marrow of the left thigh; disappears while sitting (during menstruation),[3].—Twitching pain in the thighs,[1].—*Knee.* A sensation in the bend of the right knee on walking, as if the tendons were too short; it disappears dur-ing sitting,[3].—Pain, as if screwed together, in the right knee, when stand-ing, with a sensation as if the leg would be bent together, in the evening,[3].—Cramp in the right knee, when walking,[1].—Painless drawing in the bend of the right knee; it pains when stretched out; disappears after long-con-tinued motion,[3].—[570.] Sensitive stitches in the hollow of the left knee, while walking,[2].—Tearing in the knee at night, which disappeared on ris-ing,[1].—Tearing and crawling stitches in the right knee, that after rubbing extend down into the tibia, which is only transiently relieved by rubbing,[3].

—Tearing above the right knee, also above the left, as if in the bone, which is only transiently relieved by rubbing,[3]—Sore pain in the knee on bending it, day and night,[1]—Sore pain in the right knee, worse when walking,[1] —**Leg.** *The legs as far as the calves go to sleep, during the day,*[1]—Sudden pain at night, on waking and turning the leg in bed, as if the legs were broken, after which the leg was as heavy as lead,[1]—* Cramp in the forepart of the lower leg near the tibia, when walking,*[1]—Painless drawing up the left leg at night,[1]—[580.] Painful stitches in the right leg, when rising up after kneeling; they shoot through the whole body and make her start,[3]—Tearing in the right leg, especially in the knee and ankle,[1]—Tearing in the lower part of the left tibia, and also on the outer surface of the right leg, and afterwards in the great toes,[3]—Pain in the tibiæ at night, which had disappeared in the morning on waking,[1]—Jerklike drawing in the tibia,[2]—Pressure in the tibia, while walking,[1]—Bruised pain in the tibia, while walking; the pain was intermitting, with tension in the calves,[1]—Painful cramp in the calves after walking,[1]—* Painful tension in the calves, when walking,*[1]—Cramp in the calves, in the morning, for several days,[1]—[590.] Cramp in the calves disturbed the quiet sleep at night,[1]—Painful contraction of the tendo Achillis, frequently repeated, in the evening (third day),[3]— **Ankle.** Loss of power in the ankle, while walking, so that it turned over,[1]—A feeling of stiffness in the ankle, in the morning, on rising,[1]—Inflammatory swelling of the feet, which begins on one toe,[1]—Swelling and tension of the feet,[3]—The feet give out while walking, as from weakness in the joints,[1]—*Very cold feet* from 9 A.M. till 3 P.M.,[1]—The feet burn while walking, and swell while sitting,[1]—A stitchlike crawling in the feet, as though going to sleep, in the morning,[1]—[600.] Tension in the back of the foot, as if the tendons were too short; the next day the place is sore and sensitive to touch,[3]—Sharp stitches penetrating the left sole,[3]—Drawing and tearing in the tendons of the right heel,[3]—Pain, as of suppuration, in the heels,[1]—**Toes.** Swelling of the ball of the great toe in the morning; there is much heat in it, and it pains as if it had been frozen and ulcerated,[1]—Violent cutting-burning in the toes, especially in the little toes,[1]—Frequent cramp in the toes during the day; while walking in an uneven path it seems as if they would give out,[1]—Pain, as if sprained, in the last toe-joints, while walking and on every motion,[1]—Tearing in the right great toe,[3]—It becomes easily sore between the toes,[1]—[610.] *Corns appear, which are painful to touch,*[1]—Stinging in a corn, for many days,[1].

General Symptoms.—Spasm; vertigo; she screamed, opened the mouth, and bent backwards and to the right side, and threw up the hands,[4]. —She came near falling, opened the mouth, and raised her eyes, with heat over the whole body, sweat on the face, and whining mood,[4]—Indolence, and disinclination for mental or physical labor, the whole day,[1]—He becomes tired from eating,[1]—Tired and sleepy, after walking,[1]—Walking is very fatiguing; she soon became weary, especially in the hypochondrium,[1]. —Very much fatigued, on waking in the morning, after a good sleep,[1]— In the morning on rising, very weary, with such sadness that she had to cry,[1]—[620.] He eats and drinks, but still becomes weaker every day,[4]— Weak and bruised, especially in the lower limbs, in the morning,[3]—General weakness in the forenoon, even to sinking down,[1]—*After the appearance of the menses, such great weakness that she could scarcely speak, with yawning and stretching,*[1]—* Weakness and want of energy of the body, with confusion of the head,*[1]—Great prostration in the whole body, at night, as if bruised,[3]—Great exhaustion in body and mind after an emission, and very apprehensive that something evil would happen,[1].—He is easily exhausted, while walking,[1].—Uneasiness and hastiness,[1].—On account of anxiety he was obliged to move constantly back and forth on his chair,[1].—[630.] Less sensitive than usual to the cold winter air (secondary effect),[1].—Pressive pain in the joints and muscles,[1].—Stitches in the scar of a burn,[1].—Throbbing and biting in the whole body, worse in the evening,[1].—All the joints of the body feel bruised, and pulled apart, and powerless,[1].

Skin.—*Eruptions*. Coppery eruption on the face,[5].—Hard, elevated, itching spots across the forearm near the wrist,[3].—Hard pimples upon the forehead,[1].—*A large number of pimples on the face*, without sensation,[1].—*Eruption, like red spots, on the cheeks*,[1].—[640.] Small red pimples on the chin, with yellowish tips,[3].—Several small pimples on the wrist, on the neck, and on the back of the foot, which itch severely, with burning-itching after scratching; they disappear after three days,[3].—White itching pimples on the backs of the hands, which, after scratching, burn and become red,[3].—*Moist.* Blisters on the lips,[1].—He becomes easily excoriated on the nates from riding, after which large blisters appear,[1].—*Pustular.* Eruption of small pustules on the left cheek and forehead,[3].—A boil in the anus (after sixteen days),[1].—*Sensations.* Biting in the whole body like flea-bites, which always change to another place after scratching,[3].—The skin of the face is painful, especially on the cheeks, and about the mouth and chin (after shaving),[2].—Dryness and desquamation of the skin on the tip of the nose,[3].—[650.] Unpleasant tension of the skin of the limbs, with a feeling of burning or icy coldness,[1].—Itching spread over the whole body, especially in the evening, in bed,[1].—Itching in the upper lid, which disappears on scratching,[3].—Itching on the tip of the nose, not relieved by scratching,[3].—Itching on the inner surface of the right forearm, where, after three days, an itching eruption appears, which covers a large surface,[3].—Itching on the backs of the hands and fingers, for many days,[1].—Itching in the warts of the fingers,[1].—Severe itching in the toes, which had been frozen (after twenty-four days),[1].

Sleep and Dreams.—*Sleepiness*. *Sleepiness, with frequent yawning, the whole forenoon*,[3].—Sleepiness, with photophobia, in the evening (first days),[1].—[660.] He seems as if in a slumber the whole day, and on account of it, indolent, hard of hearing, with obscured vision, fretful and gloomy,[1].—*Sleeplessness.* He was unable to sleep at night on account of heat and restlessness,[1].—She tossed about the whole night, anxious and restless, without finding rest, with frequent waking,[3].—She was unable to sleep in the evening, and had generally only very light sleep,[3].—Was unable to sleep at night until 5 A.M., and was refreshed after waking from a two hours' sleep,[1].—Very restless sleep, with frequent waking,[1].—Very restless at night; could find no quiet place in the bed,[1].—Restless night; sleep had left by 2½ A.M., on account of internal uneasiness,[1].—Very uneasy sleep; he was very much excited and was unable to sleep before 2 o'clock,[1].—Starting up on going to sleep as if she would fall,[1].—[670.] Frequent starting up on falling asleep in the evening,[3].—Loud talking in the sleep,[3].—Groaning in the sleep,[3].—Crying at night in the sleep and sobbing on waking,[1].—*Dreams.* Sleep full of vivid fancies,[1].—Very vivid dreams at night,[2].—Vivid dreams about scientific subjects; in his thoughts he made literary compositions and spoke aloud,[2].—Vivid frightful dreams, for seven nights in succession,[1].—Very fanciful and confused dreams at night, so that he scarcely slept at all,[1].—Anxious dreams at night with screaming and

crying, followed by sad and then by voluptuous dreams, with emissions,[1].—
[680.] Dreams of murders,[3].

Fever.—Chilliness. Shivering, with thirst, followed by very violent dry heat, so that she believed that fiery sparks were darting before her
eyes, every other day towards evening, followed by a little sweat at night,[4].
—Shivering, after a stool, in the evening,[3].—Chilliness for a long time after
dinner,[3].— *Great chilliness during the day,*[1].—During the febrile stage she
could not bear being uncovered, because she immediately became chilly,[3].
—Always chilly, with ice-cold feet,[3].—He became very chilly when a little
air entered the room,[3].—Chill in the evening, without thirst, followed by
heat after lying down,[3].—A chill and cold creepings in the afternoon and
trembling as from within outward, without thirst, for three hours, followed
by some thirst, burning in the skin of the whole body, and in the eyes,[1].—
[690.] Chill in the evening in bed, followed by sweat during sleep,[1].—
Chill with goose-flesh from 5 till 8 in the evening, afterwards at 11 P.M.,
waking with profuse sweat, lasting till 2 o'clock, during which she could
not tolerate the bed covering,[3].—Chill in the whole body at 9 P.M., followed
after lying down by heat, during which she fell asleep; she was, however,
frequently awakened by thirst; sweat towards morning,[3].—*A febrile chill
awoke her at night in bed,*[1].—Chill while in bed (first day),[1].—Internal chill
on beginning to eat,[1].—He was scarcely able to get warm,[1].—Shivering
down the back, which seems to commence in the chest, every afternoon
(after four weeks),[4].—Cold limbs during the day,[1].—Cold hands and feet
in the evening,[1].—[700.] Cold feet while walking, in the forenoon,[1].—
Very cold feet in the evening when she went to bed (after ten hours),[1].—
Extremely cold feet, also in the evening, long after going to bed,[1].—*Heat.*
Frequently rising heat, with redness and burning of the cheeks, in the evening,[3].—Heat at night, with moisture of the skin,[1].—Heat and thirst at
night, without severe chill and without being followed by sweat,[3].—Anxious
heat before menstruation,[1].—Easily heated the whole day,[1].—Orgasm of
blood without heat,[1].—Heat in the face and head, in the afternoon,[1].—
[710.] At night in bed the head and upper part of the body were hot, but the
limbs were cold, and only gradually became warm towards morning,[3].—
Frequent flushes of heat in the cheeks, with redness,[1].—Burning heat in
the left hand in the evening, as he went from the room into the open air and
sat down,[3].—Troublesome heat in the palms, in the morning,[1].—Very hot
feet,[1].—*Sweat.* Sweat in the morning after waking (second day),[3].—He
breaks out into an excessive sweat as soon as he closes the eyes,[4].—*Profuse night-sweat,*[1].—Exhausting night-sweat,[4].—*Offensive night-sweat,*[4].—
[720.] Sweat when eating,[1].—Sweat when eating and when walking,[1].—Much
sweat while walking in the open air,[1].—Profuse sweat when walking and
when eating warm food,[1].—*Sweat, which colors the linen yellow,*[1].—Sweat on
the head at night,[1].—Sweat in the hollows of the knees, with swelling of
the fingers, on waking after midnight,[1].—Profuse sweat of the feet,[1].

Conditions.—Aggravation.—(*Morning*), On waking, melancholy,
etc.; felt abandoned, etc.; on waking, fretful; confusion, etc.; vertigo,
etc.; on rising, vertigo, etc., returned; *heaviness in head,* etc.; on waking,
headache; after rising, headache in forehead; after rising, sticking, etc., in
inner canthus; on rising, lachrymation; on waking, stopped coryza; *when
sitting, nose-bleed;* nose-bleed; dryness of lip; mucus in mouth; after waking, sour taste; *bitter taste;* foul taste; on waking, feeling of mucus in
throat; hunger; after rising, nausea, etc.; on waking, gurgling in stomach;
in bed, pinching above navel; mostly early, in bed, pinching in upper ab-

domen; pain along urethra; *after rising, rawness, etc., in larynx;* cough; anxiety in chest; in bed, contraction of chest, etc.; when sitting, compression of the chest; stitches, etc., in left chest; on waking, palpitation; heaviness in limbs; cramp in calves; on rising, feeling of stiffness in ankle; crawling in the feet; swelling of ball of toe; weak, etc.; heat in the palms. —(*Forenoon*), Stupid, etc.; heat, etc., in forehead; pressure in parietal bones; agglutination of left eye; stoppage in left nostril; stopped coryza; passage of flatus; cutting in abdomen; tearing in thighs; general weakness; sleepiness, etc.; while walking, cold feet.—(*Afternoon*), Depressed, etc.; apprehension, etc.; nose-bleed; drawing in back teeth; 9 A.M. to 3 P.M., cold feet; chill, etc.; heat in face, etc.—(*Toward evening*), Qualmishness in abdomen; every other day, shivering, etc.—(*Evening*), Anxious, etc.; frightened; about 7 o'clock, vertigo, etc.; in bed, heat in head; stitches in vertex; tearings in the occiput; tearing, etc., on side of occiput; weakness of the eyes; by a light, pressive pain in eyes; photophobia; before going to sleep, saw frightful images; after 7 o'clock, swelling of periosteum behind ear; caries, etc.; fluent coryza; sensation in nose; in bed, looseness of teeth, etc.; throbbing in the teeth; in bed, tooth pains; after lying down in bed, pressure in stomach; *burning in rectum;* soreness of anus; hard stool, etc.; hoarseness; especially in bed, hacking cough; after going to sleep, cough; in bed, fear of suffocation; in bed, rattling, etc., in chest; palpitation of the heart; trembling of the limbs; in bed, right arm goes to sleep, etc.; when standing, stitches in middle of thigh; when standing, pain in knee; contraction of tendo Achillis; throbbing, etc., on whole body; in bed, itching over whole body; sleepiness, etc.; restlessness; after stool, shivering; chill, etc.; in bed, chill, etc.; 5 to 8 o'clock, chill; 9 o'clock, chill in whole body, etc.; cold hands, etc.; on going to bed, *cold feet;* heat; heat in hands.—(*Night*), Anxiety, etc.; heaviness in head, etc.; pain in head, etc.; ringing in ears; coryza, etc.; nose-bleed; as often as she waked, drawing in the teeth; inclination to waterbrash; pain in bladder; *frequent passage of urine;* urine scanty, etc.; when lying on right side, *dry cough;* back painful; after lying down, right leg goes to sleep; cramp in thighs, etc.; tearing in outer side of thigh; tearing in knee; drawing up left leg; pain in tibiæ; cramp in calves; prostration; *febrile chill;* heat; heat, etc.; in bed, head hot, etc.; *sweat;* offensive sweat; sweat on the head.—(*After midnight*), Tearing in right upper arm; on waking, sweat in hollows of knees.—(*Open air*), Ringing in ear; griping in teeth.—(*On blowing nose*), Whistling in ear.—(*Breathing*), Stitch in small of back.— (*Deep breathing*), Stitch above small of back.—(*Cold drinks*), Throbbing toothache.—(*During dinner*), Heat, etc., in face; eructations.—(*After dinner*), Chilliness.—(*Dust from dusty clothes*), Pressure in parietal bones.—(*On beginning to eat*), Internal chill.—(*While eating*), Fatigue in chest, etc.; sweat.—(*After eating*), Sensation in the nose; empty eructations; pressure in stomach; immediately, boring in right abdomen; dyspnœa; anxiety in chest; palpitation; anxiety, etc.—(*After an emission*), Exhaustion.—(*Lying*), Pain on end of spine; pain in ligaments of elbows, etc.—(*Before menstruation*), Anxious heat.—(*During menstruation*), Abdomen distended; pressing in groin, etc.—(*After warm milk*), Rumbling, etc., in lower abdomen.— (*During motion*), Stitches in sternum; bruised sensation in loins; fingerjoints painful; tension in finger; pain in toe-joint.—(*While moving head*), Stupefaction; brain feels loose.—(*Pressure*), Throbbing in teeth; pain in female breast.—(*During rest*), Hands go to sleep.—(*Rising after kneeling*), Stitches in right leg.—(*Rising after sitting*), Pain in loins.—(*On rising after stooping*), *Vertigo;* stitches into chest.—(*When singing*), In church, palpitation.—(*When sitting*), Vertigo; cutting in right flank; pinching in abdomen, etc.; pain in small of back; pain on end of spine; *stitches in hip;* tearing in thighs.—(*When sitting and writing*), Stitching below the right breast.—(*After sitting*), Stiffness of the limbs.—(*During sleep*), Flow of saliva.—(*While spinning*), Headache in forehead.—(*While standing*), Tearing in right thigh.—(*During stool*), Cutting in hæmorrhoids; sticking in anus; *pain in sacrum.*—(*On stooping*), Heaviness in forehead.—(*After supper*), When walking, passage of flatus.—(*When swallowing*), *Pressure in throat.*—(*Walking*), Stupefaction; throbbing pain, etc., in vertex; burning in abdomen; pain in region of kidneys; profuse urine; shoulders, etc., seem oppressed; pinching in hip; sensation in knee; cramp in knee; stitches in knee; pain in right knee; pressure in tibia; bruised pain in tibia; *tension in calves;* loss of power in ankle; sweat.—(*When walking fast*), Splashing in brain.—(*After walking*), Profuse urine; pain in calves.—(*In wet weather*), *Pain in vertex.*—(*When writing*), Headache in neck.

Amelioration.—(*Morning*), Anxiety, etc.—(*Open air*), Headache in forehead; pressure in parietal bones.—(*During dinner*), All symptoms of forenoon disappeared.—(*Eating and drinking*), Pain in throat.—(*After eating*), Tickling in trachea.—(*Lying upon arm*), Digging down arms.—(*Motion*), Tearing in shoulder.—(*Pressure with hands*), Tearing, etc., in head.—(*Rising after sitting*), Pain in loins.—(*After rising*), Pain in throat.—(*Rubbing*), Sticking, etc., in left canthus; tension between shoulder-blades; tearing in shoulder.—(*Walking*), Stitches in right side; pinching above navel; cutting in right flank.

CARBO VEGETABILIS.

Preparation. Triturations of any well-prepared charcoal (Hahnemann used charcoal from birch for his own provings; some of the other provings were made with charcoal from the red beech).

Authorities. 1, Hahnemann, Chr. K., 3; 2, Adams, ibid.; 3, Von Gersdorff, ibid.; 4, Caspari, ibid.

Mind.—Emotional. Very much excited in the evening, with distended veins,[1].—Immoderately jovial, though easily put out of humor,[2].—Sensitive weeping mood,[1].—Great weeping, in which he wished to shoot himself,[1].—He became lachrymose; everything frightened him, and he seemed to despair,[1].—She feels unhappy, with very little pain,[1].—She desired death, she felt so unhappy,[1].—*Anxiety, as if oppressed, for several days,*[1].—Trembling anxiety in the morning on waking,[1].—[10.] Inexpressible anxiety every afternoon from four to six,[1].—Increasing anxiety for several hours in the evening, with heat in the face,[1].—Anxiety in the evening after lying down, as from oppression of the chest, with heat in the head, heat in the hands, and sweat on the forehead; she was unable to remain in bed on account of a sensation as if the heart would be pressed downward; objects about her seem to become constantly narrower and smaller, and when the room was dark horrible visions passed before her sight,[1].—*In the evening after lying down he was attacked with anxiety, so that he could scarcely remain lying* (after nineteen days),[1].—Anxiety during and after eating,[1]—Anxiety after a stool, with sensation of trembling and involuntary movements,[1].—Great anxiety and heat with the pains,[1].—Anxiety as in fever; the hands become cold and she trembles,[1].—Discouraged and frightened,[1].

—Very sensitive and morose (after four hours),[3].—[20.] Sensitive, easily irritated mood, which was easily excited to foolish mirth; when laughing the muscles of the arms and hands became relaxed,[3].—Out of humor after eating,[2].— *Great irritability*,[1].—Violent irritable mood,[1].—Very irritable through the day, inclined to vexation,[1].—Exceedingly irritable; she seems to be overhurried in her business,[1].—Very irritable and out of humor; he cried easily over sad events, and just as easily laughed over the slightest trifles till the tears came to his eyes,[1].—Irritable and out of humor, with mental exhaustion (after ten hours),[4].—Irritability and sensitiveness,[2].—Peevishly irritable the whole day (second day),[1].—[30.] *Very peevish, irritable, and inclined to anger*,[1].—Peevish, impatient, desperate; he would like to shoot himself,[1].—Peevish irritability, with confusion of the head,[3].—Impatience,[1].— *Violent and irritable*, in the forenoon,[1].—Involuntary outbreaks of anger (after thirty-six hours),[1].—Indifferent, not interested in anything,[2].—*Indifference; he heard everything without feeling pleasantly or unpleasantly about it, and without thinking of it*,[1].—Music, of which he is fond, does not interest him the whole day,[2].—***Intellectual.*** Mental freedom, lightness, and general well feeling (curative action after great confusion of the whole head, as with a coryza, and general heaviness of the limbs and body), (after four hours),[4].—[40.] *Ideas flow slowly;* they constantly turn about one object, with a sensation as if the head were tightly bound,[2].— *Want of memory, periodic*,[1].—Sudden loss of memory; he could not even recollect what he had just spoken or what had just been told him,[2].

Head.—Confusion and Vertigo. *Confusion of the head, which makes thinking difficult*,[1].—Confusion of the head for several days, without pain,[1].—*Great confusion in the head, in the morning immediately after rising; he was unable to think easily, and was obliged to make a great exertion, as of rousing himself from a dream; after lying down again it disappeared*,[3].—Confusion of the head in the evening after walking (after nineteen hours),[1].—Confusion of the head after dinner,[4].—Confusion in the head, with pressure in the forehead,[1].—* *Vertigo, so that he was obliged to hold on to something* (after fifteen days),[1].—[50.] An attack of vertigo in the forenoon, with nausea and obscuration of vision, ringing in the ears, trembling, warm sweat over the whole body, which stood in drops on the forehead; shortly before this attack a few drops of nose-bleed,[1].—Vertigo on the slightest motion,[1].—Vertigo on sudden motion of the head,[1].—Vertigo only when sitting, as though the head reeled to and fro,[1].—* *Vertigo when stooping, as though the head reeled to and fro*,[1].—Vertigo on stooping, on turning in bed, and on gargling,[1].—Vertigo after waking from sleep,[1].—Vertigo and staggering when walking,[1].—Vertigo when walking or sitting (fourth day),[1].—Paroxysm as follows: In looking out of the window he was suddenly attacked by a sickening vertigo; he fell down in consequence and lay for several minutes, and when he recovered consciousness it seemed as if he had lain in a deep sleep from which he could scarcely arouse himself; after waking, nausea, which obliged him to lie down for two hours, and which returned on rising; after this he was extremely lachrymose and despondent (after six days),[1].—[60.] Dizzy, befogged (third day),[1].—Dizzy in the evening after sleeping while sitting, with trembling and quivering of the whole body and feeling of faintness on rising from sitting, which, even after lying down, lasted a quarter of an hour,[1].—Dizziness in the head, as after intoxication, spreading forward from the occiput, worse in the evening, and involving the whole head, with aggravation on walking,[2].— *Whirling in the head* the whole day,[1].—***Sensations.*** Buzzing in the head, as from bees,[1].

—Dulness of the head after waking from the midday nap,[2].—*Heaviness of the head,[1].—*The head feels as heavy as lead,[1].—At night after falling asleep he awoke several times with a sensation as if blood rushed to the head, with bristling of the hairs, anxiety, accompanied by shivering and a sensation as if some one stroked the body with the hand, and a kind of formication of the skin on every movement in bed; together with such sensitive and acute hearing that the slightest noises re-echoed in the ear,[1].—Rush of blood to the head,[1].—[70.] Rush of blood to the head, with hot forehead and confusion of the head,[1].—Great rush of blood to the head, with confusion of the head and hot forehead (after six hours),[4].—Headache, as in the beginning of coryza,[1].—Severe headache for five days; on stooping it seems to press outward in the occiput and forehead,[1].—Severe headache, which contracts the eyes, during menstruation,[1].—Headache at night,[1].—Headache after eating,[1].—Headache from sudden change from warmth to cold,[1].—Headache, which rises from the stomach into the head and destroys her senses for a short time,[1].—Burning and violent pressing headache, evenings, in bed, especially on the vertex, and extending forward to the forehead,[3].—[80.] Pain in the head, as if it were too full,[1].—Tension in the brain, more like a confusion than a pain,[1].—Spasmodic tension of the brain,[1]. —Contracting pain in the head, especially on motion,[1].—*Headache, as from contraction of the scalp,[1].—Headache, as from contraction of the scalp, especially after supper,[2].—Compressive headache,[1].—Drawing, affecting the whole head, arising from the occiput (after half an hour),[4].—Drawing headache here and there, especially in the forehead, extending to just above the root of the nose,[3].—Dull headache, with heaviness in the forehead,[3].— [90.] Pressive pain in different places in the head in slight attacks, which soon passed off and seemed to be associated with flatulence (after forty-eight hours),[4].—Paroxysmal pressure and drawings in the head,[1].—Sticking headache in the evening, in bed, extending into the occiput (after sixteen hours),[1].—Stitches here and there extending into the head, with general painfulness of the surface of the brain,[1].—*When coughing, painful stitches through the head,[1].—Tearing pain in the head (after twenty-four hours),[1].— Tearing through the whole head, starting from a small spot in the occiput,[3]. —A tearing pain in the head, sometimes starting from the limbs, and seeming to end in the head,[4].—Throbbing headache in the afternoon,[1].—Throbbing headache in the evening, in bed, with difficult breathing,[1].—[100.] Painful throbbing of the head during respiration, and in the teeth,[1].—Was awake several times at night on account of pulsation in the head, as if he would be attacked with apoplexy, with anxiety; soon after waking he came to his senses and felt that it was an illusion, for the beating of the head had disappeared; as he looked for further development of this symptom while in a state of slumber, the limbs and knees were drawn involuntarily upward and the back was bent, and he felt that if he longer postponed waking he would faint,[1].—Jerking headache,[1].—Severe shocks in the head from reading,[1].—*Forehead.* Heat and burning in the forehead,[1].— Burning in the forehead, with heat in the mouth, with pains in the eyes,[1]. —Boring and pressive headache in the forehead,[1].—Tearing-drawing in the upper part of the anterior portion of the head,[3].—Tearing-drawing through the head above the right eye,[1].—Pressive headache in the forehead, which disappears and returns,[4].—[110.] Pressive headache over the eyes extending into them,[3].—*Pressive headache in the forehead, especially just over the eyes,* which are sore on motion, the whole afternoon,[3].—Pressive pain in a small spot, formerly wounded, in the right side of the forehead (after four hours),[3].—Sticking headache above the right eye,[1].—Stitches in the ... head above the right external canthus (after two hours),[2].—*Violent tearing in the forehead, in a small spot near the temples*,[3].—Pulsating headache in the forehead after eating, with pressure in the occiput, heat in the head, and eructations,[1].—***Temples.*** Tension and pressure in both temples and in the forehead; he was unable to hold the lids open,[1].—Boring headache beneath the left temple,[1].—Pressure in the left temple, from within outward, for several hours,[2].—[120.] *Pressure in both temples*, and on the top of the head,[1].—Tearing in the temples, extending to the back teeth,[3].—Tearing pains, in frequent attacks within the head, extending to the right temple,[3]. —Throbbing in the temples and fulness of the brain, after waking from a long deep sleep in the afternoon,[2].—***Vertex.*** Headache over the whole vertex, in the morning, in bed, with painfulness of the ears, which disappeared after rising,[1].—Pressure, as if something were lying upon the vertex, or as if the integuments of the head were drawn too tightly together, which also extended to the forehead,[2].—Pressure on the top of the head every afternoon,[1].—*Pressive pain on the vertex, with soreness of the hair to touch*,[3].—Pressure on the top of the head, followed by drawing about the whole head, though more pain on the left side,[1].—Severe stitches in the top of the head,[1].—[130.] Stitches in the upper part of the head, extending to the temples,[1].—Stitches in the upper part of the head from reading,[1].— Tearing headache in the vertex and temples, by paroxysms,[3].—***Parietals.*** Dull tearing stitches from side to side, deep in the brain, on one side of the head, as from a nail driven into it,[1].—(Pain in the right side of the head when shaking it),[1].—Headache involving the whole of the right side of the head and face, with chill, coldness, and trembling of the body and the jaws,[1].—Biting-pressive headache, like a sensation in the nose from a suppressed sneeze, in the morning on waking, in the right half of the head on which he lay, and in the occiput; on raising the head the pain was relieved; on rising from bed it disappeared entirely,[3].—Pinching and cutting headache above and behind the left ear,[3].—Tearing pain in the left side of the head over the temples,[3].—Tearing in the left half of the head, starting from the left half of the nose,[3].—[140.] Tearing in the left half of the head, with drawing in the left arm,[3].—Severe tearing through the whole left side of the head,[4].—***Occiput.*** Crackling in the occiput while sitting,[1].—Confusion in the occiput, as after intoxication (after half an hour),[2].—Confusion in the occiput, like a tension from within (after half an hour),[2].—Much severe pain in the occiput and boring in the forehead at night, with sweat and pale face, cold, trembling hands, and nausea of the stomach,[1].—Pinching pain in the occiput,[1].—Frequently repeated short drawing pains in the right side of the occiput (after two hours),[3].—*Drawing and tearing in the left side of the occiput*,[3].—*Dull headache in the occiput*,[3].—[150.] Pressive pain in the occiput, from time to time,[1].—*Violent pressive pain in and on the occiput, in the lower portion*,[3].—*Pressure in the occiput*, especially after supper,[2].—Pressive headache in the upper part of the right side of the occiput, with pressure in the eyes,[3].—Pressive headache, first in the neck, then in the forehead, followed by lachrymation of the eyes, with closure of the lids,[1].—A burning-sticking in a small spot on the occiput,[3].—Tearing in the right side of the occiput (after four hours),[3].—Short tearing pains in the right side of the occiput,[4].—Frequent tearing pain, here and there, for example, in the left side of the occiput, left half of the face, left shoulder, left thigh, etc., with severe pressure in the arms and legs,[3].—Throbbing headache, very violent in the occiput, as if suppurating, from morning till evening (after nine days),[1].—***External Head.*** [160.] *The hairs fall out*,[1].—A place on the head as large as the hand is very hot to the touch, with continued headache,[1].—Drawing pains, here and there, over the head, externally,[3].—*The hat pressed upon the head like a heavy weight, and he continued to feel the sensation even after taking it off, as if the head were bound up with a cloth*,[2].—Tearing in an old scar of a cut on the top of the head,[3].—Crawling on the scalp, as if the hairs moved,[2].

Eye.—Objective. Inflammation of the right eye,[1].—Swelling of the left eye,[1].—***Subjective.*** *Burning in the eyes*,[1].—The eyes ache, in the evening, after lying down,[1].—[170.] Dull pain in the left eye,[3].—Pressure in the eyes, with confusion of the head (after six hours and a half),[1].—Pressure, as from sand in the right eye, with feeling of soreness in the canthi (after thirty-six hours),[4].—Pressure, as from a grain of sand, with sore pain, especially in the canthi, with biting in the eye,[3].—A tearing pressure on the left eye,[3].—*A heavy weight seemed to lie upon the eyes, so that he must make a great exertion, when reading and writing, in order to distinguish letters*,[1].—Severe stitches in both eyes,[1].—Pain in the eye, as if it would be torn out, with headache,[1].—Itching in the right eye (after thirty-six hours),[4].—Itching in the right eye, with great dryness of the lid (after fourteen days),[1].—[180.] Itching in the left eye, with biting in it after rubbing, especially in the inner canthus,[3].—Biting-itching, especially in the right external canthus,[3].—***Orbit.*** *The muscles of the eye pain when looking up*,[3].—Itching about the eyes,[1].—***Lids.*** Trembling of the upper lid,[1].—Twitching of the left lid (after nine days),[1].—She was unable to open the eyes at night, even when unable to sleep,[1].—The eyes are agglutinated, in the morning,[1].—The left lid seemed agglutinated, which was not the case,[1].—Drawing in the right lid (after thirteen days),[1].—[190.] Pressure in the upper lids and in the upper half of both eyeballs, on motion in the open air,[2].—Biting in the lids, with some redness of the margins (after twenty-four hours),[4].—*Itching in the margins of the lids*,[1].—A biting pressure in the external canthus of the right eye,[3].—Biting in the left canthus,[3].—Itching in the left inner canthus,[3].—***Lachrymal Apparatus.*** Severe lachrymation, and biting of the right eye (after twenty-four hours),[3].—***Ball.*** Sensitive pressure in the right eyeball from above downward (after half an hour),[3].—***Vision.*** Very short-sighted; he could only recognize people within a few steps (after three days),[1].—*He became short-sighted after exerting the eyes for some time*,[1].—[200.] Flickering before the eyes in the morning, immediately on rising,[3].—Rings surrounding an internal brighter field before the eyes,[1].—*Black floating spots before the eyes*,[1].

Ear.—Objective. A thick brown substance comes out of the right ear,[1].—*Discharge of a thick, flesh-colored, offensive moisture from the right ear*,[1].—***Subjective.*** Something heavy seems to lie in front of the ears, as if two sand-bags were there,[2].—*Something heavy seems to lie along and in front of the ears; they seem stopped*, though without any diminution of hearing (after half an hour),[2].—*Heat and redness of the left ear, every evening*,[1].—Tearing-burning pain in the lobule of the left ear,[3].—Fine pinching in the left ear,[4].—[210.] Stitches extending inward in the left meatus (after forty-eight hours),[4].—Tearing within the right ear,[3].—Tearing pain in the fossa behind the right ear,[3].—Twinges coming out of both ears (after seventeen days),[1].—Twinges in the right ear, in the evening,[1].—Twinges in the left ear,[3].—Pulsating in the ears,[1].—Tearing jerks, or some stitches, in the right inner meatus,[3].—Itching in the ears, with inclination to relieve it by swallowing,[1].—Severe crawling-itching within the right ear, after boring in with the finger, suddenly returning,[3].—*Hearing.* [220.] Loud speaking is unpleasant to the hearing,[2].—Severe humming before both ears,[1].—Crackling in the ears, as from straw, on every motion of the jaws (during breakfast),[1].—Chirping in the ears, as from crickets (after seven days),[1].—*Ringing in the ears,*[1].—Fine ringing in the left ear, in the afternoon (after forty hours),[4].—Ringing in the left ear, with whirling vertigo,[1].—*Roaring in the ears,*[1].—Illusions of hearing at night; he thought he heard some one walking who stepped up to his bed; he awoke immediately, with anxiety,[1].

Nose.—Objective. Trembling in the skin and muscles on the right side of the root of the nose,[1].—[230.] Incomplete attempts to sneeze, sometimes severe, sometimes slight,[3].—*Ineffectual attempts to sneeze, with crawling in the left nostril,* which became moist; after blowing the nose, the right nostril was stopped, with a catarrhal crawling and biting in the left side of the palate (after five hours),[3].—Repeated severe sneezing (after five hours),[4].—Very frequent sneezing, without coryza,[3].—Continual sneezing at night,[1].—Sneezing, followed by severe biting pain, when blowing the nose,[3]. —*Frequent sneezing, with constant and violent crawling in the nose,* with catarrhal roughness in it, and in the upper part of the chest, at night,[3].— Sneezing, with lachrymation of the left eye, followed by biting in the inner canthus,[3].—Sneezing, with burning over a large portion of the right side of the abdomen,[3].—Sneezing, with stitches in the abdomen,[3].—[240.] Increased moisture in the nose, preceded by stoppage of it (after three hours),[4]. —Discharge of mucus from the nose, with crawling in the left nostril, followed by severe sneezing, lachrymation of the right eye, and coryza,[3].— Discharge of green mucus from the nose,[1].—Catarrh; also, he could scarcely speak aloud (after eight days),[1].—*Coryza, with catarrh* (after seven days),[1].—Severe coryza, with hoarseness and rawness in the chest (after two days),[1].—Profuse fluent coryza,[1].—Fluent coryza every evening,[1].— Fluent coryza, with sneezing (almost immediately),[3].—*Dry coryza,*[1].—[250.] Dry coryza for several days,[1].—Dry coryza, with scraping in the throat,[1]. —Severe nose-bleed, which could scarcely be stopped (after forty-eight hours),[1].—Severe nose-bleed, in the morning in bed, immediately followed by pain in the chest,[1].—Nose-bleed every forenoon, ten to twelve drops,[1].— *Nose-bleed at night,* with orgasm of blood (after fifty-two hours),[1].—*Severe nose-bleed several times daily for two weeks, with great paleness of the face before and afterwards, every time,*[1].—Stoppage of the left nostril (after one hour and a half),[4].—Stoppage of the left nostril for an hour,[3].— Stoppage of the left nostril after sneezing,[3].—*Subjective.* [260.] Sensation of commencing coryza in the root of the nose,[2].—Catarrhal irritation for several days, night and morning, on waking; it disappeared during the day, with the exception of an occasional sneeze,[3].—Feeling of heaviness in the nose,[1].—*Drawing in the root of the nose,*[1].—Pressing in the root and bones of the nose, as in a severe coryza, though he could draw air through it,[2].—Continual crawling in the left side of the nose, in the evening,[1].—Formication in the nose for two days,[1].

Face.— Objective. *Great paleness of the face,*[1].—*Color of the face grayish-yellow,*[1].—**Subjective.** *Drawing pain in the upper and lower jaw* on both sides, with drawing in the head and confusion of it (after two hours),[3].—Tearing in the face,[1].—[270.] Twitching pain in several portions of the face,[1].—*Soreness of the facial bones of the upper and lower jaws,*[1].—**Cheeks.** Swelling of the cheeks,[1].—Glowing heat of the cheeks, after sitting a short time,[1].—Pain in the left cheek, as from a boring-burning in it, at intervals (after six days),[1].—Drawing pain in the cheeks, for two days,[1].—Twitching-drawing pain in the cheeks and jaw (after one day),[1].—Fine tearing stitches in the right check (after three hours),[3].—*Tearing pain in the face, in the left cheek,[1].—*Jerklike tearing in the left zygoma, in front of the ear, in the evening, in bed,[3].—[280.] Jerklike tearing pain in the upper jaw, on the right side,[3].—Lips. Swelling of the lips,[1].—*Swelling of the upper lip and cheek, with jerking pain,[1].—The right corner of the mouth is ulcerated,[1].—Twitching of the upper lip,[1].—Tearing pain in the left corner of the mouth, extending thence to the cheeks,[3].—Chin. Swelling of the face about the chin, for two hours,[1].—Drawing, extending from the right corner of the mouth to the chin,[1].—Cramplike pain in the lower jaw (after thirteen days),[1].—Tearing-jerking of the left lower jaw (after four days),[4].

Mouth.—Teeth. [290.] *Bleeding of the teeth when cleaning them,[1].—Bleeding of the teeth and gum for several days,[3].—Bleeding of the teeth and gum when sucking them with the tongue,[3].—Toothache in the anterior sound incisors,[2].—Toothache; the teeth seem to protrude, with a pain as if the teeth were touched by the tongue, as from an ulcer; the pain was renewed by eating,[1].—Toothache, as from acids, especially in the gum, as often as she ate anything salt,[4].—Toothache, with dry lips,[1].—Pinching pain in the right lower back teeth,[3].—Aching of the roots of the teeth, upper and lower,[1].—Drawing pain in the upper incisors,[3].—[300.] A biting-drawing pain in the upper and lower incisors, more in the gum,[3].—Slight drawing in the right back teeth, with violent jerking,[3].—Drawing pain in the hollow tooth,[1].—Frequent drawing in a hollow back tooth (after three days),[4].—Frequently returning drawing pain in the otherwise sound teeth,[4].—Gnawing and drawing pain in a hollow tooth, with swelling of the gum,[1].—Pressive toothache on the left side, in the upper back teeth,[1].—Sticking pain every moment, in perfectly sound teeth, which soon disappears and gives place to a short sticking pain in the abdomen (third day),[1].—A tickling-sticking and drawing in the first upper left back tooth,[3].—Drawing-tearing toothache in all the back teeth,[3].—[310.] Sore pain, with drawing in the first back teeth of the left side of the upper jaw,[3].—Sudden throbbing in the teeth, while eating,[1].—Violent drawing-jerking in a hollow back tooth,[3].—Gums. Swelling of the gum about a hollow tooth,[1].—*Some pustules on the gum,[1].—Retraction of the gum from the upper and lower incisors (in a young girl; removed by mercury),[4].—Retraction of the gum from the incisors, the roots are laid bare (removed by mercury), (after six days),[4].—*The gum retracts from the lower incisors,[1].—*The gum becomes loosened from the teeth, and sensitive,[1].—*Very profuse bleeding of the gum,[1].—[320.] Bleeding of the gum after sucking it (after two days),[4].—Heat in the gum,[1].—Drawing pain in the gum,[1].—*Sore pain in the gum during the day,[1].—*The gum was painfully sensitive when chewing,[1].—Tongue. *The tongue was coated white,[4].—*Yellowish-brown mucus coats the tongue,[1].—The tongue is difficult to move, with difficult speech,[2].—Heaviness of the tongue and stiffness, so that speech became very difficult,[1].—Heat and dryness of the tip of the tongue,[1].—[330.] Cramplike pain on the left side of the root of the tongue,[1].—Stitches in the tongue,[1].—Fine tearing pain in the right side of the tongue,[1].—*Sensitiveness of the tongue, with rawness in it,[1].—Soreness of the right side of the tongue, with sticking pain,[1].—General Mouth. Quite cold breath; also coldness in the throat, mouth, and teeth,[1].—Offensive breath,[1].—A blister in the upper part of the palate,[1].—*When sucking the gum, pure blood flows into the mouth, in the forenoon, returning several days at the same time (after five days),[4].—Dryness of the mouth, without thirst,[1].—[340.] Dryness of the mouth in the morning,[1]—Great dryness of the mouth, in the morning on waking,[1].—Sensation in the mouth and on the tongue, as after drinking wine freely in the evening (after ten hours),[4].—*Heat in the mouth*, especially in the upper lip,[1].—*Heat in the mouth, with rawness and dryness of the tip of the tongue* (after one and two days),[4].—*Pressive pain on the posterior part of the palate*,[3].—*Saliva.* *Increased collection of saliva in the mouth* (after a quarter of an hour),[4].—Bitter mucus in the mouth in the morning,[1].—The mouth is filled with mucus by eructations, always only a few hours after dinner,[1].—*Taste.* Flat, watery, offensive taste in the mouth (after two days),[1].—[350.] Salty taste in the mouth, the whole day,[1].—Sour taste after eating,[1].—*Bitter taste before and after eating*,[1].—*Bitterness on the palate, with dryness of the tongue*,[1].—Bitter taste, with eructations,[1].—When sucking the gum with the tongue, a taste of blood in the mouth, and the saliva becomes bloody (after fifty-one and eighty-five hours),[4].

Throat.—Inflammation of the throat, with a sensation as if something were sticking in it, with stitches,[1].—*Much hawking of mucus*,[1].—Much mucus constantly passes from the posterior nares,[1].—Sensation of dryness in the throat and posterior nares,[1].—[360.] Sensation of dryness in the throat, when swallowing,[1].—Sensation of roughness in the back part of the throat (after three days),[4].—Sensation of coldness in the lower portion of the throat,[1].—Sensation of constriction and internal swelling of the throat,[1].—Pressive pain in the throat (after six days),[1].—Violent pressive pain in the muscles of the throat, on the right side,[3].—Scratching in the throat,[1].—*Pressive tearing in the muscles of the throat*,[3].—Sore throat, as from swelling on the palate, with painful swallowing, for four days,[1].—Sore pain in the throat, when eating,[1].—[370.] *Scraping in the throat*,[1].—Scraping in the throat (after three days),[4].—Scraping in the throat, in the evening and morning, which provokes a dry cough,[1].—Severe scraping and crawling in the throat and fauces, soon transiently relieved by hawking,[3].—*Scraping and rawness in the throat*, for several days,[1].—Scraping in the throat, with some cough, which causes lachrymation, particularly of the left eye,[3].—Severe crawling in the throat, only transiently relieved by hawking, with much accumulation of saliva,[3].—Sticking-itching in the throat and neck, with red spots in it (after thirty-eight hours),[4].—*Uvula.* Inflammation and swelling of the uvula, with sticking in the throat,[1].—*Fauces and Pharynx.* Much tenacious mucus in the fauces, which he was obliged to raise,[1].—[380.] Mucus of an unpleasant taste and odor in the fauces,[1].—*Burning in the upper part of the fauces*,[3].—Burning in the fauces and back part of the throat, as in coryza (after ten hours),[4].—Contracting sensation deep in the pharynx,[1].—Pressive pain in the fauces, just behind the palate,[1].—Tearing pressure in the back part of the fauces, and in the left side of the root of the tongue,[3].—Frequent biting and burning in the fauces and palate,[3].—Biting posteriorly in the fauces, as in the commencement of coryza, though a more acrid biting,[3].—*Swallowing, coughing, or blowing the nose causes pain in the fauces and posterior nares, as if sore*,[1].—Painful hiccough in the pharynx, after eating,[1].—[390.] Frequent sensation, in the forenoon, as if something hot and sharp arose along the pharynx,[1].—*Sensation in the pharynx as if it were contracted or drawn together*,[1].—Pressure in the pharynx, when not swallowing, as if it were contracted or constricted,[3].—A kind of pressure and fulness in the pharynx, extending in the stomach, almost like heartburn,[1].—*Swallowing.* Painless impediment when swallowing; the saliva that was swallowed passed down on gradually,[3].—*The food cannot be easily swallowed; the throat seems constricted with spasms, though without pain,[1].—**Throat Externally.** Great swelling of the parotid gland, as far as the angle of the jaw,[1].

Stomach.—Appetite. Hunger, with, however, aversion to usually agreeable food,[1].—Longing for sweet and salt things,[1].—Very soon full and satisfied, after a moderate breakfast,[4].—[**400.**] Diminished appetite, toward noon, with nausea (after five days),[1].—Little appetite at noon, with slight cutting in the abdomen (after four days),[4].—Little appetite; she is soon satisfied; aching in the pit of the stomach, and sensation of emptiness in the stomach, for half an hour,[1].—Slight appetite, with heat in the mouth and rawness and dryness on the tip of the tongue (after forty-two hours),[4]. —Appetite slight, with no taste, as in catarrh,[1].—Loss of appetite, with frequent eructations, and confusion of the head,[1].—Complete loss of appetite, with coated tongue and great weariness,[4].—Want of hunger; he would like to go without eating,[3].—She could eat nothing at all in the morning till noon, then relished her food, but could eat nothing in the evening,[1].— The want of appetite is associated with a sensation of relaxation and weakness of the muscles in the limbs,[4].—[**410.**] Loss of desire for coffee,[1].— *Aversion to fat meat,[1].—Aversion to butter,[1].—*Aversion to milk, which makes her flatulent,[1].—**Eructations and Hiccough.** *Eructations, (after one hour and a half),[4].—*Violent, almost constant, eructations,[1].— Very frequent eructations, as well before as after eating, mostly in the afternoon, for eight days (after four days),[4].—Eructations, after eating and drinking,[1].—*Frequent empty eructations, the whole day, mostly in the afternoon,[3].—Empty eructations after soup and every time after drinking,[1].— [**420.**] Frequent empty eructations, preceded by transient gripings in the abdomen,[3].—The eructation is always empty, and accompanied, especially in the afternoon, with much accumulation of flatulence in the abdomen,[4]. —Sweet eructations,[1].—Sour eructations in the open air, towards evening,[1].—Sour eructations, after taking milk,[1].—Sour eructations with burning in the stomach,[1].—Bitter, scraping eructations,[1].—Constant sensation as of heartburn; acidity constantly rising into the mouth,[1].—Waterbrash,[1]. —Great inclination to hiccough from the slightest cause,[1].—[**430.**] Hiccough, after a moderate dinner,[4].—Hiccough, especially after every motion,[1].— **Nausea.** Momentary attacks of nausea,[1].—Nausea in the morning, an hour after waking, with qualmishness in the stomach,[1].—Nausea, every forenoon, about 10 or 11 o'clock,[1].—Nausea, at night,[1].—Nausea, before every meal,[1].—Nausea with every meal,[1].—Nausea, even to retching, before dinner,[1].—Nausea, with pressure in the stomach, after eating, followed by violent dragging-down pain about the navel,[1].—[**440.**] Nausea and loss of appetite, even when fasting, still more after eating, with anxiety, dizziness, obscuration before the eyes, and white tongue; he was obliged to lie down towards evening, without sleepiness (after six and seven days),[1].—Constant nausea, without appetite and without stool,[1].—Sickening nausea (fourth day),[1].—*Frequent qualmishness; he did not vomit, however,[1].—**Stomach.** Heaviness in the stomach, and sensation of trembling in it,[1].—*He feels acidity in the stomach, when lying on the back and when walking,[1].—Painfulness of the stomach, when walking or standing; it feels heavy and hanging down,[1].—Pain in the pit of the stomach, in the evening, with sensitiveness to touch, together with nausea and aversion, even on thinking of eating,[1]. *Burning sensation in the stomach,[1].—Continued burning in the stomach,[1]. —[**450.**] Fulness, eructations, general heaviness, after a moderate supper; writing is slow and difficult,[4].—*The stomach feels tense and full,[1].—Tension and pressure above the stomach, extending from the ribs,[1].—Constrictive pain beneath the pit of the stomach, which is increased by pressure of the finger,[2].—*A contractive sensation beneath the stomach,[1].—Contractive pain near the pit of the stomach, on the right side, in the morning and afternoon,[1].—*Griping in the pit of the stomach, as from flatulence,[1].—Cramp in the stomach, and cardialgia in a nursing woman,[1].—*Contractive cramp in the stomach, even at night, extending up into the chest, with distension of the abdomen; she was obliged to bend double, and could not lie down because it became worse; the pain was paroxysmal, and took away her breath,[1]. —Clawing in the stomach, extending up to the throat, like heartburn,[1].— [460.] Gnawing in the stomach, in the morning, when fasting,[1].—Cramp in the stomach, with incessant acid eructations,[1].—Pressive sensation beneath the pit of the stomach (after twenty-four hours),[4].—An anxious pressure in the pit of the stomach (after four days),[1].—Pressure in the stomach, as from something sore; worse on touch,[1].—Continued painful pressure in the pit of the stomach and in the upper abdomen, as if in the stomach, in the evening, after 7,[3].—Pressure beneath the stomach, at night, with uneasy sleep and anxious dreams,[1].—Pressive sensation in the region of the stomach, disappearing on passing wind, with rumbling,[4].—Pressure in the stomach follows rumbling in the abdomen,[1].—*Very much oppressed and full,[1].—On stooping, it seems as if sausages were lying on the right and left sides, near the stomach,[1].—*The epigastric region is very sensitive,[1].— Throbbing in the pit of the stomach,[1].

Abdomen.—Hypochondria. [470.] Painful sticking-tearing in both hypochondria, starting from a point just below the pit of the stomach, and extending to both sides,[3].—*Both hypochondria are painful to touch,[1].— *Every piece of clothing about the hypochondrium oppresses him and is unendurable,[1].—Transient but violent pain in the right hypochondrium,[3].— Pressive pain in the left hypochondrium,[1].—Violent sticking in the region of the liver (after forty-eight hours),[1].—*Tension in the region of the liver, as if it were too short there, on waking from the midday nap,[1].—*The region of the liver is very sensitive and painful to touch,[1].—Pressive pain in the liver, when walking in the open air,[1].—Violent tearing in the liver, causing cries,[1].—[480.] Bruised pain in the liver,[1].—Drawing pain beneath the left ribs,[1].—Pressure beneath the short ribs, after breakfast,[3].—*Umbilical.* Audible rumblings in the umbilical region,[2].—Burning in the umbilical region,[3].—Burning pain in the skin near the navel, frequently returning (after four hours),[3].—Severe griping about the umbilical region, after eating a little harmless food; soon disappears after eructations or passage of wind,[3].—Griping about the navel, extending into the stomach, for four days and nights (first in the morning, on rising); she was obliged to lie down, could not stand erect on account of the pain, and could not sleep at night, with constant chilliness; on the second night, diarrhœa, which was worse at night (after six days),[1].—Pressive pain in the umbilical region,[1].—Sore pain in a spot below the navel,[3].—*General Abdomen.* [490.] *Abdomen distended by flatulence, in the afternoon,[4].—*Abdomen very much distended, after dinner (ninth day),[1].—*Distension of the abdomen, with rumbling in it, after eating a little,[2].—After a stool, the abdomen is swollen, like an induration (second day),[1].—Movings about in the abdomen (immediately),[3].—Much motion in the abdomen, and frequent passage of loud, or noiseless, or moist flatus,[3].—Incessant noise in the abdomen, without urging to stool,[1].—*Audible rumbling moves slowly about the abdomen (after three hours),[3].—Loud rumbling and noise in the abdomen, for eight days,[4].—

*Audible rumblings in the abdomen, with some griping,[2].—[500.] Fermentation in the abdomen, followed by diarrhœic stool, with passage of moist offensive flatus,[1].—Complete emptiness of the abdomen after stool, especially noticed when walking,[4].—*Much flatulence and distension of the abdomen, caused by things which usually digested easily,[1].—Much flatulence, with rumbling and loud movings in the abdomen, in the afternoon,[4].—Accumulation of flatus in the right side of the upper abdomen, more towards the back, with pinching pains,[1].—Flatus moves about the abdomen, and causes here and there stitches, especially in the left side, under the ribs,[3].—Suddenly, a great quantity of flatus, in the afternoon, which passes without difficulty (after thirty-six hours),[4].—*Offensive flatus (after one hour and a half),[3]. —*Very much offensive flatus (after one hour),[4].—Passage of much wind after the rumbling,[2].—[510.] *Passage of offensive, at last moist, flatus, with painful dragging towards the sacrum, and thence toward the abdomen (after two hours),[3].—Enormous passage of odorless flatus, in the morning, on waking,[1].—Passage of some odorless flatus, with much moving of flatus in the abdomen (after half an hour),[4].—Passage of much loud odorless flatus, with frequent eructations (after four days),[4].—Great anxiety in the abdomen,[1]. —Heaviness in the abdomen,[1].—*The abdomen seems very heavy,[1].—*Sensation as if the abdomen hung down heavily; she was only able to walk quite bent,[1].—Pain in the abdomen, as from lifting a heavy weight, even when slightly raising her arm for the purpose of doing some work with the hand; the same pain is felt when touching the abdomen,[1].—*Pain in the bowels, as from lifting or a sprain, as soon as she lies upon the side; mostly in the left side of the abdomen,[1].—[520.] Burning in the abdomen,[1].—The abdomen is full and pressed, as if overloaded with food, day and night, with eructations,[1]. —If he eats or drinks, the abdomen feels as if it would burst,[1].—Tension in the abdomen,[3].—Pain over the whole abdomen, as far as the pubes, as though all the muscular fibres were drawn tense or hardened, which made him very anxious,[1].—Tensive and pressive pain in the right side of the upper abdomen, extending across the whole stomach,[1].—*Tension in the abdomen from accumulated flatus, but it is passed copiously and easily, in the afternoon,[4].— Tensive and pressive pain over nearly the whole abdomen, with constant uneasiness and weeping, as from despair,[1].—Constrictive sensation in the abdomen,[1].—Continued pressive pinching in the upper abdomen,[3].—[530.] While sitting bent over, fine pinching in the abdomen, on the left side of the spinal column,[4].—Griping in the bowels, with natural stool,[1].—Griping pains in various places in the bowels, which are frequently transient,[4].— Griping in the abdomen, during and after eating,[3].—Fine griping in the abdomen, when sitting bent,[4].—The griping in the abdomen, comes on almost only in the afternoon and evening, and appears to be caused by flatulence; it disappears after passing it,[4].—Colic before the stool,[1].—Colic, as after taking cold; it was worse before passing flatus, and relieved after it,[1].—Colic-like cramp, from morning till evening, before menstruation,[4].— Colic, during a diminished flow of the menses, with pain in all the bones, as if beaten,[1].—[540.] Flatulent colic, with passage of odorless flatus,[3].— Frequent colic, extending to the small of the back and bladder, afterwards a stool, almost as after rhubarb,[3].—Frequent pinching colic, especially in the right side of the abdomen,[3].—Dragging or griping colic, after a stool,[3].— Pressive colic, with rumbling and passage of moist, warm, odorless flatus, whereupon it ceased,[3].—Pressive colic, with urging to stool and passage of hot flatus, which relieved it,[3].—Cutting colic,[1].—Pain drawing across the abdomen, before the stool,[4].—Disagreeable pressure in the abdomen, so that she was obliged to hold it constantly with the hand,[1].—Pressive pain in the left side of the abdomen; movings about in the abdomen, with griping,[1].— [550.] Dull pressive pain on a small spot in the abdomen,[3].—Cuttings in the abdomen, momentarily, but very often,[1].—Cuttings in the abdomen that shoot through like lightning,[1].—Cuttings in the bowels, like colic, in the evening,[1].—Sticking pain in the left side of the abdomen and chest, increased by breathing,[3].—Dull pinching-stitchings, as from below upwards, in the abdomen,[3].—Bruised pain in the abdominal muscles,[1].—*Hypogastrium and Iliac Region.* Movings deep in the lower abdomen,[3].— *The flatus collects here and there in the abdomen, under the short ribs, in the hypogastric region, causing pinching and pressure, and very gradually passing down into the rectum, with sensation of heat,*[4].—Gurgling in the left side of the lower abdomen,[3].—[560.] Griping and sticking pains in the left lower abdomen,[3].—*Pinching colic in the lower abdomen,*[3].—A violent pinching labor-like colic, which especially pressed upon the sacrum (and the bladder), with rumbling of the bowels, on waking, at 3 A.M., from an uneasy sleep, with many anxious dreams,[3].—*Pressive colic in the lower abdomen,*[1].— Tearing-aching in the lower abdomen, extending up to the navel,[3].—Pinching pressure in the lower abdomen,[3].—Pinching pressure deep in the right side of the lower abdomen, extending towards the hips,[3].—Cutting pains in the lower abdomen, during menstruation,[1].—A crawling creeping-sticking in the lower abdomen (after twenty-eight hours),[3].—After a hard scanty stool, in the morning, pinching stitches in the left side of the lower abdomen, with incomplete desire for stool, like a pressure upon the rectum, throughout the whole day (after four days),[3].—[570.] A sore pain, externally, in the lower portion of the abdomen, even on touch (after four hours),[3].—Griping pain in the right inguinal region,[3].—Pressive pain in the inguinal region, in the right side,[3].

Rectum and Anus.—Passage of much mucus from the rectum, for several days in succession,[1].—*Discharge of acrid, corrosive moisture from the rectum* (after twenty-four hours),[1].—Discharge of pure blood from the rectum, with tearing pain for several days (in a young woman who had never had the like before), (after seven days),[4].—Sensation as if the stool would come, with burning in the anus and passage of flatus,[3].—*Tenesmus in the rectum,*[1].—*Gnawing in the rectum, when not at stool,*[1].—*Crawling in the rectum and complaints of ascarides,*[1].—[580.] Swollen, painful hæmorrhoids,[1].—Tickling-itching in the hæmorrhoids,[1].—Moisture of the anus, with tenesmus, when urinating,[1].—*A glutinous moisture of a musty odor exudes in considerable quantity from the anus, at night,*[1].—*Bleeding from the anus, during stool,*[1].—Rush of blood to the anus,[1].—*Burning in the anus after a stool,*[1].—Burning and sticking in the anus,[1].—Burning in the right side of the anus (after six hours),[3].—Burning in the anus, during the stool, which consists of small, hard, fecal masses,[4].—[590.] Burning in the anus, with unpleasant sensation of dryness in it (after seven days),[4].—Pinching in the anus, when not at stool,[1].—Pressive pain in the anus,[3].—Cutting in the anus, during stool,[4].—Cutting pain in the anus. with a hard stool,[3].— *Sticking in the anus, during stool, as with needles,*[1].—*Stitches towards the anus,*[1].—A few stitches in the anus, in the evening,[4].—A very painful stitch through the anus and rectum, starting from the coccyx, as with a hot needle (after six days),[4].—Biting in the anus,[3].—[600.] *Soreness of the anus,*[1].— Itching in the anus, in the morning, in bed, aggravated by scratching, and followed by burning,[4].—Itching in the anus, increased by scratching, and changing into a burning, on waking from a long sleep (after thirty-two hours),[4].—Itching in the anus, and, after rubbing, burning in it,[3].—Stitching pain in the perinæum, near the anus,[3].—*Soreness of the perinæum, with painful itching when touched,*[1].—**Soreness, with itching and moisture of the perinæum at night,*[1].—Urging to stool, after breakfast, which though not hard is only evacuated with much pressure,[3].—Sudden urging to stool, as from fulness in the rectum, but little passes, however,[2].—Great urging to stool, which is scanty and difficult to evacuate,[3].—[610.] A feeling of urging to stool, from a sensation in the abdomen and small of the back, without result,[3].—Ineffectual urging to stool (after eighty hours),[3].—Ineffectual urging to stool, in the evening (after thirty-six hours),[1].—**Ineffectual urging to stool; only wind passes with painful pressure in the rectum,*[1].—Excessive desire for stool, with crawling in the anus, and pressure in the bladder towards the small of the back, like a hæmorrhoidal colic, at intervals; instead of a stool, violent bearing-down pains in the lower abdomen, in front and back, with burning in the anus, and sensation as in diarrhœa; after the pain, a scanty passage of fæces, consisting of soft pieces, with great exertion, with relief of the pains,[3].

Stool.— Diarrhœa. Diarrhœa (after forty-eight hours),[1].— Stool twice (after fourteen hours),[4].—Stool at 10 P.M., unusually late in the day, with rumbling in the abdomen (after forty-four hours),[4].—Stool thinner than usual, with urging thereto,[4].—Stool tenacious, scanty, not cohering properly, with inactivity of the rectum (after six days),[4].—[620.] Hard stool,[3].—Hard stool, for two or three days,[1].—Stool hard, delayed, with much exertion (after thirty hours),[3].—Acrid stool, with coated tongue,[1].— The stool passes with loud passage of flatus,[3].—Passage of stool with burning in the rectum,[1].—Mucus precedes the stool, followed by hard, then by soft fæces, with cutting colic; during the first week,[1].—Much passage of mucus with the stool,[1].—**Passage of mucus, with urging in the anus,*[1].— *Filamentous yellowish mucus envelops the stool; this mucus is entirely bloody in the last portions of the fæces,*[2].—[630.] Discharge of blood with every stool,[1].—A child cries aloud, for six or seven minutes, whilst bloody mucus passes from him, instead of a stool,[1].—Passage of ascarides,[3].—*Constipation.* Complete constipation (after sixty-seven hours),[4].—The first week, stool seldom and hard, only for two or three days,[1].—One day no stool, the next day two stools,[1].

Urinary Organs.—Bladder. Pressing pain in the bladder, frequently during the day, though she was able to retain the urine,[1].—The urine is passed with pressive pain in the bladder,[1].— *Urethra.* Burning in the urethra, when urinating,[1].—Extremely painful burning and twinging in the urethra, when urinating,[1].—[640.] Contraction of the urethra, every morning,[1].—Pinching pains in the urethra (almost immediately),[1].— Frequent tearing in the urethra, when urinating; the last drops consist of mucus, and are painful to pass,[1].—Tearing and drawing in the urethra, after urinating, in the morning,[3].—Was awaked very early in the morning, by desire to urinate,[1].—Urging to urinate, nearly every hour,[1].—Frequent inclination to urinate, though it passes slowly,[1].—He was obliged to rise frequently at night to urinate,[1].— *Micturition.* Passage of much urine, after drinking a little (after six hours),[3].—Urine very scanty (after forty-eight hours),[3].— [650.] Some thick, milky urine is passed at the close of urinating,[1].— *Urine.* Very strong odor of the urine,[1].— Profuse, clear yellow urine (after twenty-four hours),[4].—Dark-colored urine,[1].—*Reddish, turbid urine,*[1].—*Dark-red urine, as if it was mixed with blood* (after two days),[1].—*Dark-red urine*, with roughness of the throat,[3].—*Red sediment to the urine*,[1].—The urine remains clear, though it deposits some gravel,[1].

Sexual Organs. — Male. Frequent erections (after twenty-four hours),[4].—[660.] Frequent continuous erections, for three days together,[1]. —He awoke every hour, with erections,[1].—Constant erections, at night, without voluptuous sensations or fancies,[3].—Great itching soreness, and a vesicle on the inner side of the prepuce,[1].—Itching and soreness of the prepuce,[1].—Swelling of the scrotum, which feels hard,[1].—Crawling in the testicles, and on the scrotum,[1].—Increased sexual desire (after forty-nine days),[1].—Complete loss of sexual desire, in the morning, not even excited by sensual thoughts (after twenty-four hours),[3].—Frequent emissions, without much sensation,[1].—[670.] Emissions, without dreams,[1].—Emission too soon on coition, followed by roaring of blood in the head,[1].—Excessive emissions, which painfully shake the nerves, followed by violent burning in the forepart of the urethra, with severe cutting and burning when urinating, which continues a long time and is renewed on slight external pressure,[3].— Discharge of prostatic fluid, when straining at stool,[1].—**Female.** Discharge of white mucus from the vagina (after four days),[1].—Leucorrhœa appeared after urinating (first day),[1].—*Much very thin leucorrhœa, in the morning, on rising, and not again during the whole day*,[1].—*Milky leucorrhœa, which is excoriating* (twelfth day),[1].—*Red sore places on the pudenda, looking like ulcers*, which do not pain, only itch, with leucorrhœa,[1].—*Aphthæ of the pudenda*,[1].—[680.] Burning in the pudenda,[1].—Heat and redness of the pudenda,[1].—Sticking in the pudenda, when urinating,[1].—*Itching in the pudenda and anus*,[1].—Itching in the pudenda on urinating,[1].—Great soreness in the pudenda, towards the forepart, in the evening,[1].—*During the leucorrhœa, soreness and rawness in the pudenda*,[1].—Smarting pain in the pudenda, with leucorrhœa, for two days; followed by appearance of the menses, which have been suppressed for many months; they flow for three days, but are quite black, followed by a very little leucorrhœa, without smarting,[1].—Great itching on the mons veneris,[1].—*Menses five days too soon* (after twenty-one days),[1].—[690.] Menses six days too soon (after two days),[1].—Menses five days too late (secondary action), (after fifty-five days),[1].—Menses six days too late; they are biting and make the parts sore,[1].—*The menstrual blood is too thick*, and of a strong odor,[1].

Respiratory Organs. — Larynx and Trachea. *Great roughness in the larynx, with deep rough voice, which failed if he exerted it, though without pain in the throat*,[3].—*He is obliged to clear his throat so often, in the evening, that the larynx becomes raw and sore*,[1].—*When coughing, severe pain in the larynx and in the region of the thyroid cartilage, as if ulcerated*,[1].—Crawling and itching in the larynx, with whistling when breathing; with tightness of the chest and a dry cough, in the evening after lying down,[1]. —*Unusual sensation of dryness in the trachea, not relieved by hawking, for several days* (after three days),[4].—Pressure in the trachea, on inspiration,[1]. —[700.] Crawling in the upper part of the trachea, as if something were tightly seated there, provoking cough (after three hours),[3].—Irritation to cough, frequently returning, in the back part of the throat, with short cough,[3]. —Irritation to cough, as from sulphur fumes, with retching,[1].—**Voice.** Slight roughness of the voice, as if oppressed by fatigue, by speaking (after three days),[4].—*Hoarseness and roughness in the larynx, so that she could not speak aloud without great exertion*,[1].—Hoarseness in the evening (after twelve days),[1].—Suddenly great hoarseness in the evening, so that he could scarcely speak a loud word, with great dyspnœa, so that he was scarcely able to breathe, when walking in the open air (after sixth day),[1].—Paroxysm as follows: The boy became hoarse, distorted his eyes (as if something were sticking in them) when he wished to speak, with lachrymation; this was followed by red cheeks, pain on swallowing, loud breathing when asleep, cough, vomiting of milk; he was obstinate and screamed frequently (after a few hours),[1].—*Almost voiceless in the morning,*[1].—*Cough and Expectoration.* Cough after the slightest cold, in the morning on rising from bed, or if she goes from a warm room into a cold one,[1].—[710.] Cough, from irritation and crawling in the throat, in a few deep paroxysms, on account of which the chest is painful, as if pressed in,[3].—Cough, which causes vomiting and retching, in the evening,[1].—*Cough in the evening, in bed, before going to sleep,*[1].—Cough every time as soon as she has eaten sufficiently,[1].—Frequent cough caused by irritation in the upper part of the chest, with roughness and scraping in the throat (after three days),[4].— Slight attacks of cough, in a few shocks (after five minutes); repeated on the third day at the same time,[4].—Repeated paroxysms of cough at night, with constantly returning irritation thereto,[1].—Short cough in the evening,[1].—Frequent paroxysms of short cough,[3].—*Spasmodic cough in three or four paroxysms daily,*[1].—[720.] *Spasmodic cough in the evening* for five hours (from walking too rapidly?), (after sixteen days),[1].—*Half-involuntary, rough cough, caused by constant roughness and crawling in the throat,*[3]. —Violent tickling cough, with whitish expectoration, in the morning after waking,[1].—Fatiguing cough, with dyspnœa and burning in the chest,[1].— Dry cough after every expectoration, which causes warmth and sweat,[1].— Rough cough, without any expectoration,[1].—Severe cough, with much yellowish, purulent expectoration, and sticking pain in the left hypochondrium on breathing, followed by severe stitches in the upper part of the left side of the chest,[1].—*Cough, caused by itching in the larynx (with tenacious, salty expectoration), in the evening on going to sleep, and in the morning after waking,*[4].—*Expectoration of mucus from the larynx, caused by short, hacking cough,*[1].—Expectoration of entire pieces of green mucus,[1].—*Respiration.* [730.] Desire for deep breathing, with moaning,[1].—He was obliged to fetch a deep breath, with exhaustion of the chest, of the abdomen, back, neck, and head, together with lifting of the feet,[1].—Shortness of breath, with anxiety on the chest; he was unable to sit, and was obliged to walk about constantly for ten days,[1].—If the tearing-drawing, burning pains attack the external chest, even for a short time, they are constantly accompanied by a sensation of oppression of breathing,[4].—Great dyspnœa, on account of which she was obliged to walk slower than usual,[1].—Difficult breathing, worse when sitting,[1].—Difficult breathing from oppression of the chest,[1].—Difficult breathing in the evening when lying, with throbbing of the head,[1].—*Difficult breathing, fulness of the chest, and palpitation on the slightest motion,* mostly towards evening,[1].—She gets out of breath on turning over in bed,[1].—[740.] Respiration stopped entirely on falling asleep, with increased vertigo,[1].

Chest.—Rush of blood to the chest, with burning in it,[1].—Rush of blood to the chest, in the morning on waking, with coated tongue,[1].—Warm rush of blood to the chest, with anxiety caused by accumulation of flatulence in the abdomen (after nine days),[4].—It constantly seemed as though the blood were rushing to the chest, with which she felt cold within the body,[1]. —*The chest feels weary on waking,*[1].—***Sensation of weakness and fatigue of the chest,***[1].—Roughness in the chest, with frequent irritation to cough,[3]. —Pain on expanding the chest,[1].—Pain in the chest, as from incarcerated flatulence,[1].—[750.] Pain in the upper part of the chest, with rough cough,[3]. —*Severe burning in the chest, as from glowing coals, almost uninterruptedly,[1].—Constriction of the chest in frequent attacks, with impediment of respiration,[1].—Tightness in the chest in the morning after rising, like a catarrh, and he was obliged to cough very hard, which caused a painful shooting through the head,[1].—Sensation as if compressed in the chest and shoulders, in the morning after rising from bed,[1].—Pinching pain in a small spot on the chest, caused by flatulence,[4].—Painful drawing in the chest (the shoulders and arms), more on the left side, with sensation of heat and rush of blood to the head, with which she feels cold to the touch,[1].—Oppression of the chest and short breath, as from flatulence pressing upward (after forty-one hours),[3].—Sensation of oppression of the chest, immediately relieved after eructations,[1].—Tight, oppressive sensation on the chest, as if coming from the abdomen, and caused by flatulence,[4].—[760.] *Chest very much oppressed and weak on waking,[1].—*After the disappearance of the coryza the chest was much oppressed, with wheezing and rattling in it; he was unable to remain in bed on account of want of air, and the cough, which affected him even to vomiting, and was difficult to loosen,[1].—Spasmodic oppression and contraction of the chest, for three or four minutes,[1].—Frequent oppressive-pressive pain in the chest,[3].—Very sensitive stitches through the chest, impeding respiration, on going to sleep,[3].—Pain in the chest, as if the flesh were raw, when coughing,[1].—Pulsation in the chest, with uneasiness and anxiety; she felt the heart beat distinctly with the hand,[1].—Itching internally in the chest,[1].—*Front.* Dull pain on the sternum in a small spot just above the pit of the stomach, as if caused by stooping forward or touching the part,[3].—*Sides.* Dull pain in the right side of the chest (after six hours),[3].—[770.] Drawing rheumatic pain in the right short ribs,[3].—Pressing rheumatic pain in the right side in the short ribs, lasting a quarter of an hour,[3].—*Pressive pain in the upper part of the right side of the chest,* extending through to the right shoulder-blade,[3].—Sticking pain in the right side of the chest and abdomen, increased by inspiration,[3].—Deep stitches in the right side of the chest during deep breathing,[3].—Violent dull stitches, like shocks, from within outward, deep in the lower part of the right side of the chest,[3].—Tearing in the right side of the chest,[3].—Burning in the left side of the chest and in the right side near the pit of the stomach,[1].—Dull pain, first in the left, then in the right side of the chest, more perceptible during expiration than inspiration,[3].—Pressure on the left side of the chest,[3].— [780.] Tearing pressure in the left side near the hip, extending to the back,[3].—A pain externally on the left breast, on touching it, like a pressure and tension,[1].—Sticking beneath the left ribs, and extending thence into the abdomen, pit of the stomach, and chest; pressure upon the larynx, aggravated by breathing, and when it disappeared renewed by pressure upon the abdomen, in the morning, in bed,[3].—Pressive-sticking pain beneath the left breast,[1].—Severe stitches below the left breast; she was unable to sleep or walk on account of them; they continue while sitting (without chill or heat),[1].—*Dull stitches in the left side of the chest, extending into the short ribs,[3].—Constrictive stitches below the left breast, which impede breathing (after three days),[1].— *Oppressive tearing in the left side of the chest* (after twenty-six hours),[3].

Heart and Pulse. — Pain, rather of a burning than sticking character, in the præcordial region,[1].—Twitching pain in the præcordial region (seventh day),[1]. — [790.] Dull, sticking, oppressive pain in the region of the heart, which goes off with audible trembling of the left side,

like the escape of incarcerated flatus (after three hours),[3].—***Heart's
Action.*** *Frequent palpitation;* very rapid beats,[1].—*Excessive palpitation for several days,[1].—Palpitation, with intermitting pulse, in the evening on going to sleep, for several days,[1].—*Palpitation, mostly when sitting.*[1]
—Great palpitation, after eating,[1].— ***Pulse.*** Rapid pulse (after two
hours),[4].—*Pulse weak and faint,[1].

Neck and Back.—Neck. The neck and head shake and tremble,
by paroxysms,[1].—* *The cervical glands are swollen and painful, especially the
posterior ones, near the neck,*[4].—[800.] Pressive and tensive pain in the neck,
as if in the cervical vertebræ,[1].—Dull, burning pain in the muscles of the
neck,[4].—Sensitive pressive pain in the muscles of the neck (after four
days),[4].—* *Tearing in the muscles of the neck,*[3].—*Tearing pain in the musc'es
of the neck,* on the left side, especially on moving it (after three days),[4].—
Pressive-tearing in the muscles of the left side of the neck, for two days
(after three days),[4].—*Drawing pain in the nape of the neck, which extends
up to the head, in which the same drawing is felt, accompanied by nausea and
rush of water from the mouth,[1].—***Back.*** Twitches in the muscles of the left
side of the back,[3].—Weakness of the back,[1].—Heaviness in the back, and
oppression in the chest,[1].—[810.] Heaviness of the back and limbs, at night,
as if weary,[1].—Painful stiffness in the back, in the morning on rising,[1].—
Pain in the side of the back, as if bruised,[1].—Burning in the upper part of
the left side of the back,[1].—Sensitive pinchings near the spine,[1].—Drawing
pain in the back, in the evening,[1].—*Drawing pain in the back,* mostly when
sitting,[1].—Drawing in the back and in the feet, only when sitting,[1].—
Rheumatic drawing in the back, especially when stooping, for several days,[4].
—Tearing, extending from the chest to the back, in the morning, in bed,
extending into the arms and the left ear, with internal heat, especially in
the head,[1].— ***Dorsal.*** [820.] Rheumatic sensation in the whole left
shoulder-blade, when writing (after six hours),[4].—Rheumatic pain in the
upper part of the left shoulder-blade, after the usual washing with water
(not cold),[4].—*Burning on the right shoulder-blade,*[3].—Sticking between the
shoulder-blades, even causing arrest of breathing, at night,[1].—Violent tearing in the left shoulder-blade, on bending back the arm,[3].—***Lumbar.***
Sensation of coldness in the small of the back, numbness and tension,[1].—
*Severe pain in the small of the back; she was unable to sit; it then felt like a
plug in the back; she was obliged to put a pillow under it,[1].—Tensive pain
and stiffness of the small of the back,[1].—Drawing pain in the small of the
back, abdomen, and left side of the back, extending into the arms; it caused
the left side to be bent quite over,[1].—Drawing pain from the lower abdomen
into the small of the back just before menstruation,[1].—[830.] Drawing-
pressive pain in the small of the back, extending down into the coccyx
(after twenty-four hours),[4].—Tearing pressure in the small of the back,[3].—
Tearing pain in the small of the back, which sometimes extends down to
the hips (after three days),[4].—Pain above the right loin, which takes away
the breath,[1].—***Sacral.*** Pressive pain near the lowest portion of the back,[1].
—*Pinching-pressive pain near the lowest portion of the spine,[1].—Tearing in
the lower portion of the back, near the sacrum,[3].—*Pressive sore pain
beneath the coccyx,[3].

Extremities in General.—Severe twitching of the arms and legs,
several evenings, in bed, which for a long time prevented her going to
sleep,[1].—The limbs go to sleep,[1].—[840.] *The limb upon which he lies goes
to sleep easily,[1].—Great heaviness of the left arm and leg, as if paralyzed,[1].—
Uneasiness of the limbs, in the evening, in bed; she was obliged to stretch

them out frequently,[1].—Slight burning pain gradually follows the drawing and tearing pains in the limbs,[4].—Burning in the hands and soles of the feet during menstruation,[1].—Tension in the knees and left hand, as if they had been overworked by severe motion,[1].—Burning sensation in both limbs, in the evening, in bed,[1].—*Drawing pain in the limbs,[1].—Drawing pain in the hands and feet,[1].—All the limbs feel bruised,[1].—[850.] Severe bruised sensation in the joints, on account of which stretching out the limbs hurts, in the morning in bed after waking; it gradually disappears after rising,[3].

Superior Extremities.—The arms and hands frequently go to sleep during the day, but especially at night, so that she does not know where she shall put them in the bed,[1].—The arms are heavy and exhausted, on motion (after four hours),[4].—Heaviness of the arms, with drawings in the back,[1].—Cramp in the arms,[1].—Drawing in the right arm,[1].—*Drawing pain in the arm upon which he is lying at night,[1].—Bruised pain in the right arm,[1].—*Shoulder.* Paralytic weakness of the right shoulder and right arm (after one-quarter of an hour),[4].—*Burning on the right shoulder,[3].—[860.] Drawing pain in the shoulder,[1].—Rheumatic drawings in the right shoulder,[3].—Stitches in the right shoulder, day and night,[1].—Tearing, in the morning, on waking, in the left shoulder, then in the right hand, then in the right upper jaw, in the incisors,[3].—Burning on the shoulder-joint (after three hours),[3].—Drawing pain in the left shoulder-joint,[3].—Sensitive drawings in both shoulder-joints, both on motion and in rest (after sixteen hours),[4].—Tearing pain in the shoulder-joint (after ten hours),[4].—Violent tearing pain in the right shoulder-joint, especially on motion, with drawings in the humerus,[3].—Paralytic tearing in the right shoulder-joint, frequently repeated,[1].—[870.] Burning pain in the right axilla,[3].—Pressive drawing pain beneath the right axilla, especially noticed on motion,[3].—*Arm.* The upper arm seems especially heavy,[4].—Burning on the upper arm (after five days),[4].—Drawing pain from above downward in the right upper arm (after four hours),[4].—Drawing pain, with burning, in the upper arm,[3].—Dull drawing on the right upper arm (after four hours),[4].—Tearing in the left upper arm (after five hours),[3].—Tearing in the left upper arm, in several paroxysms (after four days),[4].—Violent tearing in the right upper arm, especially on motion (after five days),[4].—*Elbow.* [880.] *Pain in both elbow-joints, as if bruised,* in the morning, in bed,[1].—Burning on the right elbow,[3].—*Forearm.* Drawing pain in the right forearm, extending along down the ulna, towards the wrist (immediately),[4].—Drawing and tearing in the forearm, extending to the hand and fingers, especially on motion,[4].—Tearing in the whole of the forearm,[4].—*Drawing-tearing in the left forearm, from the elbow to the hand* (after forty-eight hours),[3].—Drawing-tearing in the upper side of the left forearm, near the elbow; the place is painful to pressure upon the bone (after three hours),[3].—Drawing-tearing in the left radius (after fourteen hours),[4].—*Wrist.* A small swelling on the flexor surface of the wrist,[1].—Paralytic pain in the wrist, on moving it,[1].—[890.] Sensation in the left wrist, as if the tendons were too short, on certain motions,[1].—Drawing pain in the wrist,[1].—Drawings in the joints of the wrist, elbow, and shoulder, especially in the wind, in the morning, disappearing on motion,[1].—*Tearing in the right or left wrist,[3].—*Hand.* Ice-cold hands (after forty-eight hours),[3].—Sensation in the hands as though the muscular power was weakened, especially noticed when writing (after six hours),[3].—He could only write slowly and with difficulty (after one hour and a half),[4].—The hands are inclined to become numb,[1].—Sensation, in the morning, on washing, as if the hands would go to sleep,[1].—The hands go to sleep,[1].—[900.] A kind of pain, as from a sprain, in the right hand and wrist, as if one had made great exertion by severe grasping (after three days),[4].—Spasmodic contraction of the hands,[1].—Drawings in the right metacarpal bones (after three-quarters of an hour),[4].—Pressive pain in the back of the hand (after four days),[4].—Violent stitching in the hands (in the evening), after which the second and third fingers were drawn spasmodically across each other, and caused the others to stand far apart,[1].—Tearing in the inner portion of the left hand, extending into the base of the little finger,[3].—Bruised pain in the back of the left hand,[3].—Throbbing pain in the hand, in the metacarpal bone of the middle finger,[2].—**Fingers.** Gouty pain in the last joint of the thumb,[1].—Stitches in the ball of the thumb, starting from the wrist,[1].—[910.] Tearings under the thumb-nail,[3]. —Fine tearings in the right thumb, as if in the bone,[4].—Fine burning-tearing in the tip of the right thumb,[3].—A slow throbbing pain in the ungual phalanx of the thumb,[2].—Repeated pulsation on the back of the thumb,[4].—The tips of the fingers are cold and sweaty,[1].—Paralysis and weakness of the right fingers, when grasping anything,[4].—Stitches in a finger, when rising from sitting,[1].—Tearing pains in several fingers, in the evening,[4].—Tearings in the fingers of the right hand (after six hours),[3].— [920.] *Tearings in the fingers of the left hand,*[1].—Tearing-sticking in the middle joint of the fingers,[1].—Cold burning in the first (metacarpal) joint of the right middle and ring fingers,[3].—Boring pain in the middle joint of the left index finger, when at rest; but on moving or bending it a fine sticking as from a splinter, for six hours,[2].—Severe tearings in the last joint of the left index finger,[3].—Fine tearing in the middle joint of the right index finger,[3].—Fine stitches in the skin of the right index finger, renewed by bending the arm (after two hours),[4].—Drawing in the right index finger, extending towards the tip,[1].—Swelling of the ungual phalanx of the left middle finger, with drawing pain in it,[4].—Boring pain in the lowest joint (nearest the palm) of the middle finger and thumb,[2].—[930.] Stitches in the lowest joint of the left middle finger (after one hour and three-quarters),[4].—Sudden deep stitches in the first joint of the right middle finger (after forty-one hours),[4].—Fine tearings in the second middle finger of the right hand,[3].—Tearings in the joints of the two last fingers,[3].— Stitches as from a splinter in the ungual phalanx of the fourth finger,[4].— Tearings in the right little finger, increased by motion,[3].—Tearing in the tip and beneath the nail of the left fourth finger (after forty-eight hours),[3].

Inferior Extremities.—The legs are relaxed, so that he cannot raise them, from noon till evening,[1].—Weariness and paralytic sensation in both lower limbs (after forty hours),[4].—The joints seem unable to sustain the body (after five days),[4].—[940.] On rising, after sitting a long time, the limbs feel heavy and stiff, which disappears after walking a little,[1].— Both legs pain, especially the lower legs, when sitting or lying, so that he did not know where to rest them,[1].—Drawing sensation in the legs, especially in the lower legs,[3].—Tearing in the upper and lower leg,[3].—Tearing in the right leg, from the thigh down through the lower leg,[4].—Tearings in the legs, which seem to be aggravated by a great accumulation of flatulence,[4].—Rheumatic pain extending from the left ribs into the hip,[3].—Violent burning, externally, on the right hip,[3].—Tension in the joints of the hips and knees, while walking,[1].—*Drawing pain in the hip-joints, extending down the thighs, worse when walking,*[1].—[950.] Tearing in the hips, by paroxysms (after three days),[4].—Tearings in the right hip,[3].—*Tearing-pressive pain near and beneath the left hip, extending to the back and sacrum, frequently repeated,[3].—*Thigh.* Muscular twitches on the posterior portion of the left thigh, in the morning, in bed,[3].—Numbness of the thigh, when walking,[1].—Uneasy sensation in the right thigh and lower leg, which constantly obliged him to change his seat,[4].—Burning in the thigh, at night, in bed,[1].—Burning sensation in the upper part of the outer side of the thigh,[1].—Tension in the thigh, and a drawing, as if it were paralyzed or sprained (first four days),[1].—Tension in the thighs, above the knees, in the morning, on rising,[1].—[960.] Contractive pain in the thigh, extending to the knee, so that she has to bend the knee inward, when walking,[1].—Cramp-like pain in the outer side of the left thigh, in the lower part, when walking, and especially when raising the thigh and ascending steps, with painfulness of the part to touch (after thirty-five hours),[4].—Rheumatic drawing in the left thigh, in the evening, in bed, relieved by lying upon it,[3].—Stitches shoot down through the thigh, when walking (twelfth day),[1].—Dull stitches in the upper part of the thigh,[3].—Tearing pain in the middle of the thigh, frequently repeated,[3].—*Knee.* Weariness and sensation of unsteadiness in the knees, when walking or standing,[3].—Stiffness and weariness of the knee,[1].—Paralyzed sensation in the knee-joint, after walking,[1].—Pain in the knees, when going upstairs,[1].—[970.] Paralytic pain in the knees, when sitting or rising from sitting, and when lying, if she turns over or stretches out the knees,[1].—Burning pain in the inner side of the left knee,[4].—Severe burning in the right knee,[3].—Tension in the knees and ankles (after five days),[1].—Tension in the hollow of the knee, as from weariness, without previous motion,[1].—Drawing pain in the knees, when standing,[1].—Pressive-tearing in both knees and lower legs,[1].—Stitches in the knee-cap, after rising from sitting, with a sensation as if the knee were swollen,[1].—In the knee, a moderate blow makes the bone very sore,[1].—*Leg.* Tickling restlessness in the lower leg, in the evening,[1].—[980.] The legs go to sleep (after three days),[1].—Numbness and loss of sensation in the legs,[1].—*Heaviness of the legs* (after five days),[1].—*Sensation of stiffness in the legs, after an evening nap, so that he was unsteady while walking until he had walked a little,*[1].—*Paralyzed sensation in the left lower leg,*[1].—Flatulence causes a sensation of paralysis in the left leg by paroxysms (after five days),[4].—Severe cramp in the whole lower leg, at night, in bed, especially in the soles of the feet,[1].—Severe cramp in the lower leg, especially in the soles of the feet, when walking in the open air,[1].—Drawing in the left lower leg, with uneasiness in it,[4].—Drawing sensation from the knee down the lower leg,[3].—[990.] *Severe paralytic drawing pain extending from the abdomen down into the left leg,*[3].—Rheumatic drawing in both lower legs, extending to the metatarsal bones (after forty-five hours),[4].—Drawings and jerkings in both lower legs; he was unable to lie still, and must at one time stretch them out, at another time draw them up (for half an hour),[1].—Tearings in the right lower leg,[3].—Tearings in the lower leg, extending from the calf downward into the inner malleolus,[3].—Swollen places on the calf, painful to touch,[1].—Stitches in the calf (in a node),[1].—*Ankle.* A stitch sometimes in the left ankle, as if burnt,[1].—Tearings in the bone, below the left malleolus,[3].—*Foot.* Profuse sweat of the feet (after nine days),[1].—[1000.] Great heaviness of the feet, after every dinner (for eight days),[1].—Uneasiness of the left foot; he was obliged to move it back and forth,[1].—Pain in the metatarsal bones, as if they would be torn, on stepping upon them,[1].—Burning in the soles of the feet, after standing,[1].—Burning in the soles of the feet, when sitting and walking,[1].—*Cramp in the soles of the feet,* in the evening, after lying down; it makes the toes crooked,[1].—Drawings in the feet, mostly when sitting,[1].—**Toes.** Swelling of the toes,[1].—Pain in the joint of the great toe,[1].—A stitch shoots through the right great toe,[1].—[**1010.**] Tearing pain in the toes of the right foot, increased when walking,[3].—Tearing in the middle toes of the right foot,[3].—Severe tearing under the toenails, from evening till into the night, extending into the soles (first four days),[1].—Pain under the nail of the right great toe,[3].—Pressive pain in a corn, at night, in bed,[1].—Sticking in a corn on the left little toe,[1].

General Symptoms.—Objective. Trembling from uneasiness and anxiety; was unable to remain in any place,[1].—The whole body trembled from uneasiness and anxiety every afternoon; it seems as though he had committed a great crime; this terminated by violent weeping, even in the street in the presence of strangers,[1].—Trembling of the body, with prostration,[1].—At night he started up on account of noises, with shivering of the back,[1].—[**1020.**] A wound from a stab began to bleed again at various times,[1].—Disinclination for physical exertion,[4].—*Debility and Faintness.* Indolence, disinclined to think (after ten hours),[4].—Indolent, weary, and trembling in all the limbs, and sweating easily, in the morning (second day),[4].—Indolence, sleepiness, and indisposition, in the evening,[1].—*Weariness,* especially in the limbs,[2][3].—Weariness in the morning, in bed,[3].—Sensation of great weariness in the morning, in bed, especially in the joints, disappearing after rising,[3].—*Great weariness and stretching of the limbs in the morning,*[1].—Sensation of weariness in the morning, with trembling of the limbs and a feeling about the stomach as after drinking too much wine (after twenty-four hours),[3].—[**1030.**] Weariness in the evening,[1].—Weariness after dinner (after four days),[1].—Great weariness after the pains,[1].—After the pains had lasted two days, they were followed by excessive weariness of the affected parts,[4].—*The weariness is especially noticed when walking; less when sitting, mostly in the arms when writing,*[4].—*Weariness after a short slow walk in the open air,*[3].—Sudden weariness while walking in the open air, which, however, soon passed away (after three days),[1].—Weary and unrefreshed in the morning on rising from sleep, but after a few hours she became stronger,[1].—Weakness in the forenoon, as from stupefaction,[1].—Weakness after breakfast,[1].—[**1040.**] Tremulous weakness after stool,[1].—Sensitive weakness of the body, in the evening, as after great loss of blood,[1].—*Attacks of faintlike weakness,*[1].—Loss of energy of muscular action (after one hour),[4].—General prostration towards noon, inclination to lean the head against something and to rest; the head feels empty, with sensation of hunger (after twelve hours),[4].—Exhaustion after a stool,[1].—Very frequent momentary attacks of faintness, even to sinking down, also with vertigo, followed by colic and griping in the bowels, as in diarrhœa, though he had an ordinary stool (after twenty-four hours),[1].—*Restlessness.* Uneasiness the whole day,[1].—Uneasiness in the evening,[1].—Uneasiness at night, with drawing pain in the limbs,[1].—[**1050.**] She is unable to rest in any other position than with the limbs drawn up against the abdomen,[1].—*Subjective.* Sick and weary, as if he had just risen from a serious illness,[1].—Every member of the body hurts, as also the back, with much headache and great weakness,[1].—Drawing pain in almost all parts of the body, especially below the breast, in the neck and arms,[1],—*Rheumatic drawings in the whole body, with coldness of the hands and feet,*[3].—Fine slight stitches over the whole body, when she became warm in bed,[1].—Itching stitches on the side on which he was lying, in the evening, in bed,[1].—*Tearing in various parts of the body* at night, in bed,[1].—*Tearing and* *drawing pain in various parts of the body*,[3].—If she spoke in the presence of others all parts throbbed, the usually pale face became puffy and bluish-red,[1].

Skin.—Eruptions, Dry. [1060.] Nettle-rash for several weeks (after four days),[1].—The tip of the nose scurfy,[1].—Some scattered, red, uneven spots on the neck, with sensitive itching, in the evening (after forty-eight hours),[4].—Eruption in the angle of the wings of the nose,[1].—Eruption in the left corner of the mouth, like an itching tetter,[1].—Eruption on the chin; ulcers beneath the jaw and in front of the ear,[1].—Painful eruption on the upper lip; the red portion is full of pimples,[1].—Itching eruption on the neck and shoulders just before menstruation,[1].—*Fine itching eruption on the hands*,[1].—Painless, papulous eruption on the forehead (after five days),[1].—[1070.] Red, smooth, painless, papulous eruption, here and there in the forehead,[3].—Papulous eruption on the temples,[1].—Much papulous eruption in the face and on the forehead,[4].—Papulous eruption on the neck,[1].—Itching nettle-rash on the calves,[1].—Small white pimples on the skin of the forehead, like glands (after three days),[4].—Red pimples on the forehead, near the hairs, that pain only on touch,[3].—Some white pimples on both temples (after four days),[4].—White itching pimples about the nose,[1].—White pimples on the lower part of the cheek,[1].—[1080.] A large red pimple close to the anus, with a blackish tip, itching somewhat,[1].—**Moist.** Itching eruption on the nose, with increased moisture (after seven hours),[4].—*Itching on the thigh near the scrotum;* the place is moist (after twenty-four hours),[1].—Itching vesicular eruption on the knee,[1].—A place which had been rubbed sore, and which was nearly covered with skin again, began to be denuded anew, and became moist,[1].—**Pustular.** Pustules, with burning sensation, below the red portion of the upper lip,[1].—A large boil on the upper arm, surrounded by many itching pimples (after seven days),[1].—An ulcer on the fontanelle exuded a corrosive moisture,[1].—An ulcer that had already healed broke out afresh, and discharged, instead of pus, lymph mingled with blood; the place was hard and painful to touch,[1].—*The pus from an ulcer was offensive, like asafœtida,[1].—**Sensations.** [1090.] *Burning in various places in the skin*, at night, in bed,[1].—*Slight burning pain in various places on the skin*,[4].—Crawling in the whole body,[1].—Itching over the whole body, day and night,[1].—Itching and sticking in several parts of the body,[4].—Severe itching of a tetter before menstruation,[1].—Sticking-itching, as from fleas, in several parts of the body,[4].—Burning on the skin as from a mustard-plaster, here and there, on the back, sides, on the right side of the abdomen, etc. (after twelve hours),[3].—Tension and pressure about an ulcer (on the lower leg),[1].—Itching behind the ear,[1].—[1100.] Itching in the upper part of the outer ear, which afterward became hot,[1].—Itching about the nostrils,[1].—Itching and burning in various places in the skin on the back, chest, on the navel, on the thighs, etc.,[3].—Stitching-itching in the region of the coccyx in the evening, in bed,[1].—Itching, moisture, and soreness in the axillæ,[1].—Severe itching in the right axilla,[1].—Severe itching on the arms, hands, and between the fingers, so that he was unable to sleep at night, though without eruption,[1].—Biting-itching, constantly repeated, on the lower portion of the inner side of the left upper arm, only transiently relieved by scratching (after fifty-four hours),[4].—Burning-itching in the forearm near the elbow,[3].—Severe itching in the palms at night,[1].—[1110.] Severe itching on the outer side of the left thumb,[1].

Sleep and Dreams.—Sleepiness. Yawning,[2].—*Much yawning* *and stretching,*[3][4].—*Frequent yawning and stretching, which seem to do good* (after five days),[4].—Inclined to sleep very early in the evening,[1].—Inclination to sleep after dinner, without being able to sleep,[1].—*Sleepiness increased by motion in the forenoon while sitting and reading,*[2].—Sleepiness after supper, with red heat of the face,[1].—Sleepiness, with frequent yawning,[3].— *Great sleepiness during the day; he was obliged to sleep before and after noon; at night his sleep was full of fancies* (after eight days),[1].—[1120.] Overpowering sleepiness after dinner, with burning of the lids on closing the eyes (seventh day),[1].—Overpowered with sleep in the evening,[1].—Overpowered with sleep after eating,[1].—Intoxicated with sleep after eating,[1].— Sleep after eating, uninterrupted for an hour, but uneasy on account of anxious dreams,[2].—*Sleeplessness.* She was unable to sleep at night, but could not open the eyes,[1].—Is unable to sleep at night, although the eyes seem full of sleep,[1].—She was unable to sleep at night on account of heat in the blood,[1].—*Loss of sleep on account of uneasiness in the body,*[1].— *Falls asleep late,* not until 1 o'clock,[1].—[1130.] Uneasy sleep and frequent waking at night,[1].—Uneasy, unrefreshing sleep; prostration in the morning,[1].—On falling asleep he started up as in fright,[1].—Much coherent talking in the sleep awakens him, when he remembers the dreams,[1].—Uneasy sleep with frequent waking, and in the morning in bed headache, with burning here and there in the body,[3].—Awakes early in the morning, about four,[1].—*Frequent waking at night, with coldness of the limbs and knees,*[1].— He was frequently awakened at night, with heat and thirst,[1].—*Dreams.* Very many dreams (first night),[4].—*Night full of dreams* (after ten hours),[3]. —[1140.] Vivid dreams,[1].—Vivid dreams, which are not remembered,[3].— Very vivid dreams, causing restlessness (second night),[4].—Very vivid, lascivious dreams (second night),[1].—Anxious dreams, with uneasy sleep,[3]. —Anxious, frightful dreams,[1].—Extremely anxious dreams,[3].—Tormenting dreams disturb the sleep,[1].

Fever.—Chilliness. Chilliness in the evening,[1].—Frequent chilliness; especially at night, chilliness and coldness,[1].—[1150.] With the irritation to cough, in the evening, chilliness and drawing in the cheeks,[1].— Shivering, frequently lasting an hour,[1].—*Shivering in the evening, with weariness* and flushes of heat, before going to sleep (after ten hours),[1].— Febrile chill in the morning, with thirst, chattering, *and blue finger-nails,* lasting till afternoon; then in the evening heat and sweat, without thirst,[1]. —*Chill with thirst,*[1].—Internal chill, with great thirst,[1].—Feverish coldness in the evening; he does not feel the warmth from the stove,[1].—Coldness of the left arm and left leg,[1].—*Very cold hands and feet in the evening,*[1].—She could not get the feet warm, in the evening, in bed, before 1 o'clock,[1].—[1160.] Chilliness and heat towards evening (after twelve days),[1].—Chill at 11 A.M. for several days; heat in the evening at 6,[1].— *Heat.* Heat at night in bed,[1].—Sensation of heat, with great anxiety, in the evening, although she was cold to touch all over,[1].—General burning heat in the evening, with great weariness and fantasies at night,[1].—A little wine heats him very much,[3].—Warmth in the spine rising up to the throat,[1].—Great orgasm of blood,[1].—Orgasm of blood, with congestion to the chest, with hoarseness and hawking,[1].—Much heat the whole day, though with constantly cold feet,[1].—*Sweat.* [1170.] Much inclined to sweat,[4].—Increased sweat in the morning on waking (after three days),[4].— Profuse sweat of the body, and even of the head, before midnight,[1].—General sweat after a moderate breakfast,[1].—Warm sweat in the morning (after twenty-nine hours),[4].—Sour-smelling sweat (after eight days),[1].—Sweat of an offensive odor at night,[1].—He sweat easily on the upper part of the body in a warm room, and then again became just as easily chilled,[1].— Sweat on the forehead while eating,[1].—Frequent profuse sweat on the face (in a boy two years old),[4].—**[1180]**. Heat on the balls of the hands,[1].— Sweat of the feet when walking,[1].

Conditions.—**Aggravation.**—(*Morning*), On waking, anxiety; immediately after rising, confusion of the head; in bed, headache over vertex; on waking, headache; eyes agglutinated; immediately after rising, flickering before eyes; in bed, nose-bleed; on waking, catarrhal irritation; dryness of mouth; on waking, dryness of mouth; bitter mucus in mouth; scraping in throat; an hour after waking, nausea, etc.; pain near pit of stomach; on waking, passage of flatus; in bed, itching in anus; contraction of urethra; tearing, etc., in urethra; very early, desire to urinate; on rising, leucorrhœa; almost voiceless; on rising from bed, cough; after waking, cough; on waking, rush of blood to chest; after rising, tightness in chest; after rising from bed, sensation in chest; in bed, sticking beneath ribs; on rising, stiffness in back; tearing from chest to back, etc.; in bed after rising, sensation in joints; on waking, tearing in shoulder, etc.; in bed, *pain in elbow-joints;* especially in the wind, drawing in wrist-joint, etc.; on washing, sensation in hands; in bed, twitches in left thigh; on rising, tension in thighs; indolent, etc.; in bed, *weariness, etc.;* on rising from sleep, weary, etc.; prostration; in bed, headache, etc.; febrile chill, etc.; on waking, sweat; warm sweat.—(*Forenoon*), Violent, etc., attack of vertigo, etc.; nose-bleed; when sucking gum, blood flows into mouth; sensation in pharynx; about 10 or 11 o'clock, nausea; weakness; 11 o'clock, chilliness.—(*Toward noon*), Diminished appetite; general prostration, etc. —(*Noon*), Little appetite, etc.—(*Afternoon*), 4 to 6 o'clock, anxiety; throbbing headache; *headache in forehead;* pressure in top of head; ringing in ear; eructations; accumulation of flatulence; pain near pit of stomach; abdomen distended; flatulence, etc.; great quantity of flatus; tension in abdomen; griping in abdomen; noon till evening, legs relaxed; body trembled, etc.—(*Toward evening*), In open air, sour eructations; difficult breathing, etc.; chilliness, etc.—(*Evening*), Excited, etc.; anxiety; after lying down, anxiety, etc.; after walking, confusion of head; after sleeping while sitting, dizzy, etc.; dizziness; in bed, headache; in bed, throbbing headache; after lying down, eyes ache; heat, etc., of left ear; twinges in right ear; fluent coryza; crawling in the side of nose; in bed, tearing in left zygoma; sensation in mouth, etc.; scraping in throat; pain in pit of stomach, etc.; after 7 o'clock, pressure in pit of stomach; griping in abdomen; cutting in bowels; stitches in anus; soreness in pudenda; obliged to clear throat, etc.; after lying down, crawling, etc., in larynx; hoarseness; when walking in open air, hoarseness; cough; in bed, short cough; spasmodic cough; on going to sleep, cough; when lying, difficult breathing; on going to sleep, palpitation, etc.; drawing pain in back; in bed, twitching of the arms, etc.; in bed, heaviness of the limbs; in bed, drawing sensation in limbs; pains in fingers; in bed, drawing in thigh; restlessness in lower leg; after lying down, *cramp in soles;* indolence, etc.; weariness; weakness of body; uneasiness; in bed, stitches on the side; red spots on neck; in bed, sticking-itching in region of coccyx; chilliness; with the irritation to cough, chilliness, etc.; shivering, etc.; feverish coldness; cold hands, etc.; in bed, before 1 o'clock, could not get feet warm; at 6 o'clock, heat; burning heat.—(*Night*), Headache; pain in occiput, etc.; unable to open eyes; illusions of hearing; sneezing; *frequent sneezing, etc.; nose-bleed;* catarrhal irritation; nausea; pressure beneath stomach, etc.; diarrhœa; moisture from anus; paroxysms of cough; heaviness of back, etc.; sticking between shoulder-blades; arms go to sleep; in bed, burning in thigh; in bed, sensation in left leg; in bed, cramp in leg; tearing under toenails; in bed, pain in corn; uneasiness, etc.; *tearing in various parts;* in bed, burning in skin; itching on the the palms, chilliness, etc.; in bed, heat; offensive sweat.—(*After midnight*), Profuse sweat.—(*When walking in open air*), Most pains appear; pain in liver; numbness of thigh; cramp in lower leg.—(*Ascending steps*), Pain in left thigh; pain in knees.—(*On bending back arms*), Tearing in shoulder-blade.—(*After breakfast*), Pressure beneath short ribs; weakness; general sweat.—(*Breathing*), Pain in abdomen, etc.—(*During deep breathing*), Stitches in right side.—(*On going from a warm room into a cold one*), Cough. —(*When coughing*), *Stitches through the head;* pain in larynx, etc.; pain in chest.—(*Before dinner*), Nausea.—(*After dinner*), Confusion of head; pressure in lids, etc.; mouth filled with mucus; *abdomen distended;* for eight days, heaviness of feet; weariness; inclination to sleep; sleepiness, etc.— (*After drinking*), Empty eructations.—(*While eating*), Anxiety; toothache; throbbing in teeth; sore pain in throat; griping in abdomen; sweat on forehead.—(*After eating*), Anxiety; out of humor; headache; headache in forehead, etc.; sour taste; *nausea*, etc.; distension of the abdomen, etc.; griping in abdomen; palpitation; *overpowered with sleep.*—(*After eating and drinking*), Eructations.—(*After every expectoration*), Dry cough.— (*On gargling*), Vertigo.—(*Inspiration*), Pressure in trachea; pain in right chest, etc.—(*When lying*), Legs pain; if she turns over, or stretches out the knees, pain in knees.—(*Lying on side*), Pain in bowels.—(*When lying on back*), Acidity in stomach.—(*Before every meal*), Nausea.—(*With every meal*), Nausea.—(*Before menstruation*), Itching of a tetter.—(*During menstruation*), Headache; pains in lower abdomen; burning in hands, etc.— (*After taking milk*), Flatulence; sour eructations.—(*On motion*), Vertigo; pain in head; in open air, hiccough; pain in right shoulder-joint; tearing in upper arm; drawing, etc., in forearm.—(*On sudden motion of head*), Vertigo.—(*Raising thigh*), Pain in thigh.—(*From reading*), Shocks in head; stitches in upper part of head.—(*During respiration*), *Throbbing of the head.*—(*On rising after sitting*), Limbs heavy; pain in knees.—(*Salt food*), Toothache.—(*When shaking head*), Pain in right side of head.—(*When sitting*), Vertigo; crackling in occiput; difficult breathing; palpitation; *pain in back;* drawing in back, etc.; legs pain; pain in knees.—(*While sitting bent*), Pinching in abdomen; griping in abdomen.—(*After sitting*), Heat of cheeks.—(*After soup*), Empty eructations.—(*Standing*), Painfulness of stomach; weariness, etc., in knees; pain in knees; burning in soles of feet.—(*Before stool*), Drawing across abdomen.—(*After stool*), Anxiety, etc.; emptiness of abdomen; colic; burning in anus; tremulous weakness; exhaustion.—(*On stooping*), Vertigo; headache; drawing in back.—(*After supper*), Headache; pressure in occiput; sleepiness, etc.—(*Touch*), Pressure in stomach.—(*On turning in bed*), Vertigo.—(*When urinating*), Sticking in pudenda; itching in pudenda.—(*After waking from sleep*), Vertigo; dulness of head; throbbing in temples, etc.; itching in anus; chest feels weary; chest oppressed, etc.; stiffness in legs.—(*Walking*), Vertigo; dizziness in head; acidity in stomach; painfulness of stomach; emptiness of abdomen; tension in hip-joints, etc.; pain in hip-joints; pain in thigh; stitches through thigh; weariness, etc., in knees; sensation in knee-joint; pain in right toes; sweat of the feet.—(*On becoming warm in bed*), Stitches all over body.—(*Writing*), Sensation in left shoulder-blade; sensation in hands; weariness in arms.

Amelioration.—(*Eructation*), Sensation of oppression of chest.—(*Lying down*), Confusion in head; drawing in left thigh.—(*On motion*), Drawing in wrist-joint, etc., disappears.—(*On passing wind*), Pain in region of stomach disappears.—(*Raising head*), Headache.—(*After rising*), Head ache, etc., disappears.—(*Rising from bed*), Headache.

CARBOLIC ACID.

Acidum carbolicum, Phenol, Monoxybenzene, Phenyl-alcohol. C_6H_5OH.
Preparation, Solution in alcohol.

Authorities. 1, T. Bacmeister, M.D., proving with the 1st dilution, *from Dr. Hoyne's Monograph*, Chicago, 1869; 2, ibid., proving with the 12th dilution; 3, T. S. Hoyne, M.D., provings with the 6th and 3d dilutions, ibid.; 4, Miss G. H., proving with the 6th dilution, ibid.; 5, Mrs. T. S. H., proving with the 6th dilution, ibid.; 6, J. T. H., proving with the 6th dilution, ibid.; 7, T. C. Duncan, M.D., proving with the 12th dilution, ibid.; 8, ibid., effects of inhaling the fumes; 9, Mrs. T. C. D., effects of the fumes, ibid.; 10, Mrs. E. J. Duncan, effects of the fumes inhaled while menstruating, ibid.; 11, S. P. Hedges, M.D., provings with the 6th dilution, ibid.; 12, C. W. Boyce, M.D., effect of local application to the hand, ibid.; 13, Chas. H. Hæseler, M.D., proving with 1 to 20 drops of the crude acid (36 drops taken in three days), Hahn. M., 5, 171; 14, Mr. X. Y. Z., effects of crude drug. ibid.; 15, girl of 11, effects of 4 drops of pure acid, ibid.; 16, Chas. H. Hæseler, effects of the 3d dec. dilution, ibid.; 17, S. Lilienthal, M.D., proving with the 1st dec. dilution, and two doses of tincture, Trans. of Hom. Med. Soc., State of N. Y., 1870, p. 232; 18, Mrs. S. A. F., M.D., proving with 1st dec. dilution, ibid.; 19, Mrs. C. L., M.D., provings with 1st cent. dilution, and one dose of the 30th dilution, ibid.; 20, Mrs. A. W., proving, ibid.; 21, E. C. Price, M.D., Am. Hom. Obs., 1871, p. 148, proving with 3d dilution, 3d dec. dilution, and 2d dec. dilution; 22, T. D. Pritchard, M.D., Trans. Hom. Med. Soc. State of N. Y., 1874, 136, effects of inhaling the vapor; 23, J. N. Mitchell, Am. J. of H. M. M., N. S., 1, 354, effects of Carbolic acid put into a tooth; 24, W. M. Williamson, M.D., Trans. Penn. Hom. Med. Soc., 1871, effects of the vapor; 25, Taylor, Guy's Hosp. Rep., 1868 (Hahn. Month., 5, 169), poisoning of a child of $1\frac{3}{4}$ years by two teaspoonfuls; 26, H. W. Fuller, M.D., Brit. Med. Journ. (H. M., 5, 170), effects of doses of from three minims upward; 27, Machin, El. Crit. Med. (N. Am. J. of Hom., 18, 155), effects on three women who had washed in Carbolic-acid water; 28, Dr. Oyston, B. Med. J., 1871, effects of swallowing 1 to 2 ounces of raw Carbolic acid from a flask (thinking it brandy); 29, Dr. Pinkham, Med. and S. Rep., 19 (H. M., 5, 168), general effects; 30, Pinkham, l. c., effects of an enema containing 145 grains on a young lady; 31, Sutton, Med. Times and Gaz., April, 1868 (H. M., 5, 169), poisoning by one ounce; 32, Kline, Phil. M. and S. Rep., 1870; 33, Michelas, Wien. Med. Presse, 8, 1867 (Schmidt's Jahrb., 146, 273), effects of clyster containing 145 grains for ascarides, administered to a woman aged 22; 34, Ibid., effects on a boy of 10 years, of a clyster containing $\frac{9}{10}$ths gramme; 35, Wallace, Br. J., 1870, effects after being applied to an abscess; 36, Ph. M. and S. Rep., 1867, a nurse, 32 years old, drank half an ounce (S. J.,

151); 37, Dr. White, N. Y. Med. Gaz., 1872, effects when applied to a necrosed tibia; 38, Kohler, effects of an application to scabies (S. J., 155, 275); 39, ibid., general statement of effects; 40, Welander, Hygea, 36 (1874), Am. Hom. Obs., 1874, effects of a teaspoonful of a solution containing 25 or 30 centigrammes; 41, omitted; 42, Danion, Recherches sur l'acide phenique, Rapport an der Med. Fakult, zu Strassburg, 1869 (extracted from Dr. C. G. Rothe, Die Carbolsäure in der medicin, monograph, Berlin, 1875), proving of 1 gramme, afterward 2 grammes, afterward 4 grammes, in three portions; 43, Rothe, l. c., proving of 1 gramme in 20 parts of water; 44, Husemann, S. J., 155, p. 275, general effects of poisoning by small quantities; 45, Mosler, Br. Med. J., 1872, effects of 2 or 3 drachms; 46, Unthank, Br. Med. J., 1872, effects of the fumes; 47, Warren (New Remedies, 4, 178), effects of drinking some from a flask, mistaking it for whisky.

Mind. — Emotional. Delirium,[30] [44].—Delirium like intoxication, often lasting half an hour,[38].—Deliria, irritability, and rage, with copious perspiration,[40].—During the evening felt unusually cheerful,[3].—Feeling of sadness, with disposition to sigh and yawn (soon after 20 drops),[13].—Not in humor to think or speak,[17].—*Very irritable*,[17].—Cross; loses control of temper readily (second day),[7].—Appeared morose, and much less brilliant in conversation than usual,[14].—[10.] Affection bestowed seemed distasteful (third day),[7].—A fear of impending sickness came over him as soon as he retired to bed,[17].—*Intellectual.* Mind clear and active (second day),[7]. —Strange to say, although so affected by reading, my mind seemed unusually on the alert, and, although using it very much, nearly set me crazy with the confusion and pains in my head, yet I saw through any proposition with unusual quickness, and was desirous of intellectual work,[23].— *Disinclination to mental efforts, even to read*,[17].—*Disinclination to mental exertion* (as studying cases, preparing copy, etc.), (third day),[7].—*Entire disinclination to study; what he had accomplished seemed very trifling* (evening),[2].—Mental and bodily laziness; do not wish to exert myself in any way,[17].—Could not concentrate the mind upon anything (soon after 20 drops),[13].—I would get into an absent-minded abstracted condition, from which I would start when any one spoke to me, and would find myself at times in a nervous tremor when spoken to suddenly,[23].—[20.] When reading, cannot fix my attention on the subject so as to retain it in memory (fifth day),[17].—Want of acuteness in thinking (soon after 20 drops),[13].— Feels dull and stupid (after one hour and five-sixths),[3].—Loss of memory (soon after 20 drops),[13].—Unconscious,[32].—Unconscious for four hours; then first opened eyes, moved arm and leg,[28].—Unconsciousness, with stertorous breathing,[28].—Complete unconsciousness (after five minutes),[36].—Lost all knowledge of what passed around them,[27].—Insensibility,[29].—[30.] Nearly or quite insensible,[30].—Reclining in a chair, insensible (after five minutes),[31]. —Lay insensible to all external objects, but in a short time recovered itself,[25]. —Became insensible, falling down suddenly as if in a fit; on his recovery, said he remembered nothing whatever after tasting the liquid (immediately),[47].—Stupor,[44] [46].—Slight stupefaction,[42].—Quite comatose,[46].

Head.—Confusion and Vertigo. Transient confusion of the head,[43].—Confusion and heaviness of the head,[41].—[40.] Confusion and pain in head, pain located over right eye,[14].—Confused feeling in head (third day),[7].—Brain felt confused and painful (soon after 20 drops),[13].—Head feels muddled, although no severe pain,[17].—Muddled and confused, and could collect thoughts only with an effort,[13].—Vertigo,[38] [44].—Vertigo, with trembling,[17].—Easier in the afternoon, being much exposed to wind, which cools the heated brain, but vertigo returns as soon as he enters a room,[17].— Very dizzy from the slightest motion (after five minutes),[6].—Very dizzy; things look as if they were moving backwards and forwards (after five minutes),[4].—[50.] Giddiness,[29][46].—A giddiness and fulness, or peculiar feeling in the head (after two to eight minutes),[26].—My giddiness was better when walking fast in the open air, but as soon as I would sit down, would become so bad that I would have to hold on to something to prevent falling,[23]. —Head swimming, and he felt as if staggering like a drunken man (soon after 20 drops),[13].—Staggering as if drunk,[38].—*General Head.* Rush of blood to head (second day),[7].—Felt like rubbing head and eyes constantly (soon after 20 drops),[13].—Feeling as though I had suffered from headache, for three days before (third day),[11].—Dulness in head (third day),[7].—Dull feeling in head (after a few moments),[3].—[60.] Head felt heavy (after half an hour),[18].—Head very heavy,[17].—Heaviness of head, when leaning forward (after two hours and one-third),[3].—Heavy pain in head, running from forehead to occiput (after half an hour),[5].—Headache,[29][44].—Complained of headache,[28].—Headache, worse on left side,[17].— Headache, worse when bending head forward (after one hour and five-sixths),[3].—Headache disappeared soon after breakfast (second day),[3].— Drinking a cup of green tea relieved somewhat the headache, but not the sense of smell,[10].—[70.] Slight headache,[17].—Severe headache, with nausea (after half an hour),[10].—In morning, awoke with a hard headache confined to the upper half of the head (second day),[3].—Had a hard headache most of night, and has it this morning; feels as if a band was around the forehead (second day),[6].—Pain and fulness in head, which seemed to locate itself especially over right eye,[16].—Head hot (after thirty-five minutes),[3]. —Fulness of the brain,[17].—Fulness of head all over the brain, with dull pain,[17].—Expansive pains in head, with swimming before eyes; hardly able to write,[17].—My head felt as if inclosed in a band, which at times would seem to be compressed and crushing in my head. This pressing feeling was especially noticeable in both temples,[23].—[80.] Dull constricting headache at 7.30 A.M., about half an hour after rising, continuing and increasing until noon, when I gave up to it. It did not locate anywhere particular, but was as bad in the forehead as anywhere else. Pressure relieved for about one minute, but if continued longer increased the pain. However, if the pressure was removed, if only for an instant, and then reapplied, it would bring relief for a moment. My head seemed to swell and feel hot, even as though it radiated heat as a hot stove. These sensations seemed confined to the cranium, not coming below the base of the skull proper; continued until I went to sleep at night (second day),[11].—Dull, hot, constricted feeling in the head, especially in the forehead, on waking at 6.30 A.M., severe enough to become an ache at times (relieved by pressing the head with the hands), lasted all day and until late in the night (second day),[11].—Dull headache (second day),[38].—Dull headache, running from forehead to occiput (after five minutes),[6].—Headache, as if somebody was jagging a sword in and out all around the head; she could hardly keep the eyes open; aggravation from the least noise, and from light; desires to have head tightly bandaged (after one hour),[15].—Sore feeling, as though I had suffered from headache (third day),[11].—Head feels sore when moving it (after one hour and a quarter),[3].—The head-pains are the most severe, and are *worse on right side* (after thirty-five minutes),[3].—While smoking after tea, the head-pains are very much better (after two hours and a half),[3].—*Forehead.* Frontal headache, worse in a hot room,[17].—[90.] Headache in forehead and temples,[20].—Frontal headache and oppression of chest, beginning on left side and going over to right (after fifteen minutes),[17].—Headache in the forehead of a neuralgic character (second day),[3].—Forehead feels hot, and the pressure of a cold hand on it gives some transient relief,[17].—Burning headache in forehead (after twenty minutes),[5].—Severe burning pain in brain over the eyebrows,[17].—Full feeling in frontal lobe of cerebrum, which increased to a severe headache,[8].—A pressing fulness in the forehead,[17].—*Feeling of tightness across forehead directly above frontal sinuses,*[18].—Aching pain in forehead (transient),[3].—[100.] Slight aching in forehead, left side (after one hour),[1].—Dull aching pain in left temple and back of head, when leaning forward (after one hour and a quarter),[3].—Dull pains through the forehead (after thirty-five minutes),[3].—*Dull frontal headache in centre of forehead,*[19].—*Dull frontal headache, as if an india-rubber band was stretched tightly over the forehead,*[17].—Woke in morning with a dull frontal headache and burning in throat (second day),[17].—Does not know whether he has taken cold or not; the same dull frontal headache, with general lassitude (fifth day),[17].—Dull frontal headache, with chilliness (very soon),[17].—Dull frontal headache, somewhat relieved in the fresh air (after three hours),[17].—*Temples.* Pain extends to temple (from over right eye), with sense of soreness of the eyeball,[24].—[110.] Burning pains in right temple and top of head (after thirty-five minutes),[3].—*Feeling of tightness, as if an india-rubber band was stretched from temple to temple,*[17].—Bandlike constrictions from one temple to the other, followed by a dull, heavy headache, greatly aggravated by a walk in the open air (after half an hour),[18].—Slight aching in left temple (soon after),[17].—Dull, heavy pain in left temple during the day (fourth day),[17].—*Dull, heavy pain through the temples, with tight band across forehead, and tightness in the nose between the eyes,*[20].—When I read for any length of time the pressing in my temples became fearful, and my whole head would feel somewhat in the condition known as "asleep" in a limb,[23].—*Vertex.* I felt, on top of my head, as if my brain was swashing about,[23].—Burning pain in top of head,[3].—Constant aching pain in right side of head (after twenty minutes),[3].—*Parietals.* [120.] Neuralgic pain in left side of head (after one hour and a quarter),[3].—Beating pain in right side of head (after thirty-five minutes),[3].—Pains in head of a sharp, darting, neuralgic character, changing their situation from one side to the other, affecting the eye of the painful side so much that it was difficult to keep it open (soon after 10 drops),[13].—*Occiput.* Occipital pressure,[17].—Dull, pressing, occipital headache,[17].—Dull aching pain in back of head and right side and temple. The pains in head are constant, and similar to those felt when making the first proving (after one hour and a half),[3].—Back of head feels sore (after one hour and five-sixths),[3].—*External Head.* *Small pustulous vesicle a little to left of vertex* (third day),[21].—*Itching of scalp* (after one hour and a quarter),[3].—Itching of scalp (after fifteen minutes),[6].—[130.] Itching of scalp, first on right side, then on left,[3].

Eye.—Eyes rigid, insensible to light, pupils much dilated,[34].—Eyes heavy (second day),[7].—Burning pain in eyes, worse in left (after two hours),[3].—Burning pain in left eye (transient),[3].—*Orbit.* Pain over the right eye, which continued for an hour after being out in the air, then passed off, but returned upon returning to the room and smelling the acid again, but passed off again in the open air,[24].—A very slight pain for a few minutes, at two different times, over right eye,[21].—*Very severe orbital neuralgia over the right eye,[23].—*Slight pain over right eyebrow; the same kind of pain, but in a milder degree, under right patella, both of short duration (after half an hour),[21].—Acute piercing pain in the left supraorbital ridge, in a spot as large as a silver ten-cent piece, lasting only five or ten minutes and ceasing on rising, but leaving the spot where it had been sore to the touch for more than one day (second day),[11].—*Lids.* [140.] Eyes open, turned upward,[32][36].—Lids closed,[28].—*Ball.* Neuralgic twitching in eye-balls and through temples (soon after 20 drops),[13].—*Pupil.* Contraction of the pupils,[28][30], etc.—Pupils contracted (after five minutes),[31].—Pupils contracted and insensible to light,[25].—Pupils dilated, but showed reaction to light (after two hours),[40].—*Vision.* Eyes sensitive to light,[8].—Cannot see across room (after five minutes),[4].—[150.] Reading is impossible, as the letters look blurred and fade one in the other,[17].—While writing, the letters seem to run together, so that it is with difficulty I can read what is written (after thirty-five minutes),[3].—Swimming before the eyes,[17].—Things seem to be moving before the eyes (after three-quarters of an hour),[5].—A constant dark spot in front of the left eye,[23].

Ear.—Pressing pain in left ear (transient), (after fifteen minutes), returning from time to time (after twenty minutes),[3].—Beating pain, with a humming sound, in both ears (after six hours),[3].—Roaring in the ears,[42].—Troubled all the time with a constant humming-buzzing sound in my ears, although my hearing did not seem affected,[23].

Nose.—Both nostrils plugged up (fourth day),[7].—[160.] When blowing nose the mucus was bloody, bright-red blood (after four and one-sixth hours),[3].—Feel as if I had a cold in the head; right nostril plugged up, right eye watery (third day),[7].—Nose tight and stopped up, with full tight feeling across forehead,[20].—Left nostril stinging, with constant watering of the left eye, and watery discharge from nose,[20].—Sensation at left wing of nose as of fine electric sparks; wants to rub the part repeatedly (after fifteen minutes); during first hour same sensation on sternal end of right clavicle; later on middle finger of left hand; later on vertex. This sensation, during the time it was felt, changed slowly to a pricking-itching, with desire to rub the part, and relief from it,[2].—Tickling in right nostril, with sneezing (after one hour and one-third),[3].—*Smell.* Sense of smell very acute,[8].—Sense of smell exceedingly acute, for five days (after half an hour),[10].—Smell more acute, very decidedly; soon after watery discharge from both nostrils while in the open air; when indoors it ceases; comes again after entering a cold room (after twenty minutes),[1].

Face.—*Objective.* Pale and unconscious,[34].—[170.] The boy was very pale, weak, and cachectic,[35].—Face blanched and bathed in perspiration (after five minutes),[31].—*Face pale,*[37].—Face pale and covered with cold perspiration,[25].—Face pale or livid,[44].—Face and neck livid,[46].—Face livid, with cold, clammy sweat,[32].—Face livid, covered with cold, clammy sweat,[36].—Face flushed (second day),[7].—Face flushed, and "burns" (after fifteen minutes),[6].—[180.] Slight lividity of the lips and tips of the fingers (after five minutes),[31].—State of intense trismus (after eighteen minutes),[45].—At the attempt to examine his throat he closes his teeth tightly,[40].—*Subjective.* Pain in face and neck (after seven hours),[46].—Drawing pain in jaw, right side,[3].

Mouth.—*Teeth.* Aching in teeth of right upper jaw (after a few moments),[3].—*Tongue.* Burning on the tongue, especially on the tip,[17].—Biting sensation on tongue (immediately),[17].—*Mouth.* Mucous membrane of mouth, lips, throat, white,[28].—Swelling and soreness on internal side of left cheek opposite the molars; the cheek is in the way of the teeth when biting (the whole day), (after two days),[2].—[190.] Strong tarry odor to the breath,[25].—Burning mouth,[44].—Burning on lips, throat, and œsophagus, with heat rising up from the stomach (immediately),[17].—*Saliva.* Hypersecretion of saliva, and he could not help spitting all the time, the spittle having a bluish-white, frothy appearance,[13].—Constant discharge of saliva from the pale lips,[34].—Mouth open, filled with mucus,[32].—*Taste.* Very sharp taste; tongue burned and tingled, and felt as if a thousand pins were sticking in it (immediately),[15].—Nasty taste in mouth,[3].—Horrid taste in mouth, pungent and metallic, which he could not get rid of; it made him feel sick and squally all over (immediately),[14].—Taste of carbolic acid in mouth and throat (after seven hours),[47].—[200.] Coppery, metallic taste on tongue and upper palate,[17].—*Speech.* Inability to speak or to walk,[28].

Throat.—A good deal of hawking of clear white mucus while in the open air (second day),[7].—Pain in throat on swallowing (after one and five-sixths hours),[3].—Choking feeling in throat, with disposition to hawk up phlegm,[14].—Irritation of throat (for some days),[45].—Irritation of throat causing short, dry cough (after one hour and five-sixths),[3].—Burning in throat and œsophagus (immediately),[40].—Sense of burning in throat on swallowing the draught,[26].—Pricking-burning in throat, as if she had eaten something strong (after half an hour),[5].—[210.] Very sharp stitches in throat; the pain grows worse and worse; it is sharp and pricking (after fifteen minutes),[3].—Weather changed (?); throat sore, felt some hoarse, as if had taken cold (second day),[7].—Evening, throat some sore, right side (second day),[7].—Soreness of throat on empty deglutition (after fifteen minutes), passed off after one and one-sixth hours, except when swallowing and pressing on the upper larynx; worse on the right side,[3].—Throat sore only when swallowing (after two hours and five-sixths),[3].—While smoking, after tea, throat better for a time; not so sensitive to pressure (after two and a half hours),[3].—*Fauces. Pharynx, and Œsophagus.* Much mucus in pharynx (fourth day),[7].—Hawking from pharynx and posterior nares of much white mucus (third day),[7].—In morning, on waking, pharynx and posterior nares very dry indeed (fifth day),[7].—Burning in the œsophagus and stomach,[17].—[220.] Spasmodic contraction of œsophagus,[32].—Spasmodic contraction of the œsophagus prevented the insertion of the stomach-pump,[36].—Spasmodic and painful contraction of the œsophagus just behind the pomum Adami; while drinking ice-water, was painful for several minutes,[21].—Feeling of constriction about midway of the œsophagus (from 20 drops),[13].—Spasmodic stricture of the œsophagus prevented the patient from swallowing, and caused great difficulty in introducing the tube of the stomach-pump,[31].—*Swallowing.* Inability to swallow,[44].—Could not take medicine,[40].—*External Throat.* While walking rapidly after dinner had *spasm of carotid artery* (common, left), (third day),[7].

Stomach.—Appetite. More appetite, but not normal yet; more appetite in morning (fourth day),[7].—Unusual appetite for supper,[21].—[230.] Wanted to smoke a cigar, and thought that would relieve him,[14].—Diminished appetite,[18].—*Loss of all appetite,[35].—*Total loss of appetite, which had previously been excellent,[19].—Anorexia,[8].—Not so much appetite for dinner (second day),[7].—No appetite for tea,[3].—No appetite for tea (supper), (after half an hour),[10].—No appetite for supper,[5].—*Thirst.* Thirst,[28].—[240.] *Felt as if a little more whisky would do him good (habits perfectly temperate),[14]

—Eructations and Hiccough. Eructations,[42] [43].—Eructation of tasteless air (second day),[3].—Eructations after a light breakfast (second day),[17].—Headache disappears while moving about, but the eructations became more frequent (after one hour),[3].—Constant disposition to rift up, but could not (from 20 drops),[13].—Belching (after three-quarters of an hour),[5].—*Belching up of wind* (after a few moments),[3].—*Belching up of wind* (after one hour and a half),[3].—*Belching of wind from stomach* (after ten minutes). *Constant belching* (after fifteen minutes),[6]. — **[250.]** *Constant belching up of wind from stomach* (after two and five-sixths hours),[3].—*Constant belching up of large quantities of wind* (after twenty minutes),[3].— Regurgitation from stomach, which tastes like buttermilk and cabbage. (At dinner drank glass of milk; milk never disagrees with him), (after thirty-five minutes,[3].)—Ate heartily at lunch, but, though the stomach is full, the heat keeps rising from the stomach, with the taste of Carbolic acid,[17].—In afternoon, after dinner, long-continued hiccough,[2].—*Nausea and Vomiting.* Nausea at stomach (after fifteen minutes),[4].—Nausea most of the morning (second day),[3].—After tea, nausea returned, and was increased by taking a little sherry wine. The nausea lasted until noon next day,[5].—After tea, the nausea was much better, but she was very drowsy, which was unusual (after twenty-five minutes),[4].—Nausea, with desire to eructate (very soon),[17].—**[260.]** Nausea and vomiting,[44].—Slight nausea in throat (after thirty-five minutes),[3].—Slight nausea, with prostration,[8].—*A great deal of nausea;* shuddered and shook her head, made wry faces, *spat frequently,* etc.,[15].—Intense nausea (immediately), which continued with but little abatement for nearly an hour, and until he had drank several copious draughts of water (from 1 drop). Again the nausea followed, and almost reached the point of vomiting (from 5 drops),[13].— Aggravated feeling of sickness about stomach (soon after 10 drops),[13].— * *While eating a little breakfast, felt every now and then as if he had to get up and vomit* (from 20 drops),[13].—Vomiting and dysphagia,[35].—*Stomach.* Slight gastritis (for some days),[45].—An attack of acute gastritis followed the immediate symptoms,[47]. — **[270.]** Slight gastric catarrh, for several days,[43].—Wind in stomach very troublesome; better after raising a sort of sweetish-sour liquid,[3].—Dull uneasy feeling in stomach (after one hour and a half),[3].—Uncomfortable feeling in region of stomach and liver (soon after),[20].—Distress in stomach, as from indigestion,[18].—For about two days, his feelings represented a first-class type of acute dyspepsia (from 20 drops),[13].—Instead of feeling hungry at meals, an empty, gone feeling in the stomach, with a fulness in the throat, and a constant desire to swallow,[19]. —A great deal of gastric irritation (after seven hours),[46].—Pain and dragging feeling in stomach and low down in abdomen,[14].—Warmth in the stomach,[43].—**[280.]** Sensation of warmth in the epigastrium,[42].—Burning in the stomach,[17].—Burning in the stomach (after twenty minutes),[5].—The burning feeling in the stomach, as from a corrosive acid, is felt all the time; still the appetite is good and food digests well,[17].—Burning feeling in stomach, steadily increasing, with heat rising up the œsophagus (after three hours),[17].—Burning, ulcerating feeling in stomach and œsophagus, with nausea; this sensation reminded him of lobelia or tobacco; in fact, he had been smoking his pipe before going to bed,[17].—Stomach seems full of wind (after a few moments),[3].—Sensation as if stomach was filled with wind which ought to come up,[3].—Aching pain in stomach (after a few moments),[3]. —Felt as if he had eaten too much, and was suffering in consequence,[14].— **290.]** Appetite good, but food lies heavily on the stomach (second day),[17].

—Feeling of pressure at pit of stomach (very soon),[17].—Heavy weight in the epigastrium, as though burdened with flatulence, with a constant inclination to relieve himself by fruitless efforts at eructation, or by pressing the hand into the pit of the stomach,[13].

Abdomen.—Hypochondria. Dull pressing pain in hypochondria,[17].—Soreness of hypochondria, aggravated by motion (very soon),[17].—*Pain in right hypochondrium; also in iliac region of both sides,*[15].—Aching feeling over right hypochondrium and along back (from 20 drops),[13].—Premonitions of pain in region of liver,[20].—Dull pain in right side, over the region of the liver, and in the back, across the fifth, sixth, and seventh dorsal vertebræ,[13].—*General Abdomen.* Abdomen bloated, especially in the epigastric region, but neither hard, nor tense, nor sensitive to pressure,[40].—Bowels bloated and full of flatus after (three hours) a meal (second day),[7].—[300.] Rumbling in bowels; a feeling as if diarrhœa would come on, after walking about,[3].—*Rumbling and rolling in abdomen,* with a sense of distension (after one hour),[3].—Emission of large quantities of flatus all the evening,[3].—Emission of fetid flatus (after one hour and a half),[3].—Emission of large quantities of putrid flatus (third day),[3].—Sinking feeling all over the abdomen, a feeling of goneness, with yet a heavy weight about the stomach (from 20 drops),[13].—Pain in bowels,[20].—Sensation of fulness, with burning on outside of abdomen (soon after),[20].—Constantly a sensation of distension in the abdomen as if it were full of wind, but I was never able to discharge any,[23].—Bowels feel bloated and sore (third day),[7].—[310.] Feel as if the gas in the abdomen was incarcerated (after one hour),[3].—Abdominal muscles feel sore (second day),[7].—Bowels feel sore on walking,[17].—Jolting during riding affects unpleasantly the abdominal parietes also, which feel hot and sore,[17].—*Hypogastrium and Iliac Regions.* Burning pain in lower part of abdomen and top of head (after fifteen minutes),[3].—While sitting, crampy stitch in left inguinal region (after two hours),[1].

Rectum and Anus.—The anus itches and feels as if the skin was rubbed off (after forty-five minutes),[3].—Desire for stool all day, though he had had a natural movement in the morning (third day),[3].—Constant feeling of desire to pass a stool, and a sensation as if there was a quantity in the rectum, but I never had more than one regular stool every morning,[23].

Stool.—Diarrhœa. Diarrhœa; three watery evacuations within a short space of time, accompanied with pain and sick stomach,[16].—[320.] Ever since beginning of proving, and for some time after, two natural stools per day, which is very unusual with the prover, having generally but one passage in two days,[2].—In evening, copious and consistent stool, entirely free from pain, though the stools had been constipated and painful for some time previously,[13].—Towards evening, evacuation from bowels copious and consistent, but almost inodorous,[15].—*Constipation.* Bowels rather constipated, which is unusual (seventh day),[17].—Bowels seem torpid, but not costive (fourth day),[7].—My bowels moved regularly every morning, but the stool was insufficient, and they seemed somewhat more sluggish than normal,[23].

Urinary Organs.—Micturition. Frequent micturition,[18].—The urine was voided about once in two hours, and was large in quantity, quality normal (second day),[11].—Passed urine oftener than usual during the night, but observed no change in color (second day),[3].—Slept well, but had to rise about 5 o'clock to urinate, a very unusual thing, also passed a larger quantity than usual,[21].—[330.] Unusually free flow of urine, normal in color, in odor, and quality (third day),[11].—Copious flow of limpid color-less urine, which lasted several hours. The amount of the urine was enor-mous, though no measurement was resorted to. Its odor was slight, but peculiar, not that of Carbolic acid nor that of normal urine (after fifteen minutes),[30].—During the night, passed a large quantity of pale urine, nearly three quarts (fifth day),[22].—During day the urine was increased in quantity, and had a very strong smell (second day),[3].—Urine less in amount (fourth day),[7].—Urine diminished in quantity and heightened in color,[24].—Straining at passing urine, followed for two hours by uncomfort-able feeling,[24].—Fruitless efforts to urinate,[28].—Ineffectual attempts to pass urine,[28].—*Urine.* Greenish tinge in the urine, and disappearance of all deposits of lithates,[26].—[340.] *Urine very dark-colored*,[28].—*A dark greenish-brown color to the urine* is a characteristic sign of the incipient poisoning,[42]. —*Urine dark smoky color, alkaline;* it deposited a sediment of granular urate of ammonia; it also showed a mixture of different colored pigments, which apparently came from the coloring-matter of the dissolved blood-corpuscles; this pigment appeared always after an application of Carbolic acid, and disappeared after the removal of it,[35].—The urine passed the day after the accident *was almost black*, but was free from turbidity, and no trace of Carbolic acid, blood, or albumen could be detected in it,[47].—By nitric acid there is deposited a large quantity of brown pigment in the urine,[35].—Evacuation of offensive very dark-colored urine, depositing urate of ammonia, sometimes phosphates, but no albumen,[35].—Urine smells strongly of carbolic acid,[37].—Urine more acid than normal,[46].—Urine alka-line, dark-brown,[42].

Sexual Organs.—Male. Prickling pains through the glans penis and in urethra,[24].—[350.] During all this time I noticed my sexual organs to be in an unusually relaxed, weakened state during the day, but regu-larly every night I would have lascivious dreams, with seminal emissions, which weakened me greatly and filled me with horror,[23].—After going to sleep, was awakened by unusually strong sexual excitement, which contin-ued some time (first night),[11].—Sexual appetite very much decreased (second day),[7].—Loss of sexual desire for thirteen days,[21].—*Female. Pain in region of left ovary, when walking in the open air, soon subsiding*,[18].—Menses more profuse than usual,[10].—Menses much more profuse and darker-colored than usual, followed by headache and great nervous irritability for twelve hours (sixth day),[10].—Menses came on two days later than usual, and were more profuse,[5].

Respiratory Organs.—Larynx and Trachea. Inflam-matory condition set in, with much soreness of respiratory organs, and more hoarseness (third day),[22].—Feeling of soreness in larynx and bron-chial membrane, with some hoarseness (second day),[22].—Left side of larynx very sore when pressed upon, not true of the right side (after one hour and a quarter),[3].—Constant inclination to cough (after one hour and a quar-ter),[3].—Tickling-irritating sensation in upper part of trachea and fauces, which excited an occasional short, hacking, dry cough,[13].—*Cough and Expectoration.* [360.] Cough (fourth day),[22].—*Short hacking cough, with tickling in the throat (after one hour and a quarter),[3].—Cough, with-out expectoration (sixth day),[22].—Some cough and expectoration (eleventh day),[22].—Coughed to clear the bronchi; expectorated a little (fourth day),[7]. —Expectoration of large quantity of thick whitish mucus (second day),[3].— *Respiration. Stertorous respiration*,[28 30], etc.—Breathing stertorous (after eighteen minutes),[45].—Respiration stertorous and rapid (80),[44].—Respira-

tion stertorous, and smelling strongly of the fluid (after five minutes),[31].
—[370.] Respiration accelerated,[28].—Respiration agitated,[27].—Respiration free and deep; inclination to take a deep breath,[1].—Respiration difficult,[37].—Respiration much impeded,[25].—Room feels close and hot (second day),[7].

Chest.—Dull pain through the upper lobes of lungs,[18].—While walking out of doors, feeling of expansion (of lightness) in the lungs, also in the nasal passages (after five minutes),[1].—Tight feeling in both lungs, especially in the centre of the chest,[17].—*Feeling of narrowness in the chest, as if the diaphragm depressed the lungs,*[17].—[380.] Chest feels as if compressed, or as if a load were pressing in front, with a desire to dilate it (second day),[17].—Oppression of chest,[17].—Oppression of chest, requiring great effort to fully inflate the lungs,[18].—*Front.* Dull pressure under the sternum., in the region of the sixth rib (after three hours),[17].—Compressed feeling across lower end of sternum,[14].—*Sides.* Transient dull pain under left clavicle,[18].—*Slight uneasy pains in right lung (after one hour and a half),[3].—Dull aching pain, whole left side of chest and abdomen, running around to shoulder-blades (after two hours and five-sixths),[3].

Heart and Pulse.—Præcordium. Stitches, region of heart (after one hour and a quarter),[3].—*Heart's Action.* The beat of the heart, as well as the pulse, could not be felt,[40].—[390.] Heart's action irregular (after eighteen minutes),[45].—*Pulse.* Pulse rapid, irregular, undulating,[28].—Pulse very rapid,[35].—Feeble, intermittent, rapid pulse,[29].—Pulse quick, 95 (after five minutes),[4].—Pulse very quick, 100 (after twenty-five minutes),[4].—Pulse accelerated, 82 (after thirty-five minutes),[3].—Pulse small, frequent, and intermitting,[44].—Pulse 75 (after one hour and a half),[3].—Pulse 82 (after twenty minutes),[5].—[400.] Pulse rises from 66 to 75, intermittent (after five minutes); pulse 90 (after ten minutes); pulse 80 (after fifteen minutes); 9 A.M., pulse 100, regular (second day),[6].—Pulse risen from 70 to 82 (after one hour and a quarter),[3].—Pulse risen from 70 to 84 (after fifty-five minutes),[3].—Pulse 86 (after two hours and a half),[3].—Pulse 88 (after seven hours),[46].—Pulse 90 (after half an hour),[5].—Pulse 100 per minute, feeble, and very intermittent (after five minutes),[31].—Pulse 120 per minute, and very weak; could be counted with great difficulty,[25].—Sinking pulse and temperature,[44].—Pulse 68 (after one hour and five-sixths),[3].—[410.] Pulse 68, rather slow (after three hours and one-twelfth),[3].—Pulse 68 (third day),[7].—Pulse 68, small,[38].—Pulse 64 (after half an hour),[5].—Pulse weak and fluttering,[33].—Pulse weak and flickering,[30].—Pulse very weak,[37].—Pulse scarcely perceptible,[46].—Pulse scarcely perceptible (after eighteen minutes),[45].—Pulse and heart-beat almost imperceptible,[32].—[420.] Pulse imperceptible,[34].—Pulse imperceptible, and the beat of the heart scarcely noticed,[36].

Neck and Back.—Neck. Neck feels lame and stiff when moving head (after one hour),[3].—While smoking, after tea, lameness in back of neck and shoulders (after two hours and a half),[3].—One of the most painful sensations, and one which remained a very long time, was a very great sense of a weight on my neck, with a tenderness even to the touch, over the seventh cervical vertebra,[23].—Drawing in muscles of right side of neck, think in *splenitis capitis* (after one hour),[7].—Awoke with stitching pain in right side of neck, which increased during day (seventh day). Pain in neck very severe, with twinges of pain that would last a few seconds, then wear off; in five seconds it would return as before. This condition lasted some eight hours (ninth day),[22].—Soreness of muscles of neck (*splenitis capitis*), (third day),[7].—Back weak and sore (second day),[17].—*Back.* Good deal of pain in back and right side,[14].—[430.] *Soreness of muscles of back and limbs* (third day),[7].—Pains in small of back, and it hurts to straighten himself, and they became still worse by riding, where jolting aggravates,[17].—Aching pain across the small of back and in the lower limbs (after one hour),[3].—Severe aching pains in small of back, somewhat relieved by pressing the hand against it (fifth day),[17].—Tired sensation in renal region,[17].—The first two doses of the acid of the first centesimal dilution, taken three hours apart, relieved a severe pain in the lumbo-sacral region, which had existed more or less, mostly during the latter part of the night, for two years,[19].—Having another attack of backache, took a dose of Carbolic acid, 30th dil., which relieved the pain like magic, and have had no other attack up to date (about three weeks). Health in every respect excellent,[19].

Superior Extremities.—Shoulder. Drawing pain in left arm, from shoulder to elbow (transient),[3].—Lameness and soreness of right shoulder, when walking (second day),[3].—Rheumatic pain in right shoulder-joint nearly all day. He regarded it as an attack of rheumatism in the shoulder, having suffered with several attacks during the last eighteen years; they never lasted less than three or four days; this passed off suddenly in the evening, like all the other Carbolic acid pains (second day),[21].—[440.] Acute but transient pain in right shoulder-joint (after one hour and a half),[3].—Aching pain in right shoulder, when bending forward,[3].—Aching pain in hip has gone to left shoulder-joint; although not very severe; he is reminded of it from time to time (second day),[3].—*Arm.* *Constant tired, heavy feeling in left arm,[3].—Aching pain in left arm and right wrist (after one hour and a quarter),[3].—*Soreness of muscles of right arm* (after one hour and one-third),[3].—*Forearm.* *Aching pain in left forearm* (after fifteen minutes),[3].—*Hand.* The hand very much swollen, so that he could not write,[38].—Trembling of hands (cannot write steadily),[17].—A peculiar feeling of stiffness and discomfort (pricking) of the entire hand. This discomfort remained on the middle finger until night. At one spot it never left until there appeared a small pimple, which increased in size until it became a sore resembling a carbuncle. The flesh suppurated until a probe could be passed nearly through the finger. For several days the sore hand was intensely painful, and prevented sleep for several nights. It healed finally, but was a serious sore,[12].—[450.] Contracting pain in palm of right hand (after two hours and one-third),[3].—*Fingers.* Pain in second phalangeal joint of middle finger, right hand (after two hours and five-sixths),[21].

Inferior Extremities.—Cannot walk straight (after twenty-five minutes),[4].—*Lower extremities feel heavy as lead* (fifth day),[17].—Draggy sensation about lower extremities, which occasioned a little unsteadiness in walking (from 20 drops),[13].—*Hip.* Occasional pains in hips and shoulders (third day),[3].—Aching pain in both hips (after forty-five minutes),[3].—Transient pains in right hip (after one hour and a half),[3].—Aching in right hip (transient), (after thirty-five minutes),[3].—Transient aching pain in right hip and left knee (after two hours and a half),[3].—[460.] Hard, aching pain in right hip, like a sciatic pain, which slowly moved along the course of that nerve, and at night was in the bend of the knee, and then ceased altogether (fifth day),[22].—Very severe aching pain in right hip-joint, felt only when walking (second day),[3].—*Thigh.* Transient pain in muscles of right thigh (after a few moments),[3].—Deepseated muscular pain, on inside of upper third of left thigh, that almost made him walk lame; lasted from five to ten minutes (after half an hour),[21].—The dull aching pains extend from the spine down the posterior muscles of the thigh,[17].—Drawing in right thigh and right zygoma (very soon),[17].—His thighs feel bruised (second day),[17].—About 7 P.M., while walking, bruised pain in the middle of anterior part of right thigh, deepseated and lasting only for a few minutes (second day),[21].—*Knee.* In the night, pain for a few minutes on inside of left knee-joint (fourth day),[21].—Pain on inside of left knee-joint, lasting for a considerable time (third day),[21]. — [470.] *Aching soreness beneath left patella, all day up to about 4 o'clock P.M.; feels as if it would be stiff and sore to move it, but on the contrary during motion it is not felt at all* (second day).[21].—*Leg.* Sensation just below the knee, on the shin, as if the part was touched with a piece of ice (after forty-five minutes),[3].—*Aching pain to the left of middle of left shin-bone* (after two days),[2].—*Sharp pain in left shin* (after one hour and a half),[3].—Cramps in the calves,[42].—Severe bruised pain beneath left tendo Achillis close to posterior part of tibia, as if struck with a club; in a few minutes it disappeared for a short time, when he had a sharp pain in middle joint of large finger of left hand; this pain was only momentary, when it went back (but less intense) in the leg again (after one hour and a quarter),[21].— *Ankle.* Dull pain in right ankle and left knee, most of the morning (second day),[4].—Aching pain in right ankle, and in lower part of abdomen (after one hour),[3].—Pain in left outer malleolus (after three hours and one-fifth),[21].—*Foot.* His feet, though he was lying flat on his back, felt as though they could not support his body, even by a strong effort of the will,[17].—[480.] Feet feel heavy (after fifteen minutes),[4].—The feet feel as if bruised, all the time,[17].—*Toes.* Pain in right great toe as if pressed upon,[3].—Pain in under surface of big toe of left foot (after three hours),[21]. —Pressing pain in left great toe (after fifteen minutes),[3].—Tingling in left great toe, followed by a feeling as if pressed on (after a few moments),[3].— Sharp, stinging pain through corns (third day),[7].

General Symptoms.— Objective. Body much swollen before death,[31].—Trembling,[29].—Slight tremor over whole body, steadily increasing (after ten minutes),[40].—[490.] Muscles relaxed,[32].—Muscles completely relaxed,[36].—Loss of involuntary motion and speech,[44].—Became convulsed,[30]. —Convulsed (immediately),[45].—Convulsions,[29].—Violent convulsions, with trismus, and blood passing from the mouth in consequence of the teeth having wounded the tongue,[46].—She fell to the ground in convulsions, was delirious and without consciousness,[33].—Disinclined to work; even correcting proof is fatiguing (second day),[7].—Feeling of languor, enervation, indisposition to attend to professional duties, and drowsiness, with uncomfortable feeling of fulness in the head, varied occasionally by a passing pain through the forehead, or right or left temple,[13].—[500.] Feel languid; must lie down to rest after a light day's work (second day),[7].—Languid and sleepy; retired early (fourth day),[7].—*Great languor,*[8].—*Easily fatigued by the least walk* (am usually a good walker),[17].—*Complains of being very tired* (after twenty-five minutes),[4].—Very tired at night, and *not at all amiable* (third day),[7].—*Weakness,*[44].—Physical exhaustion (second day),[18]. —Great prostration,[29].—*Profound prostration,*[27].—[510.] Faint feeling, spreading from the thighs all over the body,[17].—Administered chloroform in large quantity (one-third of a pound), to a patient during an operation, and was thereby affected nearly as much as the patient; obliged to go into the fresh air in order to keep from fainting (fourth day),[17].—Fell insensible (immediately),[45].—Fell from her seat to the floor,[30].—Extreme syncope,[47].—

Complete anæsthesia,[34].—Complete anæsthesia, even of the conjunctiva,[44].—Numbness of skin of hands,[8].—***Subjective.*** Physical and mental exhilaration,[18].—Shuddering sensation when he took it in his mouth; imagined he could taste the acid,[21]—[520.] General feeling of dulness and heaviness,[20].—Felt badly the whole day, especially from a burning in the stomach, with a sore feeling to the touch (second day),[17].—Said he felt mean, and left for home before his usual time,[14].—Feels as if he had taken a violent cold (second day),[6].—Soreness, as if he had taken cold (thinks he has not), (third day),[7].—General soreness, worse in back, abdomen, and chest (third day),[7].—All the muscles prominently used are sore and stiff (fourth day),[7].—All symptoms go from the head downward,[17].—Pain felt only on right side,[22].—The pains seem to affect the right side first, and afterwards the same parts of the left (after thirty-five minutes),[3].—[530.] The pains appeared most frequently on left side; came and went very suddenly, and generally lasted but a short time; they generally affected the muscles and joints, but not the bones,[21].—*I became thoroughly unfit for study, as every exercise at reading increased all my symptoms, especially the pressing at the occiput,[23].—Relief of symptoms, except frontal headache, after a hearty lunch,[17].

Skin.—Eruption. Moist. Slight eruption of a vesicular character all over the body (third day),[5].—****Vesicular eruption on hands and all over body, which itches excessively; better after rubbing, but leaving a burning pain,[6].†***—*A small vesicle formed on centre of nose (fourth day),[3].—***Pustular.*** Vesicle on nose converted into a pustule, which was opened (fifth day); opened again (sixth day); opened again, and healed up (ninth day),[3].—Slight pustular eruption on right side of face (second day),[18].—***Sensations.*** Burning in the skin (second day),[38].—Tingling in lower extremities,[17].—Formication in the extremities,[42].—[540.] Itching of scalp and lower part of abdomen, as if bitten by something (after two hours and five-sixths),[3].—Itching of right ear (after thirty-five minutes),[3].—Itching of the face (after fifty-five minutes),[3].—Itching of right cheek, and sharp pain about the centre of cheek, as if bitten by a mosquito. So sudden and peculiar was this pain that I expected to find something had really bitten me (after thirty-five minutes),[3].—Itching of the back of neck and of the nose (after twenty minutes),[3].—Itching of left shoulder and right cheek (after thirty-five minutes),[3].—Itching of left elbow (after one hour and a half),[3].—Itching of left elbow (after fifteen minutes),[3].—Itching of right forefinger (after one hour and a half),[3].—Itching about the left hip (after forty-five minutes),[3].—[550.] Itching of outside of thigh and of the genitals (after one hour and five-sixths),[3].—Itching of inner part of thigh and scrotum, relieved by scratching, but it soon returns,[3].—Itching inner side of left knees (after one hour and a quarter),[3].—Itching of ankles, arms, back of neck, calf of leg, and other parts of body (after fifteen minutes),[6].—Itching of various parts of body, right thigh, buttocks, back, shin, etc. (after one hour and a quarter),[3].—Intense burning-itching of the genitals (after one hour and a half),[3].—Tingling-itching in right little finger, soon after in the left,[3].

Sleep and Dreams.—Sleepiness. Yawning (very soon),[17].—

---

† Arsenicum had no effect on the eruption. Prover had the itch some eight or nine years ago, which was cured by the external application of Sulphur. The present eruption looks very much like the itch, but the insect is wanting. *Rhus* and *Sulphur* were given, but exerted very little influence over the eruption. It gradually got better without treatment, and disappeared in about three weeks.

Yawning (after thirty-five minutes),³.—Yawned now and then, and took long inspirations,¹⁴.—[560.] Yawning constantly (after twenty minutes),⁶. —Incessant yawning (after fifty-five minutes),³.—Sleepiness (after half an hour),¹⁸.—Sleepiness, constant inclination to yawn,¹⁸.—Sleepiness, with desire to stretch,¹⁷.—Sleepy (second day),⁷.—Felt sleepy in afternoon, but could not fall into sound sleep,¹⁵.—Sleepy and chilly, although sitting in a room with a good fire,¹⁷.—I was constantly heavy and sleepy, but when I would lie down to sleep would be perplexed with dreams, and would wake up unrefreshed, with coated tongue and nausea,²³.—Became drowsy,¹⁴.— [570.] Soon lapsed into a sound and quiet slumber,¹⁶.—Had a very refreshing sleep; awoke earlier than usual, amiable (second day),⁷.—Slept soundly all night, and awoke greatly refreshed in morning,¹³.—Slept heavy; awoke sore all over, especially the legs (gluteal muscles), back, chest, and arms (fourth day),⁷.—Instead of the tremors a somnolent state set in (after two hours),⁴⁰.—Riding lulls him to sleep, and walking is an exertion,¹⁷.— *Sleeplessness.* Slept well last night, but woke often; no dreams (second day),³.—Restless sleep the whole night, with busy dreams,¹⁷.—At midnight, after waking, could not get to sleep again ; the smell of Carbolic acid seemed to keep her awake,⁹.—*Dreams.* Sleep not refreshing ; dreamed much, but cannot now (A.M.) recall the subjects (third day),⁷.—[580.] During night had a great many dreams, some amorous, others he was unable to recall when awake (third day),³.—Dreamed of great mental activity ; awoke with clear intellect ; can work (fifth day),⁷.—Slept well as usual, but dreamed of travelling, which is unusual,³.—Slept well, but dreamed of fire ; so vivid was the dream that he was awakened ; found that he was quite feverish, although the window was open and the room quite cold (second day),³.— Dreamed she could not get to sleep on account of thinking about the body I had embalmed ; thought she tossed about, and then tried to wake me, to give her some medicine to stop thinking ; she thought she could not wake me, and pulled me out of bed ; and that I was bathed in perspiration ; face pale ; thought I was dead. The fright awoke her ; she found herself lying on her back, with her mouth wide open, apparently paralyzed with fear ; she aroused me and begged in a whining tone for something to make her go to sleep. Could not at first be persuaded she had been asleep. Gave her a dose of *Nux*, and she dropped to sleep at once, and slept soundly ; awoke perfectly well in the morning,⁹.

Fever.—*Chilliness.* Diminished temperature about $\frac{1}{16}$ C.,⁴².— Skin cold and moist,³³.—Surface cold and clammy,²⁵·²⁹.—Surface cold and moist,³⁰.—Slight chilliness, while sitting in a warm room (74° F.), (after five hours),³.—[590.] 9 A.M., chilly sensations; pulse 78 (second day),³.— Soon chilly (second day),⁷.—Chilly sensations while at breakfast (second day),³.—Very chilly when in the open air (second day),⁷.—Extremities and surface of body cold,⁴⁶.—At times, when I would stoop, a sensation was felt of coldness in one spot, somewhat similar to the cold sensation experienced when a nerve in a tooth is touched, and was always followed by a clammy sweat,²³.—In a hot room a momentary chill runs from the face downward,¹⁷. —Extremities cold,³⁷.—Extremities cold (after eighteen minutes),⁴⁵.—Creeping-shuddering or horripilation in left forearm, running upwards (after one hour and one-third),²¹.—*Heat.* [600.] Great heat of body (second day),¹⁸.—Feverish and flurried, pulse 90,¹³.—Complained of heat and closeness of room, though that was airy, and thermometer 70° F., yet his pulse was normal,¹⁴.—Slight heat of face and forehead, especially left side, with pressure in left temple, seemingly on the surface of brain (soon after),².—

Sweat. Woke up in middle of night, and found he was bathed in perspiration (second day),[6].—Cold sweat,[44].—Skin covered with cold sweat,[34]. —When the giddiness was severe there were, in some instances, cold, clammy perspiration and feeble pulse,[26].—Cold, clammy sweat over face and hands,[2].

Conditions.— **Aggravation**. —(*Morning*), On waking, dryness of pharynx, etc.—(*In open air*), Discharge from nostrils.—(*Walking in open air*), *Pain in region of ovary;* feeling in lungs, etc.—(*In cold room*), Discharge from nostrils.—(*While drinking ice-water*), Contraction of œsophagus.—(*Hot room*), Frontal headache.—(*Jolting when riding*), Pains in small of back.—(*Leaning forward*), Heaviness in head; pain in temple, etc.; pain in shoulder.—(*Light*), Headache.—(*Motion*), Dizziness; soreness of hypochondria.—(*Noise*), Headache.—(*Continued pressure*), Headache.— (*Reading*), All symptoms.—(*In room*), Vertigo returns.—(*While sitting*), Stitch in inguinal region.—(*Walking*), Bowels feel sore; lameness, etc., of right shoulder; pain in right thigh.—(*After walking about*), Rumbling in bowels, etc.

Amelioration.—(*Morning*), More appetite.—(*Fresh air*), Amelioration; frontal headache.—(*After breakfast*), Soon, headache disappeared.— (*Indoors*), Discharge from nostrils ceases.—(*After hearty lunch*), All symptoms, except frontal headache.—(*While moving about*), Headache disappears.—(*Pressure*), Feeling in head; pains in small of back.—(*Momentary pressure*), Headache.—(*After raising liquid from stomach*), Wind in stomach.—(*On rising*), Pain in supraorbital ridge ceases.—(*Smoking*), Head-pains, sore throat.—(*Green tea*), Headache.—(*Wind*), Cools heated brain.

CARBONEUM.

Amorphous Carbon; lampblack; obtained (for this proving) from the chimney of a coal-oil lamp.

Authority. Dr. W. H. Burt, N. Am. J. of Hom., 9, 273, proving with repeated doses of the first trituration.

Head.—During the spasms had a dull heavy ache in the forehead, exactly in the organ of benevolence; it lasted two days and a half (third day).

Nose.—Very profuse secretion of a thick yellow mucus from the nose, which lasted about eight days (fourth day).

Mouth.—In morning tongue coated white (third day).

Throat.—4 A.M. Throat felt so very sore that he got up and put a wet towel around it, and took a dose of Aconite (second day).

Stomach.—Loss of appetite; could not eat breakfast (third day).— Entire loss of appetite (fourth day).—Appetite began to return, with a great craving for acids, which he could not allay (fourth day).

Stool.—Bowels very costive (fourth day).

Heart and Pulse.—Pulse from 80 to 90, weak and irregular; after the third day, it fell to 70, and was very weak.

Back.—[10.] Back and limbs ached very much (second and third days).

General Symptoms.—Spasms; commencing in the tongue, passing down the trachea to the lungs, which prevented him from breathing for about two minutes; then gradually left, and went to stomach, arms, hands and legs. It took four persons to hold him, two at his hands, and two at his feet. They were both tonic and clonic spasms. The spasms lasted two hours, and then gradually ceased. The hands had no feeling in them; they were closed and could not be opened; wrists perfectly pulseless; hands shrivelled and cold (third day). 2 P.M., the spasms came on very suddenly, the same as they did the first time, but not quite so violent. They did not affect the lungs at this time, but were much harder in the stomach. They lasted three hours, then gradually ceased. He seemed at the point of death. The spasms left him so weak that he could not raise his hand to his head nor sit up (fourth day).—Morning, on rising, felt very weary (third day).—In afternoon began to feel very weary (second day).

Skin.—About every ten or fifteen minutes a tingling, prickly sensation passed all over the body, which gradually increased, especially the numb, tingling sensation, until 2 P.M., when he went into spasms.

Sleep and Dreams.—Very restless night (second day).

CARBONEUM CHLORATUM.

Carboneum chloratum, Tetrachloride of Carbon, CCl_4. (A colorless liquid, soluble in alcohol.)

Authorities. 1, Sir J. Y. Simpson, Pharm. Journ., 24, 416; 2, Nunneley, Brit. Med. Journ., 1867; both are statements of the effects of the vapor.

Head.—Full pulsation in head and limbs,[2].—Full and hot sensation in head (after one hour and a half),[2].

Stomach.—Sinking and nausea at the stomach (after one hour and a half),[2].

Abdomen.—Feeling of distension,[2].

Respiratory Organs.—Since inhaling the vapor, a relaxed condition of the bronchial mucous membrane, with expectoration every morning of three or four lumps of carbonaceous mucus, and some during the day, has altogether disappeared, and the little irritation of the membrane has also gone,[2].

Heart and Pulse.—The depressing influence upon the heart greater than that of Chloroform,[1].—Failing in the action of the heart, which became weak, and not more than forty-eight per minute, with great lassitude in the limbs (after one hour and a half),[2].—The pulse becomes extremely feeble and weak,[1].—Pulse weak and rapid during the greatest degree of anæsthetic sleep,[1].

General Symptoms.—[10.] Great muscular lassitude and indisposition to move,[2].—Its primary effects are similar to those of Chloroform, but it takes a longer time to produce the same degree of anæsthesia, and generally a longer time to recover from it,[1].

Fever.—Sensation of heat all through the system,[2].

Sleep and Dreams.—Sleepiness, with a sort of passive wish to proceed with the inspiration, but as if even this were too much trouble,[2].—Bad night, with little continuous sleep till morning; lay half dreaming, with a hot skin, a swimming feeling in the head, nausea at the stomach, a very dry tongue sticking to the palate, a taste of the Tetrachloride, and a weak pulse, with a feeling like sea-sickness; restlessness, with a disinclination to move,[2].

CARBONEUM HYDROGENISATUM.

Carboneum hydrogenisatum. Carburetted hydrogen, Ethene, Olefiant gas, C_2H_4. This gas is sparingly soluble in water, but considerably soluble in alcohol.

Authorities.† 1, Sir H. Davy, from Paris's Life of Davy (Lond. Med. Gaz., 7, 563), inhaled the pure gas from a bag; 2, Sedillot, Gaz. de Strast., 1845 (S. J. Suppl., vol. 4), *poisoning by illuminating gas;* 3, Seitz, Deutsch. Kl., 1852 (S. J., 76, p. 187), ibid.; 4, Gærtner, Wurt. Corr. Bl., 1853 (S. J., 79, p. 288), ibid.; 5, Cless, Wurt. Corr. Bl., 1854 (S. J., 86, p. 34), ibid.; 6, Jaushet, L'Union, 1857 (S. J., 95, p. 76), *suffocated by coal damp;* 7, Otho, Gaz. Sarda. 1858 (S. J., 98, 171), *poisoning by illuminating gas;* 8, Leopold, V. f. Ger. Med., 1858 (S. J., 100, 293), ibid.; 9, Mayer, Om. Schr. f. Geburt, 1858 (S. J., 104, 189), poisoning of two pregnant women by illuminating gas; 10, Schumacher, Henke Zeit., 1862 (S. J., 113, p. 292), poisoning by illuminating gas; 11, Sieveking, Lancet, 1869, ibid.; 12, Wallichs, Deutsche Klin., 1869 (S. J., 151, 273), ibid.; 13, De Chaumont, Lancet, 1873, poisoning by coal gas; 14, William Taylor, M.D., Monograph on poisoning by coal gas, Edinb., 1874; 15, Tourdes (six cases, five fatal) from Taylor's work; 16, Maclagan, cases from Taylor's work.

Mind.—Emotional. An extraordinary sensation of contentment, so that life seems exalted; all his thoughts appear in a moment as if seen in an inner mirror,[4].—She occasionally gave loud cries,[4].—Only replied by monosyllables,[15].—*Intellectual.* Answers questions slowly but correctly,[5].—Some confusion of mind,[16].—Ideas confused for forty-eight hours,[15] —Intellectual faculties a blank,[15].—Complete loss of sensibility,[6].—Insensibility,[13].—[10.] Lost all power of perceiving external things, and had no distinct sensation except that of a terrible oppression on the chest,[1].—Loss of consciousness,[5 10].—Complete loss of consciousness,[4].—Consciousness completely lost,[15].—Completely unconscious,[7].—Fell unconscious to the ground,[2]. —Suddenly fell down unconscious,[7].—Fell heavily on the floor, yet the shock of the concussion did not rouse her to consciousness; but when the room was broken into, she heard the first words that were pronounced, and recognized one of the doctors who came to her help,[15].—Lying on back, unconscious, mouth widely open, and breathing audible, with a subdued stertor,[14].—Stupefaction,[5 8].—[20.] Coma,[5].—Deep coma,[12].—Deeply comatose,[14].—Entirely comatose,[16].

Head.—Confusion and Vertigo. Confusion of the head continues a long time,[4].—Vertigo,[4 8 9 10].—After making a few steps into the open air, his head became giddy, his knees trembled, and he had just sufficient power to throw himself on the grass,[1].—Slight giddiness,[1].—Extreme giddiness,[13].—The giddiness returned with such violence as to oblige him to lie on the bed; it was accompanied with nausea, loss of memory, and

---

† To the proving of Sir Humphrey Davy are added some selected cases of poisoning by *illuminating gas;* this latter gas is of complex and somewhat variable composition, containing marsh gas, olefiant gas, hydrogen, carbonous oxide, nitrogen, vapors of volatile hydrocarbons, and vapor of carbonic sulphide; it thus occupies a position between carbonous oxide and carbonic sulphide; the cases here collected possess sufficient interest to justify their insertion, though obtained from such a variable source.

deficient sensation (after two hours and a half),[1].—*General Head.*
[30.] Heaviness of the head,[10].—Head heavy and exceedingly painful (second day),[6].—Pain in head,[1].—Pain and pressure in the head,[10].—Headache,[5].
—Great headache,[13].—Severe pressure in the brain,[4].—*Forehead.* Frontal headache,[4].—Excruciating pain in forehead and between eyes (after four hours),[1].

Eye.—Eyes sunken,[7].—[40.] Eyes distorted,[4].—*Lids.* Eyes half closed,[14].—*Conjunctiva.* Conjunctiva red,[3].—Conjunctivæ slightly injected,[15].—*Ball.* The eyeballs oscillated from side to side, with a lateral, or perhaps obliquely lateral motion ; this rolling was as nearly as possible synchronous with the breathing ; it was continuous and simultaneous, both eyes moving in the same direction at the same time. It was uninfluenced by the presence or absence of light, and was unvarying in its regularity, whether the eyelids were open or closed. No individual symptom was more remarkable than the steady and extreme oscillation of the eyeballs. These traversed laterally the extreme area of motion, as if the patient were anxiously looking as far as he could to the right, then as far as he could to the left ; and neither light nor darkness, irritation nor repose, nor the internal conditions which governed the varying sensibility of the pupils, seemed in any way to modify the constancy of this motion, or relieve the monotony of its rhythm. Even when once or twice we thought that, by means of the active stimuli employed, we awakened a slight response, it only took the character of a groan, together with a momentary half-knowing look. The eyeballs never rested,[14].—*Pupil.* Pupils dilated, insensible to light,[3].—Pupils widely dilated, insensible,[5].—Pupils contracted,[15].—Pupils contracted, insensible,[4].—[50.] Pupils insensible and partially dilated,[14].—*Vision.* Dark bodies moving before the eyes (second day),[6].

Ear.—Roaring in the ears (second day),[6].

Face.—Staring look,[5].—Had quite the expression of being in a profound slumber, the mouth being relaxed, hanging down, and the saliva overflowing it,[14].—Face soiled with blackish purulent matter, which was spurted about him,[15].—Face scarlet,[4].—Face red, turgid,[5].—Face bluish,[10].
—Face cyanotic,[12].—[60.] Pale face,[5 6 9 15].—Face pale, sunken, with blue eyelids and lips,[10].—Face, neck, and upper part of forehead congested and livid, the purple of the forehead forming a broad band, which deepened over the eyebrows, and shaded off towards the scalp, which was natural in color,[14].—Face drawn, wrinkled,[7].—Face distorted in trismus,[3].—Features distorted, and mouth covered with foam,[15].—*Lips.* Lips blue,[9].—*Cheeks.* Cheeks puffy,[4].—The teeth being kept apart by a wooden gag in one side of the mouth, the opposite cheek, on the free side of the mouth, was flaccid, and flapped loosely with every breath,[14].—First complaint was of pain in her cheek and the right side of head,[15].—*Chin.* [70.] Jaws tightly clenched,[12].—Jaws firmly closed, the one against the other ; deglutition impossible,[15].—Teeth firmly clenched,[14].—When the current of air reached the sleeper, his teeth became firmly clenched, and his lips tightly closed over them. The breathing was then less full than formerly, and immediate suffocation seemed inevitable,[14].—On removing some tenacious mucus from the depending side of the mouth, his teeth snapped my finger, and remained closed for about a minute. They afterwards relaxed and opened,[14].—Trismus,[10].—Slight degree of trismus, frequently interrupted by yawning,[4].—A high grade of trismus,[5].—A very great degree of trismus,[4].—The trismus increases ; clonic cramps set in ; repeated every four or five minutes,[3].

Mouth.—[80.] Foam from the mouth,[10].—Bloody froth from the mouth,[5].—Breath had a faint, sickly, stomachy fetor,[14].—Yellow-tinged froth collected at the mouth,[14].

Throat.—Every time the feather was introduced in tickling the fauces, it came away loaded with glairy, pinkish, sero-sanguineous discharge, the source of which seemed almost inexhaustible,[14].

Stomach.—Nausea and Vomiting. Nausea,[8].—Nausea for everything,[4].—Inclination to vomit,[9].—Vomiting,[5 8 10].—Vomited once,[15].— [90.] Violently sick,[13].—*Stomach.* Digestion is impaired,[4].—Violent cramps in the stomach,[4].

Stool.—Involuntary passage of stool and urine,[3 15].—Thin rice-water stools, for some time after the attack,[4].—Stool frequent, consisting of thin fæces, mixed with dark blood and mucus,[4].†

Respiratory Organs.—Voice. Voice very feeble and indistinct,[1]. *—Cough.* Slight cough, which did not last long,[15].—Violent paroxysms of cough,[9].—*Respiration.* Mucous râles at bases of lungs,[14].—[100.] Stertorous breathing,[15].—Breath smelling strongly of gas,[16].—Breath strongly impregnated with gas,[14].—Respiration accelerated,[5].—Respiration rapid, rattling,[5].—Breathing quick, and interrupted by profound inspirations and sighs,[15].—Respiration frequent, superficial,[9].—Respirations 48 (second day),[14].—Respirations 30–36,[16].—Respirations 28 (seven hours after being found),[14].—[110.] Respiration 16–18 per minute (two hours after being found),[14].—Respiration irregular, stertorous, intermitting,[3].—Respiration short, stertorous, slow,[7].—Breathing feeble and irregular,[15].—Respiration very weak, at long intervals,[4].—Breathing labored, fluctuating, interrupted,[14].—Difficult respiration,[12].—Dyspnœa,[8].—Sensation of suffocation,[4 13].—Threatened suffocation,[1].—[120.] After bleeding, the breathing appeared easier, the patient made a movement with the head, and executed a profound inspiration, which he followed by a noisy inspiration; soon the breathing became embarrassed; mucous râles were heard,[15].

Chest.—Congestion of the lungs,[6].—Sounds of the heart scarcely audible on account of mucous râles in the chest,[5].—Sort of numbness and loss of feeling in chest and about pectoral muscles,[1].—Oppression of the chest,[14].—Transient pains in chest and extremities,[1].—Very violent tearing pains in the thorax,[4].

Heart and Pulse.—Heart's Action. Beating of the heart scarcely noticed,[3].—*Pulse.* Pulse strong, rapid, and regular,[6].—Pulse much quicker and more feeble,[1].—[130.] Pulse threadlike, and beating with excessive quickness,[1].—Pulse small, rapid,[12].—Pulse 96 (seven hours after being found),[14].—Pulse 100,[11].—Pulse 112, small and weak (second day),[14].—Pulse 120, and very feeble,[1 16].—Pulse small, 120,[15].—Pulse small and weak, 95,[3].—Pulse 78, soft (six hours after being found),[14].—Pulse 72–75, less regular, intermissions occasionally as often as 1 in 4 (four hours after being found),[14].—[140.] Pulse steady, but feeble (two hours after being found),[14].—Pulse and respiration extremely weak,[10].—Pulse scarcely perceptible,[7].—Pulse 60, scarcely perceptible,[4].—Pulse almost imperceptible,[14].—Pulse imperceptible,[15].

Neck and Back.—Violent spasms of the extensors of the back,[5].

Extremities in General.—Extremities flexed,[4].—Extremities relaxed,[7].—All the members in a state of resolution, as if paralyzed,[15].—

---

† This character of the evacuations is doubtless dependent upon the extensive ecchymosis of the intestinal canal.

[150.] Loss of motion of the limbs,[12].—Spasmodic stretching and trembling of the limbs,[10].—Weariness of the limbs,[8].—Limbs felt paralyzed; they staggered (two cases),[11].

Superior Extremities.—Arms flexed on elbow-joints,[5].—The arms are flexed on elbows; can only be stretched out by force,[4].—Arms semi-flexed in front of the body; hands resting on abdomen,[14].—Trembling of the hands,[11].—Fingers constantly flexed,[4].

General Symptoms.—Objective. Whole appearance betokened speedy dissolution, reminding one very much of the appearances presented when a patient is dying from the effects of an overdose of chloroform,[14].—[160.] The symptoms throughout bore a strong resemblance to those of apoplexy, and even the copious perspirations had a like fatal import,[14].—One very marked characteristic was the rapidly fluctuating nature of the conditions which presented themselves. These were alternately encouraging and discouraging, the system at one time striving vigorously to work off the poisonous load, and anon sinking exhausted with the effort. Thus the periods of hopeful tranquillity, when the pulse was steady and the breathing regular, were always followed by intervals of shorter duration when all these functions were deranged,[14].—Remained immovable, lying on her back,[15].—Remained immovable, lying on her back; at 4 o'clock the immobility was less complete, but she seized objects with the left hand; could not move the right hand nor leg,[15].—Lying as if dead, cold and pale; as soon as the window was opened, violent convulsions set in,[3].—On vene-section, the blood, of a dark-red color, dribbled at first, but at length jetted freely,[15].—Trembling,[2].—Occasional but slight convulsive indications, which became more frequent and perceptible, affecting the trunk and limbs only, not the head or face,[14].—Weakness,[16].—Excessive weakness,[15].—[170.] Considerably weakened, and strength only came back slowly,[15].—Movements weak and incomplete,[15].—General exhaustion continues several days,[4].—At last she was not able to rise on account of prostration and weakness,[9].—Loss of muscular power,[10].—Momentary loss of voluntary power,[1].—During night, became agitated and feverish, tormented with thirst and with painful dreams,[15].—Anæsthesia,[8].—Skin insensible,[4].—Skin completely insensible,[6].—*Subjective.* [180.] Seemed sinking into annihilation,[1].

Skin.—Skin white, veins seem dark-colored,[4].—Skin livid,[11].—Painful tingling sensation in right leg,[15].

Sleep and Dreams.—Fell asleep, and from that moment lost all consciousness for forty hours; only remembered a sensation as of a painful dream,[15].—Sleep prolonged and very deep, interrupted by cramps in the jaws and in the toes,[4].

Fever.—Chilliness. Cold skin,[5].—Body cold and feebly rigid,[14].—Skin icy cold,[15].—Skin generally cold, excepting the head,[3].—[190.] Chilliness,[10].—Shaking chill,[5].—Shaking with chill,[9].—Violent attacks of chill,[5].—Limbs cold,[2].—Extremities cold,[5].—Extremities icy cold,[11].—*Sweat.* Sweating copiously; sweat smells of gas,[14].—Skin covered with profuse clammy sweat,[7].—Great drops of sweat over the whole body, especially on the head,[4].

CARBONEUM OXYGENISATUM.

Carboneum oxygenisatum, Carbonous oxide, CO. This gas may be obtained, in a state of purity, by the action of Sulphuric acid upon Ferrocyanide of Potassium ; it is soluble in water (about two per cent. at ordinary temperatures).

Authorities.† 1, Meglin, Journ. de Med., 1786 (Frank's Mag., 1, 765), five cases of poisoning from coals in an open vessel in a room ; 2, Berthold, Hencke Zeit., 1830 (Fr. Mag., 3, 224), several cases, same cause as the last ; 3, Schrœder, Rust's Mag., 1830 (Fr. Mag., 1, 553), several cases, same as last; 4, Wagner, Hufeland's Journ., 1836 ; 5, Hergenrother, Med. Corr. Bl., Bayer, 1841 (Schmidt's Jahrbucher, 34, p. 26) ; 6, Mark, Bayer. Corr. Bl., 1843 (S. J. Suppl., Bd. 4) ; 7, Demeures, Bull. d. l. Soc., homœop. de Paris, 1849 ; 8, Buchner, All. Hom. Zeit., 28, 158, 1850 ; 9, Piorry, Gaz. des Hop., 1851 (S. J., 70, 175) ; 10, Chenot, a chemist, L'Union, 1850, poisoning, from inhaling the pure gas ; 11, Gaz. des Hop., 1857, poisoning of three women ; 12, Jachimowicz, Zeit. f. Ver. Oest., 1857 ; 13, Ozanam, L'Union, 1857 (S. J., 94, p. 26) ; 14, Freund, Om. Schr. f. Geburt., 1858 (S. J., 104, 190), poisoning of a woman seven months pregnant ; 15, Siebenhaar and Lehmann, S. J., 101, p. 274, 1858 ; 16, Thompson, Edinb. Med. Journ., 1860 ; 17, Hasse, Pr. Ver. Zeit., 1859 (S. J., 105, 41), poisoning of five soldiers ; 18, Brit. Med. Journ., 1862 ; 19, Oest. Zeit., 1862 (All. Hom. Zeit., M. B., 7, 34) ; 20, Leudet, Virch. Archiv. (S. J., 127, 24), 1865 ; 21, Klebs, Virchow's Archiv., 1865 (S. J., 127, 17) ; 22, Leudet, as last ; 23, Pirain, S. J., 127, p. 24, 1865 ; 24, Huber, All. Milit. Zeit., 1865 (S. J., 127, p. 162) ; 25, Gull, Lond. Lancet, 1866 (S. J., 133, p. 33) ; 26, Faure (S. J., 92, 220), Archiv. Gen., 1856, general treatise on asphyxia ; 27, Maclagan, Edin. Med. Journ., 1868, three cases ; 28, Linas, Gaz. Med. de Paris, 1869 ; 29, Sulzer, All. Hom. Zeit., 1873 (Hahn. Month., 8, 519) ; 30, Hirt, in Ziemssen, Handbuch der Spec. Path. and Therap., Band 1, general statement ; 31, Martin, Casper's Vjhschft., 25, 197, several cases; 32, Prof. Leeds, Phil. Med. Times, 1870, inhaled about a gill of the pure gas.

Mind.—Emotional. Condition resembling intoxication the whole day,[24].—A woman was found upon the street half unconscious, talking senselessly, screaming violently, only able to say that several of her family were similarly affected ; after she got to the house was taken with a violent shaking chill, followed by decided heat,[4].—Spasmodic crying,[2].—Screaming and convulsions,[26].—Patient depressed and stupid,[25].—Sadness and despondency,[10].—Frightful anxiety, and instinctive impulse to seek change of air, while he felt powerless to overcome the paralysis of his muscles and move from where he sat,[2].—Great anguish,[29].—Apathetic,[17].—[10.] With the lassitude, an unusual apathy, and indisposition for any muscular exertion,[28].—After supper, felt buoyant and in good humor, an effect never produced by tea ; this mental sensation soon passed over into an irritable and sarcastic one, so that I sharply criticized an article in a medical journal,

---

† But two of the authorities selected refer to the action of the chemically pure gas, viz., Nos. 10 and 32, the others refer to the effects of gas from smouldering coal, a mixture of the Carbonous oxide, and Carbonic dioxide, with some vapors of volatile carbon compounds ; the effect of the gas is due to the very poisonous property of the carbonous oxide. The attention of therapeutists is particularly called to the peculiar headache, the trismus, and the hemiplegia caused by this substance.

which a few hours ago I hardly thought worth that trouble, and threw away in disgust a book of reference, as flat and superficial, which I highly value at other times,[29]. — *Intellectual.* Mental inactivity,[3]. — Mind sluggish,[20].—Very contracted range of ideas,[7].—Incapacity to draw inferences, or to compare ideas,[7].—Confused ideas,[2].—Felt in a very confused and stupid state,[27].—Confusion and stupefaction of the senses and intellectual faculties, amounting at last to complete unconsciousness,[15].—Answers only with difficulty,[23].—[20.] On attempting to describe their sensations (according to letters left by suicides) the first few lines are well written, afterwards phrases are incomplete, and at last there are only words and letters,[26].—Dull and ever-changing images passed before my mind, but I felt unable to concentrate my mind on any one,[29].—Memory much impaired; remembered nothing of his attack; could not answer questions correctly for two days, and was not able to resume his occupation for a month (after three days),[31].—Memory completely lost for five days,[16].—Stupor and imbecility,[1].—Fell to the ground stupefied,[16]. — Unconscious,[19]. — Quite unconscious till the third day,[31].—Consciousness disappears,[10].—Complete loss of consciousness,[22].—[30.] Consciousness is sometimes suddenly lost, as if the person had been struck upon the head,[15].—Unconsciousness and piteous moaning,[24].—Shortly became insensible,[18].—Struck senseless to the floor (after one moment),[32].—Coma,[22].—Comatose,[3].—Could not be aroused,[4].

Head.—Confusion and Vertigo. Gloomy confusion of head,[12]. —*Inclination to turn in a circle,*[26].—Tendency to vertigo, and to turning in a circle,[26].—[40.] *Vertigo,*[3 9 15], etc.—Vertigo, to staggering and falling,[28].—Vertigo, with flickering before the eyes,[21].—Vertigo, and turning black before eyes,[2].—Vertigo, and temporary darkness before the eyes,[13].—Continual vertigo, especially on rising after lying down,[12].—Giddiness,[16].—Giddiness and trembling, so that he fell to the ground,[31].—On rising up, staggered, was obliged to hold fast to something, and sank exhausted into a chair,[29].— *General Head.* Heaviness of the head,[28].—[50.] Heaviness of the head, without vertigo,[7].—Excessive heaviness in the head,[12].—Dull heaviness of the head,[29].—On rising, heaviness of head, which lasted all day (second day),[7].—Sudden pain in head,[31].—*Headache,*[1 3], etc.—Headache and vertigo, for several days,[4].—Headache, especially in the temples, together with violent pulsation of the temporal arteries,[21].—Headache, beginning in the morning, and spreading throughout the whole head, but felt chiefly in the occiput, which seems pressed outwards. The nape of the neck seems swollen when touched; the whole posterior portion of the head from about the summit of the occipital bone to the base of the neck seems tense, swollen; the head can hardly be moved,[7].—Headache commenced generally with confusion and heaviness of the head, and dull undefined pressure in the temporal region, it then gradually increased and extended from the temples forward and backwards, encircling the whole head; usually it increased rapidly to an extreme severity,[16].—[60.] The headache, which is the first symptom, is also the last; in a young girl it continued with great severity for more than a month, almost without interruption,[28].—Violent persistent headache,[2].—Symptoms commenced with violent headache, which soon became very intense,[26].—Violent and constant headache, worse in the frontal region and accompanied with a sensation of tightness and constriction towards the temples,[28].—Dull headache,[24].—Pressive headache,[8].—In brain, severe pressure,[10].—Painful sawing pain through middle of head, which feels congested,[8].—*Forehead.* Intolerable pain in the forehead,[11].—Frontal headache, extending over the whole head, but chiefly felt in the forehead, which seems pushed out,[7].—[70.] Constant frontal headache (second day),[7]. —Pressing pain at the forehead and parietal bones,[29].—A severe pressing frontal headache, as if the brain were compressed, and simultaneously severe palpitations of the heart, with which I am never troubled,[29].—Weight across forehead,[18].—Throbbing pain in forehead and temples,[12].—*Temples.* The attack commences with a vague, dull pain in the temporal region, which gradually extends forward and backward, encircling the head; it becomes exceedingly intense,[26].—Headache characterized by compression of the temples,[2].—Sticking in temples,[8].—Throbbing in temples,[2].—*Vertex.* Dulness and oppression in the crown of the head,[32].—*External Head.* [80.] A small red spot (similar to the streak on the arm), on the right temple, near the outer margin of the orbit,[22].

Eye. Eyes weak and dim, sunken,[8].—Eyes wild, staring,[2].—Eyes weary-looking,[12].—Eyes distorted in the orbits,[10].—Eyes fixed and insensible,[1].—Eye hyperæmic,[25].—Eyes half-open, staring,[3].—The eyes are contracted and sunken,[7].—Eyes staring and protruding,[1].—Idiotic staring at one point,[29].—*Lids.* [90.] Lids and lips bluish-red,[5].—*Conjunctiva.* Vessels of conjunctiva injected,[1].—Conjunctiva dull red,[3].—*Pupil.* Pupils dilated,[8 22 25]. —Pupils somewhat dilated,[17].—Pupils dilated and insensible,[31].—Pupils contracted, insensible,[16].—Pupils become insensible to the light, and the conjunctiva to foreign substances,[26].—*Vision.* Dim sight,[12].—Almost constant dimness of sight and vertigo,[26].—[100.] Dimness of vision, with flickering and fluttering before the eyes,[15].—Vision obscured,[2].—Flickering before the eyes, with vertigo,[30].

Ear.—Noise in ears,[18].—After a short time, confused sounds in the ears, which are exceedingly painful; afterwards there is a continuous dull vibrating, similar to the noise of a wagon, mingled with pulsating sounds, which at first seem to be indistinct and distant, but gradually become stronger; whilst lying in deep stupor, there is an incessant humming, which gradually disappears as consciousness returns,[26].—Ringing in the ears, with various kinds of illusions of hearing,[15].—Roaring in ears,[2 12 26].—Troublesome roaring and singing in the ears,[28].

Nose.—Violent inflammation of the nose and throat, which makes swallowing very difficult (second day),[16].—Bleeding from the nose,[25 27].

Face.—[110.] Looks anxious,[3].—Face pale,[16 22].—Pale face, warm to the touch,[12].—Very pale face, continued for several days,[4].—Face livid,[2].— The complexion had assumed the livid hue of death,[32].—Cyanotic,[19].—Face red,[12].—Face red (four children),[4].—Face red and puffy,[3 25].—[120.] Face bluish-red,[6].—Face tumid,[8].—Face puffy and reddish-brown,[1].—Features distorted,[3].—Convulsions of the facial muscles,[11].—Lips bluish,[12].—Lips and tongue rosy-red,[9].—**Jaws firmly clenched,**[6] (and others).—*Trismus,*[19]. —Trismus, with epileptic convulsions,[5].

Mouth.—Tongue. [130.] Paralysis of the tongue,[11].—*General Mouth.* Mouth drawn,[1].—*Saliva.* Froth from mouth,[19].—Foaming at the mouth,[16].—While eating, flow of a slightly acid water into the mouth, which mingles with the food without causing disgust,[7].—After supper, the mouth is lined with mucus so viscid that, on trying to spit it out, it sticks to the lips,[7].—Excessive sensitiveness of taste and smell, which lasts four days, and goes on diminishing, until, in six days, these two senses are duller than formerly,[7].—Appetite as usual at dinner, but bread and all sorts of food had a foul taste, even sugared rice-cake (second day),[7].

Throat.—Dryness of the throat,[26].—Pain in the throat, from swallowing saliva; lasted all night,[7].—[140.] The sore throat continues, and extends to the right ear (second day),[7].—Violent burning pain in the fauces,[26].

Stomach.—Appetite and Thirst. In the afternoon, three hours before supper, sudden paroxysm of hunger, which soon ceases without eating (second day),[7].—No inclination to eat,[7].—Anorexia,[20].—No appetite, but food relished well,[7].—Disgust for everything,[10].—Thirst,[20].—**Nausea and Vomiting.** Felt sick, and retched once or twice,[18].—Nausea,[9 16].—[150.] Slight nausea,[32].—Nausea and vomiting,[3 25 29].—Nausea and vomiting every now and then; the stomach could bear only liquids in very small quantities,[28].—Vomiting,[26 27 31].—Repeated vomiting,[14].—Vomiting after meals,[28].—Vomiting, caused by the smallest quantity of food,[28].—The stomach was so irritable that everything taken was immediately vomited (second day),[16].—Pressing on abdomen causes vomiting of a yellowish, almost fecal-like fluid,[1 9].—**Stomach.** Digestion disturbed,[10].—[160.] Very severe and obstinate pain in the epigastric region,[28].

Abdomen.—Pains in the abdomen,[5].—Frequent crying out that they had pains in the abdomen; it, however, was not distended or tense,[4].—Violent pains in the bowels,[4].

Stool.—Involuntary evacuations,[21 27].—Stools thin, painless,[20].—Constipation,[28].

Urinary Organs.—Kidneys and Bladder. Pains in kidneys,[1].—Paralysis of the bladder,[17].—Bladder remains paralyzed a long time,[17].—[170.] Paralysis of the bladder lasted nine days after the attack,[26].—**Micturition.** Involuntary evacuation of urine and fæces,[26].—Urination from the first became more and more scanty,[28].—**Urine.** Urine contained sugar,[17].—Sugar is found in the urine (Sneff),[30].—Urine contains a trace of sugar,[25].

Respiratory Organs.—Larynx, Trachea, and Bronchi. Rattling of mucus in air-passages,[1].—Bloody mucus is raised from the bronchi,[26].—**Respiration.** Respiration audible, almost rattling, slow, stertorous,[3].—Respiration rattling,[19].—[180.] Respiration rattling, now and then intermitting,[6].—Stertorous breathing,[31].—Expired air of a peculiar smell,[19].—The expired air felt, to the back of the observer's hand, cooler than usual,[28].—Respiration is for a long time quiet, but afterwards it becomes accelerated, frequently with extraordinary energy and rapidity; expiration is quick, inspiration deep, rattling; later there occur periods of complete intermission, followed by four or five inspirations,[26].—Respiration slower,[8].—Respiration slow,[19].—Respiration slow, frequently interrupted by yawning and sighing,[28].—Respiration very soon becomes slow and stertorous,[30].—Breathing now rapidly, now slowly (four children),[4].—[190.] Respiration 24 (after one hour),[25].—Respiration 20 to the minute,[25].—Respiration short and rapid,[5].—Expiration greater than inspiration,[1].—Respiration oppressed,[12].—Respiration difficult and interrupted,[1].—Respiration very labored,[1].—Somewhat impeded respiration,[12].—Sense of suffocation,[2 10].

Chest.—The chest had ceased to expand and contract,[32].—[200.] Emphysema of the lungs, with some bloody sputa,[23].—Remarkably weak vesicular murmur on auscultation,[28].—Felt as if a stream of warmth passed from the abdomen into the chest, and thence into the head; it roared in his ears, it affected his respiration; he rose, and after tottering a few steps, fell down, attacked by sudden vertigo,[12].—Complained now and then of anguish and anxiety in the chest,[28].—Sense of a burden on the chest,[19].—On breathing, feeling as if a heavy load on chest,[2].—In chest, severe tearing pain,[10].

Heart and Pulse.—Præcordium. Intolerable pain in the region of the heart,[11].—Præcordial anxiety,[26].—*Heart's Action.* Palpitation,[3].—[210.] Violent palpitation,[2].—Violent palpitation on exertion,[2].—Pressure in præcordial region produced violent palpitation, a rapid, weak, trembling contraction and expansion,[3].—Desire to loosen clothing on account of palpitation,[2].—The action of the heart and of the lungs gradually decreased,[26].—Feeble action of the heart,[12].—Action of the heart slow and weak,[28].—Beating of the heart alternately increases and diminishes,[26].—The beating of the heart is at first increased, but afterwards it becomes slower,[26].—Beating of the heart at first strong, frequent, even amounting to palpitation, although associated with slow respiration; at last it becomes irregular and intermitting,[15].—[220.] The action of the heart is at first strong and rapid; it afterwards becomes very irregular, so that there is an intermission after four or five pulsations; the intermissions become prolonged on the approach of death, and afterwards become more frequent, so that they intermit every three or four beats,[26].—*Pulse.* At night, in bed, pulse high, rapid, 120 beats occupying a short time,[7].—Pulse 100,[25].—Pulse regular, 80, weak,[25].—Pulse 72 (after one hour),[25].—Pulse rising and falling (varying between 144 and 88),[17].—Pulse small, rapid,[22].—Pulse rapid, very small,[19].—Pulse slow and full,[8].—Small, slow pulse,[12].—[230.] Pulse small and slow, scarcely to be felt,[1].—Pulse full, 68,[16].—Pulse 64 (after thirty minutes),[25].—Pulse 56,[20].—Pulse 56, soft, compressible, undulating,[28].—The pulse is at first accelerated, afterwards retarded,[30].—Pulse very variable (four children),[4].—Pulse weak, wavy,[3].—Pulse small,[11].—The pulse had stopped beating, or beat so feebly that in the agitation of the moment it was imperceptible,[32].

Neck and Back.—[240.] Soreness of all the cervical muscles while exerting the brain (second day),[7].—Burning pain at the right scapula, which soon ceases (second day),[7].

Extremities in General.—Extremities flexed,[10].—Feeling as if the left upper and lower extremities had gone to sleep and could not be moved,[24].—Inclination to stretch the extremities,[29].—Clonic cramps in the extremities,[25].—Clonic spasms of the extremities,[31].—Trembling of limbs,[1].—Convulsions in limbs and stiffness in joints,[2].—All limbs convulsed,[1].—[250.] Great weariness of the limbs,[9].—Paralysis of the left arm and left leg continues after the attack,[9].—Complete paralysis of the right foot and right hand, and also of the muscles of the right half of the face; persisted after the attack,[26].—Pains in the extremities, followed by paralysis,[15].

Superior Extremities.—Arms flexed, could not be extended,[6].—Tossing about of the arms,[16].—The chorea-like movements of the right arm continued for some days, only on waking,[20].—The arms and hands are without strength (second day),[7].—Spasm of flexors of forearm,[19].—A remnant of pain in the left knuckle-joints, caused by a fall on the ice six months before, returned with increased severity, and extended to the corresponding parts of the right hand (second day),[7].—[260.] Fingers clenched,[6].—Numbness of three fingers of the right hand; the fingers can only be extended with difficulty,[22].

Inferior Extremities.—Trembling of legs,[2].—Attempted to rise, but was unable to do so; legs stiff and powerless,[27].—The legs can scarcely sustain the body (second day),[7].—The weakness in both legs continued to increase, to complete paralysis of the right and incomplete paralysis of the left,[20].—*Thigh.* Occasional shooting pains in the right nates, just where the ischiatic nerve emerges; there was noticed at this point an elliptical red spot half as large as the hand, without any trace of blisters, only the skin seemed to be somewhat puffy and elastic, without fluctuation,²⁰.— When sitting on a low chair, the gluteal muscles are painful, us if he had just got up after a severe sickness and was much emaciated (second day),⁷. —*Leg.* Extension of the right leg became difficult (second week),²⁰.— When putting on his garters in the morning, they cause pain, and he is obliged to tie them so loosely that they slip down (second day),⁷.—[270.] The pains in the nates extended along the sciatic nerve, and the external popliteal nerve, down to the foot; no pain on pressing on the os ilium or on moving the leg,²⁰.—*Toes.* Toes could not be moved (second week),²⁰.

General Symptoms.—Objective. Extreme emaciation followed the attack,¹⁷.—The first effect is a stage of complete rest,¹³.—The second stage is one of excitation, characterized by contractions and convulsions,¹³. —Trembling of whole body,¹.—Body stiff,¹.—Hemiplegia (persistent).²¹.— Paralysis of the sphincters,³⁰.—Sphincters relaxed,¹.—[280.] Cramps,¹⁶.— Tonic cramps,¹⁶.—Spasms, without loss of consciousness,²⁵.—Spasms, returning every five minutes, with loss of consciousness and loss of speech; the head was drawn spasmodically backwards, the arms stiffly extended; the spasms especially affected the cervical muscles,²⁵.—Violent spasms,².—Violent spasms, at first usually clonic, afterwards generally tonic, becoming tetanic,¹⁵.—Tonic spasm of most of the muscles of trunk and extremities, so that it is difficult to make patient sit or lie,¹⁹.—Repeated convulsions,¹⁷. —Epileptiform convulsions, which were renewed every time the patient was touched or spoken to, although he lay quite still and apparently unconscious,²⁵.—Disinclination to labor,²⁹.—[290.] Great lassitude in hands and feet,¹².—Weakness,¹⁸.—Weakness of the muscles,²⁶.—Extraordinary weakness,¹⁶.—General debility and malaise,²⁹.—Felt his strength fail him,¹⁸. —Every voluntary movement, even speaking, difficult,⁸.—Rising and walking seemed a most tremendous exertion,²⁹.—In morning could not rise up,⁸.—Prostration,¹³.—[300.] Great prostration,¹⁷.—Complete prostration,¹¹. —Inclination to faint,³.—Fainting,².—Suddenly fell to the ground, as if struck by lightning,¹⁰.—Very restless,².—An enormous restlessness, with anguish and oppression, forced me to get up and walk in another room where the window was open,²⁹.—Constant motion, continually flexing and extending the right arm with considerable force,²⁰.—The father was constantly moving about and complaining of his head,⁴.—Continually tossing about,¹⁶.—[310.] Four children were lying in bed senseless, tossing to and fro,⁴.—Extraordinary sensitiveness,¹⁰.—The third stage is one of anæsthesia, characterized by partial or absolute insensibility,¹³.—General insensibility,²². —Tactile sensibility was greatly diminished; patient evinced no pain when pinched and pricked quite severely,²⁶.—Sensibility of sight, hearing, smell, and taste also greatly lessened,²⁸.—Blunted sensibility of the whole skin,²⁰. —Anæsthesia of the skin (persistent),²¹.—Anæsthesia of the skin, *but the slightest touch with a hot iron recalls the sensibility,*²⁶.—The sensibility of the skin is completely lost, especially to mechanical irritation; only a glowing hot iron causes a reaction; this insensibility is at first noticed on the extremities, whence it gradually extends to the trunk, last of all involving the mammary glands and the fossæ under the clavicle and in the axilla,²⁶. —[320.] Complete anæsthesia,¹⁶.—*Subjective.* Felt very tired and fatigued,²⁷.—Generable, indefinable malaise; feeling of painful weariness; dull pain in the limbs and loins,²⁸.—Dread of every noise or jar, which shoots through the body like an electric shock; continues for several minutes; this condition gradually changes to a kind of insensibility, which is especially noticed in the tips of the fingers, and it varies in intensity with the condition of the atmosphere,[10].—Body all sore,[27].—Whole body sore to touch,[7].—Soreness of all the muscles, as after excessive fatigue (second day),[7].

Skin.—General. Skin bloodless; the veins show through it blackish,[10].—Surface of body reddish-livid,[27].—Bluish, cyanotic color of the entire skin, especially of the face, neck, antero-superior portion of the chest and back of the hands; on all which parts the skin was actually slate-colored; this color was also noticed on the mucous membrane of the lip,[28].—[330.] The skin assumes a violet color; the veins are swollen; the lips and conjunctiva are cyanotic,[26].—Purple maculation of the skin,[27].—The skin had lost its normal tone and elasticity; when pinched, the folds remained for some seconds and disappeared slowly,[28].—Along the course of the radial nerve in each forearm a linear redness, without swelling of the subcutaneous cellular tissue, more on the right than on the left side,[22].—Circumscribed spots on the anterior surface of the left forearm and on the inner surface of the left lower leg, which were totally insensible to pricking and pinching (sixth day),[24].—A brownish ecchymosis, as large as the palm of the hand, on the lower portion of the sacrum,[22].—*Eruptions, Moist.* The whole skin was covered with large and small vesicles of pemphigus (sixth day),[17]. —Herpetic vesicles on the temple in the place where the redness had been noticed,[22].—Herpes zoster on the left side of the face along the course of the trigeminus; vesicles on the forehead, above the orbit, along the course of the ramus frontalis, on the cheek below the orbit, along the terminal filament of the infraorbital nerve of the chin, along the mental nerve (eleventh day after the poisoning),[23].—A dozen herpetic vesicles, as large as a pin's head, on the inner portion of the right forearm, somewhat externally to the place where the redness had been noticed; the subcutaneous tissue seemed to be somewhat swollen,[22].—[340.] About twenty herpetic vesicles, as large as a pin's head, along the course of the right sciatic nerve, situated upon a slightly red base; from them some red streaks extend up to the right nates, and from the point of exit of the sciatic nerve to the crest of the ilium,[22].—Abscesses form upon the chest and upon the left nates, caused by subcutaneous ecchymosis,[17].—*Sensations.* Burning sensation in the skin, especially of the cheeks, without intense redness, and without elevation of temperature (very soon),[21].—Formication on both legs,[20].

Sleep and Dreams.—Sleepiness,[16]. — *Great sleepiness· for several days*,[4].—Drowsy, but unable to sleep on account of the headache and pains in the stomach,[28].—Somnolence,[23].—Sound sleep (third night),[7].—Sleep deep and prolonged, interrupted by cramps in cheeks and toes,[10].—[350.] Never slept so long before,[27].

Fever.—Chilliness. Cold, mottled skin,[5].—The temperature of the body was rapidly falling,[32].—Bodily temperature remarkably lowered; skin cold, giving to the touch an impression like that caused by contact with a corpse some hours after death, before it is quite cold.   Temp. in the axilla, + 34.6° ; in the mouth, 35.2°,[28].—Temperature 38° Cent.,[25].—Coldness,[10].—Sensation of coldness in the whole body,[24].—The attack is followed by long-continued sensation of coldness and general trembling, which may last for weeks,[26].—Severe chill, with chattering,[2].—Violent febrile chill, for several days,[4].—[360.] Violent and continued shaking chill,[14].—Daily repeated chills, with a sensation of a heavy dragging up of the abdomen when walking and standing,[14].—Chilly all day,[7].—Cool extremities,[12].— Extremities cold,[1 22].—Extremities cold and numb,[11].—Hands and feet cold,[5].—Hands icy cold,[12].—*Heat.* Febrile symptoms,[57].—At night, in bed, burning heat all over, without thirst; despite this heat and fever, slept lightly until 1 A.M., after which increase of heat, with thirst and dry mouth; the thirst was satisfied by drinking only a little; the heat, as well as the thirst and fever, now gradually diminished, and the bed, which had hitherto been too warm, was now too cold, so that he had to have more covering; sleep returned,[7].—[370.] Sensation of warmth in chest and abdomen, similar to that caused by spirituous liquors, but the hands and feet remained cold,[12].—*Sweat.* Skin covered with sweat,[25].—Beads of sweat over whole body,[10].—A little sweat on the upper half of the body, in the morning, in bed,[7].—Slight frontal sweat,[12].

Conditions.—**Aggravation.**—(*Morning*), On rising, heaviness of head; in bed, sweat on upper half of body.—(*Night*), In bed, heat.—(*In open air*), Felt worse.—(*On breathing*), Feeling of load on chest.—(*While eating*), Flow of saliva.—(*After meals*), Vomiting.—(*On rising, after lying down*), Vertigo.

Amelioration.—(*Fresh air*), Marked relief, especially to heaviness on chest.

CARBONEUM SULFURATUM.

Carbon bisulphide, CS_2. (Alcohol sulphuris, Alcohol Lampadii.) *Preparation,* Dilutions prepared with alcohol.

Authorities. 1, Knaf, Inaug. Diss. Prag., 1835 (*translated from the daybooks given in Pemerl's collection, All. Zeit. für Hom., supplement*), provings with repeated doses of 2 to 20 drops of the crude oil; 2, J. Buchner took 3 drops, afterward $\frac{1}{25}$th and $\frac{1}{50}$th of a drop (ibid.); 3, M. H., a woman, aged 24, took repeated doses of 1 to 2 drops crude (ibid.); 4, Dr. Held took 2 drops on the first day, 2 on the second, 1 on the third, 1 on the fourth, 1 on the fifth, 1 on the sixth (ibid.); 5, Anna Gasberger was cured of severe toothache, with swelling of the gum and pains in that (right) side of the head, face, and neck, by Carb. sulf., so that only some swelling of the gum was left; she continued to take the drug, however, until she took more than half a drachm of the crude oil, and developed new symptoms (ibid.); 6, Dr. Konigshœfer, aged 36, took the 2d dilution, and afterwards the 1st, repeated doses (ibid.); 7, Mrs. K., aged 26, took repeated doses of the 1st dilution (ibid.); 8, L. M., a man, aged 60, took repeated doses of the 2d dilution, afterwards the 1st dilution (ibid.); 9, Dr. Prims took the 6th dilution daily for four days, afterward the 4th and the 1st (ibid.); 10, Dr. Prims took 1, 3, 5, and 6 drops of the crude oil (ibid.); 11, Dr. Pemerl, aged 36 (formerly, five years ago) had hæmoptysis, and now has a tendency to pulmonary congestion) took the 1st dilution at 7 A.M. (three provings), afterward the 3d dilution (two provings), (ibid.); 12, Dr. Moser took 50 drops of the 1st dilution on several successive days, and afterward 1 to 10 drops of the tincture (ibid.); 13, Dr. Quaglio took 2, 3, and 4 drops of the crude (ibid.); 14, Dr. A. W. Koch, N. Am. J. of Hom., 2, 374: *a*, took the $\frac{1}{100000}$th, 3 drops four times a day for three days, 10 drops on fourth day, and 3 drops on tenth day; *b*, took the 2d dilution seven times in twelve days; *c*, 1st dilution 3 to 10 drops, nine times in thirteen days; *d*, $\frac{1}{100000}$th, 10 drops, in six ounces of water, nine tablespoonfuls in nine days; *e*, $\frac{1}{4}$th dilution, 5 drops five times in eight days; 15, Delpech, L'Union, 1855, effects of the vapor of Carb. sulf. on workmen in rubber factories, cases

cited in L'Art. Med., 4, 83, also in Zeit. f. hom. Aezt. Oest., 1, 121, also in
Ziemssen, Pathol. und Therapie, Band 1, etc.; 16, Sir J. Y. Simpson, L.
and E. M. J., 8, 743, effects of vapor on self and many others; 17, A.
Turnbull, Lond. Med. Gaz., 1, 178, effects of local application to the eye
and to enlarged glands; 18, Bergeron and Levy, Gaz. Med. de Paris, 1864,
p. 584, effects on the eye; 19, Bienhardt, Berlin Kl. W., 1871 (S. J., 143,
149), effects of inhaling the fumes in a rubber factory; 20, P. H. Van der
Weyde, statement of effects (from Hering's Monograph); 21, "S. P." (from
Hering); 22, Miller, Elements of Chemistry, vol. 2; 23, Dr. Radziejewski,
Virchow's Archiv, 53, p. 370, effects of inspiring a small quantity of the
Oxysulphide of carbon.

Mind.—Emotional. Very much excited during the night,[16].—Inhalation of the vapor caused a condition resembling intoxication from alco-
holi stimulants; this often reached such a degree that one could scarcely
walk without reeling,[11].—Raging delirium; he fell on his father and tried
to bite him (child),[18].—Depressing and disagreeable visions (in several
cases),[16].—Particularly cheerful and free from care (fourth day),[14b].—Inclination to sing (curative),[14b].—Sadness,[15].—Mood depressed, rather obstinate,[4].—Mood depressed, easily irritated,[3].—[10.] Sudden ebullitions of a
fretful mood (third day),[11].—Morose mood, inclined to get angry,[4].—Disposition very changeable; sometimes he had turns of extravagant gayety;
sometimes he flew into a passion from the most trivial causes, and in these
fits of unreasonable anger smashed everything about him,[15].—*Intellectual.* Increased activity of mind,[1].—At first the intellectual faculties are
excited; persons talk more than usual; there is an increased liveliness,[15].
—Distraction of mind,[11].—Distraction of mind; it is difficult to fix the
mind upon what one is reading,[11].—Distraction of mind; he is unable to
fix his attention upon his reading,[11].—Could not find the right words while
speaking,[15].—Frequently she did not know what she was to do with the
things she was holding in her hands,[19].—[20.] Stupidity (secondary action),[15].
—Peculiarly idiotic and childish,[19].—Loss of memory,[19].—Loss of memory,
and mental alienation,[20].—Weakness of memory (secondary action),[15].—
Memory so poor that he kept forgetting where he had placed his tools when
he had occasion for them,[15].—*Confusion and Vertigo.* Confusion of
the head,[2 5], etc.—Confusion of the head (third day),[10].—Slight confusion of
the head,[1].—Great confusion of the head,[7].—[30.] Long-continued confusion of the head, as from excessive use of spirituous drinks,[4].—Head confused, with stitches here and there in the forehead, and frequently a transient jerking pain in it,[12].—Confusion of the forehead, and vertigo,[2].—The
whole head is confused and painful, as in catarrho-rheumatic headache; it
lasted till noon, after he had produced perspiration by constant walking
(third day),[14a].—Confusion of the forehead, with sensation of constriction
of the cerebral hemisphere,[2].—Inclination to vertigo,[23].—Vertigo,[2 5].—Vertigo (after two hours),[2].—Frequent attacks of vertigo, while sitting,[4].—
Vertigo, in the afternoon, while sitting,[4].—[40.] Vertigo in the forehead,
with tendency to fall forward,[2].—Momentary vertigo,[4].—Intense vertigo,[15].
—Such violent vertigo that he was unable to stand,[23].—A reeling in the
head,[12].—*General Head.* Great dulness of the head,[21].—Head heavy,[12].
—Head heavy and confused, for several weeks,[12].—Heaviness of the head,[1].
—Heaviness of the whole head,[3].—[50.] Whole head painful and confused
after breakfast (second day),[14b].—Headache (wife),[15].—Headache when reading,[7].—Headache and giddiness,[16].—Headache commences about 9 A.M.;
the whole head is confused, and thought is difficult,[3].—Violent headache,[15].

—Violent headache (third day),[14d].—Violent headache towards 10 P.M. (second day),[14a].—Violent headache, especially in the forehead and over the eyes, the whole forenoon,[14d].—Dull headache, becoming worse towards evening,[15].—[60.] Pressure in the head,[23].—Pressive headache, in the forenoon,[7].—Head very painful, especially on top, as if it were all sore there, on brushing the hair,[14d].—Throbbing headache the whole day, aggravated by moving the head (third day),[14e].—The headache, which had disappeared during the afternoon, returned towards evening,[10].—*Forehead.* Slight pains in the forehead,[10].—Slight pain in the forehead, which soon extended to the left parietal bone, where it lasted two hours,[9].—Slight pain in the forehead, on waking (second day),[10].—Slight flitting pain in the forehead, which gradually extended to the left temple (a few minutes after taking),[10]. —Headache in forehead all day,[14d].—[70.] Confused headache in the forehead,[3].—Dull, confused headache in the forehead, with nausea,[3].—10 P.M., tensive headache in forehead,[14a].—Tensive headache in the forehead, with eructations,[14b].—Dull pain in the forehead and temples, especially a pressive pain in the right temple,[6].—Sensation of pressure in the forehead, extending to the orbits and temples,[1].—Pressure in the forehead, with slight dull pain in it, transient,[12].—Slight painful pressure in the forehead, and a little digging in it,[12].—Dull pressure in the forehead and temples, with inclination to sleep,[6].—Pressive pain in the frontal region, with sensation of heat, lasting two hours,[10].—[80.] Pressive pain in the forehead, extending from the frontal eminence to the left temple, with some tearings in that direction,[10].—Slight pressive pain in the forehead,[9].—From time to time dull pressive pain in the forehead, extending down towards the eyes,[7].— Slight pressive headache in the forehead, especially increased by reading or stooping,[7].—Pressive frontal headache the whole day, with little interruption,[6].—Pain in the forehead, tearing, appearing after half an hour, and lasting in a slight degree until afternoon, gradually disappearing, extending to the temples,[4].—Ulcerative headache in forehead (second day),[14a].— Ulcerative headache in forehead the whole day, with burning in eyes,[14d].— *Temples.* Pain in both temples, in the afternoon, especially caused or aggravated by shaking the head, or by stepping hard,[6].—Drawing pain in the temples,[7].—[90.] Drawing pain in the left temporal region,[6].—Drawing and tearing pain, extending from the forehead to the temples, lasting the whole day, better in the open air than in the room, and during rest,[3].— Pressive pain in the temples,[10].—Pressure at the insertion of the temporal muscles,[4].—Pressing inward in the temples; the pressure afterwards extending to the vertex,[2].—Stitches in the left temple, extending to the occiput,[10].—Tearing in the left temporal region,[7].—Transient tearing pains in the temples,[6].—Transient tearing in the right temple, when stooping,[7].— Violent pulsating pains in the temple (*migraine*), at 6 A.M., on waking, so that he could not lie quiet; continued until breakfast at 7.30 A.M. (second day),[14b]. —*Vertex.* [100.] Pressing pains in the vertex, often lasting all day,[15].—*Parietals.* Semilateral headache returned when walking, with great dulness and confusion in head (almost immediately),[14b].—Pressure on the right parietal bone,[9].—Severe pain in right parietal bone, as though it were violently pressed upon with a hard body,[14a] —*External Head.* Sore pimples, painful to touch, on the scalp (sixth day),[11].—Itching of the head,[3,21].

Eye.—Eyes sunken, with strongly marked gray rings around them (noon),[14a].—When applied to the eye, the vapors occasion intense prickling heat and flow of tears,[17].—Pressure upon the eyes,[10].—Pressure upon the

eyes, with inclination to close them,[12].—Severe pressure upon the eyes,[12].—
[110.] Itching pressure in the eyes, together with burning on the upper
lids and the development of a small pustule, which itches a great deal,
with secretion of much whitish-yellow mucus in the eye; this pustule lasted
four days,[4].—Stitches in the right eye, when reading (fifth day),[11].—Some
stitches in the right eye (second day),[11].—Jerking stitches in the right eye,
in the region of the superior rectus muscle,[11].—*Orbit.* Sensation of pressure in the orbits,[1].—Sore pain in the orbicularis of the left eye towards the
external canthus, especially on moving the lids (fourth day),[11].—Jerking-
stitching pain, paroxysmal, apparently alternating in various muscles of
the right eye (fifth day),[11].—Some dull stitches in the right eye, when
reading (second day),[11].—*Lids.* Twitching of the eyelids,[6].—Heaviness of
the eyelids,[3].—[120.] Burning in the margin of the lids, which are somewhat red,[7].—Biting in the right lower lid,[7] [21].—Itching in the eyelids,[21].—
Lachrymal Apparatus. Lachrymation while reading,[10].—*Ball.*
Pressure on the left eyeball, with sensation of heat in it,[10].—Great itching
of the eyeball,[4].—Insensibility of the cornea in a high degree, without disturbance of vision,[18].—*Pupil.* Pupils dilated,[5].—Pupils slightly dilated,[3].
—Momentary dilatation of the pupil (soon after taking one drop),[3].—
[130.] It generally contracts the pupil, and very seldom dilates it,[17].—
Vision. Weak vision; objects seemed to fade away on account of a mist
which spread out before them,[15].—Sight became so weak that he could
work only a few hours at a time,[15].—Dimness of vision,[3].—Obscuration of
vision,[11].—Lost the power of vision,[19].

Ear.—Left ear somewhat painful, and as if stopped,[14b].—Boring in the
right ear (after eight hours and a half),[11].—Pressive pain in the right ear,
repeated at times, just as if one were thrusting a dull instrument into the
tympanum,[10].—Sticking in the left ear (after two hours),[7].—[140.] Some
stitches in the right ear, in the afternoon (second day),[10].—Stitches in the
right ear,[10].—The stitches in the right ear became worse towards evening,
when they lasted nearly a quarter of an hour,[10].—Some stitches in the right
ear, after dinner, which were repeated at intervals of a quarter of an
hour,[10].—Stitches in the left ear (fourth day),[14a].—Stitches in the left ear,
in evening,[14e].—Fine jerking stitches in the left ear (after five hours),[11].—
Some fine stitches in the ear (after four hours),[11].—Stitches in the left ear,
as if an insect were in it, 9 P.M.,[14b].—Violent stitches and griping pain
(transitory) in left ear, which awoke him in the night (second day),[14a].—
Hearing. [150.] Ringing before the ears, lasting several days,[4].—Buzzing and singing of the wind in the right ear, like an Æolian harp, when walking in the morning,[14d].—Deafness, so that he had to be shouted to; it gradually lessened and disappeared spontaneously after some time,[15].

Nose.—Objective. End of nose red and burning, sore (second
day),[14b].—Stoppage of the nose,[3].—Some catarrhal stoppage of the nose
(second day),[11].—Nose was stopped,[4].—Sneezing,[11].—Sneezing, with traces
of blood in the nasal mucus,[11].—*Subjective.* Burning in the root of the
nose and in the throat,[10].—[160.] Prickling in the tip of the nose, like an
irritation to sneeze,[11].

Face.—Face red, puffy,[5].—Great paleness,[15].—Face as if bloated (third
day),[14a].—Lips dry,[4].—Compressive feeling in the muscles of the under jaw,
particularly alongside the larynx (immediately),[14a].—Drawing pain in the
left lower jaw,[10].

Mouth.—Teeth. Sensation of bluntness of the teeth,[1].—Toothache in
the molars of the right under jaw,[14d].—Toothache in every tooth, from

cleansing the mouth with cold water in the morning (third day),[14a].—[170.] Slight sticking in the root of a carious tooth, upper right side (after two hours),[11].—Jerking-sticking pain in a carious tooth at 9 A.M. (second day),[11].—Dull drawing-sticking toothache in a carious upper back tooth, and also in a lower tooth opposite it, at 6 A.M., lasting in the first tooth till after rising (for half an hour), (second day),[11].—Stitches extending from the crown to the root of a sound double tooth of the lower right side (after three hours),[11].—Toothache reappeared in the afternoon, tearing, and at the same time drawing; it increased during the afternoon, and was only somewhat relieved after midnight; it was intolerable in great cold,[4].—Throbbing pain, with burning in the left back teeth, not violent, coming on in the evening and lasting through the night,[4].—The toothache of yesterday is increased, and is accompanied by swelling around the painful tooth, which extends towards the palate; chewing causes no pain, but only itching and tension,[4].—The toothache overpowered all other symptoms; it lasted the whole day, and was worse at night; on account of this I was unable to observe properly my other symptoms,[4].—*General Mouth.* Twitches in the corners of the mouth,[5].—Clammy mouth, with bad taste and frequent spitting,[15].—[180.] Irritability of the mouth and pharynx, with sensation of constriction of the larynx, provoking cough, which amounts to retching, with expectoration of mucus,[2].—Burning in the mouth,[2].—Violent burning on the lips and tongue, and in the throat (immediately),[13].—Most excessive burning in the mouth and pharynx, which are extremely painful,[5].—*Tongue.* Tongue coated (noon),[14a].—Sensation of coldness on the tongue, soon changed to a sticking-burning, followed by persistent sensation like that caused by an acrid and astringent substance, as, for example, pepper (immediately),[1].—Burning, like pepper, on the tip of the tongue and in the throat (soon after the one-tenth),[6].—Fine burning upon the tongue (papillæ), (immediately),[14b].—Sharp burning pain on the tongue, as if from oil of peppermint, with peculiar oniony and garlicky taste (immediately),[14c].—Sticking-burning on the tongue,[2].—[190.] Pricking sensation on the tip of the tongue,[19].—The mucous membrane of the mouth and throat was very anæsthetic,[19].—*Saliva.* Increased secretion of saliva,[1 5 10].—Very much increased secretion of saliva,[10].—Salivation, with nausea,[15].—Saliva glutinous,[2].—Accumulation of water in the mouth (second day),[11].—Accumulation of water in the mouth, together with frequent attacks of nausea,[11].—Accumulation of water of a sweetish taste in the mouth,[6].—Increased spitting,[1].—*Taste.* [200.] Taste extremely repulsive, acrid, and scraping; swallowing caused burning in the throat and along the œsophagus,[4].—Taste sweetish, offensive,[2].—Pasty taste in the mouth,[13].—Nauseous, pasty taste in the mouth (after three hours),[11].—Metallic taste in the mouth,[10].—Metallic, sulphur-like taste,[1].—Peculiar saltish sourish taste all the forenoon, since the commencement of the próving,[14d].—Bitter sour taste in the morning,[4].—Constant bitter taste,[19].—Awoke with a very bitter taste in mouth, which disappeared after breakfast (second day),[14c].—[210.] A glass of beer, taken between 5 and 6 P.M., has not its usual taste,[14s].—Taste blunted, frequently herby,[2].

Throat.—Salty taste of the mucus raised from the throat,[11].—Continual oniony taste and smell in the throat,[14c].—Much hawking, with inclination to vomit (after one hour and a half),[11].—Dryness of the throat,[7].—She constantly complained of dryness of the throat,[19].—Great dryness in the throat compelled her to drink enormous quantities of water,[19].—Sensation of a hair in the throat,[2].—Sensation in the throat like that caused by an acrid substance (immediately),[1].—[220.] (Pains and burning in the throat, with profuse catarrh, caused by cold, wet weather),[3].—Burning in the throat,[16].—Burning pain in the throat,[10].—Burning in the throat, extending to the stomach,[3].—Burning and scraping in the throat and œsophagus,[10].—Scraping in the throat,[11].—Scraping sensation in the throat, causing cough,[6].—A scraping, raw pain (as from a foreign body) in the left side of the throat; on swallowing, it extends to the left ear; lasts one to two minutes (third day),[11].—Scraping rough sensation in the throat, with fine transient stitches,[6].—Rawness in the throat,[11].—[230.] Roughness and scraping in the throat (second day),[11].—Constant scratching and scraping in the throat, as from catarrh, all day,[7].—Burning in the soft palate (after three-quarters of an hour),[2].—Tickling in posterior part of palate, exciting a hard dry cough, soon after lying down,[14a].—Rough scraping sensation in the fauces (after one hour),[11].—Burning and scraping in the whole pharynx,[5].—Swallowing difficult,[5].

Stomach.—Appetite. Increased appetite,[1].—Desire for food, with increased secretion of saliva,[1].—Hunger, together with aversion to eating (second day),[11].—[240.] Hunger, though with aversion to the food set before him; it, however, had real relish (after five hours),[11].—Sensation of hunger, with, however, aversion to food (second day),[11].—Appetite diminished,[13].—Little appetite,[11] [14c].—Little appetite, especially for meat (third day),[11].—Loss of appetite,[19].—Appetite is lost (after repeated doses),[1].—Constant anorexia,[15].—Constant satiety, for several weeks,[12].—*Thirst.* Desire for drinks,[3].—[250.] Thirst great, especially for beer,[4].—*Eructations.* Eructations,[2] [10] [13].—Eructations, with nausea,[19].—Eructations and inclination to vomit,[10].—Eructations, extraordinary in quantity and loudness, and very fetid flatus, in afternoon,[14a].—Eructations of air,[7].—Eructations of wind (immediately),[14c].—Eructations of a very bitter fluid, at 10 P.M. (third day),[14a].—Eructations of an acid, corrosive fluid,[14c].—Eructations of nauseating, disgusting fluid,[14b].—[260.] Empty eructations,[6].—Empty eructations, tasting and smelling of the remedies (soon after the $\frac{1}{10}$),[6].—Insufficient eructations (second day),[11].—Frequent acid eructations,[3].—Frequent eructations of air, as after eating radishes,[11].—Frequent noisy eructations, followed by amelioration (as in *neuralgia cœliaca*), (second day),[14a].—Frequent odorless eructations of air, with burning in the pit of the stomach,[11].—Continual sour eructations without vomiting,[5].—Copious, noisy eructations (second day),[14a].—Copious eructations of wind and discharge of flatus,[14d].—[270.] Nauseous eructations,[1].—Slight sourish eructations, one hour after drinking coffee, at 8 A.M. (fifth day),[11].—Burning, sour eructations twice (after one hour),[11].—Burning, sour, corrosive eructations, in the afternoon, one to two hours after eating (fourth day),[11].—Heartburn the whole day, especially after smoking,[14d].—Severe heartburn, exciting cough,[14c].—Violent heartburn the whole day, especially in the forenoon and at every eructation,[14d].—Uprising of milk that had been eaten, without nausea and vomiting,[7].—*Nausea and Vomiting.* Nausea,[10] [19].—Nausea, with pressive frontal headache,[6].—[280.] Nausea and inclination to vomit,[6].—Nausea, and greenish vomiting several times daily,[15].—Nausea, with pressure in the stomach, lasting only a short time,[6].—Nausea, pressure, and sensation of coldness in the stomach (after 2 drops),[3].—Great nausea and inclination to vomit,[7].—Attacks of nausea (after three hours),[11].—Attacks of nausea, with collection of water in the mouth (after four hours),[11].—Attacks of nausea, with collection of water in the mouth, lasting several minutes and recurring at short intervals, appearing after three-quarters of an hour, and frequently repeated till after dinner,[11].—Attacks of nausea, with uncomfortable movings about in the lower abdomen (after two to three hours),[11].—Slight attacks of nausea (after three hours),[11].—[290.] During its use was occasionally sick, and vomited several times,[14].—General sick feeling the whole afternoon, with sensation of nausea, slight colic, aversion to beer, etc.,[11].—Inclination to vomit,[2 13].—Inclination to vomit, frequently preceded by nausea, like a faintness,[12].—Inclination to vomit, relieved by eructations,[2].—Inclination to vomit, which was especially noticed on entering a room, or on going from the room into the open air; the symptom was always transient,[12].—Vomiting of a small quantity of bitter water (after one hour),[7].—Vomiting green and bilious, with nausea, cold sweat, and prostration,[15].—*Stomach.* Frequent indigestion,[15].—Well-developed *status gastricus,* viz., headache, discomfort, coated tongue, indisposition to exertion, and general feeling of ill-humor (second day),[14a].—[300.] Flatulence rises from the stomach, having the acrid smell and taste of the drug, frequently repeated (soon after taking),[1].—Sensation of emptiness and discomfort in the stomach,[12].—Uncomfortable sensation in the stomach (soon after taking),[7].—Sensation of discomfort in the epigastric region, with nausea, frequent eructations of air having the taste and smell of the drug,[12].—Region of stomach more or less painful all day (second day),[14a].—Pain in the stomach, after breakfast, especially worse on deep breathing,[7].—Heaviness in the stomach, extending over the whole epigastric region,[2].—Warmth in the pit of the stomach, extending upward through the whole of the chest,[1].—A pleasant warmth diffuses itself throughout the whole stomach (soon),[1].—[310.] The warmth in the stomach increases and spreads downward throughout the lower abdomen; it is also increased in the chest and in the perspiring face and palms of the hands,[1].—Burning in the stomach and region of the liver, increased by pressure,[10].—Burning in the pit of the stomach and in the stomach,[5].—Burning in stomach up through the œsophagus, in the forenoon,[14e].—Burning sensation in the stomach, which was increased by pressing upon it,[10].—Fulness in the stomach,[9 10].—Fulness of the stomach, with eructations,[2].—Extraordinary fulness and inflation in gastric region,[14e].—Pinching in gastric region,[14d].—[320.] An uncomfortable constrictive sensation in the stomach, with good appetite,[10].—Pressure in stomach,[14a 14b 12].—Pressure in stomach and abdomen, with pains in loins (second day),[14b].—Pressure in stomach, half an hour after breakfast, followed by eructations of wind and alleviation,[14a].—Pressure in stomach, two hours after dinner; this pressure never ceases altogether, and stretches downwards into the abdomen (second day),[14a].—Pressure in stomach after stool, followed by headache and cramplike sticking in both ears (second day),[14a].—Pressure in stomach, from whatever he eats or drinks, even from beer and sugar (second day),[14a].—Pressure in stomach, with eructations of wind, after drinking beer,[14a].—Transitory pressure in stomach (third day),[14a].—Slight pressure in the stomach,[1].—[330.] Frequent slight pressure in the stomach,[7].—Some pressure in the stomach after dinner, with constriction and sticking pressing pains in chest (second day),[14a].—Very severe pressure in stomach, as from a heavy weight,[14a].—Violent pressure in stomach one hour after breakfast,[14b].—Pressive sensation in the stomach,[9].—Pressive pain in the epigastric region,[6].—Pressing pain beneath the scrobiculus (immediately),[14b].—10 P.M. Violent sticking pain in stomach through to back, when resting the epigastrium on the window-sill and taking a deep inspiration; repeated with every deep inspiration,[14e].—Transitory, pressing-sticking pains in the scrobiculus, radiating from a single point into the cardiac region (second day),[14a].—Transient stitches in the epigastric region,[6].—[340.] Stomach sensitive to pressure (second day),[10].—Stomach painful to external pressure (second day),[14a].

Abdomen.—Hypochondria. Indefinite, unpleasant, painful sensation in the region of the left lobe of the liver (second day),[11].—Sticking, colic-like symptoms in the hypochondria, after sitting a long time (sixth day),[11].—Paroxysmal, sticking pains in the region of the small lobe of the liver precede the stool (fifth day),[11].—Jerking-sticking pain, first in the right, afterwards in the left hypochondrium, continuing but a few minutes on either side, aggravated neither by pressure nor by motion, at 9 A.M. (fourth day),[11].—Stitchlike jerkings in the left hypochondrium,[11].—*Umbilical.* Pinching twinges in a small spot three fingers' breadth to the right of the navel, lasting half a minute (from the 3d dec. dilution), in the same place where the same sensation was noticed from the 1st dilution,[11].—Griping pain in the umbilical region, with urging to stool, followed by nausea and accumulation of water in the mouth,[6].—Dull stitches in the right side of the umbilical region, extending into the cœcal region, with passage of flatulence in the morning, in bed (second day),[11].—[350.] Cutting colic about the navel, with slight attacks of nausea, one hour after dinner,[11].—Some fine tearings from the right side of the umbilical region to the bladder; they frequently return until dinner,[11].—*General Abdomen.* Distension of the abdomen (after two hours),[2].—Distension of the abdomen, with sensation of soreness,[10].—Distension of the abdomen, after eating,[12].—Abdomen full and tense,[2].—Increased peristaltic motion,[1].—Increase of the peristaltic motion, rumbling, passage of flatulence,[1].—Movings about in the abdomen,[6].—Movings, like flatulence, in the abdomen (after a quarter of an hour),[11].—Rumbling of the abdomen,[2].—Rumbling in the abdomen, without pain,[6].—[360.] Rumblings and movings in the intestines,[6].—Audible rumbling in the abdomen,[5].—Flatulence,[13].—Much flatulence, and frequent passage of flatus from the rectum having the smell of the drug,[12].—Great quantity of flatus both up and down, on waking in morning (second day),[14a].—Very offensive flatulence,[13].—Passage of flatus,[7].—Passage of flatus, with sensation of itching in the rectum,[3].—[370.] Increased passage of flatus,[6].—Many and noisy passages of flatus upwards and downwards (second day),[14a].—Discharge of much flatus upward and downward,[14a].—Extraordinary discharge of wind both upward and downward, when walking (second day),[14c].—Sensation of discomfort and slight nausea in the abdomen, followed by a soft fecal stool (second day),[11].—Sensation of discomfort in the abdomen by paroxysms, also returning after a stool (second day),[11].—Sensation of discomfort in the abdomen, with accumulation of saliva in the mouth, and paroxysms of slight nausea (after four hours),[11].—Pain in the abdomen, after dinner,[3].—10 P.M., feeling in bowels as if about to have diarrhœa,[14a].—Pain in the abdomen, as though diarrhœa would follow,[8].—[380.] Pressive constrictive pain in the abdomen, with discharge of much flatus upward and downward (after one hour),[14b].—Griping here and there in the abdomen, with passage of flatulence (second day),[11].—Griping pain in the small intestines, with passage of flatus,[6].—Griping, with rumbling and rolling in the intestines, as though diarrhœa would follow,[8].—While sitting and writing, pressive pain in the abdomen seemed to cause attacks of nausea; it was relieved in the open air (second day),[11].—Slight flatulent twinges in the abdomen (fourth day),[11].—Cutting paroxysmal pain in the upper abdomen, by the right false ribs, at 6 A.M. (third day),[11].—Jerking-sticking pain in the cœcal region (second day),[11].—Pinching-sticking in the cœcal region

(second day),[11].—Slight itching-sticking pain on the right side of the abdomen below the navel, followed by semifluid stool (fourth day),[11].—[**390.**] Dull itching-sticking pain in the cœcal region as yesterday, only that the attack continues rather longer, lasting from one to two minutes (after two hours),[11].
—Stitches here and there in the abdomen,[12].—Occasional stitches in the left side of the abdomen (fifth day),[11].—Pinching stitches in the right side of the abdomen, frequently during the day (fourth day),[11].—Tearing pains here and there in the intestines,[1].—Slight colic-like pains,[10].—Tearing colic-like pain in the abdomen,[5].—Colic,[7][15].—Colic (after three-quarters of an hour),[7].—Colic, with movings about like flatulence, aggravated by inspiration, with stitching pain on pressure; the flatulence seems to accumulate in the cœcal region, moving from one side to the other; pressing upon the abdomen increases or renews the pain, at 4 A.M. (after two to three days),[11].—[**400.**] Slight colic after eating,[11].—Frequent slight colic pains,[1].—Severe colic,[15].—Severe cutting colic, followed by urgent stool, in the evening, after eating a very little salad,[11].—Pain in the abdomen on pressure,[6].—Abdomen painful to pressure,[7].—Sensation of soreness of the walls of the abdomen (second day),[10].—Dull jerking pains in the muscles of the abdomen from time to time, during the afternoon,[11].—*Hypogastrium.* Feeling of discomfort in the lower abdomen, with paroxysms of nausea, aggravated by stooping or by motion (after three hours),[11].—Slight cutting in the lower abdomen, followed by partly softish, partly crumbly stool, after drinking coffee; the same cutting pain was soon afterwards again experienced without the stool,[11].—[**410.**] Slight cutting pains in the lower abdomen; stooping, or resting the arm against the abdomen is unpleasant; the former seemed to cause the attacks of nausea, the latter the colic, even if these symptoms had disappeared,[11].—Stitchlike twinges in the left side of the lower abdomen,[11].—Dull sticking pain on pressing upon the lower abdomen,[6].—Slight colic in the lower abdomen, as if diarrhœa would follow, at 10 A.M. (second day),[11].

Rectum and Anus.—Burning and itching in the rectum,[10].—Transient stitches in the rectum,[6].—Violent burning and itching in the anterior commissura ani, which is found to be sore to the touch, in afternoon, after a stool (second day),[14a].—Urging to stool,[10].—Urgent desire for stool, at noon,[2].—8 P.M., urging to stool, which was pappy and accompanied and followed by a feeling of weakness and tremulousness (second day),[14a].

Stool.—Diarrhœa. [**420.**] Diarrhœa at night of a yellow, frothy, sour-smelling fluid, with colic-like pain in the abdomen, especially in the umbilical region, with which the navel was drawn inward; with tenesmus, which soon disappeared without returning (this returned every four or five weeks, and lasted one or two days),[3].—Sudden diarrhœa set in after dinner, with colic; this was twice repeated during the afternoon,[10].—Slimy diarrhœa, in the afternoon (second day),[10].—Watery diarrhœa twice,[10].—Transient, offensive diarrhœa, alternating with constipation,[15].—Diarrhœic stool after breakfast (second day),[14a].—Two stools in quick succession,[7].—Two small pasty stools at 11 A.M. (fifth day),[x].—Two stools, the first in part pasty, in part crumbly, the last one thin, fluid, between 9 and 10 A.M. (third day),[11].—Stool, with relief of colic,[7].—[**430.**] Stool, preceded by griping colic, which was relieved after the stool,[6].—Stool, followed by pinching-sticking pain in the cœcum (fifth day),[11].—Stool, with mucus, and discharge of cherry-red blood (in the morning, two days after, connected with the headache), (fifth day),[14c].—Immediately on waking, at 5.30 A.M., was obliged to go to stool, and had a copious, thin, yellowish evacuation, with subsequent burning at the anus, as if from acridity,[14e].—Stool at first solid, then soft, followed by rumbling in the abdomen, as if another stool would occur,[11].—Stool soft,[2].—Stool soft, having the peculiar odor of the drug,[12].—Having been three days without an evacuation, on going to stool, in the morning, after breakfast, without any special call, had a soft stool, with a considerable discharge of cherry-red blood (third day),[14b].—Soft, pasty stool, preceded by colic, soon after breakfast (second day),[11].—Insufficient soft stool at 10 A.M. (fourth day),[11].—[440.] Pasty stool (second day),[11].—Stools always pappy and scanty,[14c].—A pappy stool escaped involuntarily when making water in the afternoon,[14c].—Thin, pappy stool after breakfast (third day),[14].—Semifluid stool at 10 A.M. (fourth day),[11].—Insufficient, soft, liquid stool, preceded by slight colic,[11].—Stool at first solid, afterwards liquid, with burning in the anus (after one hour and a half), followed (after three hours) by another stool, with burning in the anus (second day),[11].—Very watery stool, as after a purge (after three hours),[11].—Considerable discharge of blood with the pappy stools,[14d].—Stool scanty, small, and even if fluid, still evacuated with difficulty in consequence of the inactivity of the bowel, in the evening,[11].—[450.] Stool dryer than usual (after five hours),[11].—An insufficient hard stool, with a slight urging towards evening,[11].—*Constipation.* Constipation (second day),[11].—No stool during the day,[14b].—Three days without an evacuation or going to stool,[14b].—Some workers suffer from constipation, some from diarrhœa,[15].

Urinary Organs.—Bladder. Violent stitchlike, crampy pain in the bladder and neck of bladder, at midnight, when making water, on coming home, after taking a glass of wine, extending forwards into the urethra, and accompanied by a similar pain in the anus and rectum; this pain is hardly bearable while it continues,[14b].—*Urethra.* Slight irritation of the mucous membrane of the urethra,[15].—Tickling in forepart of urethra, and sensation as though something were about to run out of it (after dinner),[14a].—Desire to pass urine,[1].—[460.] Great desire to pass urine,[1].—Sudden transient desire to urinate, arising from the fossa navicularis, without real urging or necessity for urinating,[1].—*Micturition.* Involuntary passage of urine,[19].—*Urine.* Urine smells of sulphur,[15].—Increase of carbonates and sulphates in the urine,[15].

Sexual Organs.—Male. The sexual organs were relaxed during the whole of the proving,[2].—Penis much shrivelled and shrunken (eighth day),[14b].—Erections in the afternoon (second day),[10].—Erections, with nightly emissions,[10].—Violent erections, with burning in the urethra,[10].—[470.] Complete impotence, with atrophied testicles, soon followed its administration,[20].—No sexual appetite since the proving begun,[14b].—Scrotum and penis shrunken from the commencement,[14c].—Left testicle and epididymis somewhat swollen (second day),[14a].—Left testicle more swollen and harder than usual, also much more painful, even when at rest,[14a].—No pain in the tumor testiculi, though the epididymis is very much swollen (fifth day),[14c].—Fine sticking-burning pains in left spermatic cord, running deep into abdomen; these pains returned in the evening, when in bed,[14e].—Jerking-sticking pain in the left testicle, continuing about two minutes (after five hours and a half),[11].—Stitches in the left spermatic cord, in the evening,[14e].—Sexual desire increased (in both sexes),[15].—[480.] Sexual desire and erections ceased; this impotence was so decided that his wife, herself diseased, gave it as a reason for leaving him,[15].—Copious emission during the night,[14d].—*Female.* Almost entire obliteration of ovaries,[20].—Menstruation five days too early, without trouble,[3].—Menstruation irregular,[15].

Respiratory Organs.—Larynx. Irritability of the larynx,[2].—Inclination to cough,[13].—Inclination to cough all day,[14c].—Desire to cough, rising from the bifurcation of the bronchi (followed after the hoarseness and irritation in the larynx),[2].—Heat in the larynx,[2].—*Voice.* [490.] Husky voice,[11].—Voice somewhat husky, though without other catarrhal symptoms (fourth day),[11].—Rough, husky voice (second day),[11].—Hoarseness,[14b].—Hoarseness, lasting two hours,[9].—Hoarseness from the larynx, with much irritation to hawk, especially on its posterior wall, seldom provoking cough, lasting thirty-six hours,[2].—Some hoarseness at noon, as if from a catarrh,[14c].—*Cough.* Violent cough, immediately after lying down in bed, at 10.30 P.M., caused by a continual and very troublesome tickling high up in the pharynx, exactly as if snuff had lodged upon the uvula, straining the chest and making it sore; convulsive and dry, lasting half an hour (sixth day),[14c].—More or less tormenting cough, without characteristic sputa,[15].—Dry cough,[6].—*Respiration.* [500.] Breath smelt of Sulphide of Carbon,[15].—Increased warmth of the expired air,[2].—Hot breath,[2].—Inspiration deep and slow,[23].—Respiration accelerated,[2].—Respiration somewhat oppressed,[6].—Oppression of breathing, with pressure on the sternum,[2].—"Seemed to have lost his breath,"[23].

Chest.—Sensation of warmth in the chest,[5].—Constriction of the chest, as though expiration were impeded. I was obliged to inspire deeply, and only obtained relief after continued deep respirations in the open air,[23].—[510.] Fulness of the chest and oppression of breathing seem to arise from the anterior portion of the right side of the diaphragm,[2].—Pressive-tensive pain in chest, stomach, and abdomen,[14b].—Oppression of the chest is increased in impure air and in a room which had not been aired in the morning, when it was also associated with anxiety,[2].—Some transient stitches in the chest and below the left short ribs (third day),[11].—The symptoms of congestion of the lungs are perceptible, and seem to involve the upper lobes of the lungs (second day),[2].—*Front.* Sensitiveness of the anterior wall of chest when sneezing, in the evening,[2].—Pressure under the sternum,[9].—Transient stitches near the left side of the sternum (second day),[11].—Violent stitches under the middle of the sternum, extending upwards like lightning (soon after),[14e].—*Sides.* Burning in the left half of the chest and beneath the sternum,[10].—[520.] Dull pressive pain in the right side of the chest,[6].—Paroxysmal pressive-sticking sensation in the region of the right last ribs, about four fingers' breadth from the pit of the stomach, at 5 P.M. (second day),[11].—Dull jerking-sticking in the lower portion of the right side of the chest (after three hours),[11].—Stitches in the left half of the chest, without cough (second day),[10].—Itching stitches in the right nipple,[11].—Chest symptoms aggravated by ascending steps,[2].

Heart and Pulse.—Heart's action accelerated,[15].—Pulse accelerated,[1 3 4].—Pulse 90 to 95,[5].—Pulse 80, and increasing (second day),[14a].—[530.] Pulse accelerated, 92 (usually 76); this, however, lasted only ten minutes, after which it was again regular,[3].—Pulse reduced to 52 beats (one case),[15].

Neck and Back.—Neck. Very marked intermittent bruit de souffle in the cervical vessels,[15].—Stiffness of neck prevented me from turning the head, toward the left particularly; continued all day (sixth day),[14b].—Painful stiffness in the nape and neck (fifth day),[14b].—Violent sticking constrictive pains in the neck, near the commencement of the œsophagus, as though there were a bone sticking there; this pain returned several times during the day,[14c].—Drawing pain in the right musc. sterno-cleido-mastoideus,[6].—Itching-sticking pain in the right sterno-cleido-mastoid muscle (fourth day),[11].—*Dorsal.* Feeling in back as though a heavy weight were lying across shoulders and weighing him down, so that his head sank forward; at noon, when walking,[14a].—*Lumbar.* Lumbar pains (hæmorrhoidal),[14c].—[540.] Lumbar pains, continuing until morning,[14b].—Persistent lumbar and sacral pains through the day (second day),[14c].—Violent lumbar and sacral pains on waking in the morning (third day),[14a].—Dislocated pain in right lumbar region, 10 P.M.,[14b].—Jerking stitches in the right lumbar region, at 7 P.M.,[11].—Tension in the small of the back, especially on ascending steps, together with occasional jerks extending towards the hip-joints,[2].—Drawing in the small of the back, in the afternoon (second day),[10].—Tearing and pressure in the small of the back,[10].—*Sacral.* Continual sacral pains,[14b].—Sensitive pain in the right tuber ischii and in the flexor side of the foot, in the afternoon, when riding,[11].

Extremities in General.—[550.] Dwindling of the limbs and of the whole muscular structure,[15].—Severe pains in the limbs,[15].—Pains in the limbs, like chronic rheumatism, with formication and general prickling,[15].—Jerking-sticking pains in several joints (third day),[11].—Intermitting dull sticking pain (sensitive twitching in single muscle-fibrillæ) in several places as large as the tip of the finger, on the inner side of the upper arm and thigh (after one hour and a quarter),[11].—Jerking-sticking transient pains on the back of the left foot and in the right wrist,[6].

Superior Extremities.—10 P.M., paralytic pain in left arm, from holding newspaper to read in bed,[14a].—Violent rheumatic pain in right arm and shoulder, in forenoon (fourth day),[14a].—Pressive pain in the right arm (third day),[10].—Slight attacks of itching-sticking pains, in places as large as the tip of the finger, on the inside of the right arm (soon after taking),[11].—[560.] Frequent slight stitches in the arms, extending from the shoulder-joint to the wrist (second day),[3].—Diminished sensibility on the arms and hands,[15].—The left arm goes to sleep, with pain and sensation of weariness in it,[10].—*Shoulder.* Jerking-sticking pain in the right shoulder-joint,[11].—*Arm.* Rheumatic pain in left upper arm, occiput, and nape,[14b].—Violent rheumatic pain in left upper arm to the bones, in the evening,[14b].—Paroxysmal itching-sticking pain in the left deltoid muscle (sixth day),[11].—Jerking stitches in the upper arm and shoulder-joint (third day),[11].—*Elbow.* In evening, frightful rheumatic pain in left elbow-joint, so that he could not move the arm without crying out; when quiet, it was painless (sixth day),[14b].—Slight stitches in the right elbow-joint, along the course of the extensors to the wrists, transient, frequently returning during the day,[3].—[570.] Tearing pain in the left elbow and in the left shoulder (these parts had formerly been the seat of a rheumatic affection); the pains were transient,[8].—Jerking in the region of the elbow (after eleven hours),[11].—*Forearm.* Trembling of the left forearm, with sticking in it, especially about the wrist,[10].—Pressive pain in the left forearm, when touching it or leaning upon it,[9].—Pressive pain in the left forearm, aggravated by leaning upon it, lasting half an hour,[10].—Jerking-stitching pain at the tendinous insertion of the biceps of the forearm, paroxysmal, going and coming, during the afternoon and night (fourth day),[11].—*Wrist.* Pain in the left wrist,[9].—Sticking in the left wrist,[10].—Transient jerking pain in the wrist, at one time in the left, at another in the right, lasting only a few seconds, frequently repeated during the day (third day, and noticed for several weeks),[12].—**Hand.** The hands (as in lead-poisoning) were held in pronation and hanging down, on account of the greater weakness of the extensors, although the flexors were also enfeebled,[15].—[**580.**] With the weakness, a kind of cramps or transient contractions of the extensor muscles of the hands, which, for a short time, entirely prevented the fingers from bending,[15].—Piercing pains in metacarpal bones of left hand, when in bed,[14a].—Insensibility of the hands; she did not notice deep needle stitches in various portions of the hands,[19].—**Fingers.** Dull sticking in the metacarpal joint of the left index finger (after three hours),[11].—Jerking-sticking in various joints of the fingers,[11].—Jerking-sticking in the metacarpal joint of the index finger,[11].—Intermitting jerking-sticking pain in the third phalanx of the left fourth finger, frequently returning (after four hours, and lasting the whole day),[11].—Prickling-sticking feeling in the fingers, especially of the left hand, and in the feet at noon, continuing more or less all day,[14c].—Very violent piercing-stitching pains through the middle and ring fingers of the right hand, several times at noon,[14b].—Jerking stitches in the joints of the left thumb (second day),[11].

Inferior Extremities.—[**590.**] Weariness of the lower extremities (from the 1st dil.),[13].—**Hip.** Itching in the region of the left hip and pelvis, obliging him to scratch (third day),[11].—**Thigh.** Violent (rheumatic) pains in the muscles of the thigh after rising (sixth day),[14a].—Violent muscular pains in the thigh the whole day, but especially in the ankle; can scarcely walk (sixth day),[14a].—Drawings from the left hip to the knee-joint (after half an hour),[4].—Drawing pain in the left thigh while walking (after half an hour),[7].—Dislocated pain in right thigh when walking in forenoon; the same in left foot near tibia (fourth day),[14c].—Jerking-sticking pain in the middle of the thigh, like a pain in a nerve, lasting half an hour, and very painful, repeated during the next forenoon; in the afternoon the same pain is felt between the tibia and fibula, after dinner,[2].—Jerking stitch in the middle of the right thigh,[11].—**Knee.** Pain in the hollow of the knee (second day),[11].—[**600.**] Tensive pain in the right popliteal space, when walking or stretching out the foot,[6].—Drawing pain in the knee-joints (from the 1st dil.),[13].—Sensation in the left knee-joint as though it were sprained,[4].—Dislocated pain in knee and sole when walking in the forenoon, as if he had made a misstep,[14c].—Dislocated pain in right knee, repeated several times during the day (second day),[14c].—Tearing pain in the right knee and ankle in the afternoon,[10].—Itching, sticking pain in the hollow of both knees, at the point of insertion of the tendons of the gracilis and sartorius muscles, and also in the tuber ischii,[11].—A peculiar, itching-stitching pain on the external tendons of the left popliteal space, more severe than formerly, and lasting several minutes (third day),[11].—**Leg.** Rheumatic (?) pain in left tibia,[14a].—Cramps in the legs and thighs (these cramps frequently occurred when weary),[8].—[**610.**] Stitches extending from the inner side of the left knee to the great toe,[4].—**Ankle.** 10 P.M., great painful lassitude in ankles and soles of feet,[14a].—Pain in the ankles, as from great fatigue caused by long walking,[12].—Frequent transient, jerking pain in the ankles,[12].—**Foot.** Frequent pain in left metatarsal bones when walking, as though they would be dislocated by a false step,[14b].—Severe pains in the joints of the foot, as if dislocated, in morning, in bed; walking is very troublesome at first after getting up, but becomes easier by walking (sixth day),[14a].—Burning and digging pain in the joints of the feet,[12].—Tearing pain in the left foot, especially in the tarsal bones, transient,[6].—Prickling feeling (*formicatio*) through both feet, as if from electric currents, while sitting on a perfectly soft sofa ; 5.30 p.m. The same sensation afterwards in the arms,[14b].—Pain at the insertion of the tendo Achillis in the os calcis on ascending steps (after nine to eleven hours),[11].—[620.] Jerking stitches at the point of insertion of the left tendo Achillis in the heel,[11].—Dull pressive pain in the left heel,[6].—Great painful lassitude and weariness in the soles after dinner (third day),[14e].—Violent cramp in the right sole, relieved by stepping firmly upon it,[11]. — *Toes.* A single, violent, sticking, piercing pain from the metatarsal bones into the toes, in the forenoon, when walking.[14b].—Some jerking stitches in the balls of the right toes (second day),[11].—Seldom jerking stitches in the toes, and in the muscles of the thighs (fourth day),[11].

Generalities.—Objective. Considerable emaciation,[15].—Deranges the whole nervous organization,[20].—Serious nervous disturbances occur after inhaling the vapor,[20].—[630.] Muscular contraction was inefficient and tremulous ; the fingers could not be closed with any degree of force ; on extending the arm for a few seconds, there was a well-marked trembling of the muscular fibres,[15].—Its vapor, breathed, produces great depression, followed by coma,[22].—Disinclination for every work, together with sleepiness, and pressure upon the eyes, lasting several weeks,[12].—Unusual weariness,[6].—General painful weariness,[15].—Weariness of the whole body, especially of the left arm, in the morning, which disappeared towards noon (second day),[10].—Painful weariness and bruised sensation in all parts of the body, especially in the back, loins, and joints of the feet (second day),[14e].—Weakness,[3].—Great weakness and prostration,[12].—Muscular debility (wife),[15].—[640.] Rapid decline of strength ; could scarcely walk, and could only work sitting ; walked with a cane, and on going upstairs, had to stop at each landing-place. This debility affected the upper as well as the lower limbs,[15].—If raised from bed she sank on to her knees and gradually slid down to the ground,[19].—On coming out of the attacks of fainting she could not walk or remember anything of her condition ; she was very much confused, and even demented ; on attempting to speak she frequently stuck out her tongue like a child, stretched the lower jaw far forward and gnashed it against the upper one ; she frequently stared at her hands and fingers with a vacant look,[19].—Prostration, weakness of the body, for several weeks,[12].—Prostration and weakness of the feet,[12].—Frequent attacks of faintness,[19].—Cannot long remain quiet in one place,[12].—Hyperæsthesia (one case),[15].—Anæsthesia of various portions of the skin, as also of the mucous membrane of the mouth, eyes, ears, and nose,[19].—*Subjective.* General excitement of the whole body (after two minutes),[4].—[650.] General feeling of illness (second day),[14a].—Indisposition and bitterness in the mouth on waking,[14d].—Indisposed on going to bed in evening, with discharge of much warm flatus,[14d].—Rheumatic pains in all parts of the body, especially the muscles of fingers and toes, very painful in left hand,[14b].—Wandering rheumatic pains all day (fifth day),[14a].—Dull sticking or itching pains in various parts of the body throughout the whole day,[11].—Peculiar jerking-sticking pains are felt at times, now in the hollow of the right knee, now in the lower abdomen, now in the spermatic cord, lasting till after dinner (after five hours),[11].—Itching-sticking pain in various parts of the body, especially in the tuber ischii and at the point of insertion of the gracilis and sartorius at the knee (second day),[11].—Jerking stitches in various parts of the body, especially in the muscles of the right eye (fourth day),[11].—Itching stitches in various parts of the body, continuing throughout the forenoon (third day),[11].—[660.] Jerking pain,

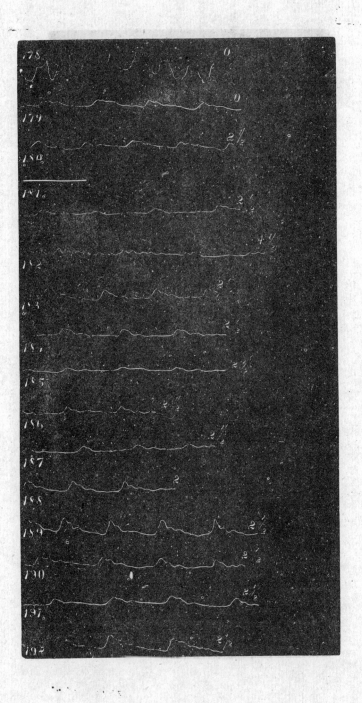

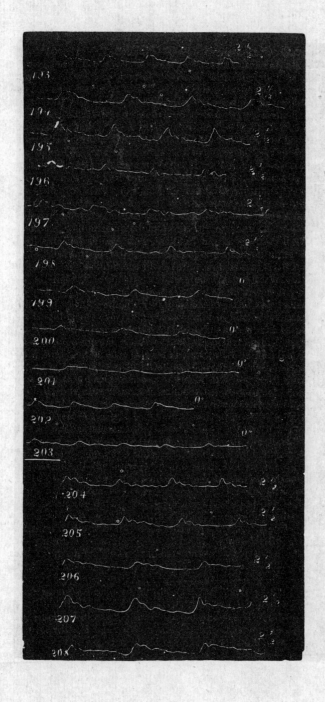

now in the forehead, now in the joints of the feet, now in the joints of the arms, lasting several weeks,[12].—Sensation of throbbing and trembling of the whole body occurred after the disappearance of the anæsthesia,[19].—When applied to enlarged glands, the part felt very cold, but immediately after, a gradual heat, accompanied with great prickling; the heat increasing the longer the medicine was kept in contact with the part, until it could no longer be endured. On removing the glass the part was red to an extent two or three times greater than the part inclosed,[17].—Symptoms generally disappear within two to four hours after taking the drug,[6].

Skin.—Objective. Eruptions, Dry. Eruption on the face after shaving in the morning,[14d].—Red, somewhat raised eruption on both cheeks and across nose and on alæ nasi at 2 P.M., after shaving; it resembles the acne potatorum or the soreness of the nose accompanying catarrh, with burning of nose and lips; it had not disappeared when he went to bed. A medical friend whom he met asked him if he had herpes on his face (second day),[14a].—Eruption on face became strongly developed after drinking two glasses of beer at noon (second day),[14b].—Small scales visible on the parts of the face formerly occupied by the eruption (fourth day),[14a].—Little scales upon the cheeks (third day),[14b].—Violently itching pimples (like nettle-rash) on the back of the right forearm, obliging him to rub and scratch it (after four hours),[11].—Several isolated papules on the right forearm which itch when touched,[11].—*Eruptions, Moist.* [670.] Small boil on left thigh,[14b].—*Subjective.* On applying this substance to the skin there is first experienced a piercing sensation of cold, owing to its rapid evaporation; this is afterwards followed by burning pain, as though the part had been dipped in hot water,[1].—Crawling along both forearms, often alternating with slight stitches (second day),[3].—Crawling from the left elbow to the tips of the fingers (excepting the thumb),[3].—Slight crawling over the whole of the right arm, with sensation as if the arm would go to sleep,[3].—Pricking-sticking feeling over the whole skin, particularly in the hands and feet,[14b].—Fine itching stitches in various parts of the skin (after three-quarters of an hour),[11].—Fine prickings in various parts of the body in the evening; 10.30 P.M.,[14b].—Itching in various parts of the body (fourth day),[11].—Itching on various parts of the body,[15].—[680.] Itching and itching stitches at intervals during the day (third day),[11].—Itching of the abdomen, after rising and washing in cold water (second day),[11].—Itching on the chest, on the right side of the back as far up as the region of the kidneys, and on the right forearm; on examining the places some colorless pimples are noticed, which itch more and are more irritable after scratching, and become red after mechanical irritation; they become pointed and at last an itchlike eruption forms; after scratching, this eruption bleeds easily and burns, in the morning after waking (fourth day),[11].—Itching of the skin on the back and on both thighs, lasting four days,[4].—Itching on the right forearm and upper arm, in the bend of the left elbow and on the thighs (third day),[11].—Itching, causing scratching, in a small spot on the right forearm, followed by the appearance of small pimples,[11].—Itching and stinging of the hands, especially between the fingers, where he discovered little vesicles filled up with lymph (fifth day),[14a].—Itching on the legs, on going to bed in the evening (second day),[11].—Itching on the calves and lower legs (second day),[11].—Yawning,[2].—[690.] Frequent yawning,[12].—Sleepiness,[4].—Sleepiness commences after 2 o'clock,[3].—Unusual sleepiness in the evening while in society,[6].—Remarkable sleepiness, with heaviness of the upper lids, which would fall,[7].—Great sleepiness during the evening,[12].—Great sleepiness in the afternoon, and though she could only fall asleep late in the evening, the sleep was uneasy and interrupted by vivid dreams,[3].—Great sleepiness after 3 P.M., though it was a long time before she could go to sleep in the evening,[3].—Great sleepiness during the whole day,[12].—Became very sleepy after taking a glass of wine in the evening, but when he went to bed could only doze, and was a long time before he could go to sleep,[14d].—[700.] Overpowering sleepiness,[15].—The morning sleep was, throughout the proving, sound and refreshing,[3].—Slept well and long during the night,[14b].—Sleep quiet through the night, with many dreams towards morning (third night),[11].—*Sleeplessness.* Rather restless night,[14a].—Very restless night (fourth day),[14c].—Sleep at night was restless,[12].—Sleep at night restless on account of many unpleasant dreams, with weeping,[7].—Sleep restless, with constant tossing about in bed, especially throwing the head about, for several weeks,[12].—Very restless sleep at night,[14b].—[710.] Night very restless; continual dreams of what I read about in the evening,[14d].—Night very restless, frequent waking, alternating with dreams (second night),[10].—Sleep uneasy at night, interrupted by many dreams,[4].—Sleep much disturbed,[19].—Sleep late in the evening, restless and frequently interrupted at night by slight stitches extending from the inner side of the left knee to the great toe,[4].—First part of night slept well; after that did nothing but toss about,[14a].—Sleep much interrupted and full of unpleasant dreams, after midnight,[2].—Difficulty in going to sleep,[15].—She did not go to sleep for a long time at night.[3].—Startings from sleep in a fright, followed by prostration during the day,[15].—[720.] Sudden waking, from bad dreams or nervous starting,[15].—Night good, but awoke early, with many dreams,[14a].—Awoke tired (second day),[14c].—Sleeplessness,[15].—Frequent insomnia,[15].—*Dreams.* Restless dreams,[15].

Fever.—Chilliness. 7 P.M., chills (second day),[14a].—With the nightly restlessness, shivering, followed by heat and profuse sweat,[15].—Chilliness,[3].—Slight chilliness all day,[14a].—[730.] Unusual sensation of coldness, chilliness, and anxiety from within outward,[7].—Icy coldness, which lasted for hours, and left him in a state of painful weariness, as if he had been beaten, or had taken a forced march,[15].—Unpleasant sensation of coldness in both cheeks during the complaints in the abdomen (second day),[11].—Cold feet,[7].—Coldness of the forepart of the foot (after three-quarters of an hour),[2].—*Heat.* Fever seldom, mostly at night,[15].—Skin hot, with burning, like nettles, in various places,[12].—Heat over the whole body, with slight headache and full pulse,[8].—The heat over the whole body towards five in the morning left great prostration, after which he slept; when he awoke after an hour he felt entirely well,[8].—Momentary orgasm of blood, with accelerated pulse,[8].—[740.] General warmth of the upper part of the body (after three-quarters of an hour),[2].—Warmth spread from the pit of the stomach up through the chest to the head, and also downward to the navel,[1].—Heat in the head and face,[10].—Forehead hot (after one hour and a half),[5].—Sensation of heat on the forehead, with moderate pressive pain and constant desire to rub the forehead with the hand,[10].—Warmth of the face and hands, especially of the palms,[1].—Heat in the face, especially in the cheeks, in the afternoon,[7].—Heat of the cheeks, lasting three-quarters of an hour (soon),[2].—*Sweat.* Perspiration checked,[12].—The skin was dry for several weeks, with suppressed perspiration,[12].—[750.] Dryness of the skin and oppressive heat did not allow him to sleep; he sponged off his body with cold water, and lay down again in bed in order to promote perspiration, but could not accomplish it; the sleep was always restless and the head heavy,".

Conditions.—Aggravation.—(*Morning*), Bitter, sour taste.—(*Forenoon*), Headache.—(5.30 A.M.), Diarrhœa.—(6 A.M.), Toothache; violent pain in temples on walking.—(9 A.M.), Headache; pain in carious tooth.— (10 A.M.), Colic in lower abdomen.—(12 M.), Desire for stool.—(*Afternoon*), Heat in face; eructations, etc.; general sick feeling.—(5 P.M.), Pain in last ribs.—(*Evening*), Headache worse; pain in teeth; stitches in left ear.— (8 P.M.), Urging to stool.—(10 P.M.), Headache.—(*Night*), Diarrhœa; stitches in left ear; fever.—(*Ascending steps*), Chest symptoms.—(*Beer*), General symptoms; confusion of head; eruptions on face; burning of nose. —(*Breathing deeply*), Pain in stomach.—(*Cold or cold water*), Toothache. —(*After dinner*), Diarrhœa; stitches in ear.—(*After eating*), Distension of abdomen; eructations; pressure in stomach.—(*Lying down*), Cough.— (*Lying on forearm*), Pain in it.—(*Motion*), Headache; discomfort in abdomen.—(*Motion of head*), Headache.—(*Pressure*), Burning in stomach.— (*Reading*), Headache; lachrymation; stitches in eye.—(*Close room*), Oppression of chest.—(*Shaking head*), Pain in temples.—(*Sitting*), Vertigo.— (*After sitting*), Colic.—(*Scratching*), Itching.—(*After smoking*), Eructations. —(*Stepping hard*), Pain in temples.—(*Stooping*), Headache; discomfort in abdomen.—(*Tobacco*), Symptoms in general.—(*Urinating*), Pain in bladder; involuntary stool.—(*Walking*), Headache.—(*Washing in cold water*), Itching of abdomen.—(*Wine*), General symptoms.

Amelioration.—(*Open air*), All symptoms; pain in head, in abdomen, etc.—(*After breakfast*), Bitter taste.—(*Cold*), All the symptoms.— (*After eating*), All symptoms.—(*Eructation*), Nausea.—(*Rest*), Pain in head. —(*Stepping firmly*), Cramp in sole.—(*Sunlight*), Pains in the limbs.

CARDUUS BENEDICTUS.

Cnicus benedictus, Linn. (Centaurea benedicta, Linn.) *Natural order*, Compositæ. *Preparation*, Tincture of the whole plant when in flower.

Authorities. Noack and Trinks, A. M. L. (from Prakt. Mitthl. d. Corr. Gess. Hom. Aezt., 1826).

Mind.—Anxiety, fear, starting up at every noise, frequent breaking out into a cold sweat.—Fretful mood.—Fretful during the fever.

Head.—Confusion of the head, with stitches in the temples.—Vertigo on raising the head, aggravated by stooping.—Continual sensation of heaviness in the head.—Sensation of heaviness in the head and limbs, as from paralysis, worse during the fever.—Pressure in the forehead, especially on stooping.—Sharp pressure in the temporal region, afterwards in the whole head, with a feeling of heaviness.—[10.] Pain in the occiput.—Pressive pain in the occiput, starting from the crown.

Eye.—Sensation in the eye as if it were pressed outward, rather a pleasant than a painful feeling.—Very painful tickling in the eye.— Cutting pain over the eyes.—*Lids.* Twitching in the lids.—Trembling motion in the canthi.—Sticking pain in the inner canthus, with lachrymation.—*Ball.* The eyeballs feel larger than usual.—Pressure in the eyeball from within outward.—*Vision.* [20.] Vision dim, distorted.—Gray spots move about before the eyes.—Flickering before the eye of small fiery stripes, disappearing after repeated opening and closing of the eye.— Transient blackness before vision.

Ear.—Sensation as if something were lying before the ears, also a feeling as if something burst like a bubble, and afterwards frequent humming.—Roaring and ringing before the ears.

Nose.—Constant feeling of gnawing and frequent tickling in the nose, followed by sneezing and drawing in the nose, as in impending coryza.

Mouth.—Teeth. Pain in the teeth, more of a drawing than sticking character, with simultaneous tickling on the upper surface of the tongue, more towards the root, which after a few minutes changed to a jerking stitch.—***Tongue.*** Tongue much furred during the fever.—Tongue sensitive, as if it were swollen, during the fever.—***Mouth in General.*** [30.] Continual sensation as if the mouth were contracted and drawn together, slowly increasing and decreasing, disappearing for some time after every meal.—Mouth very dry, with thirst, in the morning and evening.—***Saliva.*** Constant accumulation of saliva in the mouth.—Taste nauseous during the fever.—Clear, acid taste.—Taste sour, always worse in the forenoon, becoming offensive and almost sulphurous, relieved for a time after eating.

Throat.—Swallowing difficult, uncomfortable.

Stomach.—Unusual, voracious appetite.—Appetite slight.—***Eructations.*** Eructations after eating a little food.—[40.] Nausea.—*Vomiting.*—Sensation of fasting, although the stomach seems to be full.—A bitter burning as from an excessively disordered stomach, constant in the afternoon and evening.

Abdomen.—Slight griping in the abdomen.—Drawing, cutting pain in the abdomen.

Stool.—*Diarrhœa.*

Respiratory Organs.—Contraction and closure of the air-passages, causing sudden whistling inspiration, and forcible expiration.—Pain in the air-passages, as after a long-continued, obstinate cough, constantly increasing in severity, so that the whole of the air-passages became inflamed, and the inspired air seemed very cold.—Larynx rough ; hoarseness; rough voice. — [50.] Frequent, entirely toneless, rough cough, sounding like whispering, which constantly increases for several days, and then diminishes, with relief of the breathing ; singing, long-continued speaking, or reading became possible only after several days.—Constant dry hacking cough.—Difficult, accelerated respiration.

Chest.—Dull stitches in the side over the hip, now in the right side, now in the left, at first only on stooping, and on motion, but afterwards continuing when breathing and when not.—Stitches beneath the left breast.

Extremities in General. Cracking of the joints, with difficult mobility.—Paralytic-like heaviness of the limbs, worse during the fever.—Sensation when touching the limbs as if there were sore bruised spots.

Superior Extremities.—Contraction in the elbows and arms.—Tension on the inner surface of the elbow, as if it had been kept bent for a long time.—[60.] Sensation in the forearm, as if in the veins, as of a long thrust with a knife, with continued burning.—Trembling of the hands.

Inferior Extremities.—Weakness and giving way of the knees, when walking, especially during the fever. — Pinching, burning, and paralytic weakness in the bones of the knees, neck, and hands, aggravated by external pressure.—Weakness of the feet, after sitting.—Sensation as if the soles of the feet were sore.

General Symptoms.—Tension in the tendons.—Aching of all the bones, especially after stretching the limbs.—Aching and slight swelling of the veins.

Skin.—Eruption of painless rash, like nettle-rash ; a gooseskin, rather pointed, hard, preceded by cold creeping over the whole body, accompanied by feverish symptoms, lasting several days and slowly disappearing.—[70.] Small red spots on the finger, lasting several days, followed by a yellow spot lasting a long time.

Sleep and Dreams.—Constant yawning and hiccoughing.

Fever.—Chilliness.—Febrile chill, with gooseflesh, several days from noon till evening, at times appearing earlier.—*Fever.* Fever, consisting of flushes of heat in the face ; after eating, over the whole body, without thirst, with dimness of vision and pressure in the eyes, hot breath, hot lips, hands, and feet.—Burning on exerting the arms.—Burning under the skin in the face, afterwards in other parts of the body:—Much heat in the face.—*Sweat. Slight general sweat.*—Sweat, followed by burning heat in the hands.

Conditions.—**Aggravation.**—(*Morning and evening*), Mouth dry, etc.—(*Forenoon*), Sour taste.—(*Afternoon*), Febrile chill.—(*Afternoon and evening*), Burning in stomach.—(*After eating*), Eructations ; flushes of heat all over.—(*On exerting arms*), Burning.—(*During fever*), Fretful ; sensation in head ; tongue sensitive ; taste nauseous ; heaviness of limbs ; weakness of knees.—(*After sitting*), Weakness of feet.—(*Stooping*), Vertigo ; pressure in forehead.—(*After stretching limbs*), Aching of all the bones.

Amelioration.—(*After eating*), Sour taste.—(*After every meal*), Sensation in mouth disappears.—(*After repeated opening and closing of the eye*), Flickering before the eye.

CARDUUS MARIANUS.

C. marianus, Gaertn. *Nat. order,* Compositæ. (Old generic name, Silybum.)

Preparation, Tincture of the seeds.

Authority. Reil, proving with 5 to 50 drops of the tincture, and with repeated doses of an infusion of the seeds, Hom. Vierteljahrschrift, 3, 453 (translated in N. Am. J. of Hom., 3, 379).

Head.—Slight dulness of the head.—*Dulness of the head,* the whole day.—Occasionally transitory headache in the forehead and temples.—A dull headache in the forehead might have been referred to some catarrhal affection, but no catarrh followed (fourteenth day).

Mouth.—Tongue coated white in the middle ; red at the tip and edges. —*Accumulation of saliva* in the mouth, after taking coffee and milk, half an hour after the first dose.—Bitterness in the mouth after the dose.

Stomach.—Appetite *small.*—Loss of appetite.—[10.] Empty eructations, after food taken against inclination.—Nausea and inclination to vomit.—Some nausea immediately after the morning dose, repeated after every subsequent one, and ending in a feeling of inflation in the stomach ; a horseback ride of three hours in the afternoon increased the inflated feeling of the abdomen.—*Very decided nausea* after the first dose, which compelled me to take the remaining three each in a wineglassful of water, which moderated the symptom very much.—Great nausea, but no vomiting.— Violent nausea (very soon after).—Such severe and persistent nausea that I was obliged to produce vomiting by means of warm water and tickling the fauces.—Painful retching and vomiting of acid, green fluid (after ten minutes).—Increased sensation of uneasiness in the epigastric region, but no pain.—Pains in the stomach, lasting two hours, aggravated by bread and milk; meat-broth sat well at noon.—[20.] Painful griping in the stomach and cutting in the bowels, here and there, with rumbling.

Abdomen.—The feeling of fulness in the hypochondrium became less after stool, but was still perceptible enough, obliging me to draw a long breath.—The feeling of inflation in the abdomen was so strong, especially in the right side, that I expected to discover a great enlargement of the liver by percussion, but it was not so; but pressure was painful over the whole hepatic region.

Rectum and Anus.—No stool, but inclination to one.

Stool.—Stool at 8 A.M., of moderate size, pappy, loamy, destitute of bilious coloring (twenty-second day).—The morning evacuation was harder than usual.—A hard stool at 9 P.M.; formerly it took place between 7 and 8 A.M., and was rather pappy.—At 10 A.M. a hard scanty stool; at 11 a copious pappy one, but little colored by bile, more of a chocolate color, preceded by violent rumbling, with pains in the abdomen.—A very hard evacuation at a quarter to 9; a similar one, unsatisfactory, at a quarter before 7 P.M.—A very *hard, unsatisfactory, difficult evacuation of brown knotty fæces*, immediately after dinner.—[30.] Unsatisfactory, hard, loamy stool at 6 P.M.—No stool (seventeenth, nineteenth, twentieth, and twenty-third days).

Urinary Organs.—Urine scanty, brownish; two experiments, both with syrup and sulphuric and nitric acids, indicated the presence of the coloring matter of the bile in the urine.—Urine *cloudy, without sediment, golden-yellow, acid.*—Urine *wheyey, yellowish-brown, diminished in quantity,* acid (twentieth day); the next day the same, but after standing from six to eight hours, it deposited a sediment, consisting chiefly of common salt and lime; experiments with solution of sugar and sulphuric acid gave traces of the *coloring matter of the bile in the urine.*

Respiratory Organs.—Frequent urging to deep breathing, followed by painful sensations of an undefined sort in the abdomen.

Chest.—Every sudden and violent movement of the body was painful, both in the chest and abdomen.

General Symptoms.—Great debility all day.

Sleep and Dreams.—Restless at night, with frequent waking; lying on the back produced nightmare, which woke me twice.—Restless, dreamy night.

Conditions.—Aggravation.—(*Bread and milk*), Pains in stomach.—(*After coffee with milk*), Accumulation of saliva.—(*Lying on back*), Produced nightmare.—(*Riding on horseback*), Inflated feeling of abdomen.

Amelioration.—(*After stool*), Feeling of inflation of abdomen.

END OF VOLUME II.